PHYSICAL REHABILITATION

FOR THE

PHYSICAL THERAPIST ASSISTANT

Michelle H. Cameron, MD, PT, OCS
Oregon Health & Science University
Portland VA Medical Center
Portland, Oregon

Linda G. Monroe, MPT, OCS
John Muir Health
Walnut Creek, California

Carla Gleaton PT, MEd
Director, Instructor
Physical Therapist Assistant Program
Kilgore College
Kilgore, Texas

Susan M. Schmidt, AA
Physical Therapist Assistant
Oregon Health & Science University
Portland, Oregon

ELSEVIER
SAUNDERS

3251 Riverport Lane
St. Louis, Missouri 63043

PHYSICAL REHABILITATION FOR THE PHYSICAL   ISBN: 978-1-4377-0806-6
THERAPIST ASSISTANT

Notices

Knowledge and best practice in this field are constantly changing. As new research and experience broaden our understanding, changes in research methods, professional practices, or medical treatment may become necessary.

Practitioners and researchers must always rely on their own experience and knowledge in evaluating and using any information, methods, compounds, or experiments described herein. In using such information or methods they should be mindful of their own safety and the safety of others, including parties for whom they have a professional responsibility.

With respect to any drug or pharmaceutical products identified, readers are advised to check the most current information provided (i) on procedures featured or (ii) by the manufacturer of each product to be administered, to verify the recommended dose or formula, the method and duration of administration, and contraindications. It is the responsibility of practitioners, relying on their own experience and knowledge of their patients, to make diagnoses, to determine dosages and the best treatment for each individual patient, and to take all appropriate safety precautions.

To the fullest extent of the law, neither the Publisher nor the authors, contributors, or editors, assume any liability for any injury and/or damage to persons or property as a matter of products liability, negligence or otherwise, or from any use or operation of any methods, products, instructions, or ideas contained in the material herein.

Library of Congress Cataloging-in-Publication Data

Physical rehabilitation for the physical therapist assistant / [edited by] Michelle H. Cameron, Linda G. Monroe.
    p. ; cm.
  Includes index.
  ISBN 978-1-4377-0806-6 (pbk.)
  1. Physical therapy—Textbooks. 2. Physical therapy assistant—Textbooks. I. Cameron, Michelle H. II. Monroe, Linda G.
  [DNLM: 1. Physical Therapy Modalities. 2. Rehabilitation—methods. WB 460 P577645 2011]
  RM700.P4726 2011
  615.8′2—dc22

                    2010021614

Senior Editor: Kathy Falk
Developmental Editor: Megan Fennell
Publishing Services Manager: Catherine Jackson
Project Manager: David Stein
Design Direction: Maggie Reid

Printed in China

Last digit is the print number: 9 8 7 6 5

Contributors

Diane D. Allen, PhD, PT
Adjunct Assistant Professor
Department of Physical Therapy
Samuel Merritt College
Oakland, California

Nancey A. Bookstein, EdD, PT
Associate Professor, Director of Physical Therapy
    Admissions
Physical Therapy Program
School of Medicine
Senior Instructor
Cellular and Developmental Biology
University of Colorado at Denver, Health Sciences
    Center
Denver, Colorado

Lawrence P. Cahalin, MA, PT, CCS
Clinical Professor
Department of Physical Therapy
Northeastern University
Boston, Massachusetts

Cynthia Chiarello, PhD, MPT
Associate Director
Physical Therapy Program
Columbia University
New York, New York

Debra Clayton-Krasinski, PhD, PT
Assistant Professor, Clinical Physical Therapy
Program in Physical Therapy
Columbia University
New York, New York

Vanina Dal Bello-Haas, PhD, PT
Associate Professor
School of Physical Therapy
University of Saskatchewan
Saskatoon, Canada

Jennifer Dekerlegand, MPT
Heart Failure Coordinator, Research Team Leader
Hospital of the University of Pennsylvania
Division of Occupational and Physical Therapy
Philadelphia, Pennsylvania

Robert L. Dekerlegand, PT, MPT, CCS
Assistant Professor
Department of Developmental and Rehabilitative
    Services
School of Health Related Professions
University of Medicine and Dentistry of New Jersey
Stratford, New Jersey

**Christopher J. Durall, DPT, PT, MS, SCS, LAT,
    CSCS**
Graduate Faculty
Director of Physical Therapy
Student Health Center
University of Wisconsin–LaCrosse
LaCrosse, Wisconsin

Lisa L. Dutton, PhD, PT
Associate Professor, Dean
College of Health Professions
The University of Findlay
Findlay, Ohio

Joan E. Edelstein, MA, PT, FISPO
Special Lecturer
Program in Physical Therapy
Columbia University
New York, New York

Ahmed Samir Elokda, PhD, PT, CLT-LANA
Associate Professor, Director
Department of Physical Therapy
New York Institute of Technology
New York, New York

Donna K. Everix, MPA, PT
Physician Services Manager
Mills-Peninsula Health Services
Burlingame, California

Linda Fieback, MS, MA
Professional Associate
Mercy College
Dobbs Ferry, New York

Ginny Gibson, MS, OTR/L, CHT
Assistant Professor
Department of Occupational Therapy
Samuel Merritt College
Oakland, California

Susan Grieve, MPT, MS
Senior Physical Therapist
Department of Rehabilitation Services
Kaiser Permanente
Richmond, California

Rose Little Hamm, DPT, PT, CWS, FCCWS
Assistant Professor of Clinical Physical Therapy
Department of Biokinesiology and Physical Therapy
University of Southern California
Los Angeles, California

Kevin Helgeson, DHSc, PT, SCS
Assistant Professor
Department of Physical and Occupational Therapy
Idaho State University
Pocatello, Idaho

Mohamed Ibrahim, DSc, PT, MS, NCS
Physical Therapy Program
State University of New York, Downstate
Brooklyn, New York

Debra H. Iwasaki, MSPT, SCS, ATC, CSCS
Associate Head Athletic Trainer and Rehabilitation
    Coordinator
Department of Intercollegiate Athletics
University of California, Los Angeles
Los Angeles, California

Susan Klepper, PhD, PT
Assistant Professor of Clinical Physical Therapy
Department of Rehabilitation Medicine
Columbia University
New York, New York

L. Vince Lepak III, DPT, PT, MPH, CWS
Assistant Professor
Department of Physical Therapy
The University of Oklahoma
Tulsa, Oklahoma

Robert C. Manske, DPT, PT, MEd, SCS, ATC, CSCS
Assistant Professor
Department of Physical Therapy
Wichita State University
Teaching Associate
Department of Family Medicine
Via Christi Sports Medicine Fellowship Residency
    Program
Staff Physical Therapist
Via Christi Sports and Orthopedic Physical Therapy
Wichita, Kansas

Victoria Merrell, MPT
Boise, Idaho

Christiane Perme, PT, CCS
Senior Physical Therapist
Department of Physical Therapy and Occupational
    Therapy
The Methodist Hospital
Houston, Texas

Brian K. Peterson, MPT, MA
Jefferson County Hospital
Fairfield, Iowa

Julie A. Pryde, MS, PT, OCS, SCS, PA-C, ATC
Adjunct Assistant Professor
Samuel Merritt College
Oakland, California
Physician Assistant
Muir Orthopedic Specialists
Walnut Creek, California

Lori Quinn, EdD, PT
Clinical Faculty Associate
Program in Physical Therapy
New York Medical College
Valhalla, New York

Michael P. Reiman, PT, MEd, ATC, CSCS
Assistant Professor
Department of Physical Therapy
Wichita State University
Wichita, Kansas

Pamela Scarborough, PT, MS, CDE, CWS, FCCWS
Director of Education
PARKS Institute
Wimberley, Texas

Amy Selinger, PT, MS, OCS
Assistant Clinical Professor
Graduate Program in Physical Therapy
University of California San Francisco, San Francisco
    State University Joint Program in Physical Therapy
Owner, Chief Physical Therapist
Back to Life
San Francisco, California

Lynda L. Spangler, MS, PT
Assistant Professor
Department of Physical Therapy
The College of St. Scholastica
Duluth, Minnesota

Bonnie J. Sparks-DeFriese, PT, RN, CWOCN, CWS
Wound Ostomy Continence Nurse Clinician/Instructor
Wound Ostomy Continence Nursing Educational Center
School of Medicine
Emory University
Atlanta, Georgia

Jan Stephen Tecklin, MS, PT
Professor
Department of Physical Therapy
Arcadia University
Glenside, Pennsylvania

Toni Tyner, MHSL, BS
Assistant Professor
Department of Physical Therapy
California State University, Fresno
Fresno, California

R. Scott Ward, PhD, PT
Professor, Chair
Division of Physical Therapy
The University of Utah
Salt Lake City, Utah

Robert Wellmon, PhD, PT, NCS
Assistant Professor
Institute for Physical Therapy Education
Widener University
Chester, Pennsylvania

Preface

We were inspired to write *Physical Rehabilitation for the Physical Therapist Assistant* by physical therapist assistants who use Michelle Cameron's book *Physical Agents in Rehabilitation* and who, after reading *Physical Rehabilitation: Evidence-Based Examination, Evaluation, and Intervention*, wanted a version tailored to the physical therapist assistant. This book is designed and written specifically for physical therapist assistant students and clinicians. Together with its ancillaries it provides clear, concise recommendations for evidence-based physical therapy interventions for patients with any physical therapy diagnosis.

Physical Rehabilitation for the Physical Therapist Assistant is based on our physical therapists' textbook, *Physical Rehabilitation*. With the help of physical therapist assistant practitioners, educators, and students we reviewed and adapted the content of the original book and its ancillaries to address the unique needs of physical therapist assistants. The information on physical therapy examination and evaluation is condensed and the focus is on pathology and interventions. All chapters include clearly organized, easily followed descriptions of pathology; the rationale and evidence for intervention selection; and instructions for how to apply and document selected interventions. All chapters are thoroughly illustrated in full color and are supported by a wealth of online ancillary materials.

We use the American Physical Therapy Association's *Guide to Physical Therapist Practice, Second Edition* (the *Guide*) as a framework for this book, but unlike the *Guide*, we focus on evidence-based recommendations for interventions by the physical therapist assistant.

This book provides information for the generalist as well as for the specialist providing care beyond his or her area of expertise. The case studies in each chapter demonstrate how the presented information is applied within a clinical context. The additional case studies, and a variety of student exercises on the website, allow readers to practice their clinical problem-solving and test-taking skills.

The first chapter introduces the rest of the book and its overall concepts. The second chapter discusses evidence-based practice in physical therapy. These introductory chapters are followed by one chapter devoted to each preferred practice pattern (physical therapy diagnosis) presented in the *Guide*. There are also three additional chapters describing interventions that are common to many preferred practice patterns, such as assistive devices and gait assessment and training.

The structure, sequence, language, and concepts presented in this book are based on the *Guide*. The first four parts of the book are the same as the *Guide's* categories of preferred practice patterns: the musculoskeletal system, neuromuscular system, cardiovascular/pulmonary systems, and integumentary system. Then, each chapter addresses pathology and interventions for a particular preferred practice pattern. The last part of the book covers interventions that overlap many preferred practice patterns. All of the chapters have the same style and format to make information clear and readily accessible and to promote learning and recall. In addition, all chapters are thoroughly referenced with up-to-date primary research, include lists of additional resources about the specific area of practice, and have a complete glossary of useful terms and concepts.

The website accompanying this book, evolve.elsevier.com/Cameron/PTA, provides all the reference citations, with live links to Medline for the reader to obtain the article abstract and full text if available, and also links to all listed additional resources. The website also includes additional case studies; printable, modifiable forms related to the content of the chapter; animations demonstrating procedures or body processes; and a variety of other useful tools and information. Instructors using this book for teaching also have access to a complete online electronic image collection as well as all of the student resources.

This is the clearly written, up-to-date, evidence-based resource every physical therapist assistant needs for optimal patient management in rehabilitation.

Acknowledgments

We wish to thank the many people without whom this project would not have been possible.

First, we want to thank Susan Schmidt and Carla Gleaton, the physical therapist assistant subject matter experts for this text. These two experts added clarity, focus, and function to our original vision. Susan Schmidt brought her many years of clinical experience to this project right from the beginning. Carla Gleaton then added her expertise as a PTA educator. Thank you also to the original chapter contributors who gave so willingly of their knowledge and expertise. Thank you all for sharing your knowledge to improve physical therapy and to better the lives of patients beyond those you treat yourselves.

Thank you to the Elsevier team who supported and led us through the publication process, had faith in us, and reassured us that this really would all come together. We especially thank Megan Fennell, Developmental Editor, who was endlessly patient with us, took care of all the details, and answered our frequent questions and concerns calmly and efficiently. Thank you, Megan. We also thank Kathy Falk, Executive Editor, for encouraging us to move forward with this project and for putting together a great team to take this project through to production.

We also acknowledge the support of the manufacturers and other outside sources that provided us with illustrations and permission to use their images, questionnaires, forms, and other materials. All these components add to the richness of this resource.

Finally, we recognize and appreciate the endurance of our friendship. It is a testament to the strength of that bond that we took on another project together, never once becoming impatient with each other, and that somehow one of us was always strong and ready to take the lead when the other needed to rest or divert.

Michelle H. Cameron
Linda G. Monroe

Contents

Contents

Introduction

Michelle H. Cameron

OBJECTIVES

After reading this chapter, the reader will be able to:
1. Describe physical rehabilitation and the roles of those involved in providing physical rehabilitation.
2. Understand the Nagi and World Health Organization disablement models.
3. Understand the role of the *Guide to Physical Therapist Practice*.
4. Easily access information in this book regarding pathology, examination, evaluation, diagnosis, prognosis, and interventions for patients involved in physical rehabilitation.
5. Access the ancillaries provided with this book, including useful printable forms, practice boards–style test questions, and electronic links to references and resources.

This textbook provides clear explanations of the concepts essential for safe, effective evidence-based physical rehabilitation **interventions** for a wide range of patients. It is intended to be read and used by physical therapist assistant students and practicing physical therapist assistants. This introductory chapter briefly describes what **rehabilitation** is and who does it. It also provides an overview of the special features of this book, particularly its adherence to the *Guide to Physical Therapist Practice* (the *Guide*),[1] the consistent structure of each chapter, and features in and accompanying each chapter. This chapter concludes with a summary and glossary of terms used.

By reading and applying the information presented in this book, in conjunction with participating in didactic teaching and hands-on practice, the reader will learn to provide physical rehabilitation care at the level expected from a graduate of a physical therapist assistant training program. This is a broad-based, entry-level textbook that provides sufficient information for the generalist to provide care in many areas. This book will be valuable to students during their professional training and will continue to prove its value to practicing rehabilitation professionals throughout their career.

PHYSICAL REHABILITATION

Rehabilitation is a goal-oriented **treatment** process intended to maximize independence in individuals with compromised **function** that results from primary pathological processes and resultant **impairments.** Rehabilitation generally addresses the sequelae of **pathology** rather than the pathology itself. Physical rehabilitation focuses particularly on sequelae that impact physical functioning and activity and uses interventions that are noninvasive and physical in nature to promote progress toward functional **goals.** For example, physical rehabilitation may focus on impairments in mobility and **functional limitations** associated with musculoskeletal and neurological **diseases** or injuries, such as fractures or strokes, and treating them with exercises and hands-on mobilization techniques. Rehabilitation is not directed at curing disease, and physical rehabilitation, in the context of this book, does not include the use of medications or surgery as therapeutic interventions.

> ◎ *Clinical Pearl*
>
> Physical rehabilitation focuses on improving impairments and functional limitations, not on curing disease.

PHYSICAL REHABILITATION PROVIDERS

A wide range of professionals are involved in providing physical rehabilitation services. These include physicians, licensed and certified allied health care professionals, and assistants. **Physiatrists** are physicians who specialize in physical medicine and rehabilitation. Physiatrists often oversee the care of patients requiring rehabilitation, referring them to various other physicians and allied health care professionals and following up on the outcome of these referrals. Physiatrists may also provide direct patient care, including **examination**, specialized testing, and a variety of medical interventions, particularly medications. **Physical therapists** (PTs) and **occupational therapists** (OTs) and their assistants, **physical therapist assistants** (PTAs) and certified occupational therapist assistants (COTAs), are the allied health professionals who specialize in providing physical rehabilitation. In addition to these physical rehabilitation specialists, patients involved in physical rehabilitation may also be cared for by nurses, speech-language pathologists, and neuropsychologists.

According to the *Guide*, PTs "diagnose and manage movement **dysfunction** and enhance physical and functional abilities."[1] They "restore, maintain, and promote not only optimal physical function but optimal wellness and fitness and optimal quality of life as it relates to movement and health." They also "prevent the onset, **symptoms**, and progression of impairments, functional limitations, and disabilities that may result from diseases, **disorders**, conditions, or injuries."[1] PTAs work under the direction and supervision of PTs. They focus on providing interventions and may document the patients' responses to interventions and report the outcome of interventions to the PT. PTAs usually have formal training.

> ### Clinical Pearl
> Physical therapist assistants (PTAs) focus on providing interventions under the direction and supervision of physical therapists (PTs).

Patients with a wide range of needs and problems typically receive physical rehabilitation. Most have a disease, disorder, condition, or injury with consequent impairments, functional limitations, and disabilities. The conditions underlying these limitations may involve any physical system, including the musculoskeletal, neuromuscular, cardiopulmonary, and integumentary systems. For example, patients with fractures, stroke, heart failure, or pressure ulcers commonly receive physical rehabilitation services. Physical rehabilitation may also be provided preventively in patients at risk for developing impairments, functional limitations, and disabilities. For example, clients with osteoporosis may receive **physical therapy** to reduce their risk of fractures and falls.

GOALS OF PHYSICAL REHABILITATION

The goals of physical rehabilitation are to optimize patient function at home, in the community, and at work. Although these outcomes are commonly measured in terms of impairments, ideally they should be focused on changes in functional limitations and disabilities and centered on the patient's own goals for functional improvement.[3] A wide range of outcome measures may be used to assess a patient's progression toward these goals.

DISABLEMENT MODELS

Two related conceptual frameworks that help guide examination, **evaluation,** and interventions for patients in rehabilitation are disablement models, particularly the World Health Organization (WHO) and the Nagi models, and the *Guide*. These conceptual frameworks are described in the following sections.

THE WORLD HEALTH ORGANIZATION MODEL

Disablement models are approaches to thinking about the impacts or sequelae of disease on human functioning. A number of classification schemes have been proposed to categorize these sequelae. In 1980, WHO published the first classification scheme, the International Classification of Impairments, Disabilities and Handicaps (ICIDH).[4-6] This scheme, based primarily on the work of Wood, classified the sequelae of pathology as impairments, disabilities, and handicaps.[7,8] Shortly thereafter, Nagi published a similar model that used the classifications of impairments, functional limitations, and disabilities.[9] In 1993, the National Center for Medical Rehabilitation Research (NCMRR) published a classification scheme that combined concepts from the Nagi model with the original ICIDH model.[10] Most recently, in 2001, WHO revised their classification scheme to produce the International Classification of Functioning, Disability and Health-2 (ICF) scheme.[11]

Disablement model revisions are intended to reflect and create changes in perceptions of people with disabilities and meet the needs of more involved groups of people. The original models were intended to differentiate disease and pathology from the limitations they produced and were developed primarily for use by rehabilitation professionals. The newly expanded models try to have a more positive perspective on the changes resulting from pathology and disease and are intended for use by a wide range of people, including community, national, and global institutions that create policy and allocate resources for persons with disabilities. Specifically, the NCMRR model added a category of societal limitations to the functional problems associated with **disability** and abandoned the previous linear modeling approach to reflect the frequently nonsequential nature of the relationships between categories. The ICF has tried to change the perspective of disability from the negative focus of "consequences of disease" used in the 1980 model to a more positive focus on "components of health." Thus, while the first ICIDH model used categories of impairments, disabilities, and handicaps to describe sequelae of pathology, ICF uses categories of health conditions, body functions, activities, and participation to focus on abilities rather than on restrictions and limitations. More detailed information on the WHO disablement models is available on the ICF web site at www.who.int/classification/icf/en.

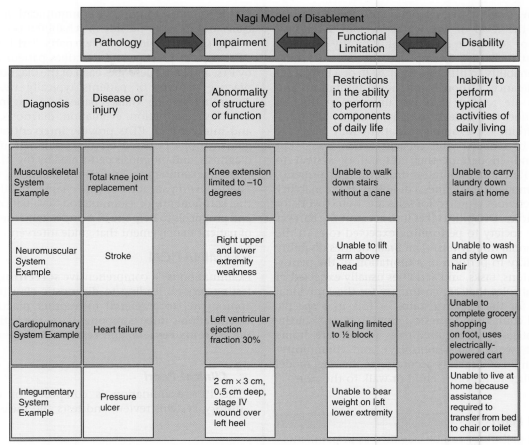

Nagi Model of Disablement							
	Pathology		Impairment		Functional Limitation		Disability
Diagnosis	Disease or injury		Abnormality of structure or function		Restrictions in the ability to perform components of daily life		Inability to perform typical activities of daily living
Musculoskeletal System Example	Total knee joint replacement		Knee extension limited to −10 degrees		Unable to walk down stairs without a cane		Unable to carry laundry down stairs at home
Neuromuscular System Example	Stroke		Right upper and lower extremity weakness		Unable to lift arm above head		Unable to wash and style own hair
Cardiopulmonary System Example	Heart failure		Left ventricular ejection fraction 30%		Walking limited to ½ block		Unable to complete grocery shopping on foot, uses electrically-powered cart
Integumentary System Example	Pressure ulcer		2 cm × 3 cm, 0.5 cm deep, stage IV wound over left heel		Unable to bear weight on left lower extremity		Unable to live at home because assistance required to transfer from bed to chair or toilet

FIG. 1-1 The Nagi model of disablement. *Data from Nagi S: Disability concepts revisited. In Pope AM, Tarlov AR (eds):* Disability in America: Toward a national agenda for prevention, *Washington, DC, 1991, National Academy Press.*

THE NAGI MODEL

This book uses a scheme consistent with the terminology and framework of the *Guide,*[1] which is based on the Nagi disablement model (Fig. 1-1). The *Guide* adopts Nagi's disablement model, stating that this "disablement model typifies physical therapist practice and is the model for understanding and organizing practice." The *Guide's* preferred practice patterns are based on the pathologies of four systems and their related impairments.[1]

According to the Nagi model and the *Guide,* the sequelae of pathology are classified as impairments, functional limitations, and disabilities.[1,4,9] Pathology refers to the alteration of anatomy or physiology that is due to disease or injury and describes a specific disease process or **diagnosis**. The *Guide* defines pathology as "an abnormality characterized by a particular cluster of **signs** and symptoms and recognized by either the patient or practitioner as abnormal. Pathology is primarily identified at the cellular level." Examples of pathology, as described by the Nagi model, include the diagnoses of cerebral vascular accident or stroke, lumbar disc herniation, or joint inflammation.

Knowledge of pathology does not provide sufficient information to guide either examination or procedural interventions in rehabilitation. For example, different individuals with a stroke may have wide-ranging alterations of motor and cognitive performance resulting in the need for different levels, approaches, and focus of both examination and interventions. Variation in the etiology, severity, and location of a stroke, as well as variation in other aspects of the patient's biopsychosocial health, may result in a range of impairments, functional limitations, and disabilities, from undetectable change from baseline to extreme change in all functional abilities and tremendous disability.

Impairments are defined by the Nagi model as disruptions in anatomical, physiological, or psychological structures or functions as the result of some underlying pathology,[6,11] and by the *Guide* as "a loss or abnormality of anatomical, physiological, mental, or psychological structure or function."[1] An impairment is a measure at the organ or organ system level and is equivalent to a sign or an objective measure. For example, decreased cervical range of motion, diminished deep tendon reflexes, reduced force production or endurance, and absent sensation are all impairments.

Impairments may lead to functional limitations. A functional limitation, as defined by the Nagi model, is a restriction in the ability to perform an activity in an efficient, typically expected, or competent manner or, as stated in the *Guide,* "the restriction of the ability to perform, at the level of the whole person, a physical action, task, or activity in an efficient, typically expected, or competent manner."[1] Examples of functional limitations are an inability to lift more than 20 lb or a limitation in sitting tolerance. Although functional limitations and impairments are related, it is not uncommon that an impairment does not, at least initially, result in any functional limitation. For example, a patient may have the impairment of reduced vital capacity when tested but never demand enough of their respiratory system to encounter a functional limitation from this impairment.

The Nagi model then defines a disability as the inability to perform activities required for self-care, home, work, or community roles. Disability takes into account the barriers presented by society to performing expected roles in the face of functional limitations.[9] The *Guide* defines disability as "the inability to perform or a limitation in the performance of actions, tasks, and activities usually expected in specific social roles that are customary for the individual or expected for the person's status or role in a specific sociocultural context and physical environment."[1] In the *Guide,* the categories of required roles are self-care, home management, work (job/school/play), and community/ leisure. Examples of disability according to the Nagi model are the inability to lift one's child or walk to the store.

Clinical Pearl

Sequelae of pathology can be classified as impairments (disruptions in structure or function), functional limitations (restrictions in the ability to perform activities), and disabilities (limitations in performing social roles).

Medical treatment is generally directed at the underlying pathology or disease, whereas rehabilitation focuses primarily on reversing or minimizing associated impairments, functional limitations, and disabilities. It is therefore essential that rehabilitation professionals assess and set goals not only at the level of impairment, such as pain, decreased range of motion, or hypertonicity, but also at the level of functional limitation and disability as they relate to the specific patient's goals. Improvements in functional limitations along with disabilities will be most important to patients and those individuals involved with their care.

THE *GUIDE TO PHYSICAL THERAPIST PRACTICE*

The *Guide,* the second and most recent edition of which was published in 2001, was developed by the American Physical Therapy Association (APTA) "to encourage a uniform approach to physical therapist practice and to explain to the world the nature of that practice."[1] This document took close to a decade to develop and forms a framework for describing the scope and content of PT practice using standardized terms and a standardized practice model. Its consistent conceptual approach to patient

care is intended to improve communication among clinicians and to those outside of rehabilitation.

The *Guide* is divided into two parts. Part 1 delineates the PT's scope of practice and describes patient management by PTs, and Part 2 describes each of the diagnostic preferred practice patterns of patients typically treated by PTs. According to the *Guide,* patient management by PTs involves examination, evaluation, diagnosis, **prognosis,** and intervention. PTAs provide interventions under the guidance of PTs based on the examination, evaluation, diagnosis, and prognosis performed by the PT. PTAs do not perform examination, evaluation, diagnosis, or prognosis. The following sections of this chapter briefly summarize the components of examination, evaluation, diagnosis, and prognosis to help the PTA understand the components of patient management that guide interventions.

EXAMINATION

Examination is "a comprehensive **screening** and specific testing process leading to diagnostic classification or, as appropriate, to a referral to another practitioner." The examination's three components are the patient **history,** the **systems review,** and **tests and measures.**

Clinical Pearl

The PT's examination is composed of the patient history, systems review, and tests and measures.

Patient History. The patient history is a systematically gathered collection of information focused on why the patient is seeking care, as well as past and current functional status and activity level. The patient history may also include information about the patient's general demographics, social history, employment or work, growth and development, living environment, general health status, social and health habits, family history, medical and surgical history, medications, and results of previously performed clinical tests. This information may be collected through interviewing the patient, caretakers, or family members and by review of prior medical records. The patient history, particularly the pattern of symptoms, will give the clinician an idea of the nature of the patient's problem and indicate the most efficient course for the rest of the examination.

Systems Review. The systems review is the first "hands-on" component of the examination. It involves a "brief or limited examination of the status of the cardiovascular/pulmonary, integumentary, musculoskeletal, and neuromuscular systems and the communication ability, affect, cognition, language, and learning style of the patient."[1] This brief review is used to target areas requiring further examination and define areas that may cause complications or indicate a need for precautions during the tests and measures and intervention processes.

Tests and Measures. The patient history and systems review are used to generate diagnostic hypotheses. Specific tests and measures of the musculoskeletal, neuromuscular, cardiopulmonary, and integumentary systems, as well as tests of patient function, are then selected to rule in or rule out causes of impairment and functional limitations. The results of these tests are used to establish a diagnosis, prognosis, and **plan of care** and to direct selection of interventions.

EVALUATION, DIAGNOSIS, AND PROGNOSIS

Evaluations are clinical judgments based on the data gathered during the examination. The evaluation involves synthesizing the findings from all of the components of the examination to establish the patient's diagnosis and prognosis. According to the *Guide*, PTs use diagnostic labels that "identify the impact of a condition on function at the level of the system (especially the movement system) and at the level of the whole person."[1] PTs assign a diagnostic label by classifying patients or clients within a specified preferred practice pattern.

◎ *Clinical Pearl*

Preferred practice patterns are the diagnostic labels used by PTs. Preferred practice patterns identify the impact of a condition on function.

According to the *Guide*, the prognosis is the "determination of the predicted optimal level of improvement in function and the amount of time needed to reach that level, and also may include a prediction of the improvement that may be reached at various intervals during the course of therapy." The prognosis should also include a plan of care that specifies "anticipated goals and expected outcomes, predicted level of optimal improvement, specific interventions to be used, and proposed duration and frequency of the interventions that are required to reach the anticipated goals and expected outcomes."

INTERVENTION

Interventions are "the purposeful interaction of the physical therapist with the patient using various physical therapy procedures and techniques to produce changes in the condition that are consistent with the diagnosis and prognosis."[1] Interventions may include coordination, communication, and documentation; patient/client-related instructions; and procedural interventions such as therapeutic exercise and physical agents.

Part 2 of the *Guide* includes sections on each of the diagnostic preferred practice patterns. These practice patterns are divided into four categories of conditions: musculoskeletal, neuromuscular, cardiovascular/pulmonary, and integumentary, with a number of preferred practice patterns within each of these categories. For each preferred practice pattern the *Guide* provides inclusion and exclusion criteria for the diagnostic classification, *International Classification of Diseases, Ninth Revision, Clinical Modification (ICD-9-CM)* codes that may relate to the practice pattern, and descriptions of the examination, evaluation, diagnosis, prognosis, and interventions related to the management of patients within this preferred practice pattern.

STRUCTURE OF THIS BOOK

This textbook is structured around concepts presented in the *Guide*.[1] By adopting the structure of the *Guide*, this book promotes clinical integration of the *Guide's* concepts.

This book is divided into five parts. The first four parts are the same as the *Guide's* categories of preferred practice patterns: musculoskeletal, neuromuscular, cardiovascular/pulmonary, and integumentary (Table 1-1). Most of the chapters within the first three parts of this book parallel the preferred practice patterns presented in the *Guide*. However, Part 4, preferred practice patterns related to the integumentary system, is organized according to wound etiology, which is more commonly done in clinical practice and research, rather than according to wound depth as in the *Guide*. Part 5 covers interventions that overlap many practice patterns and are therefore most effectively discussed together rather than repetitively in many other chapters.

In addition to the parts and chapters of this book paralleling the structure of the *Guide*, the structure of individual chapters also follow the recommendations of the *Guide*. A summary of typical examination findings by the physical therapist (including history, systems review, and tests and measures), followed by the therapist's evaluation, diagnosis, and prognosis, is provided. This is followed by detailed descriptions of interventions, which is the focus of the PTA's practice. This book also uses the language and concepts of the *Guide*. For example, the activities of physical rehabilitation are described using the terms *tests and measures* and *interventions*, rather than the more traditional terms *objective examination* and *treatment*, respectively. This is intended to help meet one of the stated purposes of the *Guide* of: "standardizing terminology used in and related to physical therapy practice."[1] Additionally, the practice of physical rehabilitation is described using the Nagi disablement model.

As with the *Guide*, the purposes of this book include improving quality of care, enhancing positive outcomes from physical rehabilitation interventions, enhancing patient satisfaction, and increasing the consistency, efficiency, and cost-effectiveness of health care.

STRUCTURE OF CHAPTERS

To facilitate learning of the presented ideas and their application in clinical practice, each chapter has a similar consistent structure (Box 1-1). This structure parallels recommendations of the *Guide*, makes information clear and readily accessible, and promotes learning and recall for the student and quick access to specific information for the experienced clinician.

EVIDENCE-BASED EXAMINATION, EVALUATION, DIAGNOSIS, PROGNOSIS, AND INTERVENTION

Although the *Guide* forms a framework for describing and implementing clinical practice, it does not evaluate or recommend specific approaches for patient management. In contrast, this book gives specific, detailed, evidence-based information on the pathology, etiology,

TABLE 1-1	Comparison of Preferred Practice Patterns from the *Guide to Physical Therapist Practice* with Chapters in This Book

Preferred Practice Patterns in the *Guide to Physical Therapist Practice*	Chapters in *Physical Rehabilitation for the Physical Therapist Assistant*
CATEGORY **PATTERN NUMBER: TITLE**	**PART: TITLE** **CHAPTER: TITLE**
Musculoskeletal	**1: Musculoskeletal System**
4A: Primary prevention/risk reduction for skeletal demineralization	3: Skeletal Demineralization
4B: Impaired posture	4: Posture
4C: Impaired muscle performance	5: Muscle Weakness
4D: Impaired joint mobility, motor function, muscle performance, and range of motion associated with connective tissue dysfunction	6: Connective Tissue Dysfunction
4E: Impaired joint mobility, motor function, muscle performance, and range of motion associated with localized inflammation	7: Localized Inflammation
4F: Impaired joint mobility, motor function, muscle performance, range of motion, and reflex integrity associated with spinal disorders	8: Spinal Disorders
4G: Impaired joint mobility, muscle performance, and range of motion associated with fracture	9: Fractures
4H: Impaired joint mobility, motor function, muscle performance, and range of motion associated with joint arthroplasty	10: Joint Arthroplasty
4I: Impaired joint mobility, motor function, muscle performance, and range of motion associated with bony or soft tissue surgery	11: Soft Tissue Surgery
4J: Impaired motor function, muscle performance, range of motion, gait, locomotion, and balance associated with amputation	12: Amputations and Prostheses
Neuromuscular	**2: Neuromuscular System**
5A: Primary prevention/risk reduction for loss of balance and falling	13: Balance and Fall Risk
5B: Impaired neuromotor development	14: Impaired Neuromotor Development
5C/5D: Impaired motor function and sensory integrity associated with nonprogressive disorders of the central nervous system—congenital origin or acquired in infancy or childhood	15: Pediatric Nonprogressive Central Nervous System Disorders
5D: Impaired motor function and sensory integrity associated with nonprogressive disorders of the central nervous system—acquired in adolescence or adulthood	16: Adult Nonprogressive Central Nervous System Disorders
5E: Impaired motor function and sensory integrity associated with progressive disorders of the central nervous system	17: Progressive Central Nervous System Disorders
5F: Impaired peripheral nerve integrity and muscle performance associated with peripheral nerve injury	18: Peripheral Nerve Injuries
5G: Impaired motor function and sensory integrity associated with acute or chronic polyneuropathies	19: Polyneuropathies
5H: Impaired motor function, peripheral nerve integrity, and sensory integrity associated with nonprogressive disorders of the spinal cord	20: Nonprogressive Spinal Cord Disorders
5I: Impaired arousal, range of motion, and motor control associated with coma, near coma, and vegetative state	21: Disorders of Consciousness: Coma, Vegetative State, and Minimally Conscious State 22: Vital Signs
Cardiovascular/Pulmonary	**3: Cardiopulmonary System**
6B: Impaired aerobic capacity/endurance associated with deconditioning	23: Deconditioning
6C: Impaired ventilation, respiration/gas exchange, and aerobic capacity/endurance associated with airway clearance dysfunction	24: Airway Clearance Dysfunction
6D: Impaired aerobic capacity/endurance associated with cardiovascular pump dysfunction or failure	25: Congestive Heart Failure
6E: Impaired ventilation and respiration/gas exchange associated with ventilatory pump dysfunction or failure	26: Respiratory Failure
6F: Impaired ventilation and respiration/gas exchange associated with respiratory failure	
6H: Impaired circulation and anthropometric dimensions associated with lymphatic system disorders	27: Lymphatic System Disorders
Integumentary	**4: Integumentary System**
7B: Impaired integumentary integrity associated with superficial skin involvement	28: Tissue Healing and Pressure Ulcers 29: Vascular Ulcers
7C: Impaired integumentary integrity associated with partial-thickness skin involvement and scar formation	30: Neuropathic Ulcers 31: Burns
7D: Impaired integumentary integrity associated with full-thickness skin involvement and scar formation	
	5: Interventions Common to Many Conditions Requiring Rehabilitation 32: Gait Assessment and Training 33: Assistive Devices for Mobility 34: Orthotics

---

BOX 1-1   **Standard Chapter Outline**

- Objectives
- Pathology
- Typical Examination Findings
  - Patient History
  - Systems Review
  - Tests and Measures
- Evaluation, Diagnosis, and Prognosis
- Intervention
- Case Study
- Chapter Summary
- Additional Resources
- Glossary

---

examination, evaluation, diagnosis, prognosis, and intervention for patients involved in physical rehabilitation.

The typical examination findings section of each chapter includes a summary of the patient history and appropriate tests and measures for each preferred practice pattern. Since the systems review is essentially similar for all patients, this is not discussed further within the individual chapters. The tests and measures are presented in categories, as recommended by the *Guide*.

The sections on intervention within each chapter include rationales for selection of interventions and in many cases explanations of how and when to apply recommended interventions. Where possible within the context of such a broad text, sufficient detail is provided to allow the reader to develop and execute an effective plan of care. Where such detail cannot be provided, the reader is directed to other specific sources for more detailed descriptions of how to apply the recommended methods and techniques.

CLINICAL PEARLS, CASE STUDIES, ADDITIONAL RESOURCES, AND GLOSSARY

This book includes a number of special features with all chapters. Clinical pearls are included throughout to emphasize important concepts. Almost all chapters include a case study demonstrating the application of the principles and techniques described and a glossary of important terms. Each chapter also includes recommendations of other books, web sites, and organizations for further information.

The book includes an Evolve site where additional case studies, direct electronic online links to useful resources and all listed references, printable forms related to the chapter, vocabulary-building exercises, and boards-style examination questions. Instructors using this text may also obtain online access to electronic versions of all figures in the text.

CHAPTER SUMMARY

This text is intended for use by physical therapist assistants. It applies the Nagi disablement model and concepts from the *Guide to Physical Therapist Practice,* in conjunction with evaluation of the current evidence, to derive summaries of typical patient examination and evaluation and recommendations for intervention, for each preferred practice pattern managed by physical therapists and physical therapist assistants. All information is presented in a clear and consistent manner in each chapter, and chapters include the special features of clinical pearls, a case study, clinically useful resources, and a glossary of terms used. The Evolve site that compliments this book provides additional case studies, study questions, printable forms for clinic use, and direct online links to listed references and resources.

ADDITIONAL RESOURCES

For links to these and additional web-based resources, see the Evolve site.

International Classification of Functioning, Disability and Health-2 (ICF)

American Physical Therapy Association (APTA)

GLOSSARY

The definitions given in this glossary and throughout this book are consistent with definitions given in other rehabilitation documents. Definitions for terms vary among sources, including other textbooks, medical and general dictionaries, and the *Guide*. These differences are likely the result of differences in audience with respect to level of detail and complexity, as well as focus. General dictionaries avoid technical medical terms, whereas medical texts and dictionaries refer to other medical concepts in their definitions. Rehabilitation-oriented documents, including this textbook, use definitions that focus on functional abilities and physical interventions.

Diagnosis: A process and a label. The diagnostic process includes integrating and evaluating the data obtained during the examination to describe the patient condition in terms that will guide the prognosis, the plan of care, and intervention strategies. Diagnosis as a label denotes the disease or syndrome a person has or is believed to have and the use of scientific or clinical methods to establish the cause and nature of a person's illness.[13] PTs use diagnostic labels that identify the impact of a condition on function at the level of the system (especially the movement system) and at the level of the whole person.[1]

Disability: The inability to perform or a limitation in the performance of actions, tasks, and activities usually expected in specific social roles that are customary for the individual or expected for the person's status or role in a specific sociocultural context and physical environment. In the *Guide*, the categories of required roles are self-care, home management, work (job/school/play), and community/leisure.[1]

Disease: A pathological condition or abnormal entity with a characteristic group of signs and symptoms affecting the body and with known or unknown etiology.[1] A condition marked by subjective complaints, a specific history, and clinical signs, symptoms, and laboratory or radiographic findings.[12]

Disorder: Derangement or abnormality of function (anatomical or physiological); pathology.

Dysfunction: Disturbance, impairment, or abnormality of function of an organ.

Evaluation: A dynamic process in which the clinician makes clinical judgments based on data gathered during the examination.

Examination: A comprehensive screening and specific testing process. The examination has three components: Patient history, systems review, and tests and measures.

Function: Those activities identified by an individual as essential to support physical, social, and psychological well-being and create a personal sense of meaningful living.

Functional limitation: The restriction of the ability to perform, at the level of the whole person, a physical action, task, or activity in an efficient, typically expected, or competent manner.

Goals: The intended results of patient management. Goals indicate changes in impairment, functional limitations, and disabilities and changes in health, wellness, and fitness needs that are expected as a result of implementing the plan of care. Goals should be measurable and time limited. (If required, goals may be expressed as short- and long-term.)

History: A component of the examination. A systematic gathering of data—from both the past and the present—related to why the patient is seeking rehabilitation services. The data that are obtained (through interview, review of the patient record, or from other sources) include demographic information, social history, employment and work (job/school/play), growth and development, living environments, general health status, social and health habits (past and current), family history, medical/surgical history, current conditions or chief complaints, functional status and activity level, medications, and other clinical tests. While taking the history, the clinician also identifies health restoration and prevention needs and coexisting health problems that may have implications for intervention.

Impairment: A loss or abnormality of anatomical, physiological, mental, or psychological structure or function.

Intervention: The purposeful interaction of the clinician with the patient and when appropriate, with other individuals involved in patient care, using various procedures and techniques to produce change in the condition.

Occupational therapy: Therapeutic activities used to develop, regain, or maintain the skills necessary for health, productivity, and independence in everyday life. It may include the use of assistive technologies or orthotics to enhance function or prevent disability. Therapy by means of activity; especially creative activity prescribed for its effect in promoting recovery or rehabilitation.[13]

Occupational therapist (OT): A person trained in or engaged in the practice of occupational therapy.[13]

Pathology/pathophysiology: An abnormality characterized by a particular cluster of signs and symptoms and recognized by either the patient or practitioner as abnormal. Pathology is primarily identified at the cellular level.

Physiatrist: A physician who specializes in physical medicine.[13]

Physical therapist (PT): A person who is a graduate of an accredited physical therapist education program and is licensed to practice physical therapy. The terms *physical therapist* and *physiotherapist* are synonymous.[1]

Physical therapist assistant (PTA): Physical therapist assistants work under the direction and supervision of physical therapists. They may assist in developing treatment plans and providing interventions. They may also document the progress of treatment. PTAs usually have formal training.

Physical therapy: Examination, evaluation, diagnosis, prognosis, and intervention provided by a physical therapist.[1] The treatment of disease and movement-related dysfunction by physical and mechanical means such as massage, regulated exercise, water, light, heat, and electricity.[13]

Plan of care: Statements that specify the anticipated goals and expected outcomes, predicted level of optimal improvement, specific interventions to be used, and proposed duration and frequency of the interventions required to reach the goals and outcomes. The plan of care includes anticipated discharge plans.

Prognosis: The determination of the predicted optimal level of improvement in function and the amount of time needed to reach that level.[1] The act or art of foretelling the course of a disease or the prospect of survival and recovery from a disease as anticipated by the usual course of that disease or indicated by special features of the case.[13] The possible outcomes of a condition and the frequency with which they can be expected to occur.[14]

Rehabilitation: A set of actions designed to restore, following disease or injury, the ability to function in a normal or near-normal manner.[14] Rehabilitation is a goal-oriented treatment process that is intended to maximize independence in individuals with compromised function due to primary pathological processes and resultant impairments.

Screening: Determining the need for further examination or consultation.

Signs: Objective evidence of physical abnormality.

Symptoms: Subjective evidence of physical abnormality.

Systems review: A component of the examination. The systems review is a brief and gross examination, or "quick check," to identify information not presented in the patient history and to identify if other health problems should be considered in the diagnosis, prognosis, and plan of care or indicate the need for referral to another health provider.

Tests and measures: A component of the examination. Specific standardized methods and techniques used to gather data about the patient after the history and systems review have been performed.

Treatment: The sum of all interventions provided by a clinician during an episode of care.

Evidence-Based Practice

Michelle H. Cameron

OBJECTIVES

After reading this chapter, the reader will be able to:
1. Define evidence-based practice.
2. Apply the concepts of evidence-based practice to the clinical practice of rehabilitation.
3. Locate and identify high quality evidence for the clinical practice of rehabilitation.

DEFINING EVIDENCE-BASED PRACTICE

Evidence-based practice (EBP) is defined by Sackett, the originator of the term, as "the conscientious, explicit, and judicious use of current best evidence in making decisions about the care of individual patients."[1,2] EBP is based on the application of the scientific method to clinical practice. EBP requires that clinical practice decisions be guided by the best available relevant clinical research data in conjunction with the clinician's experience, while also taking into account what is known about the pathophysiology of the patient's condition, the individual patient's values and preferences, and what is available in the clinical practice setting.

The goal of EBP is to identify and provide the best possible patient care. The best care is the care with the greatest likelihood of producing the best outcome for the patient. Although this may appear to be a simple and implicit goal of all patient care, it is actually complex, can be difficult to achieve, and requires integration of information from multiple sources. The best outcome requires consideration of the values of each patient within the context of their society and an ability to assess the outcome. Good outcome measures are needed to determine if an outcome has been achieved. These measures must be valid (measure what they claim to measure) and reliable (produce the same result each time they are applied) and quantify and communicate changes in patients that may result from clinical interventions. Once the clinician has identified goals and measures for **outcomes,** to apply EBP the clinician must also know what is most likely to produce the best outcomes. This requires evidence, which is described in detail later in this chapter.

Clinical Pearl

Evidence-based practice (EBP) requires that clinical decisions be guided by the best available relevant clinical research data, the clinician's experience, the pathophysiology of the patient's condition, the individual patient's values and preferences, and what is available in the clinical practice setting.

TRADITIONAL APPROACHES TO CLINICAL DECISIONS

Traditionally, a number of other approaches based on logical, rational thinking and clinician experience have been used to direct clinical practice and make clinical decisions. The most common of these is experience-based practice. An example of this approach is if most of a clinician's patients with low back pain and weak abdominal muscles had less pain a few weeks after being instructed in abdominal strengthening exercises, then the clinician would continue to apply this approach. Although this approach is appealing, it is limited. The patient's goals and expectations are not assessed, and the natural course of symptoms is not distinguished from the effects of interventions. Do we know if these patients get better because of the exercises or just because most back pain resolves

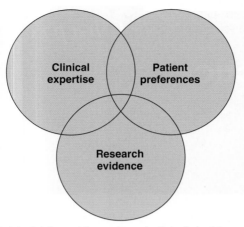

FIG. 2-1 Model for evidence-based clinical decision making.

spontaneously over time? This approach also fails to distinguish luck from probable outcome; for example, did these few patients just happen to respond well to this intervention when most would not have?

ORIGIN OF EVIDENCE-BASED PRACTICE

In contrast to prior methods, EBP uses the best evidence in conjunction with clinical expertise and patient values to make clinical decisions (Fig. 2-1). Decisions may be made about examination, diagnosis, and **prognosis,** as well as preventive and treatment interventions. The ideas of EBP originated in mid-nineteenth century Paris but did not rise to the fore until the 1980s when they were reintroduced, primarily in Canada by Dr. David Sackett and in the United Kingdom by Dr. Archie Cochrane. EBP has continued to gain popularity, although not without resistance. EBP addresses the desire of patients and payers for the most up-to-date therapies while taking into account the need for cost containment. EBP takes advantage of the growing mass of research data, including outcomes data, and improved access to this data through advances in information systems to closely monitor and analyze research studies, practice patterns, and clinical outcomes. The American Physical Therapy Association, the American Occupational Therapy Association, and the American Medical Association, as well as many other groups, support the principles of EBP. Although EBP is still in its infancy in the rehabilitation professional's culture, its application can guide practitioners to the most efficient, effective, consistent, and highest quality clinical practice.

EBP requires a clinician's expertise and the best external clinical evidence. Although evidence derived from clinical research is a crucial component, **patient preferences,** clinical circumstances, and the clinician's experience and judgment are also essential to clinical decision making. Clinical expertise is the proficiency and judgment that each clinician acquires through experience and practice. Those with greater expertise may demonstrate better practice in many ways, including most often more effective and efficient diagnosis and more thoughtful identification and effective integration of individual patients' predicaments, rights, and preferences in making clinical decisions

about their care. However, clinicians with more experience may also practice more poorly by allowing their own personal experience to inappropriately outweigh high quality evidence.

The best external clinical evidence is clinically relevant, unbiased research. Although this research may be basic science, the most useful research for EBP comes from patient-centered clinical studies evaluating the **validity** and **reliability** of clinical tests and measures, the power of prognostic markers, and the **efficacy** and safety of therapeutic or preventive interventions. External clinical evidence can invalidate previously accepted measures or interventions and can replace them with those found to be more reliable, accurate, safe, and effective.

APPLYING EVIDENCE-BASED PRACTICE TO REHABILITATION

EBP requires clinical expertise and an appreciation of clinical research evidence. Clinical expertise is developed over time through interactions with patients. For an appreciation of research evidence, the clinician must take a systematic approach, frequently extending beyond the time spent directly with patients or in the clinic. Just reading a journal regularly or attending continuing education courses is not sufficient for EBP. EBP requires the critical application of research evidence to each specific patient problem. Clinicians must find and critically appraise the relevant published evidence and combine these findings with their own clinical expertise and the patient's circumstances and values to determine a course of clinical care. Having chosen this course, the clinician must execute it and follow this with evaluation of the patient's outcome. EBP should be applied to all aspects of the clinical interaction, including selection of valid and reliable tests and measures, determination of an accurate diagnosis and prognosis, and application of effective interventions.[3]

EBP requires a shift in the thought processes of many clinicians. Although clinical advice may rely on clinical experience, expert opinions, collegial relationships, pathophysiology, common sense, community standards, published material, and other sources, when practicing EBP the clinician must always ask, "What evidence is there to support or refute this advice?"

Applying EBP to rehabilitation is particularly challenging because trials evaluating rehabilitation interventions cannot always meet the methodological standards applied to other types of clinical trials.[4] In particular, subjects, treaters, and evaluators frequently cannot be **blinded** to the application of a rehabilitation intervention because many interventions used in rehabilitation, such as manual therapy techniques, depend on the skill of the person applying them and thus necessitate at least nonblinding of the person providing the treatment. Other rehabilitation interventions, such as exercise, depend on the cooperation of the subject and thus cannot be applied without subject awareness. In addition, interventions used in rehabilitation can be difficult to describe and are frequently, by necessity, individualized. Therefore they are often not described in sufficient detail to allow a complete understanding of the intervention or replication of the study if desired. Many rehabilitation interventions also cannot be standardized because they vary with the skill, training, and experience of the provider.[5] Although these limitations may be addressed by training all providers similarly before providing an intervention, standardizing interventions, and designing similar sham interventions, complete blinding in rehabilitation studies is rare.

TYPES OF EVIDENCE

All research evidence is not equal and the evidence to be used in EBP can be classified and evaluated on a number of factors, including the study design, the types of subjects, the nature of controls, the outcome measures used, and the statistical analysis applied. One approach evaluates the quality of the question being asked by a study. All well-built questions should have four parts that can be readily remembered using the mnemonic PICO:

P: Patient or population. The question should apply to a specific population (e.g., adults with low back pain, children with lower extremity spasticity that is due to spinal dysraphism).

I: Intervention. The intervention should be specific (e.g., specified exercises applied for a specified period of time at a specified frequency).

C: Comparison intervention/measure. The intervention (or measure) should be compared to some current commonly used treatment (or gold standard measure) or to no intervention if no intervention is usually provided.

O: Outcome. The outcome should be defined as precisely as possible, ideally using a clinically relevant, reliable, validated measure (e.g., walking speed, level of independence with activities of daily living [ADLs]).

Study Design. The simplest research design is the case report. A case report is a detailed description of a patient's clinical presentation, the course of treatment, and the changes in clinical presentation that occurred during and generally after that course of treatment. A case report is generally the first type of formal evaluation of a treatment approach performed. It is most valuable for describing new methods for treating a condition when little other information is available. When **case reports** are well written, they provide information about all aspects of the patient's presentation and care in detail, and they only require the investigator to describe an individual's course of treatment and presentation. The primary disadvantage of case reports is that they only provide information about what was done to a particular patient and what happened to that patient, without clearly indicating what caused the observed changes. Therefore one cannot be certain which, if any, of the intervention(s) in question caused the observed changes or if these changes occurred independently of the interventions. Caution should be observed when considering applying the findings of a case report to other individuals because the changes that occurred in the subject of the report may have been unique to that individual. Case reports are therefore considered the least strong evidence for the **effectiveness** of an intervention for a particular problem. However, they can provide valuable information to guide controlled research studies.

A controlled research study is one in which the effects of an intervention are compared with some alternative, the control. The simplest controlled study uses only one subject whose status when an intervention is applied for a period of time is compared with the status when the intervention is not applied. This type of study provides better information about the effects of an intervention than a case report. In contrast to case reports, single-subject studies can differentiate the effects of time alone from the effects of the intervention under investigation without the time and expense of studies involving groups of subjects. Single-subject studies also eliminate the differences in initial status or individual characteristics that can confound the interpretation of studies involving groups of subjects. Studies using single subjects are particularly suitable for investigating the effects of interventions on uncommon problems where large groups of subjects may not be available and for analyzing the effects of interventions on problems whose normal progression is so variable as to obscure any effects of an intervention using a group design. Although single-subject studies have a number of advantages over case reports, because they only evaluate the response of a single individual to an intervention, caution should be applied in generalizing the findings of such studies to other subjects.

In most situations, comparing the effects of providing an intervention to one group of subjects with withholding it from another group more clearly demonstrates the effects of that intervention than a single-subject study can. Well-designed studies involving groups of subjects can provide strong evidence about the effectiveness of an intervention. Studies with large homogeneous groups are preferred because they minimize the risk of failing to detect the true effects of an intervention. Unfortunately, because large groups of individuals with similar characteristics are difficult to recruit, many studies in rehabilitation, particularly those involving human subjects, use small, heterogeneous samples and may thus erroneously conclude that treatments are ineffective. This is known as a type 2 error or a **false-negative** result.

Although well-designed and controlled studies may be able to detect small, statistically significant effects of treatment, when considering applying the findings to clinical practice the **clinical significance** of these effects must also be taken into account. For example, although a study may find that applying heat before stretching the knees of patients who have had a total knee arthroplasty results in a statistically significantly greater gain in flexion range of motion than stretching without prior heating, if the difference in gains is only a few degrees, this may not be clinically significant if it does not affect patient function. A slight acceleration of recovery may also be statistically significant while not justifying the use of an intervention in general clinical care. For example, even if applying traction is found to decrease the recovery time from a low back injury from 40 days to 39 days, in most cases the cost of applying this treatment will not be justified by this small effect.

Types of Subjects. Having selected the appropriate study design based on the effect being studied and the quality and availability of prior studies, an investigator must also select suitable research subjects. Subject selection depends on what is being studied, the type of outcome data desired, and subject availability. Studies may be carried out in vitro, which means "within glass." This term describes studies that are carried out in a container or in a test tube rather than within a living organism. In vitro studies use various nonliving materials or cell cultures as subjects. In vitro studies can generally be replicated accurately and allow for very close control of subject and intervention variability; however, given how different these set-ups are from patients, caution should be exercised in applying findings of these studies directly to clinical situations.

Using animals as research subjects overcomes some of the limitations of in vitro studies by allowing evaluation of the effects of rehabilitation interventions on the physical properties of tissue within a normal physiological environment. Although animal studies may support the application of clinical interventions, their evidence is limited because humans may respond differently and because these studies generally cannot provide information about the effect of an intervention on functional limitations or disabilities.

Studies using human subjects provide the best evidence for the effects on a patient's functional abilities and disabilities. Ideally, studies use patients with pathology rather than subjects without pathology because this provides information that is most readily applicable to other patients. However, because of limitations in access to subjects with problems of similar types and severity, as well as financial and ethical constraints in applying interventions with unknown effects or withholding potentially effective care from control patients, many studies are performed using human subjects without pathology. These studies may provide information about the physical and physiological effects of interventions, such as their impact on tissue length, muscle strength, or blood circulation, and may be used to investigate the effects of interventions on experimentally induced dysfunction such as pain. However, caution must be used in applying the findings of such studies to patients with pathology. For example, although electrical stimulation may not increase muscle strength more effectively than exercise in normal subjects, it has been found to augment strengthening when applied after knee surgery. Studies using groups of patients provide the best evidence about the effects of rehabilitation interventions on functional patient outcomes.

Controls. Because changes in subjects can occur whether an intervention has or has not been applied, the outcome of subjects who have received an intervention must be compared with the outcome of subjects who have not received that intervention. The subjects who do not receive the intervention being evaluated are known as controls.

Controls are needed to differentiate the effects of chance, normal progression of the outcome variable, and nonspecific effects of treatment from specific effects of the intervention being evaluated. Without appropriate controls, it is difficult, if not impossible, to determine if the changes observed in subjects were solely due to time or nonspecific effects or were caused by the intervention

being studied. Most of the treatments provided by rehabilitation clinicians have nonspecific effects. Paying attention to the patient may increase the patient's motivation, monitoring progress may improve the patient's compliance, and touching the patient, either directly or with a device, may provide a sensory stimulus to block pain transmission. To control for these effects, sham interventions with similar nonspecific effects to those from the intervention being studied are applied to control subjects. Such alternative interventions are known as **placebo** interventions.

Without appropriate controls, although much time, effort, and expense may be expended, study results will not clearly show if an intervention has a specific effect and therefore will not readily improve patient care. It will not be known whether the treatments being evaluated are effective and should be used with patients or whether any observed changes in subject status were the result of chance, normal progression, or nonspecific effects of the intervention.

To most accurately determine the effects of an intervention, neither the subjects of the study nor the individuals applying the intervention should know if an active or a placebo treatment is being applied. Additionally, the choice of true or placebo intervention should be random. This is known as double-blind random application. A double-blind, **randomized controlled trial** (RCT) is the gold standard for research design. Unfortunately, it is challenging, if not impossible, to apply many rehabilitation interventions in a double-blind fashion.

◎ *Clinical Pearl*

A double-blind, randomized controlled trial (RCT) is the gold standard for research design.

Outcome Measures. In addition to evaluating a study for its design and controls, the outcome measures should also be evaluated. Outcome measures should be reliable, valid, and clinically relevant. A measure is considered to be reliable if the same or a similar result is produced when the measure is repeated. For example, goniometric measurement of active knee flexion range of motion is reliable if the same or a similar angle is reported when active knee flexion range of motion is measured repeatedly. Studies should use measures whose reliability in the population being tested is proven, and the measures' reliability should be clearly documented in all research reports.

◎ *Clinical Pearl*

Reliability is the consistency or reproducibility of data. A reliable test gives the same result when applied in the same situation.

In contrast to reliability, which relates to the reproducibility of a measure, validity relates to its usefulness and the degree to which it represents the property it claims to measure. For example, for a questionnaire to be a valid measure of disability in a population, it must actually measure the reduced ability of this population to perform normal activities.

Clinical Pearl

Validity is the extent to which an instrument measures what it intends to measure.

In addition to being reliable and valid, outcome measures should relate directly to the goal(s) of treatment and should be clinically relevant and therefore include measures of the effects of interventions on impairment, functional limitations, and disability. For example, a study on the effects of exercise for patients with knee pain should include measures of functional outcomes, such as walking speed and work participation, not just lower extremity strength and knee range of motion. These types of outcomes allow prediction of functional outcome in response to interventions and therefore most effectively guide practice and support reimbursement for rehabilitation.

Cost-effectiveness studies may also guide EBP. Cost-effectiveness studies evaluate the costs of achieving the benefits of an intervention. They present the costs of providing the intervention and the potential benefits and savings associated with reducing the duration and severity of a patient's disability. Potential benefits may be improved quality of life and monetary savings such as reduced loss of income to the patient, reduced employer costs associated with replacing a member of the workforce, and avoidance of costs associated with providing further care to the patient. For example, providing traction to patients with low back pain for 10 visits may cost $500; however, if it is shown that this accelerates their return to work by an average of 1 week, this treatment may be cost-effective if the costs to those patients, their employers, and their insurance carriers associated with not working for 1 week are greater than $500 and other interventions take longer or are less effective.

Integrative Summary Reports and Studies. In some areas, there are a number of original research studies with the same purpose. The findings of studies in a particular area may be summarized and evaluated in integrative summary reports. The simplest integrative summary report is a nonsystematic review or narrative report, which is a descriptive general summary of research selected by the author of the review. The methods used to collect and interpret data are often informal and subjective rather than systematic or exhaustive, with the reviewers frequently selecting studies that support their own perspective, opinion, or clinical experience. The method of study selection is generally impossible to replicate and is frequently **biased.**

A **systematic review** is a summary of primary studies selected with a rigorous and predefined method, with precise **inclusion** and **exclusion criteria.** Published studies concerning a specific question are systematically searched for using an unbiased selection procedure. These are then abstracted, critically appraised, and synthesized, and the findings summarized. A systematic review is a comprehensive and unbiased integrative descriptive report that provides an overview of the published research on a topic. It is a scientific rather than a subjective summarization of the literature on a subject and can reveal new evidence, help deal with the volume of literature, and produce evidence to help with decision making.

In contrast to the systematic review, which is a qualitative report, a **meta-analysis** is a quantitative review. A meta-analysis combines and analyzes the numerical data from individual primary RCTs that meet rigorous predefined standards to determine the efficacy of an intervention. Meta-analyses have a precise protocol for selection and analysis of trials.

A meta-analysis involves a sequence of systematic steps, as follows:

1. The research question is precisely defined.
2. A protocol defining the objectives of the review and the eligibility criteria for trials is established.
3. An exhaustive search of the literature to find all trials that meet the eligibility criteria is performed.
4. More than one blinded investigator tabulates the characteristics of each RCT identified and assesses its methodological quality, excluding articles not meeting the eligibility criteria.
5. The results of eligible trials are analyzed with statistical tests.
6. A critical summary of the review describing the methods of the analysis, results, potential biases, and areas for potential further study is prepared.

The quality of a meta-analysis is evaluated (as is an original study) for relevance and validity, including completeness of the search, appropriateness of the selection criteria and combination of results, and importance of the results to a specific patient.

Systematic reviews of the literature and meta-analyses regarding the efficacy of rehabilitation examination measures, prognosis, and interventions frequently report that there is insufficient evidence to support current practice. This is generally because of poor study design, including low subject numbers and poor descriptions of tests and interventions. When there are sufficient data available for a meta-analysis or systematic review to come to clear conclusions, these are the ideal source of evidence because they quickly provide an unbiased, systematic evaluation of the data from many high quality studies.

Statistical Analysis. With any type of study, except for the case report, if outcomes are examined with a quantifiable measure, the **statistical significance** of the results may be assessed with statistical tests. Most statistical tests evaluate the likelihood that a given result occurred as a result of chance alone rather than a true effect of the variable or intervention being evaluated. A finding is generally considered statistically significant if there is less than a 5% chance that it occurred as a result of chance alone. The **probability** of any difference being purely a result of chance is called the **p-value.** Some statistical tests, particularly those applied to studies of examination approaches, evaluate the degree of **correlation** between the test being evaluated and the current "gold standard." Other statistical tests are applied to studies of interventions and compare the outcome of the intervention being tested with that of a control.

> ◎ *Clinical Pearl*
>
> A finding is generally considered statistically significant if the p-value is <0.05. This means that there is less than a 5% probability that the results occurred as a result of chance alone.

The usefulness of tests and measures may also be evaluated by calculation of their **sensitivity** and **specificity.** Sensitivity is the probability of a positive test result in a person with the condition (a/(a + c)). This is also known as the true positive rate. Specificity is the probability of a negative test result in a person without the condition (b/(b + d)). This is also known as the true negative rate.

	Test Positive	Test Negative
Condition present	a	b
Condition absent	c	d

Ideally, a test has both high sensitivity and high specificity. If a test has high sensitivity but low specificity, it will be positive in most people with the condition but will also be positive in many people without the condition. In contrast, a test with a low sensitivity but high specificity will be negative in most patients without the condition but will also be negative in many patients who actually do have the condition.

The value of an intervention can often be evaluated by the **number needed to treat** (NNT), which is the number of patients needed to be treated for one to benefit. The lower the NNT the more useful a treatment may be; however, this must be considered in the context of the value of the outcome.

$$\% \text{ with outcome with new intervention} -$$
$$\% \text{ with outcome with control intervention} =$$
$$\text{absolute risk reduction}$$
$$\text{NNT} = 100/\text{absolute risk reduction}$$

EFFICACY AND EFFECTIVENESS

Studies examining the value of an intervention may focus on its efficacy or effectiveness. Efficacy is the benefit of an intervention applied under ideal and highly controlled conditions. Effectiveness is the benefit of an intervention applied under circumstances that more closely approximate the real world.[6] Although efficacy may be easier to evaluate with research because it involves the application of a standardized intervention, effectiveness may be more relevant to the clinical setting where patients and clinicians vary in how they carry out interventions. For example, one could evaluate the effectiveness of a set group of exercises performed in the clinic under observation or the efficacy of a prescribed home exercise program that the patient may or may not perform as instructed.

> ◎ *Clinical Pearl*
>
> Efficacy is the benefit of an intervention under ideal conditions. Effectiveness is the benefit of an intervention in real-life, nonideal circumstances.

EVALUATING AND GRADING EVIDENCE

There are a variety of ways to evaluate research evidence. When evaluating the quality of a single study, one should consider the clinical relevance of the research question, the internal (avoiding bias) and external (generalizability) validity of the study, the appropriateness of data analysis and presentation, and the ethical implications of the tests or interventions evaluated. Are the subjects in the study similar to the patients to whom you would want to apply the test or intervention? Are objective or reproducible diagnostic standards applied to all participants? Will the conclusions, if true, have an impact on the health of your patient? Are the outcome measures known or likely to be clinically important? To assess validity one should consider if the study is peer reviewed, whether an interested party sponsors it, and if there is concealed random allocation of patients to a **comparison group.** One should evaluate if the trial is an RCT, and if so, how the groups were randomized and whether the study and **control group** are similar. Were both groups treated in exactly the same manner except for the intervention being evaluated? Were observers and subjects appropriately blinded to exposure? Are the outcomes clearly defined, objective, and clinically, as well as statistically, significant? A system may be used to collect information about the quality of a study (Table 2-1).

If a study shows no significant results, the clinician should consider whether it was adequately powered to detect an effect. If a study is inadequately powered, a type 2 error is likely. A type 2 error occurs when a study concludes that the **null hypothesis** is true (i.e., there is no effect of the intervention), when there actually is an effect. This type of error often occurs when the number of

TABLE 2-1	System for Evaluating the Quality of Studies		
Citation	Yes	No	Comments
Question study is trying to answer			
Peer-reviewed publication?			
Type of trial (RCT, other define)?			
Appropriate control group?			
Appropriate randomization?			
Outcomes clearly defined?			
Measured outcomes relevant to the question being asked?			
Outcomes clinically significant?			
Outcomes statistically significant?			
Power analysis performed?			

RCT, Randomized controlled trial.

subjects is too small and is common in clinical studies with patients. To avoid a type 2 error, the investigators should have performed a power analysis to determine how many subjects are needed to detect the size of effect they consider likely and relevant.

A number of grading schemes have been proposed for rating the overall quality of evidence available to support a particular intervention. The Agency for Health Care Research and Quality (AHRQ) (previously known as the AHCPR—Agency for Health Care Policy and Research) uses the following A to C rating scheme in its clinical guidelines:

A: Results of two or more RCTs in humans provide support.
B: Results of two or more controlled clinical trials in humans provide support, or when appropriate, results of two or more controlled trials in an animal model provide indirect support.
C: This rating requires one or more of the following: (1) results of one controlled trial, (2) results of at least two case series/ descriptive studies on pressure ulcers in humans, or (3) expert opinion.

Another commonly used scheme ranks evidence between levels 1 and 3, as follows[2]:

Level 1 Evidence from at least one RCT.
Level 2a Evidence from well-controlled trials without randomization.
Level 2b Evidence from well-designed cohort of case-controlled analytic studies.
Level 2c Evidence from multiple time series with or without intervention. This also includes dramatic results from uncontrolled experiments (e.g., penicillin for treatment of infections in the 1940s).
Level 3 Opinions of experts based on clinical experience, descriptive studies, case reports, or reports of expert committees.

Although these schemes vary, all give the highest ranking to RCTs, with more RCTs being better, and give the lowest ranking to expert opinion or case studies, with other types of trials falling in between. These schemes or other similar schemes may be used to rank evidence to guide clinical practice.

CLINICAL PRACTICE GUIDELINES

Clinical practice guidelines are systematically developed statements that attempt to interpret current research to guide practitioners' and patients' decisions about appropriate health care for specific clinical circumstances.[7] Clinical practice guidelines recommend diagnostic and prognostic measures and preventive or therapeutic interventions. For any of these, the specific types of patients or problems, the nature of the intervention or test, the alternatives to the intervention being evaluated, and the outcomes of the intervention for which these guidelines apply will be stated. For example, there are guidelines for the treatment for acute low back pain and for the treatment of pressure ulcers that include evidence-based recommendations for tests and measures, interventions, prevention, and prognosis. Often, such recommendations are classified according to the strength of the evidence supporting them[8]:

Classification of recommendations
A Established as effective, ineffective, or harmful for the given condition in the specified population.
B Probably effective, ineffective, or harmful for the given condition in the specified population.
C Possibly effective, ineffective, or harmful for the given condition in the specified population.
U Data inadequate or conflicting given current knowledge; treatment is unproven.

Application of clinical practice guidelines to an individual patient depends on the similarity of the clinical circumstances of the patient to those for which the guideline was developed, the availability and feasibility of implementing the recommended intervention(s), and the value of the expected outcome(s) to the patient.[9]

◎ *Clinical Pearl*

Clinical practice guidelines are systematically developed statements that attempt to interpret current research to guide practitioners' and patients' decisions about appropriate health care for specific clinical circumstances.

FINDING REHABILITATION EVIDENCE

Clinicians may directly search the literature for individual studies related to a clinical question using a variety of databases (Table 2-2). Systematically searching for and appraising articles found in such databases is often challenging and time consuming and may yield many publications that are neither relevant nor of sufficient quality to guide clinical practice. The assistance of a librarian can be invaluable for optimizing a search strategy, but the articles will still need to be read and evaluated for their applicability and quality.

Instead of searching directly for individual studies, a search of specialized databases of systematic reviews and meta-analyses of medical and/or rehabilitation-related research can be more effective. These specialized databases offer the expertise of their authors in searching and appraising research literature and can save the clinician much time and provide a valid answer to a clinical practice question. However, many clinical questions are not addressed by these databases and must be searched for and appraised by the individual clinician. The specialized databases of systematic reviews and meta-analyses of medical and rehabilitation-related research are the Cochrane Database of Systematic Reviews, Database of Abstracts of Reviews of Effects (DARE), and Patient-Oriented Evidence that Matters (POEMS). Table 2-3 provides information on the content of these databases.

From a perspective of scientific evidence, physical therapy and rehabilitation in general are still-developing fields; the scientific evidence needed to perform a review and make an evidence-based decision is frequently inadequate or unavailable. In such circumstances the clinical decision will involve more of the clinician's expertise and less evidence. In this book, every attempt has been made

TABLE 2-2	Databases of Primary Medical and Rehabilitation Research*
Database	**Contents**
Medline	Primary database of research published in medical journals. Can be searched using a number of search engines, including Medline Plus and Pub MED.
Cumulative Index to Nursing and Allied Health Literature (CINAHL)	Similar to Medline but with an allied health focus.
PEDro	Australian database that critically reviews articles related to physical therapy practice but does not provide a systematic review or recommendations for practice.

*Links to these databases can be found on the Evolve site.

TABLE 2-3	Specialized Databases of Systematic Reviews and Meta-Analyses*
Database	**Contents**
Cochrane Database of Systematic Reviews	Systematic reviews and meta-analyses of medically related RCTs focused on specific patient problems and interventions.
Database of Abstracts of Reviews of Effects (DARE)	Structured abstracts of systematic reviews from a variety of medical journals. DARE is produced by the National Health Services' Centre for Reviews and Dissemination (NHS CRD) at the University of York, United Kingdom. DARE records cover diagnosis, prevention, rehabilitation, screening, and treatment.
Patient-Oriented Evidence that Matters (POEMS)	Family practice database that appraises and summarizes articles related to specific medical problems.

RCTs, Randomized controlled trials.
*Links to these databases can be found on the Evolve site.

to provide evidence for recommendations and to clearly indicate where suggestions are made based on common practice when evidence is limited or unavailable.

EBP is a fact of professional life for all medical professionals. Although there will be modifications as the concept evolves, it is likely and reasonable that to continue doing and being reimbursed for patient care, clinicians will be asked to demonstrate with evidence the effectiveness of their clinical practice.

CHAPTER SUMMARY

This chapter describes evidence based practice (EBP), the different types of available evidence, and how to apply EBP to rehabilitation. Evidence from individual studies can be differentiated by their study design, the subjects, the controls, and the outcome measures. A number of studies on one topic may also be presented together in integrative summary reports. The chapter concludes with information on how to find evidence related to the clinical practice of rehabilitation.

ADDITIONAL RESOURCES

For links to these and additional web-based resources, see the Evolve site.
Guyatt G, Drummond R: *Users' guides to the medical literature: A manual for evidence-based clinical practice,* Chicago, 2002, AMA Press.
Centre for Evidence-Based Medicine
Hooked on Evidence (through the APTA)

GLOSSARY

Bias: A systematic tendency to produce an outcome that differs from the underlying truth. There are many different types of bias.

Blinded: The participant of interest is unaware of whether patients have been assigned to the experimental or control group. Patients, clinicians, those monitoring outcomes, judicial assessors of outcomes, data analysts, and those writing the paper can all be blinded.

Case reports: Descriptions of individual patients.

Clinical practice guidelines: Systematically developed statements to assist practitioner and patient decisions about appropriate health care for specific clinical circumstances.

Clinical significance: The importance of a finding within a clinical context.

Comparison group: Any group to which the index group is compared. Usually synonymous with control group.

Control group: A group that does not receive the experimental intervention. In many studies, the control group receives either the standard of care currently delivered in the community or the best care that is available on the basis of the current evidence.

Correlation: The magnitude of the relationship between different variables or phenomena.

Effectiveness: How well an intervention works in real-life, non-ideal circumstances.

Efficacy: How well an intervention works in ideal circumstances.

Evidence-based practice (EBP): The conscientious, explicit, and judicious use of current best evidence in making decisions about the care of individual patients. EBP requires integration of individual clinical expertise and patient preferences with the best available external clinical evidence from systematic research.

Exclusion criteria: Conditions that preclude entrance of candidates into an investigation even if they meet the inclusion criteria.

False-negative: In a study, if a treatment is considered ineffective when it actually is effective.

Inclusion criteria: Criteria that define who will be eligible for a study.

Meta-analysis: An overview that incorporates a quantitative strategy for combining the results of several studies into a single pooled or summary estimate.

Null hypothesis: In the hypothesis-testing framework, the starting hypothesis, generally that an intervention has no effect, and that the statistical test is designed to consider and possibly reject.

Number needed to treat (NNT): The number of patients who need to be treated over a specific period of time to prevent one bad outcome or cause one good outcome.

Outcomes: Changes in health status that may be associated with exposure to an intervention.

Patient preferences: The relative value that patients place on varying health states and intervention options.

Placebo: Intervention without known or expected biological effects.

Probability: Quantitative estimate of the likelihood of a condition existing or of subsequent events.

Prognosis: The possible outcomes of a condition and the frequency with which they can be expected to occur.

P-value: A measure of how much evidence there is against the null hypothesis. The smaller the p-value the less likely the null hypothesis is true and the more likely that an intervention had an effect.

Randomized controlled trial (RCT): An experiment in which individuals are randomly allocated to receive or not receive an intervention and are then followed to determine the effect(s) of the intervention.

Reliability: Consistency or reproducibility of data.

Sensitivity: The proportion of people who truly have a designated disorder and are so identified by the test.

Specificity: The proportion of people who are truly free of a designated disorder and are so identified by a test.

Statistical significance: A result is statistically significant if the null hypothesis is rejected. That is, the probability of the observed results falls below an arbitrary predefined threshold, most often 0.05 (i.e., 5%).

Systematic review: A critical assessment and evaluation of research (not simply a summary) that attempts to address a focused clinical question using methods designed to reduce the likelihood of bias.

Validity: A study or measure is valid when its findings or results represent an unbiased estimate of the underlying truth. The extent to which an instrument measures what it is intended to measure. Internal validity of a study refers to the integrity of the experimental design. External validity of a study refers to the appropriateness by which its results can be applied to non-study patients or populations.

Chapter **3**

Skeletal Demineralization

Nancey A. Bookstein

CHAPTER OUTLINE

OBJECTIVES

After reading this chapter, the reader will be able to:
1. Describe and differentiate among the types of skeletal demineralization.
2. Identify modifiable and nonmodifiable risk factors for skeletal demineralization throughout the lifespan.
3. Discuss tests and measures of bone density and skeletal demineralization.
4. Apply rehabilitation interventions to clients with or at risk for skeletal demineralization.

Skeletal demineralization refers to a loss of mass and calcium content from the bones. Skeletal demineralization can vary in severity. Less severe bone loss is called **osteopenia,** and more severe bone loss is called **osteoporosis.** Skeletal demineralization may be a primary disorder or may be secondary to a variety of other diseases or disorders such as **osteomalacia** and hyperparathyroidism. Osteomalacia is a disorder in which osteoid, the new organic matrix of bone, does not mineralize correctly. Unlike other causes of bone demineralization, osteomalacia is associated with proximal muscle weakness and dull, persistent bone pain that worsens with activity. With hyperparathyroidism, the excess of parathyroid hormone causes calcium to be leached from the bones into the bloodstream, thereby causing skeletal demineralization.

Skeletal demineralization of any etiology is caused by an imbalance between bone formation and bone resorption.[1,2] When bone loss exceeds bone formation, the resultant net loss of bone mass causes skeletal fragility due to trabecular thinning and discontinuity, loss of horizontal bridges, and the occurrence of trabecular microfractures (Fig. 3-1). Although skeletal demineralization is not a disease and does not cause symptoms, individuals with less than normal bone mass are at increased risk for fractures, and these fractures can be symptomatic and impair function.

Skeletal demineralization can have many causes through the lifespan, including genetics, lack of proper nutrition, hormonal imbalances, and inadequate physical activity.[3,4] Although genetics account for much of the variance in potential **peak bone mass,** life choices, disease and health challenges, socioeconomic circumstances, and environment play important roles in both the attainment of peak bone mass and in bone loss. This chapter describes the physiological mechanisms underlying skeletal demineralization and the examination, evaluation, and interventions for patients at risk for skeletal demineralization. Postural deformities, fractures, and pain are covered in Chapters 4, 9, and 22, respectively.

> ◎ **Clinical Pearl**
> Skeletal demineralization can be caused by genetics, poor nutrition, hormonal imbalances, disease, and inadequate physical activity.

PATHOLOGY

NORMAL BONE PHYSIOLOGY

The bones of the body form its skeleton. They provide structural support and act as a store for minerals,

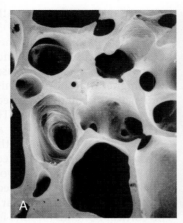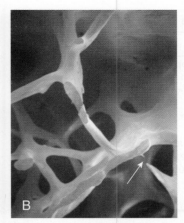

FIG. 3-1 Normal **(A)** and osteoporotic **(B)** bone. Arrow on osteoporotic bone shows a trabecular microfracture. *From Patton KT, Thibodeau GA:* Anatomy and physiology, *ed 7, St. Louis, 2010, Mosby.*

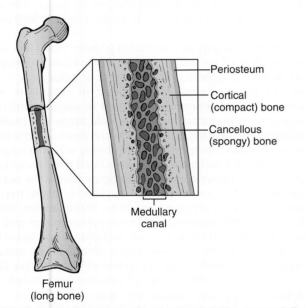

FIG 3-2 Cortical and cancellous bone, periosteum, medullary canal.

particularly calcium and phosphorus. The skeleton can be divided into appendicular and axial portions. The appendicular skeleton includes the bones of the upper and lower limbs; the axial skeleton includes the bones of the cranium, vertebral column, ribs, sternum, and pelvis. All bones have cortical bone on the outside and trabecular bone on the inside. Cortical bone is dense and solid and made up of lamellae, or compact plates (Fig 3-2). Approximately 80% of the mass of the skeleton is cortical bone.

Trabecular bone, also known as cancellous bone, has a honeycomb structure with horizontal and vertical bars filled with marrow and fat.[5] These bars of bone form struts called trabeculae, giving this type of bone its name. The axial skeleton, the pelvis, and other flat bones, as well as the ends of the long bones of the appendicular skeleton, are composed primarily of trabecular bone. Trabecular bone is responsible for about 70% of the volume of the axial skeleton, although only 35% of its weight

is trabecular bone.[3] Trabecular bone is more metabolically active than cortical bone and responds both more quickly and to a greater degree to changes in mineral homeostasis.[6,7]

Clinical Pearl

All bones are made up of a cortical dense outer layer surrounding trabecular honeycomb bone.

Bone is a dynamic living tissue that undergoes constant remodeling with coupled phases of bone resorption and formation throughout the lifespan.[8] Bone remodels in response to the demands placed on it. Bone increases in length and diameter during development, responds to mechanical stresses placed on it, and repairs itself after structural damage from trauma, fatigue, or mechanical failure.[9] Approximately 3% of cortical and 7% of trabecular bone remodels each year.[10] This tissue renewal helps maintain the skeleton's structural integrity and keep blood calcium and phosphorus levels within the appropriate range. As long as there is a balance between bone resorption and bone formation, **bone mineral density (BMD)** stays stable. A combination of mechanical stress and metabolic and nutritional support helps the system maintain this homeostatic equilibrium. Skeletal demineralization occurs when the processes are not balanced; when bone resorption exceeds bone formation, there is a loss of bone mass.

Bone remodeling involves the balanced activity of three types of cells: osteoclasts, osteoblasts, and osteocytes. Osteoclasts resorb bone and form resorption cavities in areas of bone turnover. Osteoblasts synthesize new bone matrix and osteoid to fill the cavities created by the osteoclasts. This matrix and osteoid then mineralize to form new bone. When the osteoblasts become surrounded by mineralized bone, they no longer produce matrix or osteoid and are known as osteocytes.

Bone remodeling is controlled by levels of circulating hormones, including estrogen, testosterone, **calcitonin**, **parathyroid hormone**, and **1,25-dihydroxyvitamin**

TABLE 3-1	Types of Involutional Bone Loss	
	Type I	Type II
Population affected	Postmenopausal women	Both genders
Mechanism	Hormone-driven	Age-related after 70 years of age
Bone primarily affected	Trabecular bone	Cortical and trabecular bone
Typical fractures	Vertebral and wrist fractures	Hip fractures
Typical features	Onset >50 years of age	Increased morbidity and mortality

D, and by ongoing mechanical stresses from gravity, weight bearing, and the pull on the bones by contracting muscles.[8] Typically, during middle adulthood, **osteoblastic** and **osteoclastic** functions are balanced and bone mass does not change significantly in men or women. During the years of skeletal growth, from birth to the late twenties, bone formation exceeds bone resorption so that absolute bone mass increases and both bone length and bone diameter increase. Increases in bone length stop when the epiphyses close, which generally occurs between the ages of 13 and 25 years.[11] Bone diameter continues to increase into the twenties or thirties when peak bone mass is reached.[12] Peak bone mass is then generally maintained for the next few decades until the biochemical environment of the body is affected by the hormonal changes associated with aging. Age-related bone loss begins between the ages of 45 to 50 years as the phases of bone remodeling become uncoupled and bone resorption exceeds bone formation.

Clinical Pearl

Generally, bone mass increases until the third or fourth decade, stabilizes until age 45 to 50 years, and then starts to decline.

PATHOPHYSIOLOGY

Age-related bone loss occurs in both cortical and trabecular bone. This type of bone loss, which is not caused by immobilization, is called involutional bone loss. Involutional bone loss is a long, slow, continuous process that occurs in both men and women beginning at around age 35 to 40 years.[13] This loss accelerates in women after menopause. Osteoblast activity starts to decrease and osteoclast function starts to increase in midlife. Together, these changes cause bone resorption to outpace bone formation.

In 1986, Riggs and Melton defined two involutional bone loss syndromes based on clinical features and disease patterns (Table 3-1).[12] Type I, postmenopausal osteoporosis, is a high turnover state that affects women after menopause, whereas type II, senile osteoporosis, is a low turnover, or slow state, that affects both genders after the age of 70 years.[12]

In type I involutional bone loss, although the rate of cortical bone loss is slightly increased, the rate of trabecular bone loss is greatly increased and may be up to three times higher than normal. This loss puts postmenopausal women at particularly increased risks for fractures of bones that are mostly trabecular. Thus vertebral compression fractures, which cause pain and spinal deformity, and Colles' fractures (fractures of the distal radius at the wrist) are associated with type I osteoporosis.

In contrast to type I involutional bone loss, which primarily involves loss of trabecular bone, type II bone loss affects cortical and trabecular bone loss almost equally. The cortical bone loss results in hip fractures and wedged vertebral fractures, as well as fractures of the proximal humerus, pelvis, and proximal tibia. The trabecular thinning causes gradual vertebral collapse, anterior wedging of thoracic vertebrae, and gradual and usually painless spinal deformities in the elderly such as the classic "dowager's hump."

Osteoporosis may be considered primary when it occurs independent of any other disease. Alternatively, osteoporosis may be a secondary consequence of a disease, condition, or the treatment for a disease or condition. For example, the **glucocorticoids** used to decrease inflammation or immune response in a wide range of diseases, including rheumatoid arthritis (RA) and asthma, can cause osteopenia and osteoporosis by inhibiting osteoblast function.[14] Thus RA and asthma are associated with secondary osteoporosis. Other conditions associated with the development of osteoporosis include hyperthyroidism, hyperprolactinemia, hyperparathyroidism, malignancies, renal failure, diabetes mellitus, and Down syndrome, as well as the use of drugs such as alcohol, marijuana, and heparin.

Poor availability of food, eating disorders, or malabsorption syndromes can result in low calcium uptake and thus osteoporosis due to loss of calcium from bones. In addition to primary, secondary, and dietary causes of osteoporosis, immobilization also reduces BMD. Prolonged bed rest has been shown to decrease bone mineral content and total body calcium. With reambulation, these increase at a similar rate to their loss.

RISK FACTORS FOR SKELETAL DEMINERALIZATION

Modifiable and nonmodifiable factors associated with the development of skeletal demineralization and osteoporosis and their sequelae are listed in Box 3-1. Female gender is associated with an increased risk of skeletal demineralization. Presently, five women are diagnosed with osteoporosis for every one man.[15] This is probably due in part to increased recognition of osteoporosis in women and to the fact that, in general, females are at higher risk at an earlier age. Although women risk rapid loss of bone during and immediately after menopause as a result of estrogen deficiency, both genders lose bone mass at about the same rate after age 70. The earlier menopause begins, the longer the duration of estrogen deficiency and the greater the amount of bone loss and risk for fracture.

BOX 3-1	Modifiable and Nonmodifiable Risk Factors for Low Bone Mass
Modifiable Risk Factors for Low Bone Mass	**Nonmodifiable Risk Factors for Low Bone Mass**
Low calcium intake	Gender
Low vitamin D	Age
Estrogen deficiency	Race
Physical inactivity	Body size
Excessive alcohol intake	Early menopause
Cigarette smoking	Family history
Use of specific medications	
Prolonged overuse of thyroid hormone	

BOX 3-2	Risk Factors Associated with Low Bone Mass

- Old age
- Residence in cold geographic area
- Vitamin D deficiency
- Gastrectomy
- Intestinal malabsorption associated with the following:
  - Diseases of the small intestine
  - Cholangiolitic disorders of the liver
  - Biliary obstruction
  - Chronic pancreatic insufficiency
- Long-term use of the following:
  - Anticonvulsants
  - Tranquilizers
  - Sedatives
  - Muscle relaxants
  - Diuretics
  - Antacids containing aluminum hydroxide
  - Corticosteroids
- History of the following:
  - Hyperparathyroidism
  - Chronic renal failure
  - Renal tubular defects (decreased reabsorption of phosphate)

From Goodman CC, Fuller KS: *Pathology: Implications for the physical therapist,* ed 3, St Louis, 2009, Saunders.

Race and body proportions also affect an individual's risk for skeletal demineralization; those of European and Asian descent and those with slender, small frames are at greater risk than others.[16]

Dietary factors, primarily low calcium intake, increase the risk for skeletal demineralization. Low calcium intake causes removal of calcium from its stores in the bones and teeth to meet physiological demands. Low calcium intake during childhood and adolescence results in low peak bone mass because of continual leaching of calcium from bone. The National Institutes of Health (NIH) currently recommend that all men under the age of 65 and premenopausal women, as well as postmenopausal women taking hormone replacement therapy (HRT), consume 1,000 mg of calcium each day. Postmenopausal women not taking HRT, men over the age of 65, and people with osteopenia or osteoporosis should consume 1,500 mg of calcium daily.[17] Calcium intake includes calcium from all sources, including diet and supplements. Calcium intake up to a total of 2,000 mg per day appears to be safe in most individuals. However, too much supplemental calcium can increase the risk for kidney stones.[18]

Vitamin D, a fat-soluble vitamin, is essential for calcium absorption. Vitamin D is found in food and can be synthesized by the skin after exposure to ultraviolet (UV) rays from the sun. An adequate intake of 200 international units (IU) for children, 400 IU for those aged 51 to 70 years, and 600 IU for the healthy adult after age 70 is recommended. This level can be provided by 15 minutes of sun exposure per day.[17,19] However, many recommend much higher daily levels for optimal health. Exposure must not be compromised by sunscreen or long sleeves. In areas where there is insufficient sunlight to produce an adequate amount of vitamin D during the winter months, people should be sure to include vitamin D in their diet. Although little vitamin D occurs naturally in most foods, many countries fortify basic foods, such as milk, bread, cereals, and margarine, with vitamin D to assure adequate intake. Since the 1930s, when the federal government introduced a mild fortification program to reduce the incidence of rickets, almost all of the milk produced in the US is fortified with 400 IU of vitamin D per quart. Although milk, bread, and ready-to-eat cereals are usually fortified,

products made from milk, such as ice cream and cheese, may not be.

Estrogen deficiency is also a risk factor for skeletal demineralization and osteoporosis. Estrogen deficiency has many causes, including delayed puberty, hypogonadism, amenorrhea, oligomenorrhea, and menopause without HRT. Therefore clinicians generally include questions regarding age of menarche, activity level, menstrual regularity or irregularity, parity, age at menopause, type of menopause (i.e., natural versus surgical), and use and type of HRT, including over-the-counter and herbal preparations, when taking the history of a patient with skeletal demineralization.

A reduction in mechanical loading due to lack of physical exercise,[20] immobilization, and/or long-term bed rest decreases bone density because bone requires stress for maintenance and growth.[21] Furthermore, even with activity, reduced gravitational forces cause a reduction in bone volume and density.[22-26]

Cigarette smoking and excessive alcohol intake are also risk factors for low bone mass. Smoking accelerates bone loss in both men and women and is a risk factor for hip fracture in women.[27-29] The effects of smoking on bone density begin to reverse 10 years after smoking cessation.[29] Excessive alcohol consumption predisposes individuals to hip fracture by increasing the risk of falls, as well as loss of bone density.[30]

Certain disease processes are associated with low bone mass. The more common of these are included in Box 3-2. These associations may be due to direct effects of the diseases themselves or effects of medications used to treat them. For example, corticosteroids used to treat RA and anticonvulsants used to treat epilepsy cause low BMD as a side effect and primary hyperparathyroidism directly causes calcium to be leached from bone.

◎ *Clinical Pearl*

There are modifiable risk factors (changes that can be made to reduce risk factors) and nonmodifiable risk factors (risk factors one cannot control) for skeletal demineralization.

TYPICAL EXAMINATION FINDINGS

PATIENT HISTORY

The patient history will include age and gender, past medical and surgical history, family history, functional status, present and past activity levels, history of the present condition, and the patient's goals. The clinician will also ask about current and past medication use, including prescribed, over-the-counter, and herbal preparations, because many drugs can affect bone metabolism, thereby contributing to changes in bone density.

TESTS AND MEASURES

Musculoskeletal

Posture. Postural screening is very important in patients with osteoporosis. Most osteoporotic fractures do not cause symptoms but may result in increased or increasing thoracic kyphosis. Spinal curvature may be assessed by x-ray or without x-ray, by physical examination using a **Debrunner's kyphometer** (Fig. 3-3, *A*) or a surveyor's **flexicurve** (Fig. 3-3, *B*).

Kyphotic posture can predispose people to back pain and can also increase the risk of falls.[31] Thoracic flexion also increases the load on the vertebrae, increasing

fracture risk. A detailed description of the examination of posture is provided in Chapter 4.

Anthropometric Characteristics

Height Loss. Vertebral compression fractures are the most common manifestation of osteoporosis. Although approximately two-thirds of these fractures are asymptomatic and do not cause pain, most will cause height loss. Height loss is suggestive of low bone mass and one or more vertebral compression fractures. More than 1 inch of height loss should prompt further evaluation by a physician so that patients with low bone mass or fractures are identified early, in time to be treated to decrease their fracture risk before another fracture occurs. In addition, all patients at risk for or diagnosed with osteopenia or osteoporosis should have their height measured at baseline, and changes in height should be followed during the course of intervention.

Range of Motion. Changes in posture may be due to more than changes in spinal curvature from vertebral fractures. Typically, specific soft tissue changes occur as patients develop increasing kyphotic posture. Loss of flexibility and tightness in anterior soft tissue structures commonly cause decreased range of motion (ROM) in shoulder flexion and external rotation, hip extension, knee flexion, and ankle dorsiflexion.[32,33] Decreased ROM of the cervical spine, shoulders, hips, knees, and ankles can also add to postural deformity and contribute to balance deficiencies.

Muscle Performance. Patients with skeletal demineralization often also have weak muscles. The muscles most commonly affected are those on constant stretch such as the shoulder depressors and retractors, the hip and knee extensors, and the ankle dorsiflexors. In addition, the spinal extensors, as well as the abdominals, may be weak from disuse. Grip strength, tested by dynamometer, may correlate with overall bone density[34,35] and fracture risk.[34] Strength testing should be performed with additional caution in this population to avoid positions that increase fracture or fall risks (see Chapter 5).

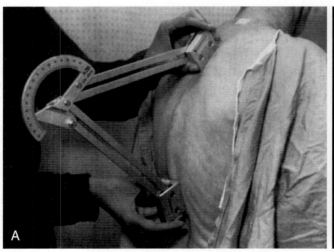 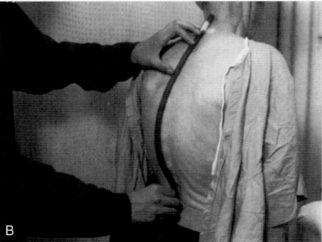

FIG. 3-3 **A,** Debrunner's kyphometer. **B,** Flexicurve. *From Lundon KM, Li A, Bibershtein S: Spine 23(18):1978-1985, 1998.*

Neuromuscular. When thoracic vertebral fractures cause pain in patients with skeletal demineralization, the pain usually follows a dermatomal pattern around the trunk. Anatomically, when the vertebral body collapses anteriorly, the shape of the intervertebral foramen changes and can put pressure on the dural sleeve of the exiting spinal nerve, causing pain to radiate around the anterior thoracic or abdominal wall. Patients may complain of chest pain, rib pain, shortness of breath, scapular pain, or even visceral pain, depending on the spinal nerve level affected.

Cardiovascular/Pulmonary. Thoracic kyphosis, if severe, can produce a decrease in aerobic capacity as the result of reduced lung/chest volume. Chapter 23 includes methods of measuring and managing cardiorespiratory endurance.

Function. Balance and gait are examined in all clients with or at risk for osteoporosis because falls in this population can easily result in fractures. Patients with osteoporosis appear to have altered balance as a result of kyphosis, which may decrease stability during activities of daily living (ADLs), putting them at increased fall and fracture risk.[36] The Tinetti Assessment Tool[37] measures both balance and gait. It was designed for elderly populations, is easy to administer, and has demonstrated good to excellent reliability (see Chapters 13 and 32).

Medical Tests of Bone Mineral Density. Various tests are available to assess BMD, including screening tests readily available to the public and medical diagnostic tests. Screening tests can identify individuals whose BMD may lie significantly outside the normal range. The primary screening tests are finger densitometry and heel ultrasonography. Although these tests are inexpensive and widely available, they are not very accurate. All results from screening tests suggesting low bone mass should be followed up with an accurate medical diagnostic test to guide treatment decisions and to establish a baseline from which to judge treatment results.

The current gold standard for measuring bone density is **dual-energy x-ray absorptiometry (DXA).** DXA relies on bone-absorbing or attenuating x-rays, but the radiation exposure is very low. DXA can measure hip and spine bone density, as well as total body bone density, with high precision and accuracy. DXA provides both absolute measures of BMD and scores that can be compared with average age-matched scores and with scores expected for young women with peak bone mass.[38]

DXA usually provides measures of BMD in g/cm^3. This information can then be converted to T-scores and Z-scores. The **T-score** is the number of standard deviations (SDs) the subject's score is away from that of a normal young female. The **Z-score** is the number of SDs the subject's score is away from that of an age-, weight-, ethnicity-, and gender-matched person.

EVALUATION, DIAGNOSIS, AND PROGNOSIS

For most individuals who fall into preferred practice pattern 4A: Primary prevention/risk reduction for skeletal demineralization, examination findings may include loss of height, thoracic kyphosis, and decreased ROM and muscle strength.[39] Individuals with a history of fracture may have chronic pain from changes in soft tissues. Complaints of acute pain will often be a result of a new fracture. Individuals, especially the elderly or those with chronic medical conditions, may also present with decreased balance and endurance (Table 3-2).

INTERVENTION

Rehabilitation intervention for patients with skeletal demineralization is intended to increase bone mass, slow bone loss, and/or reduce the risk of fractures. There are a few large, randomized controlled trials (RCTs) and a number of small clinical studies evaluating the effects of a variety of interventions in this population; however, interpretation of the findings of most of these studies is

TABLE 3-2	Evaluation and Prognosis Associated with Preferred Practice Pattern 4A: Primary Prevention/ Risk Reduction for Skeletal Demineralization		
Examination Findings	**Evaluation/Likely Diagnosis**		**Prognosis Based on Outcome Research**
Height loss >1 inch	Possible asymptomatic bone loss; postural dysfunction		At potential risk for bone loss and vertebral compression fractures; improve with exercise, patient education.
Thoracic kyphosis	Potential to compromise cardiorespiratory system; decreased balance; possible single or multiple vertebral compression fractures		Can be improved or maintained with exercise, bracing, patient education; at increased risk for possible additional fractures.
Pain: Acute	Possible new fracture; decreased physical performance and function		Self-limited over 6-8 weeks; can be decreased by intermittent bed rest, modalities, positioning, bracing.
Pain: Chronic	Changes in soft tissues: tightness, weakness		Can decrease with compliance to appropriate education, exercise program, bracing.
Decreased ROM	Chronically shortened soft tissues		Can be modified with exercise.
Muscle weakness	Chronically lengthened; atrophied soft tissues		Can be modified with exercise.
Decreased balance	Increased potential for fracture from falls		Can be improved with balance training.
Decreased endurance	Compromised cardiopulmonary function; decreased mobility		Can be improved with endurance training.

Data from Itoi E, Sinaki M: *Mayo Clin Proc* 69:1054-1059, 1994; Kanis JA, Johnell O, DeLaet C, et al: *Bone* 35(2):375-382, 1994; Lui-Ambrose T, Eng JJ, Khan KM, et al: *J Gerontol A Biol Sci Med Sci* 58:M862-866, 2003.
ROM, Range of motion.

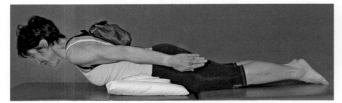

FIG. 3-4 Weighted back extension.

TABLE 3-3	Effect of Type of Spinal Exercises on the Number of New Fractures in Patients with Spinal Osteoporosis

Type of Exercise	Number of New Fractures
Spinal extension	16%
Spinal flexion	89%
Combined flexion and extension	53%
No exercise	67%

confounded by small effect sizes, questionable compliance with test or control protocol, and high drop-out rates. The next section describes rehabilitation interventions, including aerobic exercise, resistance training, and weight-bearing activities, that have been shown in some studies to improve outcomes in patients with skeletal demineralization. These interventions are followed by a brief review of medical interventions, including diet, medications, and surgery, used to improve outcomes in this population.

AEROBIC EXERCISE

Aerobic exercise, particularly when coupled with weight bearing, can improve function and increase BMD in patients with osteoporosis. For example, running 15 to 20 miles a week has been found to be associated with increased BMD in men. It is not clear if the aerobic component and/or the weight bearing associated with running or other activities are the primary cause of the increased BMD associated with these activities.

RESISTANCE TRAINING

Resistance training, including a range of exercises, such as back extension and flexion; hip flexion, extension, abduction, and adduction; knee flexion and extension; leg press; bench press; biceps curl; and lateral pull down, has been shown to enhance BMD in adults of all ages. In addition, a recent study found that progressive resisted back extension (Fig. 3-4) was associated with stronger back extensor muscles and a lower incidence of vertebral fractures up to 8 years after the termination of the exercise program.

However, one study found that significantly more fractures occurred in patients performing only spinal flexion exercises than in those performing only spinal extension exercises, combined flexion and extension exercises, or no exercise at all (Table 3-3). Therefore, in patients with or at risk for skeletal demineralization, resisted spinal extension exercises are recommended, whereas spinal flexion exercises should not be performed unless they are combined with spinal extension exercises.

Site-specific strengthening exercise should focus on the muscles supporting the trunk, hips, and upper extremities because these are areas at greatest risk for fracture. Strength training can maintain bone density and also improve postural control and stability to decrease the risk of falls. The increase in muscle mass produced by muscle strengthening may also reduce fracture risk by providing additional protection should a fall occur.

The effect of swimming on BMD is controversial. However, whether swimming does or does not increase BMD, it continues to be recommended for patients with osteoporosis because the water is a relatively safe environment in which to achieve the other benefits of exercise for those at high fracture risk.

WEIGHT-BEARING EXERCISE

In general, the evidence on the effects of weight-bearing exercise for patients with or at risk for skeletal demineralization indicates that this type of exercise primarily affects BMD at the spine, although there may also be some effect on hip and forearm BMD. Lower extremity weight bearing can be achieved through a variety of activities such as walking, running, jumping rope, dancing, skiing, stair climbing, Tai Chi, and others. Walking and stair climbing activities can easily be developed into progressive programs that patients can follow. Weight-bearing activities can also be done at differing speeds and varying intensities. The literature suggests that higher intensity weight-bearing activities have more impact on bone density but may put clients at increased risk for falls.

Weight-bearing impact exercise, such as jumping or high impact aerobics, should begin early, during the normal growth period, because it can increase peak bone strength and bone mass by as much as 30%.[40] This type of exercise should then be continued during adulthood to preserve maximum bone mass and reduce the risk of osteoporosis and its sequelae in later life. Although exercise later in life has only a small impact on BMD, being physically active does reduce the incidence of hip fracture by as much as 50% in people over the age of 65, likely due to improved balance and strength and thus a reduced incidence of falls.

BODY MECHANICS TRAINING

To avoid the increased risk of spinal compression fractures associated with spinal flexion, patients with skeletal demineralization should learn to keep the trunk in a relatively neutral position for bending and lifting activities in everyday life. Exercises or functional activities that put patients into flexed postures should be modified or avoided if possible.

Posture correction and training will address walking, standing, and sitting as tall as possible. Core stability, maintaining both a level pelvis and tension in the pelvic floor during activity, may also be included. Photographs can be an effective way for patients to learn to self-adjust their posture in standing, sitting, and during activity. Patients can begin to correct posture in a supine position

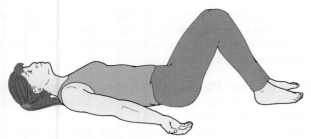

FIG. 3-5 Decompression exercise. *Redrawn from Visual Health Information, courtesy Sara Meeks Seminars.*

with knees bent and feet flat, arms flat against the supporting surface slightly away from the trunk, and palms up (Fig. 3-5). In this rest position, the patient can work on head and neck position while unloading the neck and finding the position of a neutral spine. Patients can learn to elongate the spine, as well as the extremities, while maintaining neutral positions. Maintaining good posture in sitting and standing requires constant self-monitoring. The concept of a hook attached to the top of the head and pulling the patient up from the waist may be a useful teaching tool.

While corrected posture is becoming habitual, the patient can work on gait, balance, and body mechanics with a different proprioceptive foundation. Patients should learn to use a hip hinge for all pushing, pulling, reaching, or bending activities, as well as log rolling for moving about in bed. Patients should be taught to maintain excellent body mechanics and posture while working at a desk, doing household chores, climbing stairs, getting in and out of a car, and performing other patient-specific activities.

MEDICATIONS AND DIET

Prescribing medications, giving dietary advice, and performing invasive procedures are not generally within the practice of most rehabilitation practitioners. But since these types of interventions can be critical components of the prevention and treatment of bone demineralization, they are discussed briefly.

Most medications prescribed for people with skeletal demineralization are antiresorptive agents such as estrogen, **bisphosphonates**, **selective estrogen receptor modulators (SERMs)**, calcitonin, and more recently, parathyroid hormone. Supplemental calcium is also often recommended with these medications, especially for those with poor dietary intake such as lactose-intolerant individuals and women who limit dietary intake because of concern with caloric content. Regardless of the type of compound used, the goal of any drug therapy used for this population is the prevention and reduction of fractures.

In the past, estrogen replacement was the primary therapy for the prevention of postmenopausal osteoporosis. Estrogen has the additional advantages of controlling menopausal symptoms and was thought to prevent or delay cardiovascular disease. However, data from the Women's Health Initiative (WHI) revealed that estrogen-progestin therapy does not reduce the risk of coronary heart disease and may increase the risk of breast cancer, stroke, and venous thromboembolic events.[41] Although estrogen does decrease bone loss,[42] because of its associated risk, its use is generally not recommended at this time except for short-term control of symptoms associated with menopause.

Calcium consumption may be the most important modifiable factor for preventing osteoporosis.[43] Calcium intake may be increased through diet modification or oral supplements in pill, chewable, or liquid form. Diet modification should be easy, but personal taste, caloric restriction, or financial hardship makes better dietary choices difficult for some patients. Emphasizing the importance of calcium for its wide range of functions often encourages patients to be more attentive to their calcium intake. Sufficient vitamin D is also necessary to convert calcium into a usable form. Vitamin D intake can come from oral supplements or by sun exposure to the skin. Fifteen minutes of unfiltered sunlight daily is necessary if the patient is not taking any supplement.

OSTEOPOROTIC SPINAL FRACTURE INTERVENTIONS

Conservative Measures. After a painful spinal compression fracture, bed rest and narcotic analgesics are generally recommended for pain control, although this increases the risk of pneumonia, further bone loss from disuse, and deconditioning. Because of these adverse effects of bed rest, some medical practitioners have tried to use bracing to decrease pain so that patients can stay mobile during the acute recovery phase. However, patient compliance with this intervention is often poor because most spinal braces are bulky and uncomfortable. Recently, a lightweight, low-profile, adjustable brace has become available for this purpose.[44] It is designed to stimulate back extensor muscle activity, decrease pain, and improve mobility in patients with spinal compression fractures; however, its effectiveness awaits scientific testing. Others have resisted using braces for fear that patients would become dependent and stop using what muscle control they did have. Bracing continues to be used for pain relief for patients with glucocorticoid-induced osteoporosis such as posttransplant patients. For patients dependent on antirejection drugs over a lifetime, bracing may be the only way to improve mobility.

Invasive Measures. Surgical procedures known as vertebroplasty and kyphoplasty have been developed to address the effects of skeletal demineralization on the spine. These procedures are performed percutaneously, most commonly in an outpatient setting, by injecting bone cement into the body of collapsed vertebrae. Vertebroplasty includes only the injection of bone cement, whereas kyphoplasty is done by inflating a collapsed area of bone and then elevating the end plates before the bone cement is injected.[45] The effectiveness of these procedures has not yet been established from RCTs, but case studies and nonrandomized trials suggest that these procedures can result in significant improvements in quality of life and functional status.[46,47]

CASE STUDY 3-1

OSTEOPOROSIS, T11 FRACTURE, AND BACK PAIN

Patient History

AB is a 79-year-old woman with osteoporosis and vertebral compression fractures who has withdrawn from most of her normal activities. She was a schoolteacher until she retired 15 years ago and enjoyed hiking, playing golf, and skiing. Since her husband died 5 years ago, she has developed back pain and has dramatically changed her lifestyle to accommodate her pain. She does not walk or do any other form of physical activity. She is referred to physical therapy after her last visit to the metabolic bone clinic. The physician's goals for her physical therapy treatment are to increase her strength and decrease her pain. The patient reports that both her mother and grandmother became "humped over" with age.

Tests and Measures—Significant Findings

Musculoskeletal

- Kyphotic thoracic spine with a flattened lumbar curve.
- Lower ribs are approximating the iliac crests and are lower on the right than on the left.
- AB is 5 feet 2 inches tall as measured in the **stadiometer**. AB states that she was 5 feet 4½ inches tall when she was younger. She weighs 97 lb with clothes.

Neuromuscular

- Pain level is 7/10 during the visit and ranges from 4 to 9/10 during a typical week.
- Lying down reduces low back pain for a while but then causes rib pain to increase.

Function

- Gait is slow and deliberate. There is almost no time between heel strike and foot flat and a shortened swing phase on each side.
- Tinetti Assessment Score for gait is 12/16 and for balance is 9/12.
- AB could not complete a 6-minute walk test because of fatigue after 4 minutes.

Diagnosis

Preferred practice pattern 4A: Primary prevention/risk reduction for skeletal demineralization.

Interventions

- Educate patient on how to decrease fracture risk.
- Plan for increasing physical activity using a walking program 5 to 6 days a week, adding at least 1 to 3 minutes each day. AB can progress to a goal of comfortably walking 1 mile daily.
- Posture awareness training, posture control training, and postural stabilization.
- Balance training, flexibility exercises, active and resistive exercises, and upright endurance training.
- A home exercise program.

- Safety awareness in terms of body position and body mechanics during self-care and home management, coupled with injury prevention education both inside and outside the home environment.

Role of the Physical Therapist Assistant

- What functional training exercises would help this patient in her ADLs?
- Write written instructions for the patient's walking program.
- Write written instructions for flexibility exercises the patient should perform at home.
- How could this patient's interests (hiking, skiing, and golf) be incorporated into her treatment program?

Additional Information

For the full version of this case study, including detailed examination results, interventions, and outcomes, see the Evolve site that accompanies this book. A case study describing the examination, evaluation, and intervention for a patient with osteoporosis and osteopenia is also included on the Evolve site.

CHAPTER SUMMARY

Skeletal demineralization affects a large and growing segment of the population. Although skeletal demineralization does not directly cause symptoms, it causes problems by increasing the risk of fractures.

The best treatment for skeletal demineralization is prevention through appropriate physical activity and diet during early childhood to maximize bone accretion during growth. Preventive measures include weight-bearing activities and resistive exercise regimes. Weight-bearing activity can include walking, running, stair climbing, dancing, tai chi, or virtually any activity that requires upright mobility against gravity. Resistive exercise should be site-specific, exceed normal daily loading, and be progressive. Strengthening back, hip, and knee extensor muscles and ankle dorsiflexors; stretching tight anterior structures; and elongating the trunk can improve posture and balance, reducing fracture risk. Specific balance training activities can also contribute significantly to reducing fall risk and thus fracture risk in those with low BMD.

Rehabilitation can help people with or at risk for skeletal demineralization throughout the lifespan through education, exercise, pain management, and postural correction. Education and general exercise information can also keep exercise and ADLs safe for this potentially fragile population, thereby keeping people with skeletal demineralization safe as well as active.

ADDITIONAL RESOURCES

For links to these and additional web-based resources, see the Evolve site.

Nelson ME: *Strong women, strong bones,* updated edition, New York, 2006, Perigee Trade.

Meeks S: *Walk tall! An exercise program for the prevention and treatment of osteoporosis,* Gainesville, FL, 1999, Triad Publishing.

International Osteoporosis Foundation

National Institutes of Health Osteoporosis and Related Bone Disease—National Resource Center

National Osteoporosis Foundation

GLOSSARY

1,25-dihydroxyvitamin D: Physiologically active form of vitamin D that stimulates absorption of calcium and phosphorus by the gut.

Alendronate: Fosamax; a bisphosphonate delivered by tablet.

Bisphosphonate: Group of antiresorptive compounds used for the prevention and treatment of osteoporosis in postmenopausal women and in men, as well as those patients with Paget's disease or steroid-induced osteoporosis.

Bone mineral density (BMD): Amount of bone mass present; typically measured in the lumbar spine and hip.

Calcitonin: Hormone (usually salmon) used for treatment of postmenopausal osteoporosis and pain from vertebral compression fracture; Miacalcin is delivered by nasal spray.

Debrunner's kyphometer: Metal device, similar to an inclinometer, used to measure kyphosis.

Dual-energy x-ray absorptiometry (DXA; DEXA): Gold standard measurement of BMD.

Flexicurve: A 48-cm strip of lead covered with synthetic rubber used to map the kypholordotic curve.

Glucocorticoid: Medication used to decrease inflammation in chronic conditions, such as RA, and as an antirejection drug after organ transplant.

Osteoblastic: Bone forming.

Osteoclastic: Bone removing.

Osteomalacia: Lack of mineralization of the organic bone matrix.

Osteopenia: Bone mass between 1.0 and 2.5 SD below the mean for young normals.

Osteoporosis: Bone loss greater than 2.5 SD below the mean for young normals; decreased bone mass with disruption of normal architecture resulting in increased fragility and increased risk of fracture.

Parathyroid hormone (PTH): Hormone produced by the parathyroid gland that controls blood calcium levels.

Peak bone mass: Greatest amount of bone accrued by the body.

Risedronate: Actonel; a bisphosphonate.

Selective estrogen receptor modulator (SERM): Compounds that act like estrogen on bone without affecting breast or uterine tissue.

Stadiometer: Measurement device to examine height; can be mounted on the wall or be free-standing.

T-score: Approximate amount of bone compared to a normal, young adult female.

Z-score: Approximate amount of bone present compared to age- and gender-matched controls.

Posture

Amy Selinger

OBJECTIVES

After reading this chapter, the reader will be able to:
1. Describe ideal posture in sitting and standing.
2. Differentiate between anatomical position and standard (or ideal) posture.
3. Describe the position of the head, neck, shoulder, pelvis, hip, knee, and ankle in optimal erect posture.
4. Explain the difference between static and dynamic posture.
5. Provide interventions to patients with impaired posture.

*P*osture is the relative alignment of body parts. Impaired posture is any postural abnormality that affects function. This chapter discusses normal and impaired posture in adults, the terminology used to describe posture, and interventions intended to optimize posture. Rehabilitation clinicians assess posture and intervene with the goal of changing posture to improve patient function, although there is no universally agreed upon ideal posture[1] and little research supporting a relationship between musculoskeletal pain and postural alignment.[2] This chapter makes suggestions for postural assessment and intervention based on the best available evidence.

Posture includes the relationships of body parts to each other and their relationships to the body's **base of support**. The base of support is the area of the body in contact with the supporting surface.[1] In typical standing, the base of support is the area between the outer edges of the feet (Fig. 4-1).

> ### Clinical Pearl
>
> In typical standing the base of support is the area between the outer edges of the feet.

Posture can be observed statically, with the body at rest, or dynamically, with the body in motion. Static posture can be observed in a variety of positions, including standing, sitting, lying, or in a specific task-associated position. Dynamic posture can be observed during a variety of activities, including walking, lifting, pushing, carrying, throwing, and cycling, or when moving from one position to another such as from lying to sitting or from sitting to standing. Because static posture is thought to be the basic posture from which other postures and movements stem, this chapter focuses on postural assessment and intervention for patients with functional problems related to changes in static posture.

Posture is controlled by the central nervous system (CNS), which integrates sensory information from the visual, proprioceptive, and vestibular systems to direct the muscles to achieve balance (see Chapter 13 for a more detailed discussion of balance and postural control).

IDEAL ALIGNMENT

The human body can be positioned in many static postures, including standing, sitting, kneeling, quadruped, lying, and stooping. Within these basic positions there is also a range of variations, such as standing on one leg or two; sitting with legs together, crossed, or apart; kneeling on one knee or two; or lying on one's side, supine or prone. For each of these positions the body is controlled for stability and orientation to the environment; this is

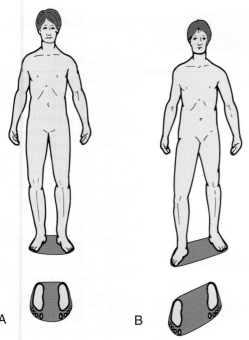

FIG. 4-1 Base of support. **A,** Feet hip width apart. **B,** Note increased base of support with one foot forward and feet further apart.

postural control. Postural orientation is the ability to maintain the appropriate relationship between body parts and between the body and the environment during the performance of a task. The human body's unique ability to maintain an erect bipedal stance allows use of the upper extremities for fine and gross motor tasks but standing erect has the disadvantages of a small base of support, a high **center of gravity (COG),** and high pressures on the vertebral column, pelvis, and lower extremities.

Ideal body part alignment, also known as **good posture,** ideal posture, **ideal alignment,** or neutral posture, is the position in which the body's weight is centered over its base of support. Ideal posture is thought to minimize the risk of injury or progressive deformity to supporting structures in all functional positions. Ideal posture requires minimal, although not the least possible, energy expenditure to maintain balanced alignment. The least amount of energy is expended in a slumped posture in which ligaments rather than muscles stabilize the weight-bearing joints.[3] Ideal posture should permit efficient mechanical joint action and limit wear and tear on the joints. As such, ideal posture requires that other conditions be normal, including muscle tone, flexibility, neuromuscular control, and reflexes.[4] Poor posture, in contrast, results in increased strain on the supporting structures and inefficient balance over the base of support.[3,4]

Anatomical position is not ideal alignment. It is the specific alignment of the body used as the position of reference for describing the anatomical planes and axes. In anatomical position the body is erect with the head and torso upright. The arms are at the sides of the torso with the shoulders in neutral rotation, elbows extended, the

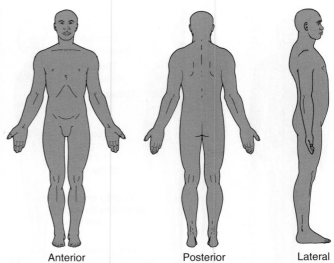

FIG. 4-2 Anatomical position.

cubital fossae of the elbow and the palms face forward, the fingers are extended, and the thumbs are adducted with the pad of each thumb facing forward. The lower extremities are straight and parallel, with the second toe facing straight forward (Fig. 4-2). From the anatomical position, three planes and three axes may be used to describe position, alignment, and motion of the body. In addition, the positions of the joints in anatomical position are considered the zero position for measurements of joint range of motion (ROM) for most joints.[5]

Clinical Pearl

Ideal alignment is the position in which the body's weight is centered over its base of support and can be described for standing, sitting, or other positions or activities. Anatomical position is a position of reference for describing the anatomical planes and axes.

STANDING POSTURE

Despite individual differences in body size and proportions, certain standards are proposed for ideal standing posture. These standards provide general indicators of a goal for ideal alignment and a standard for comparison when examining standing posture, regardless of the individual's body size or proportions.[3,5] Variations from these standards form the foundation of postural examination and evaluation. Ideal standing posture is shown in Fig. 4-3 and is described in Tables 4-1 and 4-2.

Standing in ideal alignment, one appears to be standing completely still but is actually constantly swaying forward and back and from side to side. This motion is called **postural sway.** Postural sway may vary with body morphology[6,7] and gender.[7] Some have proposed that sway may act as a pump to aid venous return.[3] Studies have shown that standing postural sway increases with fatigue[8-12] and may also increase in the context of low back pain,[13] increasing age,[14] stroke,[15,16] osteoporosis,[17] and alcohol consumption.[14,18,19] Sway may be minimized by

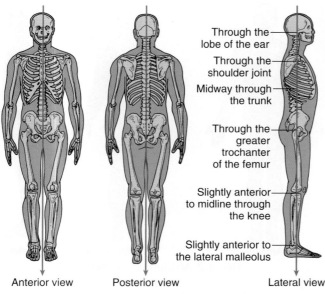

Through the lobe of the ear

Through the shoulder joint

Midway through the trunk

Through the greater trochanter of the femur

Slightly anterior to midline through the knee

Slightly anterior to the lateral malleolus

Anterior view   Posterior view   Lateral view

FIG. 4-3 Ideal standing posture. Anterior, posterior, and lateral views.

TABLE 4-1	Ideal Standing Posture from Anterior or Posterior View
Landmarks	**Ideal Alignment**
Eyes	Horizontally level.
Shoulders	Horizontally level. Superior angle slightly below the horizontal axis through T1.
Scapulae	Flat against the thorax, 30° anterior to the frontal plane, approximately 6 inches apart (or each approximately 3 inches from midline) with the medial border parallel to the spine.
Elbows	Neutral or slight **carrying angle** for males, slight to moderate carrying angle for females.
Wrists	Neutral. In neither flexion nor extension.
Hands	Face medially, toward the body.
Ribs and sternum	Ribs and the lateral contours of the rib cage symmetrical, the infrasternal angle is 90°.
Pelvis	ASISs and PSISs horizontally level.
Hips	In neutral rotation, neutral abduction and adduction.
Knees	The patellae face directly forward. Popliteal crease faces directly forward. **Q angle** approximately 13° in males and 18° in females.
Feet	Neither pronated nor supinated. Toes relaxed without **varus** or **valgus.** Calcaneus in mild valgus.
Spine	Vertically straight with occiput directly over sacrum.

Data from Kendall FP, McCreary EK, Provance PG: *Muscles: testing and function,* ed 4, Baltimore, 1993, Lippincott Williams & Wilkins; Sahrmann S: *Diagnosis and treatment of movement impairment syndromes,* St. Louis, 2002, Mosby; Winter D: *Biomechanics and motor control of human movement,* ed 3, New York, 2004, Wiley. *ASIS,* Anterior superior iliac spine; *PSIS,* posterior superior iliac spine.

TABLE 4-2	Ideal Standing Posture from Side View
Landmarks	**Ideal Alignment**
Cervical spine	Slight **lordosis.** Supports head with minimal muscular effort without upward, downward, or sideways tilt, rotation, or **retraction.**
Humerus	Less than one-third of humeral head anterior to anterior aspect of acromion. Proximal and distal ends are in the same (frontal) plane.
Elbow	Extension or slight flexion. Antecubital fossae face anteromedially and olecranon faces posteriorly.
Thoracic spine	**Kyphosis** 34° for adults and 38° for adolescents (average based on x-ray).
Ribs and sternum	Contours of ribcage symmetrical in frontal plane. No rotation of ribcage.
Lumbar spine	Lordosis 64° for adults and adolescents (average—based on x-ray).
Pelvis	ASISs in same vertical plane as pubic symphysis.
Knee	Knee is in neutral position: neither flexed nor hyperextended.
External auditory meatus, bodies of cervical vertebrae, midline of acromion, bodies of lumbar vertebrae, center of greater trochanter, point slightly anterior to midline at knee, point slightly anterior to lateral malleoli	All in vertical alignment.
Spine	Bodies of cervical vertebrae are in vertical alignment with bodies of lumbar vertebrae.

Data from Kendall FP, McCreary EK, Provance PG: *Muscles: testing and function,* ed 4, Baltimore, 1993, Lippincott, Williams & Wilkins; Sahrmann S: *Diagnosis and treatment of movement impairment syndromes,* St. Louis, 2002, Mosby; Winter D: *Biomechanics and motor control of human movement,* ed 3, New York, 2004, Wiley. *ASIS,* Anterior superior iliac spine.

intention,[20] lightly touching a stable object,[21,22] and by visual cues.[11,23,24] Postural sway is greater in unsupported sitting than in standing, although the amount of sway depends on the individual and the particular sitting position.[25]

SITTING POSTURE

As with standing, there are many potential sitting postures. Ideal sitting posture can be affected by where a person is sitting, their habits, and the task being performed.[26] Three basic sitting postures have been described when sitting in a chair: Anterior, middle, and posterior.[26] Anterior sitting (Fig. 4-4, *A*), also known as **forward sitting,** is a posture with either anterior rotation of the pelvis or increased kyphosis of the spine so that more than

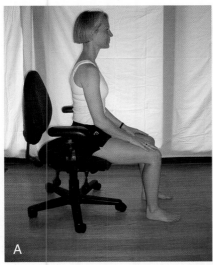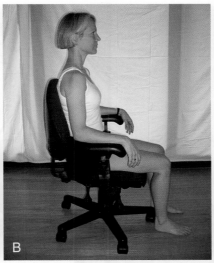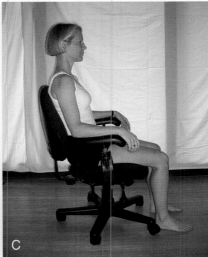

FIG. 4-4 **A,** Forward sitting. **B,** Middle (erect) sitting. **C,** Posterior sitting.

25% of the body's weight is transmitted through the feet to the floor and the COG is anterior to the ischial tuberosities. **Middle sitting** (Fig. 4-4, *B*), also known as erect sitting, is sitting with the COG directly over the ischial tuberosities with approximately 25% of the body's weight transmitted through the feet to the floor. **Posterior sitting** (Fig. 4-4, *C*) is a posture in which the COG is behind the ischial tuberosities and less than 25% of the body's weight is transmitted through the feet to the floor.[26]

Intradiscal pressure is higher in all sitting positions than in standing.[26] The primary difference between standing and any sitting posture is that sitting involves more flexion at the hips and knees. In most sitting postures, the pelvis rotates posteriorly and the lumbar lordosis reduces. The smaller the thigh-torso angle, the more the lumbar lordosis decreases. Sitting with the knees higher than the hips usually makes the lumbar lordosis reverse. Sitting on a kneeling chair (otherwise known as a **Balans chair**), with the knees lower than the hips, more closely approximates standing and promotes maintenance of the lumbar lordosis (Fig. 4-5).[27] To decrease strain on the lumbar spine and reduce lumbar intradiscal pressure, many therapists recommend that the knees be lower than the hips and the backrest be reclined to maximize the thigh-torso angle and help maintain a lumbar lordosis in sitting. This is effective for some but not all patients. Providing support for the lumbar spine when sitting or reclining the backrest also reduces intradiscal pressure and can help control low back pain in sitting.

Clinical Pearl

Many, although not all, patients are more comfortable sitting with their knees below their hips, a position that reduces intradiscal pressure.

Two postures, perching or **active sitting,** are recommended for people who are more comfortable sitting with a lordosis and for activities appropriate to anterior sitting.

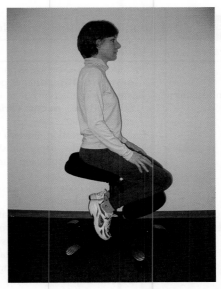

FIG. 4-5 Person in kneeling (Balans) chair.

Perching is sitting with an open thigh-torso angle by sitting at the forward edge of a seat, sitting on a seat that can tilt forward, sitting on a tall stool, or sitting on a gym ball or a specialized chair (Fig. 4-6, *A*). Active sitting involves sitting at the front of the chair with the torso leaning forward, placing the COG anterior to the ischial tuberosities with the lower extremity muscles actively supporting the sitting posture. This posture allows the spine to be in the ideal position found in standing and provides a wide base of support to stabilize the spine when static and during repetitive movement and loading (Fig. 4-6, *B*).

PATHOLOGY

Impaired or poor posture is posture that deviates from the ideal. Ideal posture is thought to contribute to optimal functioning of the human movement system, whereas impaired posture is thought to contribute to pain or

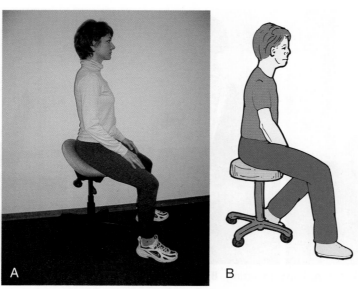

FIG. 4-6 **A,** Perching. **B,** Active sitting.

TABLE 4-3	Common Variations from Ideal Alignment
Body Area	**Variations**
Spine	Forward head, excessive kyphosis, excessive lordosis, **kyphosis-lordosis**, **swayback** (hips anterior to the **line of gravity (LOG)**, posterior pelvic tilt and reduced lordosis), flat back, scoliosis.
Rib cage and sternum	Asymmetry of the rib cage in the frontal or sagittal planes, barrel chest, **pectus excavatum** (also referred to as **recurvatum**), **pectus carinatum** (also referred to as **gallinatum**), increase or decrease in the infrasternal angle from 90°.
Scapulae	Elevation, depression, upward tilt, downward tilt, abduction, adduction, winging, anterior tilt
Shoulder	Forward shoulder, depressed shoulder, abduction, medial rotation, lateral rotation, flexion, extension, elevated humeral head, subluxed humeral head, humeral head more than 50% anterior to the anterior aspect of the acromion.
Elbow	Flexion, hyperextension, excessive carrying angle.
Forearm	Pronation, supination.
Wrist	Flexion, extension, ulnar deviation, **radial deviation**.
Hand/Fingers	Ulnar drift, boutonnière deformity, swan neck deformity.
Hip/Femur	Femoral anteversion (ante-torsion), femoral **retroversion** (retrotorsion), coxa vara, coxa valgum, femoral medial rotation, femoral lateral rotation.
Knee	Flexion, hyperextension, Q angle greater than 13° for males and greater than 18° for females, **patella alta**, **patella baja**, "squinting" patellae.
Tibia	Tibial medial torsion, tibial lateral torsion, tibial varum.
Feet	**Pes planus, pes cavus,** calcaneal varum, excessive **calcaneal valgus.**
Toes	Hallux valgus, hammer toes, claw toe(s), mallet toe(s), overlapping toe(s), Morton's toe, bunion(s).

dysfunction. Postural deviations may have a variety of causes and effects. The causes of impaired posture may or may not be modifiable. Modifiable causes of impaired posture include changes in muscle length and strength, alterations in joint ROM, muscle spasm, and positioning due to pain or habit. Nonmodifiable causes of impaired posture include structural variations and damage to the basic components that maintain posture, including the bones, joints, muscles, and nervous system. Examples of structural variations include leg length discrepancy, fixed spinal **scoliosis,** and excessive femoral **anteversion** (Table 4-3). Damage to the basic components that maintain posture may be caused by injury, such as a vertebral

compression fracture, or diseases, such as rheumatoid arthritis (RA) or osteoarthritis. CNS disorders, such as cerebral palsy, traumatic brain injury, or stroke, may also impair posture by altering muscle tone, strength, control, and/or sensation.

Changes in muscle length can result from lack of variety in movements and positions or the frequent performance of repetitive activities. Kendall proposes that muscle length and strength affect postural alignment and muscles that are shorter or longer than ideal length may cause postural deviations.[5] Muscle shortness can bring parts too close together to allow for ideal alignment. For example, an excessively short rectus femoris could pull the anterior

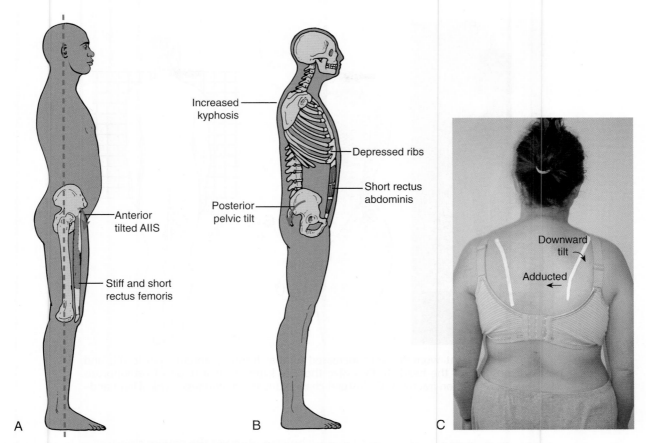

FIG. 4-7 **A,** Short and stiff rectus femoris producing an anterior pelvic tilt. **B,** Short rectus abdominis producing a posterior pelvic tilt. **C,** Scapular adduction and downward tilt.

inferior iliac spine toward the femur, producing an anterior pelvic tilt (Fig. 4-7, *A*). Similarly, a short rectus abdominis could produce a posterior pelvic tilt, a depressed ribcage, an excessively flexed thoracic spine, or any combination of these, depending on the influence of synergistic muscles and the opposing influence of **antagonist muscles** (Fig. 4-7, *B*). Excessive muscle length may allow parts of the body to separate or move too far apart. For example, a lengthened serratus anterior may allow adduction and/or downward tilt of the scapula because of the unopposed pull of the shorter rhomboids (Fig. 4-7, *C*). Muscle spasm or contracture may have similar effects to muscle shortening. For example, unilateral paravertebral muscle spasm may cause a functional scoliosis.

A variety of conditions can contribute to postural changes that can be difficult to modify. For example, increased lumbar lordosis, anterior pelvic tilt, and posterior positioning of the head are common during pregnancy and are thought to be related to changes in weight distribution, muscle length, and ligament laxity (Fig. 4-8, *A*).[28] Osteoporosis, aging, and ankylosing spondylitis are commonly associated with increased thoracic kyphosis (Fig. 4-8, *B*), and chronic obstructive pulmonary disease (COPD) is commonly associated with a **barrel chest.** Hand dominance often correlates with a typical pattern of left-right asymmetry, with the shoulder on the dominant side being slightly lower and the hip on the dominant side being slightly higher (Fig. 4-8, *C*).

Kendall proposed that there are three common types of impaired postures: Kyphosis-lordosis, **flatback,** and swayback (Fig. 4-9).[5] Kyphosis-lordosis posture is characterized by increased lumbar lordosis and thoracic kyphosis, anterior pelvic tilt, and forward head. Associated faulty joint postures may include abducted scapulae, forward shoulders, and either knee flexion or hyperextension. Flatback posture includes reduced lumbar lordosis, posterior pelvic tilt, and hip and knee hyperextension. It is common to find reduced thoracic kyphosis, cervical lordosis, and gluteal prominences. Swayback posture, like flatback posture, is characterized by a reduced lumbar lordosis and a posterior pelvic tilt, but in contrast to the flatback posture, in swayback posture the hips are anterior to the humeral heads and the lateral malleoli. It is common to find hyperextension of the knee, increased thoracic kyphosis, and abducted scapulae associated with swayback posture. The head is forward in all of these impaired postures.

TYPICAL EXAMINATION FINDINGS

PATIENT HISTORY

For the patient with impaired posture, the history will likely include information about the nature, location, severity, progression, and duration of symptoms, as well as information about the patient's current and past functional abilities.

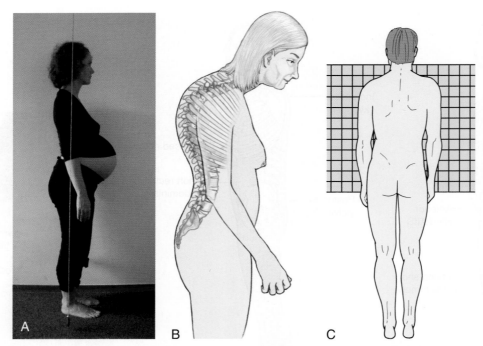

FIG. 4-8 **A,** Pregnant woman. Note increased lumbar lordosis, anterior pelvic tilt, and posterior position of the head. **B,** Excessive thoracic kyphosis as a result of osteoporosis and spinal compression fractures. **C,** Postural change due to handedness. Typical left hand–dominant posture.

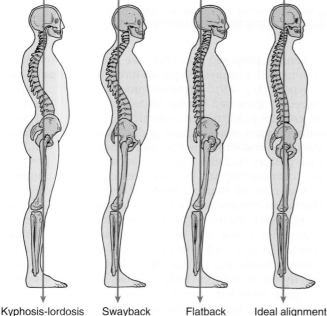

Kyphosis-lordosis   Swayback   Flatback   Ideal alignment

FIG. 4-9 Faulty postures: Kyphosis-lordosis, swayback, and flatback compared with ideal alignment.

TESTS AND MEASURES

It is particularly helpful for the clinician to begin observation when the patient is unaware that the examination has begun. In this circumstance the patient is likely to be much more relaxed and in his or her "usual" posture. The clinician observes the patient's posture as he or she walks in and sits down. The clinician can also observe whether the patient uses an assistive device and whether the patient demonstrates guarding, limitation of movement, or compensatory movements.

Specific tests and measures related to posture begin with inspection or observation. Although tests and measures are described in the standard sequence used throughout this book, in the clinical setting, tests may be grouped together by patient position for the convenience of the patient and the clinician. Standing is a good position to begin the examination. After completing tests performed with the patient standing, the clinician may progress to tests performed in sitting and then lying.

Musculoskeletal

Posture. Postural assessment is typically the first component of the tests and measures for any patient with a musculoskeletal dysfunction. The therapist observes the patient from the front, the back, and the sides. The patient's vertical reference maybe measured standing near a plumb line or in front of a grid of evenly spaced horizontal and vertical lines or the clinician may imagine a vertical line against which posture may be evaluated.

Posture is evaluated relative to ideal alignment. Postural deviations from ideal are described in terms of how the body parts have moved away from that ideal posture to achieve their current position. Anatomical position is used as the reference position from which anatomical planes and axes, as well as expressions of ROM of individual joints or parts, are described. The movements of the body, occurring in a plane about an axis, are described here in detail, using specific terminology.

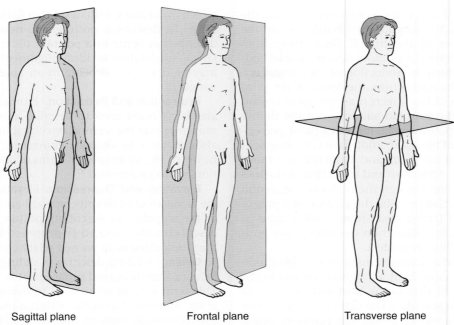

Sagittal plane   Frontal plane   Transverse plane

FIG. 4-10 Sagittal, frontal, and transverse planes.

The terms used to describe movements and positions of the body are based on the principle that movements occur in a plane around a given axis. For the sake of clarity, these planes and axes of reference are described briefly here. There are three types of planes and axes of reference: sagittal, frontal (or coronal), and transverse (or horizontal) planes (Fig. 4-10) and sagittal, coronal, and longitudinal axes. A sagittal plane passes from front to back (or back to front; the plane does not have a direction). The midsagittal plane passes through the midline of the body dividing it into left and right halves. A coronal plane passes from side to side, dividing the body into front and back. A horizontal plane divides the body into top and bottom portions. The point at which the three midplanes intersect is the COG of the body. The line of gravity (LOG) is the vertical line formed by the intersection of the midsagittal and midfrontal planes.[3,5] Movements occur in a plane and around (or about) an axis that is perpendicular to that plane (see Fig. 4-10). Shoulder flexion, for example, occurs in a sagittal plane that passes through the shoulder joint.[3]

Axes are imaginary lines through the body at right angles to each other. A sagittal axis passes through the body from front to back. Movements of abduction and adduction occur in a coronal plane about a sagittal axis. For example, shoulder abduction occurs in a coronal plane about a sagittal axis (the coronal plane passes through the humeral head from side to side and the sagittal axis passes through the humeral head from back to front). Flexion and extension occur in a sagittal plane about a coronal axis. Shoulder flexion, for example, occurs in a sagittal plane about a coronal axis that passes from one humeral head to the other. The third axis, the longitudinal axis, passes from top to bottom when passing through the trunk and from proximal to distal when passing through

an extremity. Rotation and horizontal adduction and abduction occur in a transverse plane around a longitudinal axis. Shoulder rotation occurs in a transverse plane about a longitudinal axis that extends along the center of the humerus.

Joint Positions and Motions

Flexion and Extension. Flexion and extension are movements in the sagittal plane about a coronal axis. Flexion can also be described as rotation of a bony lever around a joint to approximate the ventral surfaces (for most joints). When flexed, the distal components joined at the shoulders, elbows, wrists, fingers, and hips and the proximal components joined at the neck and torso are anterior to their anatomical or ideal position. Flexion of the knees and toes moves the distal components posteriorly. Extension is a motion of joints in the opposite direction to flexion. Anterior motion of the foot at the ankle (flexion) is called *dorsiflexion*. Posterior motion of the foot around the ankle (extension) is called *plantarflexion*. Flexion and extension of the thumb occur in the metacarpophalangeal and interphalangeal joints and are movements in an ulnar and radial direction, respectively. Hyperextension is extension beyond the normal range or position of extension. A part may be described as being in flexion, if it is in a flexed position relative to ideal alignment, or as being in extension, if it is in an extended position relative to ideal alignment.

Abduction and Adduction. Abduction is a movement where the distal portion of a segment of the body moves away from the midline in the frontal plane about a sagittal axis. Abduction may also be used to describe a motion in which the distal portion of a segment of the body moves away from the midline in the horizontal plane about a longitudinal axis and is then referred to as horizontal abduction. Adduction is the opposite of abduction and is thus a movement of the distal component toward the midline of the body. An exception to this rule is when the torso or head moves in the frontal plane away from midline, which is referred to as *lateral flexion* (or sidebending) rather than abduction. Abduction of the fingers is a spreading apart of the fingers from the center of the third digit, and adduction of the fingers is a movement toward the same point. Abduction and adduction of the thumb take place at the carpometacarpal joint in a plane perpendicular to the plane of the palm. Adduction is a movement of the thumb toward the palm, and abduction is a move away from the palm. Abduction and adduction of the toes take place around a line through the center of the second toe. Abduction may also describe the posture of a part of the body positioned farther away from midline than in ideal alignment, whereas adduction describes a part positioned closer to midline than ideal.

Rotation. Rotation describes turning about a longitudinal axis. Rotation occurs about a longitudinal axis in the transverse plane for all areas of the head and torso except the clavicles and the scapulae. The clavicles rotate about a coronal axis in the sagittal plane. The scapulae, which lie flush with the ribcage and as such are not in the frontal plane, rotate about a sagittal axis in a plane approximately 30 degrees anterior from the frontal plane. Rotation of the neck or pelvis is generally described as to the right or left. Rotation of the pelvis may also be described as clockwise or counterclockwise. Rotation of the extremities occurs about an axis through the length of the long bone in that segment, with the exception of the femur. Rotation of the femur is described around an axis that connects the center of the femoral head with the center of the knee joint.[5] Extremity rotation is described as medial or internal rotation when the rotation is toward the midline, and lateral or external rotation when the rotation is away from the midline. Internal rotation may be used to describe the posture of a part of the body positioned with more rotation toward midline, and external rotation may be used to describe the posture of a part of the body positioned with more rotation away from midline compared to ideal alignment.

Tilt. Tilt may describe movements of the head, pelvis, or scapulae. The head and pelvis may be tilted anteriorly, posteriorly, or laterally. The scapulae tilt anteriorly. In addition, when there is weakness, the scapulae may tilt so that the spinal border of the scapula moves away from the ribcage. This is called **scapular winging.** Anterior tilt of the head is a forward movement of the head accompanied by flexion or flattening of the cervical spine. Posterior tilt of the head is a rearward movement of the head accompanied by cervical extension or increased lordosis. Lateral tilt of the head is a sideways movement (also called *lateral flexion*) that is accompanied by sidebending and rotation of the cervical spine to the same side as the head. In the pelvis, anterior tilt is a downward movement of the anterior superior iliac spines (ASISs) and an accompanying upward movement of the posterior superior iliac spines (PSISs). Anterior pelvic tilt is accompanied by extension of the lumbar spine or an increase in the lumbar lordosis. Posterior pelvic tilt is an upward movement of the ASISs and an accompanying downward movement of the PSISs,

which occur along with flexion, or flattening of the lumbar spine. In describing posture, the head or pelvis may be described as being in a position of anterior, posterior, or lateral tilt relative to ideal alignment, and the scapulae may be described as being in an anterior tilt or to have winging.

Protraction and Retraction. Protraction and retraction are terms often used to describe anterior and posterior movements at the sternoclavicular joint. These terms may also be used to describe movements of the scapulae; however, the more specific terms of abduction and adduction are recommended.[5]

Elevation and Depression. Elevation and depression are terms used to describe upward and downward gliding of the scapulae. In describing posture, a scapula may be described to be elevated or depressed if it is in a position that is elevated or depressed relative to ideal alignment.

Gliding. Gliding describes a sliding motion usually of a flat or slightly curved surface relative to another surface. This term is most often used to describe the arthrokinematic motions that occur within a joint, rather than the osteokinematic motions that are described in this chapter and as such will not be further described here.

Positions and Motions of Specific Joints. Most positions and movements of the body can be described using the previous terms; however, certain joints move or can be positioned in unique ways and are then described with unique terms. General, as well as unique, joint movements and positions are listed in Table 4-4.

The position of the spine is critical to the examination of posture and is therefore described in additional detail here. There are a number of unique terms used to describe spinal position and posture. These include lordosis, kyphosis, and scoliosis. Lordosis is a curve that is convex anteriorly. The cervical spine and lumbar spine have a lordosis in the ideal standing position. Kyphosis is a curve that is convex posteriorly. The thoracic spine has a kyphosis in the ideal standing position. These normal curves of the spine, especially lumbar lordosis, are essential for maintaining upright posture.[29] Scoliosis is a lateral curvature of the spine. It is not normal to have any scoliosis, and therefore scoliosis is not considered a normal spinal curvature (Fig. 4-11). A scoliosis may be present in any portion of the spine. It may be confined to one portion of the spine or may extend through two or more portions of the spine. It may be a single C curve that is convex to the right or left or a "double" curve (also known as an S curve). Less frequently, scoliosis may have more than two curves.

Movements and positions of the spine as a whole include flexion, extension, sidebending (lateral flexion), and rotation. Flexion of the spine is a forward movement in the sagittal plane. In the cervical and lumbar spine, flexion first flattens the normal lordotic curve and then reverses the direction of this curve. In the thoracic spine, flexion increases the normally kyphotic curve. Extension of the spine is backward movement in the sagittal plane that increases the lordosis of the cervical and lumbar spine and flattens the kyphosis of the thoracic spine. Lateral flexion is sidebending movement of the head or torso to the right or left in the coronal plane. There is less lateral flexion possible in the thoracic spine than in the cervical

TABLE 4-4	Joint Positions and Movements
Joint	**Positions and Movements**
Sternoclavicular	Protraction, retraction, elevation, depression, upward rotation, downward rotation.
Glenohumeral	Flexion, extension, abduction, adduction, medial rotation, lateral rotation, horizontal abduction, horizontal adduction, **circumduction**.
Acromioclavicular	Protraction, retraction, gliding.
Scapulothoracic	Elevation, depression, abduction, adduction, anterior tilt, upward (or superior) rotation, downward (or inferior) rotation.
Elbow	Flexion, extension.
Radioulnar	Pronation (medial rotation of forearm—the palm faces posteriorly), supination (lateral rotation of the forearm—the palm faces anteriorly).
Wrist	Flexion, extension, adduction (or ulnar deviation), abduction (or radial deviation), circumduction.
Carpometacarpal	Gliding. Between trapezium and first metacarpal: Flexion, extension, abduction, adduction, slight rotation, circumduction, and opposition. Between hamate and fifth metacarpal: Flexion, extension, and slight rotation.
Metacarpophalangeal (MP)	Flexion, extension, abduction, adduction, circumduction. Thumb MP: Flexion, extension, slight abduction, adduction, and rotation.
Interphalangeal	Flexion, extension.
Pelvis	Anterior tilt, posterior tilt, lateral tilt, rotation.
Hip	Flexion, extension, abduction, adduction, medial rotation, lateral rotation, circumduction.
Knee	Flexion and extension with slight medial and lateral rotation in relation to femur during flexion and extension.
Ankle	Flexion (plantarflexion) and extension (dorsiflexion).
Subtalar and transverse tarsal joints	Supination, pronation, abduction, **inversion** (combination of adduction and supination), **eversion** (combination of abduction and pronation).
Tarsometatarsal	Gliding.
Metatarsophalangeal	Flexion, extension, abduction, adduction.
Interphalangeal	Flexion, extension.
Spine	Flexion, extension, sidebending (lateral flexion), rotation.

Scoliosis

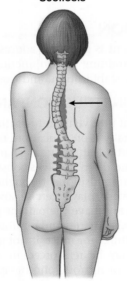

FIG. 4-11 Scoliosis. *From Patton KT, Thibodeau GA: Anatomy and physiology, ed 7, St. Louis, 2010, Mosby.*

and lumbar spine because the ribcage restricts thoracic motion in this direction. Spinal rotation occurs in the transverse plane. In the neck, rotation is described as rotation to the right or to the left and is determined by the direction that the face has turned. In the torso, rotation

is described as clockwise (left side forward) or counterclockwise (right side forward). Lateral flexion and rotation of the spine occur together as coupled movements. As a result, scoliosis always has both sidebending and rotational components. In some segments of the spine, rotation occurs in the same direction as the lateral flexion. In other spine segments, rotation occurs in the opposite direction from the sidebend (see Chapter 8). The same terms used to describe spinal movements may also be used as with other parts of the body to describe the position of the spine relative to ideal alignment.

Alignment by Region. In ideal alignment, the lower extremities are in the optimal position for weight bearing. The pelvis is in neutral, allowing it to support the abdomen and spine in an optimal position while also assisting in the proper positioning of the lower extremities. The cervical spine is positioned vertically above the lumbar spine, with the spinal lumbar and thoracic curves supporting the ribcage in a position that permits optimal functioning of the cardiopulmonary organs. The head is balanced in the center of the torso so that minimal activity is required of the neck muscles. The following section describes ideal alignment in standing by region.

Ankle. The ankle should be in 0 degrees dorsiflexion (and 0 degrees plantarflexion), and from a lateral view, the line of reference should pass just anterior to the lateral malleolus.[5,30] Because the LOG passes anterior to the joint line, there is a dorsiflexion moment. The gastrocnemius and soleus therefore work to prevent forward motion of the tibia when standing in ideal alignment.

Knee. From a lateral view, the line of reference passes slightly anterior to the center of the knee joint. Because the LOG passes anterior to the joint line, there is an extension moment at this joint. The hamstrings therefore work to prevent hyperextension of the knee.

Hip. From a lateral view, the line of reference passes slightly posterior to the hip joint and nearly directly through the center of the greater trochanter. Because the LOG passes posterior to the joint line, there is an extension moment at this joint. The quadriceps and other hip flexors therefore work to prevent posterior rotation of the pelvis.

Pelvis. In ideal alignment, the ASISs are in the same coronal plane as the symphysis pubis. Opposing pulls of muscles on the ASISs and pubic symphysis help maintain this position. Anteriorly the rectus abdominis pulls the pelvis superiorly, while the gracilis and adductor longus pull the pelvis inferiorly. The external abdominal oblique, internal abdominal oblique, and transversus abdominis stabilize the ASISs from above, and the rectus femoris, tensor fascia lata, and sartorius stabilize from below. Posteriorly, the erector spinae and quadratus lumborum pull superiorly and the hamstrings pull inferiorly.

Shoulder. From a lateral view, the plumb line passes approximately through the center of the acromion process. According to Sahrmann, the humeral head should be positioned so that no more than 25% of its diameter is anterior to the anterior-most portion of the acromion.[31]

Spine. From the posterior view, the spine should be vertically straight. The center of the occiput should be aligned with the center of the sacrum. From the lateral view, the spinal curves should be such that the bodies of the cervical vertebrae align vertically with the bodies of the lumbar spine. Those vertebral bodies should also be aligned with the external auditory meatus and the center of the humeral head, and a vertical line continuing inferiorly should fall just posterior to the center of the hip joint, just anterior to the knee joint, and just anterior to the lateral malleolus.

Various other criteria for ideal spinal alignment have been proposed. One such criterion suggests that, in standing, the C7 vertebral body aligns with (or is just posterior to) the S1 vertebral body.[29] Pelvic alignment has been proposed to be one of the most essential elements for assuming and maintaining ideal alignment of the spine and other body parts; alignment thereof is considered to be ideal when the ASISs are in the same coronal plane as the pubic symphysis.[5,31,32]

Following the examination of posture in standing, the clinician may also observe the patient's sitting posture. This examination should focus on deviations from ideal sitting posture and should include observation of where in the chair the patient sits, the tilt of the pelvis, and the alignment of the spine. The clinician should also note if and how the patient uses the backrest of the chair, as well as how and where the feet are positioned.

Range of Motion. For patients whose postural examination reveals impairment, ROM measurements of the cervical, thoracic, and lumbar spine and involved peripheral joints should be performed. ROM measurements are necessary to determine whether the patient has sufficient range available to be able to assume ideal, or at least more ideal, posture. ROM measurement technique is covered in detail in other texts.[33]

Muscle Performance. For patients with impaired posture, strength should be measured in the involved areas using manual muscle tests (see Chapter 5). Strength is measured to determine whether the patient has sufficient strength to assume an ideal posture, or at least a posture that more closely resembles ideal.

EVALUATION, DIAGNOSIS, AND PROGNOSIS

The diagnostic category for impaired posture is preferred practice pattern 4B: Impaired posture. Many factors may affect the prognosis for patients with impaired posture, which is usually one of several musculoskeletal impairments that the physical therapist will find on examination. In general, the more musculoskeletal dysfunctions that exist concurrent with the postural impairment, the longer the time required for the desired outcome. Other diagnoses will also affect the outcome and sometimes make the goals of independence or ideal posture unattainable. For example, a patient with ankylosing spondylitis may have a goal of independence in positioning for sleep, sitting, and standing without risk that the functional activity or position itself will exacerbate the progression of the disease, but ideal alignment will not be a goal because it will not be attainable. Other factors that may affect prognosis include age, length of time the patient has had the postural impairment, preexisting conditions or diseases, and the ability of the patient to adhere to the intervention.

INTERVENTION

Postural impairment is generally addressed by education, instruction, and training in conjunction with stretching and mobilization, stabilization, and exercise.

EDUCATION, INSTRUCTION, AND TRAINING

The initial focus of intervention for patients with postural impairment generally is on education. Education includes information about ideal body mechanics during functional activities and often involves consideration of a person's activities and positions throughout the day and night, including work, play, exercise, and sleep. The clinician will describe and have the patient practice ideal postures for their usual activities and reinforce the importance of using ideal postures for most, if not all, of these activities. Education may be reinforced in a variety of ways including the use of mirrors, photographs of the patient during functional activity, handouts, or even computer-based, frequently timed reminders.

STRETCHING AND MOBILIZATION

If the evaluation reveals soft tissue shortening, interventions that assist the lengthening of these tissues may be employed. Soft tissue length may be limited by passive components, such as scar tissue or contracture, or by active components, such as muscle spasm or spasticity.

These limitations may be managed with a variety of interventions, including the following:

- Massage[34-36]
- Myofascial release[37,38]
- Specific stretching exercises[36,39]
- Exercises that activate (contract or shorten) the muscles opposing restricted tissues[31]

Studies show that intermittent stretching programs and the proprioceptive neuromuscular facilitation (PNF) techniques of contract relax and hold relax can lengthen a variety of soft tissues, including muscles.[39-42] A severely shortened muscle is best lengthened gradually with a low-load stretch as can be provided by prolonged immobilization in a splint or cast.[40,43] The effectiveness of lengthening interventions may be enhanced with modalities. Modalities that increase tissue temperature, including ultrasound, diathermy, paraffin, and hot packs, have been shown to increase tissue extensibility and thus increase the lengthening obtained from a stretch.[44-50] Cryotherapy may be used before lengthening tissues in the presence of pain, muscle spasm, or inflammation and may also be used after lengthening procedures to assist in limiting the response (pain, muscle spasm, or inflammation) of the body to the tissue trauma produced by the procedures themselves. Electrical stimulation may also be used to minimize pain, inflammation, and muscle spasm before or after other interventions, as well as for neuromuscular reeducation during or after an intervention.[50]

Joint motion restrictions may be addressed with joint mobilization,[51-54] splinting,[40,55] exercises designed to use muscles that will encourage motion of the limited joint, and stretching of the joint into the direction of limited joint motion.[39,47,56] These techniques may also be assisted by therapeutic heat. Cryotherapy and electrical stimulation may be used before or after these techniques to facilitate joint motion if inflammation is present. Cryotherapy and electrical stimulation may also be used to minimize pain and inflammation after techniques used to increase joint motion.

STABILIZATION

If the evaluation reveals joint laxity, joint instability, or muscle weakness, interventions that provide stabilization to the soft tissues such as proprioceptive rehabilitation and strengthening of the surrounding muscles may be employed. Stabilization may be accomplished with splinting and education regarding proper positioning and avoidance of vulnerable positions.[5] Splinting, proprioceptive training, and strengthening exercises have been shown to improve joint stability and performance.[57-59] It is important to determine from the examination which muscles require strengthening and which do not. Posture and stability may be improved by strengthening weak muscles[5]; however, further strengthening of strong muscles in the same region may need to be avoided.[31]

EXERCISE

Few studies have studied the effects of exercise on posture. Two studies with interesting outcomes provide important information to consider when determining the intervention(s) to be used. Increasing back extensor strength with back strengthening exercises was found to reduce excessive thoracic kyphosis in otherwise healthy women aged 49 to 65 years.[60] However, the back extensor muscles, specifically the multifidi and erector spinae, were found in one study to extend the back, as well as to generate compressive and shear forces.[61] The effects of these forces should be considered when prescribing exercises for patients with poor posture and back pain. For example, exercises that activate the thoracic and lumbar erector spinae and multifidi are not recommended for individuals with intervertebral disc compression injuries because they may exert excessive compressive forces on the spinal discs. Exercises that isometrically activate the back extensor muscles may be deleterious to patients with translatory instability, particularly at L5, because of shear forces.

CASE STUDY 4-1

CHRONIC NECK PAIN

Patient History

AD is a 31-year-old man who reports neck and upper trapezius region pain for the past 10 years, which he associates with computer use. He works 45 to 60 hours per week primarily at his computer. AD bicycles 15 to 20 minutes to and from work 3 to 4 days each week and bicycles for 1 to 1½ hours once or twice each weekend for exercise. He notes pain and a sensation of coldness in the region of the right medial palm and the tips of digits 4 and 5 with soreness over the pisiform and at the elbow in the region of the ulnar groove, the medial epicondyle, and the olecranon process. He reports pain primarily with use of his computer input devices and some discomfort with writing and with movements involving thumb opposition.

Tests and Measures—Significant Findings

Musculoskeletal

- Reduced lumbar lordosis, excessive thoracic kyphosis from C7 to L2, low right shoulder, bilateral shoulder internal rotation, bilateral scapular depression (the superior medial angle was level with T3), bilateral scapular abduction, with more than 50% of the humeral head anterior to the acromion bilaterally, and left rotation of the cervical spine.
- Active shoulder flexion on the right causes C6 to rotate to the left and tingling in the right forearm and hand. Simultaneous flexion of the right and left shoulders causes C6 and C7 to rotate to the left.
- Tested in the hooklying position, the external abdominal obliques could not prevent the lumbar spine from extending when the hip was flexed or when the arms were raised from the relaxed position of arms resting by the sides.

Function

- When working at his desk, AD's thoracic and lumbar spine are markedly flexed (to bring his forearms down to the desktop where they rested for support). Cervical spine is extended (to see his monitors). Right shoulder is flexed approximately 30 to 40 degrees and his right wrist is slightly extended with his hand on the mouse. Left shoulder is flexed 40 to 45 degrees and wrist extended 20 to 30 degrees using the keyboard.

- AD often changes which arm he uses for keyboarding and mousing because of right upper extremity discomfort. In fact, he reports using the mouse with his left hand and the keyboard with his right hand most of the time now.

Diagnosis

Preferred practice pattern 4B: Impaired posture

Interventions

- Instruction in a home program of exercises and postural training.
- AD was advised to discontinue the exercises he was doing at home that encouraged flexion, including sit-ups, push-ups, and standing and sitting toe touches. He was instructed in exercises to strengthen his interscapular and abdominal muscles, reduce his thoracic kyphosis, and increase his shoulder ROM.
- At work, he was instructed to modify his position so that he would keep his arms at his sides with his shoulders in neutral flexion.

Role of the Physical Therapist Assistant

- What seating and computer modifications would help this patient improve his posture and control his pain?
- What did this patient's work, commute, and exercise postures have in common?
- Describe two exercises that would help this patient strengthen his trunk and scapular muscles and help him improve his posture.

Additional Information

For the full version of this case study, including detailed examination results, interventions, and outcomes, see the Evolve site that accompanies this book.

CHAPTER SUMMARY

Posture is the relative alignment of body parts. It can be observed and assessed statically or dynamically in various positions including standing, sitting, and lying. This chapter describes ideal posture and commonly observed types of impaired postures and explains factors that commonly contribute to postural impairment. The chapter also describes typical examination findings for a patient with impaired posture and gives detailed explanations of the terminology used to define positions and motions of different joints and body parts. This is followed by a general overview of interventions designed to bring posture closer to ideal, alleviating symptoms and maximizing function, and then a case study with specific interventions based on the specific findings in an individual patient.

ADDITIONAL RESOURCES

For links to these and additional web-based resources, see the Evolve site.

Sahrmann S: *Diagnosis and treatment of movement impairment syndromes,* St. Louis, 2002, Mosby.

Kendall FP, McCreary EK, Provance PG, et al (eds): *Muscles: testing and function,* ed 5, Baltimore, 2006, Lippincott Williams & Wilkins.

The Secret of Good Posture

GLOSSARY

Active sitting: Sitting with the ischial tuberosities at the forward edge of the seat, the pelvis and lumbar spine in a neutral position, the feet spread apart (either forward and back or side to side), and a slight forward lean at the hips.

Anatomical position: Erect standing posture with face forward, arms at sides of the torso, forearms supinated so that the palms face anteriorly, fingers in extension, and thumbs adducted with the pad of each thumb facing forward. Used as reference for terms relating to planes, axes, surfaces, joint motion, and directions of motion. Also the zero position for the measurement of most joint motions.

Antagonist muscles: Muscles that act in opposition to agonist muscles.

Anteversion: Anterior tipping of an organ or part. In the femur, an angle of more than the normal 15-degree anterior angulation of the femoral neck to the long axis of the shaft.

Balans chair: A kneeling chair.

Barrel chest: An increase in the anteroposterior diameter of the ribcage.

Base of support: The area of the body in contact with the supporting surface.

Calcaneal valgus: The calcaneus is angled with the inferior portion lateral to the superior portion; calcaneal eversion.

Carrying angle: A valgus angle of the elbow that may be seen clearly when the arm is positioned with the shoulder in neutral flexion/extension and full external rotation with the elbow extended.

Center of gravity (COG): A point about which gravity and the weight of a body act on one another to maintain equilibrium.

Center of mass (COM): A point that is at the center of the total body mass.

Circumduction: The movement of a limb in a circular motion.

Eversion: To turn outward, as in the foot.

Flatback: A posture of diminished lordosis of the lumbar spine.

Forward sitting: Sitting in a posture with the lumbar lordosis diminished or reversed or an increased kyphosis of the spine.

Good posture: Ideal body part alignment.

Ideal alignment (ideal posture, neutral posture): The position in which the center of mass is directly over the base of support.

Inversion: To turn inward, as in the foot.

Kyphosis: A posterior spinal curve or a spinal curve with a posterior convexity.

Kyphosis-lordosis: A posture with excessive thoracic kyphosis and excessive lumbar lordosis.

Line of gravity (LOG): A vertical line dropped from the body's COG.

Lordosis: An anterior spinal curve or a curve that has an anterior convexity.

Middle sitting: Sitting in a "middle position" (compared to anterior or posterior sitting) with the COM above the ischial tuberosities and the feet transmitting approximately 25% of the body weight to the floor.[26]

Patella alta: The patella is positioned more proximal than normal.

Patella baja: The patella is positioned so that the distance between the inferior pole of the patella and the tibial tubercle is less than two-thirds of the length of the patella.

Pectus carinatum/gallinatum: Excessive prominence of the sternum.

Pectus excavatum/recurvatum: Excessive depression of the sternum.

Pes cavus: Exaggerated height of the longitudinal arch of the foot.

Pes planus: Reduced height of the longitudinal arch of the foot.

Posterior sitting: Sitting characterized by less than 25% of the body weight transmitted to the floor by the feet and the COM above or behind the ischial tuberosities.

Postural control: The ability to provide for stability and orientation to the environment regardless of position or posture.

Postural orientation: The ability to maintain the body in a position appropriate for a task, including the relationship between body segments and the relationship between the body and the environment.

Postural sway: The normal movement of a body from front to back and from side to side in standing.

Q angle: The angle formed from the intersection of a line drawn from the ASIS through the center of the patella and a line drawn from the center of the tibial tubercle through the center of the patella.

Radial deviation: A movement of the wrist in which the lateral border of the hand moves toward the radius. In anatomical position the movement occurs in the frontal plane.

Retraction: Posterior movement of the clavicle or scapula.

Retroversion: The tipping backward of an organ or part.

Scapular winging: A prominence of the vertebral border of the scapula.

Scoliosis: A lateral deviation from the normally straight vertical line of the vertebral column.

Squinting (or convergent) patellae: Patellae that appear tilted medially (toward one another).

Swayback: A posture with the pelvis in posterior tilt and the hips swayed forward in relation to the feet resulting in hip joint extension.

Valgus: The distal boney segment is aligned laterally in comparison with the proximal segment.

Varus: The distal boney segment is aligned medially in comparison with the proximal segment.

Chapter 5

Muscle Weakness

Robert C. Manske, Michael P. Reiman

OBJECTIVES

After reading this chapter, the reader will be able to:
1. Describe the normal anatomy and physiology of skeletal muscle.
2. Differentiate between various causes of muscle weakness.
3. Apply appropriate tests and measures to examine muscle performance, including strength, power, and endurance.
4. Apply interventions to safely and effectively increase muscle strength.

*M*any ailments may cause impairments in muscular performance, reducing **strength**, **power**, and **endurance**, and result in muscle weakness. Therapists often examine and provide rehabilitation to patients with muscle weakness caused by muscle strains, disuse atrophy, and muscular diseases. Impaired **muscle performance** may result in minor problems, such as localized muscle

discomfort, or major functional problems, such as the inability to stand or ambulate. Muscles control the movement of body segments around joints and provide stability by resisting the movement of joint surfaces through joint approximation.[1] Improving muscle strength, power, and endurance are constant mainstays of physical rehabilitation. This chapter describes the anatomy and physiology of normal skeletal muscle and common pathologies that result in muscle weakness. It also discusses the examination of patients with muscle weakness and describes principles and methods for muscle strengthening interventions.

MUSCLE STRUCTURE

The three types of muscle tissue in the body are skeletal muscle (also known as *voluntary muscle* or *striated muscle*), smooth muscle, and cardiac muscle. This chapter only discusses skeletal muscle. Skeletal muscle can be thought of as being made up of bundles within bundles. A single skeletal muscle may contain many thousands of multinucleated muscle cells known as myofibers or muscle fibers. Each myofiber is surrounded by a cell membrane known as the *sarcolemma* and then by a thin yet strong layer of connective tissue known as **endomysium.** Each myofiber contains hundreds or thousands of **myofibrils**; organelles, such as ribosomes and mitochondria[1]; and substances, such as glycogen, enzymes, and fat.[2] The myofibrils contain overlapping parallel filaments of **actin** and **myosin** that create the appearance of alternating light and dark bands or stripes under a light microscope, giving skeletal muscle fibers a striated appearance.[3] The myofibers are bundled together in groups to form fascicles. Each fascicle is covered by an outer, thicker layer of connective tissue known as **perimysium.** Groups of fascicles are held together by another strong layer of connective tissue known as **epimysium** to form the muscle itself (Fig. 5-1).

The functional unit of the contractile system is the **sarcomere.** The sarcomere includes the actin and myosin filaments and proteins that bind them together. The thin actin filaments are made up of a long pair of molecules that form a helix.[1] A groove between this pair of molecules houses two long strands of **tropomyosin** and a smaller molecule, **troponin,** which is attached to the tropomyosin. The troponin and tropomyosin bind the actin and myosin filaments. Each myosin filament is composed of a globular head and a long tail.

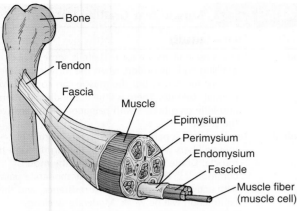

FIG. 5-1 Structure of skeletal muscle.

Skeletal muscle, unlike cardiac and smooth muscle, is under voluntary control.

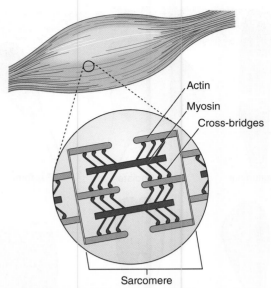

FIG. 5-2 Cross-bridge formation within muscle fibers.

PHYSIOLOGY OF MUSCLE CONTRACTION

Muscle contraction is controlled by input from motor nerves. Each motor nerve innervates a number of muscle fibers. One motor nerve and all of the muscle fibers that it innervates are known as a **motor unit.** When an electrical impulse, known as an **action potential,** reaches the end of the motor nerve that goes into the muscle, acetylcholine is released from the nerve terminals. The acetylcholine binds to receptors on the muscle fiber, and this evokes an action potential in the muscle fiber. This action potential spreads through the entire muscle fiber and results in the globular head of the myosin binding with the actin molecules to form cross-bridges (Fig. 5-2). The globular head of the myosin cross-bridge pulls on the actin filament, causing the actin and myosin filaments to slide past each other, making the muscle contract. During any muscle contraction, the filaments move repeatedly so that at any given moment only about half of the cross-bridges are actually generating force.

FACTORS AFFECTING MUSCLE PERFORMANCE

Many factors affect muscle performance, including the muscle fiber type and size, force-velocity relationships, **length-tension relationships,** muscle architecture, neural control, fatigue, the age of the individual, cognitive strategies, and various medications, particularly corticosteroids.

Muscle Fiber Type. Muscles are made up of two general types of fibers: type I and type II, and in most muscle, one fiber type predominates. Type I muscle fibers are **slow-twitch fibers** that resist fatigue and can sustain low levels of force for long periods of time. Type I muscle fibers predominate in postural muscles and patients with low back pain and injuries tend to have selective wasting of type I muscle fibers.

Type II muscle fibers are **fast-twitch fibers.** Type II fibers can exert a large force for a short amount of time and then rapidly fatigue. Muscles that produce faster, explosive movements are made up predominantly of type II fibers.

Some early studies suggested that fibers could transform from type I to type II with exercise training.[4,5] However, it is now generally accepted that this kind of change does not occur in response to training performed in rehabilitation or fitness programs.[6]

Resistance exercise can increase muscle fiber size but does not change the type or increase the number of muscle fibers.

Muscle Fiber Size. Muscle fiber size can change in response to muscle activity, becoming larger in response to exercise.

Force-Velocity Relationships. With concentric (shortening) contractions, the amount of force generated by a muscle is inversely related to its speed of movement. When the muscle shortens more quickly, it produces less force. In contrast, with eccentric (lengthening) contractions, the amount of force generated initially increases when the muscle lengthens more quickly but then quickly levels off.[7,8]

Length-Tension Relationships. A muscle's capacity to produce force also depends on its length or the amount of tension in it. Muscles can produce the most force at their normal resting length, when the most cross-bridge sites are available between the actin and myosin filaments. Fewer sites are available when the muscle is in either a shortened or lengthened position.

Muscle Architecture. Muscles can have different shapes, or architecture (Fig. 5-3). A pennate muscle has

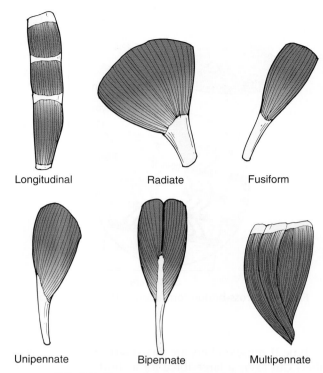

Longitudinal   Radiate   Fusiform

Unipennate   Bipennate   Multipennate

FIG. 5-3 Types of muscle fiber pennation.

TABLE 5-1	Muscle Tear Grading Categories

Grade	Characteristics
Grade I	A few muscle fibers are torn. There is some minor swelling and discomfort when the muscle contracts against resistance, but the muscle can contract with normal strength. There is little if any discoloration, and little pain occurs with palpation of the area of the strain.
Grade II	Also known as a partial tear. Moderate tearing of muscle fibers without complete tearing through the muscle. Grade II muscle strains are the most common.[18,19] This injury will cause moderate pain with active contraction against resistance, and the contraction will be weak. Moderate swelling, moderate pain with palpation, and pain with passive stretching will be present.
Grade III	Complete muscle rupture. Because the muscle fibers no longer form a continuous muscle, there may not be pain when contraction is attempted, but there will be profound weakness. Severe swelling and discoloration will be present and possibly a palpable gap in the muscle belly.

fibers arranged in a feather-like pattern. A pennate muscle can use the length-tension relationship more effectively than a longitudinal muscle. Pennate muscles can be unipennate, bipennate, or multipennate.

Neural Control. Muscle strength generally increases as more motor units are involved in the contraction, when larger motor units contract, and when the frequency of action potentials is higher.[9] Proper coordination of movement among agonist, synergist, and antagonist muscle groups is also necessary for optimal control and function.

Fatigue. Fatigue is the reduction in force production by a muscle that occurs after repeated contractions. Fatigue of one muscle or muscle group can lead to substitution by other muscle groups or muscle injury.

Individual's Age. Muscle performance changes throughout the lifespan. Muscle strength and endurance increase with age, and muscle mass increases in parallel with body mass, from childhood until puberty. The ability to increase strength rapidly accelerates during puberty, especially in boys. Strength potential is at its highest between 18 and 30 years of age. Muscle mass peaks in women between the ages of 16 and 20 years and in men between the ages of 18 and 25 years. After the third decade of life strength declines by 8% to 10% per decade through the fifth or sixth decade, with the rate of decline accelerating to 2% to 4% per year beginning in the sixth to seventh decade.[10,11]

Age-related loss of muscle strength is not uniform for all muscle groups, muscle fibers, or types of contractions. In general, lower extremity muscle strength declines more quickly than upper extremity muscle strength and

dynamic strength declines more quickly than isometric strength.

Cognitive Strategies. Positive cognitive strategies, such as arousal, attention, imagery, and self-efficacy, are associated with enhanced muscle strength and performance,[12] whereas some types of mental preparation, such as relaxation-visualization training, have a negligible or negative impact on strength performance.[13]

Corticosteroids. Prolonged use of high doses of corticosteroids, as may be prescribed for their antiinflammatory and immunosuppressant effects, cause muscle atrophy and weakness, particularly in the limb muscles.[14]

PATHOLOGY

MUSCLE STRAIN

A muscle strain is a stretch or tear of a muscle. Muscle strains most commonly occur at the musculotendinous junction, which is the weakest area of the muscle.[15,16] Muscle strains are common and account for approximately 50% of athletic injuries.[17] A muscle strain can occur acutely, when a muscle exerts a single high load intrinsic force, or gradually, as the result of repetitive low load overuse. Additionally, a muscle strain can be caused by excessive extrinsic passive stretching of a muscle. In some instances, a strain may result from a combination of excessive intrinsic and extrinsic force. The gastrocnemius may be strained when someone lands from a jump and the foot and ankle move into dorsiflexion, extrinsically stretching the muscle, while the gastrocnemius is also contracting eccentrically, placing an intrinsic force on the muscle. This type of movement occurs frequently during many athletic and recreational activities.

Muscle strain injuries are generally graded on a 3-point scale (Table 5-1). Factors that contribute to muscle strain injury include inadequate muscle flexibility, inadequate strength or endurance, synergistic muscle contraction, insufficient warm-up, and inadequate rehabilitation from previous injury.[20-22]

Clinical Pearl

Muscle strain is common with athletic injuries and can take place acutely after a single high load intrinsic force or can happen gradually as a result of repetitive, low load overuse.

DISUSE ATROPHY

Disuse muscle atrophy refers to wasting or loss of muscle as a result of lack of use. Disuse atrophy is associated with various conditions, including illness, surgery, and certain disease processes (heart conditions, cancer). Most of these conditions have one thing in common—a certain amount of convalescence. With this convalescence comes muscle disuse, as well as cardiovascular deconditioning (see Chapter 23).

Loss of muscle performance after injury or surgery is often rapid and dramatic. This can be especially debilitating for patients with impaired muscle performance before their injury or surgery. Complete cessation of training will in most instances cause an immediate decline in strength.[23] If bed rest or limitations in activity are required, or if there is inflammation after trauma or surgery, this decline in strength can be compounded.

Type II fibers degenerate and lose their ability to produce force before type I fibers, most likely because type II fibers require a high recruiting stimulus that is not achieved during reduced use and early in rehabilitation, when contractions are weak, whereas type I fibers are activated with almost all activity.

MUSCLE DISEASES

Myopathies are disorders of the muscle fibers that cause muscle weakness. Myopathies are generally classified as hereditary or acquired. One of the more common hereditary myopathies is muscular dystrophy. In this condition, depending on the subtype of the disease, weakness can occur at any age but usually starts in childhood and progresses gradually over time. Most types of muscular dystrophy are thought to have a genetic origin and are characterized by symmetrical muscle wasting without neural or sensory deficits.[24]

NEUROLOGICAL DISEASES AFFECTING MUSCLE PERFORMANCE

Many progressive and nonprogressive neurological diseases of the central and peripheral nervous system affect muscle performance. For example, cerebral palsy, which is caused by a nonprogressive lesion of the developing brain, causes a persistent and changing disorder of movement and posture that appears early in life and is often associated with muscle weakness. Myasthenia gravis, a disorder that prevents efficient transmission from the nerves to the muscles, causes weakness primarily characterized by fatigue. Peripheral nerve injury, as exists with carpal tunnel syndrome, causes weakness of the hand muscles innervated by the median nerve.

Clinical Pearl

Muscle weakness and atrophy can be caused by muscle disuse, myopathies (disorders of the muscle fibers), or neurological conditions.

TYPICAL EXAMINATION FINDINGS

PATIENT HISTORY

For the hospitalized patient, much of the history will be obtained through a review of the medical chart. In an outpatient setting, the therapist will generally obtain information regarding the patient's age, sex, race, employment, arm and leg dominance, general health status, past medical history including surgeries, and present functional status directly from the patient. Psychosocial issues related to educational level, cultural beliefs, caregiver resources, and living environment will also be discussed. Information regarding medications, laboratory or diagnostic tests, or other clinical findings will be noted.

The patient's expectations and goals for therapy will be discussed because they can affect compliance with recommendations and satisfaction with treatment outcomes.

SYSTEMS REVIEW

The systems review is used to target areas requiring further examination and to define areas that may cause complications or indicate a need for precautions during the examination and intervention processes.

A musculoskeletal scanning examination will include gross tests of range of motion (ROM), strength, and relative flexibility and include observation of body size, proportion, and symmetry. The review of the neuromuscular systems may include gross examination of coordination, balance, reflexes, sensation, skin integrity, and orientation to person, place, and time.

TESTS AND MEASURES

Musculoskeletal

Anthropometric Characteristics. Limb circumference can be used to approximate muscle size. Limb circumference is often assumed to correlate with muscle power and strength, with greater circumference and muscle bulk indicating greater strength. Although limb circumference and muscle strength do decrease with muscle atrophy, the correlation is not consistent.

Joint swelling, generally estimated by measurement of joint circumference, can inhibit muscle contraction. As little as 20 ml to 60 ml of knee joint effusion can inhibit quadriceps muscle contraction.

Range of Motion. Both active ROM (AROM) and passive ROM (PROM) will be measured during the examination of a patient with suspected muscular weakness. Muscle weakness will not affect PROM but may reduce AROM if strength is substantially decreased. If muscle injury or atrophy has affected strength enough to impair

TABLE 5-2	Muscle Testing Grading Categories	
Grade	Contraction Strength	Movement
5	Normal (100%)	Complete ROM against gravity with maximal resistance
4	Good (75%)	Complete ROM against gravity with some (moderate) resistance
3+	Fair +	Complete ROM against gravity with minimal resistance
3	Fair (50%)	Complete ROM against gravity
3−	Fair −	Some but not complete ROM against gravity
2+	Poor +	Initiates motion against gravity
2	Poor (25%)	Complete ROM against gravity eliminated
2−	Poor −	Initiates motion if gravity is eliminated
1	Trace	Evidence of slight contractility but no joint motion
0	None	No contraction palpated

Adapted from Magee DJ (ed): *Orthopedic physical assessment*, ed 5, St Louis, 2008, Saunders.
ROM, Range of motion.

lifting against gravity, the patient may have decreased AROM that is readily observed during functional activities and with specific measurement of AROM. An inability to move a given segment through full AROM when PROM is full and painless generally indicates muscle strength impairment.

Muscle Performance. Patients with muscle weakness have reduced muscle performance, which is the capacity of a muscle to do work.[25] Weakness can impair strength, power, and endurance. Strength is the ability of a muscle to exert a maximal force or torque at a specified or determined **velocity.** Power is the rate of work, or amount of work per unit time, and endurance refers to the ability to perform low intensity, repetitive, or sustained activities over a prolonged period of time without fatigue. Because optimal muscle performance and patient function relies on the balance and interplay between strength, power and endurance, muscle performance testing often includes testing of all three of these variables.

Manual Muscle Testing. **Manual muscle testing (MMT)** is used to test the strength of individual muscles or muscle groups. MMT is performed by applying manual resistance to a limb or body part. This resistance is typically applied to the limb at a point in the limb's ROM in which the muscle being tested is most efficient. Muscle strength is graded on a 0 to 5 numeric scale. All the grades above 1 may be scored as the number alone or with a score of the number with a + or −. Definitions of these scores are given in Table 5-2.

The MMT scale is easy to apply, but it is important to realize that these scores are not equally spaced. A score of 4 does not indicate that a muscle is twice as strong as one with a score of 2. Furthermore, validity of high scores may be limited by the strength of the clinician performing the test. MMT is the fastest and most efficient way to assess muscle strength in the clinical setting.

Clinical Pearl

Manual muscle testing (MMT) is the fastest and most efficient way to assess muscle strength in the clinical setting.

Hand-Held Dynamometers. Hand-held dynamometers may also be used to test the strength of individual muscles or muscle groups. A dynamometer is a device that can measure force. The hand-held dynamometer is a small device that fits in the examiner's hand and is placed at precise locations on a subject's limb in an effort to assess the force generated by various muscles or groups of muscles. Hand-held dynamometers are inexpensive, convenient, and lightweight; require minimal set-up time and training; and can be used in a wide variety of settings.[26]

Isokinetic Testing. Isokinetic strength testing measures force production during fixed velocity movement with an accommodating resistance.[27] Isokinetic strength testing is performed using an electrically powered device that maintains a chosen velocity of movement while maximizing the resistance throughout the ROM. There are many isokinetic strength testing devices available. All have components to allow testing of movement of different joints and in some instances, for testing during open and closed kinetic chain movements.

Isokinetic measures can be compared with normative data for a given population or compared to the uninvolved side to determine if muscle performance is normal or abnormal. Advantages of isokinetic strength testing include its ability to measure the strength of concentric and **eccentric contractions** and its high reliability when applied in a standardized manner.[28] Isokinetic testing can provide information about subtle changes in strength that may not be detectable by MMT.

Joint Integrity. Although joint integrity does not generally limit muscle strength, limitations in joint mobility will affect joint movement and measurement of muscle strength and performance. For example, even with full strength, a patient with a severely swollen knee will probably be unable to force the knee through full AROM as a result of pain inhibition.

Neuromuscular

Arousal, Attention, and Cognition. In patients with weakness, changes in arousal, attention, or cognition are generally apparent and will be grossly assessed during the patient history. The patient's ability to maintain attention and their alertness and orientation will affect the ability to obtain a thorough and complete history and may affect cooperation both with strength testing procedures and therapeutic interventions.

Pain. Pain can inhibit muscle contraction, giving the impression of muscle weakness. With prolonged inhibition and the resulting prolonged disuse, pain can at times also lead to significant muscle atrophy and true weakness. There are many ways to measure pain, including visual analog scales, questionnaires, and pain diagrams, as described in detail in Chapter 22.

Peripheral Nerve Integrity. Peripheral nerve integrity can be examined and evaluated clinically through a combination of strength, sensory, and reflex testing as described in Chapter 18. Nerve conduction studies and electromyography may also be used to examine and evaluate peripheral nerve integrity.

Sensory Integrity. Sensory integrity will be examined as described in Chapter 18.

> ### ◎ *Clinical Pearl*
>
> Special care should be taken to protect the skin and soft tissue in patients with sensory impairment from injury during strengthening interventions.

Cardiovascular/Pulmonary

Circulation, Ventilation, and Respiration/Gas Exchange. Vital signs checked during the systems review will generally indicate if the patient with muscle weakness has cardiovascular or pulmonary problems. Vital signs of heart rate, blood pressure, and respiratory rate should be checked at the beginning of each session involving muscle exercise in patients with cardiovascular or pulmonary problems (see Chapter 22).

Aerobic Capacity and Endurance. Because aerobic capacity depends on the function of large muscle groups, aerobic capacity and endurance can be decreased in patients with muscle weakness. (See Chapters 23 and 26 for information on measurement of aerobic capacity and endurance.) This is especially true for sedentary individuals with large muscle group atrophy or weakness that results from chronic disuse.

Function

Gait, Locomotion, and Balance. Gait is often affected by lower extremity muscle weakness. Gait assessment and intervention are discussed in detail in Chapter 32.

Assistive and Adaptive Devices. Depending on the extent of muscle weakness, the patient may need to use an assistive or adaptive device (see Chapter 33). If MMT reveals the strength of lower extremity to be less than ⅗, an assistive device may be warranted to ensure safe ambulation. Crutches, a cane, or even a walker may be needed to balance and ambulate safely and efficiently.

Orthotic, Protective, and Supportive Devices. Orthotics and protective devices can improve function and safety for individuals with muscle weakness. These devices generally support a joint, or joints, to substitute for the weak muscle. The patient's current strength, functional abilities, and lifestyle will dictate which orthosis will work best for the particular situation. For example, patients with weak dorsiflexors may benefit from an ankle-foot orthosis (AFO) and those with weakness of the quadriceps and dorsiflexors may benefit from a knee-ankle-foot orthosis (KAFO)[29] (see Chapter 34).

EVALUATION, DIAGNOSIS, AND PROGNOSIS

According to the *Guide to Physical Therapist Practice*,[30] rehabilitation for patients in the preferred practice pattern 4C: Impaired muscle performance may take from 2 to 6 months with an expected range of 6 to 30 visits to achieve optimal performance. This range is wide because many factors may affect the frequency and duration of physical therapy visits such as accessibility and availability of resources, age, caregiver consistency or expertise, cognitive status, co-morbidities, concurrent therapeutic interventions, nutritional and overall health status, psychological and socioeconomic factors, and social support.

INTERVENTION

Interventions to reduce muscle weakness are based on the overload principle and the selective adaptation to imposed demands (SAID) principle. Training should also take into account the concepts of individuality, frequency, intensity, and duration.

OVERLOAD PRINCIPLE

The human body can continually adapt to external stimuli. If an individual encounters a load greater than usual, they will, if possible, adapt to this load by increasing strength, power, or endurance, depending on the nature of the load. This adaptive response to increased training load is called the *overload principle*. Once a body adapts to a given workload, it will not change further unless the workload continues to increase. Therefore, to continually improve performance, the load must be progressively increased to promote progressive adaptation.[31] Although the body initially responds to overload with fatigue, its gradual adaptation to the increased load can be used therapeutically in rehabilitation to increase strength and fitness.[32]

SAID PRINCIPLE

A systematic approach to progression of the load applied during exercise will optimize improvements in muscle performance and resultant functional ability. According to the SAID principle, the body adapts according to the demands placed on it. Therefore exercise for patients with muscle weakness should emphasize strength, power, and endurance according to the functional goals and needs of the individual patient.

Several factors are considered when designing a strengthening program, including the patient's age, sex, medical history, previous training background, injury history, the body's structural integrity, functional goals, motivation, and any healing restraints related to their injury or surgery. A rehabilitation training program to reduce muscle weakness will also consider the following: primary energy source used, muscle(s) actions, the mechanism of resistance, and velocity of movement required.

Energy Source. Aerobic and anaerobic energy sources may be used to produce muscle actions, depending on which component of muscle performance is mostly required. Anaerobic energy sources are used predominantly for short, intense activities, and aerobic energy sources are used predominantly for longer duration, less intense activities.

Muscle Action. Muscle action refers to whether a contraction is dynamic (produces movement) or isometric (does not produce movement). Muscle action during rehabilitation exercises should match the muscles' intended action during functional activities. Exercises may include groups of muscles working together to mimic function or may focus on specific muscles when functional activities are limited by weakness in an isolated muscle or muscle group.

Mechanism of Resistance. Resistance can be applied with open-chain (with the distal extremity free) or closed-chain (with the distal extremity fixed) exercise. Strengthening programs should include activities with the same mechanism of resistance as used during for the patient's functional activity goals.

Velocity of Movement. Training is also velocity specific. Therefore high velocity training is used to improve performance of activities that require high velocity movement, and slower velocity training is used to improve performance of activities that require slow velocity movement. This velocity specificity is likely based in part on fiber specificity, with type II fibers activated more for fast movements and type I fibers activated more for slow, sustained contractions.

EXERCISE PRESCRIPTION

There are several ways to progressively overload a muscle to improve muscle performance.[33] Exercise to improve muscle performance is most readily described and prescribed according to its frequency, intensity, time, and type (the **FITT formula**).

Frequency. Frequency refers to how often exercise should be performed. The ideal frequency of exercise depends on the goals of the treatment and stage of recovery from injury or surgery. During the acute stage of healing, exercise can occur more frequently but most likely with less duration and intensity than in more advanced strengthening stages. In later advanced stages of strengthening, the frequency of training should be reduced to allow for sufficient recovery to avoid excessive fatigue, decreased performance, and overtraining.[33,34]

Intensity. The intensity is the amount of resistance used for a specific exercise and is generally set as a percentage of the individual's maximum ability for that particular exercise. The training volume is the total amount of work performed, whether in a particular session or in some set period of time.[33] As rehabilitation or training progresses, either the intensity or the volume of the exercise should be increased while the other is initially decreased.

◎ *Clinical Pearl*

The maximum amount of weight an individual can lift a specified number of times is known as the **repetition maximum (RM)**. For example, 10 RM is the most weight the individual can lift 10 times.

Duration/Time. Duration is the total number of weeks or months during which a resistance exercise program is carried out. Duration depends on multiple factors, including stage of healing, progress in rehabilitation, initial functional level, prognosis, functional goals, and presence or absence of co-morbidities. In addition, duration for a maintenance program will by definition be much longer than for a recovery or rehabilitation program.

Type/Mode of Exercise. Type of exercise relates to the specific activity being performed, including the mode of resistance (e.g., free weights, elastic band, or water) and type of activity being performed (e.g., **isotonic,** isometric, isokinetic, open chain, or closed chain). Different modes of resistance and types of exercise are discussed in greater detail later in this chapter.

NEUROMUSCULAR ELECTRICAL STIMULATION

Neuromuscular electrical stimulation (NMES) can be an effective component of a rehabilitation program for muscle weakness. NMES can help when the client is either unable or unwilling to volitionally elicit strong muscle contractions. NMES has been shown to accelerate functional recovery after surgery, prevent disuse atrophy, reduce ROM deficits, and improve motor control in patients with strength deficits of various etiologies.[35-37]

For NMES to increase muscle strength the electrical current must produce contractions that are at least 50% of the maximum volitional isometric contraction (MVIC) force for the targeted muscles.[38] NMES preferentially strengthens type II muscle fibers because it recruits motor units with type II fibers before those with type I fibers, which is the opposite order from voluntary contractions in which type I fibers are recruited first. NMES recruits type II muscle fibers first because the axons of their motor units are larger and more superficial and offer lower resistance to electrical stimulation.[39] It is proposed that this is why NMES can accelerate strengthening and shorten rehabilitation times.[39] NMES is most effective when used in conjunction with volitional muscle contractions. This promotes strengthening of both type I and type II muscle fibers and facilitates integration of motor performance into functional use.

ADAPTATIONS TO RESISTANCE TRAINING

Resistance training produces increases in strength, changes in muscle size and metabolism and a range of other effects. Initially, in the first 4 to 6 weeks of training, strength increases mostly because of neural adaptation (learning and improved coordination). Later in training, strength increases mostly because of muscle **hypertrophy.**

Training that focuses on strength and power uses more anaerobic metabolism and thus improves anaerobic capacity while also increasing muscle girth and muscle fiber size. In contrast, endurance training causes muscles to improve their aerobic metabolic capacity and efficiency and also causes selective hypertrophy of type I muscle fibers.

Strength training is also associated with the following:

- Increased neuromuscular efficiency[40,41]
- Increased bone strength and density[42,43]
- Increased ligament and tendon strength and thickness[44]
- Improved balance and decreased the risk of falling[45]
- Increased gait stability and efficiency[46]
- Improved stair climbing and chair rising ability[46]
- Decreased resting blood pressure, glucose tolerance, and insulin resistance[47,48]
- Decreased body fat and increased basal metabolic rate[47]

PRECAUTIONS AND CONTRAINDICATIONS TO MUSCLE STRENGTH TRAINING

When implementing a resistive exercise plan for the treatment of muscle weakness, additional care should be taken in very young and very old patients and in patients with co-morbidities. ROM and tissue stresses should be limited as needed to respect tissue healing constraints.

The Valsalva maneuver (an expiratory effort against a closed glottis) should be avoided during muscle contractions because this increases intrathoracic and intraabdominal pressure and leads to decreased venous return of blood to the heart. This decrease in venous return leads to a decrease in cardiac output, a temporary drop in arterial blood pressure, and an increase in heart rate. Increased heart rate with resistive exercise is especially contraindicated in high risk patients, such as those with a history of cerebrovascular or cardiovascular problems (cerebral vascular accident, myocardial infarction, heart failure, and hypertension) and the elderly. The increase in intraabdominal pressure can also injure patients with recent abdominal surgery or abdominal wall hernias. To prevent the Valsalva maneuver, instruct patients not to hold their breath and to exhale when performing a contraction. The patient may be asked to count, talk, or breathe rhythmically during exercise.

Try to assure the patient that strengthening exercises activate the intended muscles. When too much resistance is applied, muscle substitution is common. For example, if trying to improve deltoid strength through resisted shoulder elevation, when too much resistance is applied, the levator scapula will contract to assist. Close supervision, proper exercise instruction, and the use of a mirror for patients to monitor themselves can all help to reduce muscle substitution.

Dynamic resistance exercises are contraindicated when a muscle or joint is inflamed or swollen because exercise may provoke further inflammation or swelling and further damage the muscle or joint. However, low intensity **isometric exercise** can be performed if the activity does not cause pain. Patients should be carefully monitored for their immediate response to resistance exercise and for their response over the following 24 to 48 hours. If severe joint or muscle pain occurs during the activity or within the 24 to 48 hours after exercise, the activity should be eliminated or substantially reduced and the cause of the pain should be determined.

Exercise-induced muscle soreness is muscle soreness that develops during or directly after strenuous exercise performed to the point of fatigue.[49] This response is attributed to a lack of blood flow and oxygen with a temporary buildup of metabolites, such as lactic acid and potassium, in the exercising muscle.[49] This normal response often subsides quickly after exercise when adequate blood flow and oxygen return to the muscle. Implementing an appropriate cool down period of low intensity exercise (often referred to as an *active recovery*) can facilitate recovery from exercise-induced muscle soreness.[50]

Delayed-onset muscle soreness (DOMS) is soreness that occurs after vigorous or unaccustomed exercise or muscular overexertion. It often presents as a temporary stiffness and tenderness occurring approximately 12 to 24 hours after completion of the exercise and is clearly linked to eccentric activity.[2] Although the time course varies, the signs and symptoms can last up to 10 to 14 days and gradually dissipate.

Acute or delayed exercise–induced muscle soreness can be avoided by gradually and systematically progressing the rehabilitation program. The American College of Sports Medicine recommends that changes in total training volume should be made in small increments of 2.5% to 5% per session.

Strengthening exercises should also be modified for patients with osteoporosis. High resistance, explosive, or twisting type movements should be avoided, and endurance exercises or low intensity strength training should be emphasized. (See Chapter 3 for further information on exercise in patients with osteoporosis.)

MUSCLE STRENGTH TRAINING INTERVENTION

Rehabilitating muscle performance deficits is a multidimensional process. The most effective type or mode of training intervention depends on the stage of rehabilitation, the degree of muscle weakness, which muscles and types of muscle fibers are primarily involved, and the primary functional task requirements of each individual client. The primary types of muscle strength training interventions and their respective advantages and disadvantages are outlined in the next section.

Isometric Muscle Strength Training. Isometric exercises (also known as *static exercises*) are performed by increasing tension in a muscle while keeping its length constant. To perform an isometric exercise, joint motion must be prevented. This can be achieved by pushing against an immovable object such as a wall (Fig. 5-4), immobilizing the patient with an isokinetic device or with a restraint, or when the therapist can exert sufficient force, by the patient pushing against unmoving resistance provided by the therapist. Isometric exercises against resistance provided by the therapist are often preferred early in rehabilitation because they do not involve joint movement and the intensity of muscle contraction can be more closely monitored by the clinician. However, when isometric exercises are performed against other types of resistance, high forces may be exerted, making this type of exercise unsuitable early after any injury to the musculotendinous unit.

Isometric exercises can increase muscle strength, but these increases are somewhat joint angle–specific. Isometric exercises increase strength the most approximately 10

BOX 5-1	Advantages and Disadvantages of Isometric Strengthening

Advantages	Disadvantages
• Can be used early in rehabilitation because there is no joint movement. • Retards atrophy and increases "static" muscular strength. • Helps to decrease swelling. • Prevents neural dissociation. • Joint angle–specific strengthening. • Can be performed anywhere. • No special equipment needed. • Short periods of training time. • 20° strengthening overflow throughout ROM.	• Strengthening is limited to specific joint angles. • Limited to no improvement in dynamic muscular performance. • No eccentric work. • Blood pressure concerns with Valsalva maneuver. • Patient motivation is likely to be less. • Less proprioceptive and kinesthetic training. • No contribution to muscular endurance. • Can create an ischemic response in muscles.

Modified from Davies GJ: *A compendium of isokinetics in clinical usage,* Onalaska, WI, 1992, S & S Publishing.
ROM, Range of motion.

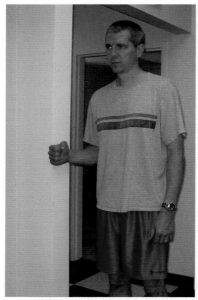

FIG. 5-4 Isometric shoulder external rotation at 0 degrees abduction.

degrees on either side of the joint angle at which the exercise is performed.[33,51-55] Therefore, with isometric strengthening, exercise should be performed at multiple angles every 20 degrees to achieve strength throughout the ROM. The advantages and disadvantages of isometric strengthening are listed in Box 5-1.

Clinical Pearl

Isometric exercise most increases strength within 10 degrees of either side of the joint angle at which the exercise is performed.

Isotonic or Dynamic Muscle Strength Training. Isotonic contractions are performed by lifting a constant weight. This contraction involves movement and is therefore also known as *dynamic muscle strengthening.* Isotonic contractions can be performed using free weights or weight machines and can be approximated with manual resistance by the therapist

Dynamic contractions can be concentric or eccentric. **Concentric contraction**s are shortening muscle contractions, and **eccentric contractions** are lengthening muscle contractions. Eccentric contractions can produce more tension per contractile unit at a lower metabolic cost than concentric contractions.[56,57] This is because eccentric contractions use elastic elements in the muscle and metabolic processes more efficiently and require fewer motor units to be active to produce the same force as a concentric contraction. Therefore eccentric contractions can be used early in the rehabilitation process, even if a patient cannot contract concentrically throughout the available AROM. In these situations, eccentric contractions can be introduced to allow some form of strengthening in this ROM. An example is the use of eccentric straight leg raises (SLR) in a knee rehabilitation program. Immediately after surgery, the first exercise would be quadriceps sets (an isometric contraction of the quadriceps against gravity) followed by eccentric SLRs. This exercise can be accomplished by having the rehabilitation specialist passively lift the leg and then guide the eccentric contraction as the patient lowers the leg to the starting position. In this situation the quadriceps are performing an isometric contraction and the iliopsoas is performing an eccentric contraction. Advantages and disadvantages of isotonic strengthening exercises are listed in Box 5-2.

Isokinetic Muscle Strength Training. Isokinetic training refers to muscle contractions performed at a constant angular velocity with varying resistance. The isokinetic dynamometer provides maximum resistance throughout the entire ROM. This type of resistance is referred to as accommodating resistance.

Consistent with the specificity principle, several studies have demonstrated that isokinetic strengthening produces the greatest gains in peak torque at the velocity used during training but that significant gains also occur above and below this training velocity, except when the velocity is very slow (30 degrees per second or less).

BOX 5-2	Advantages and Disadvantages of Isotonic Strengthening

Advantages	Disadvantages
• Dynamic constant external resistance that may be an advantage or disadvantage, depending on the situation. • Can improve muscular endurance. • Concentric and eccentric muscle action. • Use of free weights allows for multiplanar training. • Can use a variety of resistive devices (e. g., exercise machines, free weights, elastic tubing/bands). • Can use body weight for resistance. • Can exercise through full ROM. • Use of functional movement patterns. • Provides motivation from achievement. • Inexpensive and readily available with most types of resistive devices. • Can use manual resistance from rehabilitation specialist—allowing for specific tactile input and improved proprioceptive and kinesthetic awareness. • More objective documentation capabilities than with isometrics. • Various components of the program can be manipulated to maintain workload (repetitions, sets, weight). • Can increase muscle strength with few repetitions.	• Can maximally load the muscle at its weakest point in the ROM, especially with elastic tubing or bands. • The contracting muscle is only maximally challenged at one point in the ROM with free weights and some machines. • Not safe if someone has pain during movement because patient must maintain resistance. • At fast speeds of movement, there may be an increased risk of injury. • Difficult to exercise at fast functional velocities. • Does not provide reciprocal concentric exercise. • Does not allow for rapid force development. • Exercise-induced muscle soreness and DOMS. • Unable to spread entire workload evenly over the entire ROM.

Modified from Davies GJ: *A compendium of isokinetics in clinical usage,* Onalaska, WI, 1992, S & S Publishing.
ROM, Range of motion; *DOMS,* delayed-onset muscle soreness.

Advantages and disadvantages of isokinetic training are shown in Box 5-3.

Plyometric Muscle Strength Training. Plyometrics are high intensity, high velocity exercises such as jumping and bounding with the lower extremities and ballistic push-ups off a wall with the upper extremities (Fig. 5-5). Plyometrics are intended to develop muscular power and coordination. **Plyometric exercise** employs high velocity eccentric and concentric muscle loading, reflexive reactions, and functional movement patterns. Because this type of training places high mechanical demands on the body, it should only be introduced when the patient has good strength and endurance and should therefore be reserved for later, higher levels of rehabilitation.

Although plyometric type movements are used in basic activities, such as walking and running, plyometric exercise may be helpful for all patients. High velocity, low resistance (approximately 30% of maximum) dynamic weight training has been found to increase vertical jumping and isokinetic-tested leg extension strength at high speeds more than plyometric training, suggesting that, as long as the movement is fast, plyometrics may not be necessary to optimize functional outcome.

Plyometric drills should be preceded by a warm-up period to prepare the patient's cardiovascular and musculoskeletal system for the demands of this type of exercise. With lower extremity plyometrics, bilateral activities should precede unilateral activities, and low intensity jumps should precede higher level jumps.

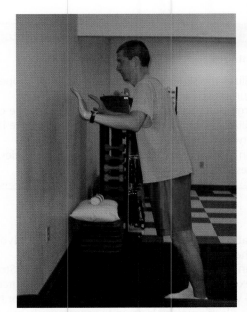

FIG. 5-5 Upper body push-up off the wall.

Plyometric training is proposed to reduce the risk of future injury by training muscle coactivation through neuromuscular adaptation. This is particularly relevant for reducing the risk of anterior cruciate ligament (ACL) tears by training quadriceps and hamstring muscle

---

BOX 5-3   **Advantages and Disadvantages of Isokinetic Strengthening**

Advantages

- Reported to cause little muscle soreness.[58]
- Concentric and eccentric strengthening of same muscle group can be performed repeatedly, or reciprocal exercise of opposing muscle groups can be performed—one muscle group always rests.
- Reliable measures with the equipment.
- Helps force development (time rate of torque development).
- Efficiency of muscular contractions.
- Can exercise at a wide range of velocities.
- Computer-based visual and/or auditory cues for feedback.
- Can provide maximum resistance at all points in ROM.
- Can safely perform high- and low-velocity training.
- Accommodates for painful arc of motion.
- Can continue exercise as patient fatigues.
- Decreased joint compressive forces at high speed.
- Short duration of joint compression.
- Physiological overflow.
- Neurophysiological "pattern" for functional speeds and movements.
- Isolated muscle strengthening.
- External stabilization.

Disadvantages

- Many physical activities far exceed the angular velocities that can be produced by isokinetic testing devices.
- Large and expensive equipment.
- Requires assistance and time for set-up.
- Cannot be incorporated into a home program.
- Most units only provide open chain movement patterns.
- Most exercise performed in a single plane and at constant velocity.
- Cannot duplicate reciprocal speeds of movement used during most daily and functional activities.
- Eccentric loading can cause DOMS.
- Lack of personnel trained in use or interpretation of isokinetic testing and rehabilitation.
- Availability of equipment.
- Time consuming, if more than one joint is exercised/assessed.
- Some artificial parameters until the tested limb reaches the velocity of the dynamometer or decelerates.

Modified from Davies GJ: *A compendium of isokinetics in clinical usage,* Onalaska, WI, 1992, S & S Publishing.
ROM, Range of motion; *DOMS,* delayed-onset muscle soreness.

BOX 5-4   **Advantages and Disadvantages of Plyometric Strengthening**

Advantages

- Utilizes the series elastic and stretch reflex properties of the neuromuscular unit.
- Large potential influence on velocity of muscle contraction.
- Utilizes dynamic muscle co-activation for more balance between antagonistic muscle groups.
- Can involve lower extremities, upper extremities, and trunk.
- Uses functional movements.

Disadvantages

- More advanced techniques requiring a high level of muscle performance capabilities prior to initiation.
- Higher risk of injury if not properly supervised.
- Usually reserved for more advanced stages of rehabilitation and for more advanced patients.

---

coactivation. Advantages and disadvantages of plyometric strengthening are listed in Box 5-4.

Strengthening Against a Variable Load. Strengthening exercises can also be performed against forces that provide varying resistance, such as elastic bands or tubing, or water. Elastic materials provide progressively more resistance as they are stretched and can provide differing amounts of resistance, depending on their composition and thickness. Because resistance is a function of how much the elastic material is elongated, to provide consistent resistance between sessions the patient must always grasp the band or tubing in the same place.[59] Water provides resistance proportional to the relative speed of movement of the patient and the water and the

cross-sectional area of the patient in contact with the water (Fig. 5-6).

INTERVENTION PROGRESSION

Several approaches have been proposed for progression of exercises to optimize muscle performance. Two of the more popular and earliest approaches are the DeLorme technique and the daily adjustable progressive resistive exercise (DAPRE) technique. The DeLorme technique was the first well-documented approach to exercise progression for muscle strengthening (Box 5-5).[60] Using this technique, exercises are performed as three sets of ten repetitions, starting with a load equal to ½ of the 10 RM and increasing to a load equal to ¾ of the 10 RM for the

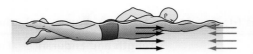

Fast-moving body results
in high resistance

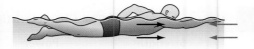

Slow-moving body results
in moderate resistance

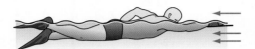

Paddles and fins increase frontal
area and increase resistance

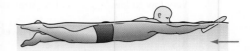

Limbs straight in front decrease
frontal area and decrease resistance

FIG. 5-6 Water resistance properties.

BOX 5-5	DeLorme Technique

Progressive Resistive Exercise
- Determine 10 RM.
- Patient then performs:
  - 10 reps at ½ of 10 RM
  - 10 reps at ¾ of 10 RM
  - 10 reps at the full 10 RM
  - Built-in warm-up
- Strength progressed weekly.

RM, Repetition maximum; *reps,* repetitions.

TABLE 5-3	Daily Adjustable Progressive Resistive Exercise (DAPRE) Technique

1. Determine initial working weight (6 RM)
2. The patient then performs the following:
   - Set 1: 10 reps of ½ working weight.
   - Set 2: 6 reps of ¾ working weight.
   - Set 3: As many as possible with working weight.
   - Set 4: As many as possible with adjusted working weight according to the number of reps performed in Set 3.*
   - The number of reps done in Set 4 is used to determine the weight for the next day.

Reps in Set	*Adjusted Working Weight for Fourth Set	Next Exercise Session
0-2	Decrease by 5 to 10 lb	Decrease 5 to 10 lb
3-4	Same weight or decrease by 5 lb	Same weight
5-6	Same weight	Add 5 to 10 lb
7-10	Add 5 to 10 lb	Add 5 to 15 lb
>10	Add 10 to 15 lb	Add 10 to 20 lb

---

second set and equal to the full 10 RM for the final set of 10 repetitions.

The DAPRE technique was proposed as a more adaptable progressive resistive exercise program than the DeLorme technique.[61] With the DAPRE technique, a 6 RM is used to establish the initial working weight and the weight or load is increased in future sessions based on the performance during the previous training session (Table 5-3). The frequency and amount of weight increase are less arbitrary with this technique than with the DeLorme technique.

Because muscle performance encompasses three often very different components (strength, power, and endurance), training for each of these components should be progressed individually. Training that focuses on strength should involve progression of the resistance, and training that focuses on power should involve progressive changes in both resistance and speed of movement. In general, strength should be focused on before power because power requires good strength. Endurance training should use lower loads with more repetitions than strength or power training. The speed of motion is also not a focus of endurance training. Table 5-4 highlights the recommended general training parameters for each respective component of muscle performance.

More recently, the Norwegian physiotherapist, Oddvar Holten, introduced the **medical exercise training/ therapy (MET)** approach to muscle training.[62] This approach involves use of the Holten diagram to guide exercise progression. This diagram depicts the relationship between the maximum number of repetitions that can be performed and the percentage of maximal resistance in regard to muscle strength, strength/endurance, and endurance (Box 5-6). The diagram helps determine the muscular effort (alterations in muscular strength, endurance, or both).

According to the diagram, exercise is most effective for improving endurance when 25 to 30 or more repetitions are performed at 60% to 65% of 1 RM or less and is most effective for strengthening when contractions at 90% of 1 RM are used.

In summary, when selecting exercises to improve muscle performance, the physical therapist will consider the following:
- The requirements of the activity to which the patient is returning.
- The patient's goals for return to functional abilities.
- Advantages and disadvantages of various types of exercise.

TABLE 5-4	Comparison of Training Characteristics for Developing Strength, Power, or Endurance			
	Strength	Power	Strength and Endurance	Endurance
Load/intensity (% of 1 RM)	80%-100%	Strength/force (70%-100%) Velocity (30%-45%) or up to 10% body weight	50%-70%	Circuit training (40%-60%)
Repetitions	Very low to low	1-5 (Strength)	12-25	Moderate to high (15-30[+])
	1-6	5-10 (Power)		
Sets	3-5	4-6	2-3	2-5
Rest period (minutes)	3-6	2 to 4-6	30-60 seconds	45-90 seconds (1:1 work-rest ratio)
Speed of performance	Slow to medium (speed of effort is as fast as possible)	Fast/explosive	Slow to medium (emphasize stabilization)	Medium
Primary energy source	Phosphagen Anaerobic glycolysis	Phosphagen	Anaerobic glycolysis/aerobic	Aerobic

From Reiman MP: Training for strength, power, and endurance. In Manske RC (ed): *Postoperative orthopedic sports medicine: The knee and shoulder*, St Louis, 2006, Mosby.

BOX 5-6   Holten Diagram

Dosage based off 1 RM = Repetition Maximum
Dosage: 100% = 1 RM
95% = 2 RM
90% = 4 RM strength
85% = 7 RM
80% = 11 RM
75% = 16 RM strength/endurance
70% = 22 RM
65% = 25 RM
60% = 30 RM endurance
Speed: >80% explosive
65%-80% breathing rhythm
<60% tissue related
Atrophy 30% 1 RM repetitions as tolerated
Mobility 10%-20% 1 RM high repetitions = 50
Endurance 70% 22 repetitions 3 sets
Stabilization 80% 11 repetitions 3 sets

Adapted from Faugli HP: *Medical exercise therapy*, Norway, 1996, Laerergruppen for Medisinsk Treningsterapi; Torstensen TA: *Medical exercise therapy for thoracic and low back pain-sciatica*, Course material, Oslo, Norway, Holten Institute.

- General and patient-specific precautions and contra-indications for the type of exercise considered.
- ROM requirements for the activity and any patient restrictions in ROM.
- The ideal approach to progression for optimal functional benefit.
- The patient's motivation and social support system.
- Working weak muscles before strong muscles in situations in which fatigue of the target muscle(s) could lead to synergistic muscle compensation, especially when the focus is rehabilitation of muscle weakness.

- Developing strength and flexibility before developing power.
- Using simple exercises before initiating more complex exercises.
- Developing proximal joint and trunk stability and control before working on extremity mobility.
- Starting exercises in a more controlled environment and then progressing to a less controlled environment in regards to stationary versus dynamic surface contact and external stabilization. Initially using a stationary, externally stabilized surface to perform strengthening, and as the patient progresses, using a less stable and more dynamic surface area.
- Initiating horizontal or gravity eliminated movements before vertical or antigravity movements.
- Initiating exercises in stress-free positions before stressful positions.
- Initiating unidirectional movements before multidirectional movements.[63]
- Progressing from isometric to eccentric to concentric to plyometric types of exercises.
- Incorporating activity-specific speeds of movement in relation to the patient's functional goals.
- Ongoing reevaluation of the patient and their needs and goals, as well as the treatment plan, which is essential for rehabilitation interventions to successfully return patients with muscle weakness to optimal function.

CASE STUDY 5-1

SHOULDER PAIN AND SCAPULAR MUSCLE WEAKNESS

Patient History
HA is a 21-year-old right-handed female college volleyball player with a 2-month history of right shoulder pain with overhead movements, including serving and spiking. This

pain started 2 months ago as a dull ache and has progressively worsened. She has used physical agents including ice, heat, electrical stimulation, and ultrasound in the training room, but none have helped. Radiographs and HA's past medical history are unremarkable, except for a family history of high blood pressure.

Tests and Measures—Significant Findings

- HA is a healthy, well-nourished muscular woman. She has no visible muscle atrophy around the shoulder on either side but has slightly larger muscles on the right.
- There is a positive sulcus sign indicating multidirectional laxity in both shoulders.
- The AROM and PROM of her cervical spine and bilateral upper extremities is slightly excessive. She also has several signs indicating generalized ligamentous laxity.
- Scapular dyskinesis (medial scapular border winging) is easily seen with AROM of the involved right shoulder.
- Strength testing reveals several areas of muscle weakness on the right, including the shoulder external rotators, scapular upward rotators, scapular protractor muscles, and scapular retractor muscles. MMT of the shoulder external rotators produces some discomfort.
- HA has positive impingement signs.

Diagnosis

- Preferred practice pattern 4D: Impaired joint mobility, motor function, muscle performance, and range of motion associated with connective tissue dysfunction

Interventions

- Moist heat followed by soft tissue mobilization to relax sore muscles and decrease muscle spasm produced by pain from overuse.
- Rest.
- Avoid overhead lifting, serving, setting, and spiking for several weeks while continuing with other upper extremity exercises below shoulder level, as well as trunk and lower extremity training.
- Once pain subsides, begin strengthening and endurance-training exercises.

Role of the Physical Therapist Assistant

- What strengthening and/or endurance training exercises would be helpful for this patient?
- How would you determine if the patient should increase or decrease her exercise intensity?
- What type of exercise is this patient likely to tolerate best during her first few treatments? Isometric, AROM, or resistive? Why?
- The plan of care for this patient includes strengthening shoulder external rotators. Document a treatment for this patient, including instruction in an external rotation exercise with resistance.

Additional Information

For the full version of this case study, including detailed examination results, interventions, and outcomes, see the Evolve site that accompanies this book. An additional case study describing the examination, evaluation, and intervention for a patient with low back pain caused by muscle weakness can also be found on the Evolve site.

CHAPTER SUMMARY

Muscle is the only type of soft tissue that can generate tension enabling the skeletal system to perform functions such as maintaining posture, respiration, moving limbs, and absorbing ground reaction forces during the gait cycle. A comprehensive examination can determine the type and degree of muscle performance impairment. This chapter describes the characteristics and ideal interventions for impairment of each aspect of muscle performance, including strength, power, and endurance.

ADDITIONAL RESOURCES

For links to these and additional web-based resources, see the Evolve site.

American College of Sports Medicine: *ACSM's resource manual for guidelines for exercise testing and prescription*, ed 6. Philadelphia, 2010, Lippincott Williams & Wilkins.

Baechle TR, Earle RW: *Essentials of strength training and conditioning*, ed 3, Champaign, IL, 2009, Human Kinetics.

Fleck SJ, Kraemer WJ: *Designing resistance training programs*, ed 3, Champaign, IL, 2004, Human Kinetics.

Komi PV: *Strength and power in sport*, ed 2, Oxford, 2003, Blackwell Science Ltd.

Manske R: *Postsurgical orthopedic sports rehabilitation: Knee and shoulder*, St. Louis, 2007, Mosby.

Neumann DA: *Kinesiology of the musculoskeletal system: Foundations for rehabilitation*, ed 2, St Louis, 2010, Mosby.

Shankman G, Manske R: *Fundamental orthopedic management for the physical therapist assistant*, ed 3, St. Louis, 2011, Mosby.

American College of Sports Medicine

National Strength and Conditioning Association

GLOSSARY

Actin: The thin protein of a myofibril that acts with myosin to produce muscle contraction and relaxation.

Action potential: A momentary change in electrical potential on the surface of a cell, especially of a nerve or muscle cell, that occurs when it is stimulated, resulting in the transmission of an electrical impulse.

Concentric contraction: A muscle action involving shortening of the muscle length.

Delayed-onset muscle soreness (DOMS): Pain or discomfort in muscles that comes on 12 to 24 hours after unaccustomed exercise, particularly exercise involving eccentric muscle contractions.

Eccentric contraction: A muscle action in which tension is developed as the muscle lengthens.

Endomysium: The sheath that surrounds each muscle fiber.

Endurance: The ability to perform low intensity, repetitive, or sustained activities over a prolonged period of time without fatigue.

Epimysium: The dense outer fibrous sheath that covers an entire muscle.

Fast-twitch (type II) fibers: Muscle fibers suited to quick, explosive actions. These muscle fibers are typically larger in diameter than type I fibers.

FITT formula: A systematic method of prescribing exercise according to its frequency, intensity, time, and type to improve muscle performance.

Hypertrophy: Increase in volume of a muscle produced by enlargement of existing cells usually as a direct result of resistance training.

Isokinetic: A concentric or eccentric muscle action at a fixed speed with accommodating resistance.

Isometric exercise: Exercise in which muscle contraction occurs with no appreciable joint movement.

Isotonic: A concentric or eccentric muscle action moving a constant weight through a range of motion.

Length-tension relationship: A muscle's capacity to produce force depends on the length of the muscle relative to its resting length. Muscles can produce the most force near their normal resting length.

Manual muscle testing (MMT): A quick and efficient way to assess and grade muscle strength by the clinician applying resistance to the subject being tested.

Medical exercise training/therapy (MET): A system of progressively graded exercise.

Motor unit: A motor neuron and all the muscle fibers that it innervates.

Muscle performance: The capacity of a muscle to do work (force × distance). The key contributing elements to muscle performance include strength, power, and endurance.

Myofibrils: Rodlike structures that are contained within and run the length of the muscle fiber. Myofibrils contain the contractile elements of the muscle fiber.

Myopathy: Any disease of a muscle.

Myosin: The thick protein in the myofibril that acts with actin to produce muscle contraction and relaxation.

Perimysium: A dense connective tissue sheath covering the muscle fascicles.

Plyometric exercise: Exercises involving rapid stretching of muscles by an eccentric contraction followed by a shortening of the same muscles in a concentric manner to increase muscular power and function.

Power: The work produced by a muscle per unit time (force × distance/time).

Repetition maximum (RM): The maximum amount of weight that an individual can lift a specified number of times, for example, the 10 RM is the most weight an individual can lift 10 times.

Sarcomere: A segment of a myofibril that represents the functional unit of striated muscle.

Slow-twitch (type I) fibers: Muscle fibers that are typically smaller in diameter than type II fibers and that are more suitable for long duration low force contractions.

Strength: The ability of a muscle or group of muscles to exert a maximal force or torque at a specified or determined velocity.

Tropomyosin: A muscle protein that inhibits contraction unless its position is modified by troponin so that the myosin molecules can make contact with the actin molecules.

Troponin: A complex of muscle proteins that binds to calcium to allow muscle contraction.

Velocity: Distance divided by time.

Chapter 6

Connective Tissue Dysfunction

Victoria Merrell, Donna K. Everix

CHAPTER OUTLINE

OBJECTIVES

After reading this chapter, the reader will be able to:
1. Describe the pathology and typical clinical manifestations and prognosis of nine common types of connective tissue dysfunctions.
2. Accurately and efficiently take a history of a patient with connective tissue dysfunction.
3. Apply rheumatology-specific outcome tools, tests, and measurement techniques.
4. Determine a diagnosis and prognosis for a patient with connective tissue dysfunction.
5. Apply effective rehabilitation interventions for patients with connective tissue dysfunction, including patient education, exercise, modalities, and aquatic therapy.

Connective tissue dysfunctions result from a group of diseases that generally share clinical and pathological features of widespread inflammation. These diseases are commonly known as *rheumatic diseases*. With the exception of osteoarthritis, the majority of the rheumatic diseases are chronic systemic inflammatory conditions with an autoimmune etiology. All of these diseases can cause joint inflammation, known as **arthritis,** as well as a range of other adverse effects.

Rheumatic diseases encompass over 100 different conditions with different clinical manifestations. All are characterized by chronic pain and progressive damage to joints and soft tissues resulting in functional impairment. Arthritis, or joint inflammation, is the most prevalent chronic condition in the United States and is the leading cause of disability.[1,2] Arthritis and the rheumatic diseases significantly limit the ability of more than 7 million Americans to participate in activities of daily living (ADLs) and vocational and leisure activities.[3] The prevalence of rheumatic disease is expected to rise so that by the year 2020, these diseases will limit an estimated 11.6 million individuals in their ability to perform daily activities.[3] This chapter focuses on a subset of rheumatic diseases that commonly cause connective tissue dysfunction, including rheumatoid arthritis and other inflammatory types of arthritis, disorders of soft tissue, and diffuse diseases of the connective tissues.

The care of individuals with rheumatic disease must be individualized and is founded on an early and accurate diagnosis. One of the challenges of working with patients with rheumatic disease is patients can have very different presentations, manifesting diverse signs and symptoms. Effective management requires an understanding of the disease process, a comprehensive examination and evaluation, and implementation of appropriate interventions to achieve realistic goals consistent with the patient's preferences. Since the rheumatic diseases involve multiple systems and have significant psychosocial ramifications, patients are best treated with a multidisciplinary approach.[4,5]

Rehabilitation plays a critical role in the management of patients with rheumatic disease and physical therapy has been identified as an integral component of care.[6,7]

Rehabilitation clinicians may provide a wide range of interventions that may be beneficial adjuncts to medication and surgery. These interventions may include patient education about the disease and components of management, instruction in joint protection and energy conservation, therapeutic exercise, physical agents, and aquatic therapy. This chapter includes information on pathology; examination; evaluation, including functional outcome assessment tools; and interventions for the rheumatic diseases most commonly encountered by rehabilitation professionals. These include systemic lupus erythematosus, rheumatoid arthritis, spondyloarthropathies, polymyalgia rheumatica, polymyositis and dermatomyositis, scleroderma, Sjögren's syndrome, crystal-induced arthropathies, and juvenile rheumatoid arthritis.

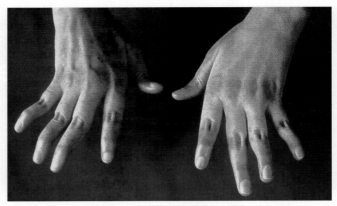

FIG. 6-1 Jaccoud's arthritis. A nonerosive deforming arthropathy of the hands that occurs in patients with systemic lupus erythematosus. *Reprinted from the Clinical Slide Collection on the Rheumatic Diseases, copyright 1997. Used by permission of the American College of Rheumatology.*

◎ **Clinical Pearl**

Rheumatic diseases are chronic systemic inflammatory conditions with an autoimmune etiology.

PATHOLOGY

SYSTEMIC LUPUS ERYTHEMATOSUS

Etiology. Systemic lupus erythematosus (SLE) is an autoimmune disease that results from the body producing antibodies directed against its own tissue (autoantibodies). In SLE, autoantibodies react with antigens to produce circulating immune complexes that deposit in tissues producing a range of effects. The clinical spectrum of SLE is broad, ranging from fatigue and mild **arthralgias** to severe and unremitting kidney inflammation **(nephritis)** that may ultimately cause renal failure. SLE may impact any or all organ systems, including the skin, oral mucosa, joints, lungs, heart, kidneys, blood, and brain, and is most damaging if there is kidney, heart, or neurological involvement. Although no single cause of SLE has been identified, numerous influential factors, including viral, genetic, environmental, and hormonal, are proposed.

Genetics. There is evidence that genetic factors predispose individuals to SLE. SLE occurs more often in relatives than in the general population. The prevalence of SLE is also three times higher in African Americans than would be expected given their representation in the general population, and SLE is more common in certain Native American tribes, particularly in females within that population.[8]

Environmental Factors. Environmental factors, including chemical exposure, ultraviolet radiation, diet, and viral infections, may trigger the expression of SLE in some individuals.[9] Drug-induced **lupus** comes on in response to a drug and resolves when the drug is no longer present. The effects of diet on SLE are poorly substantiated and are based only on expert opinion or observational studies.

Hormonal Influences. Ninety percent of patients with lupus are women, and 90% of these patients develop lupus in their childbearing years.[10] It is thought that this is because of the profound differences between the impact of female sex hormones (estrogens) and male sex hormones (androgens) on the immune system. Estrogens promote immune responses and increase the production of autoantibodies, whereas androgens are more immunosuppressive. Thus female sex hormones appear to promote both disease activity and etiology.[11]

Clinical Features. Although SLE can involve all organ systems, its most common symptoms are fatigue and arthralgia (joint pain). Arthralgias occur in 80% to 90% of patients with SLE; however, arthritis (joint inflammation) occurs in fewer than half of these cases. The joint pain and inflammation, when present, tends to be symmetrical with a predilection for the knees, wrists, and interphalangeal joints. The shoulders, hips, ankles, and elbows are less commonly involved.[10] When arthritis is present in patients with SLE, it is generally not deforming; however, 10% of patients with SLE develop a nonerosive deforming arthropathy of the hands, referred to as *Jaccoud's arthritis* (Fig. 6-1), which mostly affects the joint capsule and surrounding ligaments, causing joint instability and subluxation rather than the joint contractures and bony ankylosis associated with erosive arthritides.

Avascular necrosis occurs in 3% to 52% of patients with SLE, and involvement is frequently bilateral and asymptomatic. Avascular necrosis is thought to be caused by the corticosteroids used to treat SLE rather than by the disease itself. Prolonged corticosteroid use may also cause or accelerate osteoporosis in this population.[10]

Fatigue occurs in 80% to 100% of patients and is often the most debilitating symptom, affecting quality of life and interfering with family and social relationships.[10] Myalgias, muscle tenderness, and muscle weakness may be present in up to 69% of patients with SLE.[12]

SLE commonly causes skin rashes. The term *lupus* was derived from the Latin word for "wolf" and is used to describe the butterfly-shaped rash (Fig. 6-2) reported by 35% of patients with lupus.[13] Acute inflammatory rashes may occur on the malar regions of the face, on the trunk

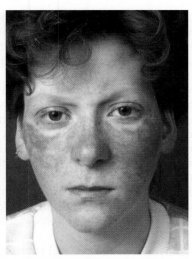

FIG. 6-2 Lupus rash. Erythematous rash (butterfly rash) extending across the malar regions of the face and across the bridge of the nose. *From Hochberg MC, Silman AJ, Smolen SJ, et al, editors:* Rheumatoid arthritis, *Philadelphia, 2008, Mosby.*

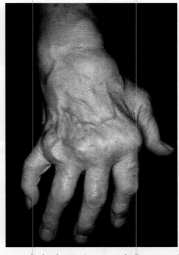

FIG. 6-3 Wrist radial deviation and finger ulnar deviation (zigzag deformity) in a patient with RA. *From Hochberg MC, Silman AJ, Smolen SJ, et al, editors:* Rheumatoid arthritis, *Philadelphia, 2008, Mosby.*

and upper extremities, or between the interphalangeal joints.

Neuropsychiatric symptoms occur in 25% to 80% of patients with SLE at some time during the course of the illness. SLE can also cause seizures, stroke, headaches, psychosis, and organic brain syndromes, but depression is the most common psychiatric disorder in patients with lupus and may be caused by the disease itself or be a reaction to the stresses associated with chronic illness.

> **⊙ *Clinical Pearl***
>
> Systemic lupus erythematosus (SLE) has a wide range of presentation from mild joint pain or fatigue to severe and unremitting kidney inflammation (nephritis) that may ultimately cause renal failure.

RHEUMATOID ARTHRITIS

Rheumatoid arthritis (RA) is a chronic, systemic inflammatory disease of unknown etiology. It is characterized by symmetrical polyarthritis of the peripheral joints, morning stiffness, malaise, and fatigue. The disease course is variable, although there are often exacerbations and remissions, and the disease may completely remit or progress aggressively to result in profound disability.

The inflammation and tissue destruction in RA are caused by complex interactions between antigen-presenting cells and T cells. RA also causes synovial proliferation, with the synovium changing from a single cell layer to a multicellular composition containing growth factors, lymphocytes, and inflammatory **cytokines.** The overgrown synovium, referred to as **pannus,** invades and destroys articular cartilage and bone.[14]

Clinical Features

Articular Manifestations. Articular manifestations of RA include morning stiffness, synovial inflammation, and structural damage. Morning stiffness correlates with the degree of inflammation and usually lasts more than 2 hours as opposed to the brief morning stiffness that occurs with osteoarthritis. Pain and swelling are key features of joints affected by RA. Acute **synovitis** may cause redness, warmth, and swelling in superficial joints; however, synovitis that affects deeper joints, such as the hips and shoulders, may be difficult to appreciate on physical examination. Persistent synovitis may lead to loss of cartilage, bony erosion, and ultimately, irreversible structural damage.[15]

Joint Specific Manifestations

Hands. The wrists and the metacarpophalangeal (MCP) and proximal interphalangeal (PIP) joints of the hands are commonly involved in RA.[15] Radial deviation at the wrist is often associated with ulnar deviation at the fingers (zigzag deformity)[16] (Fig. 6-3). This deformity is caused by chronic synovitis at the wrists and MCP joints, weakening of the extensor carpi ulnaris muscle, the ulnar bias of the power grasp,[17] and inappropriate action of the intrinsic muscles.[18]

Swan-neck deformities, which involve flexion of the MCP and distal IP (DIP) joints and hyperextension of the PIP joint, may develop as the result of persistent MCP synovitis with concomitant intrinsic muscle tightness (Fig. 6-4, *A*). Chronic inflammation at the PIP joint with avulsion of the extensor hood may lead to a **boutonnière deformity** (flexion at the PIP joint and hyperextension at the DIP joint) (Fig. 6-4, *B*).

Dorsal swelling within the synovial sheaths of extensor tendons at the wrist is also a common early manifestation of RA. Synovial proliferation may also compromise the integrity of the radioulnar joint, leading to stretching or rupture of the ulnar collateral ligament and subluxation of the ulnar head.

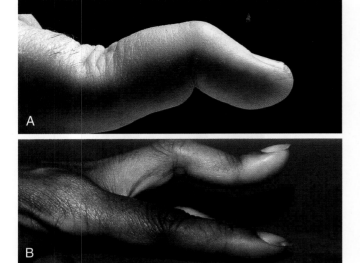

FIG. 6-4 **A,** Swan-neck deformity in patient with rheumatoid arthritis. **B,** Boutonnière deformity in patient with rheumatoid arthritis. **A** *from Ruby LK, Cassidy C: Hand clinics: Rheumatoarthritis of the hand and wrist, vol 12, no 3, Philadelphia, 1996, Saunders.* **B** *reprinted from the Clinical Slide Collection on the Rheumatic Diseases, copyright 1997. Used by permission of the American College of Rheumatology.*

Flexor **tenosynovitis** and nodule formation may compromise finger flexion, and tendons may rupture because of persistent inflammation and resulting attenuation. Tendons may also become inflamed or rupture if they rub on the jagged edges of eroded carpal bones or the ulnar styloid.

Foot and Ankle. RA can cause synovitis at the metatarsophalangeal (MTP), talonavicular, and ankle joints. Synovitis at the MTP joint weakens the joint capsules and ligaments, leading to plantar subluxation of the metatarsal heads and cock-up deformities at the toes.[15] Inflammation at the talonavicular joint results in pronation and eversion of the foot and flattening of the longitudinal arch. The tarsal tunnel may be subjected to increased stress that results from structural changes, and synovitis within the tarsal tunnel may cause compression of the posterior tibial nerve, which is manifested by paresthesias at the plantar aspect of the foot.

Hips. The hips are rarely involved in RA, and early manifestations of synovitis at the hips are difficult to detect on physical examination because of their deep location. Hip synovitis may produce pain at the groin, anteromedial knee, low back, or thigh that is reduced by positioning the hip in flexion and external rotation.[15]

Knees. Synovitis at the knee is not uncommon in RA and is easily detected on physical examination. Synovitis produces **effusions** that distend and stretch the joint capsule and contribute to ligamentous attenuation. A palpable synovial or **Baker's cyst** may also occur posteriorly in the popliteal fossa if some synovium becomes trapped and separated from the rest of the joint.

Elbows. The elbows are affected in 20% to 65% of individuals with RA. Patients may attempt to minimize pain from elbow synovitis by holding the joint in flexion

and pronation. This commonly causes flexion contractures that impair function because a loss of as little as 30 degrees of extension may interfere with performance of ADLs such as dressing, feeding, grooming, hygiene, and sit-to-stand transfers.

Shoulders. RA of the shoulder may involve synovitis at the glenohumeral joint and inflammation within the surrounding bursae and rotator cuff tendons. Standard radiographic tests of the shoulders in RA commonly reveal erosions (69%) and superior subluxation (31%).[19] Patients may not be aware of the resulting loss of motion until significant restrictions occur, since most daily activities do not require extremes of shoulder range. A person may lose as much as 50% of shoulder range of motion (ROM) before this interferes with functional activities.

Cervical Spine. RA of the cervical spine generally first presents with neck pain and stiffness. Neck pain may be caused by joint inflammation or by chronic tension in the posterior cervical muscles that results from postural strain, emotional stress, deconditioning, and altered biomechanics. Synovitis of the transverse ligament at C1, which stabilizes the odontoid process, may cause the ligament to become lax. Such ligamentous laxity or ligament rupture can cause C1-C2 instability or subluxation, which can result in cervical myelopathy (spinal cord compression).[20] Atlantoaxial (C1-C2) subluxation may initially cause pain and tenderness in the suboccipital region, as well as headaches, and progress to upper extremity paresthesias, lower extremity weakness, and instability. If not stabilized, paralysis or death will eventually occur. Patients can sometimes feel the bones sublux and report that it feels as though their head may "slip off." Atlantoaxial subluxation may also compress the vertebral arteries (the vertebral arteries pass through the foramina in the processes of C1 and C2) and induce visual disturbances (blurred vision or diplopia), loss of equilibrium, lightheadedness, dizziness, or other signs of posterior circulation stroke.[21] Inflammation at the apophyseal joints may also lead to pain and instability at multiple levels throughout the cervical spine.[15] Since C1-C2 subluxation has the potential for such bad sequelae, any examination findings suggestive of this pathology should be discussed immediately with the physician for consideration of further evaluation and management.

Systemic and Other Nonarticular Manifestations of Rheumatoid Arthritis. Systemic manifestations of RA include fatigue, malaise, subjective weakness, depression, and low-grade fever. These symptoms may precede the typical joint findings and may correlate with the degree of inflammation.

Common cutaneous manifestations of RA are rheumatoid nodules and Sjögren's syndrome. Rheumatoid nodules are subcutaneous masses, which may be soft and amorphous or firm and rubberlike, that tend to develop on the extensor surfaces of the forearm and may form within tendons or ligaments. Sjögren's syndrome, which is characterized by dry eyes and dry mouth, occurs in 10% to 15% of patients with RA. RA can also cause photosensitivity, **Raynaud's phenomenon,** and **vasculitis.**

SPONDYLOARTHROPATHIES

Ankylosing Spondylitis. Ankylosing spondylitis (AS) is a chronic systemic inflammatory disorder, primarily causing **enthesitis** and synovitis of the axial skeleton that almost always involves the sacroiliac joints. The predominant symptoms are low back pain (LBP) and stiffness that worsen with inactivity. Fatigue, malaise, weight loss, low-grade fever, and anorexia are also common. AS usually first presents between late adolescence and early adulthood, with an average age of onset of 26 years.

In AS, chronic inflammation at the enthesis (the site of ligament insertion into bone) causes fibrosis and then ossification of the ligaments and joint capsule, ultimately causing ankylosis (fusion) of the affected joints.[22] Enthesitis occurs in many areas of the spine and "squaring" of vertebrae occurs because of bony erosion at the ligamentous insertions at the corners of the vertebral bodies.[22] The term *bamboo spine* describes the typical appearance of the spine on x-ray when AS has caused complete fusion of the vertebral column (Fig. 6-5).[23] The inflammation usually progresses upward from the sacroiliac joints toward the cervical spine. Without intervention, this can result in a fixed, extremely forward flexed spine.

Etiology. AS is much more common in men than in women, with a male:female ratio of 3 to 5:1.

Clinical Features

Axial Spine. LBP is the first complaint in 75% of people with AS.[22] It can be unilateral and intermittent, but over time it becomes more persistent and bilateral. Tenderness or pain on palpation of the sacroiliac joints or LBP with hyperextension of the hip is common.[24] The back becomes stiff, and the lumbar lordosis fails to reverse with forward bending. Posture typically includes a forward head, protracted and internally rotated shoulders, increased thoracic kyphosis, and flattened lumbar spine.

Back pain combined with inactivity and stiffness can cause difficulties with sleeping, getting in and out of bed, and with dressing and grooming. As the thoracic spine and ribcage become stiff, chest expansion may be limited, requiring the diaphragm to work harder during breathing.[23] Progression to cervical spine fusion may occur, limiting cervical rotation and extension and causing difficulties with driving.[22]

Initially, the pain and stiffness associated with AS improves with exercise or a hot shower or bath, but as the joints fuse, although pain may be less, the stiffness no longer resolves.[23] Spinal fractures and spinal cord compression may occur with increased disease severity.[25]

Peripheral Joints. AS can cause arthritis in the hips, knees, ankles, and MTP joints. Hip disease is typically bilateral, and pain combined with decreased ROM may lead to contractures in the hips and knees. The upper extremity joints are rarely involved, but with increased thoracic kyphosis, the shoulders may be affected.[25]

Other. Acute anterior **uveitis** (acute iritis) occurs in 25% to 30% of patients with AS and usually subsides in 2 to 3 months. Symptoms include eye pain, increased tearing, photophobia, and blurred vision and tend to be unilateral.[22]

Reactive Arthritis (Reiter's Syndrome). Reactive arthritis, also known as **Reiter's syndrome (RS),** is a systemic disease that typically begins suddenly (within days or weeks) after a venereal infection or gastroenteritis.[26,27] Joint and eye inflammation, enthesopathy, cutaneous lesions, malaise, fever, and fatigue are common manifestations. The prognosis for reactive arthritis is good with symptoms generally fully resolving in 3 to 12 months.

Clinical Features

Musculoskeletal. Joint pain and inflammation are the principal musculoskeletal symptoms of RS. These range from mild arthralgias to severe, disabling polyarthritis.[28] Involvement is asymmetrical and usually affects the hips, knees, and ankles, but it is also common to see shoulder, elbow, wrist, and small joints in the hands and feet involved as seen in RA. Generalized stiffness often also occurs as a result of inactivity. Enthesopathy and tenosynovitis most often arise in the plantar fascia and Achilles tendon and can impair ambulation. Enthesitis may also occur at the symphysis pubis, iliac crest, greater trochanter, and anterolateral ribs.[23]

Skin and Mucous Membranes. A skin rash known as *keratoderma blenorrhagicum* (or pustulosis palmoplantaris) is the most frequent skin lesion in RS. This rash usually

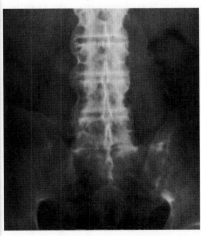

FIG. 6-5 Bamboo spine in ankylosing spondylitis. *From Gartland JJ: Fundamentals of orthopedics, Philadelphia, 1979, WB Saunders.*

occurs on the sole of the foot or the palm of the hand and initially has flaky plaques like psoriasis, but later, these lesions develop pustules and become scaly.

Psoriatic Arthritis. **Psoriatic arthritis** is an autoimmune inflammatory disorder involving chronic activation of T helper-1 (TH-1) cells. Psoriatic arthritis usually affects the skin and joints, and about one-third of patients also develop some type of eye inflammation.[29,30] Although psoriatic skin lesions precede joint manifestations in 75% of cases, the joints are affected first 10% of the time and 15% of patients have simultaneous onset of skin and joint symptoms.

When psoriasis starts in childhood, symptoms frequently resolve. In adults, the prognosis for prolonged symptoms or progression is worse if there is a family history, disease onset before age 20, erosive or polyarticular disease, or extensive skin involvement.

Clinical Features

Musculoskeletal. In psoriatic arthritis, inflammation frequently occurs where the Achilles tendon and the plantar fascia attach to the calcaneus. Spondylitis may occur and result in fusion similar to AS. Usually the arthritis associated with psoriatic arthritis affects large joints like the knees and one or two DIP or PIP joints in an asymmetrical pattern. In women, symmetrical polyarthritis, mainly affecting the small joints of the hands, feet, wrists, ankles, knees, and elbows (similar to RA), is more common; in men, involvement of the DIP joints with associated changes in the nail bed or asymptomatic and asymmetrical spinal arthritis (sacroiliitis) is more common. When there is severe involvement of the skin of the scalp, there is also often cervical spine arthritis.

Psoriatic arthritis is also associated with soft tissue swelling that creates "sausage-like" digits. **Dactylitis** (inflammation of a finger or toe), as a result of tenosynovitis and arthritis of the DIP or PIP joints, can also occur. If these joints fuse, it will cause a "claw" or "paddle" deformity.

Skin. The typical psoriatic skin lesion is a well-demarcated, erythematous plaque with a scaly appearance (Fig. 6-6). The nails are also often involved, with pitting as the most frequent characteristic. The nails can crack, turn brownish yellow (oil-drop sign), and separate from the underlying nail bed (onycholysis).

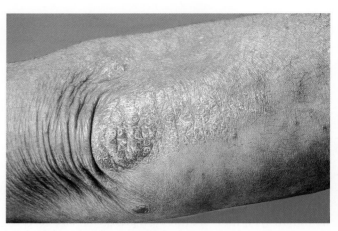

FIG. 6-6 Erythematous plaque typical of psoriasis. *Reprinted from the Clinical Slide Collection on the Rheumatic Diseases, copyright 1997. Used by permission of the American College of Rheumatology.*

POLYMYALGIA RHEUMATICA

Polymyalgia rheumatica (PMR) is a systemic inflammatory disorder that primarily causes pain and stiffness in the neck, shoulder, and pelvic girdle muscles and rarely involves the distal extremities.[31,32] Muscle biopsy reveals type II muscle fiber atrophy.[31] Low-grade fever, fatigue, anorexia, anemia, weight loss, and depression are also common in PMR. The incidence of PMR is estimated to be 10 to 53 cases per 100,000 with a peak age of onset of 60 to 80 years. The etiology of this disease is unknown, although an immunological component is suspected.[31]

Giant cell **arteritis** (GCA), also known as *temporal arteritis, cranial arteritis,* or *granulomatous arteritis,* a vasculitis of the medium and large arteries, commonly occurs together with PMR. About 50% of individuals with GCA have PMR-type complaints with muscular aches and pains. Although only 10% of patients with PMR have GCA, because GCA can cause sudden irreversible loss of vision, patients with PMR are generally evaluated for GCA.

Etiology. PMR is more common in women than men with a ratio of 2 to 3 : 1, and PMR almost exclusively affects whites, especially Scandinavians and people of northern European descent.[32,33] There appears to be a familial predisposition to PMR and GCA.[31]

Clinical Features

Musculoskeletal. Patients report stiffness after prolonged sitting and after getting out of bed in the morning and also report pain at night and with movement.[31] The signs of PMR are usually bilateral and symmetrical tenderness of periarticular structures, including bursae, joint capsules, and tendons. Synovitis of the hands, wrists, and knees may be present, and flexor tenosynovitis can lead to carpal tunnel syndrome.[32]

Vascular. PMR does not cause vascular changes, but GCA, which is associated with PMR, is primarily a vascular disease. GCA causes the vessels to initially become filled with inflammatory infiltrates. They may then become thickened, tender, and nodular, causing a diminished or absent pulse, and blood clots can develop at the sites of inflammation.[31] Frequently, the vessels in the neck and head are affected by GCA, and rarely, the ones in the brain are also affected. Without intervention, GCA causes irreversible blindness in 25% to 50% of cases as a result of occlusion of the orbital or ocular arteries. Rapid initiation of treatment with corticosteroids can prevent this visual loss.[31]

POLYMYOSITIS AND DERMATOMYOSITIS

Polymyositis and **dermatomyositis** are rare autoimmune diseases that cause chronic inflammation in striated muscle. Dermatomyositis also affects the skin. The most prominent feature of both of these diseases is proximal muscle weakness affecting the hips and shoulders; ocular and facial muscle weakness is very rare. The joints, lungs, heart, and gastrointestinal (GI) systems can also be affected.

◎ *Clinical Pearl*

Polymyositis and dermatomyositis cause muscle inflammation that results in proximal muscle weakness and pain.

Symptoms of muscle pain, morning stiffness, weakness, fatigue, malaise, chills, fever, or weight loss generally come on rapidly. In dermatomyositis, symptoms may appear briefly and then remit spontaneously without treatment. This form of **myositis** has the best functional outcome. The two age peaks are between 10 and 15 years of age for children and 45 and 60 years of age for adults.

Before corticosteroids were used to treat dermatomyositis, up to 50% of patients died from its complications. Now, the 5-year survival rate is 90%.[34] Risk factors for poor outcome include older age of onset, malignancy, delayed initiation of corticosteroids, pharyngeal dysphagia with aspiration pneumonia, interstitial lung disease, myocardial involvement, and complications from corticosteroids and other **immunosuppressive drugs.** Children with dermatomyositis have a poor prognosis if GI vasculitis and sepsis occur.[34]

Etiology. The etiology of these diseases is unknown, but viruses, infectious agents, genetic components, immune system dysfunction, and presence of autoantibodies are all proposed influences.[35] Polymyositis and dermatomyositis occur more often in women than in men, with a higher incidence in African Americans than in whites, with ratios of 2.5:1 and 3 to 4:1, respectively. Polymyositis and dermatomyositis onset is more frequent in winter and spring months, especially in children, after exposure to viral and bacterial infections.

Clinical Features

Musculoskeletal. Muscle weakness is the most prevalent clinical feature of polymyositis and dermatomyositis, with the shoulder and pelvic girdle muscles being affected most significantly. In about 50% of cases the neck flexor muscles are weak, and rarely, the ocular and facial muscles are affected.[36,34] About 50% of patients with polymyositis and dermatomyositis complain of muscle pain, but it is the muscle weakness that most impacts function, affecting tasks such as reaching overhead, dressing, toilet transfers, and stair climbing. Decreased neck flexor strength also impairs the ability to lift the head off a pillow, and pharyngeal muscle weakness may cause swallowing difficulty.[35] Muscle shortening as a result of atrophy and fibrosis can also reduce joint ROM and cause contractures that impair function.[34] Electromyography (EMG) studies are abnormal in 85% to 90% of patients with polymyositis or dermatomyositis.[35]

Skin. The rash associated with dermatomyositis has a typical erythematous or heliotrope (purple) color and presents on the upper eyelids, malar areas (cheeks), bridge of the nose, nasolabial folds, "V" areas of the anterior neck and upper chest, "shawl sign" of posterior shoulder and neck, extensor surface of the elbows and knees, and MCP and PIP joints and around the nails. The skin also has a scaly characteristic. "Mechanic" or "machinist" hands, with rough skin with cracks or fissures over the distal digital pad, are also typical of dermatomyositis.[34] As the disease progresses, the skin becomes shiny, atrophic, and hypopigmented.[34]

Cardiac. Although cardiac muscle involvement is common in polymyositis and dermatomyositis, it is generally asymptomatic until the disease is advanced. Rhythm abnormalities are the most frequent cardiac manifestations, and infrequently, congestive heart failure may occur.

Pulmonary. There are four common pulmonary effects of polymyositis and dermatomyositis. Initially, persons may be asymptomatic with only radiographic evidence of fibrosis or measurable decreased vital capacity. Later, aspiration pneumonia may occur as a result of pharyngeal dysphagia. More commonly, patients have slowly progressive interstitial lung disease that is symptomatically masked by the myopathy. A few patients develop aggressive pulmonary involvement with diffuse alveolitis, a nonproductive cough and rapidly progressive dyspnea leading to respiratory distress syndrome.[34]

Gastrointestinal. Pharyngeal dysphagia may cause nasal regurgitation and dysphonia, as well as swallowing difficulties that can lead to aspiration pneumonia. Patients report that food "sticks" (especially bread and meat) because of dysmotility of the lower esophagus.[34] Gastric reflux, heartburn, and constipation are common. The vasculitis and ischemia that occur in children can also cause life-threatening GI hemorrhage or perforation.[34]

Other. The peripheral vascular system is often affected by Raynaud's phenomenon, especially in dermatomyositis.[34]

SCLERODERMA

Scleroderma is an autoimmune connective tissue disease characterized by fibrosis of the skin and internal organs. "Scleroderma" means hardening of the skin, and taut, hidebound skin is the most characteristic feature of scleroderma.[37]

The two types of scleroderma are limited and diffuse.[38] "Limited cutaneous" or "localized" scleroderma primarily affects the skin distal to the elbows and knees and affects the lungs, although there may be some involvement of the skin of the face or neck. Fatigue and Raynaud's phenomenon are also common in this form of the disease.

"Diffuse" scleroderma or **systemic sclerosis** is the more aggressive form of the disease. In this form of the disease, there is fibrosis of the internal organs, musculoskeletal structures (tendons, muscle, joints, and synovium), blood vessels, the GI tract, lungs, heart, and kidneys, as well as much of the skin over the trunk and proximal extremities.

> ### ◎ *Clinical Pearl*
>
> Scleroderma causes thickening of the skin. The diffuse form also causes fibrosis of the organs, joints, and blood vessels.

Etiology. Scleroderma is rare in children and seldom runs in families, but there is a tendency for other autoimmune and connective tissue diseases to occur in relatives.[37] More women have the disease, with an average ratio of 3:1 women to men. The average age of onset is between 35 and 65 years.[37]

Clinical Features

Musculoskeletal. The earliest symptoms of scleroderma are often joint and muscle pain and stiffness without signs of inflammation.[39] Pain with joint motion accompanied by a tendon friction rub may indicate inflammation or fibrosis of the tendon sheaths or adjacent tissues.

Swelling and fibrosis can also limit motion, particularly in the fingers and face, and fibrosis around the carpal tunnel may result in carpal tunnel syndrome. Vascular involvement can further reduce hand function by causing pain and skin ulceration. A progressive loss of hand function may occur as pain and decreased flexibility lead to inactivity, which causes muscle weakness and atrophy and further loss of flexibility and more pain. Patients with scleroderma often cannot perform simple functional fine motor tasks such as fastening buttons or snaps, opening jars, or tying shoes.

Skin. Skin changes in scleroderma occur in three phases of varying duration. The first phase begins with puffiness and edema in the distal phalanges, sometimes together with mild inflammation, erythema, and itching. The second phase is characterized by progressive tightening of the skin leading to fibrosis, decreased flexibility, and severe drying. The fibrotic tissue binds to the deeper tissues as the skins thins out, creating a tethering effect. The third phase is characterized by skin atrophy without inflammation or fibrosis.[39]

Decreased elasticity of the facial skin can make the person appear expressionless with pursed lips, decreased oral aperture, a pinched nose, and smooth facial creases, creating a mouselike appearance **(Mauskopf)** (Fig. 6-7). In systemic sclerosis, there may also be mixed hypopigmentation and hyperpigmentation of the skin that creates a tanned or "salt and pepper" discoloration. Subcutaneous calcium deposits can also form in the fingers, forearms, or other areas of pressure in patients with limited systemic sclerosis.[39]

Vascular. Raynaud's phenomenon occurs in about 90% to 95% of patients with scleroderma.[40] Scleroderma can also adversely affect circulation by causing

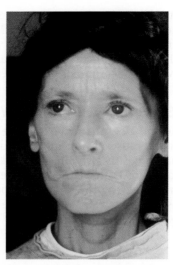

FIG. 6-7 Mauskopf appearance of the face in patient with scleroderma. *Reprinted from the Clinical Slide Collection on the Rheumatic Diseases, copyright 1997. Used by permission of the American College of Rheumatology.*

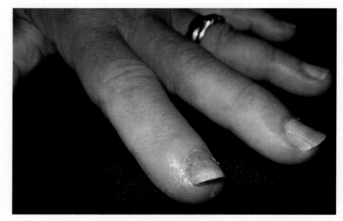

FIG. 6-8 Digital ischemia complicating scleroderma during winter. *From Walsh TD, Caraceni AT, Fainsinger R, et al, editors:* Palliative medicine, *Philadelphia, 2008, Saunders.*

proliferation of smooth muscle cells around blood vessels narrowing the vessel which can cause blood clots to form in the vessels. These vascular effects can cause arterial insufficiency and digital ischemia, leading to ulceration that can occasionally necessitate digital amputation (Fig. 6-8).[37,38,41]

Cardiac. Fibrosis of the heart and its vessels usually occurs late in the course of systemic sclerosis and is associated with a poor prognosis. The most common symptoms of cardiac involvement are dyspnea with exertion, palpitations, and chest discomfort.[39]

Pulmonary. Impaired lung function resulting from pulmonary fibrosis is almost universal in scleroderma. The most common symptom is dyspnea with exertion. Pulmonary function tests may help detect reduction in lung volumes or diffusing capacity before symptoms begin (see

Chapter 26). Pulmonary fibrosis can also lead to pulmonary hypertension, which is the primary cause of death in limited scleroderma. Less frequent pulmonary problems include aspiration caused by esophageal dysfunction, chronic cough, respiratory distress, pulmonary hemorrhage, and pneumothorax. There is also an increased prevalence of lung cancer in patients with scleroderma.[39]

Gastrointestinal. Scleroderma can cause difficulty chewing food, loss of teeth, and malnutrition because of the decreased perioral aperture, dry mucosal membranes, and periodontal disease. Heartburn, dysphagia, and dyspepsia are also common, and patients frequently have a sensation of food "sticking" because of lower esophageal dysmotility. Esophageal involvement can also lead to reflux of acid from the stomach into the esophagus, which can result in esophageal erosions, bleeding, stricture, and possibly cancer. Aspiration can also cause coughing, hoarseness, and chest pain.

Other Clinical Signs and Symptoms. Fifty percent of those with scleroderma have depression. There can also be sexual dysfunction in males as a result of neurovascular involvement, causing impotence. Sjögren's syndrome (see the next section) often accompanies scleroderma, so there is a need for fastidious dental care, as well as artificial tears for corneal lubrication. Trigeminal neuralgia may also occur, and thyroid fibrosis can lead to hypothyroidism.[39]

SJÖGREN'S SYNDROME

Sjögren's syndrome (SS) is an autoimmune disorder primarily characterized by inflammation of the exocrine glands.[42] Involvement of the salivary and lacrimal glands results in decreased production of saliva and tears, causing dry mouth **(xerostomia)** and dry eyes **(xerophthalmia)**, respectively. Additional features of SS include synovitis, neuropathy, and vasculitis. Patients with SS may present to rehabilitation because of the effects of the synovitis on their functional abilities or when they have secondary SS caused by another rheumatic disease such as RA.

The pathogenesis of SS is unknown; however, it is thought that a virus triggers the autoimmune process in genetically predisposed individuals. Because women are more often affected by SS than men, it is also proposed that hormones play a role in the development of SS.[43]

◎ *Clinical Pearl*

Sjögren's syndrome (SS) is characterized by dry eyes and dry mouth.

The cardinal features of SS are dry eyes and dry mouth. Additional manifestations include dry skin, hypothyroidism, nonproductive cough, peripheral neuropathy, lymphoid malignancy, and increased urinary frequency. Patients may also develop musculoskeletal manifestations, including myalgias, arthralgias, and arthritis.

CRYSTAL-INDUCED ARTHROPATHIES

Gout. Gout is caused by deposition of uric acid crystals in the joints and connective tissue. Although gout is

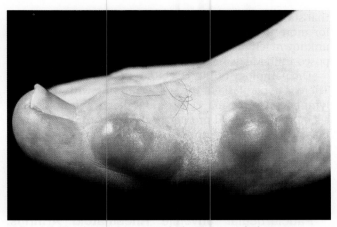

FIG. 6-9 Gouty tophi around the joints of the great toe. *Reprinted from the Clinical Slide Collection on the Rheumatic Diseases, copyright 1997. Used by permission of the American College of Rheumatology.*

related to high uric acid levels in the blood **(hyperuricemia),** many people with hyperuricemia do not develop gout. Uric acid levels are influenced by genetic and environmental factors.

Gout is characterized by three stages: hyperuricemia, acute intermittent gout, and chronic tophaceous gout. The rate and degree of progression varies among patients.[44] Clinical gout initially presents with warmth, swelling, pain, and erythema at a single joint. The pain progresses from mild twinges to intense and severe pain. The initial attack is most often at the first MTP joint.[45] Other joints commonly involved in the initial stages of gout include the ankles, heels, midfoot, and knees. The joint symptoms may be accompanied by systemic symptoms, including fever, chills, and malaise. Such acute episodes may last for hours to weeks and can recur at varying intervals.[44]

Chronic tophaceous gout may develop in individuals who have had acute intermittent gout for over 10 years. The involved joints become chronically swollen and painful. **Tophi,** which are deposits of uric acid crystals around the joints, then develop (Fig. 6-9). Tophi occur most often at the fingers, wrists, ears, knees, olecranon bursae, and Achilles tendons.[44]

Pseudogout. Pseudogout is similar to gout but is caused by deposition of calcium pyrophosphate dehydrate (CPPD) crystals, rather than urate crystals, in joints and periarticular tissues. The crystals are mostly deposited in the cartilage. Acute joint inflammation (arthritis) results from the release of CPPD crystals from the cartilage or other tissues into the joint space.

Acute pseudogout is characterized by inflammation at one or two joints that lasts for days or weeks. Fifty percent or more of the attacks affect the knees, but any joint may be involved. Acute attacks may be induced by acute illness, surgery, or trauma. Patients are generally symptom-free between bouts.

JUVENILE RHEUMATOID ARTHRITIS

Juvenile RA (JRA) is the most common connective tissue disease in children. It is a chronic inflammatory disease that starts before the age of 16 and causes joint symptoms for more than 6 weeks. Although the etiology of JRA is unknown, environmental triggers in genetically predisposed individuals have been hypothesized.[46]

The pathology of JRA resembles that of adults with RA. There is hyperplasia of the synovial lining with clusters of lymphocytes, plasma cells, and other immunologically active cells. Synovial proliferation with pannus formation may result in cartilaginous degradation, bony erosion, and subsequent joint destruction.

JRA is divided into three different subtypes based on clinical manifestations and course within the first 6 months of illness. The subtypes are **pauciarticular,** polyarticular, and systemic JRA.[47]

Pauciarticular Juvenile Rheumatoid Arthritis. Pauciarticular JRA involves four or fewer joints and is the most common form of JRA. The joint inflammation tends to be milder than in the other subtypes and extraarticular manifestations are rare. Children with pauciarticular JRA respond well to medical treatment, and joint symptoms often remit within several years. JRA commonly affects the knees, ankles, wrists, and elbows, with the knees being involved in 75% of the cases. The hips are generally spared. Chronic uveitis occurs in 20% of patients.[48]

Polyarticular Juvenile Rheumatoid Arthritis. Polyarticular JRA is the second most common form of JRA and involves five or more joints in a symmetrical presentation, including both large and small joints. As many as 20 joints may be involved at one time, including joints of the cervical spine, the costovertebral joints, and the temporomandibular joints (TMJs). The prognosis for patients with polyarticular disease is not as favorable as in pauciarticular JRA, especially in individuals who are rheumatoid-factor positive.

Systemic-Onset Juvenile Rheumatoid Arthritis. Systemic-onset JRA (SOJRA) is the least common subtype of JRA, occurring in only 10% of patients. High spiking fevers twice daily and the presence of a rash on the trunk and proximal extremities are characteristic. The arthritis may coincide with systemic features or manifest weeks to months later. Children with SOJRA often feel ill, fatigued, and lose their appetite, resulting in weight loss, with constitutional symptoms and rash being most notable during febrile episodes.

TYPICAL EXAMINATION FINDINGS

PATIENT HISTORY

Most of the key information needed for diagnosis, evaluation, and selection of interventions for patients with connective tissue dysfunctions can be identified from the patient history. Physical and psychological needs and concerns are considered to understand how the patient's condition affects their functional abilities. Medical aspects of the disease are also considered since connective tissue dysfunctions are associated with chronic, systemic processes.

The history will include the patient's experience with the disease, including their expectations and goals for treatment. Involving the patient in goal setting develops rapport, helps to gain trust and confidence and, improves adherence to treatment. The chronology of the patient's symptoms, including how and when the symptoms began and how they evolved, as well as the current presenting symptoms, is also included to assist with intervention selection and goal setting. Symptoms may include pain, stiffness, weakness, and fatigue, as well as other complaints.

The patient's past medical history (medical, surgical, rehabilitative, and alternative/complementary) and the patient's social history may also provide information relevant to the plan of care

SYSTEMS REVIEW

The systems review is used to target areas requiring further examination and to define areas that may cause complications or indicate a need for precautions during the examination and intervention processes. Chapter 1 includes details of the systems review.

TESTS AND MEASURES

Musculoskeletal. Postural assessment may initially be performed with the patient standing, with attention to deviations from normal spinal curves (see Chapter 4). As previously discussed, patients with **spondyloarthropathy** may develop forward-head positioning with increased thoracic kyphosis and loss of lumbar lordosis.

Anthropometric Characteristics. All joints will be inspected for deformities, malalignment, and swelling. Increased girth may be caused by intraarticular effusion, synovial thickening, periarticular soft tissue inflammation, or extraarticular fat pads. Warmth, a sign of inflammation, may be detected by palpation.

Range of Motion. Active ROM (AROM) and passive ROM (PROM) will be measured and recorded at all peripheral joints. Causes of limitations may include pain, weakness, muscle shortening, or swelling. Joint **crepitus** may be noted as a grinding or grating sensation that is either palpable or audible with movement of joints or supportive structures. The goniometer is the instrument of choice for measuring peripheral joint motion, and the tape measure is the most convenient instrument for measuring spinal motion.[6]

Spine ROM may initially be examined with attention to deviations from the normal spinal curves. **Schober's test** may be employed to quantify motion at the lumbar spine. In this original Schober's test, a mark is made on the patient's lower back and a mark 10 cm higher (Fig. 6-10). The patient then bends forward at the waist with the knees straight (as if trying to touch the toes) and one remeasures the distance between the marks while the patient is bent over. If the distance between the marks is less than 15 cm, there is decreased spine mobility. In a modified Schober's test, the first mark is placed 5 cm lower and a distance of less than 20 cm between the marks indicates decreased mobility. Thoracic mobility may be assessed by measuring chest circumference at the level of the nipples (T4) during exhalation and inhalation. It is normal for the chest circumference to increase by at least 5 cm from maximum exhalation to maximum inhalation.

Muscle Performance. Connective tissue dysfunction may be associated with generalized or localized weakness.

Modified Schober's test (normal: total > 20 cm)

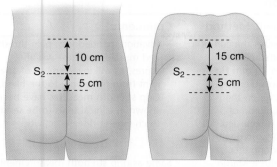

FIG. 6-10 Modified Schober's test. *From Fam AG, Lawry GV, Kreder HJ: Musculoskeletal examination and joint injection techniques, Philadelphia, 2005, Mosby.*

Muscle performance and strength deficits may be tested with functional strength assessment tools and other standardized measures (see Chapter 5). For patients with connective tissue dysfunction, it is recommended that strength be tested functionally rather than graded by manual muscle testing (MMT) because MMT may be unreliable in this population of patients who are often unable to assume standardized testing positions and in whom joint pain often limits test performance.[6]

Neuromuscular

Pain. Pain should be quantified using a visual analog scale (VAS) or other descriptive scale (see Chapter 22). Additionally, the location of painful and tender areas should be determined and documented.

Peripheral Nerve Integrity. Inflammation associated with connective tissue dysfunction may indirectly affect peripheral nerve function. For example, entrapment neuropathies are commonly seen in the rheumatic diseases, and synovitis may result in nerve compression at the carpal tunnel (median nerve), medial epicondyle (ulnar nerve), and tarsal tunnel (posterior tibial nerve). See Chapter 18 for a discussion of peripheral nerve injuries.

Integumentary. Cutaneous manifestations of connective tissue dysfunction may be a primary manifestation of the underlying disease process or a secondary manifestation of vascular insufficiency or medications. In particular, corticosteroid medications may cause skin thinning and fragility that may impact selection of rehabilitation interventions, adaptive equipment, and assistive devices. Common cutaneous manifestations of diseases that cause connective tissue dysfunction include nail changes, rashes, reduced skin elasticity, cutaneous plaques, subcutaneous nodules, ulcerations, Raynaud's phenomenon, or trophic changes.[6]

Function. Functional status and the ability to perform activities in the home, community, and at work may be assessed with a variety of validated instruments. These include the Button test, Grip Strength test, Jepson Hand Function test, Timed-Stands test, and the Keitel Index. These tests involve direct observation of the patient performing a task and all have been validated in patients with chronic rheumatic diseases and are sensitive to change. The Button, Grip Strength, and Timed-Stands tests are easy to use in the clinical environment because they are quick and the standardized equipment is inexpensive. As with other tests and measures, these functional tests can be used to indicate the patient's baseline condition and to measure progress over the course of treatment or time. Table 6-1 contains tools to measure function in this population.

Gait, Locomotion, and Balance. Gait examination is an integral part of the examination of patients with connective tissue dysfunction. All phases of gait will be analyzed with specific attention to joint position, alignment, and compensatory patterns. Patients should be examined with and without assistive devices and from all angles.

Self-Care and Home Management/Work, Community, and Leisure Integration. Most tests of self-care and home management for this population are based on self-administered questionnaires. Three self-report measures specifically designed to assess function in patients with arthritis are the Functional Status Index (FSI),[49,50] the Arthritis Impact Measurement Scale (AIMS),[51] and the Health Assessment Questionnaire (HAQ). The FSI was developed specifically for examination of patients with arthritis and has been validated in this population.[52] The AIMS and the HAQ are often used to assess functional outcome in patients with connective tissue dysfunctions and have both been extensively validated.

A few instruments were specifically developed for assessing the outcome of pediatric patients with connective tissue dysfunctions. These measures are limited by the complexities involved in working with children, including variability in developmental roles and tasks and changes in growth and behavior from infants to toddlers to adolescents.[53] The Children's HAQ (CHAQ) is used most often and includes age-appropriate activities.[54] More comprehensive indices include the Juvenile Arthritis Quality of Life Questionnaire[55] and the Childhood Arthritis Health Profile (CAHP),[56] which address not only function but also health quality of life issues such as pain, psychosocial functioning, and areas concerning family, friends, and school. The Juvenile Arthritis Functional Assessment Scale (JAFAS) includes 10 ADLs that are assessed by a health professional.[57] The Juvenile Arthritis Functional Assessment Report (JAFAR) is a longer modified version of the JAFAS designed as a self-report instrument with separate versions for proxy reports by parents or self-administration by the child.[58]

EVALUATION, DIAGNOSIS, AND PROGNOSIS

Information from all aspects of the examination, including the patient history, systems review, and tests and measures, are interpreted together by the clinician to derive a treatment diagnosis. Patients falling into the preferred practice pattern 4D: Impaired joint mobility, motor function, muscle performance, and range of motion associated with connective tissue dysfunction, as described in the *Guide to Physical Therapist Practice*,[59] typically have decreased ROM, muscle guarding or weakness, pain, swelling or effusions, joint instability, and some limitation in their ability to perform functional tasks that may require adaptive equipment or assistance from others.

| TABLE 6-1 | Standardized Measures for Evaluating Physical Functioning in Patients with Chronic Rheumatic Disorders Using Direct Observation |

Measurement Tool	Purpose	Measurement Method	Comments
Grip strength test	Measurement of hand, wrist, and forearm strength.	Patient squeezes the cuff of a sphygmomanometer inflated to 30 mm Hg as hard as possible. The highest level on the mercury column of 3 attempts is recorded. May also be measured with a Martin Vigorimeter.	Motivation, handedness, pain threshold, and muscle weakness will affect scores, as will involvement of any joint from the elbow to the hand. Grip strength measures have been shown in clinical trials to be sensitive to change in disease activity.
Thumb to index strength test	Hand and finger function.	Measured with a Martin Vigorimeter.	Same as grip strength measurement.
Time to walk 50 feet	Measurement of LE function.	Individual walks 50 feet on a flat surface using any aides or assistive devices. Time is recorded to the nearest 0.1 second.	Motivation can affect performance. Low reliability, insensitive to changes in disease activity.
6-minute walk test	Field test of fitness.	Measures the distance the patient can walk in 6 minutes.	Motivation can affect performance. Low correlation with standard laboratory tests of physical fitness. Sensitive to change in exercise clinical trial in fibromyalgia. Little information available for other disorders.
Jepson Hand Function test, Grip Ability test, Grip Function test, Arthritis Hand Function test	Various measurements of hand function tested in persons with arthritis. Activities tests are based on ADLs.	Specific tasks (e.g., picking up cards, pouring water from a jug, writing) are performed in presence of evaluator.	May be used in clinical trials of specific hand treatments, following hand surgery, and in long-term outcome studies. Some tests require special equipment.
Button test	Measurement of hand function that can be used in clinical practice.	Standard board with 5 buttons. Patients are timed while they unbutton and button using right and left hands separately, with scores from both hands averaged.	Motivation is an important factor. Useful in disorders that affect hand function (e.g., RA).
Timed-Stand test	Measurement of LE function.	Measures number of seconds it takes the patient to stand up and sit down 10 times from a chair using only the LEs.	Motivation, age, and nonmusculoskeletal co-morbid conditions may affect scores. Sensitivity to change has not been determined.
Keitel Index	UE and LE extremity function with emphasis on ROM.	Measures performance of 24 standard tasks requiring peripheral and axial joint motion. Performance is evaluated by a trained observer. Takes 10-15 minutes to complete.	Motivation may be a factor. Time and personnel to observe and score tasks are a factor in its use. Scale is sensitive to short-term change.

Adapted from Robbins L, Burckhardt CS, Hannan MT, et al (eds): *Clinical care in the rheumatic diseases,* ed 2, Atlanta, 2001, Association of Rheumatology Health Professionals.
Data from Pincus T, Callahan LF: *J Rheumatol* 19:1051-1057, 1992; Anderson JJ, Felson DT, Meenan RF, et al: *Arthritis Rheum* 32:1093-1099, 1989; Newcomer KL, Krug HE, Mahowald ML: *J Rheumatol* 20:21-27, 1993; Kalla AA, Smith PR, Brown GMM, et al: *Br J Rheumatol* 34:141-149, 1995; Sullivan M, Ahlmen M, Bjelle A, et al: *J Rheumatol* 20:1500-1507, 1993; Walker JM, Helewa A: *Physical therapy in arthritis,* Philadelphia, 1996, WB Saunders.
LE, Lower extremity; *ADLs,* activities of daily living; *RA,* rheumatoid arthritis; *UE,* upper extremity; *ROM,* range of motion.

INTERVENTION

Interventions for patients with connective tissue dysfunctions are most effective when a multidisciplinary approach that includes patient education for self-management and cognitive behavioral interventions is used in addition to medical and physical interventions. A partnership between the clinician and the patient is also critical, since success depends on ongoing participation and compliance with home exercise programs and an appreciation of the principles of pain management, rest, joint protection, use of adaptive equipment for ambulation and ADLs, energy conservation, and splinting.

This section first discusses the general approach to management of functional limitations related to connective tissue dysfunctions and **inflammatory arthritis,** including RA, psoriatic arthritis, RS, SLE, crystal-induced arthropathies, and scleroderma, with reference to disease-specific variations. Physical therapy management of the spondyloarthropathies, polymyositis/dermatomyositis, PMR, and JRA are discussed subsequently because of differences in the treatment approach for these conditions.

RHEUMATOID ARTHRITIS AND OTHER INFLAMMATORY CONDITIONS

The examination and evaluation provide the foundation for individualizing interventions and therapeutic goals in patients with inflammatory connective tissue dysfunctions. Rehabilitation interventions to reduce pain; increase and maintain joint mobility, muscle strength, and cardiovascular fitness; conserve energy and reduce fatigue; and optimize function should be started early before irreversible joint deformities occur. The interventions employed to accomplish these objectives include patient education, rest (joint protection, energy conservation, and splinting), physical agents, and therapeutic exercise.

Patient Education. Patient education is integral to promoting self-management in inflammatory arthritis. The American College of Rheumatology (ACR) guidelines for the treatment of RA include patient education as a first line of treatment.[60] Quality education for patients with arthritis should foster self-management behaviors to help patients achieve or maintain optimal health status or quality of life.[61] Patient education is most effective when it helps patients incorporate behavioral change into their lifestyles. This can be done through interactive methods that build confidence and improve skills such as decision-making, problem-solving, self-monitoring, and communication with health care providers. This may be done in groups or individually. Educational interventions that include behavioral techniques are usually more effective than interventions that rely exclusively on transmitting information, although informational education may also improve outcomes. The arthritis education program with the most substantial evidence supporting its effectiveness is the Arthritis Self-Management Program (ASMP) developed at Stanford University. This arthritis self-help course is taught through the Arthritis Foundation in the United States.

Patient education programs for connective tissue inflammatory disorders are associated with decreased pain, reduced numbers of physician visits, and significant cost savings, as well as an enhanced ability to control various aspects of the disease and promotion of self-management techniques.

Rest and Joint Protection. Rest is a key component in the management of arthritis and includes both general and joint-specific rest. The management of inflammatory arthritis requires a fine balance between activity and rest. Recommendations for rest may be included as part of the patient education program, and specific techniques may be reviewed by an appropriate health professional and practiced by patients to enhance adherence.

Recommendations for general rest during the active phases of inflammatory arthritis are for 8 to 10 hours of sleep per night with 30 to 60 minutes of rest during the day. Instruction in energy conservation techniques may help patients with pacing and planning of scheduled rest periods to avoid undue fatigue and joint flares.

Joint-specific rest is recommended for joints with active inflammation to avoid activity-related injuries, provide periods of unloading, and promote function and activity in spite of joint swelling and pain. Joint-specific rest may include activity modification, use of assistive devices or adaptive equipment, and protective or supportive splinting. Some pieces of adaptive equipment can help maintain and promote independence in people with connective tissue dysfunctions. Fig. 6-11 shows the reach zones of a patient sitting at a workspace. Adaptive equipment can make the difference between independence and relying on another person for ADLs.

Various assistive devices (Fig. 6-12), as described in Chapter 33, can also be used to aid ambulation. Device selection may be difficult in this population because of systemic disease and involvement of multiple areas including the hands. A platform crutch or walker may help to reduce lower extremity weight bearing and distribute the weight-bearing forces to a large area of the upper extremity. If a platform walker is used, it should have wheels because it will generally be too heavy and awkward to lift. Extra-depth shoes and molded insoles can also be used to decrease pain in weight-bearing activities such as standing, walking, and stair climbing. Sometimes a simple change in the physical environment, such as replacing the tap head of the faucet with a lever tap, can increase independence with household tasks.[62]

Physical Agents. Electrotherapy and thermotherapy are used in patients with arthritis to decrease pain and inflammation, reduce stiffness, and increase mobility. Some studies support the use of thermotherapy, low level laser therapy (LLLT), and transcutaneous electrical nerve stimulation (TENS) in patients with arthritis.[63] Physical agents most effectively control pain in patients with arthritis when they are combined with exercise.

Heat. Heat is the most commonly used physical agent in arthritis care by health professionals and patients. Heat has been demonstrated to reduce pain, promote relaxation, reduce muscle spasm, and enhance flexibility of muscles and periarticular structures.

The stage of the disease process must be taken into account when selecting thermal modalities for the

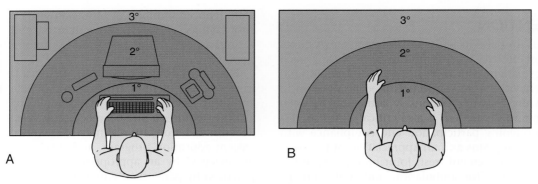

FIG. 6-11 Reach zones at a work station.

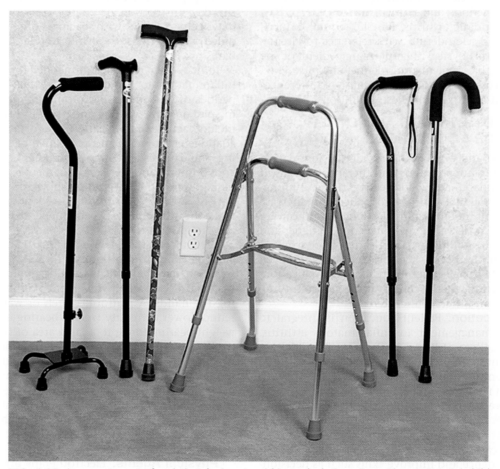

FIG. 6-12 An assortment of assistive devices to aid in ambulation. *From Pierson FM, Fairchild S: Principles & techniques of patient care, ed 4. St. Louis, 2008, Saunders.*

treatment of inflammatory arthritis. When there is acute inflammation, heat may worsen symptoms and may increase joint damage by promoting the activity of collagenase, thereby accelerating collagen breakdown.

Cold. Cold can reduce pain, inflammation, and muscle spasm in patients with arthritis. Cold may be applied with cold packs, ice massage, or cold water immersion.

Heat and Cold. There is no evidence that heat or cold alter the immunological processes in inflammatory arthritis; however, both improve function and decrease pain,

particularly when used in conjunction with an exercise program.[64]

Electrotherapy. The research on the use of TENS for inflammatory arthritis primarily focuses on RA affecting the wrist. Well-designed studies demonstrate that TENS can reduce pain and improve hand function without adverse effect in patients with RA.[65]

Low Level Laser Therapy. A number of studies show that LLLT reduces pain and morning stiffness and increases ROM in patients with RA.

TABLE 6-2	Recommendations for Health and Fitness in the Apparently Healthy Population				
Exercise Goal	**Mode**	**Frequency**	**Intensity**		**Duration**
General health	Whole body, repetitive activities	Most days of the week	Moderate (55%-70% age-predicted maximal heart rate; RPE 12-13/2-4		30 minutes accumulation (3 10-minute bouts)
Cardiovascular fitness	Rhythmic, aerobic exercise	3-5 days/week	70%-85% age-predicted maximal heart rate; RPE 14-16/4-7		20-30 minutes continuous
Muscular fitness (strength and endurance)	Dynamic, resistance exercise for major muscle groups	2-3 days/week on alternate days	Volume: 8-10 exercises; resistance adequate to induce fatigue after 8-12 repetitions, or 10-15 reps if over 50-60 years of age or frail		—
Musculoskeletal flexibility	Gentle stretching; static or PNF technique	2-3 days/week minimum	Repetitions: 3-4 repetitions for each stretch		Hold position for 10-30 seconds for static; 6-second contraction followed by 10-30 second assisted stretch for PNF

Data from *ACSM guidelines for exercise testing and prescription,* ed 6, Philadelphia, 2000, Lippincott Williams & Wilkins.
RPE, Rate of perceived exertion; *PNF,* Proprioceptive neuromuscular facilitation.
RPE scale 6-20 scale/0-10 scale.

Exercise. Connective tissue dysfunctions result in pain, stiffness, and fatigue, with a concomitant decline in function, because of decreased ROM, muscle strength, and aerobic capacity. Joint immobilization may also lead to weakening of cartilage and periarticular structures, whereas the regular joint motion and intermittent weight bearing that occurs with many forms of exercise may enhance joint health.[66] Despite previous beliefs that exercise may harm individuals with arthritis, current research has found that various forms of exercise can safely help patients with rheumatic disease.[67] People with arthritis can generally follow recommendations for health and fitness applied in the healthy population as depicted in Table 6-2, while adhering to general and joint-specific recommendations for pacing and rest. A meta-analysis found that aquatic therapy, stationary cycling, and weight-bearing exercise are safe for patients with RA and improve their flexibility, strength, endurance, function, cardiovascular fitness, and general health without increasing joint symptoms.[68]

Range of Motion Exercise. ROM exercises can alleviate stiffness, increase or maintain joint mobility, and increase the flexibility and elasticity of periarticular structures. Active and active-assisted exercise is recommended in patients with inflammatory arthritis, avoiding overstretching inflamed tissues. During periods of acute inflammation, joint ROM may be maintained by performing one to two repetitions through the full ROM daily.[69] The number of repetitions may be gradually increased as the acute joint symptoms subside. Active ROM exercise in combination with relaxation has also been shown to improve function and reduce pain in patients with RA.[70]

Strengthening Exercise. Loss of muscle strength, endurance, and power in patients with arthritis may be caused by the inflammatory disease process, disuse atrophy, side effects of medications, inhibition caused by

joint pain and inflammation, and loss of mechanical joint integrity. Studies show that muscle conditioning programs can improve strength, endurance, proprioception, and function without increasing pain or disease activity in patients with RA.[71]

Table 6-3 outlines the purpose and recommendations for isometric and dynamic muscle conditioning exercise for individuals with arthritis. Strengthening exercises for patients with RA may be static or dynamic and are recommended to be at a load of 50% to 80% of maximal voluntary contraction, 2 to 3 times per week. The exercise may be performed against body weight or using resistance training equipment such as weights or elastic bands (Fig. 6-13), with gradual progression in either a supervised clinical environment or at home with professional guidance.

Aerobic Exercise. Many studies suggest that people with arthritis can exercise regularly and vigorously enough to improve cardiovascular fitness and endurance without increasing joint symptoms.[68,72] Evidence-based recommendations for aerobic exercise in patients with RA are as follows: the goal for the intensity level of aerobic exercise should be moderate to hard (60% to 85% of maximum heart rate) and exercise should be performed 3 times weekly for 30 to 60 minutes.[73] Exercise may be either land-based or performed in an aquatic environment with progressive adjustment in intensity.

Aquatic Therapy. Aquatic therapy is physical therapy performed in the water environment and may incorporate mobility exercises, strengthening activities, aerobic conditioning, and functional tasks. Exercise performed in water can reduce pain, probably because of the sensory input from hydrostatic pressure and temperature, relax muscles, and reduce joint compression.[74] Aquatic fitness programs can improve activity level, function, mobility, strength, exercise tolerance, and mood in patients with RA

TABLE 6-3	Purposes, Recommendations, and Precautions for Isometric and Dynamic Muscle Conditioning Exercise in Patients with Connective Tissue Dysfunction	
	Isometric	**Dynamic**
Purpose	Minimize atrophy. Improve tone. Maintain and increase static strength and endurance. Prepare for dynamic and weight-bearing activity.	Maintain and increase dynamic strength and endurance. Increase muscle power. Improve function. Enhance synovial blood flow. Promote strength of bone and cartilage.
Recommendations	Perform at functional joint angles. Breathe normally, do not hold breath. Intensity: ≤70% MVC. Duration: 6 seconds. Frequency: 5-10 reps daily.	Able to perform 8-10 reps against gravity before increasing resistance. Use functional movements. Modify ACSM guidelines as appropriate.
Precautions	Decreased muscle blood flow. May increase intraarticular pressure. May increase blood pressure.	May increase biomechanical stress on unstable or malaligned joint. Need for power grip.

From Robbins L, Burckhardt CS, Hannan MT, et al (eds): *Clinical care in the rheumatic diseases,* ed 2, Atlanta, 2001, Association of Rheumatology Health Professionals.
reps, Repetitions; *ACSM,* American College of Sports Medicine; *MVC,* maximum voluntary contraction.

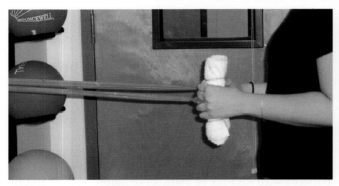

FIG. 6-13 Strengthening exercise with elastic band.

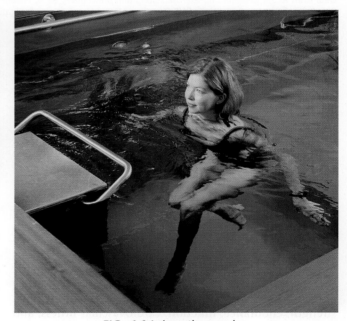

FIG. 6-14 Aquatic exercise.

(Fig. 6-14).[75,76] Community-based exercise programs like the Arthritis Foundation's Aquatic Program not only increase ROM and strength but also provide social support and camaraderie.[77]

Exercise and Juvenile Arthritis. Children with JRA have joint pain, swelling, and mobility limitations that lead to reduced physical activity, fitness, and function.[78] Various types of exercise have been shown to result in decreased disease severity and increased activity,[79] mobility,[79] strength,[80] and aerobic fitness,[79] as well as improved function in children with arthritis. In a review of the literature on exercise and physical activity in children with arthritis, the following observations were made:

1. Children with JRA may participate in either aquatic or land-based exercise programs without disease exacerbation.
2. Participation in an aquatic or land-based exercise program twice a week for 6 weeks may reduce disease activity and improve exercise endurance.
3. Studies suggest that exercise on land may promote greater gains in strength and function than aquatic exercise programs.
4. Weight-bearing exercise is necessary for developing adequate bone growth and bone density in children.
5. Individualized and supervised strengthening exercise appears to be safe and effective in children as young as 8 years of age.
6. Individualized exercise may be more appropriate for children with severe disease, whereas children with mild-to-moderate disease may benefit from group exercise programs.
7. Children with mild disease should be able to participate in most sport with proper screening and physical conditioning. However, highly competitive contact sports should be avoided during active disease.

SPONDYLOARTHROPATHIES

The few published studies on interventions for patients with AS indicate that exercise needs to be ongoing to maintain improvements and that more disabled patients are generally more motivated to exercise. Interventions that promote self-management significantly improve self-efficacy and self-reported levels of exercise and function.[81] Group exercise also more effectively improves pain, stiffness, thoracolumbar mobility, fitness, and global health scores than individual treatment sessions.[82] Hydrotherapy may also be used safely, although patients with AS may feel a sensation of chest pressure when immersed in chest-deep water.[83]

In the clinical setting, based on the limited available evidence and typical findings in the patient examination, the following interventions are recommended for patients with spondyloarthropathies. The focus of treatment is postural reeducation because these diagnoses primarily affect the spine. In AS, the inflammatory process progresses from the sacroiliac joint superiorly throughout the spine, producing a fused spine, so it is critical to keep the spine erect to minimize fusion in flexion. Flexibility exercises for the spine, hips, and shoulders should be emphasized to prevent a forward flexed posture and maintain the ability to reach overhead. With thoracic spine involvement the ribcage is also affected, so breathing exercises are recommended to optimize expansion with inhalation and exhalation movements. To maintain upright posture, the anterior axial structures, especially the pectoral and hip flexor muscles, should be stretched and the posterior spinal extensors, specifically the scapular and hip extensor muscles, should be strengthened. Abdominal muscle strengthening may also help support the spine and improve posture.

POLYMYALGIA RHEUMATICA

Currently, there is no published research evaluating the effects of physical therapy interventions on patients with PMR. The interventions recommended are those thought to lessen the impairments and functional limitations typically found during the examination. Since proximal weakness is the most significant clinical finding in PMR, the focus of treatment is strengthening exercises for the hip and shoulder girdle muscles. Depending on the duration of symptoms and flexibility limitations, ROM activities for the hips and shoulders may also be indicated. When shoulder ROM is limited, patients often complain of shoulder pain and difficulty in functional tasks, such as washing and dressing, that require reaching overhead or behind. Systemic corticosteroids, which are frequently given to treat symptoms of PMR, do not always resolve joint restrictions even though they generally relieve pain and stiffness. Soft tissue and joint mobilization may improve ROM and function in such circumstances.

Postural reeducation is usually also recommended for patients with PMR. These patients are often older women with a forward flexed posture at baseline before their diagnosis. Stretching anterior structures, especially the pectoral muscles, and strengthening the hip, spinal extensors, and abdominal muscles can reduce trunk weakness and

provide a more effective base of support and foundation for extremity motion. This can improve independence with functional activities. Proprioceptive neuromuscular facilitation (PNF) techniques may also be used to improve trunk stability and extremity strength. Aquatic therapy can safely be used to increase endurance, reduce fatigue, and strengthen the trunk and extremities.

POLYMYOSITIS AND DERMATOMYOSITIS

Historically, exercise was considered contraindicated for patients with myositis, especially in the acute stages, because it was thought that this would cause more muscle damage and increase muscle enzyme levels, potentially damaging the kidneys. However, it has been shown that although creatinine phosphokinase (CPK), the primary product of skeletal muscle breakdown, levels do rise in patients with polymyositis during isometric exercise, the CPK levels fall rapidly after the exercise ceases.[84] Furthermore, a number of studies demonstrate that exercise is safe in patients with myositis and results in increased strength, respiratory function, and aerobic capacity, as well as improved well-being and function, without significantly elevating muscle enzyme levels. Based on the current evidence, it is recommended that patients with myositis participate in vigorous strengthening and conditioning programs to address their functional deficits. Exercise programs based on PNF techniques, weight lifting, and other land-based conditioning activities, as well as aquatic exercises, can help individuals with myositis regain independence with functional tasks.[85,86]

SCLERODERMA

Because scleroderma tends to tighten the soft tissues and thus reduce joint ROM and soft tissue flexibility, interventions intended to maintain joint ROM and soft tissue flexibility are often used. Two areas to focus on are the face, especially around the mouth for activities such as eating and brushing teeth, and the fingers to maintain the ability to perform fine motor skills and ADLs. There are few published studies in this area and no randomized controlled trials; however, small studies have found that mouth opening significantly improves with mouth stretching and oral augmentation exercises. Paraffin can also improve finger, thumb, and wrist flexibility and perceived stiffness and skin elasticity in patients with scleroderma.

CASE STUDY 6-1

RHEUMATOID ARTHRITIS

Patient History

CH is a 52-year-old woman who presents with pain and mobility limitations at the shoulders, wrists, MCPs/PIPs, knees, ankles, and feet. She was diagnosed with RA 3 years ago after experiencing peripheral joint symptoms for 10 years. She was quite active before diagnosis but now reports a significant loss of function. She finds dressing and grooming activities, meal preparation, and housework difficult. Her walking is limited to one block by pain at her ankles and feet, and she climbs stairs non-reciprocally.

CH's sleep is disturbed by shoulder and foot pain, and she reports feeling stiff for 1½ hours in the morning.

Tests and Measures—Significant Findings
Musculoskeletal
- CH has swan-neck deformities at the left ring and small fingers and a Boutonnière deformity at the right small finger. Her MCP joints and ankles are swollen bilaterally. CH has bilateral calcaneal valgus positioning and bilateral forefoot pronation.
- CH has mobility limitations at the shoulders, elbows, wrists, right knee, and ankles.

Function
- CH has an antalgic gait pattern with decreased step length, decreased cadence, limited push-off at terminal stance, and accentuated pronation at midstance. Walk time for 50 feet was 35 seconds. In 1 minute, she walked 105 feet, compared with an age-adjusted average of approximately 194 feet.
- CH has difficulty with dressing (buttons, shoes, and socks), sit-to-stand transfers, and negotiating stairs. She can button 5 buttons in 1 minute.

Diagnosis
Preferred practice pattern 4D: Impaired joint mobility, motor function, muscle performance, and ROM associated with connective tissue dysfunction.

Interventions
- Instruction in joint protection and energy conservation techniques with introduction to adaptive equipment and practice within relevant contexts.
- Functional splints for swan-neck deformities and boutonnière deformities to be used during the day. Resting splints to be used at night.
- Instruction for a home exercise program, including ROM, strengthening, and aerobic conditioning exercise.
- Strengthening exercises gradually progressed from isometrics to elastic band–resisted exercises for upper and lower extremities Aerobic conditioning gradually progressed to 30 minutes of cumulative exercise to be performed 4 to 5 times per week.
- Custom foot orthotics to accommodate existing foot deformities and provide enhanced arch support were fabricated. Footwear recommendations.

Role of the Physical Therapist Assistant
- Suggest three exercises for this patient's initial home exercise program.
- Document a treatment for this patient that includes one home exercise with written instruction.
- What types of aerobic activities would be appropriate for this patient?
- What joint protection and energy conservation techniques would be appropriate to teach this patient?

Additional Information
For the full version of this case study, including detailed examination results, interventions, and outcomes, see the Evolve site that accompanies this book.

CHAPTER SUMMARY
Connective tissue dysfunctions primarily result from rheumatic diseases with various pathologies and generally autoimmune or unknown etiologies. A thorough understanding of these conditions and the effectiveness of different interventions assists the clinician in selecting appropriate, individualized interventions specific to patient needs. Since these diseases are generally chronic and progressive, patients may need frequent reexamination and modification of their home program and other interventions. Visits may need to be scheduled judiciously to accommodate restrictions in the patient's health care coverage.

Patients should be educated about their disease and instructed in activity modification, the use and benefits of adaptive equipment, joint protection, pacing, and the importance of learning to manage their disease. Interventions should emphasize enhancing function to promote independence while also managing pain. Exercise is one of the most effective interventions for people with connective tissue disorders, since increasing muscular strength to support the joints improves biomechanical efficiency and reduces pain and fatigue. Exercise can be performed at home, in a community-based setting, or in the aquatic environment. Outcome measures will help determine which interventions are most effective and enable health care providers to achieve the goal of improving the quality of life for patients with connective tissue disorders.

ADDITIONAL RESOURCES
For links to these and additional web-based resources, see the Evolve site.

Banwell BF, Gall V (eds): *Clinics in physical therapy: Physical therapy management of arthritis,* New York, 1988, Churchill Livingstone.

Firestein GS, Budd RC, Harris ED, et al (eds): *Kelley's textbook of rheumatology,* ed 8, Philadelphia, 2009, Saunders.

Klippel JH, Stone JH, Crofford LJ, et al (eds): *Primer on the rheumatic diseases,* ed 13, New York, 2009, Springer.

Melvin JL: *Rheumatic disease in the adult and child: Occupational therapy and rehabilitation,* ed 3, Philadelphia, 1989, FA Davis.

Melvin JL, Jensen GM (eds): *Rheumatologic rehabilitation series assessment and management,* Bethesda, MD, 1998, American Occupational Therapy Association.

Robbins L, Burckhardt CS, Hannan MT, et al (eds): *Clinical care in the rheumatic diseases,* ed 3, Atlanta, 2007, American College of Rheumatology.

Smolen JS, Weinblatt ME, Weisman MH, et al (eds): *Rheumatology,* ed 4, St. Louis, 2008, Mosby.

Walker JM, Helewa A: *Physical therapy in arthritis,* Philadelphia, 1996, Saunders.

American College of Rheumatology (ACR)

The Arthritis Society (Canada)

Lupus Foundation of America

Scleroderma Foundation

GLOSSARY

Ankylosing spondylitis (AS): A form of inflammatory arthritis that has a predilection for the sacroiliac joints, axial spine, and ligamentous/tendinous insertions.
Arteritis: Inflammation of the arteries.
Arthralgias: Joint pain.

Arthritis: Encompasses over 100 types of rheumatic diseases but literal translation means inflammation of the joint.

Avascular necrosis: Necrosis of bone caused by ischemia.

Baker's cyst: A cystic swelling within the popliteal space posterior to the knee as a result of mechanical irritation or synovial inflammation.

Boutonnière deformity: A finger deformity with flexion at the PIP joint and hyperextension at the DIP joint.

Crepitus: Grating, grinding, or popping sensations/sounds that occur with movement of a joint.

Cytokines: Proteins secreted by a variety of cells to help regulate immunological responses (e.g., **interleukin,** tumor necrosis factor, lymphokines, and interferon).

Dactylitis: Inflammation of a finger or toe.

Dermatomyositis: Diffuse inflammatory disease of striated muscle that leads to symmetric proximal muscle weakness with a dermatological component.

Effusion: Excess fluid in the joint resulting from joint irritation or inflammation of the synovium.

Enthesitis: Inflammation where ligaments and tendons attach to bone.

Gout: A disease characterized by acute episode of arthritis resulting from the deposition of uric acid crystals at the joint or in surrounding tissues.

Hyperuricemia: Abnormal amount of uric acid in the blood.

Immunosuppressive drugs: Substances that suppress or interfere with the normal immune response.

Inflammatory arthritis: Systemic arthritis that involves inflammation of the synovium of the joint.

Interleukin-1 (IL-1): Substance from monocytes and macrophages important in the acute phase response.

Lupus: A chronic inflammatory autoimmune disease that may affect the skin, joints, and internal organs.

Mauskopf: Loss of facial expression as the result of tightening/tautness of the skin resulting from scleroderma.

Myositis: Inflammatory disease of striated muscle.

Nephritis: Inflammation of the kidney.

Pannus: Excessive proliferation of synovial and granulation tissue that invades joint surfaces.

Pauciarticular: Involvement of few joints.

Polymyalgia rheumatica (PMR): Condition characterized by stiffness and pain at the shoulder girdle without weakness; usually seen in women over 50 years of age in conjunction with an elevated erythrocyte sedimentation rate (ESR).

Polymyositis: Diffuse inflammatory disease of striated muscle that leads to symmetric proximal muscle weakness.

Pseudogout: Synovitis caused by the deposition of calcium pyrophosphate dehydrate crystals resulting in arthritis; articular chondrocalcinosis.

Psoriatic arthritis: A spondyloarthropathy with concomitant psoriasis.

Raynaud's phenomenon: An intermittent vasoconstriction of the distal small arteries, arterioles, and capillaries that results in blanching, erythema, and cyanosis of the hands.

Reactive arthritis: Spondyloarthropathy with enteric or venereal infectious trigger (also known as Reiter's syndrome).

Reiter's syndrome (RS): Triad of arthritis, conjunctivitis, and urethritis (also known as reactive arthritis).

Rheumatoid arthritis (RA): Systemic disease characterized by inflammation of the joint synovium.

Schober's test: A measurement of spinal mobility in patients with spondyloarthropathy.

Sclerodactyly: Sclerosis and tapering of the fingers in progressive systemic sclerosis.

Scleroderma: A chronic disease of unknown etiology that causes sclerosis of the skin and organs (GI tract, heart, lungs, and kidneys) and arthritis.

Sjögren's syndrome (SS): Disease of the lacrimal and parotid glands resulting in dry eyes and mouth; frequently occurs with RA, SLE, and scleroderma.

Spondyloarthropathy: Inflammation of the spine and sacroiliac joints. Describes a category of diseases that includes ankylosing spondylitis, reactive arthritis/Reiter's syndrome, and psoriatic arthritis.

Synovitis: Inflammation of the synovium.

Systemic lupus erythematosus (SLE): Systemic inflammatory disease characterized by small vessel vasculitis and a diverse clinical presentation.

Systemic sclerosis: A chronic disease of unknown etiology that causes sclerosis of the skin and organs (GI tract, heart, lungs, and kidneys) and arthritis.

Tenosynovitis: Inflammation of the synovial lining of the tendon sheaths.

Tophi: Deposits of uric acid crystals around the joints.

Uveitis: Inflammation of the iris, ciliary body, and choroids, or the entire uvea.

Vasculitis: Inflammation of the blood or lymph vessels.

Xerostomia: Dry mouth.

Xerophthalmia: Dry eyes.

Chapter 7

Localized Inflammation

L. Vince Lepak III

CHAPTER OUTLINE

OBJECTIVES

After reading this chapter, the reader will be able to:
1. Explain the phases of inflammation.
2. Describe how various pathologies contribute to and are affected by localized inflammation.
3. Identify the signs and symptoms of localized inflammation.
4. Recognize and measures signs and symptoms associated with localized inflammation.
5. Describe evidence-based interventions for an individual with localized inflammation.

Inflammation is the body's first response to tissue damage or injury. As the first line of defense, it is critical to the survival of the human organism. Inflammation is a localized protective response elicited by injury or destruction of tissues that destroys, dilutes, or walls-off the injurious agent, as well as the injured tissue. It is not one process but rather an overlapping sequence of interactions between stimuli and the body's cellular and biochemical defenses designed to destroy offending pathogens and initiate tissue healing. The extent of the inflammatory response depends on the body's reactivity and the mode and extent of cellular injury.[1]

PATHOLOGY

According to the *Guide to Physical Therapist Practice* (the *Guide*), localized inflammation is a pathology that has a multifactorial impact on an individual.[2] The diagnostic classification associated with localized inflammation is preferred practice pattern 4E: Impaired joint mobility, motor function, muscle performance, and range of motion (ROM) associated with localized inflammation. The *Guide* lists a wide range of risk factors for this preferred practice pattern, including abnormal response to provocation, ankylosing spondylitis, bursitis, capsulitis, epicondylitis, fasciitis, gout, osteoarthritis, prenatal and postnatal soft tissue inflammation, synovitis, and tendinitis. A number of these are also risk factors for other preferred practice patterns, particularly pattern 4D: Impaired joint mobility, motor function, muscle performance, and ROM associated with connective tissue dysfunction (see Chapter 6). To separate these, this chapter focuses on inflammation that is primarily due to local insult or degeneration, whereas Chapter 6 focuses on the systemic inflammatory and autoimmune disorders. In addition, Chapter 28 provides a detailed discussion of inflammation and tissue healing particularly as they relate to wound healing.

A wide range of stimuli can provoke localized musculoskeletal inflammation. These include trauma from crush, contusion, avulsion, rupture, sprain, or strain injury, as well as infection, physical or chemical agents (thermal injury or chemical irritation), derangement of joint components, degeneration, crystal deposition, foreign bodies, immune reactions, and overuse. In response to any of these stimuli, a cascade of events, known collectively as the *inflammatory response*, occurs. This response should be balanced, first initiating inflammation and then limiting its extent and duration to avoid harm.[3] When inflammation is prolonged, it is known as *chronic inflammation*. The earliest descriptions of inflammation were derived from clinical observation, including what continue to be described as the five classic (or cardinal) signs of inflammation: rubor (redness), calor (heat), dolor (pain), tumor (swelling), and functiona laesa (loss of function).[4] Since chronic inflammation may not produce the classic signs of inflammation, chronic inflammation may not be recognized until enough tissue damage has occurred to create impairments and limit function. Chronic inflammation often persists because the body cannot resolve the initial damage or because the initial stimulus did not initiate a sufficient acute inflammatory response to trigger completion of the cascade of events needed to resolve the condition. In addition, the ongoing presence of infectious agents, foreign bodies, metabolic byproducts, exogenous irritants (mechanical or chemical), and persistent immune responses can all contribute to maintaining a chronic inflammatory state.[5]

This chapter outlines the major events of the inflammatory process in the musculoskeletal system and describes factors that can cause pathological or chronic inflammation. Inflammatory conditions commonly encountered and treated by rehabilitation professionals are described, including a summary of the pathophysiology of each. This is followed by discussion of typical examination findings, evaluation, and interventions for successfully managing localized inflammatory conditions.

◎ *Clinical Pearl*

The five classic signs of inflammation are rubor (redness), calor (heat), dolor (pain), tumor (swelling), and functiona laesa (loss of function).

STAGES OF TISSUE HEALING

The first stage of tissue healing is the inflammatory stage (phase I). This stage is designed to initiate healing; prevent further damage; rid the body of pathogens, foreign material, and nonviable tissue; and thus prepare the way for tissue repair through collagen proliferation (phase II or proliferation). Phase III, remodeling or maturation, occurs when the initial weak collagen produced during the proliferation phase is gradually replaced by stronger collagen. This phase can last 2 years or longer. Fig. 7-1 illustrates the stages of tissue healing.

Phase I—Inflammatory Phase. Inflammation usually resolves 24 to 72 hours after the initial trauma, but repeated agitation and associated risk factors can delay its completion and lead to secondary injuries.[6] Inflammation is designed to protect the body and promote repair by destroying, diluting, or sequestering the injurious agent and the injured tissue. In the first 5 to 10 minutes, a vasoconstrictive vascular response is initiated to help contain the insult. The initial vasoconstriction is quickly followed by prolonged vasodilation and increased capillary permeability. The increased capillary permeability allows more fluid, plasma proteins, white blood cells, and fibrin to enter the area.[7,8] Fibrin plugs form in the blood vessels and wall

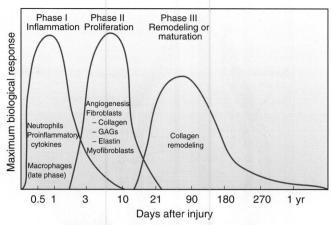

FIG. 7-1 Stages of tissue healing: Inflammation, proliferation, and remodeling. *GAGs,* Glycosaminoglycans.

off the injured area. At this point, the clinical signs of inflammation, redness, heat, swelling, and often pain appear. The rise in tissue temperature creates a favorable environment for cellular multiplication and metabolic reactions.

During the inflammatory phase, **macrophages** are the predominant cells. They rid the area of debris, microorganisms, and residual **neutrophils** through phagocytosis. A vast array of growth factors (**angiogenesis** growth factor, platelet-derived growth factor, **fibroblast** growth factor, and others) and **cytokines** (interleukin-1 and tumor necrosis factor) are also released during the inflammatory response. These facilitate tissue repair, stimulate specific immune responses, promote the release of chemotactic factors that attract fibroblasts, and help regulate the production of collagen through the release of matrix metalloproteinases (MMPs), which are primarily produced by fibroblasts.

The end of the inflammatory phase is signaled by the release of fibrinolysin, an enzyme that helps open the lymphatic channels. Pain and loss of function now occur as a result of increased sensitivity of the pain receptors, activation of neurologically mediated reflexes, and increased pressure on surrounding structures from edema.[9]

Phase II—Proliferation Phase. The proliferation phase begins as the number of fibroblasts increases and the number of macrophages decreases. Fibroblasts are the dominant cell type of the proliferation phase. They synthesize MMPs, collagen and other proteins, fibronectin, glycosaminoglycans, and elastin. Some fibroblasts differentiate into **myofibroblasts,** which are responsible for wound contraction.[6,10] Granulation and angiogenesis are also associated with this phase.

Proliferation starts a few days after the initial insult and is usually complete within 3 weeks, although it can last for as long as 6 to 12 weeks. In the early portion of this phase, type III collagen, which is fairly weak, is produced and loosely arranged in a disorganized fashion in the damaged area. Later in this phase, this collagen aligns itself to some degree with the stress imposed on it and starts to be replaced by stronger type I collagen.[6]

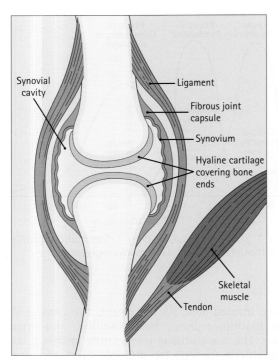

FIG. 7-2 Diagram of a simple synovial joint showing the two articulating bone ends separated from each other by synovial fluid and enclosed within a fibrocollagenous capsule. Surrounding ligaments and tendinous muscle attachments prevent excess movement. *From Stevens A, Lowe JS:* Human histology, *ed 3, St. Louis, 2005, Mosby.*

Phase III—Remodeling or Maturation Phase. Phase III, the remodeling or maturation phase, begins by day 21 after the initial injury and may continue for months or years. This phase is characterized by a continual restructuring of the collagen from weak unorganized fibers to stronger fibers (type I) that are continually being reorganized to meet the demands of imposed mechanical forces.

COMPONENTS OF THE FUNCTIONAL JOINT COMPLEX

A quick review of the functional joint complex can help the reader understand the specific inflammatory conditions of the musculoskeletal system. These generally involve synovial or diarthrodial joints because these joints' capacity for movement makes them vulnerable to injury and thus local inflammation. The typical synovial joint (Fig. 7-2) includes hyaline cartilage at the articulating ends of the bone, menisci, ligaments, a joint capsule, bursae, tendons, and muscles. In some places, particularly in areas close to bones, tendons are surrounded by tendon sheaths that form tunnels to protect the tendons and bathe them in synovial fluid. There may also be fascia that extends beyond the tendons or ligaments to provide greater strength and stability.

Lining the joint capsule of all synovial joints is a well-vascularized, well-innervated tissue known as *synovium*. Within the joint, synovial fluid facilitates movement through lubrication and nutrient exchange to adjacent,

relatively avascular tissues such as tendons and cartilage. The constituents of synovial fluid change in the presence of inflammation, and physicians may remove some of this fluid with a needle and analyze it to help with diagnosis. In addition, synovial fluid pressure may rise in response to inflammation. This rise can decrease capillary perfusion[11] and inhibit muscle activation around the joint.[12]

> ### Clinical Pearl
> Synovial fluid helps nourish articular cartilage and lubricate joints and tendon sheaths.

Cartilage. Normal adult articular cartilage is mostly composed of an extracellular matrix containing collagen and proteoglycans, within which there are a few chondrocyte cells. Chondrocytes make up only 1% to 2% of the articular cartilage and are responsible for maintaining a balance between the synthesis and breakdown of the extracellular matrix.[11] The chondrocytes synthesize the collagens and proteoglycans that make up the matrix and synthesize proteinases that degrade collagens. Unfortunately, cartilage has a limited capacity for repair.[13]

Articular cartilage is primarily made of hyaline, which is 65% to 80% water.[11] Fluid passes freely between the cartilage and the synovial fluid of the joint, hydrating the joint and providing it with nutrition. Articular cartilage generally has no blood supply or lymphatics to provide it with nutrition. Articular cartilage is elastic, compressible, and self-lubricating.

Normally, cartilage is protected from wear by a form of self-lubrication that occurs as weight-bearing gradually deforms the cartilage, pushing water out of the interior onto hydrophilic surface tissues. This produces a "squeeze-film" of lubrication that is re-imbibed by the cartilage when the pressure is removed.[11] Movement through physiological ROM helps nourish the articular cartilage by providing intermittent hydrostatic pressure changes that increase the diffusion of fluid and maintain or increase proteoglycan and collagen synthesis. However, joint motion without loading or compression does not provide enough nutrition to maintain cartilage integrity over time.[14] Immobilization and weightlessness, as well as excessive loading (obesity), developmental abnormalities (e.g., Perthes' disease), and joint incongruities, can lead to overloading or underloading of the cartilage and result in articular cartilage degradation.[15] Furthermore, damage to any of the structures that protect cartilage by absorbing excessive weight-bearing forces, including muscles, tendons, and ligaments around a joint as well as the subchondral bone, can cause wear on the cartilage to be increased.[14]

> ### Clinical Pearl
> Articular cartilage is avascular and has a limited capacity for repair.

SPECIFIC INFLAMMATORY CONDITIONS

Osteoarthritis. Osteoarthritis (OA), or degenerative joint disease, is the most common type of arthritis in the United States and the world.[16] OA is responsible for 59 million physician visits each year, is the primary reason for total hip and knee replacements (see Chapter 10), is the leading cause of lower extremity disability among the elderly, and is a leading cause of disability in persons 15 years or older.[17,18] OA can interfere with a wide range of activities of daily living (ADLs), including ambulation, bathing, dressing, eating, drinking, home maintenance, taking medication, toileting, sleeping, using a telephone, and writing.[16] The knees are affected by OA more commonly than any other joint, and this is the primary reason that individuals have difficulty climbing stairs and walking.[18]

OA is characterized by the breakdown of the joint's cartilage and change in periarticular bone (osteophyte formation and subchondral sclerosis).[19,20] OA first affects the structure of articular cartilage, causing edema or microcracks in the extracellular matrix and variability in chondrocyte quality and quantity. As destruction of the cartilage progresses, fissuring and pitting occur down to the subchondral bone. The subchondral bone can then be eroded, and subchondral microcysts may develop. Fragments of cartilage may also fall into the joint. These are phagocytosed in the synovial fluid and cause mild synovial inflammation. In OA, the synovial cells also produce a range of inflammatory mediators and cytokines that can alter the cartilage matrix and stimulate chondrocytes to synthesize destructive enzymes to further degrade the cartilage.[11,21,22] **Osteoblasts** from exposed subchondral bone may also synthesize enzymes that further contribute to the degenerative process.[23]

Eburnated bone (bone that appears polished and shiny, indicating a full thickness loss of articular cartilage)[24] attempts to regenerate, causing subchondral bone sclerosis and a build-up of bony outgrowths at the joint margins called *osteophytes*. Osteophytes are covered with poor quality cartilage.

Prolonged synovitis associated with the joint damage from OA can also cause capsular fibrosis and limitations in joint ROM.[15] Reflexive inhibition of muscle contraction that results from pain and swelling can further contribute to functional losses by causing muscle atrophy and imbalanced forces around the joint. Joint narrowing that is a result of the erosive changes in the bone may also lead to ligament instability. Together, these structural changes may lead to biomechanical instabilities that create a cycle of joint degeneration and local synovial inflammation (Fig. 7-3).

Pain-free joint motion requires an intact joint with relatively few degenerative changes. Damage or degeneration of the articular cartilage, synovium, capsule, ligamentous structure, or other components of the functional joint complex can decrease ROM, cause pain, and lead to joint instability, malalignment, or mechanical disturbances.[25] Any loss of congruency or stability in the normal complex may initiate or accelerate degenerative changes (OA), leading to loss of mobility and joint deformities.[26]

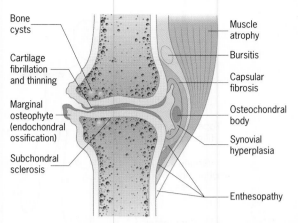

FIG. 7-3 Diagram of a knee showing early osteoarthritis. There is medial compartment narrowing owing to cartilage thinning with subarticular sclerosis and marginal osteophyte formation. *Courtesy Fleshandbones.com.*

The exact causes of OA are not known, but a variety of systemic or local risk factors are known to be associated with OA. Systemic factors include age, gender, ethnicity, hormonal status and bone density, nutritional factors, and genetics. Local factors include obesity (caused by the compressive and shearing forces applied through the weight-bearing joints), joint injury (trauma, particularly if it results in intraarticular damage), joint deformity (congenital or developmental), occupational factors, sports participation (repetitive stress), and muscle weakness.[18,27] The primary risk factors for the development of OA appear to be increased age, obesity, hip injury, congenital or developmental hip disorders, and a genetic predisposition to the disorder.[20]

The prevalence of OA increases with age.[28] Approximately 50% of people over the age of 65 years have radiographic signs of OA. This increases to 80% for persons 75 years old and older.[20]

◎ *Clinical Pearl*

Osteoarthritis (OA), or degenerative joint disease, is the most common type of arthritis. It is characterized by the breakdown of joint cartilage and osteophyte formation. The knee is the joint most frequently affected by OA.

Obesity may contribute to OA by increasing compressive and shearing forces applied through the weight-bearing joints of the body. However, factors associated with obesity other than weight bearing clearly also affect the development of OA because although the presence of obesity correlates most with the development of OA in weight-bearing joints, it also correlates with OA at other joints, including those of the hands.

Bursitis. Bursae are fluid-filled sacs located at numerous points throughout the body (Fig. 7-4). They are designed to provide a smooth gliding surface between bones, tendons, ligaments, muscles, and skin.[29] Bursae may become inflamed by trauma, overuse, or as part of a more systemic inflammatory process (e.g., rheumatoid arthritis, crystal arthropathies, or infection). Detecting the

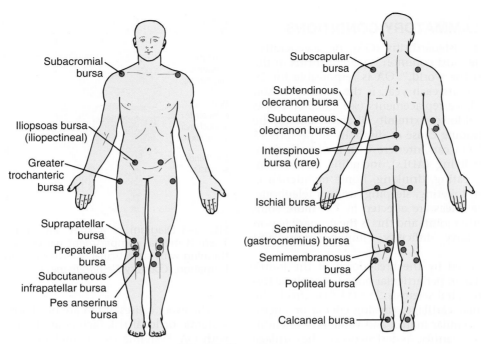

FIG. 7-4 Sites of bursae.

classic signs of inflammation with bursitis can be difficult if the bursa is deep or the response is mild. Unrecognized, chronic bursitis leads to effusion, thickening of the bursal wall, deposits of fibrin, and the development of a cartilage-like material around the bursa that may need to be surgically excised to relieve symptoms. Bursitis can cause pain that limits a person's ability to engage in normal daily activities (e.g., reaching overhead, ambulation, and participating in work or recreational activities). Bursae are widely distributed, and bursitis may occur at any bursa.

Capsulitis. Capsulitis is an inflammation of the joint capsule. Although any synovial joint capsule may be affected, glenohumeral joint capsulitis is the most common.[30] Glenohumeral joint capsulitis is often referred to as *adhesive capsulitis* of the shoulder, or *frozen shoulder*. Risk factors for adhesive capsulitis include female gender, diabetes mellitus, recent trauma to the shoulder, and immobility of the shoulder. Adhesive capsulitis occurs most commonly after the age of 40 years, and approximately 25% of those who develop adhesive capsulitis in one shoulder will subsequently develop it in the other. The four stages of adhesive capsulitis with different pathological changes, signs, and symptoms are listed in Table 7-1.

Ligament Sprain. A ligament sprain is a stretch or tear of a ligament. Ligament sprains are graded according to severity.[31]

- *First-degree sprain:* Minimal loss of structural integrity, no loss of motion, little or no swelling, and little to no functional loss, although there is usually some localized tenderness and slight bruising. Patients can generally return to activity immediately with some protection and can resume full unprotected activity within 10 days to 2 weeks.

- *Second-degree sprain:* Weakened ligament, initial loss of motion, bruising, and swelling with pain at the limits of motion. Immobilization and/or protection are necessary to prevent further injury and it may take 2 to 3 months for the patient to return to full activity.

- *Third-degree sprain:* Completely torn ligament, excessive motion, potential joint instability, significant bruising, and often bleeding within the joint.

Lower extremity sprains are more common than upper extremity or axial sprains because of the forces placed on the lower extremity. Ankle sprains and knee sprains are both common, particularly in sports participants. The history, with a focus on the exact mechanism of injury, in conjunction with a careful physical examination generally allows the therapist to isolate the specific structure(s) involved. Fractures can often occur in conjunction with ligament sprains. Therefore if the patient cannot bear weight after an injury consistent with a ligament sprain, they should be referred to the physician immediately for consideration of further work-up.[32]

Muscle Strain. A muscle strain is a stretch or a tear of a muscle and is the most common injury in sports. Muscle strains typically occur near the myotendinous junction of muscles crossing two or more joints.[33] When muscle damage occurs, force production is initially reduced due to muscle fiber disruption and inflammation. It has also been found that muscle function is reduced further approximately 24 hours after the initial injury. Although the mechanism for this delayed effect is poorly understood, it is thought to be caused by a neutrophil-mediated response that results in further muscle injury.[34] As with ligament sprains, muscle strains are categorized into three degrees according to severity. These degrees reflect similar

TABLE 7-1	Stages of Adhesive Capsulitis in the Shoulder			
Findings	Stage 1	Stage 2 Freezing Stage	Stage 3 Frozen Stage	Stage 4 Thawing Phase
Duration of symptoms	0 to 3 months	3 to 9 months	9 to 15 months	15 to 24 months
Pain	Pain with active and passive ROM	Chronic pain with active and passive ROM	Minimal pain except at end-ROM	Minimal pain
ROM	Limitation of forward flexion, abduction, internal rotation, external rotation	Significant limitation of forward flexion, abduction, internal rotation, external rotation	Significant limitation of ROM with rigid "end-feel"	Progressive improvement in ROM
Examination under anesthesia	Normal or minimal loss of ROM	ROM essentially identical to ROM when the patient is awake	ROM identical to ROM when patient awake	Data not available
Arthroscopy	Diffuse glenohumeral synovitis, often most pronounced in the anterosuperior capsule	Diffuse, pedunculated synovitis (tight capsule with rubbery or dense feel on insertion of arthroscope)	No hypervascularity seen, remnants of fibrotic synovium seen, capsule feels thick on insertion of arthroscope, diminished capsular volume	
Pathological changes	Hypertrophic, hypervascular synovitis, rare inflammatory cell infiltrates, normal underlying capsule	Hypertrophic, hypervascular synovitis with perivascular and subsynovial scar, fibroplasias, and scar formation in the underlying capsule	"Burned out" synovitis without significant hypertrophy or hypervascularity, underlying capsule shows dense scar formation	

Data from Hannafin JA, Chiaia TA: *Clin Orthop* 372:95-109, 2000.
ROM, Range of motion.

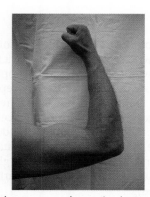

FIG. 7-5 Third-degree muscle strain (complete tear) of the biceps. Note that the muscle belly has balled up during contraction.

types of tissue damage and physical findings as in ligament sprains and cause similar functional limitations for similar periods of time.[31] One notable physical finding with a third-degree muscle strain (i.e., a complete tear) is that the muscle will not be able to generate any force and will "ball up" when contraction is attempted (Fig. 7-5).

◎ *Clinical Pearl*

Muscle strains typically occur near the myotendinous junction of muscles crossing two or more joints.

Tendinitis. Tendinitis is an acute inflammatory condition of the tendon and its surrounding structure that may lead to degeneration (tendinosis or angiofibroblastic dysplasia) if not treated appropriately (Fig. 7-6). Often, persistent low-grade inflammation and gradual weakening of the tissues are unrecognized until macrotrauma occurs (partial tear). Overuse and abnormal biomechanics are primarily responsible for eventual tendon failure.[35] Associated risk factors include but are not limited to a sudden increase in physical activity, age (peak incidence 30 to 50 years of age), decreased vascularity, abnormal joint alignment or altered ROM, and strength deficits or imbalances.[36]

Current and recent studies indicate that the chronic tendon disorders that commonly occur at the shoulder, elbow, knee, or ankle involve a degenerative process (called *tendinosis*), as well as or more than an inflammatory process (appropriately called *tendonitis*).[35,36] Since both degeneration and inflammation may occur together, some authors prefer to use the term *tendinopathy*.[36] Tendinitis (tendinosis, tendinopathy) can be divided into the following 5 stages, which range from less to more severe[31]:

• *Grade I:* Least severe pain, only occurs with activity, does not interfere with performance, generalized tenderness, and disappears before the next exercise session.
• *Grade II:* Minimal pain with activity, localized tenderness, does not interfere with activity intensity or duration.
• *Grade III:* Interferes with activity but usually disappears between sessions, localized tenderness.

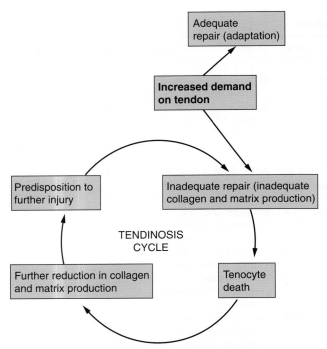

FIG. 7-6 Tendinosis cycle. *Redrawn from Leadbetter WB:* Clin Sports Med *11:533-578, 1992.*

- *Grade IV:* Interferes with intensity of training and does not disappear between activity sessions, significant localized pain, tenderness, crepitus, and swelling.
- *Grade V:* Most severe form, interferes with sports and ADLs, symptoms are chronic or recurrent, signs of tissue changes and altered muscle function.

Tenosynovitis. Tenosynovitis, or paratendinitis, refers to an inflammation of the synovial sheath. Like tendinitis, the term *tenosynovitis* is used to describe both inflammatory and noninflammatory conditions.[37] The tendons at the wrist and ankle have synovial sheaths that encompass them to help the tendons glide freely as they pass between bone and the retinaculum (Fig. 7-7). The synovial sheath produces synovial fluid to help reduce friction and protect the tendon.[37] Synovial sheaths may become damaged or inflamed as the result of systemic disease (rheumatic conditions), trauma, overuse, or retinacular thickening. This may result in the tendon sheath thickening that can cause nodular swelling or narrowing of the tendon.[37,38]

De Quervain's tenosynovitis is stenosing tenosynovitis of the synovial sheaths surrounding the abductor pollicis longus and the extensor pollicis brevis tendons just proximal to the wrist. It is one of the more common examples of tenosynovitis in the upper extremity. In trigger finger and trigger thumb, stenosis of the tendon sheath and hypertrophy or swelling of the flexor tendon lead to a snapping or locking of the digit.[38,39]

Fasciitis. In the extremities, there are two functional types of fascia: the superficial fascia and the deep fascia. The superficial layer acts as the basal layer of the skin. It is designed to allow movement of the skin, to provide support and give shape, and to protect deeper structures from excessive pressures. The deeper fascia is much thicker, and the fibers are more organized and have major muscular and bony attachments. It serves a similar function to its more superficial counterpart. The plantar aponeurosis is one of the thickest fascia in the body and is composed of superficial and deep fascia.[40]

Plantar Fasciitis. Plantar fasciitis is a localized inflammatory condition of the plantar aponeurosis. It is the most common cause of unilateral localized heel pain in sedentary or athletic adults.[41-43] The condition generally develops over 6 weeks (in patients who seek immediate care) to 12 months.[44,45]

Plantar fasciitis is thought to be caused by overuse, although the exact mechanism is unclear. Some suggest that shoes with poor cushioning, pes cavus or planus, increase in running/walking distance or intensity, or a hard running/walking surface may increase the risk for plantar fasciitis.

Currently, there is no standard for the diagnosis of plantar fasciitis except clinical symptoms (pain with weight bearing, especially during the initial steps in the morning or after sitting for prolonged periods) and signs (reproduction of symptoms with palpation at the medial tubercle of the calcaneus).

Clinical Pearl

Clinical symptoms of plantar fasciitis are pain in the heel with weight bearing, especially with the first steps of the day.

Tensor Fascia Lata Fasciitis. Tensor fascia lata fasciitis, also known as iliotibial band friction syndrome (ITBFS), is an overuse injury with a population-specific incidence. This syndrome is caused by repetitive rubbing of the iliotibial band over the lateral femoral condyle during knee flexion and extension. Perceived causes for ITBFS include certain anthropometric and biomechanical characteristics (e.g., genu varum), inadequate flexibility of the iliotibial band, weak hip abductor (gluteus medius), inappropriate footwear, and training surface conditions (hilly or crowned).[46]

Prenatal and Postnatal Soft Tissue Inflammation. The physiological changes that occur during pregnancy predispose women to a range of soft tissue inflammation conditions. During pregnancy, hormonal changes, ligament laxity, weight gain and redistribution, and soft tissue swelling place the woman at risk for musculoskeletal strains that may cause injury or exacerbate prior injuries. Common musculoskeletal impairments prenatally and postnatally include low back pain, pubic pain, hip and knee pain, carpal tunnel syndrome, and de Quervain's tenosynovitis.[47]

Pelvic pain during pregnancy generally occurs if the pubic symphysis widening causes inflammation. This usually begins during the tenth to twelfth weeks of pregnancy. Walking and bending exacerbate pain, and gait analysis may reveal an increased waddling gait.

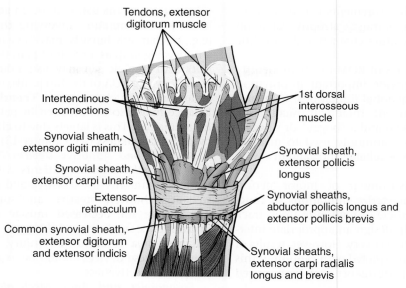

Tendons, extensor digitorum muscle

Intertendinous connections

1st dorsal interosseous muscle

Synovial sheath, extensor digiti minimi

Synovial sheath, extensor carpi ulnaris

Extensor retinaculum

Synovial sheath, extensor pollicis longus

Synovial sheaths, abductor pollicis longus and extensor pollicis brevis

Common synovial sheath, extensor digitorum and extensor indicis

Synovial sheaths, extensor carpi radialis longus and brevis

FIG. 7-7 Synovial sheaths of the wrist.

Hip pain can be the result of pubic symphysis pain, sacroiliac pain, bursitis, or hip joint pathology (**osteonecrosis** or **osteitis pubis**). Knee pain is usually the result of patellar tracking difficulties. Carpal tunnel syndrome (the second most common musculoskeletal disorder during pregnancy after low back pain) and de Quervain's tenosynovitis are the result of swelling and inflammation.

TYPICAL EXAMINATION FINDINGS

PATIENT HISTORY

The patient history will include the patient's description of his or her current condition and its evolution. This will help the clinician determine the stage and severity of the disorders and the likely structures involved. A description of the activity when the symptoms started may also indicate the mechanism of injury and the likely affected tissues. The nature of a patient's symptoms may also clarify the diagnosis. Stiffness after inactivity that eases with movement is generally thought to indicate inflammation. Stiffness that lasts more than an hour and occurs primarily in the morning is commonly associated with arthritic inflammation, although these symptoms are not always present and cannot be considered diagnostic.

A visual analog scale (VAS) can be used to establish a baseline for symptom severity before or during an activity and at rest (see Chapter 22). The responsiveness of symptoms to activity also gives an indication of severity, with pain that occurs at rest indicating a more severe problem than pain that only occurs during or after activity.[48]

General demographics should include information such as age, gender, race/ethnicity, education, and language because these can affect the probability of certain pathologies, as previously noted. Social history can elicit cultural beliefs and behaviors, resources, and support that affect the client's condition. Growth and development, living environment, general health status, prior level of fitness, family history, and past medical and surgical history are all factors that contribute to the client's reason for seeking care.[2]

An employment or work history should focus on information about repetitive movements, exposure time, environmental risk factors (temperature, humidity, or equipment), posture-related risk factors (excessive or sustained postures), and psychological stresses. All of these factors can contribute to localized inflammation.[49]

TESTS AND MEASURES

Musculoskeletal. Posture should always be examined because an individual may develop or assume an unwanted position as a result of pain arising from localized inflammation. When a part is injured, the body naturally splints the area to prevent further injury. This immobilization can lead to faulty biomechanics, which can perpetuate stress and strains on bones, joints, ligaments, capsules, and muscles.[50] Postural asymmetry or altered alignment may correlate with gait abnormalities and altered ROM.[51]

Anthropometric Characteristics. Anthropometric characteristics (palpation, girth, and volume measurements) are primarily used to measure soft tissue edema or joint effusion. Edema or effusion may take several days to develop or become apparent, and effusion can be difficult to detect and even harder to quantify. Changes are more easily appreciated in small superficial joints, such as the interphalangeal joints, than in larger or deeper joints, such as the hip and the lumbar zygapophyseal joints.

Girth[52] and volumetric measurements can be used to detect joint effusion, edema, or muscle atrophy. Palpation is also used to detect temperature changes and joint line tenderness.

Range of Motion. Measures of ROM can help identify inflamed structures and provide important information about impairments and functional limitations. If inflammation and effusion are present, there will usually be a loss of active and passive ROM and a "boggy" or sluggish end-feel.[53] A goniometer is commonly used to measure ROM and has been found to be reliable and valid in a wide range of populations.[54,55]

Muscle Performance. Assessment of motor performance is necessary to characterize limitations of functional joint use, identify muscle or tendon injuries, track patient progress, and to help design an appropriate intervention program to facilitate recovery. However, results of strength testing should be interpreted with caution in this population because motor performance may be impaired by pain.

Although there are multiple methods to assess muscle strength, manual muscle testing (MMT) is appropriate for testing muscle performance in most patients with localized inflammation (see Chapter 5). MMT results are often graded on a 5-point nonlinear scale.

Hand-held dynamometers may also be used to measure strength in this population. They provide a quantitative linear measure of strength.

Joint Integrity and Mobility. To determine joint integrity, the degree and direction of joint play, including any laxity or hypomobility will be noted and compared to the uninvolved side.

Neuromuscular. Common measurement scales, including the horizontal or vertical VAS, the verbal rating scale (VRS), verbal descriptor scales (VDS), and faces pain scales (FPS), may be used to assess pain in patients with localized inflammation (see Chapter 22). Although pain is a hallmark sign of localized inflammation, the absence of pain does not necessarily indicate that the patient does not have pathology or functional deficits.[56]

Cardiovascular/Pulmonary. Several standardized walking tests (2-minute, 6-minute, 12-minute, Shuttle, and Self-Paced) may be used to assess exercise tolerance and cardiovascular fitness in individuals with or without cardiopulmonary pathologies, including those with localized inflammation. These measures may also give the examiner insight into the individual's ability to perform ADLs.[57]

Integumentary. The examination of patients with localized inflammation will include assessment for local warmth, swelling and redness (edema or effusion), temperature changes, tenderness, and muscle atrophy or hypertrophy.

Function

Gait, Locomotion, and Balance. In a patient with localized inflammation, impairments of ROM, edema, strength, sensation, pain, or other concomitant factors can affect gait, locomotion, and balance. A person's ability to ambulate depends on their ability to develop acceleration while maintaining relative stability. Impairments may cause noticeable compensations, deviations, or substitutions in the gait pattern. In general, patients with localized inflammation involving the lower extremities (e.g., trochanteric bursitis) may have reduced gait speed or a noticeable limp as a result of pain (known as an *antalgic gait*).[57] An antalgic gait may also indicate a long-term hip pathology (e.g., OA of the hip joint), resulting in weak hip abductors and a characteristic **Trendelenburg gait.**[58,59] Balance may also be impaired in patients with localized inflammation. This is largely due to changes in gait caused by pain or weakness (see Chapter 13).

Assistive and Adaptive Devices/Orthotic, Protective, and Supportive Devices. Patients with localized inflammation commonly use assistive and adaptive devices, as well as orthotic, protective, and supportive devices, to compensate for decreased muscle performance, ROM impairments, and loss of balance and to protect an inflamed area from further injury, inflammation, and damage. These devices should be examined for fit, function, and effectiveness.

Ergonomics and Body Mechanics. Ergonomics and body mechanics are often examined in patients with localized inflammation because this may identify tasks or activities that contribute to the client's condition. The demands, frequency, duration of exposure, or position of the joints during activity can cause microtrauma over time that then causes localized inflammation. Therefore a thorough evaluation of the patient's ergonomics and body mechanics at work, home, and in the leisure environment may help to establish, reduce, or prevent the cause(s) of their condition.

EVALUATION, DIAGNOSIS, AND PROGNOSIS

According to the *Guide,* patients who fall into the preferred practice pattern 4E: Impaired joint mobility, motor function, muscle performance, and ROM associated with localized inflammation often have the following abnormal examination findings: Temperature changes, joint swelling, loss of ROM, altered function, joint line tenderness, **fluctuance,** and localized pain when the inflamed tissues are stressed.[53] These patients should demonstrate steady improvement and optimal return to function within 6 to 24 physical therapy visits over 2 to 4 months.[2] The optimal number of visits and time frames for each client is determined in part by the pathology, the duration of the event, and any associated concomitant factors that could influence management (e.g., age, cognitive status, overall health status, smoking, and social support).

Currently, there is evidence to suggest that involvement in a rehabilitation program can improve the outcomes of individuals with inflammatory conditions of the joint and surrounding soft tissues such as OA[60] and rheumatoid arthritis.[61] Rehabilitation can limit the formation of edema,[62] help control pain,[63] and allow the person to return to function earlier.[64] The rehabilitation specialist can use physical agents, manual therapy, bracing (splinting and orthotics), strengthening and stretching exercise, work-site modification (ergonomics and tool modification), and patient education to promote recovery and protect the client from further injury.

INTERVENTION

OVERVIEW

Rehabilitation management of inflammatory conditions occurs in two stages: the acute stage and the restorative stage.[9] During the acute stage, which coincides with the inflammatory phase of healing, interventions focus on controlling the inflammatory process, minimizing further injury, promoting healing, and minimizing or eliminating any associated signs and symptoms. Physical agents and bracing or wraps may be used protect the area and limit swelling. The patient should be taught joint protection, rest, and edema management principles. Other goals of treatment at this stage include reducing or eliminating pain and maintaining cardiovascular fitness. Prolonged immobilization should be avoided because this can cause weakness and loss of ROM.[65] This stage usually lasts a few days to a week, depending on the severity of the injury and the tissues involved.[9]

The restorative stage begins as the acute stage or inflammatory phase subsides. The timing of this will vary, depending on the injury and the extent of the damage. This stage coincides with the proliferative phase of tissue healing. The goals of this stage are to establish full pain-free ROM, increase or restore flexibility, improve or restore cardiovascular and muscular fitness and performance (strength, power, and endurance), and address any other neuromuscular deficits (proprioception, coordination, agility, or balance). The ultimate outcome of this stage should be to return the individual to their prior or desired level of function.[9]

PROTECT, REST, ICE, COMPRESSION, AND ELEVATION

PRICE is an acronym for protect, rest, ice, compression, and elevation. This acronym is used to describe the interventions recommended during the acute stage of localized inflammation. These interventions are intended to limit swelling and speed the client's return to activity.

Protection can be accomplished through the use of tape, bracing, an orthosis, or, in severe cases, casting. With acute soft-tissue musculoskeletal injuries a flexible or semi-rigid orthosis is preferred to a rigid cast because experimental and clinical trails have shown that controlled motion results in greater patient satisfaction, earlier recovery of ROM and less strength loss, and a quicker return to activity than does complete immobilization.[64,66] The ideal device (taping, brace, or inflatable cast) should limit the amount of torque applied to the injured area while avoiding disuse associated with prolonged immobilization. This "relative" rest is designed to limit damage to the injured structure while stimulating collagen alignment, preventing adhesions, improving circulation and proprioception, and maintaining muscle strength.[66]

Ice, compression, and elevation limit the formation of edema by reducing local blood flow to the affected area. Ice limits hemorrhaging and edema formation by causing vasoconstriction of small vessels. Ice also helps to control pain. Compression can also reduce blood flow to an area. Moderate compression (40 mm Hg) that reduces local intramuscular blood flow by about 50% is recommended.[67] Elevation of the limb is the final component of PRICE. Elevation limits hemorrhage and reduces edema by reducing the arterial pressure in the elevated limb.

> ### ◎ *Clinical Pearl*
> The interventions recommended during the acute stage of localized inflammation are protect, rest, ice, compression, and elevation (PRICE).

PHYSICAL AGENTS

Cryotherapy. Cryotherapy is the therapeutic application of cold or ice to a patient. Cryotherapy is often used to treat patients with acute localized inflammation because it reduces the formation of edema and hematoma associated with acute trauma and inflammation. Ice produces these effects by causing vasoconstriction, decreasing microvascular permeability, and reducing the rate of local tissue metabolism.[62,68] These effects may also protect the surrounding tissues from secondary trauma that results from pressure and enzymatic reactions.[69] Ice has been shown to reduce pain and the formation of edema associated with injury.

Cryotherapy may also be used during the restorative stage of rehabilitation in patients with localized inflammation. In particular, cryotherapy has been shown to help maintain improved ROM after the application of heat with stretching.[70] It is hypothesized that decreasing the viscoelasticity of the tissues in the stretched position helps maintain the new length and/or that nociceptive input is decreased, allowing tissues that were otherwise too sensitive to stretch to be engaged.[70]

Cryotherapy can be applied for localized inflammation using ice or cold gel packs, ice baths, cold compression pumps, or ice massage. Differences in the thermodynamic properties of these agents may affect their rates of cooling, particularly of the superficial tissues. Ice packs provide more rapid cooling of superficial tissues than gel packs at the same temperature,[69] since ice changing from a solid to a liquid has a greater capacity to absorb heat from the tissues. This difference in effect is less pronounced in deeper tissues because the effect is distributed over a larger volume of tissue.

Cryotherapy has been shown to improve clinical parameters in patients with localized inflammation. It has been shown to improve ROM, strength, and function in clients with radiographically confirmed OA at the knee when compared to standard treatment or a placebo. Recommendations for treatment include a 20 to 30 minute period of application and an interface (soft towel) between the subject and cooling agent, as well as a reminder that cold applied to an area of little muscle or adipose near superficial nerves should be limited to 10 minutes.[71] These recommendations are made to reduce the risk of frostbite because full-thickness skin damage may occur with prolonged application of ice and/or when there is no interface between the cold modality and patient.[72]

Cryotherapy is used in the treatment of patients with acute localized inflammation to reduce edema and hematoma associated with acute trauma and inflammation.

Thermotherapy. Thermotherapy (heat) can decrease pain, promote relaxation, decrease muscle spasm, lower skin impedance, decrease the stiffness of joints, promote collagen extensibility, increase local tissue metabolism, promote vasodilation, and accelerate healing.[73,74] However, thermotherapy should not be used in the acute stage of an injury because it may worsen edema and inflammation. There are many modalities that produce heat, including hot packs, ultrasound, diathermy, paraffin baths, fluidotherapy, whirlpools, and infrared lamps. These modalities can be divided into two broad categories of superficial (<1 cm) and deep (>1 cm) heat. Ultrasound and diathermy are the only heating modalities listed that are considered deep heaters. The rest are superficial heating agents that can be categorized as moist or dry and as having a constant or declining source of energy.[73]

When heating modalities are properly applied, metabolic, vascular, neuromuscular, and soft tissue extensibility are affected. Heat increases the rate of metabolic activity, which increases oxygen consumption and phagocytosis. Increases in tissue temperature are also usually associated with vasodilation and an increase in blood flow to the area that helps bring nutrients and red and white blood cells to that area and remove metabolites. Heat also increases capillary permeability and fluid exchange. Neuromuscular effects of heat include decreased pain, general relaxation, decreased skin impedance, decreased muscle spasm, and increases in nerve conduction velocity and neuronal firing.[73] Thermotherapy is often used to promote flexibility and soft tissue extensibility,[75] which can decrease joint stiffness in patients with chronic localized inflammation. Superficial heat may promote muscle relaxation and flexibility,[76] but it will probably not increase the blood flow to deep muscles.[73] It is recommended that the targeted tissues be heated to between 104° F (40° C) and 113° F (45° C) for 5 to 10 minutes to increase their extensibility.[73]

Thermotherapy is used to promote flexibility and enhance soft tissue extensibility.

Ultrasound. Therapeutic ultrasound (US) produces thermal and nonthermal effects. Thermal effects include increased collagen extensibility, alterations in blood flow, changes in nerve conduction velocity, increased cell membrane permeability, increased tissue metabolism, and increased pain threshold. Thermal US is recommended for use in the restorative stage of rehabilitation of localized inflammation primarily to promote increased soft tissue extensibility before stretching. It is not recommended during the acute stage of rehabilitation of localized inflammation because, as with other forms of heat, thermal US may exacerbate edema and inflammation in the early stages of healing.

Nonthermal effects of US include increased cell membrane permeability, increased intracellular calcium, increased rate of protein synthesis by fibroblasts, production of stronger collagen fibers, altered enzymatic activity, accelerated angiogenesis, increased macrophage responsiveness, accelerated bone healing, increased release of inflammatory mediators (prostaglandin E_2 and leukotriene B_4), and decreased length of the inflammatory stage of tissue healing.[77-81] Pulsed US is recommended in the acute stage of rehabilitation for patients with localized inflammation because it may help stimulate and accelerate the inflammatory phase, leading to earlier healing and resolution of pain.[77,81,82] Even in degenerative conditions that lack clinical signs or symptom of inflammation, such as tendinosis, low level pulsed US may facilitate recovery.[77]

Phonophoresis (the use of US to facilitate transdermal drug delivery) with a corticosteroid, such as dexamethasone, may also help reduce inflammation during the acute stage of rehabilitation.[78]

Selection of the optimal US treatment parameters is based on the goals of the treatment (thermal or nonthermal), the depth of the tissue involved, and the area of the tissue involved. Specific information on the application, precautions, and contraindications related to the application of US can be found in a text on physical agents.[78] For a list of suggested resources, see the Additional Resource list at the end of this chapter.

Electrical Stimulation. Electrical stimulation (ES) can be used to address the impairments (edema, pain, ROM, and force deficits) associated with localized inflammation. For reduction of edema, ES should be applied within the first 24 hours after injury, using a monophasic pulsed current with a pulse rate of around 120 pulses per second, a current amplitude sufficient to produce a strong sensation, and a treatment duration of 20 to 90 minutes, with the cathode at the site of inflammation.

Transcutaneous electrical nerve stimulation (TENS) can reduce the pain associated with localized inflammation. Reducing the pain allows increased activity levels, which lead to a quicker return to function and fewer therapy visits.[63] Two prominent theories for this effect are the gate control theory and the release of endogenous opioids. According to the gate control theory, stimulation of larger diameter myelinated sensory neurons blocks the transmission from smaller diameter pain-transmitting neurons.

There is also evidence that TENS may control pain by promoting the release of endogenous opioids. Opioids activate pathways from the periaqueductal grey and rostral ventral medulla, which inhibits transmission of nociceptive stimuli from spinothalamic tract cells.[63] Increased concentrations of endogenous opioids have been measured in the bloodstream and cerebrospinal fluid of animals and humans after the application of TENS.[63,83]

ES can also be used to promote ROM, increase muscular strength or endurance, and facilitate motor recruitment when motor nerves are stimulated sufficiently to produce muscle contractions. When used in this context, ES is referred to as *neuromuscular electrical stimulation* (NMES). NMES and voluntary exercise with similar regimens both produce significant increases in strength. Adding NMES to exercise enhances strengthening in people with strength deficits.[84-86] The optimal parameters, precautions, and contraindications for applying ES to improve muscle performance are discussed in Chapter 5 of this book.

Iontophoresis. Iontophoresis is the application of an electrical current to promote transdermal drug delivery. The principle of iontophoresis is that low–amperage direct monophasic electrical current will repel drug ions with the same charge into and through the skin to the inflamed structure. Iontophoresis has been used successfully to delivery antiinflammatory drugs, such as dexamethasone, in sufficient concentrations to provide a therapeutic effect, although in lower concentrations than typical with localized injection.[87] Human studies have demonstrated that the delivery of dexamethasone by iontophoresis can produce immediate improvements in impairments associated with localized inflammation, including improved ROM and decreased pain.[88-90]

MANUAL THERAPY

Early mobilization has been suggested to promote early ROM and prevent joint contracture in patients with localized inflammation. However, there is limited evidence to support the use of manual therapy in acute and chronic inflammatory conditions.

THERAPEUTIC EXERCISE

Therapeutic exercise does not necessarily change the course of localized inflammation but may lessen the pain and disability associated with inflammatory conditions such as OA.[91] Exercise and physical activity can increase muscle strength and endurance, retard bone loss, control joint swelling and pain, improve joint lubrication, reduce joint stiffness, maintain or improve flexibility, increase aerobic fitness and reduce fatigue, reduce postural sway, prevent exacerbations and risk factors associated with a sedentary lifestyle, and promote weight management in patients with localized inflammation.[91-97] Exercise should address muscle performance, cardiovascular conditioning, flexibility, and proprioception.

The American College of Sports Medicine (ACSM) recommends that people with arthritis begin exercise slowly and progress gradually, avoiding rapid or repetitive movements of affected joints.[93] Since no one type of exercise has been proved to be more beneficial than another, it is recommended that exercises be well tolerated by the patient, focus on areas of deficits, and address the functional needs of the patient[98,99] (see Chapters 5 and 23). Exercises should be adapted to patients with localized inflammation to avoid overuse and exacerbation of symptoms in areas with localized inflammation. For strengthening, exercise intensity may be progressed according to standard protocols.[100]

During an exacerbation of an inflammatory condition, repetitive movement involved in most strengthening exercises should be avoided. However, it is important to maintain ROM during such periods. Each joint should be moved through its full available ROM at least several times each day to prevent contractures. Static isometric exercises may also be performed to maintain strength. As inflammation resolves, isotonic or dynamic exercise may be started, initially emphasizing low resistance and high repetitions (reps).[101]

Cardiovascular fitness programs for patients with localized inflammation should use low-impact exercises that use large muscle groups in a smooth and continuous manner. Examples include walking, bicycling, swimming, and even dancing.[98,102,103] Exercise intensity is most readily guided by the patient's perceived level of exertion. A level between 11 and 16 on the Borg scale of perceived exertion is appropriate for most patients with localized inflammation.[104] (Chapter 23 includes a discussion of perceived exertion scales including the Borg scale.)

Patients with localized inflammation benefit from exercises to enhance flexibility because poor flexibility increases the risk of injury and interferes with function. Stretching of major muscle groups should be emphasized. Static stretching should be performed slowly to the point of mild discomfort and held for 10 to 30 seconds. Longer durations do not appear to significantly enhance flexibility. If proprioceptive neuromuscular facilitation (PNF) techniques are used, a 6 second contraction should be held, followed by static stretching for 10 to 30 seconds. For either method, each muscle group should be stretched at least 3 times, 2 to 3 days each week.[103,105]

Proprioception may decline with age and joint disorders such as OA at the knee.[27] Inadequate proprioception can lead to repetitive trauma at the joint. In particular, patients with a history of recurrent injuries to the same area and those reporting a feeling of instability or giving way at a joint may benefit from proprioceptive exercises.[33,106] Support sleeves have also been recommended to increase proprioceptive input to enhance a feeling of stability.[107]

Aquatic exercises can be used as an exercise regime when a client has impaired ROM, strength, muscle power, endurance, or balance. As with any other tool, it may not be appropriate for all individuals within a specified practice pattern. The physical properties of water can unload a joint if the water depth is sufficient, while providing varying amounts of resistance, depending on the speed of the movement, depth of the part, the direction of movement, viscosity of the water, and the surface area of the part being moved. The effects of the hydrostatic forces can result in physiological changes (e.g., increased cardiac output by 32%, decreased vital capacity by 8%) when the client is immersed up to their neck.[108] Therefore appropriate screening must be performed before its implementation.

◎ *Clinical Pearl*

Therapeutic exercise can improve muscle performance, cardiovascular conditioning, flexibility, proprioception, and balance.

ORTHOTICS

Orthotics, including braces, taping, and splints, are recommended for patients with localized inflammation to limit the load imposed on the affected structures. This can help the individual return to activity sooner and limit exacerbation of inflammation and local tissue damage. Shoe orthoses, or even shoes with good support, can limit excessive pronation or decrease the demand placed on the Achilles tendon. A brace, strap, or taping placed over the patellar tendon can assist in the recovery of jumper's knee (patellar tendinitis/tendinosis), although it does little to reduce the load to the tendon.[109] Other devices include straps for lateral epicondylitis, neoprene sleeves for knee OA[107] or an unloading brace for unilateral medial compartment OA,[110] compression boots[111] or stabilizing braces for lateral ankle sprains,[112] hand splints for patients with arthritis affecting the hands, orthoses for the spine, and others, depending on the patient's condition and needs (see Chapter 34).

PATIENT EDUCATION

Patient education is aimed at empowering individuals to manage their pathology and its effect on their daily life.[113] Effective education allows the patient to become their own diagnostician about what activities are harmful or helpful and allows them to recognize an exacerbation and implement an appropriate plan to manage it.

Patient education should include information about pathology, methods to reduce inflammation and pain, joint protection strategies, methods to increase function (exercise and ADL training), modification of the home and work environment, and coping strategies. Therapists may use handouts, video, or other educational methods to augment education through direct verbal communication.

JOINT PROTECTION AND TOOL MODIFICATION

Box 7-1 lists common joint protection techniques.[61] Assistive devices can also be used to reduce joint impact during ambulation. Recommendations for joint protection may range from elevating toilets and seats for those with lower extremity or spinal impairments to changing or enlarging the grips of commonly used kitchen or work appliances to providing assistive devices for getting dressed (e.g., buttonhook device). Evidence from randomized controlled trials (RCTs) supports that joint protection reduces pain and improves function in patients with localized inflammation[114] and may even slow the progression of inflammatory diseases.[61]

To optimize recommendations for joint protection to prevent or reduce functional deficits associated with localized inflammation, an assessment of environmental barriers in the home, community, and/or work is recommended. Vibration, mechanical shock, high palmar and gripping loads, external loads, hard and sharp edges, poor postures, and repetitive movements, as well as extremes of temperature, humidity, and psychological stress, may all impact the occurrence of functional limitations associated with localized inflammation.[115,116]

PACING STRATEGIES (ENERGY CONSERVATION)

Pacing strategies involve breaking down daily activities into manageable tasks and devising a strategy for accomplishing those tasks. Pacing requires finding a balance between rest and activity. If a client's symptoms are exacerbated by their current level of activity, they may still be able to complete those activities if they do small amounts at a time. For example, mowing the whole yard or vacuuming the whole house has to be done all at one time or all in 1 day. If the yard takes 3 hours to mow, the person could incorporate an hour of rest for every hour of mowing or they could mow the front yard 1 day and the back yard the next. This takes more time overall, but this strategy may allow the person to achieve their own goals without further injury.

> ### ◎ *Clinical Pearl*
>
> Instructing a patient in pacing strategies may allow a patient whose symptoms are exacerbated by their current level of activities to complete those activities and achieve their goals without further injury.

PSYCHOSOCIAL MANAGEMENT OF CHRONIC INFLAMMATORY DISEASES

Many chronic diseases, such as arthritis, have no cure and will likely have periods of exacerbation with an unpredictable course. These may necessitate day-to-day adjustments in activity, as well as long-term adaptations to a gradual decline in functional capacity, with gradually increasing economic burden over several years.[113] These factors and others can result in stress, depression, and learned helplessness.

Learned helplessness occurs when the client stops trying because they feel helpless. They lose motivation because they do not feel that their efforts affect the outcome. To combat these issues, it has been

---

BOX 7-1	**Common Joint Protection Principles**

1. Respect pain.
2. Avoid improper postures or positions.
3. Avoid staying in one position for a long time.
4. Use the strongest and largest joints and muscles for the job.
5. Avoid sustained joint activities.
6. Maintain muscle strength, joint ROM, and conditioning.
7. Use assistive devices and/or splints.

From Schwarz SP: *250 tips for making life with arthritis easier,* Atlanta, 1997, Longstreet Press.
ROM, Range of motion.

recommended that interventions for patients with chronic conditions involving localized inflammation include stress management, coping skills, cognitive restructuring, problem solving, behavior modification, altering a patient's perception and responses to pain, teaching the difference between harm and hurt, and educating family members about the patient's condition.[117]

CASE STUDY 7-1

OSTEOARTHRITIS

Patient History

JJ is a 53-year-old man who presents with right knee pain, which was diagnosed as being caused by OA. JJ had a right meniscectomy 30 years ago for a torn meniscus. He reports his knee is stiff in the morning, and he has difficulty standing for more than 1 hour, walking for long periods (>20 to 30 minutes), and getting up and down from the floor.

Tests and Measures—Significant Findings
Musculoskeletal
- Height 5 foot 9 inches; weight 200 lb. Bilateral genu varus.
- Palpation of the right knee did not reveal temperature changes. Effusion of the right knee was detectable by palpation along the medial and lateral joint lines.
- Circumferential measurements:

Area	Right	Left
10 cm above medial knee joint line	50 cm	53 cm
Knee joint line	43 cm	42.5 cm
10 cm below medial joint line	41.5 cm	42 cm

- Knee ROM.

Flexion/extension	Right	Left
AROM (sitting)	115-15°	135-0°
PROM (supine)	120-8°	140-0°

- Right knee passive accessory (joint play/component) movements in all directions were decreased compared to the left knee.

Neuromuscular
- Gross coordination and balance appear intact.
- Pain upon examination was 2/10. Pain at worst is 6/10; pain at best is 1/10.

Cardiovascular/Pulmonary
- Using a pedometer, JJ was able to ambulate 402 m (1318.9 feet) in 6 minutes with some shortness of breath. He was able to ascend 10 steps in 24.45 seconds.

Function
- During ambulation on level surfaces, JJ has a slight limp on the right, an anterior trunk lean at initial contact, and decreased stance time on right. When going up and down stairs, he is not able to use a step-over gait because of knee pain and instability. No apparent balance deficits.

Diagnosis
Preferred practice pattern 4E: Impaired joint mobility, motor function, muscle performance, and range of motion associated with localized inflammation.

Interventions
- Initially concentrate on restoring ROM and improving strength. Pain should subside as ROM and strength improve.
- Patient will be enrolled in the Arthritis Foundation aquatics program and given upper extremity strengthening exercises to promote weight loss and cardiovascular endurance.
- Patient will be prescribed a home exercise program that will be adjusted as necessary.

Role of the Physical Therapist Assistant
- Why is aquatic exercise a good form of exercise for this patient?
- Describe and document three exercises of activities that could be used in the clinic to improve R knee ROM in this patient
- What specific strength and/or endurance training exercises would be helpful for this patient?
- Write three home program activities suitable for this patient.

Additional Information
For the full version of this case study, including detailed examination results, interventions, and outcomes, see the Evolve site that accompanies this book.

CHAPTER SUMMARY

This chapter describes the inflammatory process and how various pathologies associated with localized inflammation present. An organized and detailed review of typical examination findings, evaluation, diagnosis, prognosis, and management of individuals is provided for preferred practice pattern 4E: Impaired joint mobility, motor function, muscle performance, and range of motion associated with localized inflammation. Suggestions of interventions, including physical agents and therapeutic exercises, to reduce or minimize the impact the physiology or impairments associated with localized inflammation are presented. The case study demonstrates how this information is applied to practice. This chapter is to be used in conjunction with other chapters in this text to most effectively manage clients with localized inflammation in your practice.

ADDITIONAL RESOURCES

For links to these and additional web-based resources, see the Evolve site.
Cameron MH: *Physical agents in rehabilitation,* ed 3, St. Louis, 2009, Saunders.
Arthritis Foundation

The Bone and Joint Decade
National Institutes for Arthritis, Musculoskeletal, and Skin Diseases

GLOSSARY

Angiogenesis: Development and formation of blood vessels.

Cytokines: Proteins secreted by a variety of cells to help regulate immunological responses (e.g., interleukin, tumor necrosis factor, lymphokines, and interferon).

Fibroblast: Connective tissue cell that secretes proteins (collagen, glycosaminoglycans, elastin, and glycoproteins) to help form the extracellular matrix. Fibroblasts have the ability to differentiate into other cells (e.g., osteoblasts, chondrocytes, and myofibroblasts).

Fluctuance: Abnormal condition in which the area under the skin being palpated feels "boggy" or viscous. It is an indication of pus accumulating, especially if the surrounding area is indurated.

Macrophages: Large cells whose primary role is phagocytosis and removal of pathogens. Macrophages produce a variety of substances (e.g., H_2O_2, ascorbic acid, fibronectin, lactic acid, and angiogenesis growth factor) to promote angiogenesis and wound debridement.

Myofibroblasts: Fibroblasts that differentiated to resemble smooth muscle (contains myofilaments) for the specialized function of approximating (contracting) the borders of an injury.

Neutrophils (granulocytes): Phagocytic white blood cells.

Osteoblasts: Bone-forming cell.

Osteonecrosis: Necrosis of the bone (also avascular necrosis and ischemic necrosis of the bone).

Osteitis pubis: Noninfectious inflammation of the pubis.

Trendelenburg gait: Disorder of the hip abductors caused by weakness or an inhibition. During the stance phase, the body weight is transferred to the affected side and the hip abductors on the affected side are unable to support the pelvis, resulting in a pelvic drop or tilt toward the swing limb. Although typically seen in adults, this gait pattern may be seen in children with a slipped capital femoral epiphysis.

Spinal Disorders

Cynthia Chiarello

OBJECTIVES

After reading this chapter, the reader will be able to:
1. Identify the pathophysiological and mechanical basis of selected common pathological conditions of the spine.
2. Discuss the importance of classification systems for guiding the management of spinal dysfunction.
3. Describe typical findings of scanning and detailed spinal examinations.
4. Describe the evidence to support the use of various rehabilitation interventions for the management of spinal disorders.

*M*usculoskeletal spinal disorders are an immense problem in industrialized societies resulting in tremendous personal and economic costs. Low back pain (LBP) is usually defined as pain extending from the twelfth rib inferiorly to the gluteal fold, whereas neck pain is pain between the occiput and the third thoracic vertebra.[1] It is estimated that 70% to 85% of the population will experience back or neck pain at some time in their life and between 14% and 50% of adults have LBP at some time during any single year. In the United States, LBP is the most common reason for activity limitation in individuals under the age of 45, and approximately 2% of the workforce receives compensation for LBP annually.[2] LBP is also common during normal pregnancy, occurring in 48% to 90% of pregnancies, and is two to three times more common in pregnant women than in the general population.[3-5]

It is a commonly held belief that LBP almost always resolves within 4 to 6 weeks. However, there is evidence to suggest that this is not the case. For example, one study found that only 30% of patients with back pain in primary care practices were pain-free within 4 weeks, whereas 70% to 80% still had symptoms.[6] In addition, it may appear that back pain has resolved in many patients because they do not return to their health care provider with this complaint, but this may reflect a disillusionment or dissatisfaction with the medical establishment rather than a resolution of symptoms.[6] It is reported that although up to 75% of individuals with new episodes of back pain return to work within 4 to 6 weeks, many remain symptomatic.[6] Furthermore, even if an episode of back pain passes, this does not imply a resolution of the problem, since the hallmark of LBP is recurrence, with as many as 85% of individuals experiencing multiple episodes. In fact, the strongest predictor for back pain is a previous episode of back pain.[2,7]

Musculoskeletal impairment is the most common impairment for those under the age of 65 years, and spine impairments are the most frequent subcategory of musculoskeletal impairment. LBP is the most frequent reason for referral to outpatient physical therapy, representing over 25% of outpatient discharges from both hospital-based and private physical therapy practices.[8] Because spine-related pain is such a large-scale problem, affecting much of the population, it is imperative that physical therapists (PTs) and physical therapist assistants (PTAs) are well equipped to manage spinal problems.

Physical therapy plays a critical role in the management of patients with spinal disorders. PTs are required to have an in-depth knowledge of musculoskeletal examination and evaluation in order to determine and direct the most appropriate interventions, assess outcomes, recognize serious pathology, and make referrals to other health

TABLE 8-1	The Phases of Spinal Degeneration as Described by Kirkaldy-Willis		
	Facet Joints	Clinical Presentation	Intervertebral Disc
Phase I: Dysfunction	Synovitis Minimal cartilage degeneration	Restricted movement Unilateral radicular symptoms	Circumferential and radial annular tears
Phase II: Unstable	Joint capsule laxity Facet joint subluxation Subperiosteal osteophytes	Increased movement Unilateral radicular symptoms	Tears all the way through the annulus Complete internal disc disruption Circumferential annular bulging Loss of disc height
Phase III: Stabilization	Periarticular fibrosis Osteophytes	Restricted movement Multilevel bilateral radicular symptoms	Ossification

Adapted from Kirkaldy-Willis W, Gernard T: *Managing low back pain*, ed 4, New York, 1991, Churchill Livingstone.

TABLE 8-2	Sensory, Motor, and Reflex Nerve Root Innervation		
Nerve Root	Sensory Distribution	Motor Distribution	Reflexes
C4	Top of the shoulder	Trapezius, rhomboid	None
C5	Lateral arm	Deltoid, biceps, brachioradialis	Biceps
C6	Lateral forearm, thumb, and index finger	Biceps, extensor carpi radialis longus and brevis	Brachioradialis
C7	Middle finger	Triceps, pronator teres	Triceps
C8	Medial forearm, little and ring finger	Interossei, flexor digitorum profundus	None
T1	Medial arm	Interossei	None
L2	Proximal anteromedial thigh	Iliopsoas, adductors	None
L3	Distal anteromedial thigh, knee, and upper leg	Adductors, quadriceps	None
L4	Medial leg and foot	Tibialis anterior, quadriceps	Patellar
L5	Lateral leg and dorsum of the foot	Extensor hallucis longus	Hamstring, Achilles
S1	Lateral foot, posteromedial thigh and leg	Peroneus longus and brevis, gluteus maximus,	Achilles
S2	Posterolateral thigh	Gastrocnemius, soleus, gluteus maximus	Achilles

professionals when indicated. PTAs must be familiar with typical examination findings in patients with spinal disorders and be competent at providing interventions for patients with spinal disorders. This chapter provides the reader with an overview of techniques of examination and details of intervention for patients with spinal disorders, assuming that the reader is already familiar with the basics of anatomy and spinal biomechanics.[9,10]

PATHOLOGY

PHASES OF SPINAL DEGENERATION

Progressive degenerative changes of the spine are often associated with symptoms.[11] This degeneration can be considered to occur in three phases, progressing from restricted movement during phase I (dysfunction), followed by hypermobility in phase II (unstable), and then again by stability in the final phase, phase III (stabilization) (Table 8-1).[11,12]

RADICULOPATHY

In general, a **radiculopathy** occurs when nerve conduction in the axons of a spinal nerve or its roots is impeded by compression or ischemia.[10] Numbness results when conduction is blocked in sensory nerves, and weakness occurs when motor nerves are obstructed. Signs of radiculopathy include muscle wasting, motor weakness, depressed deep tendon reflexes, and sensory changes in the distribution of the involved nerve root.[13] Symptoms commonly include central spinal pain, with or without associated pain radiating from the neck or back to the limb. When a single nerve root is affected, the signs and symptoms are limited to the specific distribution of that nerve root. The typical sensory, motor, and reflex changes caused by disturbances at individual nerve roots are shown in Table 8-2.

Encroachment on the central spinal canal or neural foramina can cause radicular symptoms (Fig. 8-1). Encroachment may have a variety of causes, including space-occupying lesions such as a bony spur or a protruding disc, osteoarthrosis of the spinal joints, degeneration of the ligamentum flavum or facet joint capsule, or nerve root sleeve fibrosis or hyperplasia. Nerves are particularly susceptible to injury at the nerve root because in this area there is no dense connective tissue between the nerve fibers and because the connective tissue covering the nerve, the perineurium, may be missing or not well developed in this area.[12,14] Nerve root encroachment may injure the nerve by mechanical and chemical means. Mechanical compression can cause direct damage, and indirectly, compression may cause damage by impairing blood flow to the nerve or by tethering it to surrounding structures, thus reducing its mobility and making it vulnerable to irritation from stretch.[14] Chemical irritation may be produced by direct contact of nucleus pulposus material from the disc with the spinal nerves. This can reduce nerve conduction and cause biochemically mediated inflammatory, microvascular, and structural injury to the nerve.[14]

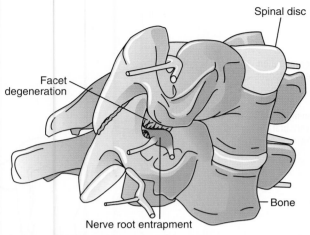

FIG. 8-1 Neural foraminal stenosis causing nerve root entrapment and radiculopathy.

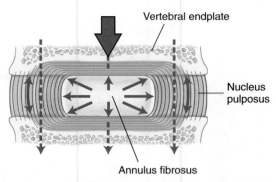

FIG. 8-2 Force distribution in the nucleus pulposus and annulus fibrosus in response to compression. *Modified from Bogduk N: Clinical anatomy of the lumbar spine and sacrum, ed 3, New York, 1997, Churchill Livingstone. In Neumann DA:* Kinesiology of the musculoskeletal system, *ed 2, St. Louis, 2010, Mosby.*

Synovial cytokines, which come from facet joint leaking, and T cells, which are present during inflammation, can also impair nerve function.[14]

INTERVERTEBRAL DISC DISEASE

Intervertebral disc (IVD) disease is responsible for a large proportion of spinal disorders. It is estimated that 5.7 million new cases of IVD disease will be diagnosed each year.[15] The IVD has a unique structure that allows for mobility at the interbody joint while maintaining weight-bearing capabilities and withstanding mechanical stress. The IVD is made up of three components (Fig. 8-2): An outer cartilaginous ring, the **annulus fibrosus (AF)**; an inner gelatinous core, the **nucleus pulposus (NP)**; and vertebral end plates (VEP) that cover the disc from above and below. In a healthy, normal IVD the interaction of these components accounts for the disc's mechanical weight-bearing properties. When the disc is loaded in compression, as occurs in standing, the weight of the head, arms, and trunk are transmitted through the VEP to the NP. Since the NP cannot be compressed, it exerts the force centrifugally in all directions, distracting the annular fibers. This annular tension prevents further expansion of the NP, and thus the weight is borne on both the NP and AF. The radial force exerted by the NP supports the AF and places pressure on the VEP, allowing for the load to be transmitted from one vertebra to the next.[9]

The unique structure of the IVD also allows for complex spinal movements. All spinal movements affect the IVD, the interbody and zygapophyseal (facet) joints, the posterior ligaments, and the muscles around the spine. During bending, including flexion, extension, and lateral flexion to either side, the IVD is compressed on the concave side of the curve and stretched on the convex side of the curve.

The NP tries to escape the compressive force by moving to the convexity.[9] For example, in spinal flexion, the anterior annular fibers buckle, the posterior annular fibers are under tension, and the NP moves posteriorly to escape the anterior compression (Fig. 8-3). The load on the disc causes the pressure within the nucleus to rise. If there are degenerative changes, such as clefts or fissures within the disc, the additional pressure may lead to rupture of annular lamellae and herniation of the NP.[9] Torsion or twisting movements occur when all points on one vertebra move circumferentially in a direction opposite to the adjacent vertebra.[9] During a twisting movement, the attachments of fibers from the AF oriented in the direction of the twist will separate and resist the motion. When stress exceeds the mechanical capabilities of the disc or when the disc degenerates, lesions may develop.[16]

A healthy disc, without any previous injury, can withstand compression without NP herniation. Under continued or excessive loading in compression or in compression with flexion, as occurs with heavy lifting in untrained individuals, or with an unanticipated fall, the VEP develops fractures. These VEP fractures may damage and break down the NP, causing a decrease in disc height and radial bulging of the annulus. The NP then herniates through fissures in the AF under the normal minor compression that occurs with daily activities involving spinal flexion or flexion together with rotation. Various types of IVD herniations are shown in Fig. 8-4. With conservative management, IVD herniations diminish in size or completely resolve and symptoms resolve.

It is difficult to distinguish normal age-related changes in the IVD from pathological degenerative changes. Over time the NP dehydrates, changing from a translucent, mucoid, gelatinous structure to an opaque, white fibrocartilaginous structure, which is barely distinguishable from the AF.[9,17-20] This dehydration changes the disc's fluid mechanical response to loading from fluid pressurization of the NP to elastic deformation of the annulus, increasing the risk for annular injury.[20] Disc degeneration also makes the disc stiffer and the annulus weaker, further increasing the risk of annular tears and fissures.[21]

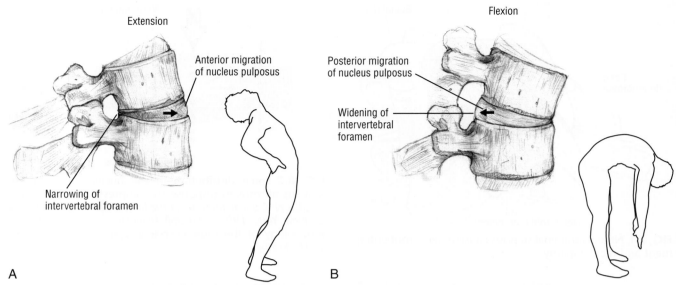

FIG. 8-3 The effect of extension and flexion on the intervertebral disc. **A,** Lumbar extension producing a sight anterior migration of the nucleus pulposus and narrowing of the intervertebral foramen. **B,** Lumbar flexion producing a sight posterior migration of the nucleus pulposus and widening of the intervertebral foramen. *From Mansfield PJ:* Essentials of kinesiology for the physical therapist assistant, *St. Louis, 2009, Mosby.*

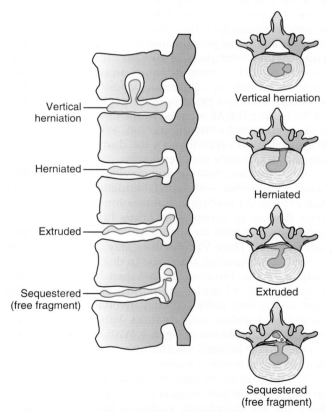

FIG. 8-4 Types of disc herniation: Vertical herniation, herniated, extruded, and sequestered.

Disc dehydration also makes the disc thinner and shorter, increasing compression of the facet joints and reducing the size of the intervertebral foramina. This increases the risk for nerve root impingement. If the IVD herniates, it may become even thinner. Loss of disc height appears to be related to degenerative changes and not age alone, since average lumbar disc height has been found to increase up to the fifth to seventh decade[22,23]; the decline in overall body height with age is due to decreased height of the vertebral bodies.[24]

The AF also dehydrates and degenerates to some degree with age. After the age of 50 years, the AF commonly has peripheral tears or rim lesions in the outer layer, circumferential tears or a split between the AF layers, and radial tears extending from the NP to the outer annulus.[25] Annular tears have been observed to occur together with mechanical changes in the vertebral bone and intervertebral joint complex,[26] suggesting that these degenerative changes may not necessarily be a function of age but rather reflect progression over time after an injury has occurred.[17]

◎ *Clinical Pearl*

Although degenerative disc changes increase with age, if the disc is injured degeneration will start early and progress over time.

SPINAL STENOSIS

Spinal stenosis is a narrowing of the spinal canal, intervertebral foramina, or radicular canals, resulting from bony or soft tissue encroachment reducing the space between the spinal cord or spinal nerve roots and the vertebral elements.[27-30] Spinal stenosis occurs most often in the elderly, may occur at one or several spinal levels, and can have a variety of causes.[27] Spinal stenosis does not always cause symptoms, and the amount of narrowing is not necessarily proportional to the intensity of symptoms.

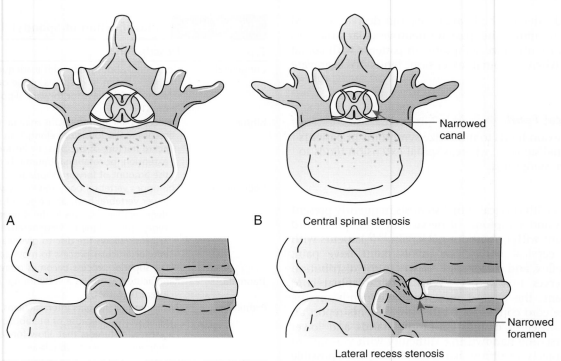

A

B   Narrowed canal

Central spinal stenosis

Narrowed foramen

Lateral recess stenosis

FIG. 8-5 **A,** Normal. **B,** Stenotic.

TABLE 8-3	Classification of Cervical Spinal Stenosis Syndromes
Clinical Syndrome	**Parts of Spinal Cord Affected**
Transverse lesion syndrome	Corticospinal, spinothalamic, and posterior cord tracts
Motor system syndrome	Corticospinal tracts and anterior horn cells
Central cord syndrome	More pronounced motor and sensory deficits in the upper extremities than in the lower extremities
Brown-Séquard syndrome	Ipsilateral motor deficits with contralateral sensory deficits
Brachialgia and cord syndrome	Radicular upper extremity pain together with motor or sensory long-tract signs

Because asymptomatic stenosis is common, as with other degenerative spinal changes, diagnosis is established by agreement between signs, symptoms, and imaging studies (Table 8-3).[27]

Cervical spinal stenosis may be classified into clinically relevant syndromes according to the portion of the spinal cord producing the symptoms.[31] Classification of lumbar spinal stenosis is based on either etiology or anatomical location. The etiology of spinal stenosis can also be further subdivided into congenital or acquired. Congenital stenosis, which is rare, is caused by idiopathic or developmental narrowing of the spinal canal and by itself does not necessarily cause compression of nerves but rather makes the patient more vulnerable to other sources of narrowing.

Congenital stenosis usually becomes symptomatic in the fourth to fifth decade. Acquired spinal stenosis, which is more common than congenital stenosis, is usually caused by degeneration of bone or ligaments and IVD protrusion. Acquired stenosis usually becomes symptomatic in the sixth to seventh decade.

Classification of spinal stenosis based on the anatomical location of the narrowing is used to guide surgical intervention. Central stenosis (Fig. 8-5, *B* top) is mainly caused by facet joint hypertrophy, buckling of the ligamentum flavum, disc protrusion, degenerative spondylolisthesis, or a combination of these anatomical changes.[27,28] Lateral stenosis (Fig. 8-5, *B* bottom), which narrows the canal through which the nerve root exits the spinal canal, involves facet joint hypertrophy and osteophyte formation, decreased disc height, and protrusion of the disc posterolaterally into the intervertebral foramen. The degenerative changes seen in central stenosis can cause lateral stenosis, or lateral stenosis may occur alone.

There is considerable individual variation in spinal cord and vertebral canal volume, size, and shape, which results in variation in the amount of space available for the cord within the bony canal. In the cervical cord, a narrow canal increases susceptibility to symptomatic stenosis. Spinal stenosis also has a dynamic component because the dimensions of the spinal canal and intervertebral foramina, as well as the volume of the spinal cord, change with flexion and extension of the spine. The spinal canal narrows with extension and widens with flexion in both normal and degenerated spines, with more narrowing occurring during extension if there is more degeneration. The spinal cord stretches with flexion, decreasing its cross-sectional area, and thickens with extension, increasing its cross-sectional area.[32] Thus spinal flexion, which increases spinal and intervertebral canal area and decreases spinal cord area, optimizes the space for neurovascular structures and tends to minimize symptoms in patients with spinal stenosis, whereas spinal extension tends to aggravate symptoms.

> ### ◎ *Clinical Pearl*
>
> Spinal flexion tends to minimize symptoms in patients with spinal stenosis, whereas spinal extension tends to aggravate symptoms.

Patients with cervical spinal stenosis frequently present with signs and symptoms of nerve root and spinal cord involvement with or without neck pain.[29,32] Patients with primarily cervical nerve root involvement have pain, sensory, reflex, and motor disturbances in the distribution of the nerves involved.[29,32] With cervical spinal cord involvement, the clinical presentation depends on the area of the cord compressed, but most patients report an insidious onset of clumsiness in the hands and lower limbs, worsening handwriting, difficulty with grasping or holding objects, or diffuse hand numbness, with possible balance difficulties and an awkward gait.[29]

Lumbar spinal stenosis is clinically characterized by disabling chronic and progressive LBP, unilateral or bilateral leg pain, and lower extremity weakness. Since the L3-4 and L4-5 segments are most often affected, cauda equina compression can produce radicular symptoms with motor, sensory, and reflex changes in the affected nerve root distributions.[27,28,30] Neurological signs and symptoms are present in only about 50% of patients during examination but may become evident in many more with symptom-provoking activities such as walking.[27]

The hallmark of lumbar spinal stenosis is **neurogenic claudication,** which is activity-dependent pain radiating into the thigh, leg, or both that increases with prolonged standing or lumbar extension and that is relieved by sitting, lying down, or lumbar flexion. Patients with lumbar spinal stenosis generally walk with a forward-stooped posture with lumbar flexion.[33] Neurogenic claudication is increased by increasing lumbar lordosis of the spine even without activity and improves with increased spinal flexion. In addition, patients with neurogenic claudication tend to have worse symptoms walking downhill because this puts the spine in extension and less pain with walking uphill as this puts the spine in flexion.

> ### ◎ *Clinical Pearl*
>
> The hallmark of lumbar spinal stenosis is neurogenic claudication, which is activity-dependent pain radiating into the thigh, leg, or both that increases with prolonged standing or lumbar extension and that is relieved by sitting, lying down, or lumbar flexion.

SPONDYLOLYSIS AND SPONDYLOLISTHESIS

Spondylolysis is a bilateral defect in the pars interarticularis of a vertebra that decreases the ability of the posterior

TABLE 8-4	Classification of Spondylolisthesis
Type	**Description**
Congenital	Congenital abnormality with inadequacy of the upper sacrum or dysplasia of the posterior arch of L5. Allows for forward slippage of L5 on S1.
Isthmic	Defect in pars interarticularis may be due to recurrent microfracture elongating the pars, acute fracture of the pars, or flexion, extension, or rotational trauma. Is graded by the amount of forward slippage.
Degenerative	The upper vertebral body moves forward on the lower vertebral body as a result of spondylotic degenerative changes in the disc and zygapophyseal joints. Degenerative facet arthrosis allows the disc to give way and the inferior articular process to move forward as the superior process becomes more eroded.
Traumatic	Rare, acute fracture in a vertebra not in the pars interarticularis.
Pathological	Weakening of the pars interarticularis, pedicle, or facet joint because of metabolic bone diseases or tumors that allow forward slippage of superior vertebrae.

Data from Esses S: *Textbook of spinal disorders,* Philadelphia, 1995, JB Lippincott; Kirkaldy-Willis W, Gernard T: *Managing low back pain,* ed 4, New York, 1991, Churchill Livingstone.

elements to stabilize the motion segment.[34] **Spondylolisthesis** occurs when a vertebra translates forward in the sagittal plane with respect to an adjacent vertebra. The intact facet joint or the pedicles usually resist this forward slippage. Spondylolysis can progress to or occur with spondylolisthesis or may occur alone. Spondylolysis and spondylolisthesis are usually diagnosed radiologically. As with other radiological findings, caution must be exercised when attributing symptoms to these abnormalities since both spondylolysis and spondylolisthesis can be asymptomatic.

Spondylolisthesis is common in the lumbar spine and rare in the cervical spine. When spondylolisthesis does occur in the cervical spine, it is usually due to defects in the pars lateralis of the pedicles of C2, C4, or C6.[32] In the lumbar spine, spondylolisthesis can be classified by etiology as described in Table 8-4 and illustrated in Fig. 8-6.[35]

Age appears to play a role in the development of spondylolisthesis. Spondylolysis and spondylolisthesis can occur during adolescence, possibly as a result of rapid growth and increased athletic participation, but symptoms usually start later in life. In adults, patients who present with pain and are found to have spondylolisthesis have similar symptoms to those with spine-related pain without spondylolisthesis.

> ### ◎ *Clinical Pearl*
>
> Spondylolisthesis describes the anterior displacement of a vertebra in relation to the vertebrae below and is commonly found in the lumbar spine but rarely in the cervical spine.

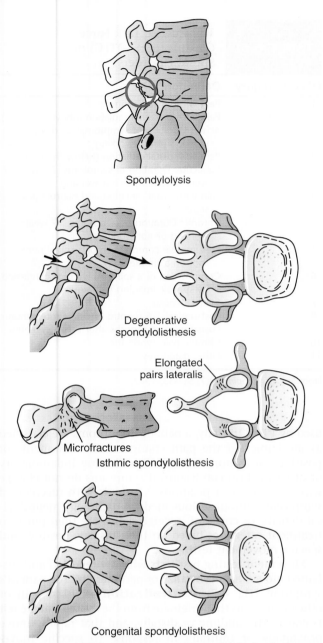

FIG. 8-6 Spondylolysis and types of spondylolisthesis: Degenerative, isthmic, and congenital.

WHIPLASH-ASSOCIATED DISORDERS

Whiplash-associated disorders (WAD) are bony or soft tissue injuries of the neck and related areas that occur after a rear or side collision in which the neck is subjected to acceleration–deceleration. Most WADs are caused by motor vehicle accidents, but WAD may also be caused by sports-related injuries and falls. WAD most commonly causes neck pain, headache, and decreased cervical spine mobility but can also cause neck stiffness and low back and shoulder pain, as well as visual disturbances and dizziness.[36,37]

Although the IVDs, facet joints, and vascular and neurological systems may sometimes be involved in WAD, the ligaments and muscles generally sustain most damage as a result of direct stretching or neuromuscular reflex contractions. With acute WAD, there is typically a decreased cervical active range of motion (AROM), more activity in the superficial neck flexors, and generalized hypersensitivity to many stimuli.

Many individuals with WAD improve rapidly, but some continue to experience significant pain and disability. Patients with symptoms at 3 months tend to continue to have symptoms for 2 years or more.[37] Several factors have been linked to delayed recovery and poor outcome, including sociodemographic status, crash-related features, litigation, and various other physical and psychosocial factors. There is strong evidence and agreement that a high initial pain intensity immediately after the injury predicts a difficult and extended recovery.[38-41]

BACK PAIN DURING PREGNANCY AND POSTPARTUM

Back pain during pregnancy is common. Large-scale studies have found that 35% to 90% of women have back pain during pregnancy and that back pain during pregnancy is 2 to 3 times more common than at other times in life. Although many factors may be associated with an increased risk of back pain during pregnancy, a history of back pain before pregnancy is the most consistent and well-substantiated risk factor.[42-46] Having back pain during pregnancy does not affect the pregnancy outcome[47] and does not appear to be associated with weight gain before or during pregnancy.[45] Back pain during pregnancy may severely limit activities of daily living (ADLs) beyond the typical limitations experienced during pregnancy and more than one-third of women who have back pain during pregnancy find that this pain limits their activities.[4,48]

Back pain during pregnancy and postpartum may originate from the lumbar spine (above the sacrum) or from the sacroiliac (SI) joint structures (also called *posterior pelvic pain* [PPP]).[43,49-51] Pain from the lumbar spine generally increases with forward flexion, causes decreased lumbar ROM, is elicited with palpation of the lumbar spine muscles, has negative SI joint provocation tests, has occurred previously, and improves with exercise and education.[43,49,51] In contrast, with PPP, which is four times more common than lumbar spine pain during pregnancy, lumbar ROM is normal; pain is located in the buttocks and posterior pelvis; is worse with walking, standing, or turning in bed; may decrease with an SI belt; is elicited with palpation of the gluteal and hip muscles; has positive SI provocation tests; and usually begins during pregnancy.[49,50] Women with PPP do not appear to benefit from back exercises and education addressing the lumbar spine.[51] Lumbar pain and PPP can coexist during pregnancy.[3-5,44]

Current evidence indicates that back pain during pregnancy is not a normal consequence of pregnancy that can be predicted to resolve with delivery. Approximately 15% to 65% of women report substantial persistent back and pelvic pain postpartum,[48] and if a woman has back pain during pregnancy, she is at increased risk of pain postpartum[5,49] and has a poor prognosis for improvement immediately after delivery. Postpartum pain does not appear to be related to the use of epidural anesthesia or to the type of delivery.[47] Some risk factors for pain persisting 2 years or more after delivery are onset of severe pain early in gestation and inability to decrease weight to prepregnancy levels.[47]

◎ *Clinical Pearl*

Back pain during pregnancy usually originates from the sacroiliac (SI) joint structures and does not appear to improve with back exercises or education for the low back but may benefit from an SI belt.

SPINAL DISORDER CLASSIFICATION SYSTEMS

Spinal disorders are not caused by a single pathological entity, and very often the precise cause of a patient's signs and symptoms is not known. Therefore a number of **classification systems** have been developed to categorize spinal disorders into syndromes based on a combination of pathology, clustering of signs and symptoms, and duration of symptoms. These classification systems can help with clinical decision making, determining prognosis, evaluating the quality of care, conducting research, and selecting interventions for patients with spinal disorders.[52] Currently, several classification systems are being investigated for clinical usefulness, reliability, and validity.

The Québec Task Force on Spinal Disorders classification system is the system most frequently referred to by physicians and the medical literature. The three classification systems most often used by PTs are the McKenzie Classification System, the Treatment-Based Classification System, and the Movement System Impairment-Based Classification.

The Québec Task Force on Spinal Disorders Classification System. In 1987 the Québec Task Force on Spinal Disorders presented a diagnostic classification system for spinal disorders that could be used to assist in making clinical decisions, determining prognosis, assessing quality of care, and carrying out scientific research.[53] Patients are classified using simple clinical criteria determined through history, physical examination, radiological tests, and reaction to treatment. This system classifies activity-related spinal disorders into 11 categories and further divides these categories by duration of symptoms and work status (Table 8-5).

The McKenzie Classification System for Spinal Disorders. The McKenzie approach to classifying patients with back pain is the system most commonly

TABLE 8-5	The Québec Task Force Classification (QTFC) of Spinal Disorders
QTFC Category	**Definition**
1	Pain without radiation
2	Pain with proximal radiation (above the knee)
	Acute: Duration of symptoms: <7 days; working or not working
3	Pain with distal radiation (below the knee)
	Subacute: Duration of symptoms: 7 days to 7 weeks; working or not working
4	Pain with distal radiation and neurological signs
	Chronic: Duration of symptoms: >7 weeks; working or not working
5	Presumptive compression of a spinal nerve root on a simple x-ray
6	Compression of a spinal nerve root confirmed by specific imaging techniques
7	Spinal stenosis
8	Postsurgical 1-6 months after the intervention
9	Postsurgical >6 months after the intervention
10	Chronic pain syndrome
11	Other diagnoses

From Spitzer W: *Spine* 12(7):S1-S53, 1987.

used by PTs.[54] Initially, a patient's symptoms are classified as mechanical if the pain changes with movements or positions or as nonmechanical, indicating inflammatory or other medical conditions, if symptoms do not change with movement or positions.[55] Patients with mechanical symptoms without serious medical pathology, neurological deficits, or constant, severe sciatica are then put into treatment categories based on their history, posture, and specific movement testing.

Movement testing first tests whether repeated and sustained movements centralize or peripheralize the patient's symptoms (Fig. 8-7). **Centralization** refers to pain or other symptoms that originate from the spine, that are felt lateral to the midline or distally, and that rapidly move proximally or centrally in response to specific movements.[56,57] Movements that cause centralization are believed to be therapeutic. Peripheralization refers to pain or other symptoms moving laterally or distally in response to specific movements. Movements that cause peripheralization should be avoided or minimized.

Back pain is then also classified into one of the following three syndromes: postural, dysfunction, or derangement. The examination findings and suggested interventions for each of these syndromes are summarized in Table 8-6. **Postural syndrome** is thought to be caused by prolonged abnormal stresses that produce mechanical deformation or vascular insufficiency and then pain in normal articular or contractile structures.[56,58,59] The **dysfunction syndrome** is characterized by pain that results from mechanical deformation of abnormal adaptively shortened soft tissue following maintenance of poor positioning after degeneration, trauma, or a derangement. This pain is intermittent and occurs with a loss of ROM

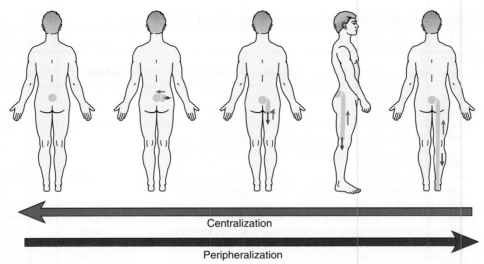

FIG. 8-7 Centralization occurs when symptoms move toward the midline or site of origin. Peripheralization occurs when symptoms move away from the midline or site of origin. *From Magee DJ:* Orthopedic physical assessment, *ed 5, Philadelphia, 2008, Saunders.*

in a specific direction. The **derangement syndrome** is characterized by anatomical disruption of the structures of the intervertebral joints. McKenzie originally attributed a derangement to internal disruption of the IVD or herniation of the NP but later stated that pain from derangement can also be caused by displacement of articular structures. In a derangement, spinal movement is painful and limited in the direction of displacement.[56,58,59]

Overall, despite conflicting reports, most of the evidence indicates that therapists can reliably categorize low back patients according to the McKenzie classification system, particularly if they have some additional training in the use of this system.

Treatment-Based Classification System for Spinal Disorders. A treatment-based classification system was developed by Delitto and colleagues. According to this system patients are categorized based on the history of their condition, the responses of signs and symptoms to movement tests, and alignment of body structures.[60,61] This treatment-based system has two to three levels reflecting the clinical decisions needed for patient classification.

The first level is based on whether the patient can be managed primarily and independently by PT or by a PT in consultation with another health care practitioner, or if referral to another health care practitioner is required. Information for classification at this level is obtained from patient self-reports, a medical screening questionnaire, a modified **Oswestry Low Back Pain Disability Questionnaire,** pain diagrams, a pain scale, and Waddell's screening for abnormal illness behavior.[52,61,62]

The second level of classification is based on the stage and severity of disability. In stage I, also referred to as *acute,*[61,63] patients cannot sit for more than 30 minutes, stand for more than 15 minutes, and walk more than $\frac{1}{4}$ mile and have an Oswestry score of greater than 30.[62] In stage II, which reflects a less severe problem, patients have an Oswestry score between 15 and 30, but their back pain

still prevents them from performing instrumental ADLs (IADLs).[62] In stage III, patients can perform IADLs and score less than 15 on the Oswestry, but they cannot perform sustained activities requiring high physical demands.[62]

The third level of classification only applies to patients with acute symptoms (stage I) and consists of four categories: immobilization, **mobilization,** specific exercise, and traction.[63] Patients are placed into these categories based on key examination findings, and each category designates specific recommended treatments.[61] Patients in the immobilization category have findings indicating lumbar segmental instability. Patients in the mobilization category have findings indicating that they need lumbar or SI mobilization or **manipulation.** Patients in the specific exercise category have centralization during the examination, and patients who appear to have nerve root compression without centralization are placed into the traction category (Table 8-7).

Patient classification may change during an episode of back pain. Thus patients receive interventions specific to their individual presentation, and these interventions are modified as the patient's presentation changes.[63]

Patient classification according to the treatment-based approach has moderate interrater reliability, and this system has demonstrated validity in directing effective treatment. In a randomized controlled trial (RCT), the outcome of patients with LBP treated for 4 weeks as directed by this classification system had greater improvement in disability, were more likely to return to work, and were more satisfied with treatment. Also, there was a trend toward lower costs than for patients treated according to clinical practice guidelines for patients with acute work-related LBP.

Movement System Impairment-Based Classification System for Low Back Pain. A movement system impairment-based classification system was developed by Sahrmann and colleagues. This classification

TABLE 8-6	The McKenzie Classification System for Spinal Disorders	
Category	Examination Findings	Suggested Interventions
POSTURAL SYNDROME		
	Lumbar posture is poor in sitting and standing but without deformity. Pain occurs only with sustained postures and is not reproduced by repeated movements.	Promote postural correction. Avoid sustained end-range positions.
DYSFUNCTION SYNDROMES		
Flexion	Poor posture with loss of movement or function. No pain or radiation with movement. Pain at end-range of flexion that does not worsen with repetition. Loss of flexion ROM. Symptoms appear stable without rapid changes.	End-range flexion exercises.
Extension	Poor posture with loss of movement or function. Pain at end-range of extension. Loss of extension ROM. Symptoms appear stable without rapid changes.	End-range extension exercises.
Adherent root	Intermittent sciatic pain. Loss of flexion ROM with deviation during range. Flexion reproduces lower extremity pain that ceases on standing.	Stretching exercises for adherent nerve root.
Side-gliding	Poor posture occurs with loss of movement or function. Loss of side-gliding ROM with intermittent central LBP at end-range of side-glide, which does not worsen with repetition.	End-range gliding exercises.
DERANGEMENT SYNDROMES		
One	Central or symmetrical LBP without postural deformity of lumbar spine. Repeated flexion may peripheralize or worsen pain. Repeated extension centralizes, diminishes, or eliminates pain.	Initially repeated extension exercises.
Two	Central or symmetrical LBP, with or without buttock or thigh pain. Lumbar kyphosis.	Initially prone lying or sustained extension position followed by repeated extension exercises.
Three	Unilateral LBP, with or without buttock or thigh pain. No postural deformity of lumbar spine. Repeated flexion may peripheralize or worsen pain. Repeated extension centralizes, diminishes, or eliminates pain.	Usually repeated extension exercises centralize pain. If not, side-glide with extension.
Four	Unilateral or asymmetrical LBP with or without buttock or thigh pain. Lateral shift postural deformity. Flexion and extension increase pain.	Correction of lateral shift followed by extension exercises.
Five	Unilateral or asymmetrical LBP with or without buttock or thigh pain. Constant or intermittent leg pain extends below the knee. Repeated flexion peripheralizes or worsens pain. Repeated extension centralizes, diminishes, or eliminates pain.	Usually repeated extension exercises centralize pain. If not, side-glide or rotation followed by extension exercises.
Six	Unilateral or asymmetrical LBP with or without buttock or thigh pain. Constant leg pain extends below the knee. Lateral shift postural deformity. Flexion and extension increase pain.	Correction of lateral shift followed by extension exercises.
Seven	Unilateral or bilateral LBP with or without buttock or thigh pain. Deformity of accentuated lordosis. Repeated flexion centralizes, diminishes, or eliminates pain.	Flexion exercises.

From McKenzie R: *The lumbar spine: Mechanical diagnosis and therapy,* Waikane, New Zealand, 1981, Spinal Publications; Razmjou H, Kramer JF, Yamada R: *J Orthop Sports Phys Ther* 30(7):368-383, 2000; Riddle DL, Rothstein JM: *Spine* 18(10):1333-1344, 1993.
ROM, Range of motion; *LBP,* low back pain.

system focuses on movement system impairments independent of symptom acuity. The fundamental principle of this system is that the habitual movements and postures individuals adopt in reaction to the stresses of functional activities differ from a kinesiological ideal to eventually cause LBP.

In this system, patients are categorized according to the direction of spinal alignment or motion that produces or exacerbates symptoms. Patients are classified into one of five mutually exclusive categories: lumbar flexion, lumbar extension, lumbar rotation, lumbar rotation with extension, or lumbar rotation with flexion.[64,65] Treatment strategies focus on limiting direction-specific motions or alignments that increase symptoms and on ameliorating

impairments in muscle force and joint flexibility thought to affect the lumbar movement dysfunction.[60]

TYPICAL EXAMINATION FINDINGS

The clinician follows a series of hierarchical steps to develop a diagnosis and plan of care for patients with spinal dysfunction. After completing the patient history and systems review, the clinician performs a scanning examination to determine which structures are involved and to establish a musculoskeletal diagnosis. The scanning examination establishes which impairments and limitations require intervention and may indicate a need for more specific examination. The clinician combines findings from the patient history, systems review, and the

TABLE 8-7	The Delitto Treatment-Based Diagnostic Classification System for Spinal Disorders	
Classification	**Examination Findings**	**Treatment**
MOBILIZATION		
SI pattern	Unilateral symptoms without signs of nerve root compression, positive findings for SI region dysfunction (pelvic asymmetry, standing, and seated flexion tests)	Joint mobilization or manipulation techniques and spinal AROM exercises
Lumbar pattern	Unilateral symptoms without signs of nerve root compression, asymmetrical restrictions of lumbar side-bending motion, lumbar segmental hypomobility	Joint mobilization or manipulation techniques and spinal AROM exercises
SPECIFIC EXERCISE		
Flexion pattern	Patient preference for sitting versus standing, centralization with lumbar flexion motions	Lumbar flexion exercises, avoidance of extension activities
Extension pattern	Patient preference for standing versus sitting, centralization with lumbar extension motions	Lumbar extension exercises, avoidance of flexion activities
Immobilization	Frequent previous episodes, positive response to prior manipulation or bracing as treatment, presence of "instability catch" or lumbar segmental hypermobility	Trunk strengthening and stabilization exercises
Traction	Radicular signs present, unable to centralize with movements, may have lateral shift deformity	Mechanical or auto-traction

Adapted from Delitto A, Erhard RE, Bowling RW: *Phys Ther* 75(6):470-485; discussion 485-479, 1995.
SI, Sacroiliac; *AROM,* active range of motion.

scanning and specific examination to evaluate the patient, determine the diagnosis and prognosis, and plan interventions.

PATIENT HISTORY

In patients with spinal dysfunction, a thorough, carefully directed history is the first step of the examination that helps to guide intervention. The history will indicate if the patient's condition is probably mechanical or nonmechanical and whether it is acute, subacute, or chronic. The patient's responses to specific questions will then direct selection of specific tests and measures. The patient history includes information about the patient's psychosocial and occupational status and relevant medical history, as well as information about the location and severity of pain, sensory changes and weakness, the effects of movement or postural and position changes on symptoms, and whether symptoms centralize or peripheralize with position changes.

During the history, the therapist also screens the patient for indicators of serious medical pathology or red flags (Box 8-1). The presence of any red flags increases the likelihood that the patient's problem is not of musculoskeletal origin, and therefore the patient should be referred to a physician for medical diagnosis and possible intervention.

Patients may also complete general health or spinal-disorder specific self-report questionnaires before the initial examination and at intervals during a period of treatment. This can save valuable clinician time and be used to evaluate progress.

SYSTEMS REVIEW

The systems review is used to target areas requiring further examination and to define areas that may cause complications or indicate a need for precautions during the

BOX 8-1	**Red Flags: Indicators of Possible Serious Medical Pathology**

- Presentation age <20 years or onset >55 years
- Violent trauma (e.g., fall from a height, traffic accident)
- Constant, progressive pain that does not change with movement or position
- Thoracic pain
- History of:
  Carcinoma
  Systemic steroid use
  Drug abuse
- Human immunodeficiency virus (HIV)
- Systemically unwell
- Unexplained weight loss
- Persistent severe restriction of lumbar flexion
- Widespread neurological symptoms (numbness, weakness)
- Structural deformity
- Test results:
  Erythrocyte sedimentation rate (ESR) >25 mm
  Plain x-ray showing vertebral collapse or bone destruction

Adapted from Waddell G: *The back pain revolution,* Churchill Livingstone, 2004, New York.

examination and intervention processes. Chapter 1 includes details of the systems review.

TESTS AND MEASURES

Many clinical tests may be used to examine patients with spinal disorders. The following section briefly describes commonly used clinical tests for the spine, including indications for the test and interpretation of findings of these tests.

Scanning Tests and Measures. A scanning examination of the spine is used to rule in or rule out involvement of various structures and to determine if symptoms are of musculoskeletal origin. Findings may indicate need for more specialized tests or a higher level of skill and experience in interpretation.

Musculoskeletal

Posture. Deviations from normal postural alignment are frequently seen in many types of spinal disorders. Although some believe that specific postural abnormalities are indicative or predictive of specific spinal disorders, evidence indicates that postural abnormalities are not pathognomonic for any specific dysfunction[66,67] and are not good predictors for the severity of back pain.[66] However, in conjunction with other signs and symptoms, postural analysis can be a useful adjunct for planning interventions for patients with spinal dysfunction. In general, interventions are directed at returning posture to ideal posture when this does not aggravate symptoms. Chapter 4 includes further details of postural examination and ideal posture.

Range of Motion. Spinal ROM is the most commonly assessed impairment in patients with spinal disorders. AROM into flexion, extension, sidebending, and rotation is usually estimated by comparison with the expected norm or measured with an inclinometer and is documented on a movement diagram indicating the plane(s) in which movement is limited and any symptoms produced at the end of range (Fig. 8-8). The quality of movement, such as any hesitancy or reluctance to complete a motion or slight deviations in movement direction, hitching, or catching, is also documented. Alterations in the smooth quality of a movement may direct the therapist to perform specific mobility examination of the involved segments.

After completing each movement, the therapist applies overpressure to the movement by applying gentle graded pressure in the direction of the movement and noting the effect on range and symptoms.

The response of symptoms to single and repeated motions is observed so that movements associated with centralization of symptoms can be recommended as part of the intervention plan while movements that cause peripheralization or aggravation of symptoms are avoided.

Passive Range of Motion of Single Intervertebral Joints. Passive physiological intervertebral mobility (PPIVM) testing is a routine part of the PT's spinal examination. PPIVM testing assesses motion at each segmental level during passive motion into flexion, extension, side flexion, and rotation. To test PPIVM, the therapist palpates each segment as it is passively moved through its normal ROM and the therapist notes whether the movements provoke symptoms, judges end-feel, and decides whether the amount of available movement is normal, reduced (hypomobile), or excessive (hypermobile). This information, along with the results from the rest of the examination, is used to determine appropriate interventions. Painful hypomobile segments may benefit from mobilization or manipulation followed by stretching and strengthening of related muscles, whereas hypermobile segments may benefit from stabilization. Precise palpation skills are required for accurate determination of PPIVM.

Muscle Length. Examination for muscle tightness or loss of extensibility precedes evaluation for weakness because tight muscles influence movement patterns. Tight muscles will limit range. Patients with cervical and thoracic spinal dysfunction may have short upper trapezius, levator scapulae, and pectoralis major muscles. Patients with lumbosacral dysfunction may have short lumbar erector spinae, hip flexor, hamstring, piriformis, quadratus lumborum, and hip adductor muscles.

Muscle Performance. Specific manual muscle testing (MMT) is completed to evaluate strength. Extremity muscles may be weak if the spinal dysfunction is affecting the spinal cord or the roots of the peripheral nerves innervating the muscles. Spinal dysfunction may cause trunk muscle weakness, and trunk muscle weakness may predispose patients to spinal dysfunction.

Mechanical Provocation Tests. Mechanical provocation tests involve application of a series of maneuvers that may aggravate or diminish a patient's presenting symptoms. A change in symptom severity indicates that the disorder is mechanical in nature and should be responsive to physical intervention. In the spine a series of specific **provocation tests,** called foraminal closure or **quadrant tests,** are used to rule in or rule out nerve root irritation and to direct intervention. These tests are not intended to identify the specific cause of nerve root irritation.

Quadrant/Foraminal Closure Tests. There are many different variations of foraminal closure tests for the cervical spine. Spurling's test involves cervical sidebending and extension together with axial compression or overpressure. Reproduction of symptoms in the neck or arm corresponding to the side of bending constitutes a positive test and is suggestive of cervical radiculopathy.

Cervical Compression. Cervical compression is used to assess for nerve root impingement that results from

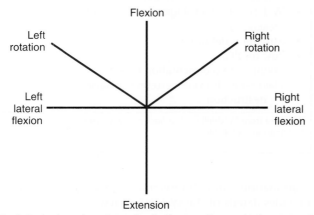

FIG. 8-8 A short-hand method of recording spinal range of motion. The therapist marks the locations of diminished range and any symptoms that occur during or at the end of motion.

encroachment on structures within the intervertebral foramen. To perform the test, with the patient sitting, the therapist clasps both hands across the top of the patient's head and applies a downward force on the head. A positive test reproduces the patient's presenting symptoms because compression mechanically constricts the intervertebral foramen.

Cervical Distraction. The cervical distraction test is a provocation test in which relief of symptoms constitutes a positive finding. With the patient sitting or supine, the therapist grasps the patient's head and to impart a distraction force, the therapist leans back to lift or pull on the patient's head.

Neuromuscular. Neurological screening is an important component of the scanning examination and is used to determine if spinal nerve function is affected in patients with spinal or radicular symptoms. Results of neurological screening tests will be documented in all patients with spinal disorders and should routinely be rechecked.

Pain. The severity, nature, and location of pain is determined by palpation of the areas overlying the spinal region being evaluated. This may help to identify which structures are causing pain.

Peripheral Nerve Integrity. Sensory modalities are screened using light touch, pin prick, and vibration in various dermatomal distributions (see Table 8-2). Motor function is assessed by testing the strength of the limb muscles that are representative of each nerve root distribution using MMT and by comparing the strength of one side with the strength of the other side (see Table 8-2).

Reflex Integrity. Deep tendon reflexes (DTRs) in the upper and lower extremity are tested. DTRs are diminished with some types of spinal nerve root impingement. To assess reflexes, the muscle tendon is tapped with a reflex hammer, and the response is compared to the other side.

Neurodynamic Tests. **Neurodynamic tests** mechanically stress nervous tissue in an attempt to determine if spinal nerve roots and peripheral nerves are causing pain. If mechanical stress on a nerve evokes pain, this suggests that the nerve has impaired mobility.[68] In all of the neurodynamic tests, the examiner carefully positions the patient and applies a tensile force to the nerve, noting symptoms. A series of **sensitizing maneuvers** are then applied in a sequential manner to successively apply additional mechanical stress to the tissues.

Straight Leg Raise Test. The most common neurodynamic test is the straight leg raise (SLR) test, which is used to evaluate for involvement of lumbosacral nerve roots and the sciatic nerve. To perform the SLR test, the patient lies supine and the opposite hip and knee are extended to stabilize the pelvis. The therapist passively lifts the test leg, keeping the leg in neutral rotation and the knee in extension. The therapist documents whether pain occurs unilaterally or bilaterally, if there is resistance to movement, the hip range when symptoms occur, and the type of symptoms elicited. Sensitizing maneuvers, such as reducing the hip flexion slightly when symptoms occur and then sequentially adding ankle dorsiflexion, medial hip rotation, and neck flexion, can be used to localize symptom etiology (Fig. 8-9). The SLR test is considered positive if symptoms are reproduced by any of these maneuvers.

Prone Knee Bend Test. The prone knee bend test is intended to mechanically stress the femoral nerve and the L2 and L3 nerve roots. Like the SLR test, symptom reproduction is thought to indicate a nerve root lesion. To perform the test, the patient lies prone and the therapist stabilizes the patient's pelvis and passively flexes the knee, maintaining neutral hip rotation. The test is considered positive when the maneuver reproduces the patient's symptoms.

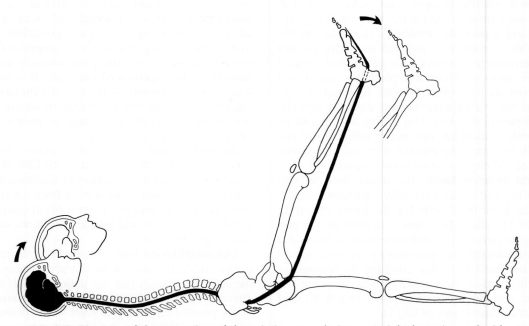

FIG. 8-9 Diagram of the excursion of the sciatic nerve during a straight leg raise and with the addition of the sensitizing maneuver of cervical flexion. *From Butler DS:* Mobilisation of the nervous system, *New York, 1991, Churchill Livingstone.*

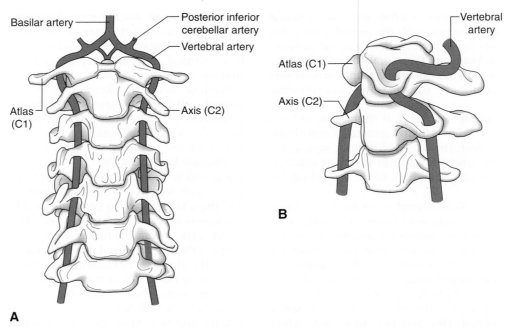

FIG. 8-10 **A,** Location of the vertebral artery within the foramen transversarium of the cervical spine. **B,** Twisting of the vertebral artery in the upper cervical spine with rotation. *Adapted from Gibbons P, Tehan P:* Manipulation of the spine thorax and pelvis: An osteopathic perspective, *New York, 2004, Churchill Livingstone.*

Slump Test. The slump test combines the extremes of the SLR test with ankle dorsiflexion and neck flexion in a sitting position with thoracolumbar spinal flexion. The patient sits with thighs fully supported on a plinth and is then asked to "slump," fully flexing the thoracic and lumbar spine without flexing the neck. The therapist exerts overpressure through the thoracolumbar spine to add further flexion. If asymptomatic, the patient fully flexes their neck and the therapist adds overpressure. The patient then sequentially extends the knee on the symptomatic side and if possible, dorsiflexes the ankle on the same side. This is a difficult position to maintain and usually the sensitizing maneuvers are added and released before progressing to a position that places the spinal cord and nerve roots on this much tension. If symptoms are provoked, the sensitizing maneuver is reversed and the effect on symptoms is noted. The slump test should be interpreted with caution because many subjects without pathology will become symptomatic with this maneuver, giving it low specificity for nerve involvement.[69]

Upper Limb Tension Tests. The upper limb tension tests (ULTTs) are the upper extremity equivalent of the SLR and prone knee bend tests for the lower extremity nerves. The ULTTs place the upper extremity nerves and the cervical spine nerve roots under mechanical stress and sequentially add sensitizing maneuvers to provoke symptoms. There are four ULTTs that combine movements of upper extremity and cervical spine to bias, stressing the median, ulnar, and radial nerves. Chapter 18 has detailed descriptions and illustrations of ULTTs.

Special Tests

Vertebral Artery Test. The vertebral artery test is used to determine whether extremes of movement of the cervical spine will compromise the vertebral artery and the cerebral circulation and should therefore be avoided during treatment. The vertebral arteries pass through the foramen transversarium in the cervical spine en route to the cerebral circulation. The arteries turn sharply at the C1 and C2 vertebrae before entering the foramen magnum (Fig. 8-10). In patients with vascular disease or significant osseous and soft tissue encroachment, there is a potential for arterial occlusion with extremes of cervical rotation and extension. There are several variations of this test, but all use combinations of cervical extension and rotation with some adding traction or compression. Given its inherent potential risk, this procedure should only be performed by an experienced clinician. If symptoms occur during any component of the test, the therapist concludes the procedure, the test is considered positive, and high-velocity or maintained end-range techniques of the cervical spine are contraindicated.

Sacroiliac Joint Tests. SI dysfunction is reported to occur in up to 30% of patients with LBP. SI dysfunction may be identified by palpation of lumbosacral and lower extremity landmarks and special tests for pain provocation, movement, and pelvic position in conjunction with a history of buttock and leg pain made worse with unilateral weight bearing.

Standing Flexion Test. The standing flexion test is used to determine the side of an iliosacral lesion. To perform the standing flexion test the patient stands with feet hip distance apart, bearing weight symmetrically. The therapist is positioned with eyes level to the posterior superior iliac spines (PSISs) and the thumbs are placed on or just under the PSISs. The patient bends forward, keeping their knees straight. The amount of cranial movement of the

PSISs is observed. The test is considered positive for restricted mobility if the PSIS on one side moves more cephalad, or moves before, the one on the other side.

Sacral Fixation Test. Like the standing flexion test, the sacral fixation test (also known as *Gillet's test,* the *marching test,* or the *stork test*) is used to test for the presence and side of an iliosacral lesion. The patient and therapist are positioned as described for the standing flexion test. The therapist places one thumb on a PSIS and the other on the adjacent part of the sacrum. The patient stands on one leg while flexing the opposite hip and knee to at least 90 degrees. The therapist palpates the PSIS on the side of the flexing leg. The procedure is repeated on both sides. A test is considered positive for restricted mobility if little or no PSIS movement occurs.

Sitting Flexion Test. The sitting flexion test is also used to test for the presence and side of a iliosacral lesion. The subject sits on a level surface with feet supported on a stool. The therapist is positioned with eyes level with the PSISs, and the thumbs are placed on or just under the PSISs bilaterally. The patient flexes the trunk fully forward until their elbows are between their knees while the therapist palpates for cranial movement of either PSIS. A test is considered positive for restricted mobility if either PSIS moves cranially.

Long Sitting Test (Supine-to-Sit Test). The long sitting test is used to examine for abnormal movement of the innominate on the sacrum and to determine the direction of innominate rotation. This test is performed with the patient starting supine and the therapist standing at the patient's feet with their thumbs just distal to the apex of the malleoli. The patient then moves into a long sitting position with knees extended, and the therapist observes for changes in the position of the malleoli. In a patient with a posteriorly rotated innominate, the limb will appear short when the patient is supine and will then appear to lengthen in long sitting. In a patient with an anteriorly rotated innominate, the lower extremity appears long in supine and shorter in long sitting.

Compression Tests. Various tests apply shearing and compressive forces through the SI joints to provoke symptoms and determine the side of involvement. These tests examine mobility and the response to provocation and are considered positive if symptoms on the side tested increase or the joint has reduced mobility.

Limb Length Inequality. Limb length inequality (LLI) is a difference in length between the two lower extremities. Anatomical or true LLI occurs when one of the bones in the lower extremity is shorter than the one on the other side.[70] Functional or apparent LLI is when one lower extremity is shorter than the other while the bones are of equal length. In functional LLI, the length discrepancy is caused by adaptive soft tissue shortening, joint contractures, ligamentous laxity, or axial malalignment. Although the relationship between LLI and back pain is controversial and is not completely supported, practically speaking, when LLI is observed in patients with LBP, correction should be attempted and implemented if it helps alleviate symptoms.

Examination of Neighboring Joints. When examining a patient with a spinal disorder, the therapist will screen neighboring joints to determine if the spine is the primary site of origin of the patient's symptoms.[68,71] For example, upper cervical spine symptoms frequently occur in patients with temporomandibular joint (TMJ) dysfunction and neck pain can be referred from the shoulder. Similarly, lumbosacral dysfunctions can be caused by hip pathologies.

Detailed Tests and Measures. The results of the scanning examination can be used to develop initial diagnostic hypotheses, prioritize the patient problem list, and develop a plan of care for most patients with spinal pain. However, some patients require more in-depth examination procedures, which are generally only performed by an experienced manual therapist, to accurately identify the cause of their symptoms.

EVALUATION, DIAGNOSIS, AND PROGNOSIS

After completing the examination, the PT has much information to synthesize in performing the evaluation component of patient management. From the history, the therapist obtains information about the severity, chronicity, and irritability of the current condition. This information guides the vigor of further testing and interventions. The history also provides important prognostic information.

Although patients with spinal disorders fall into the *Guide to Physical Therapy Practice*[72] preferred practice pattern 4F: Impaired joint mobility, motor function, muscle performance, range of motion, and reflex integrity associated with spinal disorders, a more specific understanding of their condition is usually necessary to direct optimal intervention. The classification systems of spinal dysfunction discussed earlier in this chapter provide the PT with specific criteria to place a patient into a diagnostic category to direct interventions. The plan of care is directed toward techniques that target the mechanical dysfunctions identified during the examination. Active involvement of the patient in the intervention and in setting goals will help ensure patient participation and provide the patient with information needed to reduce the risk of recurrence.

INTERVENTION

MOBILIZATION AND MANIPULATION

Mobilization and manipulation are manual therapy techniques in which skilled passive movements are applied to joints and related soft tissues at a variety of speeds and amplitudes.[72] Manual therapy is not the sole purview of a single profession and is and always has been practiced by many different practitioners. In the United States today, depending on state regulations, spinal manual therapy techniques may be applied by physical therapists, chiropractors, osteopathic physicians, medical doctors, and others. In some states, PTAs may perform spinal mobilization, whereas other states' regulations do not allow this. If your state allows you to perform spinal mobilization or manipulation, you can learn these techniques from advanced courses.

The effect of manual therapy for reducing pain and improving mobility in patients with spinal disorders is thought to be mediated by mechanical and neurophysiological mechanisms. Mechanically, joint mobilization and manipulation directly impart external forces to the joints of the spine and the overlying muscles, ligaments, and soft tissue structures. These forces may restore more normal joint play and articular relationships,[73] separate facet joint surfaces, release trapped synovial folds, break intraarticular adhesions and scar tissue, and stretch specific joint capsules and muscles. Neurophysiologically, manual therapy alters central sensory processing and thereby increases the pain threshold.[74] During mobilization and manipulation, reflex changes and altered motor neuron excitability can reduce muscle spasm by interfering with the pain-spasm cycle and may thereby improve posture and movement.[74,75]

There is has been more research investigating the effectiveness of spinal manipulative therapy (SMT) than almost any other intervention for spinal disorders. In many RCTs, SMT has been found to be more effective than placebo or no intervention for acute, subacute, and chronic spinal disorders.[72,76,77] However, when the literature is systematically examined through critical reviews and meta-analyses in which methodological quality of the research is considered, SMT, either alone or in combination with other interventions, has not been found to be any better than other approaches for treating patients with spinal disorders.[72,76,77]

Patients with musculoskeletal disorders characterized by intermittent pain, diminished ROM, and hypomobility are most likely to respond to mobilization or manipulation. Specific indications for mobilization or manipulation are listed in Table 8-8. Precautions and contraindications for mobilization and manipulation are listed in Table 8-9.

MUSCLE ENERGY TECHNIQUE

The muscle energy technique (MET) is a form of manual therapy in which the patient voluntarily contracts a specific muscle from a controlled position in an exact direction, at varying levels of intensity, against a force applied by the therapist.[78] MET can be used to relax hypertonic muscles, mobilize restricted joints, strengthen weak muscles, stretch muscles and related connective tissue, reduce local edema, and improve local circulation.[73,78,79] MET is an active technique that requires the patient to participate with the therapist to improve function.

The mechanism of METs has yet to be substantiated. Based on principles of neurophysiology and motor control, it is believed that in the presence of dysfunction, the muscles at a spinal segment are facilitated to become hypertonic in response to nociceptive input.[80] This hypertonicity restricts movement of structures innervated by that segment, leading to local circulatory congestion, changes in connective tissue mobility, and pain. Once a segment becomes facilitated, it is both hypersensitive and hyperactive so that a small, normally tolerated stimulus will cause an overactive response without selectivity for a specific muscle or organ.[79,80] MET uses postisometric relaxation and reciprocal inhibition to decrease the tone in the

TABLE 8-8	Indications for Joint Mobilization
Symptom Characteristics	**Examination Findings**
Mechanical origin	Symptoms are aggravated by certain movements or postures and are relieved by rest or other positions.
Diminished ROM	Loss of active or passive osteokinematic movement found on examination of ROM, PPIVM, and position testing.
Joint hypomobility	Diminished arthrokinematic movement determined by diminished passive mobility (PA) and position testing.
Joint asymmetry	Asymmetrical movement at individual joints as determined by PPIVM and position testing.
Tissue texture abnormality	Abnormal resistances to movement as a result of pain, spasm, trigger points, or thickened and stiff soft tissues overlying the joint.
Pain	Neuromusculoskeletal pain on movement, palpation, and elicited by provocation tests.

ROM, Range of motion; *PPIVM,* passive physiological intervertebral mobility; *PA,* posterior to anterior.

hypertonic muscles to reestablish their normal resting length and block nociceptive input.[80]

The system of muscle energy treatment depends on accurate localization and classification of the dysfunction. The dysfunction is classified according to findings from a series of specific palpatory, movement, and provocation tests. There is a specific MET for each diagnostic classification.

To perform an isometric MET the patient is positioned comfortably, permitting the operator to control all patient positions and movements. The operator moves the patient through a series of precise movements to locate the barrier to motion by palpation of movement in three planes: sagittal (flexion and extension), frontal (lateral flexion), and horizontal (rotation). After finding the barrier, the patient is moved slightly into a position just before the barrier is engaged, which is known as the *interbarrier zone.* The patient then performs a low force isometric contraction of the muscle opposing the motion for approximately 10 seconds and then relaxes for 3 to 5 seconds. The operator then repositions the patient to the new barrier and repeats the procedure.[73,79] After completion of the MET, the patient is reexamined to determine if the procedure has corrected the dysfunction.

A sample of MET procedures is found in Fig. 8-11. Contraindications to MET procedures include unstable joints, fractures, severe rheumatoid arthritis, severe osteoporosis, malignancy, cauda equina syndrome, and open wounds. Because the patient must actively participate with the operator throughout the procedure, this intervention is also not recommended for patients who cannot cooperate

TABLE 8-9	Precautions and Contraindications to Mobilization and Manipulation*

Precautions	Contraindications
MOBILIZATION	
Neurological signs	Malignancy involving the spinal column
Rheumatoid arthritis	Cauda equina lesions affecting bowel or bladder function
Osteoporosis	Spinal cord involvement
Spondylolisthesis	Active inflammatory (e.g., RA) or infective arthritis
Hypermobility	Rheumatoid collagen necrosis of vertebral ligaments
Pregnancy	Bone disease and severe osteoporosis
Previous malignancy	Instability
Dizziness	Vertebral artery disease
Steroid use	Fracture or dislocation
Cervical trauma	
Internal derangement	
Psychological issues	
MANIPULATION*	
Disc lesions	Frank spinal deformity caused by old pathology
Ankylosing spondylitis after acute stage	Generalized congenital hypermobility (Ehlers-Danlos syndrome)
Congenital anomalies	Osteoporosis
Neurological dysfunction	Lower limb neurological symptoms caused by cervical or thoracic dysfunction
Irritable conditions	Undiagnosed pain
	Protective joint spasm
	Evidence of involvement of more than two adjacent nerve roots of the lumbar spine

RA, Rheumatoid arthritis.
*Precautions and contraindications listed under manipulation are in addition to those listed for mobilization.

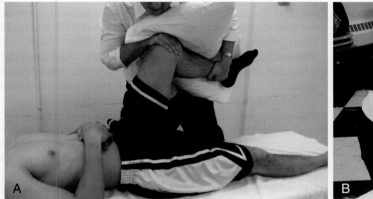 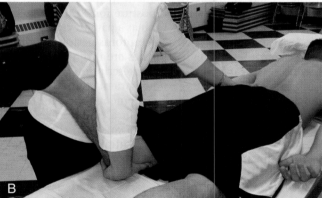

FIG. 8-11 Selected METs. **A,** Supine position for MET for an anterior innominate with barriers in flexion, adduction, and internal rotation. **B,** Prone position for MET for a posterior innominate with barriers in extension, abduction, and external rotation.

because of a language barrier, personality factors, or other reasons that preclude cooperation.

ⓒ *Clinical Pearl*

Muscle energy techniques (METs) use the patient's own muscle contractions to reduce muscle spasm and normalize muscle tone and length.

EXERCISE

Exercise is one of the most commonly used interventions for the management of spinal disorders, yet the literature on its efficacy is contradictory.[77,81-83] PTs prescribe exercises by integrating the results of the examination with their knowledge of pertinent literature and disease processes and an individual patient's functional needs. Exercises can include activities to improve impaired muscle performance, deconditioning, disuse and atrophy, endurance, hypomobility or hypermobility, neuromuscular control, balance and coordination, and posture and alignment. Exercises for patients with spinal dysfunction are not confined to the trunk and consist of programs that also train the pelvic, hip, and shoulder muscles. An individualized program is the hallmark of a physical therapy exercise prescription.

The following specific exercise intervention programs for patients with spinal disorders are most frequently employed and investigated by physical therapists.

MCKENZIE APPROACH TO INTERVENTION

The McKenzie approach to intervention, which emphasizes patient self-management through exercise and education, is one of the most popular methods of intervention among PTs for patients with spinal dysfunction and for treating patients with LBP.[54]

McKenzie's approach to intervention and management of spinal pain is integrated with the examination process in which patients are classified into subgroups for the purpose of directing treatment. During the examination the patient undergoes a series of repeated end-range test movements to determine whether a mechanical maneuver centralizes (draws toward the spinal midline) or peripheralizes (spreads distally or laterally) their symptoms. For most patients, movements toward extension will centralize symptoms; in other patients, symptoms will centralize with lateral movement in the frontal plane (called *sidegliding*); and in a very few, symptoms will centralize with other directions of movement.[56,84] The direction of the movement that centralizes or abolishes symptoms forms the basis for beginning the intervention program. Patients are advised to perform a series of 10 to 15 repetitions of each movement noted in the examination to centralize their symptoms. These exercises are repeated as frequently as every 2 hours for a patient in acute pain. Once the symptoms stay centralized, a patient in the acute stage is advised to maintain a lordotic posture for 24 to 48 hours to promote tissue healing. As soon as a patient can tolerate additional movement without symptoms peripheralizing, exercises in other movement planes are introduced.[56]

As noted in Table 8-6, exercise prescription is linked to the classification according to the patient's syndrome. For example, a patient with a derangement four syndrome would present with a lateral shift or a posture in which the shoulders are typically shifted away from the side of pain (Fig. 8-12, *A*). To produce a centralization of symptoms the therapist would instruct the patient in self-correction of the lateral shift (Fig. 8-12, *B*), and if this did not produce centralization the therapist would assist the patient with manual correction (Fig. 8-12, *C*). With repeated lateral shift correction, the symptoms would be expected to move from the leg to the lumbosacral midline, at which time extension exercises are added. This may begin with simple prone lying, followed by the patient assuming a prone on elbows position (Fig. 8-12, *D*) and continued with press-up exercises (Fig. 8-12, *E*). These movements are to be done as passive mobility exercises and with minimal contraction of the paraspinal muscles. The repetitive nature of McKenzie exercises have been shown to elicit hemodynamic stress. Patients with cardiopulmonary co-morbidities or those at risk for such disease should therefore be carefully monitored while performing repetitions of McKenzie exercises.[85]

In the McKenzie approach, passive treatment modalities, such as hot packs or ultrasound, are frowned on, with the therapist guiding the patient into an active role for symptom management. Patients gain confidence in their ability to manage pain, should symptoms recur, by gaining an understanding of the relationship between their pain and movement. Prevention of future episodes of pain is facilitated by postural education and prophylactic exercises.

> ### ◎ *Clinical Pearl*
>
> McKenzie's approach to spinal pain emphasizes the patient's self-management by implementation of an exercise program that repeats movements that cause reduction or centralization of symptoms. These movements are intended to treat current dysfunction and prevention of future episodes.

SPINAL STABILIZATION EXERCISES

Spinal stabilization exercises are designed to target the muscles that control segmental stability. Stabilization exercises are specifically designed to target the multifidus (MF) and transversus abdominis (TrA) muscles, which work together, contracting before the initiation of arm and leg movement, to stiffen the spine.[86-89] Spinal stiffness protects the spine from reactive forces to reduce the risk of spinal injury.[90]

In normal trunk function, co-contraction of the TrA and MF muscles stabilizes the spine when the limbs are moved and occurs independently of contraction of the larger, multisegmental, superficial muscles of the trunk, such as the erector spinae and rectus abdominis, which move the trunk. In patients with chronic LBP, as well as those with experimentally chemically induced back pain, motor control of the TrA has been found to be impaired, with delayed onset of contraction with limb movement.[90,91] The MF is also reflexively inhibited in patients with LBP, exhibiting weakness, loss of control, and a decreased cross-sectional area.[92-94]

The hallmark of stabilization exercises is drawing in of the abdominal wall, also called *abdominal bracing,* which generates a co-contraction of TrA and MF (Fig. 8-13). As the emphasis of stabilization exercise is motor control of the deep spinal muscles, a low level continuous contraction, less than 30% to 40% of a maximum voluntary contraction, is used. Accurate replication of the correct holding co-activates only the TrA and MF without activating other trunk muscles.[86] Control is developed through repeated practice, which allows patients with back pain to learn or relearn how to isolate TrA and MF contraction to maintain spinal stability.

> ### ◎ *Clinical Pearl*
>
> Trunk stabilization or abdominal bracing controls spinal segmental stability through co-contraction of the multifidus (MF) and transversus abdominis (TrA) muscles.

Therapists can teach patients techniques to master abdominal bracing with co-contraction. These include focusing on contracting the TrA or MF one at a time, verbal and visual cues, different postures and positions, facilitation and feedback techniques, and techniques to

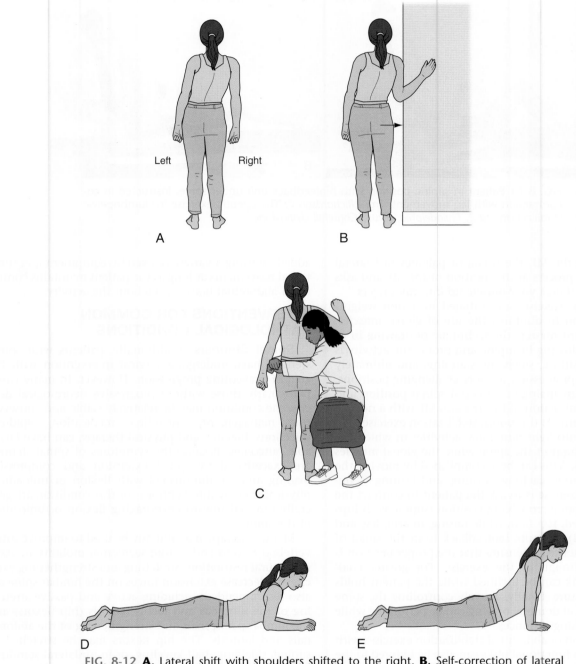

Left   Right

A   B

C

D   E

FIG. 8-12 **A,** Lateral shift with shoulders shifted to the right. **B,** Self-correction of lateral shift. **C,** Manual correction of lateral shift. **D,** Prone on elbows. **E,** Press-up.

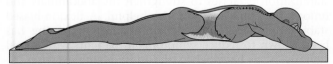

FIG. 8-13 Co-activation of transversus abdominis and multifidus.

decrease activity of overactive global muscles.[86] Verbal cues that can help elicit TrA contraction are "draw in your abdomen" and "pull your navel up and in toward your spine." The therapist can check by palpation for a contraction of the TrA and can teach the patient to self-check by palpating between the lateral border of the rectus abdominis and the anterior superior iliac spine (ASIS). Contraction of the TrA has been found to occur with contraction of the diaphragm[95] and the pelvic floor musculature.[96] Therefore, to facilitate contraction of TrA in patients who have lost the perception of muscle contraction, patients can be asked to contract their pelvic floor muscles or to deeply sigh with expiration.[86] When overactivity of global muscles interferes with local muscle contraction, electromyography (EMG) biofeedback from the external oblique and rectus abdominis muscles can help teach the patient to isolate muscle contraction. To promote an isolated

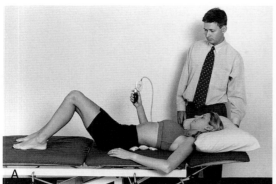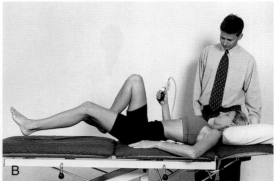

FIG. 8-14 Patient in supine position with biofeedback unit under spine. Instructed in co-contraction with leg movement. *From Richardson C:* Therapeutic exercise for lumbopelvic stabilization, *ed 2, Philadelphia, 2005, Churchill Livingstone.*

contraction of the MF, the therapist palpates just lateral to the spinous process at the location of the MF and asks the patient to "bulge your muscle up into my fingers."

Stabilization exercises are initiated in a non–weight-bearing position to diminish the use of global muscles. Once the patient masters the technique of drawing in or abdominal hollowing in supine and prone, the activity is progressed to sitting, sidelying, standing, and ultimately walking. With progression to more challenging positions, the patient must maintain a neutral spinal position and hold the co-contraction of the TrA and MF with a normal breathing pattern. At this point, stabilization exercises can be integrated into light functional activities in which the local muscles support the spine while the global muscles move the trunk. This can be accomplished by moving the extremities during reaching, turning, and leaning. A frequently used exercise is to ask the patient to contract the TrA and MF from a crooklying position (supine with hips and knees flexed, feet flat), while raising an arm, leg, and both (Fig. 8-14). Pressure biofeedback from the small of the back can be used to ensure that the proper position is maintained throughout the exercise. For greater challenges the trunk can be inclined while the patient holds an upright posture. Finally, actively controlling the spine in neutral with abdominal bracing can be performed while walking increasing distances.

Incorporation of abdominal stabilization exercises with greater loads in functional tasks can also be tailored to the demands of the patient's work, leisure, and other usual activities. External load can be increased with several types of exercises, body positioning, decreasing stability of the body position, and equipment. Therapists are urged to be creative in developing an individualized program. In a commonly used exercise, the patient extends an arm, a leg, and both to increase spinal load from a quadruped position. This can be made more difficult by placing a small ball or balance board under the hand. Bridging from a hooklying position is performed, and stability is challenged by using a single leg for support, a ball under the foot, or by increasing speed. Many exercises incorporate the use of a large gym ball to challenge stability. Exercises that train the global muscles, such as the erector spinae, quadratus lumborum, and abdominal obliques, can be added by using a variety of exercise equipment and functional movements as long as the patient maintains control of an abdominal brace throughout the activity.

INTERVENTIONS FOR COMMON PATHOLOGICAL CONDITIONS

Spinal Stenosis. Traditionally, patients with spinal stenosis have undergone surgical intervention with the goal of preventing progression. However, in many cases, particularly those without progressive neurological deficits, the condition may be relatively stable and conservative management, including medication, epidural injections, bracing, and physical therapy, can have favorable outcomes. Because the symptoms of spinal stenosis are exacerbated by spinal extension and compressive loading and are diminished with flexion or unloading, physical therapy interventions for this condition are generally directed toward encouraging flexion or unloading of the spine.

Manual therapy may initially be used to improve intervertebral flexion and restore segmental mobility to assist in postural restoration. Stretching and strengthening exercises to decrease extension forces on the lumbar spine are also recommended, including active and passive stretching of the iliopsoas and rectus femoris (hip flexors) and the lumbar paraspinals and strengthening of the abdominals and gluteals. The hip flexors may be stretched in supine, sidelying, half-kneeling, or in unilateral standing. Lumbar paraspinal stretching may be performed in supine, quadruped, or sitting. Postural awareness exercises and stabilization exercises to strengthen the abdominals and unload the spine may also be helpful. A flexion-biased stabilization program for abdominal strengthening has been shown to reduce symptoms in patients with spinal stenosis,[97,98] as have pelvic tilts and bridging exercises.[99]

Bicycle exercise is recommended for general conditioning in patients with spinal stenosis because the seated position keeps the spine in flexion. Inclined treadmill walking, which also flexes the spine, may also be well tolerated by patients with spinal stenosis, and body weight support with a harness during treadmill ambulation has been shown to increase ambulation duration and distance before the onset of symptoms in patients with spinal stenosis.[30,100] Aquatic therapy may be useful for both strengthening and conditioning as the support of the water reduces spinal compression forces. Physical therapy treatment programs in which manual therapy was reinforced with therapeutic exercise and a graded walking program have been shown to significantly improve patients' impairments, functional limitations, and disability for up to 18 months.[100,102]

> ### ◎ Clinical Pearl
>
> Exercises that decrease lumbar extension forces and unload the spine are used to diminish the symptoms of spinal stenosis.

Spondylolisthesis. Surgical stabilization to prevent the progression of slippage is generally recommended for management of patients with severe spondylolisthesis with radicular signs or significant pain and for those who fail to improve with conservative intervention. However, most patients with spondylolysis and spondylolisthesis respond well to nonoperative treatment consisting of modalities for pain relief, bracing, exercise, electrical stimulation, and activity modification. It is unclear what type of exercise provides the greatest benefit to these patients; however, most recommend that extension exercises be avoided in patients with spondylolisthesis because these can increase anterior shearing force on the vertebrae, which could result in additional slippage. In addition, some common abdominal strengthening exercises, such as supine SLRs, bent leg raises, and static cross-knee curl-ups, are not recommended because they also exert high mechanical loads on the lumbar spine. Studies have found that most patients with spondylolisthesis have good symptom relief with flexion exercises and spinal stabilization exercises.

Whiplash. The Québec Task Force on WAD reviewed published RCTs for evidence regarding interventions typically used for treatment of whiplash.[102] They found that active exercise produced both short- and long-term benefits and joint mobilization produced short-term results. In contrast, research on soft cervical collars and extended periods of rest indicates that these interventions, although commonly used clinically, encourage inactivity and delay recovery. In 2002, seven experts, using study selection recommendations from the Dutch Royal Physical Therapy Association, developed evidence-based clinical practice guidelines for the physical therapy management of WAD from published studies.[38] Their guidelines for the treatment of WAD, as shown in Table 8-10, are divided into 5 recovery phases, starting at less than 4 days after injury and progressing to more than 3 months after injury. Interventions focus on education, exercise therapy, and functional activities.

TABLE 8-10	Goals and Interventions for Patients with Whiplash-Associated Disorder	
Recovery Phase	**Goals of Treatment**	**Interventions**
Phase 1 (<4 days)	Decrease pain. Provide information. Explain the consequences of whiplash.	Education: Nature of injury, natural course of whiplash, avoid factors that lead to chronicity. Exercise therapy: Frequent cervical AROM within limits of pain. NSAIDs in consultation with physician.
Phase 2 (4 days-3 weeks)	Provide information. Improve function. Return patient to normal activities.	Education: Reassure about benign nature of symptoms. Exercise therapy: Graded activities such as muscle stabilization exercises and ROM to prevent fear of movement. Functional activities: Reaching, walking, postural control.
Phase 3 (3-6 weeks)	Provide information Explain consequences of whiplash. Improve function. Increase activities.	Education: To prevent chronicity correct pessimistic beliefs and passive coping strategies. Exercise therapy: Muscle strengthening and stabilization. Postural correction and awareness. Functional activities: Increase graded activities required for prior usual activities.
Phase 4 (6 weeks-3 months)	Provide information. Explain consequences of whiplash. Improve activity levels. Improve participation.	Education: Restore patient's confidence that symptoms do not indicate chronicity. Exercise therapy: Provide a personalized graded exercise program. Give alternative ways of performing tasks by changing frequency and speed. Functional activities: Increase activities on time-dependent basis.
Phase 5 (>3 months)	Provide information. Explain consequences of whiplash. Improve activity levels. Improve participation.	Education: Recovery may be delayed. Promote healthy behaviors. Encourage feelings of self-control and optimistic attitudes about pain. Consider the need for psychological referral if symptoms persist for this long. Functional activities: Continue graded activities.

AROM, Active range of motion; *NSAIDs,* nonsteroidal antiinflammatory drugs.

CASE STUDY 8-1

LOW BACK PAIN AND INTERVERTEBRAL DISC HERNIATION

Patient History

MJ is a 39-year-old woman who works as nurse's aide. MJ presents with a 3-month history of LBP and radiating symptoms to her right posterior thigh and lateral calf. The symptoms started when MJ was bending and lifting a food service tray from a low tray holder to a raised cleaning bin. At that time, she experienced centralized LBP progressing to her right posterior thigh and lateral calf and noticed some foot slap during ambulation. MJ had a transforaminal epidural corticosteroid injection 4 days ago, which relieved her lateral calf pain. MRI reveals the right L4/L5 IVD to have a lateral herniation with nerve root compression.

Tests and Measures—Significant Findings

Musculoskeletal
- Decreased tolerance to weight bearing on the right lower extremity (LE) with the right hip held in slight external rotation and knee flexion for comfort.
- Lumbar AROM: Flexion is 50% of normal with pain into low back, right buttocks, and posterior thigh; extension is 10% of normal with stiffness and pain.

Neuromuscular
- Pain scale: 7/10 currently. There is pain to palpation throughout the right buttock with a trigger point in the right piriformis.

Neurodynamic Tests
- SLR test: At 45 degrees on the right with symptom provocation to the right thigh.
- Prone knee bend test: Within normal limits bilaterally, slight stretching pain in the anterior thigh.
- Slump test: + with symptom provocation in the right LE.

Function
- Pain is worsened by walking and sitting for more than 5 to 10 minutes and with rising from sitting. Pain improves with lying supine, prone, and prone on elbows.

Diagnosis

Preferred practice pattern 4F: Impaired joint mobility, motor function, muscle performance, range of motion, and reflex integrity associated with spinal disorders.

Interventions
- Pain modulation with ice to the low back and right buttock and gentle joint mobilization to the lumbar spine.
- Instruction in a home exercise program that includes prone press-ups throughout the day to control pain and transversus abdominis muscle strengthening exercises in supine.

- Progress to include a more vigorous stabilization program and stretching of the right piriformis and bilateral hip flexor muscles and higher grade joint mobilizations.

Role of the Physical Therapist Assistant
- How long would you apply ice to this patient? How many minutes? How often? When?
- Document a home exercise program for this patient, including two passive extension exercises and two abdominal strengthening exercises.
- What symptoms would prompt you to contact your supervising therapist for further guidance with interventions for the patient?

Additional Information

For the full version of this case study, including detailed examination results, interventions, and outcomes, see the Evolve site that accompanies this book. Two additional detailed case studies for a patient with LBP and spinal stenosis and a patient with whiplash-associated disorder are included on the Evolve site.

CHAPTER SUMMARY

Patients with spinal disorders may have back or neck pain with or without radiation of symptoms to the extremities. Spinal disorders for which a pathoanatomical diagnosis can be made and for which physical therapy may be helpful include radiculopathy, intervertebral disc disease, spinal stenosis, spondylolisthesis, and whiplash-associated disorders. However, despite the abundance of research on the diagnosis of spinal disorders, for the overwhelming majority of patients a definitive pathoanatomical diagnosis cannot be made and therefore classification systems that are independent of pathology have been developed to direct treatment. Three of these classification systems, the McKenzie approach, the treatment-based approach, and the movement impairment–based approach, are described in this chapter. Interventions that have been shown to help patients with the spinal disorders described in this chapter include joint mobilization and specific kinds of exercise.

ADDITIONAL RESOURCES

For links to these and additional web-based resources, see the Evolve site.

Dutton M: *Manual therapy of the spine: An integrated approach,* New York, 2002, McGraw-Hill.

Lee D: The pelvic girdle: *An approach to the examination and treatment of the lumbopelvic-hip region,* ed 3, New York, 2004, Churchill Livingstone.

Richardson C, Hodge P, Hides J: *Therapeutic exercise for lumbopelvic stabilization: A motor control approach for the treatment and prevention of low back pain,* ed 2, New York, 2004, Churchill Livingstone.

Saunders HD, Saunders R: *Evaluation, treatment and prevention of musculoskeletal disorders,* ed 4, vol I, Bloomington, MN, 2004, Educational Opportunities.

Vleeming A, Mooney V, Dorman T, et al: *Movement, stability, and low back pain: The essential role of the pelvis,* New York, 1997, Churchill Livingstone.

American Academy of Orthopedic Surgeons
Journal of Orthopedic and Sports Physical Therapy
Spine Society of Australia

Useful Forms

Neck Disability Index Form
Oswestry Low Back Pain Disability Questionnaire
Roland-Morris Disability Questionnaire

GLOSSARY

Annulus fibrosus (AF): Outer component of the intervertebral disc.

Centralization: Proximal or central movement of distal pain or symptoms that originate from the spine in response to specific movements.

Classification system: A method used to categorize spinal pain disorders that are independent of pathology on diagnostic imaging. Frequently depends on the patient's presenting signs and symptoms and is related to intervention.

Derangement syndrome: One of the major categories of the McKenzie classification system characterized by anatomical disruption of the structures of the intervertebral joints.

Dysfunction syndrome: One of the major categories of the McKenzie classification system characterized by pain that results from mechanical deformation of adaptively-shortened soft tissue after maintenance of poor positioning after degeneration, trauma, or a derangement.

Limb length inequality (LLI): A difference in length between the two lower extremities. In anatomical LLI, one of the bones of the lower extremity is short. In functional LLI, shortening of one of the lower extremities occurs without shortening of the bones.

Manipulation: A manual therapy technique in which a high-velocity thrust is applied at the limits of range.

Mobilization: A manual therapy technique in which graded passive movements are imparted within the anatomical limits of joint range.

Neurodynamic tests: Manual provocation tests that mechanically stress nervous tissue to determine if spinal nerve roots and peripheral nerves are causing pain.

Neurogenic claudication: A condition characterized by aggravation of neurological signs and symptoms, such as pain, paresthesias, and lower extremity cramping with ambulation, or by increasing lumbar lordosis of the spine. Symptoms improve with a change in posture.

Nucleus pulposus (NP): Gelatinous inner core of the IVD.

Oswestry Low Back Pain Disability Questionnaire: A disease-specific self-report questionnaire that assesses pain and disability in LBP.

Passive physiological intervertebral mobility (PPIVM): A spinal examination technique in which the passive motion at each segmental level is palpated in flexion, extension, side flexion, or rotation.

Postural syndrome: One of the major categories of the McKenzie classification system characterized by pain that results from maintenance of poor posture.

Provocation tests: Tests in which a series of maneuvers are applied that may aggravate or diminish a patient's presenting symptoms. A change in symptom severity indicates that the disorder is mechanical in nature.

Quadrant tests: A series of provocation tests that compress the contents of the intervertebral foramen and neighboring facet joints.

Radiculopathy: Irritation of a nerve root at any level of the spine.

Sensitizing maneuvers: Movements sequentially added to the distal extremity during a neurodynamic test to provoke symptoms that further stretch the nerves under examination.

Spinal stenosis: Narrowing of the spinal canal or intervertebral foramina because of bony or soft tissue encroachment so that the space between the spinal cord or nerve roots and the vertebral elements is compromised.

Spondylolisthesis: Translation of vertebra forward in the sagittal plane with respect to an adjacent vertebra.

Whiplash-associated disorders (WAD): Bony or soft tissue injuries of the neck and related areas that occur after a rear or side motor vehicle collision in which the neck is subjected to acceleration-deceleration energy transfer.

Fractures

Julie A. Pryde, Debra H. Iwasaki

OBJECTIVES

After reading this chapter, the reader will be able to:
1. Describe fractures and their subtypes using the proper terminology.
2. Identify local and systemic factors affecting fracture healing.
3. Recognize fractures commonly seen in adults and children.
4. Discuss mechanisms of injury of fractures and how these relate to fracture patterns and soft tissue injury.
5. Differentiate between primary and secondary fracture healing.
6. Select and apply evidence-based interventions for patients with fractures.

Fracture treatment and rehabilitation is a challenge requiring a cooperative effort from all members of the health care team, including the physician or other health provider and the rehabilitation specialist. With the significant cost of this treatment and high potential for disability, it is imperative that the therapist and therapist assistant understand the principles of fracture healing and the biomechanical principles of fixation to optimize the patients' functional outcome.

In 2002 in the United States, over 9 million patients were seen in physician offices for fracture management. The treatment of fractures is the third most common surgical procedure for men of all ages, after cardiac catheterization and prostatectomy.[1] The cost of fracture care in the United States is substantial; nearly one-third of patients with fractures require admission to the hospital.

NORMAL BONE

Through their relationship with each other and with muscles, bones give form to the body, support tissue, protect organs, and permit movement. Mature bone is a rigid connective tissue consisting of cells, fibers, ground substance, and minerals containing elements such as calcium. Minerals give bones their inherent rigidity, and the bone cells, osteoblasts and osteoclasts, are the living part of the bone that give it the ability to grow, repair, and change shape. Osteoblasts synthesize bone, and osteoclasts reabsorb bone, primarily during the process of growth and repair.

In addition to their structural function, bones have a crucial role in chemical homeostasis since they store many minerals, including calcium and phosphate. Bones also play a major role in blood cell formation in adults because blood cells are first formed in the bone marrow.

Bone can be described as cortical (also known as *compact*) or cancellous (also known as *spongy*). These types of bone differ in their amount of solid matter and number and size of spaces. All bones have a thin outer layer of periosteum that covers the dense outer layer of **cortical bone,** which surrounds a central mass of **cancellous bone** (Fig. 9-1). Cortical bone provides strength for weight bearing and rigidity for muscular attachments. Some bones have a medullary (also known as *marrow*) canal centrally located within the cancellous bone. Blood cells are formed in the medullary canal.

There are 206 bones in the human body. Bones may be classified according to their location. The 80 bones of the axial skeleton include the bones of the skull, pelvis, ribs, sternum, vertebrae, and scapulae. The other 126 bones are part of the appendicular skeleton. Bones can also be classified according to their shape. **Long bones,** such as the

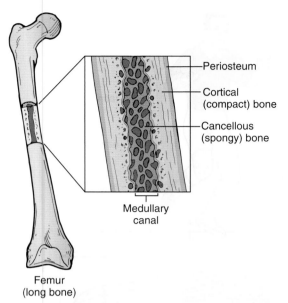

FIG. 9-1 Cortical and cancellous bone, periosteum, medullary canal.

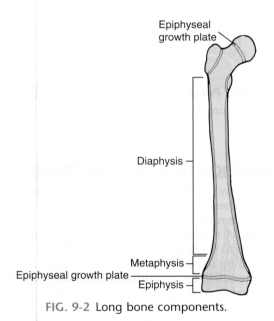

FIG. 9-2 Long bone components.

femur and humerus, are longer than they are wide. They have a tubular midportion, the **diaphysis,** which widens into a broader neck portion, the **metaphysis.** The end of the bone, the **epiphysis,** is widest in order to distribute the force of weight bearing over a wide area. In children, the epiphysis and metaphysis are separated from each other by a cartilaginous growth plate, which is the **epiphyseal growth plate** (Fig. 9-2). This plate is where the bone grows in length. After puberty, the epiphyseal plate calcifies and the epiphysis and metaphysis merge so that by adulthood, this demarcation is undetectable.

Short bones, such as the carpals and tarsals, are cuboidal in shape and are found exclusively in the ankle and wrist. They have a thin layer of cortical bone covering cancellous bone with no central medullary canal. Flat bones, such as those of the skull and pelvis, serve a protective function. These bones are made up of cortical plates that lie roughly parallel to one another and sandwich a cancellous central core. **Irregularly shaped bones** are found throughout the body and include the mandible and the vertebrae. **Sesamoid bones** develop in certain tendons in areas where those tendons cross the ends of long bones. They protect the tendon from excessive wear and increase the mechanical advantage of the muscle by changing its angle of attachment. The patella is an example of a sesamoid bone. **Accessory bones** are the supernumerary bones that develop when additional ossification centers appear and form extra bones. Many bones develop from this process but normally fuse together to form one. If one of these parts fails to fuse to the main bone, an "extra" bone appears. An accessory navicular bone is a common example of such a bone in the foot. **Heterotopic bone** may develop within soft tissue or around joints in areas where it is not normally present. Such bone often develops after blunt trauma or closed head injury.

> **Clinical Pearl**
> Bones give form to the body, support tissue, protect organs, and permit movement.

PATHOLOGY

FRACTURES AND THEIR CAUSES

A fracture is a break in the continuity of a bone. This term applies to all bony disruptions, ranging from small hairline fractures to multifragmentary or **comminuted fractures.** Bones fracture when the stress applied to them exceeds their strength. The most common cause of fractures in normal bone is trauma. This trauma may be direct or indirect, depending on whether a force is applied directly to the bone or at a distance from it. For example, with direct trauma, a bone may be fractured by an object falling on it or striking it. With direct trauma, there is often soft tissue injury around the fracture, and the fracture is often comminuted (in more than two pieces). Direct trauma is the most common mechanism of injury for fractures of the distal end of the fourth or fifth metacarpal **(boxer's fracture)** and for **transverse fractures** of the distal end of the radius **(Colles' fracture)** (Fig. 9-3, *A*). With indirect trauma, a fracture may be caused when a bending or twisting stress is applied at a distance from the resultant fracture. For example, a fall on an outstretched hand may result in a radial head fracture, whereas an inversion stress at the ankle may result in a fifth metatarsal fracture (Fig. 9-3, *B*).

The risk for a fracture and the pattern of the fracture depends largely on the nature of the applied force and the properties of the bone. A fracture may arise when a force

Clinical Pearl

Open fractures have a greater risk of complications than closed fractures because infection can enter through the broken skin.

RISK FACTORS FOR FRACTURES

The most common cause of fractures is trauma. The incidence of fractures and the types of fractures sustained vary with age, race, and co-morbidities. In the elderly, especially those with osteoporosis, the most common fractures are hip fractures; in children, forearm and leg fractures are more common.

Osteoporosis accounts for the largest number of fractures among the elderly. A woman's risk of developing a hip fracture is equal to her combined risk of developing breast, uterine, and ovarian cancer.[17] It is estimated that 8 million American women and 2 million American men have osteoporosis, putting them at risk for the pain and disability associated with fracture. Women have a higher risk of fracture than men of the same race, and whites generally have a higher risk of fracture than African-Americans of the same gender.[18] Over 90% of hip fractures are associated with osteoporosis, and most are associated with a fall.[19] Nationally, it is estimated that the direct costs for osteoporotic hip fractures was $18 billion in 2002.[20] National statistics show that 10% to 20% of people with hip fractures die within 6 months, 50% cannot walk without an assistive device, and 25% require long-term aid.[21] The most common sites of osteoporotic fractures are the vertebrae, hip, wrist, and proximal humerus.[22] Chapter 3 of this book has more information on the pathology, examination, and management of patients with osteoporosis.

Fractures in the elderly are also frequently associated with a history of poor balance and falls, especially falls to the side in which the patient lands on the greater trochanter[23] (see Chapter 13). Certain anthropometric characteristics, including tallness, long femurs, and low body weight, are also associated with increased hip fracture risk.[24] Some risk factors for fractures, such as advanced age, low body mass index, and low levels of physical activity, probably affect fracture incidence through the linked characteristics of osteoporosis, propensity toward falling, and the inability to absorb impact.[24]

Some fracture patterns occur most commonly or only in children. These include **greenstick fractures** and **torus fractures.** Greenstick fractures, as previously described, only occur in children and adolescents because these fractures only happen in somewhat elastic bones. A torus fracture is buckling of the bone that occurs most commonly in the forearm bones of children. With this type of fracture the bone becomes compressed at the point of impact, producing only a change in angulation of the cortex. Epiphyseal fractures also only occur in skeletally immature patients. When an epiphyseal fracture occurs at the end of a long bone near the joint, the disruption may halt or impair bone growth.

Certain diseases can weaken bone to such an extent that minor trauma results in a fracture. Fractures that occur under such circumstances may be called *pathological fractures.* Pathological fractures are associated with benign and malignant tumors, osteogenesis imperfecta, Paget's disease, osteomalacia, osteoporosis, and bone cysts. Approximately 75% of malignant tumors in bone are metastatic from a primary cancer elsewhere, most commonly the breast, thyroid, kidney, lung, or prostate[25]; 50% of bony metastases occur in the spine, usually in the thoracic or lumbar regions. A high index of suspicion for pathological fracture is necessary in patients with a history of cancer. Vertebral compression fractures are frequently seen in patients with advanced osteoporosis and are one of the most common pathological fractures. Because these fractures are not associated with significant trauma, they may go undetected unless there is a high level of suspicion on the part of the clinician.

Clinical Pearl

Pathological fractures are fractures that occur where the bone is weakened by another disease process such as a tumor or cyst.

FRACTURE HEALING

A fracture initiates a sequence of events that may ultimately restore the injured bone to its original state. Fractures in bone heal with like tissue without scar formation. This allows them to regain their prior mechanical and structural integrity. To understand the different processes that contribute to bone healing, it is helpful to view these events as distinct processes occurring in the bone itself and in the adjacent soft tissues. Depending on the type of fracture, its location, and the method by which it is treated, these responses may occur simultaneously or sequentially.

Clinical Pearl

Fractures in bone heal with like tissue without scar formation.

Primary and Secondary Fracture Healing. During primary healing, new bone grows directly across the compressed fracture site to unite the fracture without **callus** formation.[26] It takes approximately 5 to 6 weeks for a fracture to close by primary healing.[27] Although the healed bone is initially weak, with time and repeated static and cyclic loading, extensive remodeling occurs and the new bone regains the full strength of intact undamaged bone. Initially, when the bone is weak, the fracture site is stabilized and strengthened by the fixation device. When a rigid or stable fixation device is used, the site can be strong immediately after fixation, allowing for early initiation of weight bearing, functional activity, and rehabilitation. Early activity can shorten recovery time by reducing loss of range of motion (ROM), strength, and function.

However, surgical implantation of a fixation device, as opposed to using an external cast and avoiding surgery, subjects the tissues to a surgical procedure with its own inherent trauma and risks.

If motion across a fracture site is minimized but not eliminated, a fracture will close by secondary healing. Secondary healing, also known as *callus healing* or *indirect healing,* is an ordered process that starts with formation of a fibrous callus around the fracture site and ends with its conversion to bone. The callus initially stabilizes the fracture. The callus must be big enough to compensate for its relatively poor strength. Some motion at the fracture site is required to induce callus formation. However, there is a fine line between enough motion to induce the callus and too much motion that can prevent healing. Secondary healing occurs in fractures treated with stress-sharing devices such as casts, Kirschner wires (K wires), intramedullary rods, and external fixation devices. These devices align the bone fragments but do not compress the fracture gap, therefore allowing for some degree of motion. Secondary healing is the most common type of bone healing. Secondary healing is rapid and can bridge a gap as large as half of the diameter of the fractured bone.

Stages of Fracture Healing. Fracture healing generally occurs in three stages: inflammatory, repair, and remodeling.[28] These stages may overlap, and events that begin in one stage may continue into the following stage. The length of each stage varies with the location and severity of the fracture and associated injuries and other local and systemic factors.

The inflammatory stage of fracture healing typically lasts 1 to 2 weeks. When a bone is injured, both the bone and its blood supply are disrupted. Disruption of the blood vessels in and around the bone leads to formation of a hematoma at the injury site. The organization of this hematoma is the first step of fracture repair. The hematoma causes various molecules and cells to initiate the healing process.[29,30] Such molecules, including cytokines, interleukins, and various growth factors, regulate the early stages of healing, including cell proliferation and differentiation. Open fractures or those treated surgically may not have a hematoma at the fracture site, which may slow healing.

Soon after the hematoma forms, inflammatory cells, including neutrophils, macrophages, and phagocytes, invade the area. Along with osteoclasts, these cells remove the damaged and necrotic tissue near the distal edges of the fracture and lay the groundwork for the repair stage to begin. Radiographically, the fracture line becomes more visible as the necrotic material is removed, which is why some hairline fractures are not evident on x-ray until days after the initial injury.

The repair stage usually begins within 2 weeks of fracture occurrence and lasts several months. It is characterized by the differentiation of mesenchymal stem cells into the cell types necessary for tissue restoration. Chondrocytes and fibroblasts lay down a matrix for the callus. Initially, a soft callus composed mainly of fibrous tissue and cartilage with a small amount of bone is formed. Osteoblasts then mineralize this soft callus, converting it to a hard callus and increasing the stability of the fracture.

However, this immature bone is still weaker than normal bone, particularly in response to torque, and therefore must be protected. **Delayed union,** or **nonunion,** as described later in this chapter, generally results from errors in this phase of healing. The repair stage ends when the fracture is clinically stable. Radiographically, the fracture line begins to disappear during this stage.

During the remodeling stage, which can take months or years to complete, osteoblasts and osteoclasts replace the immature, poorly organized bone with mature, organized laminar bone, making the fracture site more stable. The ultimate goal of this stage is to restore the bone to its original strength and structure, giving it the ability to withstand the usual stresses placed on it. During this stage, areas of bone that sustain little stress are reabsorbed by osteoclasts, while more bone is laid down by osteoblasts in areas with high stress. Mechanical loading of the fracture site is needed to facilitate strong callus formation, fracture alignment, and ultimately lamellar remodeling.[31] Over time, the medullary canal inside the bone reforms and angular, although not rotational, deformities may correct. By the end of remodeling, the fracture line is no longer visible radiographically and the bone at the fracture site should have the same stiffness as normal bone and the same or greater strength than normal bone. Because a fully healed fracture is often stronger than the surrounding bone, subsequent application of an excessive load to the whole bone generally does not cause a fracture at the original fracture site but rather above or below the fracture site.

◉ *Clinical Pearl*

Because a fully healed fracture is often stronger than the surrounding bone, subsequent application of an excessive load to the whole bone generally does not cause a fracture at the original fracture site but rather above or below the fracture site.

Prognosis for Fracture Healing. Although the length of time for fracture healing varies, there is a typical rate at which fractures heal and some predictable variability based on the location and nature of the fracture and the type of fixation. For example, a distal radial fracture is expected to heal within 6 to 8 weeks, whereas healing of a midshaft femoral fracture may require 6 months.

The location and stability of the fracture can also affect how much callus forms. For example, metaphyseal fractures tend to heal with little callus formation because there is little surrounding periosteum and because the interdigitation and impaction of the fracture keeps the site stable and limits the fracture gap. In contrast, diaphyseal fractures tend to form a large callus because they are not impacted and have a larger fracture gap and more periosteum.

Fractures caused by high-speed or high-force impacts often heal slowly because there is more soft tissue and vascular damage in the area of the fracture and more fracture comminution. Open fractures also tend to heal more slowly than closed fractures because of the amount of soft tissue damage and bone loss, as well as fracture displacement and increased infection risk. Infection around a fracture not only compromises healing but may also lead to chronic infection of the bone known as **osteomyelitis.** Intraarticular fractures may also heal slowly because they can require extensive surgical intervention to assure good joint alignment.

Some fractures heal more slowly than expected or fail to heal at all. Slow healing is known as *delayed union,* and failure to heal is known as *nonunion.* Nonunion is generally defined as failing to heal after 6 to 8 months.[32] When a fracture fails to heal, cartilage or fibrocartilage forms over the fracture surfaces and the cavity between the fracture surfaces fills with fluid that resembles normal joint or bursal fluid. This false joint or **pseudoarthrosis** may or may not be painful but will always be unstable. A fibrous union formed by dense cartilage or fibrocartilage band may also be an end result and although it will stabilize the fracture site and may be painless, this union does not restore normal strength.

Common risk factors for delayed fracture healing include diabetes mellitus, smoking, long-term steroid use, nonsteroidal antiinflammatory drugs (NSAIDs) and other medications, and poor nutrition.[33] Diabetes is thought to impair fracture healing by causing a defect in collagen or collagen cross-linking.[33] Cigarette smoking interferes with osteoblast activity.[34] Nicotine can also impair healing by causing vasoconstriction and inhibiting angiogenesis, both of which can reduce blood flow to the fracture site.[35,36] Humans who smoke have been found to have more complications with fracture healing, including infections, amputations, and nonunions or **malunions,** and slower healing rates than their nonsmoking counterparts. With over 50 million smokers in the United States, it is important that the clinician and the patient take into consideration that smoking may delay fracture healing and increase the risk of complications and thus contribute to a poorer functional outcome.

Corticosteroids can delay fracture healing and increase the risk for fractures.[37,38] Delayed healing is thought to be due to decreased synthesis of organic bone matrix components and slowed differentiation of osteoblasts from mesenchymal cells. NSAIDs are also thought to slow fracture healing.

Nutrition also influences fracture repair as the energy required for the body to heal a fracture is substantial. To synthesize large volumes of collagen, proteoglycans, and other matrix constituents, cells need a steady supply of the components of these molecules—specifically proteins and carbohydrates. Fractures that would heal rapidly in well-nourished patients may fail to heal in patients with severe malnutrition.

A patient's age can also influence the rate of fracture healing. Infants have the most rapid rate of fracture healing, and the rate of fracture healing declines with age.[39] Fracture healing in adults and the elderly follows the same sequence, but in the elderly, it is often slower and less effective. For some fractures, age-related changes are significant enough to alter the treatment patterns. For example, a nondisplaced closed femoral fracture in a 3-year-old child may be effectively managed with a cast with restoration of tissue structure and function in 6 weeks, whereas a 70-year-old patient may require surgery and up to 6 months for an outcome that is much less predictable.

The amount of soft tissue damage also affects the rate of fracture healing. The time for a bone to heal is greatly prolonged in fractures that have more soft tissue stripping or damage. Studies have shown that muscle damage slows bone healing.[40] If the fracture site loses its intrinsic vascularity as a result of periosteal stripping from surgery or injury, comminution, or a large initial displacement, the extrinsic blood supply becomes imperative for fracture healing. The extrinsic blood supply of bone comes mainly from the muscles and the soft tissues that surround it.

The presence of infection can also slow or prevent fracture healing. Infection may cause necrosis of normal tissue, edema, and thrombosis of blood vessels.[41] If bone necrosis is present, healing depends entirely on ingrowth of vessels from the living side of the fracture and surrounding soft tissues. This type of healing occurs more slowly, and healing is less predictable.[42] Necrosis can be caused by irradiation, infection, surgical trauma, prolonged use of corticosteroids, and sickle cell anemia. Bone that has been irradiated often heals at a much slower rate than normal bone. This is especially important for pathological fractures treated with radiation.[43] Pathological fractures caused by malignancies also often fail to heal if the neoplasm is left untreated. This is also true of infected bone, which requires removal of the underlying infection and debridement.

The presence of osteoporosis does not impair fracture healing but may increase the time it takes to restore the mechanical strength of the bone. The decreased bone mass may also reduce the strength of the interface between a hardware implant used for internal fixation, which may lead to failure and subsequent delayed union or nonunion of the fracture site.[44]

◎ *Clinical Pearl*

Fracture healing may be delayed by diabetes, smoking, certain medications, and malnutrition.

Types of Fracture Fixation. If a fracture is inherently stable, such as occurs with a torus fracture of the radius as described previously, then a cast or a brace will exert sufficient force to limit interfragmentary motion. A cast is an externally applied circumferential plaster or fiberglass device that allows for secondary healing. Usually the joints above and below the fracture site are immobilized to prevent rotation or translation at the fracture site. Splints and braces, which are removable, can also be used for fracture stabilization. They offer the advantage of being removable for ROM and hygiene but also the disadvantage of possibly allowing for excessive motion with the noncompliant patient.

Many fractures require surgical placement of additional internal or external fixation to maintain stability while they are healing. The surgical procedure required for placement of these fixation devices may alter normal healing by injuring soft tissues, blood vessels, or periosteum around the fracture site.

A variety of techniques are currently used to surgically fix fractures. Many factors influence the selection of a fixation method, but the most crucial is the need for sufficient stability to achieve fracture healing. The biomechanics of fracture fixation is based on the principles of stress shielding or stress sharing. A stress-shielding device transfers stress to the implanted device and holds the fractured ends of bones together under compression so that no callus forms. The fracture heals by primary healing with no motion across the fracture, and all stresses in the area are absorbed by the plate. A compression plate is an example of a stress-shielding device. A stress-sharing device, such as a cast, intramedullary rod, or external fixator, absorbs only part of the forces at the fracture site. This allows for "micromotion" of the fracture site, which induces callus formation through secondary healing.

Most implanted fracture fixation devices are made of stainless steel, titanium, or occasionally a cobalt-chromium alloy. These devices can have a wide range of forms. A common device is the intramedullary rod. This is a long straight piece of metal placed in the bone. These are commonly used for fixation of fractures of long bones, most frequently the shaft of the femur, tibia, or humerus. They restore bone alignment and allow early weight bearing and mobilization of the joints above and below the fracture site. Intramedullary rods are load sharing and allow for secondary fracture healing through callus formation.

K wires hold fragments of bone together before rigid fixation. They lack sufficient mechanical stability to be used as primary support for weight-bearing bones but can be used in conjunction with other stronger wires or with other forms of external fixation such as casts or splints.

Plates are stress-shielding devices that take the load of the bone to allow for primary healing without callus formation. They are used most frequently in the upper extremity (UE) and the fibula where early load bearing is not as important. Plates are also used for periarticular and periprosthetic fractures where good alignment and lack of callus are most important. Because primary healing is slow, compression plating often requires a non–weight-bearing period, as well as secondary support such as a cast or splint, to prevent hardware failure that results from cyclic loading.

TYPICAL EXAMINATION FINDINGS

The examination of a patient who has sustained a fracture follows a format that allows the clinician to "paint" a picture of the patient and develop an intervention program that optimizes the patient's functional outcome. The examination includes a patient history, a systems review, and tests and measures.

PATIENT HISTORY

A thorough history of a patient with a fracture will include information about the patient's current presenting concerns, their prior level of function, and their goals for therapy. Direct communication with patients about their goals is important because their goals may differ from those of the physical therapist (PT) or physician.

Additionally, information from family members and other caregivers, especially when the patient is a child, is elderly, or has impaired cognitive abilities or other special needs, may allow the therapist to develop a realistic and appropriate plan of care for the patient. The patient's goals should be considered when selecting and prioritizing interventions. For example, if the patient's primary functional goal is independent toileting, then the therapist will focus on dynamic balance, safe transfers, and increasing strength or ROM to enable the patient to remove and replace clothing, as well as to achieve being able to rise from sitting to get on and off of the commode. Alternatively, if the patient's goal is to be able to sleep in his or her bed on the second floor, the therapist may need to address endurance, as well as managing stairs.

The patient history for patients with a fracture will also include demographic information and a social history, as well as information about their living environment. Attention will be paid to the presence of stairs or other environmental barriers, as well as bathroom access, especially for patients with LE fractures with a limited weight-bearing status. The PT may wish to examine the patient's home to ascertain if the patient will be able to safely negotiate his or her environment and to determine if environmental adaptations, such as hand rails, may need to be installed or if assistive devices, such as shower chairs, raised commodes, or reachers, are necessary or helpful for the patient during recovery. The availability of caregivers or family members to assist in the rehabilitation and recovery of the patient will also be noted.

The patient history will include information about when and where the fracture occurred, how it has been managed thus far, and what limitations or precautions have been recommended. The date of injury will help the clinician know the stage of healing. If the fracture involved a joint, current mobility and long-term functional outcome will more likely be affected than with an extraarticular fracture. The method and duration of fracture immobilization will influence the rate of recovery and the nature and duration of activity and weight-bearing precautions. Information about the surgery, fixation devices, as well as surgical restrictions (e.g., weight bearing or ROM) is taken from the operative report.

A general medical history may also alert the clinician to any factors that may delay fracture healing, such as diabetes, osteoporosis, or smoking, or that may delay or impair functional recovery such as a stroke. The patient's current medications may give insight into their ongoing medical problems, their pain level, and the possible risk for side effects that could delay fracture healing or functional recovery. The use and quantity of analgesic medications may give an indication of the patient's pain level. Antiinflammatory medications may impact pain and swelling, as well as the rate of tissue healing, and anticoagulants may limit the vigor of therapy. The use of other medications, alcohol, or tobacco can also be noted at this time.

SYSTEMS REVIEW

The systems review is used to target areas requiring further examination and to define areas that may cause complications or indicate a need for precautions during the examination and intervention processes. Chapter 1 includes details of the systems review.

TESTS AND MEASURES

When performing tests and measures on a patient with a fracture, it is important to follow ROM, resistance, and weight-bearing restrictions. Tests and measures start with an overall observation of the patient, their posture, and their willingness to move. Joints above and below the involved area are assessed to ensure that nothing is overlooked that may jeopardize an optimal outcome. For example, it is important to examine the wrist and shoulder in a patient that has sustained a fracture at the elbow.

Musculoskeletal

Anthropometric Characteristics. The girth around a joint and/or volume measurements, as well as observation and palpation, may be used to assess for the presence of edema. Girth and volume measurements of the involved side are compared with those of the uninvolved side to determine if a change has occurred. Edema is an indicator of inflammation and soft tissue injury. Loss of skin landmarks and wrinkles suggests moderate swelling, and a delay in capillary refill indicates severe swelling.[45]

Girth measurements around the middle of a limb segment may also be used to assess for muscle atrophy. Muscle atrophy is common after prolonged immobilization but may also occur if a peripheral nerve was injured at the time of the fracture. For example, axillary and radial nerve injuries commonly occur in conjunction with proximal humeral fractures. Atrophy that results from disuse can be differentiated from atrophy that results from nerve injury by peripheral nerve examination as described later.

Swelling in the limb may also indicate a more sinister pathology such as a deep venous thrombosis (DVT). Trauma, surgery, and prolonged immobilization are risk factors for local DVT formation.[46] In the LE, a DVT can occur proximal or distal to the popliteal artery. Proximal DVTs (PDVTs) are considered more dangerous because they are often larger and more likely to lead to pulmonary embolus. With hospitalizations getting shorter, it is more likely that rehabilitation professionals in both the inpatient and outpatient setting will see patients with DVTs. Although the Homans sign, the presence of pain in the calf when the toes are passively dorsiflexed, is often used clinically to screen for the presence of DVT, the poor sensitivity and specificity of this test make it inappropriate for clinical use.[47] It is recommended that clinicians use a clinical decision rule (CDR) (Box 9-1) that includes the presence of swelling and pain, as well as various other aspects of the patient history and physical examination, to more accurately estimate DVT risk.[48-50]

Range of Motion. Passive ROM (PROM) and active ROM (AROM) of the joint above and below the fracture, as well as muscle length, will be examined. If the fracture involves the hand, wrist, or foot, measure the ROM of the individual joints, as well as the functional range of combined movements. In addition to measuring the quantity of the motion, the PT will examine the quality of movement, including the presence of stiffness, muscle spasm, or guarding during the movement. Loss of ROM and joint

---

BOX 9-1	Clinical Decision Rule (CDR) for Proximal Deep Venous Thrombosis

- Active cancer within 6 months or diagnosis or palliative care
- Paralysis, paresis, or recent plaster immobilization of the LE
- Recently bedridden >3 days or major surgery within 4 weeks of application of the clinical decision rule
- Localized tenderness along the distribution of the deep venous system—firm palpation in the center of the posterior calf, popliteal space, and along the femoral vein along the anterior thigh
- Entire LE swelling
- Calf swelling >3cm compared to the asymptomatic LE measured 10 cm below the tibial tuberosity
- Collateral superficial veins (nonvaricose)
- Alternative diagnosis as likely or greater than that of DVT such as cellulitis, calf strain, or postoperative swelling

Score each as 1 point if positive except for the final bullet, which is scored as (−2). Interpret scores as follows:

<0: Probability of PDVT is 3% (confidence level 95%)
1-2: Probability of PDVT is 17% (confidence level 17%)
>3: Probability of PDVT is 75% (confidence level 75%)

Data from Wells PS, Anderson DR, Bormanis J, et al: *Lancet* 350:1795-1817, 1997 and Wells PS, Hirsh J, Anderson DR, et al: *J Intern Med* 243:15-23, 1998.
LE, Lower extremity; *DVT,* deep vein thrombosis; *PDVT,* proximal DVT.

---

stiffness are particularly common after an intraarticular fracture and prolonged joint immobilization.

Muscle Performance. Strength testing of the primary muscle groups around the fracture site, as well as a general screening for the strength of the involved upper or lower quarter, will be performed. The quality of the movement and any compensatory or accessory movements will be noted. For example, when testing forward flexion of the shoulder after a humeral fracture, trapezius activity instead of deltoid recruitment is recorded. Strength may be tested by manual muscle testing (MMT), hand-held dynamometry, or isokinetic means (see Chapter 5). Loss of strength because of disuse atrophy and inefficient motor recruitment is common after prolonged immobilization.

Joint Integrity and Mobility. The integrity of the joints above and below the fracture should be examined. This may be tested by accessory joint motions and ligament stability tests.

Neuromuscular

Pain. It is important for the clinician to determine if the patient has pain, and if so, its location, severity, quality, frequency, and how these symptoms change in relation to both rest and activity (see Chapter 22 for details of pain measures). Symptoms may occur not only at the fracture site but also in other areas affected by changes in biomechanics, sleeping positions, or gait changes. For example, immobilization of the UE with a sling may result in cervical pain, and gait deviations caused by a LE fracture may cause back pain. The response of symptoms to activity will give the clinician an appreciation of the severity and irritability of this patient's presentation.

Peripheral Nerve Integrity. Peripheral nerve integrity is generally determined through a combination of strength testing, sensory testing, and reflex testing (see Chapter 18). Electromyography (EMG) may also be used in select cases. Peripheral nerve integrity will often be examined in patients with fractures commonly associated with peripheral nerve injury, such as humeral shaft fractures, and in patients who report sensory changes or pain that is electrical in quality.

Integumentary. The clinician will assess the area of the fracture for any signs of inflammation such as swelling, redness, and temperature changes. These findings are normal early in fractures treated with both immobilization and surgical fixation. These findings should be differentiated from signs of infection, which often include fever and constitutional symptoms. The healing of any incision and the mobility of the scar should also be examined. Soft tissue mobility testing may be limited by tissue healing constraints, especially if the fracture was open and required skin grafts.

Function

Gait, Locomotion, and Balance. For the patient with a LE fracture, gait and balance will be examined. These tests may be limited at the initial examination by weight-bearing restrictions but should be repeated as weight-bearing restrictions are lifted.

After a LE fracture, it is common for patients to have gait deviations secondary to weight-bearing restrictions, pain, decreased strength, decreased proprioception and balance, and use of assistive devices or braces. Weight-bearing restrictions and pain with weight bearing will often cause the patient to use a "limb shortening strategy," with increased hip flexion, knee flexion, and ankle dorsiflexion, in an attempt to keep the extremity from full contact with the floor. Decreased strength or balance often results in the patient shortening his or her step length and may decrease the length of time in the stance phase of the affected extremity. Additionally, the patient may tend to shuffle his or her feet to decrease the amount of time in single limb support. A patient using assistive devices or braces may tend to ambulate with a "jerky" motion to advance his or her limb following the assistive device.

Assistive and Adaptive Devices/Orthotic, Protective, and Supportive Devices. Patients with weight-bearing restrictions will be provided with an assistive device, and the device should be checked for correct fit and appropriate use (see Chapter 33). The therapist should note if the patient is safe to use the specific device alone or with a trained individual or family member. If a brace or other protective device is used, note if the fit is appropriate, the alignment is appropriate, and it is functional.

EVALUATION, DIAGNOSIS, AND PROGNOSIS

Most patients who fall into preferred practice pattern 4G: Impaired joint mobility, muscle performance, and range

of motion associated with fracture have a history of trauma leading to fracture followed by some type of immobilization.[51] Tests and measures generally reveal decreased strength, decreased ROM, and reduced joint mobility, as well as pain and edema. For those with LE fractures, there are also often impairments in gait and balance and the patient often requires an assistive device for ambulation.

According to the *Guide to Physical Therapist Practice*,[51] the expected range of number of visits per episode of care for a patient with a fracture is between 6 and 18. Where a patient falls within this range may depend on the type of fracture and how it is managed. Fractures that are immobilized for a long period of time, involve a joint, or need surgical correction and those associated with significant soft tissue injury tend to need more physical therapy. Patient motivation may also affect the required duration of treatment.

The factors that influence prognosis for functional recovery after a fracture may be broadly placed into two categories: (1) extrinsic factors and (2) intrinsic factors. Extrinsic factors are factors not under the control of the patient that may lead to delayed healing of the bone or soft tissue, thereby delaying functional return. Intrinsic factors are factors under the patient's control that may lead to delayed functional recovery (Box 9-2).

BOX 9-2	**Extrinsic and Intrinsic Factors that Influence Fracture Healing**
Extrinsic Factors	**Intrinsic Factors**
• Type of fracture • Degree of comminution • Size of the fracture gaps • Accuracy of the reduction • Stability of the fixation • Whether the fracture was grafted • Involvement of the articular surface of the joint • Wound healing • Presence of infection • Degree of devitalization/ presence of osteoporosis • Patient's age • Events during postoperative care • Amount of surrounding soft tissue damage • Nerve damage • Vascular compromise • Presence of heterotopic ossification • Development of reflex sympathetic dystrophy (RSD) • Medications that interfere with healing • Co-morbidities	• Noncompliance with physician's restrictions • Noncompliance with home exercise program • Noncompliance with wound care management • Poor effort and lack of motivation • Smoking or use of other nicotine products • Poor nutrition

INTERVENTION

There are many intervention strategies and tools that can help a patient achieve optimal return of function after a fracture. In this section, specific interventions are identified and the reader is provided with evidence-based rationales and a clear explanation of how and when to apply each intervention. It is important to note that all interventions should be directly related to specific functional outcome goals and that these goals should be based on the limitations found during the initial examination and work in conjunction with the specific restrictions set forth by the referring physician (e.g., weight-bearing and ROM limitations).

COMMUNICATION AND DOCUMENTATION

One of the most important aspects of managing the patient with a fracture is communication between the members of the management team: the physician, the PT, the patient, and the caregiver. It is imperative that orders for rehabilitation, especially limitations and/or restrictions, be clearly delineated. It is the responsibility of the clinician to request a clarification of orders before commencing treatment. The therapist will have the initial examination, goals, plan of care, and treatment notes available for the referring physician and other members of the medical team.

EXERCISE

Aerobic Conditioning. Most fractures are caused by trauma, and many are associated with co-morbidities, multiple surgical procedures, lengthy hospital stays, and significant decreases in functional mobility. All of these factors contribute to a more sedentary lifestyle. There is little literature evaluating the specific benefits of aerobic exercise for patients with fractures, but one can extrapolate from the benefits for a sedentary population. These include lowering blood pressure, building stronger bones, improving muscle strength, improving flexibility, decreasing anxiety and depression, controlling weight, and improving functional abilities.[52-57]

The American College of Sports Medicine (ACSM) defines aerobic exercise as "any activity that uses large muscle groups, can be maintained continuously, and is rhythmic in nature." Aerobic exercise stresses the cardiovascular system above that which it is taxed at rest and makes it more efficient at delivering oxygenated blood to the working muscles and removing metabolic waste from the body (see Chapter 32). ACSM guidelines for healthy aerobic activity include the following:

- Exercise 3 to 5 days each week
- Warm up for 5 to 10 minutes before aerobic activity
- Maintain the exercise intensity for 30 to 45 minutes
- Gradually decrease the intensity of the workout
- Stretch to cool down for 5 to 10 minutes

The aerobic exercise program for a patient recovering from a fracture will reflect the restrictions placed on the patient by the physician. The therapist can be creative in implementing an aerobic conditioning program that matches the patient's current ability and can progress the program in intensity, length, and variety to most closely match the patient's desired functional outcome. Choices of aerobic training may include but are not limited to walking, treadmill jogging or running, stair climbing, elliptical training, stationary biking, dancing, swimming, and using a cross-country skiing machine, an upper body ergometer, or a rowing machine.

An example of adapting these activities for a patient with a fracture would be stationary bicycling with only the uninvolved leg (and both arms) for the patient who sustained a LE fracture and may not bear weight on that limb (Fig. 9-7, *A*). Additionally, an athlete who sustained a LE stress fracture and is training for a specific competition but has not been cleared for full weight bearing may benefit from body weight–supported treadmill jogging (Fig. 9-7, *B*) or by jogging in water, with or without the use of a vest flotation device. If the patient has pain with impact but does not have a weight-bearing restriction, he or she may benefit from cross-training on an elliptical trainer. As with all aerobic conditioning programs, it is ideal to alternate the mode of exercise, when possible, to recruit additional muscle groups, overcome plateaus in aerobic capacity, and avoid monotony of endurance training.

Balance, Coordination, and Agility Training. After a period of prolonged immobilization or altered weight-bearing after a fracture, patients may have an abnormal or altered sense of balance. The patient's body must adapt to changes in center of gravity (COG) and must modify postural reflex reactions to accommodate these changes. COG may be changed slightly by simple alterations in position such as when the UE is kept in a sling in front of the patient with a clavicle fracture. Conversely, the COG may be altered significantly when an external fixator is applied for a complex tibial fracture, and the patient is required to not bear weight on that lower extremity and must use bilateral axillary crutches.

Additionally, joint swelling after acute trauma may result in muscle inhibition. It is common for the quadriceps muscles to be inhibited and contract poorly when the knee is swollen and for the peroneus longus muscle to be inhibited when the ankle is swollen.

Other factors that may contribute to impaired coordination and balance, especially when the task demands significant strength, include disuse atrophy and altered neuromuscular control. If the task is too demanding for the patient to perform, he or she may attempt to recruit compensatory muscles to complete the task, thereby modifying his or her stabilizing posture and counterbalance force.

Most of the research on the effects of balance, coordination, and agility training on functional recovery from fractures has been conducted on elderly patients with hip fractures. There is strong evidence to support ongoing functional, weight-bearing group exercise or home exercise programs (HEPs) for elderly patients with or without cognitive impairments who have sustained fall-related hip fractures. These programs also appear to be cost-effective when weighed against the substantial cost of hospitalizations for injuries sustained from subsequent falls.

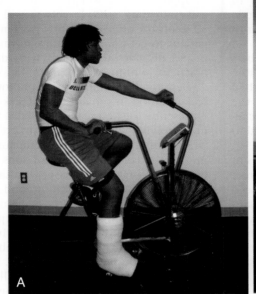 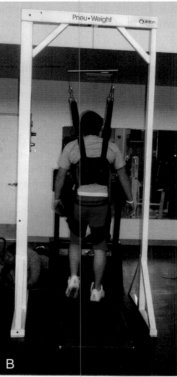

FIG. 9-7 Aerobic conditioning with fractures. **A,** Patient with a lower extremity fracture performing aerobic conditioning on a stationary bicycle. **B,** Patient with a lower extremity stress fracture performing aerobic conditioning while partially unweighted using harness and treadmill.

Stretching. After immobilization following a fracture, patients often have decreased ROM, joint stiffness, and decreased flexibility of the musculotendinous unit and surrounding fascial layers. Since long-term functional limitations are more often complicated by soft tissue dysfunction rather than the actual damage to bone, interventions should address soft tissue restrictions and lack of flexibility in the muscle groups surrounding the fracture site as early as it is safe to do so.

A number of different stretching techniques may be used to increase ROM and flexibility and reduce joint stiffness. These include ballistic, static, and passive stretching, as well as techniques based on proprioceptive neuromuscular facilitation (PNF). These techniques are described in Table 9-1.

The evidence evaluating which stretching method to use, the ideal duration of stretching, and the timing of stretching in relationship to a workout to elicit maximal gains in muscle length is contradictory. Some findings suggest that at least 30 seconds of static stretching per day, 5 times per week for 6 weeks is sufficient to increase hamstring flexibility.

In regard to timing of stretching, the ACSM's guidelines state that muscles, tendons, ligaments, and joints may be "more responsive to stretching after the endurance phase."

There are no clinical trials to date that demonstrate a correlation between stretching method and functional

TABLE 9-1	Stretching Techniques
Technique	**Description**
Ballistic	Quick, repetitive bouncing movements
Static	Slow, sustained stretching
Passive	Slow, sustained stretching by an external force
PNF	Contraction of a lengthened muscle, followed by stretching, either actively or passively; may need the assistance of a partner

PNF, Proprioceptive neuromuscular facilitation.

gains; however, many medical professionals recommend static stretching because it is relatively simple to learn, does not require a partner, and is less likely to exceed the limits of tissue extensibility than a resistive or ballistic style stretch. Additionally, static stretching may facilitate the inhibition of muscle contraction by the Golgi tendon organs (GTO), thereby allowing greater increases in hamstring length.[58]

Proponents of PNF-style stretching argue that it may produce greater gains in flexibility than other types of stretching because autogenic inhibition and reciprocal inhibition allow the muscle to relax more effectively.[59] Others propose that this approach is effective because the tactile cues involved provide a neurologically enhanced training stimulus.[60] Still others advocate a viscoelastic theory, in which increases in flexibility are caused by repeated repositioning of the collagenous and elastin fibers within the connective and contractile tissue.[59] Recent studies have shown that submaximal contractions (with contract-relax PNF programs) are sufficient to produce gains in muscle length.[61] A limitation of PNF-style stretching, however, is that it usually requires a partner to provide resistance and a subsequent stretching force.

Ballistic stretching rapidly stretches the muscle fibers activating the intrafusal muscle spindles and leading to a reflexive and protective muscle contraction of the stretched muscle.[62] This may increase the chance of injury to the muscle or tendon and may cause muscle soreness, especially in sedentary individuals who are not accustomed to the rapid stretch.[63]

Strengthening. One of the primary complications of fractures is weakness secondary to immobilization, disuse, swelling, pain, or direct muscle trauma. The PT will keep in mind restrictions in ROM, use of splints or braces, and weight-bearing status that may limit a patient's ability to perform strengthening exercises. The PT should communicate with the surgeon to ensure that sufficient fracture healing has occurred to progress through the stages of strengthening.

Chapter 5 contains general recommendations for interventions to address weakness and impaired muscle performance. Strengthening interventions will be adapted from the standard application because of the activity restrictions placed on the patient. For example, for a patient with a tibial fracture and weak quadriceps during resisted straight leg raises, resistance should be applied at the proximal leg or distal thigh rather than distal to the fracture. Similarly, a patient with a fracture of the distal radius may not be able to use hand-held weights in the initial stages of rehabilitation to strengthen his or her shoulder girdle but may be able to use an elastic band or tubing applied to the distal humerus to provide appropriate resistance.

FUNCTIONAL TRAINING

Gait Training. Many patients with LE fractures have gait deviations and may benefit from gait training (see Chapter 32). In patients with fractures, the therapist must ensure that the patient has sufficient ROM, strength, balance, and pain control before advancing gait, or they may cause the patient to adopt additional compensatory strategies that may further affect their ability to ambulate. When patients are recovering from LE fractures, it is common for a physician to advance the patient's weight-bearing status as their healing status progresses. They may start with non-weight bearing (NWB), and advance through toe-touch weight bearing (TTWB), to partial weight bearing (PWB), to full weight bearing as tolerated (WBAT). These restrictions may be based on a number of factors such as the severity of the injury, whether the fracture was stabilized, the length of time from the initial injury, and whether the bone shares weight-bearing responsibilities (i.e., fibula versus tibia). When a patient is PWB, the surgeon may give specific restrictions regarding the percentage of body weight that the patient may apply through his or her affected limb. Many patients have

difficulty determining the amount of pressure that is equal to a portion of their body weight, for example, 25% of their body weight. One solution that has been suggested to help remedy this problem is to determine what 25% of their total weight is and have them use a bathroom scale to apply the 25% weight on their affected limb as they gait train (i.e., a 200 lb patient will be allowed to apply 50 lb on the affected limb). This remedy may enable the patient to get a more accurate feeling of what 25% PWB is and provides the patient with direct feedback while practicing within his or her limitations.

Despite the number of limitations of the bathroom scale method in providing feedback for PWB training, it is presently the best readily available tool to assist patients in complying with weight-bearing restrictions.

Assistive Devices. After a fracture, a patient is usually immobilized or has other restrictions placed on him or her by the surgeon to allow proper healing. These restrictions, combined with pain, swelling, and weakness will often prevent the patient from independently performing activities of daily living (ADLs) or from participating in independent ADLs (IADLs). With an UE fracture involving the wrist or hand, the patient loses the ability to perform even simple tasks that require two hands. Similarly, if a patient has a LE fracture and cannot bear full weight on his or her extremity, the patient will need to use an assistive device for mobility, which may further encumber the use of the UEs. This patient may now need to use a backpack or other type of carrier to carry his or her belongings. There are numerous assistive devices to aid patients who are recovering from fractures with resuming ADLs and IADLs. These range from wheelchairs, walkers, and crutches to assist with mobility to reachers that enable a person to grasp something placed beyond their reach (see Chapter 33 for more information on assistive devices).

Injury Prevention. Throughout the rehabilitation process, the PT should reevaluate the patient's ability to safely negotiate his or her environment. If a patient does not have the strength, balance, or cognitive ability to safely move in his or her environment before discharge from the hospital, the PTA needs to consult with the PT. An alternate discharge plan may need to be arranged. Case management and/or social services are usually available to ensure that services are brought into the home or that the patient is discharged to the proper level of care.

Since fractures occur when external forces exceed the inherent strength of the bone, the focus of fracture prevention has been on improving bone density (with osteoporotic patients) and on reducing the incidence of falls (via balance, agility, strength training, and education programs) (see Chapters 3 and 13).

MANUAL THERAPY

Physical therapy should focus on the restoration of ROM once sufficient healing or stable fixation has occurred. Early motion will help to decrease the incidence of adhesions, decrease atrophy of articular cartilage, and help prevent capsular or ligamentous contractures.[64,65] If the patient does not have sufficient strength to perform active ROM exercises, the therapist may want to begin with PROM activities.

PROM is the amount of motion that is produced solely by an external force, without any active muscle contraction. The external force may be applied by the clinician, gravity, or an external device. If the patient is hesitant to move the extremity, the therapist may want to begin by manually moving the patient's joint into the allowed ROM while the patient lies in a relaxed position. The therapist can maintain the joint in the end-range position briefly and then slowly return the joint back to its resting position. When performing manual PROM on a patient, it is important for the therapist to provide gentle but firm contact with the patient's extremity at all times. To relax, the patient must trust that the therapist will not make any sudden moves or push into a region of pain. If the patient is fearful, he or she will tend to muscle guard and block motion from occurring.

The therapist can also teach patients how to use gravity and their opposing limb to independently perform PROM as a part of their HEP. For example, while performing supine wall slides to increase knee flexion ROM, patients can be instructed to use gravity to allow their heel to slide down the wall, thereby flexing the knee. After a brief holding period in the flexed position, patients can use the opposite LE to push the heel up the wall and assist the knee back into extension. Similarly, to obtain terminal knee extension, a patient can be taught to lie prone with the knee hanging off the edge of a bed. Gravity will produce a force on the lower leg to help achieve terminal knee extension.

A more technical device that has been developed to assist with PROM is the continuous passive motion (CPM) machine. CPM machines are electrically powered devices that provide a slow and controlled passive mechanical force to move a joint through a prescribed or preset ROM. The clinician is able to control the ROM, as well as the speed of motion (Fig. 9-8). Although many physicians continue to prescribe CPM machines after LE surgical procedures, the literature shows mixed results in terms of both short- and long-term benefits.[66,67]

ELECTROTHERAPEUTIC MODALITIES

Electrotherapeutic modalities may be used to control pain or edema associated with a fracture, facilitate specific muscle strengthening, and perhaps most importantly in patients with fractures, improve tissue healing. It is important to note that the successful use of modalities to produce the desired outcome depends on the appropriate selection and application of modality variables. Continued research is needed in this field to further define which treatment variables produce the best results.

Electrical Stimulation to Control Pain. Pain is the most common symptom associated with fractures. Clinicians debate which method most effectively controls pain with the fewest side effects. Transcutaneous electrical nerve stimulation (TENS) is one of the primary electrotherapeutic modalities that can relieve pain. A few benefits of the use of TENS over other methods of pain management are that it is noninvasive and well tolerated by most patients. TENS is thought to decrease pain, according to the gate theory of pain control, by selectively stimulating A-beta nerve fibers, thereby interfering with the transmission of noxious stimuli from the periphery to the brain via small myelinated A-delta nerve fibers and small unmyelinated C nerve fibers.

Conventional TENS (with a pulse frequency of 100 to 150 pps, a pulse duration of 50 to 80 μsec, and an intensity above sensory but below motor threshold) has been found to be comfortable and effective in decreasing pain.[68-70] TENS has also been found to cause a release of endorphins in the spinal cord.[71] Motor level electrical stimulation with a low pulse frequency of less than 10 pps has been found to stimulate the production of endogenous opiates, which have also been found to decrease one's perception of pain.[72,73]

Electrical Stimulation to Control Edema. Monophasic pulsed electrical current, particularly high voltage pulsed current (HVPC), has been studied for its effects on edema formation after trauma. Proposed mechanisms for this effect include repelling negatively charged ions and cells from the area of inflammation and decreasing the permeability of the microvascular membrane.[74] Additionally, when electrical stimulation produces muscle contractions, these contractions may reduce edema by improving lymphatic and venous return. No specific evidence to date supports the use of electrical stimulation to decrease edema or inflammation in patients with fractures.

Electrical Stimulation to Improve Strength. Neuromuscular electrical stimulation (NMES) is often used clinically as an adjunct to strengthening exercises and to retard the effects of disuse atrophy. Most studies in this area involve postoperative LE injuries, including anterior cruciate ligament (ACL) reconstructions, meniscectomies, lateral releases, and total knee arthroplasty (TKA).[75-82] The effect of this intervention is based on the fact that electrical stimulation can produce strong muscle contractions and that strong muscle contractions can increase strength, according to the overload principle. It is assumed that this increased strength will then translate to an increase in function.

Electrical Stimulation to Promote Fracture Healing. Since the 1950s, researchers have been interested in finding biological applications for electricity, especially as it pertains to the healing of fractures. Of particular interest is the potential benefit for improved fracture healing with nonunions, which account for approximately 5% to 10% of all fractures in the United States annually.[83,84]

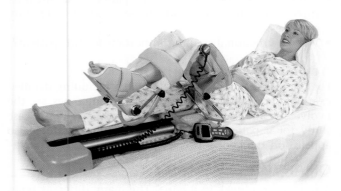

FIG. 9-8 Continuous passive motion. *Photo courtesy Chattanooga Group.*

In the laboratory, electromagnetic fields have been found to stimulate the biological processes involved in osteogenesis via stimulation of extracellular matrix synthesis, increases in proteoglycan and collagen synthesis, and inhibition of osteoclastic bone resorption.[85-87]

Currently, there are three clinical methods to deliver electrical stimulation to bone. The first method involves the application of direct current (DC) directly to the fracture site using percutaneous or surgically implanted electrodes. This invasive procedure is beyond the scope of physical therapy practice. Capacitive coupling (CC) uses external electrodes applied to the skin with conductive gel to produce an electrical field at the fracture site. Pulsed electromagnetic fields (PEMF), or inductive coupling (IC), uses electromagnetic coils placed over the fracture site without contact with the skin and can be secured to the outside of a cast.

PHYSICAL AND MECHANICAL AGENTS

Ultrasound (US) is a form of mechanical energy that can be transmitted through biological tissues, via a piezoelectric crystal, as high frequency acoustical pressure waves. PTs have used US for its thermal, as well as nonthermal, effects on soft tissues (muscles, tendons, ligaments, joint capsules, and so on) for many years. Use of US as a modality in patients with fractures, however, has been negligible in the physical therapy community because it was previously thought to be contraindicated in the area of a healing fracture.[88] However, recent evidence shows that low-intensity pulsed US (LIPUS) can promote fracture healing. The Food and Drug Administration (FDA) cleared the use of LIPUS for accelerating fresh fracture healing in October 1994 and for the treatment of established nonunions in February 2000. The FDA-approved device used in clinical trials is the EXOGEN 2000. The parameters are preset within this unit.

There are a number of proposed mechanisms for the effectiveness of LIPUS on delayed union or nonunion fractures. These include influences on gene expression at all stages of healing, increasing blood vessel formation at the site of the clot, increasing growth factor release, increasing synthesis of cartilage matrix proteins by chondrocytes, increasing cartilage formation at the fracture callus, increasing the progression of bridging at the bone gap, and increasing blood flow at the fracture site during and shortly after the US stimulus has been removed.[89-94]

CASE STUDY 9-1

COLLES' FRACTURE

Patient History

JT is a 35-year-old right-hand dominant cafeteria worker who sustained a Colles' fracture to her right UE 6 weeks ago after tripping and falling onto an outstretched arm. She was treated conservatively with a cast, which was removed yesterday. She reports no pain at rest but has a dull ache when she attempts to move her wrist. She reports that her wrist also gets sore and tired after attempting to eat a few bites with her fork in her right hand. JT's past medical history is significant for a 4-year history of cigarette smoking, but JT reports that she stopped smoking before having her children.

Tests and Measures—Significant Findings
Musculoskeletal

- Significant atrophy of right forearm musculature (both flexors and extensors). No swelling. Visible callus formation on the dorsal aspect of the radius, 2 inches proximal to the joint line.
- AROM of right wrist: Flexion—45 degrees, extension—30 degrees, radial deviation—5 degrees, ulnar deviation—8 degrees. JT also has difficulty opposing her thumb to her fifth finger.
- Grip strength on the right with hand-held dynamometer on 3 trials is 14 psi, 16 psi, 17 psi at position 3, compared to 60 psi, 62 psi, 68 psi on the left. Strength by MMT of right wrist flexion and extension is grossly 3/5 within her available range.

Neuromuscular

- Mildly decreased coordination and dexterity with quick finger opposition on the right.

Diagnosis

Preferred practice pattern 4G: Impaired joint mobility, muscle performance, and range of motion associated with fracture.

Interventions

- Joint mobilization to the radiocarpal and intercarpal joints. Static stretches.
- Strengthening exercises for the entire right UE, including the shoulder girdle, elbow, wrist, and hand intrinsics. Manual dexterity exercises with the right hand.
- Functional training.
- Apply ice after therapy.

Role of the Physical Therapist Assistant

- Why is it important for this patient to apply ice after the other therapy interventions?
- Which of the prescribed types of exercises will improve strength? Which will improve ROM? Which will improve coordination?
- Write a home program for this patient that includes three strengthening and three manual dexterity exercises.
- Why is functional training important for this patient?

Additional Information

For the full version of this case study, including detailed examination results, interventions, and outcomes, see the Evolve site that accompanies this book. A detailed case study for a patient with a delayed union fracture also appears on the Evolve site.

CHAPTER SUMMARY

A fracture is a break in a bone. The many different types of fractures are categorized based primarily on their location and the mechanism of injury. Fractures may initially be treated with immobilization and in many cases, surgical fixation, to promote healing. Fracture healing may be affected by extrinsic and intrinsic factors. Fracture healing and functional recovery may be accelerated and optimized by appropriate rehabilitation interventions, including exercise, PROM, joint mobilization, and various physical agent modalities.

ADDITIONAL RESOURCES

For links to these and additional web-based resources, see the Evolve site.

Bucholz RW, Heckman JD, et al (eds): *Rockwood and Green's fractures in adults,* ed 6, Philadelphia, 2006, Lippincott.

Einhorn TA, O'Keefe RJ, Buckwalter JA (eds): *Orthopaedic basic science: Foundations of clinical practice,* ed 3, Chicago, 2007, American Academy of Orthopedic Surgeons.

Schatzker J, Tile M: *The rationale of operative fracture care,* ed 3, New York, 2006, Springer.

The Journal of Bone and Joint Surgery

American Academy of Orthopedic Surgeons

GLOSSARY

Accessory bone: Supernumerary bones that develop when secondary ossification centers appear and form extra bones. Such bones are commonly seen in the foot and are often mistaken for fractures.

Avulsion fracture: A fracture caused by a tendon or ligament pulling off a small piece of bone to which it is attached.

Boxer's fracture: A fracture of fourth and/or fifth metacarpal often seen after the patient strikes an object or person.

Callus: A combination of cartilage, bone and fibrous tissue that fills and surrounds the fracture site during the process of fracture healing.

Cancellous bone: Spongy bone.

Closed fracture: A fracture without a break in the overlying skin.

Colles' fracture: A metaphyseal fracture of the distal radius that is dorsally angulated.

Comminuted fracture: A fracture that forms more than two pieces of bone.

Compression fracture: A fracture in which cancellous bone collapses and compresses on itself. Typically this occurs in the vertebral bodies.

Cortical bone: The dense outer layer of bone.

Delayed union: Progression of healing of a fracture that is slower than average.

Diaphysis: The central tubular portion of a long bone.

Epiphysis: The end of a long bone.

Epiphyseal growth plate: A horizontal growth plate located at the ends of immature long bones.

Fracture: A break in a bone.

Greenstick fracture: A fracture through only one side of a bone This fracture is common in children.

Heterotopic bone: Abnormal bone formation within a tendon, muscle, or joint.

Impaction fracture: A fracture in which a bony fragment, generally cortical, is forced or impacted into cancellous bone. Typically this occurs at the ends of long bones.

Irregularly shaped bones: Bones, such as those in the jaw or the spinal column, that are of various shapes—examples of which are the mandible and the vertebrae.

Linear fracture: A fracture that runs parallel to the long axis of a bone.

Long bones: Tubular-shaped bones.

Malunions: Fractures that have united with angulation or rotation to a degree that gives a displeasing appearance or adversely affects function.

Metaphysis: The part of a long bone between the diaphysis and the epiphysis where the bone starts to widen.

Nonunion: The failure of a fracture to heal.

Oblique fracture: A fracture at approximately 30 degrees to the long axis of the bone.

Open fracture: A fracture in which the skin is broken exposing the fracture site to the external environment.

Osteomyelitis: Inflammation of the bone caused by a pathological organism.

Pseudoarthrosis: A false joint that develops at the site of a fracture

Sesamoid bone: A bone within a tendon.

Stress fracture: A fracture caused by repeated, prolonged, or abnormal stress.

Torus fracture: A fracture that warps but does not completely break one side of the cortex of the bone, also known as a *buckle fracture*. This fracture is most commonly seen in children.

Transverse fracture: A fracture perpendicular to the long axis of the bone.

Chapter 10

Joint Arthroplasty

Julie A. Pryde

CHAPTER OUTLINE

OBJECTIVES

After reading this chapter, the reader will be able to:
1. List the surgical considerations and options available for joint arthroplasty and arthrodesis.
2. Understand the postoperative precautions and restrictions following specific joint arthroplasty procedures.
3. Discuss the current research on joint arthroplasty and its limitations.
4. Understand the goals of total joint replacement surgery.
5. Identify safe and effective evidence-based rehabilitation programs for patients after joint arthroplasty.

Joint arthroplasty is any reconstructive joint procedure, with or without an implant, designed to relieve pain and/or restore joint motion. Most joint arthroplasty involves a joint implant and is known as *joint replacement surgery.* Over the past 4 decades, joint replacement surgery has become the most successful surgery for patients with severe debilitating arthritis.[1] These procedures have also been used successfully in the management of joints affected by **avascular necrosis**, fractures, and tumors.[2-4]

Joint replacement procedures, such as total hip and total knee replacements, are types of joint arthroplasty.

Hip or knee joint replacements have become some of the most common procedures in orthopedic surgical practice in the United States, with an estimated 152,000 total hip arthroplasties (THA) and 360,000 total knee arthroplasties (TKA) performed in the United States in 2000.[5] The number of these procedures is steadily increasing as the population ages and the age of patients having these surgeries decreases.[6] Although the average age of a patient undergoing THA is 69 years, this procedure is increasingly being performed on patients less than 50 and more than 75 years old.[7]

Total joint replacement has emerged as one of the most successful and common procedures for the treatment of joint degeneration as a result of arthritis, and arthritis is the reason for the majority of elective joint replacement surgeries.[8] Over 21 million people in the United States have arthritis, and as the population ages, this number will undoubtedly increase.[9] Arthritis is the leading cause of long-term disability in the United States and the second leading cause of decreased physical activity.[10] As health care–related expenditures increase, joint replacement surgeries have emerged as an accepted cost-effective and efficacious treatment for the management of arthritis.[11,12] For example, the cost-effectiveness of a THA has been found to be similar to or better than that of a coronary artery bypass graft (CABG) or renal dialysis.[13]

The knee is the joint most frequently affected by osteoarthritis (OA)[14,15] and therefore is the most common joint replaced. Although many conservative measures may initially reduce the pain and disability associated with OA of the knee, with severe arthritis, TKA is necessary to optimize functional outcome.

◎ Clinical Pearl

Total joint replacement is one of the most common and successful interventions for patients with joint degeneration caused by arthritis.

PATHOLOGY

The term *arthroplasty* refers to any reconstructive joint procedure, with or without joint implant, designed to

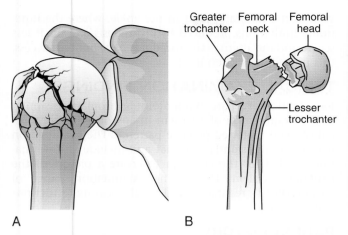

Greater trochanter Femoral neck Femoral head

Lesser trochanter

A   B

FIG. 10-1 Traumatic causes for joint replacement. **A,** Four-part humeral head fracture. **B,** Displaced femoral neck fracture.

relieve pain and/or restore joint motion. There are a number of different types of arthroplasty. Total joint replacements involve removing both the proximal and distal joint surfaces and replacing them with an artificial joint implant. The primary components of these implants are made of an inert metal, such as chromium cobalt, titanium, or stainless steel, or of ceramic. Some components of specific joint implants are made of high-density polymer plastics such as polyethylene. These include the glenoid component of the shoulder, the patella resurfacing "button" and spacer of the knee, and in some hips, the liner of the acetabulum. Implants can be attached to the bone with cement **(methylmethacrylate),** screws, or other hardware or without cement, using either biological fixation by ingrowth of bone into a porous-coated implant or by being tightly press-fit.

Hemiarthroplasty involves removing and replacing only one side of the joint, or one compartment in the case of the knee. This procedure is gaining favor and is often used when one side of a joint is damaged and the other side is intact. This often occurs with trauma that damages the long bones, causing, for example, a four-part humeral head fracture or a displaced femoral neck fracture (Fig. 10-1). Hemiarthroplasty may also be indicated for unicompartmental arthritis, avascular necrosis, or when a tumor needs to be excised. Hemiarthroplasty of the knee, shoulder, and hip is generally successful, reducing pain and improving function.

Clinical Pearl

Total joint replacement involves removing both the proximal and distal joint surfaces and replacing them with an artificial joint implant. Hemiarthroplasty involves removing and replacing only one side of a joint.

A bipolar or unipolar hemiarthroplasty can be used to treat fractures on or around the femoral neck that can not

be treated by open reduction internal fixation. In a unipolar hip arthroplasty the femoral head and neck are replaced with a prosthetic implant with a stationary head that articulates with a single bearing. This type of device is often used in elderly patients who place lower demands on the prosthesis as a result of their ambulatory and medical status. This is also the least expensive type of implant used. The more complex bipolar hip prosthesis has a fixed femoral head component capped with a plastic acetabular bearing attached to the femoral ball and a mobile metal cup attached to the plastic bearing. The metal cup can move freely along the cartilaginous acetabular surface, which is thought to lessen the potential for pain and destructive wear.

Under special circumstances, such as when there is joint infection, joint ankylosis, or failure of a prior arthroplastic procedure, a number of alternative arthroplastic procedures that do not involve replacement of the joint with an implant may be performed. These include **resection arthroplasty,** also known as *excisional arthroplasty,* which involves removal of one or both articular surfaces of a joint, allowing a fibrotic scar to form in the space that remains, and **fascial arthroplasty,** which involves debriding the joint and placing a foreign material, such as fascia, between the two joint surfaces. These procedures, although used less commonly, are still appropriate in selected cases.

In the hip, one type of resection arthroplasty, Girdlestone pseudarthrosis, which dates back to 1923, can be used as a temporary intervention or permanent treatment of joint infection or when ankylosis of the hip has placed it in an unsuitable position for function. This may be seen in some patients with spinal cord injury, severe Parkinsonism, multiple sclerosis, or head injury. In this procedure the femoral neck and head are resected at the level of the intertrochanteric line and the remaining end of the femur is left free to articulate with the acetabulum. Although this procedure improves perineal care and allows for a pain-free joint with relatively good motion, the hip generally has poor stability, and the involved lower extremity is shortened. These result in gait deviations and the need for an assistive device during ambulation. A similar procedure, the resection arthroplasty, can be performed in the knee after an infected prosthesis is removed. This also generally produces an unstable joint.

When a total joint replacement fails as a result of fracture or loosening, or in other patient-specific circumstances, **arthrodesis,** also known as *joint fusion,* may be performed. Arthrodesis is the creation of a bony union across a joint. This procedure can alleviate the pain associated with arthritis by eliminating motion across the joint. It is also used to treat fractures across a joint that can not otherwise be managed. Arthrodesis may occur spontaneously, for example, as the result of infection, or be surgically produced. Unfortunately, since arthrodesis eliminates motion, it generally also impairs function, and with spontaneous arthrodesis, functional outcomes are worse because the joint fuses in the position that produces the least pain rather than in the position that optimizes function.

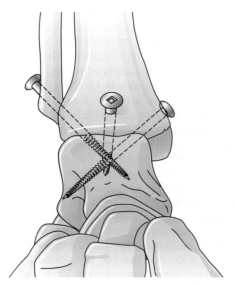

FIG. 10-2 Surgically fused ankle.

BOX 10-1   Indications for Arthrodesis

- Painful, degenerative, posttraumatic arthritis or RA that can not be helped by arthroplasty
- Avascular necrosis or osteonecrosis that can not be treated by arthroplasty
- Neurological disease that resulted in an unstable joint
- Neuropathic joints
- Infection such as chronic osteomyelitis
- Failed total joint arthroplasty caused by infection, resulting in severe bone loss, and precluding a revision arthroplasty
- Deltoid or quadriceps femoris paralysis

RA, Rheumatoid arthritis.

Surgical arthrodesis can be performed in almost any joint, including those of the spine. The most commonly fused joints are the ankle, wrist, spine, and thumb. The technique used to produce fusion is similar in all joints. The articular cartilage is removed from the joint surfaces, and the joint is positioned at an optimal angle for function and to maximize the contact area between bony surfaces for optimal stabilization and fusion. The joint is filled with autologous or cadaveric bone chips or pieces to produce a graft, and the joint position is maintained with internal fixation hardware, such as rods, plates, or screws, or by an external fixation, such as a cast or external fixator (Fig. 10-2). Over time, the bone graft solidifies to permanently immobilize the joint.

There are many indications for arthrodesis (Box 10-1). However, because of the poor functional results for most joints, this procedure is avoided if possible. For example, in the elbow, the loss of motion produced by a fusion prevents most functional uses of the extremity, including feeding and personal hygiene. However, in some joints, such as the tibiotalar joint in the ankle, where the functional limitations produced by arthrodesis are much less severe and the alternative procedures have limited success, this procedure is often used.

TYPICAL EXAMINATION FINDINGS

Examination of a patient after joint arthroplasty is similar to the examination of a patient in any of the other musculoskeletal preferred practice patterns. The examination will follow the standard format and include all information needed for the clinician to create a picture of the patient's problem. During the examination, range of motion (ROM), resistance, and weight-bearing restrictions will be noted.

PATIENT HISTORY

The patient history will begin with demographic information, a social history, and information about the patient's living environment. Information about physical barriers, such as stairs, and areas with limited access, such as bathrooms, will be considered for someone with a lower extremity arthroplasty, especially if their weight-bearing status is limited. This information will help determine the need for assistive devices, such as raised commodes, reachers, and shower chairs, during the recovery period. The availability of caregivers' or family members' assistance will also be ascertained.

◎ *Clinical Pearl*

The patient history for a patient with a lower extremity joint arthroplasty will include information about physical barriers in the home such as stairs or a bathroom with limited access.

It is important to note if the patient is currently using an antiinflammatory medication or anticoagulant because this may limit the vigor of therapy. For example, Coumadin (an anticoagulant) makes patients more prone to bleeding and bruising and therefore aggressive soft tissue mobilization should be avoided. It is also important to note any prior surgeries, injuries, or other musculoskeletal problems that may limit or impact the rehabilitation process.

Next, the therapist will establish the nature, location, and severity of a patient's current symptoms. Whatever the symptom, the therapist will note whether it is constant (all the time) or intermittent (comes and goes) or if it is varying (changes in intensity) or nonvarying (does not change in intensity). The therapist will indicate the symptom level at rest and what activities increase the patient's symptoms. In addition, the therapist will note how long it takes for symptoms to settle back to their baseline.

The therapist will document the patient's level of function before the arthroplasty and the expectations for recovery. For example, was this patient a limited household ambulator who wants to increase his or her walking in the community or does this patient plan on returning to golfing or dancing? This information will help set appropriate patient-specific goals.

SYSTEMS REVIEW

The systems review is used to target areas requiring further examination and to define areas that may cause complications or indicate a need for precautions during the examination and intervention processes. Chapter 1 includes details of the systems review.

TESTS AND MEASURES

Musculoskeletal

Posture. The position of the joint and how the patient holds the joint in relationship to his or her body may give the clinician important clues to the function of that area of the body (see Chapter 4). It is important to look at the entire upper or lower quarter of the affected side of the body to determine how this area may function. For example, a patient who holds the total shoulder adducted, internally rotated, and elevated may have had prolonged limitations in glenohumeral ROM and used compensatory shoulder hiking to achieve arm elevation. This may lead to trapezius and levator scapulae muscle overuse and spasm, which may also lead to cervical symptoms. After a total knee replacement, knee pain and effusion may result in an antalgic gait and limitations in knee extension that may then cause low back and hip pain.

Anthropometric Characteristics. Girth is measured to assess for swelling and atrophy. Increased joint girth may indicate a joint effusion, whereas reduced limb girth above or below the joint may be due to muscle atrophy. Girth measurements should be noted relative to consistent landmarks, such as the medial joint line or medial malleolus, to optimize the reliability of measurements between sessions and clinicians and to optimize sensitivity to changes over time. Measures should also be compared to the uninvolved side.

Swelling in the lower extremities may also be a sign of thromboembolic disease. Joint replacement surgery places patients at high risk for deep vein thrombosis (DVT) in the involved extremity, as well as pulmonary emboli (PE). Risk factors for DVT are shown in Box 10-2.

Range of Motion/Joint Mobility. Passive ROM (PROM) and active ROM (AROM) at the involved joint and joints above and below the involved joint will be measured. The clinician examines for the quality and quantity of motion, as well as end-feel. ROM is usually noted for both the affected and unaffected side. Joint precautions, as well as ROM restrictions, need to be respected, as noted by the physician. For the knee, the mobility of the patella will also be inspected because restrictions in its mobility may result in restrictions of knee ROM and function.

Muscle Performance. Strength testing of the muscle groups crossing the involved joint, as well as a general screening of the involved limb, will be performed. Manual muscle testing (MMT) is generally appropriate for this purpose (see Chapter 5). The restrictions and precautions from the prescribing clinician will be noted, particularly after upper extremity arthroplasty.

> ### Clinical Pearl
> ROM and strength will be measured in the involved joint and be compared to the opposite side to assist with goal setting.

Neuromuscular. The quality, intensity, duration, and frequency of pain will be noted, as well as changes with rest and activity. The location of pain should also be noted since there may be pain not only in the operative area but also in areas affected by changes in biomechanics or alterations in gait or sleeping positions. For example, an antalgic gait may cause back pain, and shoulder immobilization may cause neck pain. The types and doses of analgesic medication used may also give the clinician an indication of pain severity and how the patient's pain is responding to current interventions (see Chapter 22).

Integumentary. The healing status and mobility of the incision will also be noted. Soft tissue mobility testing may be limited because of tissue healing constraints. Obesity, diabetes, peripheral vascular disease, steroid and tobacco use, prior infection, and malnutrition all increase the risk for poor healing.

BOX 10-2	**Risk Factors for Deep Vein Thrombosis**	
Strong Risk Factors	**Moderate Risk Factors**	**Weak Risk Factors**
• Fracture (pelvis, femur, tibia) • THA or TKA • Major general surgery • Major trauma • Spinal cord injury	• Arthroscopic knee surgery • Central venous lines • Chemotherapy • CHF or respiratory failure • Hormone replacement therapy • Malignancy • Oral contraception therapy • CVA • Pregnancy: Postpartum • Previous venous thromboembolism • Thrombophilia	• Bed rest >3 days • Immobility due to sitting (e.g., prolonged air travel) • Increasing age • Laparoscopic surgery • Obesity • Pregnancy: Antepartum • Varicose veins

From Anderson FA, Spencer FA: *Circulation* 107(S):19-116, 2003.
THA, Total hip arthroplasty; *TKA,* total knee arthroplasty; *CHF,* congestive heart failure; *CVA,* cerebrovascular accident.

Function. If the patient has undergone a lower extremity joint replacement, balance and proprioception will be examined and addressed throughout the treatment (see Chapter 13). These may be difficult to examine fully during the initial examination because of pain, as well as ROM and strength deficits. Gait and transfers will also be examined and assessed.

EVALUATION, DIAGNOSIS, AND PROGNOSIS

According to the *Guide to Physical Therapy Practice*,[16] the preferred practice pattern for most patients with joint replacement is 4H: Impaired joint mobility, motor function, muscle performance, and range of motion associated with joint arthroplasty.

The results of total joint arthroplasty have improved over time; hip, knee, and shoulder procedures currently have the best outcomes. Extensive evidence shows that 85% to 90% of patients report pain reduction after TKA.[1,17,18] Patients who have had a THA have significantly increased maximum walking speed, stride length, and cadence and oxygen consumption with walking.[19] Patients who have undergone a total shoulder arthroplasty (TSA) feel that the impact of the procedure on their health is comparable to that of THA or CABG.[20] Replacement of other joints, such as the ankle, wrist, elbow, and first metatarsophalangeal (MTP), are less successful because of limited advances in technology and limited use.[21]

INTERVENTION

Preoperative patient education has been advocated for many years as important to the overall rehabilitation of patients undergoing joint arthroplasty. Many medical centers offer a multidisciplinary, team-taught, preoperative group class for patients planning to have an arthroplastic procedure and their families. These classes cover information about the procedure, the rehabilitation process, and the early postoperative period. Studies of educational programs for clients undergoing THA report fewer dislocations, fewer phone calls to surgeons, less medication use, an ability to walk sooner, and a decreased length of hospital stay.

Education, exercise, and functional mobility training, including gait training if appropriate, are the three main components of rehabilitation after arthroplasty. This postoperative rehabilitation aims to optimize function, while ensuring adherence to ROM and weight-bearing precautions and preventing complications such as DVTs and pneumonia.

TOTAL HIP ARTHROPLASTY

The first recorded total hip replacement was performed more than 150 years ago by Sir Anthony White, a surgeon at London's Westminster hospital. However, it was not until the early 1960s that Sir John Charnley, also in England, popularized what is known today as the THA. Since then, advancements in biologically compatible implants and fixation and surgical techniques have continued to produce ever better results in THA. Recent refinements include "mini" open, one-, and two-incision techniques that result in less soft tissue damage,

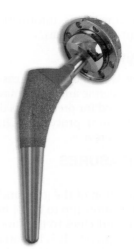

FIG. 10-3 Hip replacement components: Metal head with metal acetabular liner. *Image courtesy Biomet.*

particularly of the muscles. The two main surgical approaches to THA are the anterior and the posterolateral; the posterolateral approach is the most common. The joint may also be cemented or uncemented, depending on the patient's life expectancy, bone quality, and activity level. An uncemented acetabular component is used for most patients because it lasts longer. A cemented acetabular component is only used for the patient with a life expectancy of less than 10 years. Indications for uncemented femoral components vary with surgeon preference but are usually reserved for younger patients. Implants are modular so they can be customized to the specific anatomy of each patient. The components are usually made of metal alloy such as titanium or cobalt chrome. Highly polished ceramic femoral head components are also used in limited patient populations. In most patients, the alloy or ceramic femoral head component articulates with a polyethylene plastic acetabular insert. Metal or ceramic heads that articulate with metal liners are also available for active, younger patients (Fig. 10-3).

Pathology. The THA procedure exposes the acetabulum and proximal femur and then removes the femoral head and neck. The proximal femoral medullary canal is reamed to prepare it to accept the femoral component. The acetabulum is prepared by rasping and articular cartilage debridement. Most acetabular components just press-fit into place, but some are held in with screws. These components are rarely cemented. If the femoral component is cemented, the methylmethacrylate cement is first put into the proximal femur under pressure, and then the femoral component is inserted. If there is no cement, the proximal femur is underreamed so that the femoral component can be impacted into the femur (Fig. 10-4). Reduction and stability testing is performed before the soft tissue is closed. In some patients, the joint capsule is resected before soft tissue closure.

THA revision may be needed for a variety of reasons, including infection, component failure, or mechanical loosening. According to data from United States hospital databases, approximately 18% of all THA procedures are revisions.[22] For a revision, bone grafting, whether

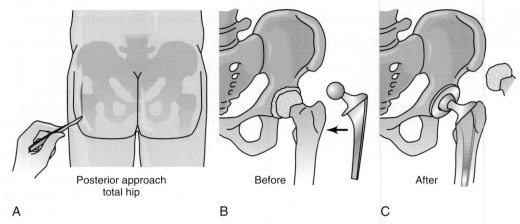

FIG. 10-4 Total hip arthroplasty procedure.

autologous or allograft, is often necessary to fill architectural defects caused by the primary arthroplasty, to fill defects made when the initial implant was removed, or if there was a fracture or poor bone stock that results from severe osteoporosis. Postoperative care must consider the unique demands of these patients and the specific limitations imposed by their surgery.

Prognosis. The primary indications for THA are pain and disability. Although some authors have attempted to define specific criteria for the appropriateness of THA, the subjective nature of patients' symptoms will always require patients to weigh the risks and benefits of such procedures according to their own values.

Common physical impairments after THA include decreased muscle strength, limited hip ROM and flexibility, and abnormalities of gait. Persistent, although improved, muscle strength deficits after THA have been documented in several studies. Leg length discrepancy can affect patient satisfaction and prognosis for overall function after THA. Many patients report a sensation that their operated leg is longer than the nonoperated leg. This may be due to a true leg length discrepancy caused by a limited amount of bone being resected from the femoral neck, the implant being longer than the patient's original anatomy, or because the acetabulum's center of rotation has changed. The perception of a leg length discrepancy, without an actual discrepancy, may also result from temporary periarticular soft tissue imbalances because of use of an abduction pillow or from years of compensation resulting from long-standing arthritis. A true leg length discrepancy of more than 1 cm will often cause patient dissatisfaction.[23]

Driving. An important activity of daily life that most patients are anxious to resume is driving. After THA, the decision to allow a patient to resume driving is based on a combination of factors, including discontinuation of postsurgical precautions, side of the surgery, reaction times, and use of narcotic pain medication. Note that the physician, not the therapist, has to decide when a patient can resume driving. Patients in the United States return to their preoperative driving reaction times with their right leg (for braking) in 4 to 6 weeks postoperatively with a right THA and as early as 1 week postoperatively with a

left THA. Reaction times of patients with OA of the hip are slower than age-matched subjects with normal hips.[24]

Athletic Participation. Athletic activity after total joint replacement depends in part on preoperative activity. Patients who have not participated in a specific sport or activity before surgery are less likely to achieve a high level of skill and may have an increased risk of injury. The technical aspects of joint reconstruction are also important predictors of functional outcome and athletic activity after joint replacement.[25] Another important consideration is implant fixation. Athletic activity increases the stress on fixation, and several studies have shown that an increased activity level contributes to the loosening and ultimately the failure of implants.[26-28]

Wear of the polyethylene liner, which depends on how much it is used, influences the survival of total joint replacements. A prosthetic joint should wear like a car tire, in that wear is a function of use or the number of cycles that the joint goes through, not how old it is. It is thought that walking is the most important physical activity affecting the wear of hip and knee replacements.[29]

Fixation of the prosthesis also affects implant success or failure. In this case, activity may improve prognosis because exercise can increase bone density and thus improve implant fixation. Some studies have shown that there is a lower rate of prosthetic loosening in active patients.[30,31] This may be because of improved bony ingrowth in noncemented implants and protection of the implant by greater hip abductor strength.[32]

Overall, the evidence suggests that there should be a balance between too little and too much activity, with too little activity leading to decreased bone density and early prosthetic loosening (before 10 years), whereas too much activity may lead to prosthetic wear and late loosening (after 10 years).

◎ *Clinical Pearl*

After a joint replacement, too much activity may lead to prosthetic wear and loosening, but too little activity may lead to decreased bone density and also contribute to early prosthetic loosening.

BOX 10-3	Activity After Total Hip Arthroplasty—1999 Hip Society Recommendations		
Recommended/Allowed	**Allowed with Experience**	**Not Recommended**	**No Conclusion**
Stationary biking	Low-impact aerobics	High-impact aerobics	Jazz dancing
Croquet	Road biking	Baseball/softball	Square dancing
Ballroom dancing	Bowling	Basketball	Fencing
Golf	Canoeing	Football	Ice skating
Horseshoes	Hiking	Gymnastics	Roller or inline skating
Shooting	Horseback riding	Handball	Rowing
Shuffleboard	Cross-country skiing	Hockey	Speed walking
Swimming		Jogging	Downhill skiing
Doubles tennis		Lacrosse	Stationary skiing machine
Walking		Racquetball	Weight lifting
		Squash	Weight machines
		Rock climbing	
		Soccer	
		Singles tennis	
		Volleyball	

From Healy WL, Iorio R, Lemos MJ: *Am J Sports Med* 29:377-388, 2001.

In a survey of 54 members of the Hip Society regarding their recommendations for athletic and sports participation for their patients who had hip replacement surgery, 42 athletic events were evaluated. Each surgeon was asked to rate the activity as recommended/allowed, allowed with experience, not recommended, or no conclusion (Box 10-3).[33]

Intervention

Postoperative Rehabilitation. After THA, inpatient rehabilitation generally follows a preset protocol, depending on the nature of the surgery, the patient, and the preferences of the surgeon. In general, the following goals should be attained before discharge to the home:

- Adhere to hip precautions and weight-bearing status restrictions
- Ambulate on flat surfaces for 100 feet with the use of an assistive device
- Attain functional transfers (toilet, bed) and activities of daily living (ADLs)
- Adhere to interventions to reduce the risk of bed rest hazards such as DVTs, pneumonia, pressure ulcers, and PE
- Obtain ROM within precaution limits and initiate strengthening of knee and hip musculature
- Attain independence in initial home exercise program (HEP)

Discharge to home may be delayed if the patient lives alone or has no resources for help, and the patient may need to rehabilitate in an interim facility before discharge. With improvements in surgical technique, pain control, and rehabilitation, anecdotally patients seem to be recovering more quickly and achieving independence sooner after undergoing THA, with most hospitalized for 3 to 5 days.

Precautions, Restrictions, and Complications. One of the most important aspects of inpatient physical therapy is to educate the patient about weight-bearing restrictions imposed by the surgeon and other precautions that must be followed after a total hip replacement. Weight-bearing restrictions after arthroplasty are not standardized and are generally based on individual surgeon preference.

Definitions of weight-bearing status are also not standardized and therefore can lead to confusion among practitioners. Full weight-bearing status implies that the patient may put all of his or her weight on the involved limb, whereas non–weight-bearing status means that they must keep all of their weight off of the limb. The confusion begins with terms such as touch-down weight bearing (TDWB) and partial weight bearing (PWB). PWB is best described by percentage of total body weight the patient may place on the affected limb. Some authors state that PWB is 30% to 50% of body weight.[34,35] TDWB generally means that the patient may touch the affected foot to the floor for help with balance only and has been described as 10% to 15% of body weight.[36]

> **Clinical Pearl**
>
> One of the most important goals of inpatient physical therapy after total hip arthroplasty is for the patient to understand and adhere to weight-bearing and other postoperative restrictions.

Reduced weight bearing is achieved by use of assistive devices such as walkers, crutches, and canes. Determination of the appropriate assistive device depends not only on the weight-bearing status but also on the individual patient. Walkers are usually the first choice for most patients after a THA because these provide the greatest stability and the largest base of support. They reduce the contact forces at the hip to 1 times body weight during ambulation and 0.5 times body weight during double leg stance.[37,38]

ROM restrictions are prescribed postoperatively to prevent dislocation of the prosthetic joint (Fig. 10-5). Patients with weak periarticular structures, such as those with collagen disease, revision surgeries, or previous dis-

No! **Yes**

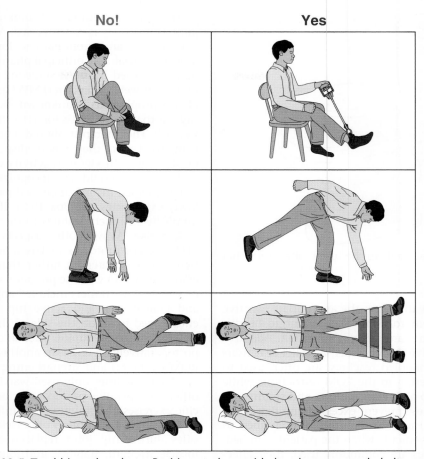

FIG. 10-5 Total hip arthroplasty: Positions to be avoided and recommended alternatives.

locations, are at the greatest risk for dislocation. Other causes of dislocation include malpositioned prosthesis, trauma, and falls. The risk of dislocation appears to be the greatest during the first week after surgery when patients are least familiar with the ROM restrictions and when the periarticular soft tissues are the weakest. The rate of prosthetic hip dislocation in the postoperative phase has been reported to be between 2.1% and 3.1% for an initial replacement and 8.3% for those undergoing revision surgery.[39,40] The rate of dislocation decreases over time and levels off between 10 to 13 weeks postsurgery.[41] How long ROM restrictions should be adhered to is not standardized. Most surgeons require that precautions be maintained for 12 weeks after the surgery, although others recommend adherence to these restrictions for the life of the prosthesis.

To avoid overstressing healing tissues and risking injury or dislocation, the rehabilitation professional should know the anatomical approach used in the surgical procedure. This will give an appreciation of which structures were structurally compromised and which motions are least stable. The movements the surgeon used to dislocate the hip during the surgical procedure will have the greatest instability and risk of dislocation after the procedure. For example, after a THA with a posterior approach, hip flexion greater than 90 degrees, hip adduction, and internal rotation should be avoided to prevent femoral head dislocation in a posterior direction. Similarly, after THA

with an anterolateral approach, the hip should be protected from extremes of extension and external rotation. With the minimally invasive anterior approach, ROM precautions are often not necessary because of the limited soft tissue damage, minimal soft tissue release, and the high degree of stability achieved intraoperatively.

Although there is sparse evidence to support specific guidelines for total joint precautions, given the risk for dislocation with excessive forces postoperatively and frequent reference to such precautions in the literature and in common practice, it is prudent for the clinician to adhere to and instruct patients in total joint precautions. These precautions should be presented to the patient in functional terms. For example, a patient who underwent a THA with a posterior approach who is told not to exceed 90 degrees of hip flexion may not realize that bending over to put on stockings or pull on pants is exceeding this limitation. Patients should be instructed to avoid low seats and toilets without risers because this will increase hip flexion and probably exceed the limitation imposed by the surgeon. It is also important to tell the patient to avoid reaching their hand past their knees. For example, patients will be unable to pick objects off the floor without the help of a "reacher." Patients should also be told that when rising up from a chair, they should slide the hips forward and then stand. Patients should be reminded to not stand with feet turned in (internal rotation) or sit cross-legged.

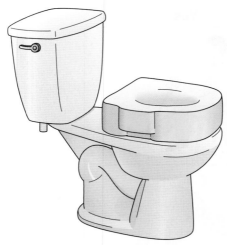

FIG. 10-6 Raised toilet seat to be used after total hip arthroplasty.

It is also important to obtain the appropriate assistive devices and equipment to allow the patient to be discharged from inpatient care safely after a THA. Adaptive equipment and assistive devices, such as toilet seat risers (Fig. 10-6) and long-handled reachers, are often used to assist patients in adhering to the ROM restrictions while performing ADLs. Hip abduction pillows and splints and knee immobilizers (these prevent excessive hip flexion by limiting knee flexion) are also commonly prescribed to prevent restricted movements when the patient is in bed. Although these devices are commonly used, their effectiveness has not been studied.

◎ *Clinical Pearl*

The risk of THA dislocation appears to be the greatest in the first week after surgery. However, many surgeons require that precautions be maintained for 12 weeks postoperatively.

Prevention of Thromboses. One of the most common causes of severe complications after joint arthroplasty is the formation of intravascular blood clots (thrombi), which generally form in the deep veins of the legs and can cause severe complications if they embolize (move) to the lungs, resulting in a PE, which is one of the most common causes of death after lower extremity arthroplasty.

Prophylaxis for thromboemboli can be broadly divided into 2 categories—nonpharmacological and pharmacological. Nonpharmacological thromboprophylaxis interventions include elastic compression stockings, early ambulation, and intermittent pneumatic compression (IPC). Early ambulation is encouraged because it is also associated with a lower incidence of symptomatic thromboembolic disease.[42] IPC devices can be helpful but are only effective if used at all times when the patient is not walking. How long each day such devices must be used is unknown, although it is presumed that the longer the better.[43]

The optimal method of thromboprophylaxis after total joint arthroplasty is controversial. A combination of pharmacological and nonpharmacological methods seems most beneficial. The principal pharmacological prophylactic agents used by most surgeons are Coumadin or low molecular weight heparin (LMWH). The optimal duration of this prophylaxis is unknown, but there is evidence to suggest that prophylaxis for THA should extend for 4 to 6 weeks.[44] The therapist should know if these drugs are being used, since they may predispose patients to bruising or bleeding with vigorous activity or mobilization.

Therapists should also recognize signs and symptoms of DVT, which include increased pain and swelling in the lower extremities (see Box 10-2). It is important to communicate any such findings to the surgeon.

Exercise. As with other aspects of rehabilitation after THA, exercise protocols are based mainly on clinical experience and preferences rather than on research-derived evidence. A THA exercise program reported as a consensus of several practitioners included ankle pumps, quadriceps and gluteal sets, and active hip flexion.[45] Patients are encouraged to sit on the side of the bed, stand with the walker, and begin supine knee and hip flexion exercises postoperatively on day 1. In another protocol, active assist ROM (AAROM) and strengthening were initiated on day 2.[46] Some facilities only used walking programs, whereas other postoperative protocols included instruction in specific exercises and functional training.[47]

The surgical disruption of muscles, ligaments, and capsules during hip joint replacement surgery can affect muscle strength, stability, and joint proprioception. Hip abductor strengthening has been described as the singlemost important exercise for the patient to return to a nonantalgic gait.[48] Hip abductor strengthening after THA has been shown to prevent a Trendelenburg gait (see Chapter 32) and improve hip stability,[49,50] and patients with greater hip abduction strength demonstrate quicker early postoperative functional progress.[51]

Muscle strengthening programs after THA must respect surgeon-imposed restrictions, as well as tissue healing and pain. This is achieved by starting with exercises that place the least amount of stress on the joint and soft tissue envelope, progressing to functional activities. A progression of isometrics followed by isotonic antigravity activities, such as knee extension exercises, then progressing to pulleys, weights, and elastic resistance bands is recommended. Closed kinetic-chain activities, such as step-ups and mini-squats, allow for a progression to functional ADLs and recreational activities. These activities most often involve some degree of weight bearing and muscle co-contraction, which often adds to joint stability. Exercises to improve balance are also recommended after THA because poor balance has been shown to be highly predictive of falls and subsequent disability in the elderly.

The evidence indicates that most of the benefits of rehabilitation are achieved by 3 to 6 months after surgery[52]; however, patients may continue to make gains for up to 2 years.

Modalities. Research on the use of modalities in the treatment of total hip replacement is very limited. For example, only one study was found that examined the use of cryotherapy after THA.[53] This study demonstrated that local cooling reduces surgery-related pain after THA. Cryotherapy is also thought to limit bleeding and swelling by constricting blood vessels and may reduce tissue metabolism and inflammation, preventing secondary soft tissue damage. Ice also has a local anesthetic effect and reduces muscle spasms. Although this local treatment does not penetrate to the depth of the hip joint and capsule, it may modulate pain by gating at the spinal cord level and by producing anesthesia of the skin in the area.

The use of ultrasound (US) over a cemented joint replacement or one with polyethylene plastic components is contraindicated since these materials may be rapidly heated by US.[54] US may, however, be used on noncemented and all metal component joints because US does not rapidly heat metal or loosen screws or plates.[55] The effect of US on cemented joints with or without plastic components is in all likelihood minimal, since little US will penetrate to the depth of most prosthetic joints; however, it is recommended that the clinician err on the side of caution and not use this modality over such materials.[56] Diathermy is contraindicated in patients with metal implants, including total hip replacements, because the metal can become very hot and damage adjacent tissues.

TOTAL KNEE ARTHROPLASTY

According to the National Institutes of Health (NIH) Consensus Study on total knee replacement, the use of rehabilitation services is the most understudied aspect of perioperative management of total knee replacement patients.[57] Postoperative physical therapy and rehabilitation "greatly influence the outcome of total knee arthroplasty."[58]

The three main types of component design used for uncomplicated primary knee replacements are the **cruciate retaining knee,** the **posterior stabilized knee,** and the **mobile bearing knee.** There are negligible functional differences between these prostheses, thus selection usually depends on the preference of the surgeon. In the posterior cruciate retention design, the posterior cruciate ligament supplements the anteroposterior (AP) stability of the prosthesis. In the posterior stabilized implant, the cruciate ligaments are resected and AP stability is provided by the conformity of the components and by a central tibial spine. A mobile bearing knee has a polyethylene insert that articulates with the femoral component and with the metallic tibial tray, thus creating a dual surface articulation (Fig. 10-7). This feature is intended to reduce the stress and fatigue wear on the polyethylene insert and possibly the **osteolysis** caused by polyethylene particles that may contribute to joint replacement failure.

TKAs also vary in their method of fixation. The prosthesis can be cemented or uncemented, or a combination of the two, known as a *hybrid.* The hybrid fixation, in which the tibial component is cemented and the femoral component is uncemented, is gaining popularity; however, cemented TKAs are still the most common.

Pathology. For the TKA procedure, a longitudinal incision of the skin is made along the anterior aspect of the knee from just proximal to the patella to just distal to the tibial tubercle. The quadriceps are then either split or

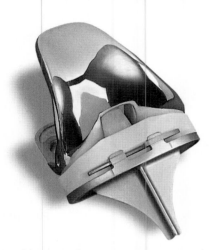

FIG. 10-7 Total knee replacement components for a mobile bearing knee. *Image courtesy Biomet.*

moved aside to expose the joint. The knee is then flexed and the entire knee joint, including the ends of the tibia and femur, as well as the menisci, anterior cruciate ligament (ACL), and possibly the posterior cruciate ligament depending on the implant, are excised and the prosthesis is placed (Fig. 10-8). If there are knee deformities, soft tissue and ligament balancing are performed to achieve optimal alignment. The wounds are then thoroughly irrigated, a drain placed, and the incision is closed with sutures.

A more recent trend in knee replacement is a minimally invasive surgical approach, in which the quadriceps muscle is either not cut or only a small 1 to 2 cm "snip" in the vastus medialis oblique muscle is made. This avoids damage to the extensor mechanism and thereby allows better quadriceps contraction than with the traditional approaches in which the quadriceps tendon is cut. The skin incision is also much shorter (3 to 5 inches versus 8 to 12 inches in the traditional TKA), which limits soft tissue trauma. The same clinically proven implants as used in the traditional total knee replacement are utilized. This modified procedure is gaining popularity because it appears to cause less pain and blood loss and results in a shortened hospital stay, improved ROM and strength, and less time on crutches or a walker. However, there is still limited research on outcomes for minimally invasive TKAs.

Another advancement in TKA is computer-assisted surgery. Although this technique is not widely used, some centers report excellent results because of improved alignment of the lower extremity when compared to the conventional technique. The potential benefits in long-term outcome and functional improvement require further clinical investigation.

Examination. The examination of the patient with a TKA is similar to that presented in the general arthroplasty examination section with a few added components specific to the knee in general such as assessing patellar mobility. It is also important to assess the extensor mechanism's extensibility, as well as its ability to generate a

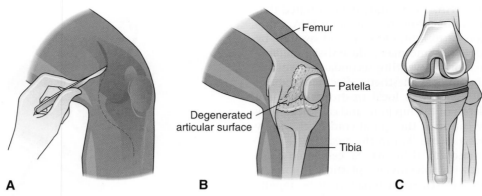

FIG. 10-8 Total knee arthroplasty procedure.

contraction and ultimately adequate force. This should be done through passive ROM and MMT, respectively.

Prognosis. Studies comparing preoperative and postoperative knee total ROM after TKA report a mean increase of 8 degrees.[59] After TKA, quadriceps strength is commonly less than it was preoperatively for up to 2 months after the surgery,[60] and generally remains below that of the uninvolved side,[61,62] and that of age-matched people without OA,[63-65] even after strength training. Weakness directly after surgery is most likely caused by pain, effusion, and soft tissue injury, as well as by muscle atrophy and limited volitional control. Quadriceps weakness impairs function and has been correlated with an increased risk of falling,[66] as well as decreased ambulation speed,[67] decreased performance in sit-to-stand transfers,[68] and decreased ability to negotiate stairs.[69]

According to one prospective study, early quadriceps weakness after TKA is due to impaired volitional control of the muscle and to a lesser extent, atrophy. Pain had surprisingly little effect on muscle activation. Thus pain control alone will not be sufficient to improve strength, and efforts must be made to directly address voluntary muscle activation early in the postoperative period, using modalities, such as biofeedback and electrical stimulation, if needed to offset these deficiencies.[70]

A survey assessed activities considered important and limiting to patients that had undergone TKA.[71] Of those surveyed, 40% felt that squatting was an important task and 75% reported some limitation in this activity. It was not noted whether this limitation was due to lack of ROM or strength, but many patients noted that it was difficult to descend stairs and participate in heavy domestic chores that are affected by lower extremity strength. Rehabilitation efforts should focus on activities that help patients improve performance of ADLs.

Athletic Participation. Indications for total knee replacement have expanded over the last decade to include improvement in athletic participation. Recommendations regarding which athletic activities patients may participate in after TKA must take into account biomechanics, joint stability, strength, prior experience, and level of participation. Tibiofemoral and patellofemoral biomechanics in the TKA have shown peak loads of 2 times body weight

with level walking and 3.1 times body weight while descending stairs.[72]

A biomechanical study tested the compressive forces generated on three different TKA implant designs during four recreational activities: Cycling, power walking, downhill skiing, and mountain hiking. The authors measured the amount of implant surface area that was loaded to the polyethylene yield point and found that cycling and power walking were the safest activities, whereas downhill skiing and mountain hiking were associated with significant overloaded areas.[73] Some activities, such as mountain hiking, may be modified to reduce the joint loads. For example, avoiding steep descents, walking slowly when going downhill, and using ski poles or hiking poles when hiking can reduce the load on the knee joint by as much as 20%.[74]

The results of a survey of 58 members of the Knee Society regarding recommendations for participation in 42 different athletics and sports activities after TKA are shown in Box 10-4.[75]

Driving. Another important aspect in returning to normal life and independence after TKA is returning to driving. Brake response time after TKA returns to preoperative level as early as 3 weeks postoperatively, and at 9 weeks postoperatively, there is a significant improvement over baseline measurements.[76] Based on these findings, surgeons generally recommend that patients undergoing TKA return to driving 6 weeks after surgery.

Intervention

Postoperative Rehabilitation. The following guidelines for rehabilitation progression should be tailored to the individual patient. The rehabilitation professional should evaluate the findings from the examination to determine when milestones are met and when rehabilitation can proceed and not rely on a "cookbook" approach or "protocol." The therapist must, however, respect tissue healing parameters and the postsurgical precautions.

Immediate postoperative recovery of the patient with a TKA centers on achieving functional milestones. Inpatient rehabilitation programs and functional milestones are similar to those of THA, including ambulation with an assistive device, independent transfers, achievement of ROM, initiation of strengthening, and understanding and

BOX 10-4	Activity After Total Knee Arthroplasty—1999 Knee Society Recommendations			
Recommended/Allowed	**Allowed with Experience**	**Not Recommended**	**No Conclusion**	
Low-impact aerobics	Road biking	Racquetball	Fencing	
Stationary biking	Canoeing	Squash	Roller or inline skating	
Bowling	Hiking	Rock climbing	Downhill skiing	
Golf	Rowing	Soccer	Weight lifting	
Dancing	Cross-country skiing	Singles tennis		
Horseback riding	Stationary skiing machine	Volleyball		
Croquet	Speed walking	Football		
Walking	Doubles tennis	Gymnastics		
Swimming	Weight machines	Lacrosse		
Shooting	Ice skating	Hockey		
Shuffleboard		Basketball		
Horseshoes		Jogging		
		Handball		

From Healy WL, Iorio R, Lemos MJ: *Am J Sports Med* 29:377-388, 2001.

performance of an appropriate HEP. Since postoperative hospital stays have become shorter, the clinician must educate the patient, family members, and other caregivers on the importance of these milestones.

Most surgeons advocate the same rehabilitation parameters after total knee replacement for implants with cemented or biological fixation, although some advocate limited weight bearing for up to 6 weeks for uncemented implants. It is customary for full weight bearing to be allowed with all primary TKAs unless certain other conditions, such as severe osteoporosis, fracture, concomitant osteotomies, or bone grafts, are present. This may not be the case with revision TKAs, especially if bone grafting or tibial tuberosity osteotomies were performed. It is always prudent to contact the surgeon if there is any doubt as to the weight-bearing status of the patient.

During the initial phase of outpatient rehabilitation, the focus should be on tissue healing and reducing pain and inflammation. It is during this period that modalities, such as cold and compression, are used to decrease pain and swelling.

The use of **continuous passive motion (CPM)** machines after TKA remains controversial. No study to date has offered conclusive evidence of the long-term benefits of the use of CPM. CPM is considered a cost-effective intervention that facilitates early knee flexion after TKA. Studies suggest that CPM promotes greater and earlier knee flexion ROM, decreased postoperative knee pain, fewer days of inpatient rehabilitation, decreased DVT incidence, and a decreased need for surgical manipulation.[77,78] Use of a CPM machine can be started immediately postoperatively, although some surgeons advocate waiting until postoperative day 2 to avoid disruption of the incision.

Achieving knee flexion early in rehabilitation allows patients more independence in ADLs, since 65 degrees of flexion is required for a normal swing phase during gait, and 105 degrees is needed to rise comfortably from sitting. Final postoperative knee flexion ROM depends on the type of implant used, the preoperative ROM,[79] and the mobility

of the patient's soft tissues. Aggressive rehabilitation and adequate pain control are also paramount to prevent postoperative contractures and optimize flexion ROM. It has been suggested that a lack of physical therapy can contribute to decreased functional ROM after TKA.[80]

To achieve optimal results, ROM activities for the patient with a TKA should be initiated soon after surgery. Patients often have a flexion contracture immediately after surgery because of irritation of the joint and hemarthrosis. This will resolve with time and appropriate rehabilitation. ROM activities can include passive knee flexion and extension, as well as active heel slides and supine wall slides. Forward and backward pedaling on a stationary bicycle can also increase flexion ROM. With the saddle of the bicycle high, a patient with limited flexion can often "rock" back and forth and ultimately complete a backward revolution. This is an excellent way for a patient to improve ROM in a safe and self-controlled manner.

⊚ *Clinical Pearl*

To achieve optimal results after TKA, activities that address both flexion and extension ROM should be initiated soon after surgery.

Full extension ROM is also essential for a normal gait pattern and for efficient function of the lower extremity. A limitation of as little as 5 degrees of extension may require a quadriceps force of 30% of a person's body weight to stabilize the knee, with more force being needed as the amount of knee flexion limitation increases.[81] Therefore a patient who cannot achieve full extension during gait will expend more energy walking. They may also have limited knee stability as a result of compromised strength of the quadriceps muscles after TKA. Full extension can be achieved in a variety of ways (Fig. 10-9). First, the patient should not sleep with a pillow under the knee, although this will be a position of comfort. To achieve full

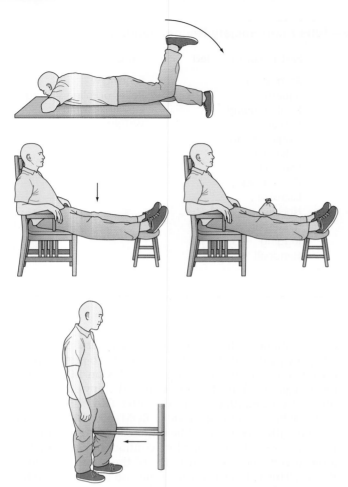

FIG. 10-9 Activities to increase knee extension.

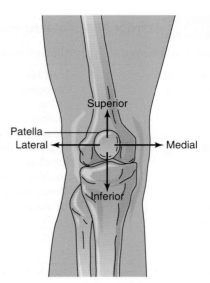

FIG. 10-10 Patellar mobilization.

extension, the patient may lie prone with the knee on the edge of the bed, allowing gravity to extend the knee. Another option is to lie supine and place a pillow under the heel, allowing the knee to extend. To further intensify this stretch the patient may use a slow-sustained pressure manually or from a small weight, such as a phone book or weighted bag, to achieve full extension. Backward walking may also help the patient who has difficulty achieving full extension. This may be done in a pool or on land.

◎ *Clinical Pearl*

Full knee extension ROM is essential for a normal gait pattern and for efficient quadriceps function to stabilize the knee.

Prevention and early recognition of ROM limitations are essential to prevent **arthrofibrosis,** a potential complication of any knee surgery. Arthrofibrosis is a process that occurs when diffuse scar tissue or fibrous adhesions form within or around a joint. This scarring can restrict flexion, extension, or patellar mobility. Manual patellar mobilization, as well as mobilization of the soft tissues of the quadriceps and patellar tendon, is critical to restoring

normal extensor mobility and ultimately a functional knee. The patella should be mobilized in all planes, mediolateral and superoinferior, and the tendons should be manually mobilized medially and laterally (Fig. 10-10). Gentle patellar and scar mobilization initiated after the incision site is stable may also help prevent contractures and promote functional ROM. Patellar mobilization is very important because the suprapatellar pouch is often where adhesions that limit ROM develop. These mobilizations should also be taught to patients so that they can be performed at home. Decreased superior mobility of the patella interferes with the ability of the quadriceps muscles to straighten the knee and may also result in an **extensor lag.** An extensor lag occurs when the range of active extension is less than the passive extension of the joint. In the case of the knee, this may also be known as a *quadriceps lag* because it is caused by the quadriceps muscles not being able to straighten the knee fully even though the patient may have full passive extension. Full inferior glide of the patella is essential to maximize flexion ROM.

If rehabilitation techniques are not effective in achieving functional ROM, it may be necessary to add bracing, such as dynamic splinting (Fig. 10-11), or have surgical intervention through arthroscopic release or manipulation under anesthesia to maximize ROM. Early motion is the key for the successful rehabilitation of the postoperative knee.

Pool therapy is an excellent adjunct for gait training, ROM, strengthening, and ultimately recreation in patients after TKA. One study in Germany with 25 patients reported that hydrotherapy was superior to the "standard rehabilitation program" in the rehabilitation of patients with TKA.[82] Another activity that often helps patients achieve full knee extension ROM is standing closed-chain knee extensions using a resistance band (or towel) placed at the distal thigh and held by the therapist for feedback. This activity will also improve extension by increasing active extension force and gently stretching the posterior capsule.

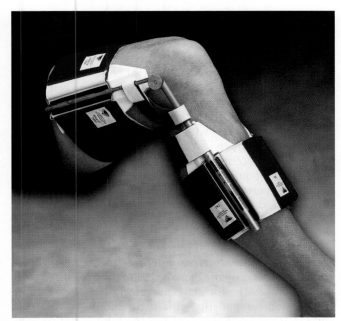

FIG. 10-11 Dynamic splinting of the knee for increased ROM. Low load prolonged stretching device that can be used to improve knee flexion or extension ROM. *Courtesy Dynasplint Systems, Inc.*

Electrical Stimulation. Neuromuscular electrical stimulation (NMES) is an alternative and potentially more effective means than exercise alone of decreasing persistent quadriceps weakness in the appropriate patient. It adds to active exercise alone by recruiting a greater proportion of type II fibers. These fibers have a higher incidence of atrophy in patients with a history of severe OA.[83] It has been shown that NMES used alone or in combination with volitional exercise is helpful in regaining functional quadriceps strength in this patient population.

Exercise. Rehabilitation after TKA must restore the function of muscles that cross the knee joint, as well as those muscles that influence the proximal and distal motion segments. During the initial stages of rehabilitation, regaining motor control of the quadriceps muscles should be emphasized. In patients with an acute knee effusion as a result of acute or surgical trauma, reflex inhibition of the quadriceps is common.[84-86] Strengthening exercise after TKA should start with quadriceps isometrics and straight leg raises. Open-chain lower extremity strengthening activities can be progressed as tolerated to promote voluntary quadriceps control. Repetitive open-chain exercises, especially in the range of 40 degrees to full extension, may increase soft tissue irritation that can occur in the early postoperative period.[72] Electrical stimulation, biofeedback, and tactile stimulation can be used for quadriceps facilitation. In addition, hip adduction and abduction strengthening exercises, as well as hamstring curls, may be added to strengthen all muscle groups around the knee joint. As strength improves and pain decreases, closed-chain strengthening should be added to improve function. Most patients with chronic knee joint arthritis have altered quadriceps function, especially for performing closed kinetic-chain activities such as stair

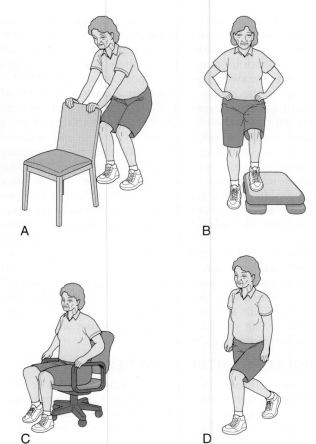

FIG. 10-12 Sample of closed kinetic chain exercises for the lower extremity. **A**, Mini-squat. **B**, Step-up. **C**, Stool pull/push. **D**, Lunges.

stepping.[87-89] Closed-chain exercises may include mini-squats, front and lateral step-ups, stool pulls, and lunges as tolerated (Fig. 10-12). These activities improve quadriceps, hamstring, and overall lower extremity strength. The patient should avoid activities that increase load on the joint because this may damage the replaced surfaces. Such activities include squats and leg presses performed at more than 90 degrees of flexion. Some rehabilitation professionals feel that TKA patients should be treated similarly to patients with patellofemoral pain syndrome, since many of these patients have very limited quadriceps strength and dysfunction of their extensor mechanism. Gym equipment may also be used for a variety of closed-chain strengthening activities. Stationary cycling, pool therapy, and a walking program may be added to achieve optimal function and allow patients to ultimately return to participation in selected recreational sports activities. However, activities that involve high impact should be avoided because these increase wear on the components and can hasten the need for revision.

◎ *Clinical Pearl*

Deep squats should be avoided after TKA because they increase knee joint loading and may damage the replaced surfaces.

Sensorimotor functions, such as proprioception, joint position sense, and balance, are all important for function of the lower extremities. Proprioception is the conscious and unconscious perception of limb position in space, including the awareness of joint position and movement.[90] Balance is the ability to maintain a posture or postural control during movement. Elderly people and patients with arthritis and with TKAs have been shown to have a poorer joint position sense than young people without OA, and reestablishing joint position sense and balance are important for optimizing patient outcomes.[91-94] Some studies have shown that proprioception and balance improve after a total knee replacement, although not consistently for all types of implants and not to levels equal to age-matched subjects without joint disease.[95-99] Some studies have postulated that improvement in joint position sense and balance after TKA is due to reestablishment of soft tissue tension and joint space, reduction of pain and chronic inflammation, and the resumption of ADLs.[99] Since balance and proprioception can impact the frequency of falls and subsequent injury, rehabilitation programs for TKA should include activities that will improve these functions (see Chapter 13).

SHOULDER ARTHROPLASTIES

Shoulder arthroplasty is not as common as THA or TKA, and most general orthopedic surgeons have limited experience with it. However, the number of TSAs has increased substantially over the past decade from approximately 10,000 in 1990 to 20,000 in 2000.[5] TSAs involve replacement of both the glenoid and the humeral head, whereas hemiarthroplasties involve the replacement of only the humeral component. Because of the need for careful soft tissue balancing and implant insertion, this procedure is considered by many to be mainly for pain relief.

Pathology. Both constrained and nonconstrained TSA prostheses are currently used. A constrained TSA has a ball and socket design that reduces humeral motion. A nonconstrained TSA more closely resembles the normal anatomical motion of the shoulder joint, allowing for more humeral motion, and is the type of prosthesis most commonly used. A semiconstrained prosthesis with a hood on the superior aspect of the glenoid that helps with stability is sometimes used for patients with irreparable rotator cuff tears. The humeral component of total shoulder replacements can be either press-fit or cemented, whereas the glenoid portion is always cemented. Symptomatic loosening of the glenoid component is usually associated with pain, whereas loosening of the humeral component is often asymptomatic. The implant may loosen if an eccentric load is placed on the glenoid by the humeral component, especially if the humeral head migrates superiorly as a result of poor deltoid or rotator cuff function from weakness or a tear. Postoperatively, 1% to 13% of patients with TSAs develop rotator cuff tears.[100]

Another less common form of shoulder arthroplasty is the Copeland surface replacement of the humeral head, which replaces only the damaged joint surface and restores the anatomy with minimal bone resection. This procedure is indicated for patients with rheumatoid arthritis (RA) and OA if the bone is strong and the joint is not severely damaged.[101]

Shoulder arthroplasty involves an incision from a point superomedial to the coracoid process down toward the anterior insertion of the deltoid on the upper arm. If the surgery is undertaken because of a humeral fracture, the soft tissue attachments of the tuberosities are preserved and reattached to the humeral shaft and stem before the wound is closed so that the rotator cuff can function. If the surgery is undertaken because of arthritis, the subscapularis muscle and the joint capsule are taken down. The humeral head is then removed and the glenoid is inspected. If it is significantly worn, it is replaced. The humeral canal is then reamed, and the humeral component is inserted, with or without cement, depending on the shoulder's condition and the surgeon's preference. The final components are then placed and the subscapularis is repaired. The deltopectoral interval and the skin are then closed (Fig. 10-13).

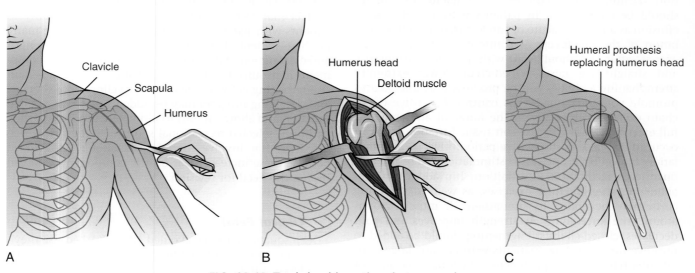

FIG. 10-13 Total shoulder arthroplasty procedure.

Prognosis. Over the past 2 decades, TSA and hemiarthroplasty of the shoulder have been successfully used to treat a wide variety of shoulder conditions. Most total shoulder replacements are performed on patients with OA, RA, avascular necrosis, or posttraumatic fractures.[102] A retrospective study indicates that patients of surgeons with a higher annual caseload of shoulder arthroplasties have fewer complications and shorter hospital lengths of stay than patients of surgeons who perform fewer of these procedures.[103] It has also been shown that centers where more of these procedures are performed have better outcomes and lower complication rates.[104]

The outcome depends on factors common to all total joint replacements, as well as those specific to the shoulder, most importantly, the status of the rotator cuff muscles. In patients with minimally retracted or nonretracted rotator cuff tears that are limited to the supraspinatus tendon, a multicenter study has shown that the outcome of shoulder arthroplasty done for OA is similar to that for patients without rotator cuff tears. However, if the infraspinatus or less importantly, the subscapularis is involved, the outcome is poorer.[105] Although patients often have limited ROM, strength, and function before surgery, TSA can primarily be expected to relieve pain rather than improve other symptoms. Meta-analyses have found that more than 90% of patients with shoulder OA, RA,[106] or osteonecrosis[107,108] and over 70% of patients with shoulder fractures do have complete or near-complete relief of pain after TSA.[109,110]

Functional results after TSA vary, depending largely on the underlying cause. Patients with OA or osteonecrosis tend to get the best ROM, reaching 75% to 80% of normal and being able to achieve an average forward flexion ROM of greater than 140 degrees and external rotation ROM of 45 degrees, as well as reaching their hand behind their back to approximately 2 to 3 levels above their presurgical ROM. Flexion after hemiarthroplasty performed in patients with humeral fractures can range from 90 to 120 degrees. Outcome is best with a well-reduced fracture, a motivated patient, and an appropriate rehabilitation program with a maximum recovery of function usually occurring within 6 to 12 months of the surgery.[111-113] Patients with RA or dislocation arthropathy have poorer functional outcomes than other patients, regaining on average 50% to 60% of normal motion because they often have poor soft tissue and bone quality. Patients with **arthropathy** that is a result of a rotator cuff tear also fare poorly, generally achieving only 33% to 50% of normal motion. Some patients who have a TSA for recurrent instability have pain and arthrosis after surgery, at times because of continued multidirectional instability, overtightening of the soft tissues, or progressive cartilage wear.[114,115]

Strength after TSA is generally sufficient to allow ADLs, as well as light recreational fitness activities such as golf, light fitness training, gardening, and swimming.

The surgeon and rehabilitation professional need to communicate and characterize the anticipated functional improvement after TSA in a way the patient can understand. Shoulder-specific functional gains in relation to preoperative shoulder function are the most effective way to present this information. TSA for the treatment of primary OA significantly increases shoulder function from 4 out of 12 to 9 out of 12 tasks.[116] Patients with better preoperative function tend to have better postoperative function, although patients with the poorest preoperative function may have the greatest improvement overall. On average, patients reported that they gained two-thirds of the functions that had been absent preoperatively. Thus TSA can provide substantial improvement in shoulder function.

TSA also significantly improves quality of life for patients with OA. Self-assessed health status improved significantly after TSA and to a similar degree as for hip arthroplasty and CABG surgery, although for none of these procedures did health status reach the level of healthy subjects without indications for these procedures.[117]

In patients undergoing Copeland surface replacement for the treatment of RA, a case series of 75 shoulders between 1986 and 1998 noted improvements of 50 degrees in flexion, to 100 degrees of total flexion motion, with 96% of patients reporting improved satisfaction compared to their preoperative status.[118]

The major complications of TSA are loosening of the glenoid component, instability, and late rotator cuff tears, although sepsis and nerve injury have also been reported. TSA failure is primarily the result of loosening of the glenoid component, which has a risk of 1% per year.[119,120]

Interventions. The rehabilitation clinician must consider a number of unique anatomical and biomechanical features of the shoulder when designing a rehabilitation program for patients after TSA. First, the shoulder is not a weight-bearing joint but still achieves joint compressive loads equal to the weight of the arm when it is abducted. Lifting a weight, tossing a ball, or swinging a racquet or golf club significantly increase this load. Second, the glenohumeral joint is quite unstable because there is little contact between the bones and because it is subjected to shear forces in many directions. Stability in a TSA is achieved through the prosthetic components and appropriate tension in the soft tissues. Patients with OA and those with generalized joint laxity may have persistent glenoid retroversion despite attempts at surgical correction and can therefore be prone to posterior instability especially with shoulder elevation and horizontal adduction.[121] The risks of anterior instability may be increased by anteversion of the glenoid or by anterior capsule insufficiency.[122] Patients with RA are more likely to have multidirectional instability as a result of rotator cuff or capsuloligamentous instabilities. An optimal functional outcome requires restoration of an optimal scapulohumeral rhythm and upper quarter length-tension relationships, as well as functional strength.

Rehabilitation begins with PROM on the day of or the day after the surgery. Early mobilization promotes appropriate collagen formation, decreases pain, and minimizes the adverse effects of immobility.[123,124] The amount of external rotation and forward flexion PROM achieved by the surgeon at the time of wound closure should guide rehabilitation.[125] Ideally, the shoulder should externally rotate 40 degrees without excessive tension on the subscapularis.[126] The extent and amount of activity allowed depends on the extent of soft tissue damage and the quality of the repair. During surgery, the subscapularis muscle is cut and then repaired. Therefore passive external rotation and active internal rotation are limited for the first 4 to 6 weeks after surgery. Elements of the surgery that may limit or alter the rehabilitation process include rotator cuff repairs and subscapularis z-plasty lengthening.

Patient-conducted flexibility programs performed several times a day after TSA to improve shoulder ROM and flexibility have been reported.[127] A home-based program that started with PROM and progressed through AAROM at week 5 and eventually to elastic-band strengthening at week 10 has also been described.[128] This program was coordinated and instructed by a PT but was completed by the patient at home. Some patients with RA, traumatic arthritis, and osteonecrosis did not maintain flexion ROM postoperatively, which may be due to weakened, thinned rotator cuff muscles or an excessive inflammatory response. Muscle weakness has been implicated as a risk factor for not regaining flexion ROM after humeral fracture and TSA.[129] Self-motivated patients with OA and no other shoulder pathology who undergo TSA may benefit from an independent home-based program coordinated and supervised by a rehabilitation professional, but patients with additional shoulder pathology may need a clinic-based program.

Current programs for TSA rehabilitation are based on experience, without research into their effectiveness or superiority. Typically there is a progression from PROM to AROM, followed by progressive strengthening and stretching. The patient is usually in a sling for 2 weeks for an uncomplicated TSA with a longer period of protection of 4 to 6 weeks if the surgery involved a rotator cuff repair or fracture. It is important to instruct the patient to take his or her arm out of the sling frequently to perform ROM exercise for the joints distal to the shoulder for a few minutes to avoid problems with stiffness in these areas. PROM, and possibly AAROM, are initiated on postoperative day 1. These activities include pendulum exercises in the standing position, as well as supine PROM flexion and PROM/AAROM into external rotation to a limit of usually 40 degrees. Pendulum or Codman's exercises facilitate relaxation and initiate early glenohumeral joint motion and scapulohumeral mobility.[130,131] This exercise is also useful as a "warm-up" activity and often helps modulate pain and spasm of the shoulder girdle musculature. It is important to teach the patient the correct way to do this activity because vigorous motion done actively can avulse the anterior capsule and subscapularis repair, or in the case of fractures, tuberosity displacement, which can have devastating complications. This exercise may be too painful for patients with generalized soft tissue laxity because of the distractive force of the hanging upper limb, which is equal to approximately 14% of total body weight.[132]

The goal of inpatient therapy is to teach patients ROM activities that they can do at home. Initially, supine PROM in the scapular plane will allow for the greatest impingement-free arc of motion with the least soft tissue stress.[133] This position allows the humeral head to be centered in the glenoid and the capsule to be relaxed with the

appropriate tension on the ligaments and the muscles. An electromyography (EMG) study of shoulder rehabilitation exercises found that the passive exercise of forward elevation and external rotation generated the least amount of electrical activity in the deltoid and rotator cuff musculature.[134] Less activity was noted in the supraspinatus and middle deltoid with elevation in the scapular plane if the elbow was bent rather than extended. These exercises should be initiated in the supine position and progressed to sitting because the supine position allows the patient to be more relaxed and is helpful in isolating glenohumeral motion and discouraging scapulothoracic substitution patterns. This should progress to AAROM as soon as possible if there are no contraindications, such as a fracture or soft tissue injury, to allow for activation of shoulder girdle muscles. In patients with rotator cuff repairs, assisting external rotation with a cane may be preferable to having the therapist assist because the latter has been found to be associated with higher levels of EMG activity in the rotator cuff muscles.[135] External rotation is one of the hardest and most painful motions to regain, but it is important to achieve good ROM in this direction because external rotation ROM of less than 40 to 45 degrees is associated with significant functional limitations. Patients are typically discharged from the hospital 48 to 72 hours after TSA surgery and are given instructions to continue with their ROM program at home.

◉ *Clinical Pearl*

Early PROM activities are essential after TSA to optimize final ROM and function.

Outpatient therapy can be started, and AROM activities can be initiated 10 to 14 days postoperatively. As pain decreases and the patient can demonstrate adequate shoulder girdle control during supine exercise, more functional upright ROM activities should be started. Upright ROM activities, such as wall walking, cane or wand activities, and pulleys, help improve functional ROM and strengthen the rotator cuff muscles.[131] The first 6 weeks should focus on regaining ROM, and once the subscapularis has had time to heal, strengthening can be initiated as tolerated. The strengthening program should start with isometric contractions in various directions and at a variety of angles and gentle scapular stabilization. Scapulothoracic strengthening can be initiated with rowing motions, serratus anterior strengthening, scapular clocks, and table-top activities such as weight shifts. To avoid straining the anterior soft tissues of the shoulder, rowing motion should only go as far back as the midcoronal line of the body (Fig. 10-14).

Shear stresses on the glenoid component of shoulder implants are thought to be the primary cause for loosening and ultimately failure of shoulder arthroplasty. Therefore it is important that the rotator cuff minimize glenohumeral joint shear. It has been shown that the glenohumeral joint reaction forces gradually increase to 90% body weight at 90 degrees of flexion,[136] and the

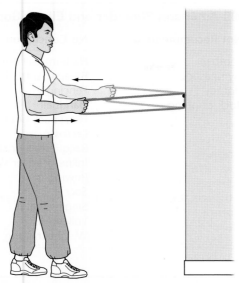

FIG. 10-14 Rowing exercise stopping at midcoronal line.

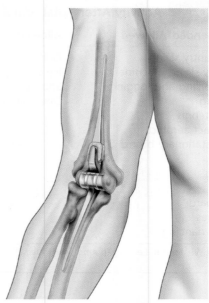

FIG. 10-15 Total elbow arthroplasty (Zimmer Coonrad-Morrey Total Elbow System). *Image courtesy Zimmer, Inc.*

humeral head migrates superiorly if the rotator cuff is weak or fatigued, loading, and ultimately causing failure of the glenoid.[137-139] It is important to strengthen but not overstress the rotator cuff during rehabilitation. Supine AROM exercises are a good way to start to strengthen the rotator cuff and deltoid muscles. In this position, the sheer forces on the glenohumeral joint are minimized.[140] This activity can be initiated 2 weeks after an uncomplicated TSA or hemiarthroplasty in patients with an intact rotator cuff and no fracture and can be progressed to standing when the patient has control of the extremity in supine. The patient should be reminded that pain-free motion below 90 degrees with NO weight can be performed throughout the day but that lifting, pulling, or pushing with the extremity should be avoided until instructed by the surgeon or rehabilitation professional.

Isometric strengthening can be initiated 1 week after TSA if done in a submaximal progression. However, because of the subscapularis repair performed as part of the TSA, internal rotation should not be performed for 6 weeks after a TSA. In patients with rotator cuff repairs, isometrics of the involved muscles should not be initiated for 4 to 8 weeks after the surgery, depending on the nature of the tear and its repair. With fractures, isometrics should not be performed for 3 to 4 weeks after the surgery to allow for a callus to form at the fracture site. Multiple angle isometrics can also improve strength in very weak patients, especially with external rotation.[141]

Isotonic rotator cuff strengthening should be initiated 6 to 12 weeks postoperatively in patients with intact rotator cuffs and 3 to 6 months postoperatively in those with rotator cuff repairs. Initially, all shoulder flexion movements should be done with the elbow flexed to reduce the upper limb moment arm. The patient may use manual resistance, hand weights, elastic bands, or aquatic therapy to provide resistance for strengthening the upper quarter. Elastic resistance training should be used primarily for midrange strengthening where it is safest and easiest to control. Aquatic activities have the advantage of

providing resistance that varies with the speed of motion, buoyancy to support the arm, and potentially the comfort of warmth if the pool is heated to a therapeutic level.

By 3 to 6 months after TSA the patient should be encouraged to continue with a HEP of stretching and strengthening because gains in strength and function may be seen for up to 18 to 24 months after the procedure.

> **◎ Clinical Pearl**
>
> Guidelines for timing of shoulder muscle strengthening after TSA depend on whether the surgery also involved repair of the rotator cuff muscles.

Athletic Participation. There is limited published research on shoulder replacement and athletic activity restrictions. Surgeons were asked to rate 42 activities as recommended or allowed, allowed with experience, not recommended, and no conclusion; their recommendations are listed in Box 10-5.

TOTAL ELBOW ARTHROPLASTY

Pathology. Total elbow arthroplasty (TEA) (Fig. 10-15) is useful when conservative management of a painful or unstable elbow, caused by OA or RA, is unsuccessful. Elbow involvement occurs in 20% to 40% of patients with RA, may be bilateral, and may significantly impair a patient's ability to work or perform ADLs. TEA may also be used for primary management of a distal humeral fracture in certain patients.

Four main designs of elbow prostheses have been developed: Constrained, semiconstrained, unconstrained, and resurfacing. Currently, a semiconstrained hinge type and an unconstrained surface replacement are used most often. The semiconstrained hinge prosthesis allows 5 to

BOX 10-5	Activity After Total Shoulder Arthroplasty—1999 American Shoulder and Elbow Society		
Recommended/Allowed	**Allowed with Experience**	**Not Recommended**	**No Conclusion**
Cross-country skiing	Golf	Football	High-impact aerobics
Stationary skiing machine	Ice skating	Gymnastics	Baseball/softball
Speed walking and jogging	Shooting	Hockey	Fencing
Swimming	Downhill skiing	Rock climbing	Handball
Doubles tennis			Horseback riding
Low impact aerobics			Lacrosse
Road or stationary biking			Racquetball or squash
Bowling			Inline or roller skating
Canoeing			Rowing
Croquet			Soccer
Shuffleboard			Singles tennis
Horseshoes			Volleyball
Ballroom dancing			Weight training

From Healy WL, Iorio R, Lemos MJ: *Am J Sports Med* 29:377-388, 2001.

10 degrees of valgus and varus tilt and axial rotation. The unconstrained prosthesis still has some inherent stability by virtue of the interlocking shape of the components.[142]

Prognosis. Relief of pain is the primary goal of TEA.[143] Improved motion after TEA is the next most important goal. Improved motion is especially important if there is concomitant disease of the shoulder because limitations in ROM of both joints will severely restrict function.

Early results of TEA were compromised by design flaws in the prostheses that led to an unacceptable number of complications. Through subsequent improvements in implant design, cement, interfaces, and high-density polyethylene bearings, the average lifespan and functional performance of these implants have improved significantly. After a TEA the patient is usually permanently restricted from lifting more than 5 lb (2.25 kg) repetitively or more than 10 lb (4.5 kg) for a single episode. TEAs generally last from 8 to 15 years.[144]

Some patients experience a loss of elbow extension strength after TEA, which may be caused by scarring and adhesions of the triceps as a result of the approach used in the surgery. This can limit many ADLs, including rising from a chair using armrests. Surgical techniques that spare the triceps may result in fewer difficulties with ADLs by improving the strength and function of the elbow.

The infection rate of TEA is high when compared to other joint replacement surgeries. Postoperative infection rates of the elbow are 8% to 12% as compared to 0.8% for total shoulder replacements.[145] This may be due to the relative subcutaneous exposure, the potential for olecranon bursa infection, and the extent of the reflection of the muscles over the distal humerus and proximal ulna.

Clinical Pearl

TEA is generally effective for relieving pain but often results in loss of ROM and strength.

Intervention. Limited information is available on therapeutic interventions after TEA. Some protocols have been published in textbooks from centers in which many of these procedures are performed; however, there is little published research in this area. The following suggestions are based primarily on expert recommendations.

Use of compressive cryotherapy has been shown to decrease postoperative swelling in patients undergoing elbow surgery.[146] Since such swelling may lead to soft tissue problems that may restrict ROM, early icing and compression are recommended. Active rehabilitation should begin 5 to 7 days after the semiconstrained TEA, when the elbow may be removed from its postsurgical extension splint. This thermoplastic extension splint should be placed anteriorly and worn at night and between exercise sessions for 6 weeks after the surgery and then be discontinued. This splint promotes elbow extension, which is often the hardest motion to maintain after surgery and the most critical for functional weight bearing on the upper extremity. Full extension may not be achieved if there were long-standing soft tissue contractures before surgery. However, many functional activities, such as reading a newspaper, drinking from a glass, pouring liquid from a pitcher, and using silverware, may be performed with limited elbow movement in midrange from 130 degrees of flexion to 30 degrees of extension and from 50 degrees of supination to 50 degrees of pronation.[147]

With the semiconstrained TEA, AAROM exercises are begun on day 7. These can include flexion-extension, as well as pronation and supination at 90 degrees of elbow flexion. Pronation and supination are performed at 90 degrees of flexion because in this position the bones, rather than the ligaments, provide the most joint stability.[148] The elbow should also be kept close to the body during all exercises to avoid stretching the newly reconstructed collateral ligaments. If patients have difficulty avoiding varus stress on the joint, a hinged elbow brace with no ROM restrictions may be used to provide lateral stability. For 6 weeks after TEA patients should also avoid ADLs that require motions in the scapular or frontal plane.

AROM and NMES for the biceps and triceps can usually be started 2 weeks after a semiconstrained TEA, unless a triceps splitting or reflecting surgical approach was used. In this circumstance, the triceps should not perform forceful extension for 3 to 6 weeks (depending on the physician) to ensure proper healing of the extensor mechanism. For patients who use an assistive mobility device, such as a cane, walker, or crutches, a platform should be added to allow upper extremity weight bearing without active elbow extension (see Chapter 33).

At week 6 (or 12, depending on the surgeon) after a semiconstrained TEA, if the joint is stable and extension ROM is good, extension splint use may be discontinued and ROM exercises may be performed away from the body. At this time, light resistance exercises for the elbow can be started, within the patient's comfort level. Some authors recommend not performing concentric or eccentric strengthening exercises but instead rely on only gentle isometrics and ADLs to increase strength.[149]

With an unconstrained TEA, splinting the elbow at between 30 to 90 degrees of flexion is recommended to prevent posterior dislocation and to promote implant stability.[150,151] The length of time and position of immobilization for optimal outcome has not been adequately studied and is therefore primarily determined by surgeon preference. When the degree of flexion immobilization exceeds 30 degrees, the residual flexion contracture worsens.[152] Therefore a 30-degree extension splint should be worn full time for 2 weeks and thereafter only at night and during high-risk activities. The goal of this splint is to encourage a flexion contracture of 30 degrees to promote stability of the implant and prevent it subluxing or dislocating posteriorly. The ROM goal for flexion is at least 130 degrees to allow for performance of most ADLs.

With an unconstrained TEA, PROM and AAROM limited to between 30 and 150 degrees of flexion should begin within 7 days after the surgery. The joint should only be moved to the point of tissue tension and aggressive PROM should be avoided. Sagittal plane precautions are also applied, and the patient should be encouraged to perform home exercises many times each day. For the first 2 to 3 months, lifting is limited to 1 to 2 lb and thereafter a lifelong limit of 5 lb is imposed. Most strength and function will return with the routine performance of ADLs. Therefore strengthening programs are generally not needed unless the patient is so severely limited that weakness prevents the performance of ADLs. In this case, only midrange isometric strengthening activities should be used because concentric and eccentric strengthening activities may adversely affect implant stability. Patients are also cautioned not to participate in any upper extremity impact sport, such as golf or tennis, after undergoing any TEA.

TOTAL WRIST ARTHROPLASTY

Although the wrist was one of the first joints to be treated with prosthetic replacement, total wrist arthroplasty (TWA) is rare in mainstream orthopedic practice.[153] This may be because symptomatic wrist arthritis is rare, because prostheses are limited, and because of the availability of other acceptable forms of treatments such as limited or complete joint fusion or other surgical procedures that relieve pain while retaining some wrist ROM.[154] Wrist implants have had trouble with component loosening, rapid wear, and breakage, especially at the distal component of the prosthesis.

TWA is generally used to treat patients with RA that affects the wrist and low functional demands. In these patients, who often have many upper extremity joints involved, TWA can preserve motion at the wrist to help compensate for loss of motion in other joints. Patients with traumatic or degenerative arthritis of the wrist usually do not have other joints of the upper extremity involved and are generally candidates for more conservative approaches. In addition, if a patient, such as a musician, needs increased motion a TWA may be warranted. If a patient wished to return to an impact sport, such as golf, he or she should anticipate the need for a revision because of the high risk of implant loosening. Patients with an arthrodesis (fusion) of one wrist and an arthroplasty on the other generally prefer the arthroplasty to the fusion because of the associated reduction in pain and deformity despite high complication rates.[155,156] Studies have shown that 75% to 90% of patients report pain relief with TWA with an average ROM of 36 degrees of extension, 29 to 41 degrees of flexion, 7 to 10 degrees of radial deviation, and 13 to 20 degrees of ulnar deviation.[157,158] It has been reported that at the wrist, 60 degrees of extension, 54 degrees of flexion, 17 degrees of radial deviation, and 40 degrees of ulnar deviation are sufficient to perform all routine ADLs; however, most activities (with the notable exceptions of perineal care and pushing off armrests to rise from a chair) can be completed with 40 degrees of flexion and extension, 10 degrees of radial deviation, and 30 degrees of ulnar deviation.[159] Appropriate candidates for TWA are those with severe pain from RA and elderly patients with severe OA.

◎ *Clinical Pearl*

TWA is rarely performed because joint fusion is often effective at relieving wrist joint pain with fewer complications.

Pathology. The TWA procedure starts with a dorsal incision over the wrist. In many cases, a dorsal tenosynovectomy of the extensor tendons is also necessary. For a rigid implant, the distal portions of the radius and ulna, some of the carpals, and a small portion of the proximal aspect of the third metacarpal are removed. A rigid stemmed prosthesis is then press-fit into the third metacarpal intramedullary canal and the distal radius. In most cases, this implant is cemented in place (Fig. 10-16).

Intervention. Since very limited information on interventions after TWA was found in the literature, the following information is based on expert opinion from texts, journals, and protocols from medical centers that routinely perform these procedures.

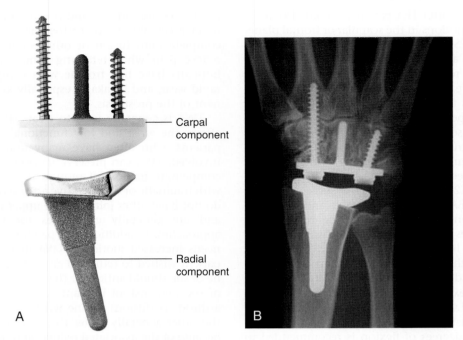

Carpal component

Radial component

A

B

FIG. 10-16 **A,** Wrist prosthesis (implant). **B,** X-ray of implanted wrist prosthesis. **A** *image courtesy KMI.*

For a TWA to be successful, the patient must have intact and functioning wrist extensor tendons, as well as a stable radiocarpal joint. If this is not the case, ligament reconstruction is often necessary.[160] Rehabilitation after wrist arthroplasty requires balancing ROM and stability needs. The duration of postoperative immobilization depends on the stability of the prosthesis intraoperatively and is usually about 2 to 4 weeks. If there is any tendency toward instability, the period of immobilization should be extended. In patients with RA, who are those most commonly having wrist arthroplasty, longer immobilization does not necessarily lead to long-term stiffness. Immobilization should be in a position of neutral flexion and extension to allow the volar and dorsal portions of the capsule to heal with equal lengths for more optimal balance of the joint. Initial placement of the forearm in supination may reduce the risk of early volar dislocation of the prosthesis.[153] Because TWA is associated with substantial postoperative swelling, the hand should be elevated and finger motion should be started early.

After the cast and sutures are removed at 2 weeks, the patient should be fitted with a molded wrist splint to be used for the next 2 to 4 weeks, during which time an active ROM program for the wrist should be initiated. This program should include active flexion, extension, pronation, and supination of the wrist. Passive ROM is discouraged for the first 8 weeks postoperatively, at which time light strengthening through isometrics may also be initiated. Unrestricted use of the hand and wrist is not allowed for the first 3 months. Long-term activity restrictions, although not well defined, should include avoidance of repetitive forceful motion and impact loading.

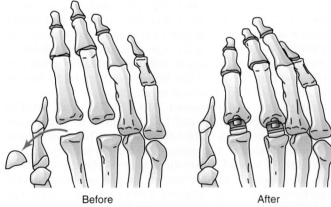

Before   After

FIG. 10-17 Metacarpophalangeal arthroplasty: Before and after. *Copyright Medical Multimedia Group, LLC.*

FINGER ARTHROPLASTY

Arthroplasty of the fingers and thumb are used to treat a wide variety of painful conditions that limit hand function. Whether the etiology is OA, RA, or posttraumatic arthritis, a wide variety of both implant and nonimplant arthroplasties can successfully improve function. Implant arthroplasty has been successful in the metacarpophalangeal (MCP) (Fig. 10-17) and proximal interphalangeal (PIP) joints, whereas ligament reconstruction tendon interposition (LRTI) has become a mainstay in the treatment of basal or carpometacarpal (CMC) arthritis, although implant arthroplasty is also used for CMC arthritis.

Metacarpophalangeal Arthroplasty. MCP arthroplasty has been performed since the 1950s.[161] Since that time, advances in technology have led to the development of a variety of techniques and implants. Implants may have a single- or two-piece hinge design, be constrained or nonconstrained, and be fixed with or without cement. Implants may be silicone, metallic, or ceramic coated; however, a hinged silastic spacer is used most commonly for MCP and PIP joint reconstruction in patients with RA.[162] This design is referred to as a "load distributing flexible hinge." It acts like an internal splint to maintain alignment. It does not simulate normal joint mechanics but does provide pain relief and a useful arc of motion.[163]

Contraindications to MCP arthroplasty include infection, inadequate bone stock or soft tissue covering, and an irreparable musculotendinous system. Patients with juvenile RA may not have large enough intramedullary canals to accept implants, so a simple resection arthroplasty may be performed on these patients.[164,165] It is also important to consider what other joints are involved in patients with complex RA deformities. For example, a fixed radial deviation of the wrist will lead to recurrent ulnar deviation of the fingers even after successful MCP arthroplasty.[166]

Many surgical approaches are used for placement of MCP arthroplasties. For example, for a single-digit arthroplasty of the MCP joint, the extensor mechanism of the finger is exposed through a longitudinal incision, whereas, if multiple joints are to be replaced, a transverse incision is more common. The extensor mechanism is dissected so that it can be relocated at the time of wound closure. If the patient has RA with ulnar drift, the drift is then corrected. If possible, the sagittal bands of the MCP capsule are preserved. The capsule is incised to expose the MCP joint. The proximal phalanx is cut to remove the articular surface, and an awl is then inserted into the intramedullary canal of both the proximal phalanx and metacarpal until the appropriate fit is obtained. Trial implants are inserted, and the joint is tested for stability and ROM. The final implant can be press-fit or cemented, depending on the prosthesis chosen. Then the extensor mechanism is relocated, and the wound is closed.

Prognosis. The goal of MCP arthroplasty is to decrease pain, enhance joint stability, and ultimately improve hand function. By restoring skeletal alignment and improving tendon mechanics, the patient should regain more effective and efficient finger function.

The final result of a finger implant arthroplasty in patients with RA is not a normally functioning joint, but a painless arthroplasty with a functional ROM.[167] The largest meta-analysis to date reviewed all the published series of MCP joint arthroplasty used for the treatment of RA and found that this procedure effectively corrected the ulnar drift deformity and improved the aesthetic appearance of the hand.[168] A goal of 70 degrees of MCP flexion is recommended. Grip strength does not increase after MCP arthroplasty, possibly because usually other joints are also invoved.[169,170] However, two studies found that hand function does improve, particularly functions requiring pinch, span, and hook grip.[171,172] Patient satisfaction with this procedure may be more affected by pain relief and aesthetic appearance than by more readily measurable outcomes such as strength and ROM.[173]

Intervention. Therapy regimens after MCP arthroplasty should protect the joint, improve ROM, and safely progress the patient back to activity. Although many articles describe surgical technique and outcomes for MCP arthroplasty, few describe their postoperative regimen with any specificity, making comparisons of therapy intervention protocols difficult.[163,174,175] For example, in a review of 64 studies that described results of MCP arthroplasty, only 5 described their postoperative regimen.[176] The main differences between rehabilitation protocols were the use of passive or active MCP extension and the splinting of the MCPs in extension[177] versus flexion.[178] One of the difficulties with performing studies of the rehabilitation for this procedure is its relative infrequency compared with other arthroplasties such as hips and knees. For example, one group took 3 years to find 43 hands to include in their research.[175]

Postoperative rehabilitation is recognized as an important factor in the successful outcome of joint arthroplasty of the hand.[179] In general, therapy regimens after MCP arthroplasty are based on the principles of tissue healing and scar formation; however, there are wide differences in splinting, exercise protocols, and time frames.[180] All of the regimens started therapy within 2 to 5 days after surgery. CPM machines are rarely used because they have not been shown to increase the ROM after this procedure.[181] Initially the goals of therapy are to monitor wound healing, decrease edema, and prevent scar adherence. Tissue healing after this procedure is often impaired because many of the patients are on long-term corticosteroid treatment for RA. Additionally, as ulnar drift is common in this population, the postoperative splint is usually fashioned in slight radial deviation to align the digits with the corresponding metacarpal. In addition, to optimize finger ROM, the PIP may be splinted in extension with the MCP in flexion. Some authors advocate using dynamic splints, whereas others recommend passive or resting splints.[180-183] Most allow patients to begin retraining the hand and begin active ROM at the MCP within 7 to 10 days after surgery. Patients may begin to use their hands for ADLs and light activities at about 1 month, although night splints are often continued for 4 months to help reduce extensor lags. It is important to obtain motion early because capsular tightness that persists beyond 3 to 4 weeks after surgery may limit final functional outcome.

Clinical Pearl

Rehabilitation after finger joint arthroplasty generally focuses on optimizing ROM and functional use for ADLs.

Interphalangeal Joint Arthroplasty. The normal PIP joint has the greatest arc of motion of any joint of the hand and therefore plays a critical role in hand function.[184] Arthroplasty of the PIP and distal interphalangeal (DIP) joints may be indicated for the treatment of pain, stiffness, deformity, instability, and loss of cartilage in the joint. Typically, these finding are sequelae of OA, RA, or trauma. An acceptable alternative treatment to arthroplasty may be arthrodesis, depending on the patient's functional needs and limitations. For example, a patient who needs a powerful grip and joint stability, such as a laborer, may be better served by an arthrodesis than an arthroplasty, which may be prone to loosening and failure. PIP function, especially of the fourth and fifth fingers, generally will significantly impact the overall function of the hand, whereas DIP function will have less functional impact. Therefore, in the fourth and fifth digits, a PIP arthroplasty may be preferred to arthrodesis.[185]

Prognosis. The primary goals of interphalangeal joint arthroplasty are to relieve pain and to improve hand function. The ROM goals for the PIP joint of the fourth and fifth fingers are 60 to 70 degrees of flexion and neutral extension. In a retrospective review of a series of 70 PIP arthroplasties in 48 patients, there were no significant changes in flexion ROM after PIP arthroplasty but extension ROM did increase, improving the functional motion of the joint.[186] Pinch and grip strength did not change significantly, but overall pain relief was good in 70% of patients. Patients who had these implants placed because of RA had poorer outcomes than those who had the procedure performed because of degenerative or posttraumatic arthritis.

Less flexion of the interphalangeal joints is needed for functional use of the index and middle finger than for the fourth and fifth fingers.[187] With DIP arthroplasty of these fingers, 30 degrees of flexion and neutral extension are acceptable. When assessing the functional outcomes from these procedures, the function of the hand as a whole should be considered. If the arthroplasty of the PIP joint is on the same finger as an MCP arthroplasty, the overall function of that finger will be more severely impacted than if the PIP was fused and the MCP was treated with an arthroplasty.[184] Patients with PIP arthroplasty with simple joint contractures or joint surface incongruity on the same digit tend to fare better than those with tendon imbalances such as swan-neck deformities.[188,189]

CASE STUDY 10-1

TOTAL KNEE ARTHROPLASTY

Patient History

MV is a 66-year-old woman with a history of right knee OA. She underwent a cemented primary TKA 2 weeks ago. She spent 4 days as an inpatient and received physical therapy and CPM. She was discharged home 10 days ago. She lives with her husband in a 2-story home with 12 stairs up to the second story. She has been referred to outpatient physical therapy with a prescription for evaluation and treatment for "s/p R TKA." Her goal for therapy is to be able to "stroll through the streets of Venice" on her upcoming trip to Europe in the fall (6 months from now). Currently, her pain is a constant 4/10 but increases to 6/10 with activity. Pain is controlled with ice and hydrocodone with acetaminophen.

Tests and Measures—Significant Findings

- Effusion of the right knee. Girth is 55 cm on the right and 45 cm on the left measured at the level of the medial joint line.
- AROM and PROM of the right knee: 10 to 95 degrees
- Strength 3?/5 hamstrings and quadriceps with poor control of the quadriceps with straight leg raise.
- MV ambulates with a front-wheeled walker with an antalgic gait and weight bearing as tolerated. She has a decreased ability to go from sit to stand and requires minimal assistance if the chair does not have arms.

Diagnosis

Preferred practice pattern 4H: Impaired joint mobility, motor function, muscle performance, and range of motion associated with joint arthroplasty.

Interventions

- PROM and AROM exercises in supine, prone, and seated to facilitate increased flexion and extension. Exercises to include activities on a stationary bicycle, as well as clinician- and patient-directed ROM.
- Soft tissue mobilization of the scar and peripatellar area, and patellar mobilizations, to improve ROM and soft tissue extensibility.
- Open and closed kinetic-chain strengthening activities to improve strength and ultimately function. If quadriceps strength is not responding to active strengthening techniques, NMES will be utilized.
- Balance and proprioception will be improved through single leg balance activities.
- Aerobic capacity and endurance will be improved through cycling and treadmill walking.
- Ice and electrical stimulation or a cryotherapy/pneumatic compression device will be used at the end of the treatment session to control pain and swelling.

Role of the Physical Therapist Assistant

- What activities could you do with this patient in the clinic to improve her ability to go from sit to stand? What could you instruct her to do at home to help her improve her sit-to-stand function and independence?
- Why do you think that the PT would emphasize regaining knee extension over flexion for this patient?
- How much knee ROM do you think is generally required to walk up and down stairs step over step? What will this patient be able to comfortably do first, walk up stairs or walk down stairs? Why?

Additional Information

For the full version of this case study, including detailed examination results, interventions, and outcomes, see the Evolve site that accompanies this book. A full case study of a patient after a shoulder hemiarthroplasty also appears on the Evolve site.

CHAPTER SUMMARY

Joint arthroplasty is most commonly used to treat pain and loss of function caused by arthritis. It is one of the most widely performed orthopedic surgical procedures in the United States and will doubtless increase in frequency with the increasing longevity of the population. Understanding and implementing appropriate rehabilitation interventions after joint arthroplasty is essential. Studies of patient outcomes, although not extensive, have demonstrated that patients who undergo joint arthroplasty have limitations in ROM, strength, proprioception, and ultimately function that are decreased by appropriate rehabilitation. Rehabilitation interventions generally focus on early safe ROM activities followed by strengthening and ultimately, functional activities.

ADDITIONAL RESOURCES

For links to these and additional web-based resources, see the Evolve site.

National Institute of Arthritis and Musculoskeletal and Skin Diseases (NIAMS)

American Academy of Orthopaedic Surgeons (AAOS)

American College of Rheumatology (ACR)

GLOSSARY

Arthrodesis: The surgical fusion of the bony surfaces of a joint with internal fixation such as pins, plates, nails, and/or bone graft.

Arthrofibrosis: Increased fibrous tissue in a joint that limits ROM.

Arthropathy: Any disease or abnormal condition affecting a joint.

Arthroplasty: Any reconstructive joint procedure with or without an implant that is designed to relieve pain and restore motion

Avascular necrosis: Death of bone cells as a result of loss of a blood supply.

Continuous passive motion (CPM): A machine that passively moves a joint at a prescribed speed and through a prescribed ROM.

Cruciate retaining (or sparing) knee: A total knee replacement in which the posterior cruciate is retained for stability.

Extensor lag: When the knee's PROM into extension exceeds the AROM into extension. This term is synonymous with quadriceps lag.

Fascial arthroplasty: Removal of the bone from one or both of the articular surfaces of a joint and allowing a fibrotic scar to form in the space that remains.

Hemiarthroplasty: Replacement of one side of a compartment of a joint. For example, in the shoulder, replacement of the humeral component only.

Methylmethacrylate: Epoxy cement used in cemented total joint surgery to attach the implant to the bone surface.

Mobile bearing knee: A total knee replacement in which a polyethylene insert articulates with the femoral component and the metallic tibial tray.

Osteolysis: Softening or destruction of bone.

Posterior stabilized knee: A total knee replacement in which both cruciate ligaments are excised and the stability of the knee depends on the implant.

Resection arthroplasty: Removal of one or both articular surfaces of a joint (also known as excisional arthroplasty).

Chapter 11

Soft Tissue Surgery

Christopher J. Durall, Robert C. Manske

OBJECTIVES

After reading this chapter, the reader will be able to:
1. Differentiate types of nonmineralized connective tissue, including bursa, synovium, cartilage, fascia, ligament, capsule, and tendon.
2. Compare and contrast the mechanical properties of the different types of nonmineralized connective tissue.
3. Discuss the effects of immobilization and remobilization on connective tissue.
4. Describe in general terms the rehabilitation process after soft tissue surgery.
5. Discuss the different types of surgeries performed on bursae, synovium, cartilage, fascia, ligaments, capsules, and tendons.
6. Explain unique elements of the rehabilitation process after surgery on bursae, synovium, cartilage, fascia, ligaments, capsules, and tendons.
7. Provide safe and effective rehabilitation to a patient after a soft tissue surgery.

$\mathcal{M}$any musculoskeletal pathologies and injuries require surgical intervention and a period of post-operative rehabilitation to maximize functional recovery. Tissues that undergo surgery are subjected to trauma, albeit controlled trauma. As with other forms of trauma, the affected tissues undergo a healing process. After surgery, there is often a period of immobilization. Thus, to most effectively manage postoperative rehabilitation, the physical therapist assistant (PTA) must understand the healing process and how immobilization affects musculo-skeletal tissues. Tissue healing is reviewed in detail in Chapter 28.

This chapter discusses the rehabilitation of individuals with impairments and functional limitations after soft tissue surgery. The effects of immobilization are described, as well as remobilization parameters and interventions for rehabilitation. This chapter includes a discussion of the unique properties of nonmineralized (or soft) **connective tissue,** an overview of soft tissue postoperative rehabilita-tion, tissue-specific rehabilitation recommendations, and case studies. Skeletal muscle, although an integral soft tissue in the musculoskeletal system, is not often surgi-cally repaired and thus is not covered in this chapter.

PATHOLOGY

NONMINERALIZED CONNECTIVE TISSUES OF THE MUSCULOSKELETAL SYSTEM

All body structures are comprised of various combinations of four types of tissue: Connective, epithelial, nerve, and muscular. Aside from muscle, the structures of the muscu-loskeletal system are all composed of connective tissues. Connective tissues perform many highly specialized meta-bolic and biomechanical functions in the body, including providing structural support and facilitating movement. All connective tissues have an abundant **extracellular matrix** but are relatively devoid of cells. The extracellular matrix, produced by the cells, consists of ground sub-stance and fibers, which give the tissues their unique char-acteristics (Fig. 11-1). **Cartilage,** for example, has a firm, yet flexible extracellular matrix, whereas bone has a rigid extracellular matrix.

The ground substance of connective tissue contains interstitial fluid, **proteoglycan molecules,** and proteins

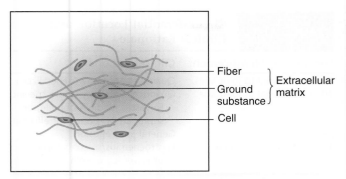

FIG. 11-1 Constituents of connective tissue.

that "glue" the cells to the matrix.[1] The proteoglycan molecules combine with water to form a fluid or semisolid gel that lubricates and creates space between adjacent fibers in the extracellular matrix. Space between fibers prevents the fibers adhering to one another.[1] The ground substance reduces friction between fibers and prevents the formation of fibrous adhesions.

The three types of connective tissue fibers are **collagen,** reticular, and elastic. All are formed from varying proportions of collagen and elastin proteins. Collagen proteins undergo little elongation in response to tensile loading, whereas elastin proteins are more extensible or rubber-like.[2] Tissues with a high collagen content, such as **tendons** and **ligaments,** resist or transmit tensile forces well, whereas tissues with a relatively high elastin content, such as skin, are more pliable.[1]

There are many different types of collagen fibers, but our discussion is limited to types I, II, and III, which are most abundant. Type I collagen, which is the most abundant, has the greatest tensile strength and is found in many connective tissues, including tendon, bone, and ligaments. The function of type I collagen is resisting tension. In contrast, type II collagen is most effective at resisting pressure and appropriately is abundant in the hyaline cartilage lining weight-bearing joints. Type III collagen, the second most abundant type of collagen, is found in skin, blood vessels, and the granulation tissue of healing wounds. Type III collagen fibers are more delicate than type I and are gradually replaced by type I collagen fibers during tissue healing.[3]

Clinical Pearl

Connective tissue binds structures together to form a framework that supports the organs and the body.

Connective tissue can be classified as dense or loose and as regular or irregular, according to the density and orientation, respectively, of its fibers. Dense regular connective tissue has a high concentration of fibers arranged in a regular or unidirectional manner. Dense regular connective tissue has a relatively poor vascular supply and therefore heals less well than other more well-vascularized tissues.[4] This is in part why tendons and ligaments, which are comprised of dense regular connective tissue, often heal slowly or incompletely. Dense irregular connective tissue, as found in joint **capsules,** has densely packed fibers with multidirectional orientation. This tissue also has relatively low vascularity and therefore heals slowly.[4] Unlike dense connective tissue, loose connective tissue has relatively few fibers and therefore relatively low tensile strength. Loose connective tissue is found in the superficial **fascia** throughout the musculoskeletal system. In contrast to dense connective tissue, loose connective tissue is relatively well vascularized and thus heals more readily.[4] **Synovium** is a specialized connective tissue on the innermost portion of the capsule of synovial joints. Synovial cells secrete fluid that is thought to serve two main purposes: Joint lubrication and nourishment of the avascular articular cartilage.[5] Synovial cavities may be contiguous with pouches containing synovial fluid known as **bursae,** which are located at frictional interfaces in the musculoskeletal system.

Bone and cartilage are also specialized connective tissues. As with other connective tissues, bone and cartilage have cells (osteoblasts and chondrocytes, respectively) that secrete an extracellular matrix. The firm, slightly yielding yet resilient matrix of cartilage is ideal for damping compressive loads and reducing friction at joints, and the rigid, calcified matrix of bone provides structural support and protection.

Although there are several forms of cartilage, articular cartilage and fibrocartilage are the forms most commonly affected by orthopedic surgery. Articular cartilage is a specialized form of hyaline cartilage that covers the ends of bones in diarthrodial joints. This type of cartilage has a high proteoglycan and water content to allow it to distribute compressive loads.[5] Fibrocartilage has properties of dense connective tissue and properties of hyaline cartilage.[2,4] It has more type I collagen and thus greater tensile strength than articular cartilage but more proteoglycan and water than dense connective tissue, so it can also tolerate pressure loading.[4,5] Fibrocartilage often forms temporarily at fracture sites and is a permanent component of the intervertebral disks of the spine, the menisci at the knee and wrist, the labrum at the shoulder, and the acetabulum at the hip.

Unlike other connective tissues, cartilage is avascular and alymphatic. It is nourished by the diffusion of nutrients from the synovial fluid and by capillaries in adjacent connective tissue. The lack of a direct vascular supply precludes an inflammatory response to injury and gives cartilage a poor healing potential. Articular cartilage far from the bony surface, which relies entirely on the diffusion of nutrients and oxygen through the cartilage matrix, has almost no ability to heal.[4,5] If articular cartilage close to subchondral bone is injured, it may heal with a mixture of hyaline cartilage and fibrocartilage.[5]

Clinical Pearl

Cartilage is an avascular, dense connective tissue found on the articular surface of bones.

EFFECTS OF IMMOBILIZATION AND REMOBILIZATION ON NONMINERALIZED CONNECTIVE TISSUE

After surgery, immobilization may be needed to prevent disruption of the surgical repair. However, prolonged immobilization results in the loss of ground substance and subsequent dehydration and approximation of the embedded fibers in the extracellular matrix.[6-8] These microstructural changes contribute to the formation of fibrous adhesions and increased friction between fibers, leading to reduced tissue length and strength.[1,8-11]

Numerous studies have shown that controlled remobilization after injury or surgery can reverse many of the adverse effects of immobilization.[12-14] Mechanical stress of the appropriate magnitude and direction can stimulate collagen synthesis and optimize its alignment,[12,15-17] whereas too much or too little stress can impair collagen synthesis.[18-21] For example, controlled muscle contraction can make collagen fibers in tendons orient in the direction of force transmission from the muscle to the skeletal attachment. This optimizes the structural integrity and functionality of the tissue.[12,17]

During tissue healing, much of the initial collagen formed is type III, which is weaker than type I collagen.[18,22] As the connective tissue matures, which may take up to a full year after a period of immobilization,[8] most of the type III collagen is replaced by type I collagen.[18] Thus healing connective tissue may be weaker than fully mature tissue for many months after an injury or a period of immobilization.[3,23] Clinically, it is important to remember that mechanical forces that may be safe for mature, healthy tissue may injure healing tissue for up to a year after the injury.

⊚ *Clinical Pearl*

Mechanical forces that may be safe for mature, healthy tissue may injure healing tissue for up to a year after the injury.

OVERVIEW OF REHABILITATION AFTER SOFT TISSUE SURGERY

Although rehabilitation after soft tissue surgery varies slightly according to the type of tissue operated on, there is considerable overlap for all tissue types, with most focusing on remobilization, increasing range of motion (ROM), decreasing edema, and returning to an optimal level of functional activity. This section describes general, non–tissue-specific postoperative rehabilitation. Unique considerations for each type of nonmineralized connective tissue are discussed in the next sections.

TYPICAL EXAMINATION FINDINGS

PATIENT HISTORY

The therapist will generally review the medical chart to gather pertinent information before meeting the patient, including information about the surgical procedure and

TABLE 11-1	Circumferential Location and Clinical Rationale
Location of Measurement	**Clinical Rationale**
20 cm proximal to joint line	Quadriceps atrophy (generalized)
10 cm proximal to joint line	Quadriceps atrophy (more specific to vastus medialis oblique) or suprapatellar pouch for effusion
Joint line	General joint effusion
15 cm distal to joint line	Gastrocnemius/soleus atrophy or lower leg edema

From Manske RC, Davies GJ: *Crit Rev Phys Rehabil Med* 15(2):141-166, 2003.

any contraindications to movement or activity. The patient's present functional status and their anticipated long-term functional goals will be discussed. Plans and expectations regarding return to activity will be brought up early so that the clinician and patient can reach agreement and fully understand each other's concerns. For instance, the patient may have unrealistic expectations regarding how quickly he or she can return to full activity. The therapist will also briefly explain the generic intervention process, as well as the specific patient's unique rehabilitation considerations based on the type of connective tissue affected.

SYSTEMS REVIEW

The systems review is used to target areas requiring further examination and to define areas that may cause complications or indicate a need for precautions during the examination and intervention processes. Chapter 1 includes details of the systems review.

TESTS AND MEASURES

Musculoskeletal

Posture. The affected limb position is observed. Patients tend to assume a position that is comfortable, but in some instances the most comfortable position, if maintained for prolonged periods, may lead to undesirable adaptive tissue shortening.

Anthropometric Characteristics. Limb circumference is often measured bilaterally at several locations around and over affected joints to assess for swelling or soft tissue atrophy (Table 11-1).

Range of Motion. ROM will be assessed both actively and passively in joints affected by the surgery. Surgical restrictions, as well as the patient's symptom response, will guide the passive motion assessment.

Muscle Performance. High-intensity strength testing is often contraindicated in the initial postoperative period, since high levels of muscle tension may damage surgically repaired tissue. However, the physical therapist may test if the patient can move the affected body segment through his or her available ROM against gravity (criteria for a "fair" [3/5] muscle grade).

Joint Integrity and Mobility. The indications and appropriate vigor for clinical stress and mobility testing varies considerably with joint structure and is typically not well tolerated after orthopedic operative procedures and may be contraindicated, depending on the type of procedure performed.

Neuromuscular

Arousal, Attention, and Cognition. The astute therapist forms an opinion about a patient's arousal, attention, and cognition while obtaining the patient history and performing the systems review as described. In essence, the patient should be able to interact meaningfully with the therapist and ideally should not be easily distracted or have difficulty following through with directions.

Pain. Pain, or other symptoms, is recorded and tracked using a visual analog or other type of scale. Qualifiers (e.g., boring, stabbing, or achy) may also be used to further describe the pain.

Peripheral Nerve Integrity. Peripheral nerve integrity is assessed through testing of reflex integrity, sensory integrity, and muscle performance.

Reflex Integrity. Deep tendon reflexes may be assessed if there are no contraindications to movement or muscle contraction.

Sensory Integrity. Superficial skin sensation may often be reduced or compromised in a patient after soft tissue surgery because of severing of superficial nerves or compression by local swelling.[24] Sensation testing should be conducted regularly to assess for nerve regeneration.

Motor Function—Control and Learning. Motor function is generally quickly assessed during the systems review by observing the patient's coordination and movement in response to simple requests (e.g., "try to straighten your knee").

Cardiovascular/Pulmonary. Vital signs are typically assessed in the inpatient setting at the beginning of each rehabilitation session (see Chapter 22). In addition, in the outpatient setting, vital signs will likely be recorded during the initial evaluation and again if the patient experiences marked or inexplicable symptom changes. It is important to regularly monitor and record vital signs in all patients with cardiopulmonary compromise. Circulation can be quickly assessed by palpating for skin temperature, pulses, and by viewing skin color and capillary refill.

Integumentary. During the initial examination and at each subsequent meeting, the surgical site should be carefully inspected for any indicators of an adverse reaction (e.g., erythema, swelling, wound drainage, or heat). The skin color and presence of scar formation should also be noted. Wound healing, as well as scar formation and compliance, should be monitored throughout the rehabilitation process. The integument in any areas subjected to prolonged pressure or shear should also be monitored regularly for the development of pressure ulcers (see Chapter 28). Because of decreased oxygen perfusion, ischemia, and low oxygen tension, soft tissue healing may be delayed in individuals with systemic diseases, such as diabetes or peripheral vascular disease, and in individuals who smoke.[25] A list of postoperative "red flags" or signs and symptoms that merit further investigation and/or physician notification can be found in Box 11-1. These warning signs and symptoms may indicate the presence of infection or disruption of the surgical repair and should be carefully documented and quickly communicated to the surgeon.

BOX 11-1	**Postoperative Red Flags: Signs and Symptoms that Merit Further Investigation or Physician Notification**

- Erythema
- Increased edema
- Colored or purulent drainage
- Increased local tissue temperature
- Fever or other systemic manifestations (e.g., hyperhidrosis)
- Unexplainable marked increase in pain
- Excessive mobility after a stabilizing procedure
- Significant loss of mobility after a releasing procedure

Function

Gait, Locomotion, and Balance. For surgeries involving the lumbar spine, pelvis, or lower extremities, gait is assessed because postoperative pain, swelling, and weakness can affect stride length, stride width, and stance time[26] (see Chapter 32). Weight-bearing restrictions imposed by the surgeon need to be clearly communicated to the patient.

Orthotic, Protective, and Supportive Devices. The therapist (or physician) determines if the patient's functional ability would improve by the use of orthotic, protective, or support devices. Previously dispensed devices should be inspected on and off the patient, and the skin should be checked to determine if the fit and usage of the device is appropriate. The patient should also be observed using any devices to ensure that the devices are used safely.

Ergonomics and Body Mechanics. Ergonomics and body mechanics are not typically assessed formally during the initial examination but may be appropriate to examine later in the rehabilitation process.

Environmental Barriers, Self-Care, and Home Management. Environmental barriers and self-care and home management are discussed during the patient history.

Work, Community, and Leisure Integration. Work, community, and leisure integration are not typically assessed formally during the initial examination but should be examined and evaluated later in the rehabilitation process.

EVALUATION, DIAGNOSIS, AND PROGNOSIS

According to the *Guide to Physical Therapist Practice*,[27] rehabilitation for patients in the preferred practice pattern 4I: Impaired joint mobility, motor function, muscle performance, and range of motion associated with bony or soft tissue surgery may take from 1 to 8 months (roughly 6 to 70 visits), although there are many factors, such as adherence to the intervention program; age; caregiver consistency and expertise; chronicity or severity of condition; concurrent medical, surgical, and therapeutic interventions; and overall health status, including nutritional status, that may require modification of the frequency and duration of physical therapy visits.[28] At present, specific evidence-based data on the prognosis or outcome of patients in this practice pattern are not available.

INTERVENTION

The process of tissue healing (see Chapters 7 and 28) consists of an inflammatory phase, a fibroplastic proliferation phase, and a maturation phase. The intervention process after soft tissue surgery is divided into three phases that roughly correspond with the three phases of healing: Immediate postoperative phase (also known as the *maximum protection phase*), the intermediate phase (also known as the *moderate protection phase*), and the advanced strengthening/return to activity phase (also known as the *minimum protection phase*). Unfortunately, the phases of healing are not punctuated with obvious beginning or end points. Likewise, the signs and symptoms indicating that a patient is ready to advance from one phase of rehabilitation to the next are often subtle. Nonetheless, some criteria can be used to guide rehabilitation progression decisions.

Although this chapter primarily addresses postoperative rehabilitation, preoperative interventions are valuable as well. Restoring or maximizing joint motion and strength before orthopedic surgery has been shown to reduce postoperative recovery time.

IMMEDIATE POSTOPERATIVE PHASE

During the immediate postoperative period, the surgically affected connective tissues undergo an inflammatory response. While the inflammatory response is necessary for healing, the associated pain and edema can impede the rehabilitation process.[29-31] Goals of the immediate postoperative period include protection of the soft tissues from harmful stress, minimizing the adverse effects of immobilization, and controlling pain and inflammation. Bracing and assistive devices (e.g., crutches, splints) can be used to protect the tissues from excessive stress after spine, pelvic, or upper or lower extremity surgery. A scale can be used to help the patient quantify their weight bearing. Aquatic therapy and unloading devices may be appropriate for patients with weight-bearing restrictions. After upper extremity surgery, slings, splints, or immobilizers can be used to protect the soft tissues.

Several interventions have been shown to be effective for pain modulation, including cryotherapy,[32] manual therapy,[33] exercise,[34,35] and electrical stimulation.[36] Cryotherapy, which causes local vasoconstriction and increases blood viscosity, or monophasic pulsed electrical current may be used to limit edema formation during the inflammatory response.[37-39]

To minimize the adverse effects of immobilization and to stimulate collagen synthesis and proper collagen alignment, movement should begin as soon after surgery as the surgeon deems safe. As discussed earlier, connective tissue must be stressed appropriately if it is to become sufficiently robust. Early motion can be achieved through either passive ROM (PROM) or active assisted ROM (AAROM).[34,35] If the surgeon has not imposed joint motion limits, the therapist may consider imposing motion limits based on the patient's pain and swelling response to

movement. Patients who take analgesic medications may have greater pain tolerance to movement or exercise, but they also may be at greater risk of iatrogenic injury and therefore should be advised to exercise below their pain threshold.

> ### ◎ *Clinical Pearl*
>
> In the immediate postoperative phase exercises or ROM should be advanced carefully. In this phase many patients take analgesic medications, elevating their pain tolerance and thereby increasing their risk of injury during therapy.

INTERMEDIATE POSTOPERATIVE PHASE

The intermediate phase begins when the acute inflammatory reaction has subsided, typically 1 week after surgery.[40,41] Goals of the immediate postoperative period include pain and edema reduction; restoration of normal functional movement patterns; increased joint motion and muscle strength; and improved neuromuscular coordination, timing, strength, endurance, and **proprioception.** During this phase, it is important to continue protecting the soft tissues with bracing, splinting, assistive devices, and gradual, symptom-limited exercise progression.

Edema remaining after the acute inflammatory response can cause pain[42] and impair muscle performance.[29-31] Interventions that have been found to be effective in reducing edema during this phase include elevation,[43] compression,[44] motor-level electrical stimulation,[45] and exercise.[46] Elevation of the edematous segment above heart level promotes venous and lymphatic return via the effects of gravity.[43] Compressive wraps or garments can reduce edema by driving extracellular fluid into the venules and lymphatic vessels.[46] Exercise can also promote proximal movement of venous and lymphatic fluid since contracting and relaxing muscles compresses and decompresses venous and lymphatic vessels, pumping the fluid proximally.[46] If necessary, motor-level electrical stimulation can be used to induce the muscle contractions and thus enhance circulation.[45]

Because dense, regular connective tissue is poorly vascularized, interventions that increase local circulation and metabolism may facilitate tissue healing.[47] Local circulation may be increased with thermotherapy[48,49] (e.g., hot packs, paraffin baths, fluidotherapy, continuous ultrasound), massage,[50] exercise,[48,51] and electrical stimulation.[45,52]

Strengthening exercises should be initiated during this phase, when the muscle-tendon unit can safely tolerate tensile loading. After tendon repairs, resistance exercise may be delayed for several weeks or months, depending on surgeon preference.[53-56] The intensity of strengthening exercises (see Chapter 5) will be progressed, based on the patient's symptom response. If joint movement is contraindicated, isometric exercises should be considered. Concentric and eccentric muscle actions should be predicated on the appropriateness of joint movement. Adjacent or synergistic motion segments should also be exercised to reduce atrophic changes from reduced activity.

Remaining functional limitations, such as gait impairments and reduced hand function, are often addressed during this phase. Activities intended to enhance position-sense (proprioception), balance (see Chapter 13), neuromuscular control, and cardiovascular fitness (see Chapter 23) should be instituted as early in the process as possible.[57] Any lingering motion deficits should be addressed with stretching and/or mobilization.

Objective and subjective criteria are used to determine when a patient is ready to progress to the advanced strengthening and return to activity phase. Based on clinical experience, it is recommended that the following criteria be satisfied (at a minimum) before advancing a patient to the advanced strengthening and return to activity phase: A stable surgical repair; no pain during activity; minimal, transient postexercise pain; no swelling; joint AROM and PROM within normal limits (or comparable to the contralateral side); and bilateral deficits less than 25% with manual muscle testing (MMT), isokinetic testing, and functional testing.

> ◎ **Clinical Pearl**
>
> In the intermediate postoperative phase therapy focuses on achieving normal functional movement patterns; increased joint motion; increased muscle strength and endurance; and improved neuromuscular coordination and timing.

ADVANCED STRENGTHENING AND RETURN TO ACTIVITY PHASE

During the last phase of rehabilitation, patients should be advanced to their maximum functional potential. Goals during the advanced strengthening and return to activity phase include restoration of full ROM, strength, endurance, and proprioception and maximization of functional ability. During this phase, more strenuous and stressful exercises are introduced. Jumping, hopping, and running may be introduced for patients recovering from lower extremity surgery, and diagonal patterns that mimic overhand sports may be initiated for patients recovering from upper extremity surgery. High-intensity sport- or work-specific activities should be introduced to prepare the patient for return to activity. To reduce the risk of reinjury, resistance exercise intensity should ultimately be consistent with the intensity of the patient's work, sport, or activities of daily living (ADLs).

Ideally, at the end of this phase, the patient will return to work, sports activities, and ADLs without functional limitations. Some patients, however, do not regain full functional ability after soft tissue surgery and rehabilitation. Despite this, every attempt must be made to maximize their functional ability.

> ◎ **Clinical Pearl**
>
> The advanced strengthening and return to activity phase is also known as the minimum protection phase.

TABLE 11-2	**Considerations After Surgery to Different Types of Soft Tissue**
Tissue	**Considerations**
Bursal	Infection
	Symptom limited
	Complex regional pain syndrome
Cartilage	Immobilization time frames
	Joint hypomobility after immobilization
	ROM limitations
	Excessive swelling
	Inability to bear weight secondary to pain
	Painful "grinding," "catching," or "popping"
	Complex regional pain syndrome
Fascial	Immobilization time frames
	Complex regional pain syndrome
Ligament	Immobilization time frames
	Joint hypomobility after immobilizations
	Active ROM limitations
	Passive ROM limitations
	Muscle flexibility limitations
	Feeling or sensation of "instability"
	Contracture
	Inadequate soft tissue mobility
	Complex regional pain syndrome
Tendon	Immobilization time frames
	Joint hypomobility after immobilizations
	Active ROM limitations
	Passive ROM limitations
	Muscle flexibility limitations
	Inadequate tendon resiliency
	Contractures
	Inadequate soft tissue mobility
	Complex regional pain syndrome

ROM, Range of motion.

The next section includes common surgical procedures performed on soft tissue and unique rehabilitation considerations for each. Table 11-2 provides information about unique signs and symptoms for each surgical procedure.

SOFT TISSUE–SPECIFIC POSTOPERATIVE REHABILITATION

Bursae or Synovium. Surgery to bursae and synovium is generally performed when these structures are pathologically inflamed or hypertrophied. Surgical procedures include incision and drainage of inflamed bursae (also known as *decompression*) and excision of chronically infected and thickened bursae or synovium (also known as *bursectomy* and *synovectomy*, respectively).

Examination. Assessment of joint mobility and strength is limited by symptoms in the surgical region. Bursae are compressed against bone by tendons, so activities that increase pressure of the tendon against the bone, such as MMTs, may still provoke pain after a bursal decompression.

Prognosis. Several studies report that outcomes after bursal decompression or bursectomy are favorable,[58-61] which is probably a result of these procedures directly addressing the symptomatic tissues.

Intervention. Postoperatively, the affected region is generally immobilized with a splint for comfort. Typically, no muscles are cut for bursal procedures so the rehabilitation can progress on a symptom-limited basis.

Cartilage Surgery. Cartilage may be treated surgically to promote repair of damage and to stimulate new cartilage growth. The procedures performed on articular cartilage include lavage (washing out of the joint to remove loose cartilage fragments and degradative enzymes), autologous osteochondral cylinder transplantation, autologous chondrocyte implantation, and various chondro-stimulating techniques.[62] Autologous osteochondral cylinder transplantation involves harvesting one or more osteochondral "plugs" from a healthy donor site and transplanting them into the region of articular cartilage degeneration. Autologous chondrocyte implantation involves obtaining a few healthy chondrocytes from the patient and then growing the cells on a culture medium to increase their number. These cells are then implanted into a region of cartilage damage in the same patient.[63] Chondro-stimulating techniques include drilling, abrasion, and microfracture. All of these are intended to stimulate mesenchymal cells in the subchondral bone to produce new cartilage.[62] Unfortunately, the mesenchymal cells synthesize primarily fibrocartilage rather than hyaline cartilage, and fibrocartilage does not distribute forces as well as the hyaline cartilage it is replacing.[64,65] It is also prone to fibrillation and breakdown over time.[66] Although not yet used clinically, some studies suggest that placing growth factors in an area of cartilage damage may also help promote repair.[67,68]

The procedures performed to repair fibrocartilage damage include debridement (removal of damaged portion of fibrocartilage), removal of the entire fibrocartilage (e.g., knee meniscectomy), repair with sutures or bioabsorbable tacks, and fibrocartilage replacement or transplant (e.g., knee meniscal allograft transplantation).

Examination. After cartilage surgery, weight-bearing restrictions are commonly imposed. The therapist should ensure that the patient adheres to these restrictions. A standard floor scale can be used to determine the amount of weight being borne on the surgical leg.

Prognosis. Favorable long-term outcomes have been reported after autologous osteochondral cylinder transplantation for the treatment of small- and medium-sized focal chondral and osteochondral defects at the knee[69] and talus,[70,71] as well as after osteochondral allograft implantations to repair articular defects in the distal femur.

Outcomes after arthroscopic repair of traumatic triangular fibrocartilage complex injury at the wrist have been reported to be favorable, with good or excellent results in most cases.[72,73] Outcomes after labral injuries at the hip depend on the stage and extent of the labral and chondral lesion[74] but appear to be favorable in many cases.[75] Glenoid labral injuries at the shoulder also appear to respond favorably to surgical fixation[76] or debridement in most cases.[77]

Regarding knee meniscal surgeries, short-term recovery and overall functional outcome are better after a partial meniscectomy than after a total meniscectomy.[78,79] However, long-term outcomes appear to be determined largely by the type of meniscal tear.[80] Outcomes after posterior horn tears appear less favorable than bucket-handle or anterior horn tears[81] (Fig. 11-2). When meniscal

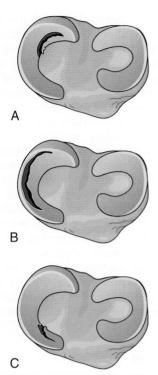

FIG. 11-2 Common meniscal tear patterns. **A,** Posterior horn tear. **B,** Bucket-handle tear. **C,** Anterior horn tear.

allografts are used, patients who receive deep-frozen meniscal transplants have less pain and swelling and can squat and climb stairs more easily than those who receive lyophilized (i.e., freeze-dried) transplants.[82]

Intervention. Aquatic therapy and/or unloading devices may be used to allow walking with reduced weight bearing. The transition from full weight bearing to impact loading should be made gradually. For instance, an elliptical exerciser can be employed for weight-bearing exercise without impact loading before transitioning to treadmill walking or jogging. Deficits in muscle performance should be addressed, but the impact of joint compression or shear must be considered when prescribing specific exercises.

Fascial Surgery. Surgery to fascial tissue is generally performed to relieve tension or pressure, to increase joint movement, or to reduce fascial compartment pressure. Orthopedic surgeries involving fascia consist primarily of fasciotomies, also known as fascial releases. **Retinaculum**—essentially thick fascia—can also be released if necessary (e.g., lateral patellar retinacular release, carpal tunnel retinacular release). After a fascial or retinacular release, new fascia develops in the space formed by the incision, resulting in physiological lengthening of the fascia.[83]

Examination. When a fascial or retinacular release is performed to increase joint ROM, joint mobility must be assessed regularly. Otherwise the examination may proceed as described in the general examination section.

Prognosis. Outcomes after fasciotomies for chronic exertional compartment syndrome of the lower leg(s) appear to be favorable in most cases.

Intervention. When a fascial or retinacular release is performed to increase joint ROM, interventions that preserve or improve mobility, such as joint-specific mobilizations and AAROM or PROM exercises, should be used. When a fascial release is performed to relieve tissue tension or pressure, the therapist should avoid untoward tissue tension or pressure throughout the rehabilitation process.

Ligament and Capsular Surgery. Orthopedic surgeries on ligamentous tissues are generally performed to repair ligament ruptures or partial ruptures and include primary repairs and reconstructions using autogenous (the patient's own) or allogenous (from a donor) tissue. Capsular surgeries are generally performed to repair torn or attenuated capsular restraints and include capsular reconstructions and capsular shortening procedures. Several synonyms have been used to describe capsular shortening procedures, including imbrication,[84] capsulorrhaphy,[85] and reefing.[86]

Intracapsular ligamentous reconstructions (i.e., grafts) undergo a process of remodeling commonly known as **ligamentization.**[87-89] The newly transplanted ligament goes through four distinct phases: (1) avascularity and necrosis, (2) revascularization, (3) cellular repopulation, and (4) structural remodeling.[89] Immediately after transplantation the graft undergoes necrosis because of its loss of blood supply. During this phase the collagen becomes disorganized and ultimately breaks down. The tensile strength of the reconstructed tissue quickly drops well below that of the original graft.[88] Extraarticular ligaments and capsular tissue heal more readily than intraarticular structures and typically do not lose much strength initially because they have more vascular perfusion. Thus the extraarticular medial collateral ligament (MCL) heals more quickly and readily than the intraarticular anterior cruciate ligament (ACL), but in both cases, the stresses applied during rehabilitation must be systematically controlled to avoid damaging the repair.

Examination. Because surgically repaired ligament and capsule can be easily overstressed early in the postoperative period, forceful testing of ROM should be avoided during this period, particularly in the direction that would stretch the repaired tissue.

After intraarticular ACL reconstruction, a ligament arthrometer can be used to assess the integrity of the repair. The KT-1000 (MEDmetric Corporation, San Diego, CA), a ligament arthrometer (Fig. 11-3), has been shown to objectively and quantitatively measure the amount of anterior translation of the tibia on the femur.[90-92]

Prognosis. Outcomes after capsular and ligamentous repairs are usually good. Because of the extensive use of ligament repairs and reconstructions throughout the body, the number of studies describing outcomes is extensive. Furthermore, many different procedures are used at each of the various locations of ligament repair. For example, numerous studies have found that patients have good functional outcomes when measured shortly after or even up to 10 years after ACL repair or reconstruction.[93-99] In general, with modern surgical and rehabilitation techniques, most patients can return to full participation in sports or other strenuous activities after ligament reconstruction.[100]

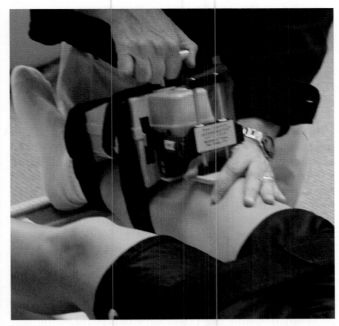

FIG. 11-3 KT-1000 used to measure anterior cruciate ligament tightness/laxity.

Intervention. During the immediate postoperative period, soft tissue healing restrictions also limit interventions. In most cases, protected ROM rather than complete immobilization is recommended to minimize capsular or ligamentous tissue stress. The exact restrictions vary, depending on the specific requirements of the repair, the stresses expected on full return to activity, the tissue quality, the type of tissue used for the repair (autograft, allograft, or synthetic), and the referring physician's beliefs regarding soft tissue healing time frames. For example, immediately after thermal capsulorrhaphy of the shoulder performed to treat shoulder instability, patients should not fully abduct or externally rotate their arm to avoid overstretching the healing tissue and making the shoulder unstable again. Similarly, after the classic Bankart repair of the anterior glenoid labrum and capsule of the shoulder, forceful full ROM should be avoided as this would jeopardize the surgical repair and fixation. In some instances, however, obtaining full ROM is an early goal, most notably for knee extension after ACL reconstruction or repair.

Because ligaments and joint capsules not only constrain and guide joint movement but also provide proprioceptive or joint position sense via mechanoreceptors embedded within the ligament or capsule,[101] surgical repair or reconstruction may quickly restore joint integrity, but joint proprioception may remain impaired unless specifically addressed in the rehabilitation program.[102,103]

Tendon Surgery. Tendon surgeries are generally performed when there are partial tears or ruptures of tendons. Tendon surgeries include tenodesis, tendon transplants, tendon primary repair, tenotomy, and tendon debridement. Although the terms *tendon transplant, primary repair,* and *debridement* are self-explanatory, the terms *tenodesis* and *tenotomy* are less clear. Tenodesis is any surgical fixation of a tendon. Tenodesis is commonly performed with the tendon of the long head of the biceps, and during this procedure the long head may be moved to a new location to help restore its functional use. Tenotomy means surgical removal of a portion of a tendon.

Examination. After surgery to a tendon, stress on the tissue should be limited during both the examination and interventions. As with ligaments and capsules, forceful examination of PROM should be avoided. In addition, strength testing of the muscle(s) attached to the involved tendon should not be performed initially as contraction of the muscle will stress the tendon and may cause it to rupture. For example, performing full active finger flexion immediately after repair of the flexor tendons may cause the tendon to rupture.

The duration and degree of force restriction depends on the specific requirements of the repaired tendon, the stresses it is expected to tolerate for full return to activity, the tissue quality, the repair tissue type (autograft, allograft, or synthetic), and the physician's beliefs regarding soft tissue healing time frames. During the immediate postoperative period, the patient should strictly adhere to soft tissue healing restrictions to optimize soft tissue healing and functional outcomes.

Prognosis. There is extensive literature concerning patient outcomes after tendon repair. A thorough review of this literature is beyond the scope of this chapter; however, a few examples follow. Many authors report that surgical reconstruction of tendons, such as the Achilles tendon, have favorable outcomes, including increased strength and function and decreased risk of rerupture.[53,55,56,104] The flexor tendons of the hands are also frequently surgically repaired or reconstructed and the outcome of these procedures varies, depending on numerous factors, including the patient's age, health, lifestyle, as well as associated damage to skin, vascular system, nerves, and skeletal structures.[105-108]

Intervention. As with the other soft tissue injuries previously described, surgical procedures to tendons generally require a brief period of immobilization to allow for tissue to form in and around the area of the repair. The duration of immobilization depends on a range of factors, including the health and age of the patient, the type of repair, which tendon was repaired, the quality of repaired tissue, and the surgeon's beliefs regarding healing times for the various tissues. For example, after flexor tendon repairs, recommendations regarding early activity vary. Some favor immobilization,[109] others favor early passive mobilization,[110,111] and yet others favor early active mobilization.[112-115]

After a lower extremity tendon rupture and repair, a brace or immobilizer is generally recommended to limit forces from weight bearing and to limit ROM during ambulation. After an upper extremity tendon rupture and repair, a splint or sling may also be needed to limit or prevent active contraction of the ruptured tendon. The duration of immobilization a surgeon recommends is likely to vary among patients and is generally influenced

not only by which tendon is repaired but also by the size of repair, the quality of the tendon, the location of the tear (muscle, tendon, or muscle-tendon junction), the type of fixation (suture, staple, or anchor), the presence of other concomitant injuries, and the age and general health of the patient.

A wide variety of immobilization protocols after Achilles tendon repair are described in the literature.[116-121] These include casting for 4 to 9 weeks, possibly using a heel lift after the cast is removed and restricting weight bearing from weight bearing as tolerated to no weight bearing during the period of cast immobilization. Since there is a risk of poor outcome when restrictions are not followed, the clinician involved in patient rehabilitation should obtain patient-specific guidelines from the referring physician regarding the nature and duration of restrictions after any tendon repair.

CASE STUDY 11-1

REHABILITATION AFTER ANTERIOR CRUCIATE LIGAMENT REPAIR (SEMITENDINOSUS-GRACILIS)

Patient History

CM is a 28-year-old man working full time in the United States Armed Forces. He ruptured the ACL of his right knee while playing football 4 months before surgery. CM underwent an arthroscopically assisted semitendinosus-gracilis hamstring ACL reconstruction (ACLR) and a partial medial meniscectomy and was seen by the physical therapist 3 days after this surgery. He was then placed in a motion-controlled, double-hinged knee brace locked in full extension for ambulation. He was ambulating weight bearing as tolerated, per the physician's orders.

Tests and Measures—Significant Findings

Musculoskeletal

- PROM: Right knee: 3-50 degrees of knee flexion. Left knee: 0-135 degrees.
- Girth measurements were as follows:

Knee	Right	Left
20 cm proximal to the knee joint line	56 cm	54 cm
10 cm proximal to the knee joint line	45 cm	43 cm
Knee joint line	39 cm	37 cm
15 cm distal to the knee joint line	41 cm	40 cm

- CM was noted to have an extensor lag during active straight leg raising.

Function

- Able to ambulate with bilateral axillary crutches on a level surface with a step-to gait.
- After instructions to weight bear as tolerated, he was measured to place approximately 50% of his body weight on his RLE without increasing his symptoms.

Diagnosis

Preferred practice pattern 4I: Impaired joint mobility, motor function, muscle performance, and range of motion associated with bony or soft tissue surgery.

Interventions

- Immediate therapy consisted of modalities for pain relief and edema control. Electrical stimulation with elevation and cold therapy were used.
- CM was instructed to use compressive hose or a compressive wrap at all times when not in therapy.
- Quadriceps strengthening and knee ROM exercises in supine.
- Begin a home exercise program that includes prone hangs and sitting with foot and ankle over a bolster.
- The hamstrings were used as an autograft reconstruction source, thus hamstring stretching was delayed for 4 weeks and hamstring resistance exercises were delayed for 6 weeks.

Role of the Physical Therapist Assistant

- What do the girth measurements indicate?
- Why was cold therapy used instead of heat therapy? What were the goals for this intervention?
- What does the extensor lag indicate?
- Write a description for the patient of the proper way to use compressive hose or a compressive wrap. What are the goals of this intervention?
- Write instructions for three exercises for quadriceps strengthening and to increase knee ROM with the patient supine.

Additional Information

Box 11-2 is an example of an ACL repair rehabilitation protocol. For the full version of this case study, including detailed examination results, interventions, and outcomes, see the Evolve site that accompanies this book. A full case study for a patient undergoing rehabilitation after knee meniscal repair and a patient undergoing rehabilitation after Achilles tendon repair also appears on the Evolve site.

CHAPTER SUMMARY

This chapter provides a framework for rehabilitation after soft tissue surgery based on available scientific evidence and clinical empiricism. Several factors are considered when designing postoperative rehabilitation programs, including the biomechanics of healing and mature connective tissue, the effects of immobilization and

---

| **BOX 11-2** | **Anterior Cruciate Ligament Repair Rehabilitation Protocol** |

General Guidelines
- Assume 8 weeks for complete graft revascularization
- Rarely use CPM
- Isolated hamstring strengthening began 6 weeks postoperatively
- Supervised physical therapy takes 3-9 months

Activities of Daily Living Progression
- Bathing/showering without brace after suture removal
- Sleep with brace locked in extension for 1 week
- Driving: Wait 1 week for automatic vehicles with left leg repair
- Wait 4-6 weeks for standard vehicles or right leg repair
- Brace locked in extension for 1 week for ambulation
- Crutches and brace for ambulation as needed for 6 weeks
- Weight bearing as tolerated immediately postoperative

Phase I: Immediate Postoperative Phase (Postoperative through 6 Weeks)
Goals
- Protect graft fixation (8 weeks)
- Minimize the effects of immobilization
- Control inflammation and swelling
- Immediate full knee passive extension
- Quadriceps activation
- Patient education

Restrictions
- Weight bearing as tolerated with axillary crutches as needed for 6 weeks
- Hamstring mobilization and stretching in 4 weeks

Brace
0-1 week: Locked in full extension for weight bearing and sleeping
1-6 weeks: Unlocked for ambulation, remove for sleeping

Therapeutic Exercises
- Gentle heel slides
- Quadriceps setting
- Patellar mobilization
- Non–weight-bearing gastrocnemius and soleus stretching
- SLR in all planes (SLR times 4) with brace locked in full extension until quadriceps prevent extensor lag
- Quadriceps isometrics at 60 and 90 degrees
- Gluteal setting
- Weight shifting
- Static balance exercises
- Heel raises—bilateral progressing to unilateral

Clinical Milestones
- Full knee extension
- SLR without extensor lag
- No limp or pain during gait
- 90 degrees of knee flexion

Continued

BOX 11-2   Anterior Cruciate Ligament Repair Rehabilitation Protocol—cont'd

- No signs of active inflammation
- No increased effusion or edema
- No increased pain

Phase II: Intermediate Phase (6-8 Weeks)
Goals
- Restore normal gait
- Maintain full knee extension
- Progress flexion ROM
- Protect graft
- Initiate **open kinetic-chain exercises** for hamstrings

Comments
Discontinue use of the brace and crutches, as allowed by the physician, when the patient has full extension and can perform SLR without extensor lag.

Therapeutic Exercise
- Wall slides 0-45 degrees, progressing to mini-squat
- Multi-Hip (4-way) machine)
- Stationary bicycling (high seat, low tension promoting ROM)
- Closed-chain terminal extension with resistive tubing or weight machine
- Heel raises
- Balance exercises (e.g., single leg balance)
- Hamstring curls
- Aquatic therapy with emphasis on normalization of gait
- Continue hamstring stretches, progress to weight-bearing gastrocnemius and soleus stretches

Clinical Milestones
- Maximize ROM
- Good quadriceps recruitment
- Maintenance of full passive knee extension

Advanced Strengthening Phase III (8 Weeks-6 Months)
Goals
- Full ROM
- Improve strength, endurance, and proprioception of lower extremity to prepare for full functional activities
- Avoid overstressing graft or graft fixation
- Protect patellofemoral joint

Therapeutic Exercise
- Continue flexibility exercises as appropriate
- StairMaster: Begin short steps, avoid knee hyperextension
- NordicTrack knee extension: 90-45 degrees of knee flexion
- Advanced closed kinetic-chain strengthening (single leg squats, leg press 0-45 degrees, step-ups begin at 2 inches progressing to 8 inches)
- Progress proprioceptive activities (slide board, use of ball, racquet with balance activities, and so on)
- Progress aquatic program to include pool running, swimming (no breast stroke)

Criteria for Advancement
- Full pain-free ROM
- No evidence of patellofemoral joint irritation
- Strength and proprioception approximately 70% of uninvolved leg
- Physician clearance to initiate advanced **closed kinetic-chain exercises** and functional progression

Return to Activity: Phase IV (9 Months?)
Goals
- Safe return to athletics
- Maintenance program for strength and endurance

Comments
Physician may recommend a functional brace for use during sports for the first 1-2 years after surgery.

Modified from Manske RC, Prohaska D, Livermore R: Anterior cruciate ligament reconstruction using the hamstring/gracilis tendon autograft. In Manske RC (ed): *Postsurgical orthopedic sports medicine: Knee and shoulder,* Philadelphia, 2005, Elsevier.
CPM, Continuous passive motion; *SLR,* straight leg raises; *ROM,* range of motion.

---

remobilization on connective tissue, and the prognosis for a successful outcome after different orthopedic procedures. The case studies provide examples of how the concepts and evidence presented may be applied to specific patients.

ADDITIONAL RESOURCES

For links to these and additional web-based resources, see the Evolve site.
Brotzman SB, Wilk K: *Clinical orthopaedic rehabilitation,* ed 2, Philadelphia, 2003, Mosby.
Lundon K: *Orthopedic rehabilitation science: Principles for clinical management of nonmineralized connective tissue,* St. Louis, 2003, Butterworth-Heinemann.
Manske RC: *Postsurgical orthopedic sports rehabilitation: Knee and shoulder,* St. Louis, 2006, Mosby.
Maxey L, Magnusson J: *Rehabilitation for the postsurgical orthopedic patient,* St. Louis, 2001, Mosby.
American Orthopaedic Society for Sports Medicine
The Physician and Sportsmedicine online (registration/charge required for access)

GLOSSARY

Bursae: Type of nonmineralized connective tissues consisting of small pouches of synovial fluid; usually located at areas of high friction in the musculoskeletal system.
Capsules: Type of dense, irregular nonmineralized connective tissue that surrounds and supports joints.
Cartilage: Type of specialized nonmineralized connective tissue that supports and cushions the skeleton (e.g., articular cartilage and fibrocartilage).
Closed kinetic-chain exercises: Exercises in which the distal limb or body part is fixed. During this form of exercise,

muscles and joints act in a predictable pattern or sequential order.

Collagen: The most abundant structural protein in the body and an integral component of connective tissue.

Connective tissue: One of the four types of tissue in the body from which all structures are derived; connective tissue supports, binds, or separates more specialized tissues and organs of the body.

Extracellular matrix: A component of connective tissue, consisting of ground substance and fibers produced by the connective tissue cells.

Fascia: Type of loose nonmineralized connective tissue that divides and binds muscles and organs in the body.

Ligaments: Type of dense, regular nonmineralized connective tissue that connects bone to bone or bone to cartilage and helps stabilize joints.

Ligamentization: The process of remodeling that an intraarticular graft undergoes. This process is broken into four distinct phases: (1) avascularity and necrosis, (2) revascularization, (3) cellular repopulation, and (4) structural remodeling.

Open kinetic-chain exercises: Exercises in which the distal limb or body part is free to move without causing any appreciable motion at another joint. During this form of exercise, muscles and joints do not act in a predictable pattern or sequential order because the distal end is free to move on its own.

Proprioception: Position sense coming from skin, ligaments, tendons, muscles, and joint capsule, integrated to maintain joint stability.

Proteoglycan molecules: Biological molecules that consist of a protein core with glycosaminoglycan side chains; a major component of cartilage.

Retinaculum: Thickened fascia (see Fascia).

Synovium: Type of specialized nonmineralized connective tissue on the innermost portion of the capsule of synovial joints. Synovial cells secrete fluid that lubricates joint surfaces and nourishes articular cartilage.

Tendons: Type of dense, regular nonmineralized connective tissue that connects muscle to bone or other tissue.

Chapter 12

Amputations and Prostheses

Joan E. Edelstein

OBJECTIVES

After reading this chapter, the reader will be able to:
1. Identify the incidence, etiologies, and levels of upper and lower extremity amputation.
2. Perform a rehabilitation examination and evaluation of patients with amputation.
3. Develop preoperative and postoperative interventions for the residual limb and the entire patient with an amputation.
4. Describe prosthetic options for patients with all levels of upper and lower extremity amputations.
5. Design a basic prosthetic training program for patients fitted with upper and lower extremity prostheses.
6. Compare the functional outcomes of patients according to etiology, amputation level, and prosthetic components.

Amputation is a specialty area in rehabilitation. In 1996, the rate of amputation in the United States was 52.4 per 100,000, with most being lower extremity amputations.[1] Most lower extremity amputations become necessary because of underlying vascular disease or diabetes, whereas most upper extremity amputations are needed because of trauma. A minority of amputations are needed because of malignancy or congenital limb anomalies. Many people with amputation are fitted with a prosthesis

(a replacement for a body part). Regardless of site or design, a prosthesis does not substitute fully for the appearance or function of the anatomical extremity.

PATHOLOGY

Acquired amputation results from peripheral vascular disease, trauma, and more rarely, diseases such as osteogenic sarcoma, meningitis, and **Hansen's disease** (leprosy). Occasionally, a patient may elect amputation to eliminate a nonfunctional extremity. Another etiology is congenital extremity absence or malformation evident at birth; sometimes the malformed extremity is revised surgically to facilitate prosthetic fitting and improve function.

The most common etiology of amputation in the United States is peripheral vascular disease (PVD), particularly arteriosclerosis.[2] The typical patient with PVD is a man in his mid-sixties with a history of diabetes, coronary artery disease, hypertension, and smoking.[3,4] Diabetes increases the risk for amputation by causing both PVD and neuropathy. Thromboangiitis obliterans, a disease characterized by inflammation and occlusion of the small- and medium-sized arteries, and thrombophlebitis, inflammation of veins, often with clotting, are primary PVDs that increase the risk of amputation. In patients with PVD, amputation is generally the last resort, after the patient has endured years of treatment for intermittent claudication (cramping in the calf after a brief period of walking), recurrent skin ulcers, and edema. The precipitating event for amputation in patients with PVD is usually skin ulceration that fails to heal followed by osteomyelitis (infection of bone) and/or gangrene (see Chapter 29).

Trauma is also a common cause of amputation, particularly upper extremity amputation. Patients who sustain trauma requiring amputation usually also sustain injury to many other systems and areas, complicating their recovery, but are generally younger than other patients who undergo amputation.[5]

In less than 1/1,000 live births the infant is born with one or more absent or abnormal extremities. This may be the result of intrauterine exposure to teratogens, such as thalidomide and x-rays, or constriction of the distal portion of the developing extremity by amniotic bands.

Congenital limb anomalies are more common in the lower than the upper extremity.[6] Limb anomalies are classified as transverse—where the distal portion is absent—or longitudinal—where the proximal portion is absent, but the distal portion is present.[7] A transverse anomaly may be further subcategorized as partial or complete, with termination through the diaphysis or through the joint (resembling a disarticulation), respectively. Since congenital anomalies occur in children, the family should be involved in all stages of habilitation, and habilitation should be structured to help the child reach developmental milestones.

Some malignancies that affect bone, such as Ewing's osteogenic sarcoma, are treated with amputation. Osteogenic sarcoma most commonly occurs at the distal end of the humerus or femur in adolescence or young adulthood. The patient may undergo shoulder or hip disarticulation, or transpelvic (hemipelvectomy), transhumeral, or **transfemoral amputation** as part of the treatment of this disease. These patients may also receive radiation or chemotherapy, or both. Radiation can affect rehabilitation because radiation can make the skin more fragile, whereas chemotherapy can reduce the patient's energy level. Radiation and chemotherapy may also reduce the patient's appetite, resulting in weight loss that can disturb socket fit.

Hansen's disease (leprosy) is caused by infection with *Mycobacterium leprae*. *M. leprae* infects sensory nerves, causing sensory loss. Sensory loss leads to ulceration from repeated trauma that is complicated by bony and soft tissue resorption. This resorption, known as *autoamputation,* may cause loss of the ends of the digits, portions of the nose, and other body parts.

Rarely, a viable body part is amputated when patients decide that their overall function would be better without it than with it. For example, a patient contracted poliomyelitis in infancy, which markedly interfered with the growth of his left leg. In adolescence, he chose to have the leg amputated above the knee and wear a prosthesis rather than wearing a shoe with an 8- to 12-inch lift for the rest of his life. Similarly, there is a published report of several men with spinal cord injury who underwent bilateral hip disarticulation, after developing deep pressure ulcers, to allow them to transfer much more easily from bed to wheelchair.[8]

Clinical Pearl

The most common reasons for amputations are peripheral vascular disease (PVD) and trauma, followed by malignancies of the bone and congenital limb anomalies.

TYPES OF AMPUTATION

Amputation surgery is classified as closed when the skin is sutured, or open when the skin is not sutured. **Open amputation** is much less common in civilian practice and is indicated when the operative site is contaminated. This procedure usually involves severing the muscle

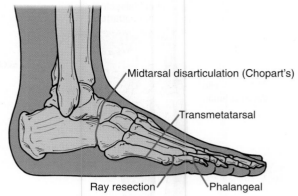

FIG. 12-1 Minor lower extremity amputations.

without suturing **(guillotine amputation).** Traction is then applied to the open edges of the skin to retain its length so that, on secondary closure, there will be enough skin for coverage. With a **closed amputation,** the skin edges are stapled or sutured together and the underlying muscles may be sutured to one another **(myoplasty)** or sutured through holes drilled in the bone **(myodesis).** The cut ends of bones are beveled to reduce the likelihood of sharp osteophytes, which can be painful. Nerves are severed under tension so that they retract within muscle bellies rather than terminating near the skin. This reduces the risk of local pain.[9]

Amputations can also be classified as minor, referring to amputations distal to the wrist or ankle, or major, referring to more proximal amputations.

Lower Extremity Amputations

Minor Lower Extremity Amputations. Partial foot amputation is removal of any portion of the foot. The most common levels for this type of amputation are phalangeal, transmetatarsal, and midtarsal disarticulation (also known as *Chopart's disarticulation*) (Fig. 12-1). Ray resection refers to removal of a metatarsal and its phalanges.

The main concern with phalangeal amputation in patients with PVD is the possibility of further amputation. **Transmetatarsal amputation** shortens the foot considerably and with the loss of the metatarsal heads, compels the patient to bear substantial weight on the calcaneus. During gait, late stance is altered by the loss of metatarsophalangeal hyperextension, and during swing phase, the shortened foot can slip from the shoe.

Ray resection creates a foot that is abnormally narrow. This reduces the base of support in standing, and the absence of one or more metatarsal heads and their muscular attachments reduces the strength of plantarflexion during terminal stance. Loss of the first ray is particularly disabling because this part of the foot usually takes much of the load when walking on level and irregular surfaces.

The Chopart's disarticulation involves amputation between the talus and navicular on the medial side of the foot and between the calcaneus and the cuboid on the lateral side of the foot. With this procedure, the triceps surae are kept intact and the dorsiflexors are transected, causing the foot to assume a plantarflexed position, unless

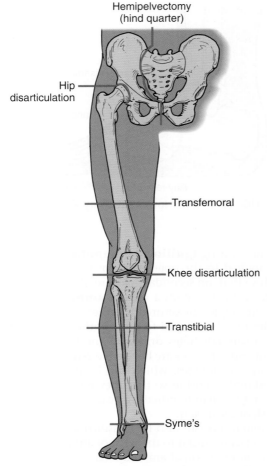

FIG. 12-2 Major lower extremity amputations.

the Achilles tendon is sectioned or otherwise attenuated. Standing on a plantarflexed foot places stress on the amputation scar, produces a very small weight-bearing area, and severely compromises terminal stance.

> ### Clinical Pearl
>
> Phalangeal amputation alters weight distribution in the foot increasing the risk for areas of high pressure and subsequent tissue breakdown and the need for further amputation.

Major Lower Extremity Amputations. A **Syme's amputation** involves transection of the distal tibia and fibula through broad cancellous bone with preservation of the calcaneal fat pad (Fig. 12-2). All the foot bones are removed, and the skin overlying the calcaneal fat pad is sutured to the anterior portion of the distal shank. The residual limb tends to be bulbous distally. Although the amputated leg is slightly shorter than the sound extremity, the patient can move short distances without a prosthesis. Walking long distances requires a prosthesis to equalize leg length and provide foot function, thereby lessening the risk of back pain.

Other major lower extremity amputations are as follows:

- Ankle disarticulation (separation of the foot at the ankle).
- Transtibial (amputation through the tibia and fibula), also known as *below-knee amputation* (any of a group of amputations and separations in the vicinity of the anatomical knee joint).
- Transfemoral (amputation through the femur), also known as *above-knee amputation.*
- Hip disarticulation (separation of the femur from the acetabulum).
- **Transpelvic amputation** (removal of any portion of the pelvis and all distal parts), also known as hemipelvectomy.
- **Translumbar amputation** (removal of the entire pelvis and all distal components), previously known as *hemicorporectomy,* requires creation of a urinary diversion, as well as a colostomy.

Unlike distal amputations, which are usually necessary because of PVD, hip disarticulation and transpelvic amputation are most often required because of a malignancy in the bone or less commonly because of trauma or soft-tissue infection.[10]

> ### Clinical Pearl
>
> Syme's amputation involves transection of the distal tibia and fibula and removal of the ankle and all the foot bones but with preservation of the calcaneal fat pad for weight bearing.

Upper Extremity Amputations

Minor Upper Extremity Amputations. Partial hand amputation or removal of any portion of the hand is a minor upper extremity amputation.

Major Upper Extremity Amputations. Major upper extremity amputations are classified as follows (Fig. 12-3):

- Wrist disarticulation (separation of the radius from the proximal carpals or separation between the proximal and distal row of carpals).
- **Transradial amputation** (through the radius and ulna), previously known as *below-elbow.*
- Elbow disarticulation (separation of the humerus from the ulna or amputation through the most distal portion of the humerus).
- **Transhumeral amputation** (through the humerus), previously known as *above-elbow.*
- Shoulder disarticulation (separation of the humerus from the scapula).
- Forequarter (removal of any portion of the thorax, together with any portion of the shoulder girdle and all distal parts).

TYPICAL EXAMINATION FINDINGS

PATIENT HISTORY

A thorough patient history is the first component of the examination. The therapist will generally obtain information regarding the patient's age, sex, race, employment, arm and leg dominance, general health status, past medical history and surgeries, and present functional status.

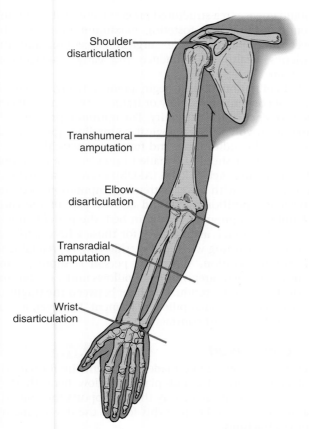

FIG. 12-3 Major upper extremity amputations.

Shoulder disarticulation

Transhumeral amputation

Elbow disarticulation

Transradial amputation

Wrist disarticulation

Psychosocial issues related to educational level, cultural beliefs, caregiver resources, and living environment, as well as information regarding medications, laboratory or diagnostic tests, or other clinical findings, are also noted. The patient's expectations of therapy will likely be discussed because these can affect compliance with recommendations and satisfaction with treatment outcomes.

SYSTEMS REVIEW

The systems review is used to target areas requiring further examination and to define areas that may cause complications or indicate a need for precautions during the examination and intervention processes. Chapter 1 includes details of the systems review.

TESTS AND MEASURES

Musculoskeletal

Posture. A patient's postural assessment focuses on pelvic alignment, scoliosis, and kyphosis (see Chapter 4). Severe postural abnormality compromises prosthetic fitting and the patient's function.

Anthropometric Characteristics. The length and the girth of the residual limb are measured because these affect the type of prosthesis and the snugness or looseness of the socket. Length and girth are measured at defined distances from stable bony landmarks. Common landmarks are the acromion and medial humeral epicondyle for transhumeral and transradial residual limbs, respectively, and the greater trochanter and medial tibial plateau

for transfemoral and transtibial residual limbs. Girth is measured over time, and final prosthetic fitting is generally delayed until girth remains stable, when edema has resolved and atrophy has peaked, so that limb volume is stable and fit will remain good.

Range of Motion. Range of motion (ROM) of all joints on the amputated and contralateral extremity will be measured. Joint ROM restrictions should be addressed early to avoid contractures from inactivity, faulty positioning, and muscle imbalance.

Muscle Performance. Strength of the entire affected extremity will be tested to determine if muscle strengthening interventions are needed to optimize function and prosthetic use.

Neuromuscular

Arousal, Attention, and Cognition. Depression is common among people with amputations. Phantom limb pain, residual limb pain, and back pain are major contributors to depression in this group.

Pain and Sensory Integrity. **Phantom sensation** and pain are among the most vexing symptoms after amputation.[8] Most patients remain aware of the missing part (phantom sensation) for the rest of their lives. The patient should be reassured that phantom sensation is a normal concomitant of amputation. There may also be pain in a portion of the residual limb (local pain) or pain may be felt in the missing body part **(phantom pain).** Because the hand has a relatively large cerebral representation, phantom sensations or phantom pains are often quite prominent after amputation of the hand. The phantom limb may feel foreshortened or otherwise distorted, and pain sensations may vary and include burning, electric shocks, or other abnormal unpleasant feelings. For most patients, phantom pain subsides within a year after amputation.

> ### ◎ Clinical Pearl
>
> Phantom pain in which pain is felt in the missing body part, generally subsides within a year after amputation.

Cardiovascular/Pulmonary. Regardless of the etiology of amputation, the remaining extremity and the residual limb must have an adequate blood supply to maintain viability. Poor circulation increases the risk of ulceration and gangrene. Routine examination for circulatory status will include visual inspection looking for color changes, palpation of all portions of the residual limb, and after a lower extremity amputation, palpation of the contralateral foot and assessment of peripheral pulses throughout the legs. Assessment of skin temperature is important because abnormal warmth suggests infection, whereas cold skin indicates circulatory insufficiency. Circulation may be further examined with Doppler ultrasound and transcutaneous oxygen assessments (see Chapter 30).

Integumentary. The skin will be examined initially and should be rechecked during subsequent treatments to assess healing and for signs of excessive or persistent pressure. Soap, lotion, or other topical preparations, as well as the sock or liner used with the prosthesis or the material of the prosthesis itself, can cause skin irritation. Redness that does not quickly resolve with removal of pressure is the first stage of a pressure ulcer (see Chapter 28).

For the person with lower extremity amputation, the skin should be inspected on the sound leg, as well as on the residual limb. After an amputation, the sound foot is vulnerable to breakdown because it has to support more weight.

EVALUATION, DIAGNOSIS, AND PROGNOSIS

According to the *Guide to Physical Therapist Practice*,[11] rehabilitation for patients with amputation is in the preferred practice pattern 4J: Impaired motor function, muscle performance, range of motion, gait, locomotion, and balance associated with amputation.

Patients with an amputation caused by PVD, particularly those with concurrent diabetes, are at high risk for another amputation. On average, for patients with diabetes, the interval between amputations is less than 20 years.[12] Future amputation surgeries may include surgical revision of the initial amputation because of poor wound healing and/or amputation of the contralateral extremity because of systemic disease effects and increased use. Using an appropriate well-fitting prosthetic may delay further amputation by distributing body weight and reducing the load on the sound side.

Walking with a lower extremity amputation and a prosthesis also increases energy consumption and reduces walking speed when compared with walking with intact extremities. This tends to result in lower activity levels. It should also be kept in mind that, given the high energy cost of ambulating with bilateral lower extremity prostheses, it is more energy efficient for people with bilateral transtibial[13] or bilateral transfemoral amputations[14] to use a wheelchair than to ambulate with protheses.

Reintegration into the work force is often delayed by problems with the residual limb, particularly wound healing. In addition, because most upper extremity amputations involve only one hand and one can do most daily and vocational activities without a prosthesis, many individuals eventually opt to discard their prosthesis.[15] Factors contributing to ongoing prosthetic use among adults include graduation from high school, employment, emotional acceptance of the amputation, and the perception that the prosthesis is expensive. Those with transradial amputation are more likely to persist with prosthetic use compared with those having other levels of amputation. Early fitting for people with traumatic amputation, as well as posttraumatic counseling, contributes to continued prosthetic usage.[16]

INTERVENTION

PREOPERATIVE AND POSTOPERATIVE MANAGEMENT

The goal of preoperative care is to prepare the patient for life after amputation surgery and to begin rehabilitation. Postoperatively, regardless of whether the patient is or is not eventually fitted with a prosthesis, the individual should engage in a structured program aimed at hastening wound healing and fostering maximum function. The level of amputation, the surgical procedure, and the patient's health all influence the early management program.

Rehabilitation should begin preoperatively, except in cases of congenital anomaly or trauma involving immediate severance of the extremity. The optimum preoperative program involves psychological counseling, joint mobility, general conditioning, and functional activities.

Every effort should be made to prevent the formation of contractures. Active ROM (AROM) exercises are helpful, and for those with lower extremity amputation, bed and wheelchair positioning should also be part of the early rehabilitation program. While in bed, the patient should lie prone as much as tolerated; for those who experience difficulty breathing when prone, sidelying is preferable to the supine position. When the person is supine, some well-intentioned caregivers place pillows under the lumbar spine, beneath the residual limb, or between the thighs to increase comfort; such pillow placement, however, fosters the development of contractures.

> ### ◎ *Clinical Pearl*
> Every effort should be made to prevent the formation of contractures. Do not place a pillow beneath the residual limb in such a way that it supports the limb in a flexed position because this fosters the development of contractures.

General conditioning exercises aimed at improving strength and endurance can help reverse deconditioning, which is common among older adults with PVD.[17] Gentle strengthening exercises for the trunk and all extremities are recommended. Functional activities provide constructive activity and foster self-care. Candidates for lower extremity amputation should be taught bed-to-wheelchair and chair-to-chair transfers before their surgery, and those who are candidates for immediate postoperative ambulation should learn three-point transfers with the aid of a walker or a pair of crutches.

The individual who is scheduled for upper extremity amputation should be encouraged to gain proficiency in one-handed activities. Most patients, while initially clumsy, achieve reasonable proficiency in one-handed dressing, grooming, and dining. Even if a prosthesis is to be prescribed, the patient will rely more on the remaining hand because it is sensate and more agile than any mechanical device. If the amputation will occur on the dominant side, early care should also address change of dominance. The patient may eventually write with the prosthesis on the preamputation dominant side; however, other activities, such as managing buttons, using a knife when cutting meat, and tying shoelaces, are generally easier with the dexterous, sensate sound hand whether it is dominant or not.

EARLY POSTOPERATIVE MANAGEMENT

The goals of early postoperative management are to foster wound healing and promote maximum function. Early rehabilitation begins as soon as the patient is medically stable after surgery and ends when a prosthesis is fitted. For the person who is not a candidate for a prosthesis, early rehabilitation ends when the residual limb is no longer painful and maximum function is achieved. In either instance, care focuses on the residual limb, as well as the patient as a whole. Residual limb care should focus on wound healing, pain reduction, edema control, joint mobility, and strengthening. Holistic care at this time includes psychosocial counseling, general conditioning, care of the remaining foot (in the case of lower extremity amputation), and functional activities.

Wound Healing. Wound healing is fundamental to recovery from amputation surgery. An open wound is vulnerable to infection, which may have serious consequences, including gangrene with subsequent reamputation, and sepsis, which can be fatal. Interventions aim to create a clean, stable wound environment to facilitate healing. Modalities that may hasten healing include electrical stimulation, ultraviolet, US, intermittent pneumatic compression, hydrotherapy, and negative pressure,[18] although not all modalities are appropriate for those with PVD. Chapters 28 through 31 provide additional information about wound care and healing.

Edema Control. Edema control promotes wound healing, reduces pain, and facilitates prosthetic fitting. The larger the extremity circumference, the more postoperative edema is likely to be present. Thus there will be more edema, followed by more volume loss, after a transfemoral amputation than after a transtibial, transradial, or transhumeral amputation. Ideally, edema control measures are introduced at the time of surgery; however, if the patient is medically unstable, edema control is sometimes delayed. Edema control measures should be used until the patient is wearing a prosthesis for most of the day, or until the wound has healed and the residual limb is no longer painful. Limb volume changes continue to occur for an average of 120 days after surgery.[19] Interventions intended to stabilize limb volume after amputation of the upper or lower extremity include soft dressings (elastic bandage and elastic shrinker socks), semirigid dressings (Unna bandage and air splints), and rigid (plaster or plastic) dressings. A thin dressing should be placed directly on the amputation wound, particularly if sutures or staples are in place.

Soft dressings are used most commonly,[20] possibly because the materials are relatively inexpensive and dressing application and removal are simple. Elastic bandages should be applied in a figure-of-eight pattern, avoiding circular turns.[21] Elastic bandages have several disadvantages. They must be reapplied several times a day because they tend to loosen as the patient moves about. Although individuals with transtibial amputation generally can bandage themselves, it is very difficult for those with transfemoral amputation to wrap the residual limb and torso effectively. If the transfemoral bandage rolls distally, the patient is apt to develop an adductor roll, a mass of tissue in the medial thigh; the roll is subject to chafing and subsequent breakdown. Furthermore, pressure beneath the dressing varies with each application, making volume stabilization relatively ineffective.[22-25]

Shrinker socks are closed-ended tubes made of fabric knitted with elastic threads. They are relatively easy to roll onto the amputation limb, and when properly applied, compress the limb uniformly.[24] The transtibial sock usually remains snugly on the distal thigh; however, the transfemoral sock requires a belt with garters for suspension. Newer versions of shrinker socks include elasticized shorts[26] and gel socks.[27]

Semirigid dressings, especially the **Unna dressing,** overcome most of the problems with soft dressing.[28-30] The Unna dressing is made of gauze permeated with zinc oxide and calamine, with glycerin and gelatin added as moisture-retention agents. The bandage is applied over a thin sterile wound dressing and is placed obliquely on the residual limb, with turns requiring cutting the bandage, rather than twisting it. This nonextensible bandage adheres to the skin, assuring suspension and constant compression, and is relatively thin, making it especially suitable for transfemoral amputations. It can be placed high in the groin to prevent an adductor roll. Rehabilitation, especially for those with transfemoral amputation, is significantly accelerated by the Unna dressing.

Usually the Unna bandage is left in place until sutures are removed, unless there are signs of infection, in which case the bandage is removed immediately. With transtibial, transradial, and transhumeral amputations, sutures are generally removed 7 to 10 days after surgery; with transfemoral amputations, sutures are usually removed slightly later, at around 14 to 18 days after surgery. The bandage can be removed by cutting it with bandage scissors.

An alternative to the Unna semirigid dressing is an air splint, which is an inflatable plastic limb encasement. It is easy to apply and remove and is self-suspending. Inflation ensures uniform pressure within the splint because a gas in a closed container distributes pressure uniformly.[31] The splint may be augmented with an aluminum frame, permitting limited weight bearing.[32,33] The drawbacks of air splints include bulkiness and susceptibility to punctures.

Rigid dressings can also be used to assist with edema reduction after amputation. These dressings are made of a series of layers. The first layer, next to the skin, is an elasticized cotton sock. Elastic plaster and then a reinforcing layer of regular plaster are wrapped over the sock. Cotton or Dacron webbing straps are plastered in place to provide suspension.[34,35] The rigid dressing remains on the residual limb until suture removal, although it may be removed if the wound becomes infected or pain is intolerable. The rigid dressing may be the foundation for an immediate postoperative prosthesis (IPOP) if a **pylon** with foot is plastered into the dressing. Compared with soft dressings, some investigators report that rigid dressings foster faster wound healing and volume stabilization with fewer surgical revisions, while also accelerating rehabilitation.[36,37] Others, however, found no difference in infection rate or time to prosthetic fitting with this type of dressing.[38] Sometimes a rectangular window is cut near the suture line to permit wound inspection. After inspection, the window is plastered in place. Alternatively, the plaster may be bivalved, so that it can be removed for wound examination.[39] Polyethylene may be substituted for plaster.[40,41] Application of rigid dressings requires considerable skill.[42] The cast is also relatively heavy, so the suspension straps must be kept taut. Suspension for a transfemoral rigid dressing requires a shoulder harness, making sitting awkward. The cast is removed with a cast cutter.

Pain Management. One of the benefits of compressive amputation limb dressings is reduction in pain.[36] However, the cause of pain or other unpleasant sensations should be removed whenever possible.[43] Local pain may respond to removal of an irritant, if one can be identified. Occasionally, a neuroma near fascia can cause either local or phantom pain. In this circumstance, excision of the neuroma may help. Directly after surgery or trauma resulting in amputation, oral or intravenous analgesics may be effective for pain control.[5] Massage, resistive exercise of the contralateral extremity, relaxation,[44] acupuncture,[45] and various modalities, such as US, transcutaneous electrical nerve stimulation (TENS),[46,47] and biofeedback, may also help with pain management.

Joint Mobility. Joint mobility should be preserved with active exercise,[48] positioning, and/or splinting. To prevent flexion contractures after transtibial or transradial amputation, the nearest proximal joint should be kept extended with a splint or a rigid or semirigid dressing. When in bed, the patient should spend as much time as tolerated in a prone position. Regardless of position, the individual should not have pillows placed under the lumbar spine, between the thighs, or under the thigh or transtibial residual limb. When in the wheelchair, the patient should sit in good posture without a pillow between the thighs; the transtibial residual limb should rest on an extension support projecting from the wheelchair seat so that the knee can be extended.

Strengthening. Strengthening the muscles of the residual limb facilitates eventual prosthetic use. The patient with an upper extremity amputation is usually a young, healthy man who can readily preserve or increase strength of the proximal musculature, including the shoulder girdle, to allow use of prostheses that are controlled with shoulder motions. Those with lower extremity amputation are often older and have more co-morbidities and are therefore less able to increase strength. Nonetheless, they should try to strengthen the hip extensors and abductors[49,50] because these muscles are important during stance phase when walking with any prosthesis at or below the transfemoral level. Individuals with transtibial amputation should also work on knee extensor strength because strong knee extension is essential for transferring from one seat to another and for best use of a prosthesis. Without active exercise, isokinetic and isometric quadriceps strength will decrease significantly.[51] Various types of resistance, including manual, active, elastic, pulley, and isokinetic resistance, can be used to increase strength of patients with amputation and to reduce energy consumption when the patient walks with a prosthesis.[52] Exercises suitable for younger and older adults with lower extremity amputation are listed in Table 12-1.

Care of the Remaining Extremity. The person with lower extremity amputation, particularly the adult with arteriosclerosis, should be instructed in meticulous care of the remaining extremity and avoidance of activities that increase the risk of poor healing and further amputation. Activities that are especially deleterious and that aggravate the effects of PVD include smoking, bathing in hot water, using a heating pad, exposing the feet to a radiator or fire, and wearing circular garters. In addition, using chemical corn or callus removers; walking barefoot; wearing a shoe without hose; wearing hose with mends, holes, or an elastic top; and wearing flip-flop sandals increase the risk of trauma and infection.

TABLE 12-1	Exercises for Adults with Lower Extremity Amputation
Exercise	**Technique**
Bridging	Lie on back with head on pillow and arms folded across chest. Towel roll under residual limb. Bend sound leg. Push residual limb into towel while lifting buttock on amputated side. Hold 5 seconds.
Hip extension	Lie on chest with arms folded under head. Keep thighs close together. Lift residual limb to clear the other thigh while keeping abdomen on mat.
Hip abduction: Sidelying	Lie on sound side, with bottom knee bent. Lift residual limb.
Quadriceps sets	Lie on back, with sound knee bent. Slowly tighten thigh muscles in residual limb while counting to 5.
Knee extension	Sit on chair. Straighten knee, holding position for 3 seconds.
Straight leg raise	Recline on back, propping yourself on your elbows. Bend sound knee. Raise residual limb 4 inches, holding position for 5 seconds. Slowly return to starting position.
Hip adduction	Sit on mat with hands bent for support. Place towel roll between thighs. Squeeze roll for 5 seconds.

Foot care should occur on a daily basis and include inspecting the foot using a mirror and looking for redness, blisters, cuts, toenail discoloration, and edema. The feet should be washed in lukewarm water and dried well, especially between the toes. The feet should be lubricated with moisturizing lotion after drying, but lotion should not be used between the toes. Toenails should be trimmed straight across, and if they are thick or the patient has sensory loss, they should be trimmed by a podiatrist. Shoes should be checked for wrinkled linings, protruding tacks, and debris.

◎ *Clinical Pearl*

It is important to teach the patient to inspect the sound foot and the residual limb for redness, blisters, cuts, toenail discoloration, and edema.

Preprosthetic Training. The person with lower extremity amputation should practice standing on the intact foot with the aid of a walker or a pair of crutches. Some therapists begin standing practice in parallel bars. If this is done, it is important to discourage the patient from pulling on the bars because this is not an effective or safe technique for using any type of assistive device.

During the early postoperative period, before the patient has a prosthesis, they may have a rigid dressing with a pylon. The pylon is fixed into the rigid dressing at one end and into a prosthetic foot at the other end to make an IPOP. The pylon should be detached whenever the patient leaves the physical therapy department to prevent unsupervised weight bearing. Until sutures are removed, the person should bear only as much weight as directed by the physician on this temporary prosthesis. This is usually a maximum of 25 lb. Loading can be monitored with a bathroom scale. The individual can progress to three-point gait and transfers during this phase.[34]

Adjustable sockets that can be attached to a pylon and foot are also commercially available for people using semi-rigid or soft dressings. The socket circumference and depth can be adjusted to fit over the dressing using straps and padding. As with the IPOP, this prosthesis can be used for practicing three-point transfers and gait with assistive devices.

Most people with lower extremity amputation use a wheelchair on a temporary or permanent basis. The wheelchair should have its rear wheels displaced posteriorly or have tip guards, so that the rearward transposition of the seated person's center of gravity will not cause the wheelchair to tip backward. The person with a unilateral amputation and no expectation for a prosthesis should have one swing-out footrest to support the sound lower extremity, and individuals who can be expected to wear a prosthesis should have a pair of swing-out footrests to support the prosthetic foot and the sound foot. To facilitate transfers, wheelchairs for patients with bilateral amputations who are not candidates for prostheses should have no footrests.

Someone with an upper extremity amputation should practice one-handed activities to foster resumption of self-care. A temporary prosthesis facilitates edema control and aids with accomplishing bimanual activities. If the dominant hand was amputated, the patient should be guided to change hand dominance to accomplish manipulative tasks. With the possible exception of handwriting, the sound hand will become the dominant extremity whether a prosthesis is provided or not. As soon as possible, the patient should be encouraged to bathe, groom, dress, feed, and toilet independently, using the sound upper extremity. Occasionally, the patient may rely on adaptive equipment, such as a combination fork and spoon, or on trunk motion to perform a particular task.

LOWER EXTREMITY PROSTHETIC OPTIONS

A prosthesis does not always benefit the person with an amputation. It is contraindicated for those with severe cardiovascular or pulmonary disease that would make the exertion needed to use the prosthesis functionally unsafe or if the prosthesis allows the individual to perform activities that place excessive strain on the heart.[53] Few patients with dementia are candidates for a prosthesis, especially if the person cannot comprehend instructions for donning the prosthesis and using it safely. Very occasionally, the individual with cognitive deficits can use a prosthesis if the caregiver is extraordinarily supportive. If the patient is not motivated, prosthetic prescription should be delayed until the person appears interested in rehabilitation (Table 12-2).

Medical factors that influence but do not preclude prosthetic prescription include neuropathy, arthritis, lack of skin integrity, contracture, and weakness.

For the patient who is a candidate for a prosthesis, the only absolute limitations to specific prescriptions are size and cost. Nearly all components are manufactured in adult size, but the options for children are much more limited.

Partial Foot Amputations. No prosthesis is necessary after a phalangeal amputation because the absence of one or more phalanges has minimal effect on standing and walking, although amputation of the first or fifth phalanges compromises late stance. However, the patient will walk more comfortably and the shoe will look better with a filler in the toe box, the distal portion of the shoe. Ideally, a custom-made filler that fits the residual foot precisely should be used to minimize the risk of abrasion that can compromise the amputation scar and cause calluses or ulceration. If the entire toe is removed, the plantar aponeurosis supports the longitudinal arch less effectively, making a longitudinal arch support helpful. With any ray resection, the patient should be provided with a custom-made foot prosthesis to restore the width of the foot and increase the weight-bearing area.

Transmetatarsal amputation shortens the foot considerably. A custom-made, total-contact resilient socket attached to a shoe-filler is recommended to protect the residual limb from abrasion. The shoe should have the fastening on the proximal dorsal surface, as well as a padded tongue, longitudinal arch support, and a cushioned- or beveled-heel rocker sole. These can restore normal function in the late stance phase of gait and avoid an unsightly transverse crease in the upper portion of the

TABLE 12-2	Lower Extremity Prosthetic Options		
Amputation	**Prosthesis**	**Balance**	**Gait**
Toe	Toe filler Longitudinal arch support	Minimal effect, may have pes planus	Late stance: Propulsion
Ray	Sole wedge	Minimal effect, tend to load the unaffected border	Minimal effect
Transmetatarsal and midtarsal	Total-contact resilient socket + toe filler Shoe with fastening on proximal dorsal surface Firm shoe counter Padded tongue Longitudinal arch support Cushion or beveled heel Rocker sole	Tend to shift posteriorly and onto contralateral foot	Late stance: Decreased propulsion during swing phase Prosthesis should remain on foot
Syme's	Syme's foot: Keel accommodates long socket Socket: Expandable, no medial opening, or medial opening	Minimal effect, if end-bearing	Comparable to transtibial

shoe. The plantar surface of the insert should also be curved to facilitate late stance.[54]

Since Chopart and similar intertarsal amputations produce a short foot, which can easily slip from the shoe during swing phase, the patient should wear a shoe that fastens high on the dorsum of the foot. Ideally, a partial foot prosthesis that replaces the forefoot and midfoot is used. Sometimes the prosthesis is attached to a posterior upright that fastens around the proximal portion of the leg.

◎ *Clinical Pearl*

With partial foot amputations, a prosthesis is not always needed; however, fillers, inserts, or specially made shoes will help normalize the gait pattern.

Syme's Amputation and Ankle Disarticulation. After a Syme's amputation or an ankle disarticulation, gait is optimized with use of a prosthesis with a foot specifically manufactured for this type of amputation and a custom-made plastic socket that encases the leg up to the level of the tibial tuberosity. The socket may have no opening on the side walls, particularly if the amputation limb is relatively streamlined. An elastic liner inside the socket facilitates donning. Alternatively, the socket may have an opening in the medial wall, especially if the amputation limb is bulbous (Fig. 12-4). The opening makes donning easier but will need to be closed after donning; a piece of plastic on the medial wall allows uniform weight bearing.

Transtibial Amputation. The transtibial prosthesis consists of a foot, shank, socket, and suspension. Prosthetic feet are mass-produced in sizes to fit 6-month-old infants to adults with very large feet. All feet support weight when the wearer stands or is in the stance phase of gait, and all absorb shock at heel contact. They respond passively to the amount and direction of the load applied

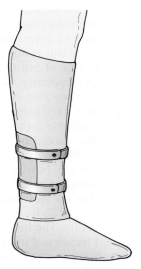

FIG. 12-4 Syme's prosthesis with opening in socket wall to permit entry of bulbous limb.

by the wearer. Feet are designed to simulate metatarsophalangeal hyperextension during late stance and remain in neutral position during swing phase. No prosthetic foot provides sensory feedback, and none plantarflexes when the knee is flexed nor plantarflexes to permit tip-toe walking. Prosthetic feet, with or without a shoe, may fail to attenuate impact force after initial contact during the stance phase of gait.[55]

Foot. Feet may be classified as nonarticulated and articulated. Nonarticulated feet have no separation between the foot and the prosthetic shank but do permit some passive motion in all planes. They may be further classified according to the amount of energy stored during stance phase and released at late stance and early swing phase. Because they have no moving parts, nonarticulated feet are relatively lightweight and durable.

The solid ankle cushion heel (SACH) foot is the basic nonarticulated foot (Fig. 12-5). It consists of a rubberlike

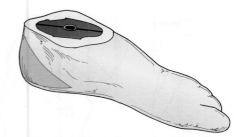

FIG. 12-5 Solid ankle cushion heel (SACH) foot.

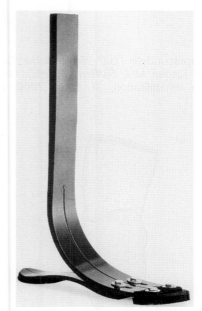

FIG. 12-6 Flex-Foot. *Courtesy Ossur North America, Aliso Viejo, CA.*

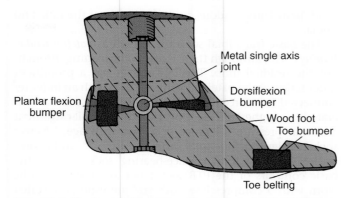

FIG. 12-7 Single-axis foot. *From Fergason J: Prosthetic feet. In Lusardi MM, Nielsen CC (eds):* Orthotics and prosthetics in rehabilitation, *St. Louis, 2000, Butterworth-Heinemann.*

axial bolts. Plantarflexion in early stance is somewhat faster than with a nonarticulated foot because once the patient applies minimal load to the rear foot, the foot moves downward. Compressible bumpers control this motion. Some articulated feet allow only sagittal plane motion (single-axis) (Fig. 12-7), whereas others allow tri-planar motion (multiple-axis).

> ### Clinical Pearl
>
> The Flex-Foot is a prosthetic foot that can absorb and store energy during midstance phase and release it at the end of stance phase.

Shank. The shank is the portion of the prosthesis between the foot and the socket. It must be rigid enough to support the wearer's weight. Most shanks are shaped to match the contour of the contralateral leg. They may be exoskeletal (crustacean), with a rigid weight-bearing plastic or wood shell, or endoskeletal, consisting of a central weight-bearing metal or plastic pylon and a cosmetic cover. The pylon allows slight adjustment of alignment, and some newer models of pylon have a shock-absorbing mechanism.[58] A torque absorber may also be installed in the shank to absorb transverse stress that would otherwise be transmitted to the skin of the residual limb. This is particularly helpful for people who play golf or walk on uneven terrain.

Socket. The socket is considered the most important part of the prosthesis because this component contacts the wearer's skin. Sockets for permanent, definitive prostheses are custom-made of plastic that is either entirely rigid or flexible on the inside with a rigid frame. The flexible plastic is thought to dissipate heat more effectively than the rigid socket; however, construction of a flexible socket and rigid frame takes more time than making an entirely rigid socket. All sockets are designed to contact portions of the residual limb. Areas of the residual lower limb that tolerate pressure best are the patellar ligament, triceps surae belly, and pes anserinus, also known as the *medial tibial flare.* Areas that do not tolerate pressure well are the tibial tuberosity, crest, and condyles, as well as the fibular

compressible heel, a rigid longitudinal support known as the **keel,** and a rubber-like toe section and overall covering. At heel contact, the wearer compresses the heel cushion. At late stance, as the person transfers weight forward, the foot hyperextends at the junction between the distal end of the keel and the toe section. The SACH foot is inexpensive and is available in the largest range of sizes and includes designs to accommodate high-heeled shoes. Other relatively simple feet have a flexible keel that yields slightly when the wearer steps on an uneven surface.

Feet that store more energy are sometimes known as *dynamic* or *energy response feet.* They are also nonarticulated but incorporate an elastic element that the wearer stresses during early or midstance and that recoils during late stance, simulating the propulsive action of the triceps surae.[56] Flex-Foot is one example of a dynamic energy response foot (Fig. 12-6). It has a carbon-fiber leaf spring extending from the toe to the proximal shank and a carbon-fiber heel section. The long leaf spring stores considerable energy as the wearer moves forward on the foot.[57] The Flex-Foot is appreciably more expensive than a SACH foot.

Articulated feet have a separation between the foot and the shank, allowing motion to occur around one or more head, hamstring tendons, and distal ends of the tibia and fibula.

The basic transtibial socket is known as *patellar tendon bearing* (PTB), although there is also some loading throughout the residual limb. The PTB socket has a prominent indentation at the patellar ligament. Tests with an indenter connected to a force transducer confirm that subjects tolerated the highest pressure over the midpatellar ligament and that pressure tolerance decreases with age.[59] Newer socket designs include total surface-bearing[60-62] and hydrostatic[63] models. Total surface-bearing sockets have the basic contours of the PTB socket but are designed to be worn with a compressible liner and are especially suited for suspension by a distal attachment. The hydrostatic design has smoother contours and is most appropriate for short, fleshy residual limbs. With this type of socket, distal tissue cushions the bottom of the socket.

Most transtibial sockets are worn with one or more interfaces or liners.[64,65] The oldest type of interface is a thermoplastic foam concentric replica of the socket. In addition to cushioning impact, the liner makes it easier to alter the size of the socket. As the residual limb atrophies, the prosthetist can add material to the inside of the socket; the flexible liner also creates a smooth surface against the wearer's skin. In addition to the liner, or in place of it, the patient wears one or more socks made of wool, cotton, or Orlon acrylic. Sock thickness is described by ply, referring to the number of threads woven together. The individual should not wear more than 15 ply socks because thicker padding obscures the concavities and convexities within the socket. A nylon sock worn next to the skin provides a smooth surface to reduce the risk of abrasion. In addition to or instead of socks and the resilient socket liner, the patient may wear a liner made of silicone[66-68] or polyurethane,[69] sometimes with gel-filled or mineral oil–filled channels to equalize pressure within the socket.

Suspension. The fourth component of the transtibial prosthesis is provision for suspension during swing phase and whenever the prosthesis is hanging such as during climbing stairs and ladders. The simplest, least expensive, and most adjustable suspension is the supracondylar cuff (Fig. 12-8) which is attached to the proximal portion of the socket and buckled or strapped around the distal thigh. Some people augment the supracondylar cuff with a waist belt and fork strap. The fork strap extends anteriorly from the waist belt to the socket and incorporates an elastic segment. Alternatively, the person may wear a rubberized sleeve from the distal thigh to the proximal portion of the prosthesis. The sleeve creates a smooth contour about the knee that makes it more attractive when the wearer sits. However, the sleeve requires two strong hands to don and will not fit a very large thigh.

A transtibial prosthesis can also be suspended using a silicone liner and a metal pin that lodges in a receptacle in the proximal portion of the shank (Fig. 12-9). Testing with force sensors reveals that during swing phase the liner squeezes proximally while creating a large suction distally.[70] This distal suction may compromise skin health. Other modes of suspension include a webbing strap or lanyard extending from the distal portion of the liner through a hole in the socket to a proximal attachment.

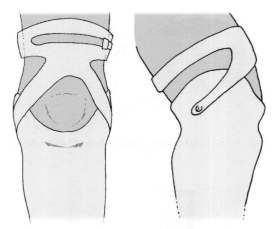

FIG. 12-8 Supracondylar cuff. *From Berke G: Transtibial prostheses. In Lusardi MM, Nielsen CC (eds):* Orthotics and prosthetics in rehabilitation, *St. Louis, 2000, Butterworth-Heinemann.*

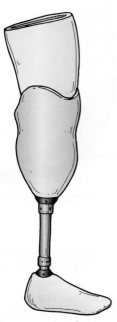

FIG. 12-9 Distal pin suspension for a transtibial prosthesis.

Alternatively, the contour of the socket brim may be designed to provide suspension. **Supracondylar suspension** features a brim extending over the medial and lateral femoral epicondyles, and the socket covers the patella to accommodate a very short residual limb (Fig. 12-10). Donning is easy because the patient does not have to fasten any straps or buckles; however, prosthetic fit is not readily adjustable.

The oldest mode of suspension is the thigh corset, consisting of a leather or flexible plastic corset around the thigh secured with straps or lacing. The corset is attached to the socket by a pair of metal side bars with single-axis hinges. This type of suspension provides mediolateral stability, is readily adjustable, and supports some weight on the thigh. However, the corset is more difficult to don than other types of suspension, can cause pressure atrophy

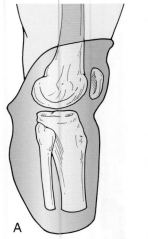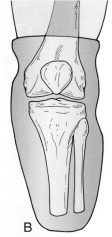

FIG. 12-10 Supracondylar suspension. **A,** Lateral view. **B,** Anterior view.

of the thigh, retains heat, is heavy, and is bulky at the knee.

◎ *Clinical Pearl*

Suspension is needed to keep the prosthesis in place during swing phase and whenever the prosthesis is hanging such as during climbing stairs and ladders.

Prosthesis Alignment. Prosthesis alignment is adjusted to optimize the wearer's stability and ease of movement. In the sagittal plane, the socket is flexed slightly to enhance quadriceps function, reduce the tendency of the residual limb to slide downward in the socket, and increase loading on the patellar tendon. The farther anterior the prosthetic foot is placed relative to the socket, the more stable the prosthesis. For a frail patient, the foot is located forward, so that the weight line passes well in front of the knee. For an athletic person, the foot is located slightly behind the socket, so that the knee is easy to flex.

In the frontal plane, the socket is adducted slightly to enhance loading on the proximal medial aspect of the residual limb. The foot is slightly medial to the socket to augment proximomedial loading and to maintain a relatively narrow walking base. Regardless of socket and foot alignment, the prosthesis should be shaped to present an attractive appearance.

Knee Disarticulation. The prosthesis for a knee disarticulation consists of a foot, shank, knee unit, socket, and suspension. Any foot and shank can be used. The knee unit should have a relatively small vertical dimension, so that when the wearer sits the prosthetic knee does not protrude noticeably. The socket covers the residual limb to the proximal thigh. Two socket designs are generally used. The older design has an anterior opening and fastens with straps or laces. It is best suited to the person with an amputation limb with a bulbous end, as is characteristic of a true disarticulation. The newer socket does not have an anterior opening; instead, it has a flexible liner, similar to that of the Syme's prosthesis. It is appropriate for the

individual with a streamlined residual limb, without protruding femoral epicondyles. This latter type of prosthesis usually does not require an additional suspension unit as the socket is usually effective at keeping the prosthesis on.

Transfemoral Amputation. The transfemoral prosthesis consists of a foot, shank, knee unit, socket, and suspension. Any foot can be included in the transfemoral prosthesis; however, the basic SACH foot and the single-axis foot are more likely to be used than more sophisticated designs. The patient who is hesitant about applying weight to the prosthesis may do better with a single-axis foot because this will plantarflex with less force than needed for a SACH or other nonarticulated foot. The prosthesis can have an endoskeletal or an exoskeletal shank. An endoskeletal shank, in addition to being adjustable and more cosmetic with its cover, is lighter in weight than an exoskeletal shank. The thigh portion, between the socket and knee unit, may have a torque absorber or a unit that enables manually locked thigh rotation, or both. However, the transfemoral endoskeletal cover is subject to considerable erosion at the knee when the wearer sits or kneels.

Many designs of knee units are available. These have different axes, friction mechanisms, extension aids, and stabilizer mechanisms (Table 12-3), although a given unit may not have all these features. All knees are designed to flex when the wearer sits.

Knee Units

Axis. The axis connects the proximal and distal parts of the unit. The single axis with a transverse bolt is most common (Fig. 12-11). It is simple in design and works well for most patients. The polycentric axis has two or more pairs of pivoting side bars arranged so that when the knee is flexed the instant center of rotation is the intersection of the longitudinal axes of the bars. Usually the intersection is posterior to the weight line, making the prosthesis stable through a longer portion of stance phase.[71] However, because it has more moving parts, the polycentric axis unit is not as durable as the single-axis version.

Friction Mechanism. A friction mechanism resists shank movement during the swing phase of gait to prevent excessive knee flexion during early swing (known as *high-heel rise*) and abrupt extension at late swing (known as *terminal impact*). Most knee units have some way to adjust the amount of friction. Either the single-axis or the

TABLE 12-3	Knee Unit Component Options
Components	**Options**
Axis	• Single • Polycentric
Friction mechanism	• Constant/sliding • Variable/fluid • Hydraulic • Pneumatic
Extension aid	• External • Internal
Stabilizer mechanism	• Manual lock • Brake

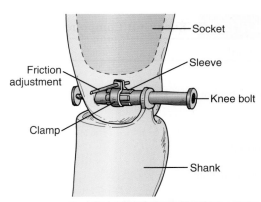

FIG. 12-11 Single-axis knee unit.

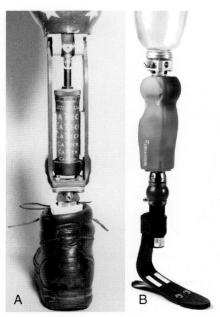

FIG. 12-12 **A,** Hydraulic knee unit. **B,** Microprocessor-controlled knee unit. **A** *from Psonak R: Transfemoral prostheses. In Lusardi MM, Nielsen CC (eds):* Orthotics and prosthetics in rehabilitation, *ed 2, St. Louis, 2006, Butterworth-Heinemann.* **B** *photo of Rheo Knee courtesy Ossur.*

polycentric axis can be combined with any type of friction mechanism. A constant, or sliding, friction knee unit is simplest. It has one or two adjustable clamps around the knee axis that keep friction constant throughout stance phase. In contrast, a variable, or fluid, friction unit provides different amounts of friction throughout swing phase, typically more at early and late swing and less at midswing. Sliding friction units use solid parts, such as a clamp rubbing on another solid structure such as the knee bolt, to generally provide constant friction. Fluid friction units have a cylinder containing either oil (hydraulic) or air (pneumatic) to generally provide variable friction. All fluid units vary friction with the speed of knee motion. When the wearer walks slowly, the friction is low, providing little restriction to shank movement. When the wearer walks quickly or runs, the unit provides more friction to resist excessive shank motion. Consequently, the motion of the prosthetic leg more closely resembles that of the contralateral sound leg at all walking speeds. There are also new computer-controlled fluid friction control mechanisms available that use information from ankle and knee motion sensors to adjust resistance according to gait velocity and alterations in terrain.[72] Hydraulic and pneumatic units are more complex, heavier, and more expensive than sliding friction units. Hydraulic units offer a greater range of cadence response, and they tend to cost and weigh slightly more than pneumatic units.

Extension Aid. An extension aid is a mechanism for extending the shank at the end of swing phase so that the wearer can be assured of a straight knee at the time of heel contact. An external elastic webbing over the knee unit, known as a *kick strap,* is the simplest type of extension aid. An internal extension aid has elastic webbing or a coil spring that recoils at late swing to extend the shank. The internal unit is more cosmetic, and when the user sits, the internal unit keeps the knee flexed. All fluid units have an internal extension aid.

Stabilizer Mechanism. The final feature of a few knee units is a stabilizer mechanism. The simplest stabilizer is a manual lock, consisting of a spring-loaded pin designed to lodge in a receptacle in the proximal shank. The locking unit provides maximum stability, not only during early stance phase, when control is needed, but also throughout the entire gait cycle.[73] With this type of device the wearer walks with a stiff knee and must unlock the unit when

sitting. A braking stabilizer is one that provides considerable friction to resist knee motion only during early stance. Braking stabilizers are available with sliding friction units, known as *weight-activated units,* as well as with several hydraulic units. The sliding friction braking unit stabilizes the knee during early stance if the wearer initiates stance phase with the knee extended or flexed less than 25 degrees. The unit is designed to protect against inadvertent knee collapse if the person should happen to catch the foot on an object or irregularity in the walking surface; however, if the wearer begins stance phase with the knee flexed more than 25 degrees, the knee will flex and may cause a fall. Hydraulic swing and stance phase control knee units (Fig. 12-12, *A*) give the patient the closest approximation of normal gait kinematics. Microprocessor-controlled stance flexion units (Fig. 12-12, *B*) increase friction at heel contact, regardless of the angle of the prosthetic knee, to absorb shock and enable the wearer to walk more normally with controlled knee flexion in early stance.

The thigh section, between the socket and the knee unit, may be equipped with a manually locked rotator unit to allow the person to sit tailor fashion. A torque absorber can also be installed in the thigh section to accommodate stress in the transverse plane.[74]

Socket. Increasingly, people with transfemoral amputation are being fitted with a flexible socket seated in a rigid frame. As compared with an entirely rigid socket, the flexible socket/frame combination is more comfortable when the person sits because the flexible plastic conforms to the contour of the chair. It is also cooler because the thin plastic transmits body heat, and it is easier to modify the flexible thermoplastic by applying heat or removing

TABLE 12-5	Exercises for Unilateral or Bilateral Transtibial or Transfemoral Prosthetic Wearers
Method	**Technique**
Side-to-side shifting	• Stand between 2 chairs or in parallel bars, feet 2-4 inches apart. Hold the chair backs. • Shift weight from the pelvis to right and left. • Do not bend at the waist.
Forward-backward shifting	• Stand between 2 chairs or in parallel bars, feet 2-4 inches apart. Hold the chair backs. • Shift weight from the pelvis forward and backward. • Do not bend at the waist.
Single-limb stance	• Stand between 2 chairs or in parallel bars, with step stool in front of the sound leg. Hold the chair backs. • Step slowly onto stool with the sound foot. Eventually remove hands from the chairs or parallel bars. • Stepping quickly on the stool reduces the effectiveness of the exercise because less time is spent bearing weight on the prosthesis.
Side-stepping	• Stand facing a sturdy table. Place hands on table for balance. • Side-step to sound side, moving from the pelvis. • Keep the torso erect without bending at the waist.
Braiding	• Stand with the feet 2-4 inches apart. • Cross the prosthesis in front of the sound leg. • Bring sound leg on line with prosthesis. • Cross prosthesis behind sound leg. • Bring the sound leg on line with the prosthesis. • Rotate the trunk while moving the legs. • Keep the torso erect.
Ball rolling	• Stand with the prosthesis next to a sturdy table. • Place a tennis ball in front of the sound foot. • Place sound foot on ball and roll it in all directions. • Keep the torso erect.
Elastic band	• Secure one end of the elastic band to a sturdy table leg. • Place the other end of rubber around the sound ankle. • Hold onto a chair while kicking sound leg backward and forward, and side to side. • Keep the torso erect and the knee on the amputated side extended.
Knee flexion/extension	• Stand with the sound leg next to a sturdy table. • Place the sound foot 6 inches in front of the prosthetic foot. • Flex the hip on the amputated side to flex the knee on the same side. • Extend the hip on the amputated side to extend the knee on the same side. • Repeat knee flexion/extension on the sound side. • Repeat with the prosthetic foot in front of the sound foot. • Keep the torso erect.
Leg swing	• Swing the prosthesis forward and backward rhythmically. • Keep the torso erect.

Heel strikes	• Start with the prosthesis behind the trunk.
	• Balance on the prosthetic toe.
	• Push on front socket wall, swing through, and then quickly push on back socket wall.
	• Coin toss
	  1. Toss coins on floor.
	  2. Hit the prosthetic heel on coins called at random.
	  3. Keep the knee on the prosthetic side extended.
	• Tiny steps
	  1. Walk with short steps, emphasizing rapid hip flexion, then extension.
	  2. Performing this exercise slowly may allow the knee to flex inadvertently.
	• Step-ups
	  1. Place stool in front of prosthesis.
	  2. Lead with prosthesis to step up on stool.
	  3. Push on back socket wall.
	  4. Performing this exercise slowly may allow the knee to flex inadvertently.

In comparison with an anatomical hand, the TD has the following limitations:

- Appearance: The shape of the human hand changes with the activity being performed, whereas prosthetic hands have a stylized shape and are covered by a glove to resemble the wearer's skin color. Some people increase the lifelike effect by adding nail polish, rings, bracelets, and even adhesive bandages to the glove. The glove is susceptible to discoloration and damage from abrasion.
- Prehension pattern: The human hand can move in a near-infinite number of positions. Although most TDs can be opened and closed, their fingers only move in one plane. The prosthetic hand has a basic

TABLE 12-6	Causes of Common Gait Deviations with a Transtibial Prosthesis		
Deviation	**Compensation**	**Prosthetic Cause**	**Anatomical Cause**
Early stance	Excessive knee flexion: Buckling	High shoe heel Insufficient plantarflexion Stiff heel cushion Socket too far anterior Socket excessively flexed Cuff tabs too posterior	Flexion contracture Weak quadriceps
	Insufficient knee flexion	Low shoe heel Excessive plantarflexion Soft heel cushion Socket too far posterior Socket insufficiently flexed	Extensor hyperflexion Weak quadriceps Anterodistal pain Arthritis
Midstance	Excessive lateral thrust Medial thrust	Excessive foot inset Foot outset	
Late stance	Early knee flexion: Drop off	High shoe heel Insufficient plantarflexion Heel too short Dorsiflexion stop too short Socket excessively flexed Cuff tabs too posterior	Flexion contracture
	Delayed knee flexion: Walking uphill	Low shoe heel Excessive plantarflexion Heel too long Dorsiflexion stop too stiff Socket too far posterior Socket insufficiently flexed	Extensor hyperreflexia

TABLE 12-7	Causes of Common Gait Deviations with a Transfemoral Prosthesis		
Deviation	**Compensation**	**Prosthetic Cause**	**Anatomical Cause**
Lateral displacements	Abduction stance	Long prosthesis Abducted hip joint Inadequate lateral wall adduction Sharp or high medial wall	Abduction contracture Weak abductors Lateral distal pain Adductor redundancy Instability
	Circumduction swing	Long prosthesis Locked knee unit Loose friction Inadequate suspension Small socket Loose socket Foot plantarflexed	Abduction contracture Poor knee control
Trunk shifts	Lateral bend stance	Short prosthesis Inadequate lateral wall adduction Sharp or high medial wall	Abduction contracture Weak abductors Hip pain Instability Short amputation limb
	Forward flexion: Stance	Unstable knee unit Inadequate socket flexion	Instability
	Lordosis: Stance	Short walker or crutches	Hip flexion contracture Weak extensors
	Medial (lateral) whip: Heel off	Faulty socket contour Knee bolt externally (internally) rotated Foot malrotated Prosthesis donned in malrotation	With sliding friction unit: Fast pace
	Foot rotation at heel contact	Stiff heel cushion Malrotated foot	
Excessive knee motion	High heel rise: Early swing	Inadequate friction Slack extension aid	
	Terminal impact late swing	Inadequate friction Taut extension aid	Forceful hip flexion
Reduced Knee Motion	Vault: Swing	Same as circumduction	With sliding friction unit: Fast pace
	Hip hike: Swing	Same as circumduction	
	Uneven step length	Uncomfortable socket Insufficient	Hip flexion contracture Instability

posture of a three-jaw chuck, in which the thumb opposes the index and long fingers. The ring and little fingers of the prosthetic hand do not move. Hooks provide finger-tip prehension.

- Grasp size: The anatomical adult hand can grasp a basketball and span an octave on the piano. TDs have a maximum grasp size of approximately 4 inches, adequate for most basic tools.
- Grasp force: Healthy young men achieve prehension forces in excess of 120 lb. Most daily activities, however, require 7 lb or less of grasp force, although vocational and avocational tasks may need more forceful prehension. Depending on TD design, grasp force ranges from 1 to 50 lb.[95]
- Sensation: The human hand has receptors that detect movement, heat, cold, light touch, and deep pressure. TDs provide no sensory feedback, other than visual cues.

TDs may be passive or active. A passive TD has a wire armature in each finger to allow the wearer to bend or straighten the digit with the other hand, or with pressure against a firm surface. This type of hand is lightweight, inexpensive, and durable and can be used to hold packages, stabilize paper while the wearer is writing, and improve overall appearance.

Active hands have a wearer-controlled mechanism to allow prehension. A myoelectrically controlled hand is one with a battery-powered motor that is activated by contraction of the remnants of forearm muscles. In the usual transradial arrangement, the person has skin electrodes embedded in the socket of the prosthesis (Fig. 12-16). One electrode lies over the forearm flexors and another electrode lies over the extensors. Isometric flexor muscle contraction generates an action potential, which is detected by the electrode that in turn transmits the signal to the motor that triggers the closing mechanism. With some versions, the longer the patient maintains the contraction, the greater the force of closure and more closely the three radial prosthetic fingers approach one another. Most myoelectric hands are designed to provide grasp forces ranging from less than 1 lb to approximately 35 lb. Relaxation of the forearm muscles causes the fingers to remain in the position they were in just before relaxation, and the hand is opened by the wearer contracting the extensor muscles.

Myoelectric hands are popular because they have a good appearance and provide useful grasp force and because most transradial prostheses with myoelectric terminal devices do not require a harness over the torso. A multicenter comparison of 120 children fitted with both myoelectric and cable-controlled hands revealed that although 78% preferred the myoelectric hands, at a 2-year follow-up, only 44% continued to wear the myoelectric TD.[96] More recently developed hands include force sensors that automatically adjust grip force to maintain grasp of a heavy object without additional muscular contraction.

Electric switch-controlled hands are also available. These have a battery-powered motor that is operated by the wearer using a pull switch or similar mechanism attached to a harness. These switch-controlled hands are less expensive than myoelectric ones but do require the patient to wear a harness.

Limitations of motorized hands are that they require occasional recharging of the battery and the relative delicacy of the mechanism requires that the patient refrain from immersing the hand in fluids. Also, the prosthesis, whether myoelectric or switch-controlled, is relatively heavy, and finger action rather slow.

Another option for hand prostheses are cable-controlled hands. Depending on the mechanism, the wearer can either close (**voluntary closing** [VC]) or open (**voluntary opening** [VO]) the three radial fingers by applying tension to a cable attached to a harness. These hands are less expensive and lighter than electric hands, but the mechanism is still relatively fragile and must be protected against immersion, debris, and rough use. Also, the grasp force with VO hands is approximately 4 lb, which is insufficient for many functional tasks.

Hooks are the primary alternative to prosthetic hands. Although a hook does not resemble the natural hand, it does provide the wearer with a versatile tool to assist in performance of many activities. Hooks are manufactured in sizes to fit 6-month-old infants to adults with moderately large hands. Cable-controlled hooks are the lightest, least expensive, and most durable TDs. Cable-controlled hooks consist of a moving tine, known as a finger, which pivots toward a fixed finger, providing pinch. A cable is attached distally to a projection on the moving finger and proximally to the harness. Hooks are made of aluminum, steel, or titanium and have neoprene-lined fingers. Most VO hooks (Fig. 12-17, *A*) have one or more rubber bands proximally that determine grasp force. An experienced wearer usually has enough bands to provide 5 to 8 lb of grasp force. The patient exerts force through the harness to open the hook, and tension of the rubber bands causes the hook to close. VC hooks (Fig. 12-17, *B*) have a mechanism that responds to the tension the wearer applies to the cable. As the wearer increases the cable tension, the grip force increases up to about 60 lb. Relaxation of cable tension allows the hook to open.

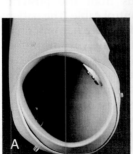
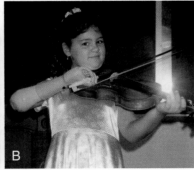

FIG. 12-16 Myoelectric transradial prosthesis. **A,** Electrode placement within the socket. **B,** Playing the violin with a myoelectric prosthesis. *A from Zenie J: Prosthetic options for persons with upper extremity amputation. In Lusardi MM, Nielsen CC (eds): Orthotics and prosthetics in rehabilitation, ed 2, St. Louis, 2006, Butterworth-Heinemann. B courtesy MH Mandelbaum Orthotic & Prosthetic Services.*

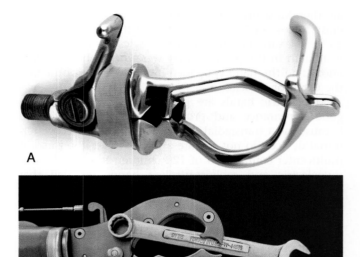

FIG. 12-17 **A,** Voluntary-opening hook. **B,** Voluntary-closing hook. **A** *courtesy Hosmer Dorrance Corporation, Campbell, CA.* **B** *courtesy T.R.S., Inc., Boulder, CO.*

The relatively slender fingers of a hook TD allow the wearer to see the object being manipulated better than with a prosthetic hand. This is important because all prostheses lack tactile sensation. One can also operate a cable-controlled hook with greater accuracy and speed than other devices, and the small contact area of the hook allows manipulation of very small objects. Hooks with myoelectric mechanism are also occasionally prescribed. These provide substantial grasp force but weigh more and are more expensive than cable-controlled hooks.

◎ *Clinical Pearl*

Although a hook prosthesis does not resemble the natural hand, it is often the preferred prosthesis because it allows for greater force generation and better visualization of objects being manipulated.

Wrist Unit. With any type of upper extremity amputation the TD is generally attached to a wrist unit that provides rotation to enable pronation and supination of the TD. With a friction wrist unit, the TD is turned by the wearer who twists it with the sound hand, or nudges it against a firm surface. A rubber washer or a clamp within the unit maintains the desired position, although there are devices with locking mechanisms to provide greater stability. With a locking wrist unit, the patient must unlock the unit, turn it, and then lock it manually. A few wrist units have a mechanism to allow the wearer to select 0, 25, or 50 degrees of palmar flexion. This feature is important to those who cannot position the TD at the midline by internally rotating the shoulder. The typical candidate for a wrist flexion unit is someone with bilateral transhumeral amputations.

Socket. The prosthesis for a patient with a transradial amputation has a plastic forearm proximal to the wrist unit that attaches to a custom-made plastic socket. The amputation limb fits into the socket. The length of the socket-forearm combination should equal the length of the sound forearm.

Suspension. An upper extremity prosthesis is secured to the patient's body either by a snugly-fitted socket or by a harness. Socket suspension requires that the proximal brim of the socket encases the humeral epicondyles; this design is known as *supracondylar suspension.* Myoelectric transradial prostheses usually have supracondylar suspension. The Muenster socket, developed in Muenster, Germany, is a type of socket that encases the epicondyles and the olecranon. This socket is indicated for short and very short residual limbs. An alternative to supracondylar or Muenster suspension is a roll-on flexible plastic suspension sleeve, with electrodes embedded in it if myoelectric control is to be used.

A harness can also be used to both suspend an upper extremity prosthesis and transmit shoulder motion to a cable-controlled TD. This harness is usually made of Dacron tape and has a transradial figure-of-eight design. The harness is made with two strips of tape riveted to the medial and lateral sides of the socket and then joined in an inverted-Y strap over the anterior aspect of the upper arm. The strap then passes through the deltopectoral triangle to the back of the torso, crossing the spine to pass under the contralateral axilla and then around the contralateral shoulder, to form an axillary loop. From there, the strap passes back over the spine to the distal portion of the scapula, where it is known as the control attachment strap because it is buckled to the control cable. The figure-of-eight harness is easy to don and is relatively inconspicuous because it does not cross the front of the chest. The figure-of-nine harness is similar, with an axillary loop and a control attachment strap, but it lacks the inverted-Y portion because the figure-of-nine harness is worn with a supracondylar or Muenster socket. Patients who cannot tolerate an axillary loop can wear a transradial chest strap harness. This type of harness includes a strap that encircles the chest and a broad shoulder saddle that lies over the ipsilateral shoulder and is attached to the chest strap. The control attachment strap extends from the posterior portion of the chest strap to the control cable. The patient must unbuckle the strap when doffing the harness. Some people complain that this type of harness is uncomfortable or unsightly.

Control Systems. Upper extremity prostheses, except passive hands, require a system to control the TD and wrist unit. For a myoelectric prosthesis the wearer uses muscles within the socket to activate electrodes to achieve finger opening and closing. Cable-controlled prostheses use a single steel cable attached distally to the TD and proximally to the control attachment strap (Fig. 12-18). This cable is encased in a steel tubular housing secured distally to the socket and proximally to the proximal portion of the socket or to a flexible plastic or leather pad placed over the triceps muscle. The housing prevents the cable from bowstringing when the wearer bends the elbow. Flexing the glenohumeral joint or abducting the

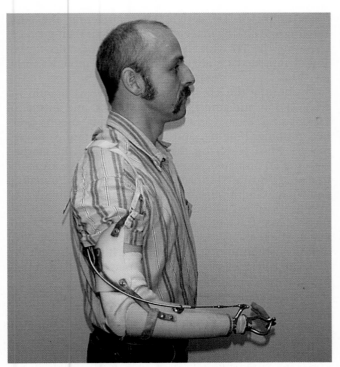

FIG. 12-18 Transradial prosthesis. *Courtesy Hosmer Dorrance Corporation, Campbell, CA.*

scapula applies tension to the cable, and this tension opens or closes the TD, depending on its mechanism.

Transhumeral Prostheses. The transhumeral prosthesis includes all of the components used in a transradial prosthesis with the addition of a forearm section and an elbow unit.

Terminal Device and Wrist Unit. Any type of TD and wrist unit can be included in a transhumeral prosthesis. Some patients with a short transhumeral or **humeral neck amputation** or a shoulder disarticulation or **forequarter amputation** may require a wrist flexion unit to position the TD close to the mouth, chest, and perineum. In all instances, the wrist unit is bonded to the distal end of the forearm arm section that is a plastic truncated cone the same length as the missing anatomical forearm.

Elbow Unit. Prostheses for amputations at the standard transhumeral level and higher require an elbow unit that enables elbow flexion and extension, locking, and rotation. The elbow unit has a turntable to provide transverse rotation. The patient can position the forearm manually by pushing it away from or toward the chest. The turntable is needed even if the glenohumeral joint is unimpaired because the cylindrical residual limb encased in a cylindrical socket would rotate inside the socket, rather than transmitting anatomical shoulder rotation to the distal portion of the prosthesis.

The elbow unit is embedded in the proximal portion of the forearm section. Elbow units provide a hinge for elbow flexion and extension; most also have a lock to secure the desired elbow angle and a turntable to allow the wearer to rotate the forearm horizontally. Young children are usually fitted with a passive elbow unit with a hinge with a friction clamp that maintains the desired elbow angle.

Older children and adults are generally fitted with a cable-controlled locking elbow unit that can be locked in seven, eleven, or more positions, depending on the design. Tension on the locking cable locks and then unlocks the unit, triggering an alternator mechanism within the unit. Tension on a separate cable flexes and extends the elbow. Myoelectrically controlled elbow units enable elbow flexion and extension, as well as locking. The elbow motor is activated by different skin electrodes than those that operate the TD. Some people are fitted with a hybrid prosthesis that combines a myoelectrically controlled hand with a cable-controlled elbow unit.

Socket. The transhumeral socket is custom-made plastic. The patient with an elbow disarticulation can be fitted with a socket that terminates at the proximal portion of the upper arm. Patients with higher amputations need a socket that extends superiorly to maintain stable fit, although such higher trim lines do somewhat restrict shoulder motion.

Suspension. Transhumeral prostheses usually require harness suspension because there are no bony prominences available for their suspension. The usual harness is the transhumeral figure-of-eight harness. This is similar to the transradial figure-of-eight harness with the addition of an elbow lock control strap and more suspension straps. A few patients are fitted with a transhumeral chest strap harness.

Control Systems. Cable control of the transhumeral prosthesis is usually achieved with two cables, each encased in steel housing. One cable extends from the control attachment strap on the back of the harness to the TD. This cable has proximal and distal housing sections. If the elbow unit is unlocked, tension on the cable causes elbow flexion; controlled relaxation of the cable allows the elbow to extend. If the elbow unit is locked, tension on the same cable activates the TD. The second cable extends from the elbow unit locking mechanism to the anterior support strap of the harness. Tension on this cable locks and unlocks the elbow unit alternatively.

Electrically powered elbow units are less commonly prescribed. These units are activated by switches in the harness, or elsewhere in the prosthesis, or by skin electrodes placed over the remnants of the anterior and posterior deltoid muscles.

Controls Training. Once the prosthesis is custom made for the patient, it should be assessed carefully. Often the therapist performs the examination and reports the findings to others on the clinical team. Controls training should not proceed until the clinical team is certain that the prosthesis fits and operates properly; otherwise, the wearer is apt to exert unnecessary effort to achieve adequate function. Controls training involves instructing the patient to operate all components of the prosthesis and to don the appliance.

Transradial Prosthesis. Donning is an essential skill. The patient first dons a T-shirt to protect the skin from irritation by the harness straps. Then the amputation limb is placed in a cotton, wool, nylon, or silicone sock. The patient then inserts the residual limb into the socket and then places the sound hand through the axillary loop. If a chest strap is used for suspension, the person should place the residual limb in the socket, wrap the chest strap around the torso, and then fasten the strap in the front.

A supracondylar or Muenster socket fits very snugly. To don this, the residual limb is first put in tubular stockinet with the distal end of the stockinet extending beyond the end of the residual limb. The patient then inserts the residual limb in the socket, taking care to place the end of the stockinet through a hole drilled through the end of the socket. The stockinet continues through another hole in the plastic forearm. The person tugs on the stockinet to draw the skin and subcutaneous soft tissue into the socket. If the socket is part of a myoelectrically controlled prosthesis, the patient continues pulling on the stockinet until it is pulled completely out of the prosthesis, so that the skin is in direct contact with the socket and its electrodes. If the socket is part of a cable-controlled prosthesis, the patient pulls on the stockinet until the socket is well positioned, then tucks the end of the stockinet into the forearm cavity.

TD operation with a myoelectrically controlled prosthesis begins before construction of the prosthesis. The therapist uses an electrode to determine where on the forearm the greatest voltage can be measured when the patient forcefully contracts the flexor or extensor muscles. The patient then practices isolated contraction of the flexors while maintaining relaxation of the extensors, and vice versa. Once optimal electrode positions are found, the electrodes are embedded in the socket so that they overlie these chosen sites. With the finished prosthesis on, the patient then practices opening the TD to different distances, as well as closing the TD with various amounts of force. The rehabilitation program emphasizes endurance exercises for the forearm musculature to reduce fatigue when the patient is engaging in a prolonged task.

Cable-controlled TD training begins with the prosthesis on the patient. The best position for early training is with the elbow flexed approximately 90 degrees because the wearer can see the TD easily and the harness and cable are in the easiest position for TD operation. The therapist resists glenohumeral flexion until the patient observes the TD open or close. If the TD is VO, it will open; if it is VC, it will close. The patient practices glenohumeral flexion until the motion can be done without external resistance and the TD operates reliably. Control motion should be confined to the amputated side because tensing the contralateral musculature can interfere with performance of bimanual activities. The next step in training involves having the patient keep the elbow flexed while attempting to operate the TD by abducting the scapula. This maneuver achieves TD operation close to the body.

With a VC TD the wearer practices closing it gently, then forcefully, and then with intermediate amounts of force. Control of a VO TD includes drills in opening the hand or hook at various distances. The patient also practices relaxing cable tension to allow the device to snap closed. The most difficult control procedure requires the wearer to close the TD partially by maintaining tension on the control attachment strap.

Regardless of TD design, after mastering the basic opening and closing maneuvers, the patient then practices operating the TD with the elbow extended, fully flexed, and at intermediate angles and with the shoulder in all positions.

Positioning the TD involves using the wrist unit. An array of soft and firm balls, cubes, disks, and prisms of various sizes, known as a *form board,* can be used to practice grasping, holding, and releasing commonly shaped objects. Most pieces on the form board can be grasped with the TD pronated. Some items, such as disks, are easier to manage if the TD is placed halfway between pronation and supination. A large, rigid ball is most readily secured in a hook turned to the supinated position; with a prosthetic hand, the ball is easier to grasp with the TD pronated. The therapist teaches the patient to rotate the wrist unit to position the TD appropriately. If the wrist unit has a locking mechanism, the wearer must unlock it, rotate the TD, and then relock the wrist unit.

Transhumeral Prosthesis. Donning a transhumeral prosthesis with a figure-of-eight harness is easiest with the prosthesis placed on a table with the harness untangled. The patient wears a T-shirt and a residual limb sock, inserts the sound extremity into the axillary loop, and then places the residual limb in the socket. If the prosthesis has a chest strap, the individual dons the socket, encircles the chest with the chest strap, and then secures it.

TD operation and positioning is taught first with the elbow lock engaged. TD and wrist unit operation are performed in the same way as a transradial prosthesis. The therapist also teaches the patient to rotate the forearm in the horizontal plane by pulling or pushing the forearm so that the elbow unit pivots at the turntable.

Elbow unit control begins with the elbow unlocked. The therapist shows the patient that the same glenohumeral flexion or scapular abduction that operates the TD also flexes the elbow because the cable connected to the TD also passes in front of the elbow hinge. To extend the elbow, the patient gradually relaxes the shoulder or scapular musculature.

The second step in elbow unit control is elbow locking and unlocking. Training should start with the prosthesis off the patient. The therapist shows the patient that the elbow lock is an alternator mechanism, that is, the first pull on the elbow lock cable locks the unit. The next pull unlocks it; a soft clicking sound occurs when the alternator engages. The patient pulls on the elbow lock cable with the sound hand until smooth, reliable action is achieved. Then, with the prosthesis on the patient, the therapist unlocks the elbow and supports the forearm with one hand while using the other hand to resist an oblique movement composed of humeral hyperextension and shoulder girdle depression until the elbow locks. Repeating the movement unlocks the unit. The patient then practices rapid elbow locking and unlocking while the therapist continues to support the forearm. The final step in elbow unit controls training requires coordination of elbow flexion and locking. The patient flexes the elbow to the desired angle, then locks it quickly. If the locking motion is done slowly, the forearm would extend. Flexion of the elbow hinge requires shoulder flexion, and elbow locking needs shoulder hyperextension.

Use Training. Use training emphasizes employing the prosthesis as an assistive device, complementing maneuvers of the sound hand. Most daily activities, such as drinking from a cup, are naturally performed with one hand. The individual who wears a prosthesis would do the same and generally hold the cup in the intact hand. A few tasks, however, are ordinarily done bimanually. These activities form the basis of use training. In general, the prosthesis performs the more stationary portion of the task. The therapist should allow the patient to experiment with various techniques, offering cues only when the individual is stymied. Techniques used by people with hemiplegia often work well for those with an amputation. Some adaptive aids can also be useful. Use training is beneficial whether the patient has an active or passive TD.

Vocations. The prosthesis serves as a useful tool to aid in the performance of the clerical aspects of most school and professional endeavors. Machinery may also be adapted, often with little cost or effort, to suit the capabilities of most people who wear a prosthesis. Unlike those with more distal amputations, people with transhumeral amputations will have difficulty reaching overhead with the prosthesis. Keyboard control can be aided by use of a keyboard designed for one-handed use. Alternatively, one can press the key with the tip of the hook or with the eraser end of a pencil held in the TD using a one-finger, "hunt and peck" technique. Driving is aided by a spinner knob bolted to the steering wheel.

Care of the Residual Limb and Prosthesis. The residual limb must be kept clean and dry. Nightly use of a moisturizing lotion should keep the skin supple. The patient should inspect the torso and both arms for signs of reddening at the margins of the prosthesis and along the path of the harness, with particular attention to the contralateral axilla.

TD care is simplest with the cable-controlled hook. The device should be kept clean and wiped dry if unintentionally immersed. One should check the neoprene lining for deep cracks, which indicate that the lining needs replacement. Rubber bands on a hook should be changed when they become brittle.

With a prosthetic hand, care of the glove includes avoiding sharp or rough textured objects. The glove can be cleaned with a slightly moistened soapy cloth. One should never place the hand on a varnished surface. The wearer should avoid exposing the glove to solvents, such as gasoline, kerosene, or turpentine, or staining agents like ballpoint pen ink, newsprint, tobacco, mustard, grape juice, and beet juice. Nail polish can be worn but must be removed by scraping rather than with acetone.

The socket should be wiped each evening with a moistened soapy cloth. Unless the prosthesis is myoelectrically controlled, one should wear a fresh sock daily. Most harnesses can be unbuckled from the rest of the prosthesis. The Dacron strap can then be laundered. If the housing on the control cable becomes unwound, it could snag clothing and possibly cause the control cable to break and then the housing would require replacement. A clean

T-shirt worn under the harness protects the skin and the harness.

> **⊚ Clinical Pearl**
>
> Rehabilitation for the person with an amputation includes instruction in daily skin inspection and cleaning of the residual limb, as well as daily inspection and cleaning of the prosthesis.

ADVANCED ACTIVITIES

Depending on the individual's stamina and motivation, the rehabilitation program may go considerably beyond basic training. For the person with lower extremity amputation, advanced activities may include climbing stairs and curbs, kneeling, stepping over obstacles, running, and jumping.

Sometimes the side of amputation is pertinent. For example, transferring into the passenger side of a car is easier for someone wearing a right lower extremity prosthesis than a left one. The person would simply swing the intact left leg into the car, then lift or otherwise move the prosthesis into place. Driving, however, is easier for the person with a left prosthesis because the individual can use the intact, sensate right foot to operate the accelerator and brake pedals of a vehicle with automatic transmission. The adult who wears a right prosthesis can cross the left leg over the right to use the sound foot for pedaling. Alternatively, the person can attach a pedal extension to enable right foot operation. People with unilateral or bilateral transtibial amputation can also operate the car with the prosthetic feet, relying on proprioception from the knee and hip for safe operation; however, it is prudent to check the state motor vehicle regulations to determine whether such operation is permissible. Hand controls are indicated for the individual with bilateral transfemoral amputations, with or without prostheses.

Bicycling is easier if a toe clip is added to the pedal on the amputated side. A prosthesis is more effective at pulling the pedal than pushing it. Some individuals with lower extremity amputations bicycle without a prosthesis. Skiing can be performed with short rudders attached to the ski poles whether the person wears a leg prosthesis or not. Individuals with bilateral leg amputation often use a sled for winter fun.

Sports that require running or jumping can be enjoyed by people with leg amputation. Even with an energy-storing prosthetic foot, the athlete gets more propulsive force from the sound leg; consequently, the individual usually runs with a hop-skip progression. Runners with bilateral amputations generally wear a pair of Flex-Feet or other energy-storing feet designed for running. Jumping also relies on the power generated by the sound leg. Regular participation in vigorous activity has been shown to be associated with positive body image.[96]

Some people with upper extremity amputation may develop considerable manipulative skill for vocational and avocational pursuits. Many musical instruments can be played by children and adults with upper extremity amputation. The most accessible are brass wind instruments because the valves are ordinarily operated with one hand while the prosthesis stabilizes the instrument. One may have to switch hands; for example, a trumpet is designed to be played with the right hand controlling the valves. It can, however, be played with the left hand. Conversely, the French horn, normally played with the left hand, can be operated in reverse. The trombone is well suited to people with amputations because most models have no valves. Guitars and other stringed instruments, ordinarily fingered with the left hand, can have the strings reversed. This may also require changing the position of the bridge, depending on the instrument. A pick or bow can be adapted so it is secured in the TD or in an elastic cuff worn on the forearm. Piano compositions for one-handed performance exist in the beginner, intermediate, and advanced repertory.

Sports are well within the reach of individuals with upper or lower extremity amputation, whether they wear regular or modified prostheses or use modified equipment. Special TDs can be exchanged for the usual one to hold a bowling ball or golf club, manage a baseball catcher's mitt, and perform gymnastic stunts. Professional football, basketball, and baseball players with limb deficiencies are role models for their skilled one-handed prowess. Accounts of athletes who overcame major impairments may inspire some patients.[97-99] Many sports organizations are open to people with disabilities. Participation is an excellent way of integrating into the community, as well as garnering the physiological benefits of exercise

CASE STUDY 12-1

CLOSED AMPUTATION LEFT TIBIA

Patient History

AB is a 72-year-old retired machinist who was diagnosed with type 2 diabetes 7 years ago. He tests his blood glucose daily and relies on diet to control his glucose levels. Four years ago he underwent a successful angioplasty to repair a blockage of the left peroneal artery. One year ago he cut his left hallux on a shard of glass, and within 2 weeks his entire foot had become gangrenous. Two vascular surgeons recommended immediate amputation at the musculotendinous junction of the left leg. AB presents 3 weeks after a closed amputation through the proximal tibia with myodesis. Postoperatively, the limb was dressed with elastic bandage compressive dressing.

Tests and Measures—Significant Findings
Musculoskeletal

- The amputation limb is 7 inches long from the medial tibial plateau to the bony end of the tibia. The circumference has smooth contours with no proximal constriction or distal tissue redundancy.

- Muscle Performance: Left: Quadriceps 3/5; hamstrings 4/5; hip musculature within normal limits. Right: Ankle, knee, and hip strength within normal limits.

Neuromuscular
- Sensation is intact on the residual left limb.

Integumentary
- Left: The amputation scar is well healed, nonadherent, and with minimal invagination. Color and temperature are normal. Ample granulation tissue is evident, with no exudate. Right: There is interdigital dermatitis and dorsal calluses on the second and third toes.

Diagnosis
Preferred practice pattern: 4J: Impaired motor function, muscle performance, range of motion, gait, locomotion, and balance associated with amputation.

Interventions
Postoperative Management
- Instruction in a ROM and general conditioning exercise program.
- Instruction to wear his temporary prosthesis 8 to 10 hours daily and continue to wear his shrinker sock at night.
- Transfer and mobility training, including 3-point transfer, ambulation, relying on bimanual support standing within parallel bars, progression to ambulation with a walker.

Prosthetic Management
- Fitting of a definitive prosthesis at 6 weeks postoperative.
- Therapy intervention to include donning and doffing of his prosthesis, balance facilitation, and gait training. Emphasis on left knee control, safe activities of daily living (ADL) performance, and increasing his endurance.

Role of the Physical Therapist Assistant
- What kinds of strength and conditioning exercises will likely be included for this patient in his first 3 weeks of therapy, and how will they be different from the strength and conditioning exercises in his last 3 weeks of therapy?
- Describe 2 quadriceps strengthening exercises that could be done as part of this patient's home program.
- Describe the steps involved in donning and doffing this patient's prosthesis.
- Initially, how often during prosthetic training should the skin of the residual limb be inspected? What will you instruct the patient to look for during skin inspection?

Additional Information
For the full version of this case study, including detailed examination results, interventions, and outcomes, see the Evolve site that accompanies this book. Full case studies for a patient undergoing rehabilitation after a left transfemoral amputation and a patient undergoing

rehabilitation after a right long transradial amputation also appear on the Evolve site.

CHAPTER SUMMARY

Amputation is a relatively infrequent occurrence in the civilian world. Lower extremity amputation is much more common than upper extremity amputation, with PVD as the principal cause. People with transtibial, transfemoral, transradial, and transhumeral amputations are most frequently seen in rehabilitation. The functional outcome of adults with unilateral lower extremity amputation depends on amputation level, as well as the individual's general health. Ambulation with a prosthesis is slower and consumes more energy per distance than able-bodied gait. People fitted with a unilateral upper extremity prosthesis can accomplish ADLs, although many tasks can also be done one-handed. Advanced activities for all patients involve maneuvering over all types of terrain and engaging in recreational activities. In all instances, the goal of rehabilitation is to enable the patient to engage in the broadest range of endeavors.

ADDITIONAL RESOURCES

For links to these and additional web-based resources, see the Evolve site.

Burgess EM, Rappoport A: *Physical fitness: A guide for individuals with lower limb loss,* Washington, DC, 1990, Department of Veterans Affairs.

Carroll K, Edelstein JE: *Prosthetics and patient management: A comprehensive clinical approach,* Thorofare, NJ, 2006, Slack.

Lusardi MM, Nielsen CC (eds): *Orthotics and prosthetics in rehabilitation,* Boston, 2005, Saunders.

May BJ: *Amputations and prosthetics: A case study approach,* ed 2, Philadelphia, 2002, FA Davis.

Meier RH, Atkins DJ: *Functional restoration of adults and children with upper extremity amputations,* New York, 2004, Demos Medical Publishing.

Mensch G, Ellis PM: *Physical therapy management of lower extremity amputations,* Gaithersburg, MD, 1986, Aspen.

Shurr DG, Michael JW: *Prosthetics and orthotics,* ed 2, Upper Saddle River, NJ, 2002, Prentice Hall.

American Association of Adapted Sports Programs

American Orthotic and Prosthetic Association

Disabled Sports USA

GLOSSARY

Closed amputation: Amputation surgery in which the skin is sutured.

Forequarter amputation: Amputation through any portions of the scapula, clavicle, and thorax.

Guillotine amputation: Amputation surgery in which all portions of the limb are severed at the same level.

Hansen's disease: Leprosy, a communicable disease caused by *Mycobacterium leprae* that may result in autoamputation of the digits, nose, and ears.

Humeral neck amputation: Amputation through the proximal portion of the humerus.

Keel: Longitudinal supporting structure of a prosthetic foot.

Myodesis: Amputation surgical procedure in which one muscle group is sutured to another group.

Myoplasty: Amputation surgical procedure in which muscles are sutured to bone through holes drilled in the bone.

Open amputation: Amputation surgery in which the skin is not sutured because of infection. Secondary closed amputation is usually planned.

Phantom pain: Discomfort experienced in the missing limb segment.

Phantom sensation: Awareness of the missing limb segment.

Pylon: Endoprosthetic vertical support substituting for the shank.

Supracondylar suspension: Mode of suspension of a transtibial prosthesis in which the brim terminates immediately above the femoral epicondyles, or a transradial prosthesis in which the brim terminates immediately above the humeral epicondyles.

Syme's amputation: Amputation through the distal portion of the tibia and fibula, with the calcaneal fat pad sutured to the distal end of the amputation limb; all tarsals and distal structures are removed.

Transfemoral amputation: Amputation through the femur, previously known as *above-knee.*

Transhumeral amputation: Amputation through the humerus, previously known as *above-elbow.*

Translumbar amputation: Amputation through the lumbar spine, previously known as *hemicorporectomy.*

Transmetatarsal amputation: Amputation through the metatarsals.

Transpelvic amputation: Amputation through the pelvis, previously known as *hemipelvectomy.*

Transradial amputation: Amputation through the radius and ulna, previously known as *below-elbow.*

Unna dressing: Postoperative limb dressing composed of gauze permeated with zinc oxide, calamine, glycerin, and gelatin.

Voluntary closing (VC): Mode of terminal device operation in which the patient volitionally closes the fingers and springs cause opening.

Voluntary opening (VO): Mode of terminal device operation in which the patient volitionally opens the fingers and rubber bands or springs cause closing.

OBJECTIVES

After reading this chapter, the reader will be able to:
1. Identify the relationship between balance disorders and fall risk.
2. Define terminology used in the physical therapy management of balance disorders.
3. Specify the central and peripheral components of postural control mechanisms.
4. Compare and contrast the roles of the visual, vestibular, and somatosensory systems in postural control.
5. Identify and differentiate between pathologies that can result in impaired balance.
6. Relate common age-related changes in postural control mechanisms to fall risk in the elderly.
7. Identify and describe typical examination findings used in the management of patients with balance disorders or who are at increased risk for falls.

8. Select and apply appropriate interventions to improve balance and reduce fall risk in patients with loss of balance or increased fall risk.

Poor **balance** and falls adversely affect the lives of thousands. More than one-third of adults aged 65 years and older fall each year.[1] When people fall, 20% to 30% sustain moderate to severe injuries, such as hip fractures or head trauma, that reduce their mobility and independence and increase their risk for premature death.[2] The risk of sustaining severe injury from a fall is higher for older adults and those with co-morbidities such as stroke, Parkinson's disease (PD), vestibular dysfunction, amputation, arthritis, and head trauma. Falls may result in pain, injury, and disability, and after falling, individuals may lose confidence in their ability to perform routine activities. A heightened fear of falling can also lead to restriction of activities.[3] Although not all falls can be prevented, the poor balance that precipitates some of them can be improved to reduce the risk for falls and their consequences.

Clinical Pearl

Falls not only cause pain, injury, and disability but also loss of confidence and fear of falling that can then lead to restriction of activities.

Balance is the ability to locate and maintain one's center of gravity (COG) within or over one's **base of support (BOS)**.[4,5] Sensory and motor systems are used to maintain an upright position during static and dynamic tasks in multiple and changing environments. Balance is sometimes referred to as **postural control** because it involves controlling the position or posture of the body at rest or when moving. The term *posture* implies holding a particular static position (see Chapter 4). The terms *postural control* and *balance,* as used in this chapter, refer to the ability to move efficiently and effectively in a variety of environments and situations without falling. Postural control involves the use of many systems to obtain information about the environment and produce appropriate

TABLE 13-1	Fall Prevention for Individuals with Increased Fall Risk
Type of Patient	**Examples of Intervention**
Individual of advanced age	Muscle strengthening and endurance program focused on lower extremities.
	Patient education in reducing environmental hazards that represent fall risk.
Individual with a history of falls	Exercise program and gait training focused on components and types of postural control that show deficits.
	Assessment and modification of patient's environment as appropriate.
Individual with CNS pathology with chronic or progressive balance deficits	Exercise program, instruction in ADLs, and gait training with assistive devices as needed.
	Patient and caregiver instruction on fall prevention and safety.

Adapted from American Physical Therapy Association: *Phys Ther* 81:9-744, 2001.
CNS, Central nervous system; *ADLs,* activities of daily living.

movements and responses. The visual, somatosensory, and **vestibular systems** relay information about the position and movement of the body, particularly the head, in relation to the environment and the position and movement of the environment in relation to the body.[3,6-9] The neuromuscular and musculoskeletal systems allow for voluntary or reactive motions in response to the sensory input. The cognitive system interprets sensory input to select and coordinate motor output in terms of posture and movement. Cognition is particularly important for functional balance because it "provides us with the collective ability to anticipate or adapt our actions in response to changing task demands and the environment."[3] Redundancy among the systems allows for compensation if a system is compromised.[2]

Postural control may need to change in response to changing task demands, such as differences in lighting, stability, or evenness of the supporting surface, or mechanical **perturbations.** To live and move freely in the environment, people need to have effective static balance, automatic and **reactive postural responses,** anticipatory control, and volitional postural movements.[4,10] A lack or dysfunction of any type or component of postural control can hinder a person's ability to meet particular task demands and increase the risk of falling.

Many pathologies and impairments can affect postural control. Therefore patients with various diagnoses in different practice settings, including acute care, long-term care, inpatient rehabilitation, outpatient practice, and community sites, may benefit from interventions to reduce their risk of loss of balance and falls (Table 13-1).

PATHOLOGY

CAUSES OF BALANCE DYSFUNCTION

Balance dysfunction during normal tasks in an ordinary environment occurs when postural control systems function inadequately. Current theories of balance are based on a systems approach that assumes that balance is controlled by many interacting systems. When one or more of these systems has a problem, the other systems adapt as much as possible to prevent falling while still accomplishing the task.

According to the dynamic equilibrium theory of balance control (Fig. 13-1),[10] sensory and motor systems interact

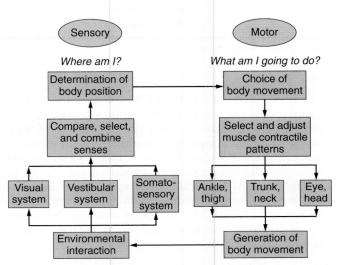

FIG. 13-1 The dynamic equilibrium model of balance control. *Courtesy NeuroCom.*

to dynamically control equilibrium and allow adjustment to displacement of a person's COG through appropriate changes in the BOS.[11] The sensory system receives information about the environment, and the neuromuscular and musculoskeletal systems allow for motor planning and motor output in response to this information. This interaction can provide the static, adaptive, anticipatory, and reactive control required for people to move in and respond to a changing environment.[11]

Various pathologies or impairments can cause problems with balance (Table 13-2). The intrinsic causes of balance problems can be grouped into the following five categories: (1) peripheral sensory, (2) central sensory, (3) peripheral motor, (4) central motor, and (5) cognitive.[12] The next section of this chapter reviews these causes of balance problems and provides examples of each.

Peripheral Sensory Impairments. Vision, vestibular sensation, and **somatosensation** all contribute to postural control, and if impaired, can result in balance dysfunction. The visual system includes the eyes with the visual receptors; the optic nerves that project, via connections, to the occipital region of the brain; and the nerves and muscles of the oculomotor system. Visual receptors detect light and differences in light patterns to allow us

TABLE 13-2		Causes of Balance Problems	
System	Area	Areas of Impairment	Consequences
Sensory	Peripheral	Visual system, receptors Vestibular system, receptors Somatosensory system, receptors: primarily lower extremities	Decreased ability to sense the position or movement of the head or body in relation to a static or dynamic environment
	Central	Cortical areas responsible for interpreting and integrating sensory information	Decreased ability to combine information from relevant sensory input; perception of space, true vertical or horizontal may be distorted
Motor	Peripheral	Muscles, joints, motor units	Decreased ability to execute balance strategies or reactions to postural sway
	Central	CNS areas responsible for planning, coordinating, and affecting motor control	Decreased ability to plan and coordinate postural control under static and dynamic conditions
Cognitive	Central	Cortical and limbic areas responsible for attention, arousal, and judgment	Decreased ability to remember previously successful strategies, judge and attend to potential dangers

CNS, Central nervous system.

to identify objects and obstacles. Vision also detects relative motion of the environment and thus provides orientation to help maintain balance. The central visual field is used most for environmental orientation to tell us where we are in space. Peripheral vision, also known as *ambient vision,* provides information about movement relative to the environment, including head movements and postural sway.[9] Vision contributes to anticipatory and responsive postural control. Any pathology that impairs vision, such as glaucoma, macular degeneration, cataracts, diplopia, or visual field cuts, can impair balance.[13]

◎ *Clinical Pearl*

Visual pathologies, such as glaucoma, macular degeneration, or diplopia, can increase the risk for falls and can impair balance.

The visual and vestibular systems work together to generate eye movements that allow observation of moving or stationary objects when the head is moving or stationary. This helps maintain upright posture and allows a person to keep track of his or her position in space.[13]

Although eye movements are a form of motor output, because of their intimate link with vision and the vestibular system, problems with eye movements are generally considered with peripheral sensory impairments. Important occulomotor functions relating to balance include conjugation, saccades, smooth pursuit, **vestibulo-ocular reflex (VOR),** and nystagmus. Problems with any of these can interfere with orientation to the environment. Eye movements should be conjugate, with the eyes moving together, so that an image always falls on corresponding points of the two retinas. Diplopia (double vision) will occur if the eyes do not move together. Saccades ensure that the gaze can move quickly from one point of fixation to another so that sensory information can be rapidly gathered and responded to. Smooth pursuit allows a moving object to be visually followed while keeping the

image on the center of the retina. The VOR, which maintains eye fixation as the head turns, is a combination of smooth-pursuit movements and saccades elicited by movement of the head. The VOR is normally suppressed when one follows a moving object while moving one's head, as when watching a moving car or a running pet. Nystagmus is involuntary back-and-forth, up-and-down, or rotating movement of the eyes that occurs in response to the environment or the body "spinning." Nystagmus that lasts for only a few beats after spinning can be normal, but spontaneous, position-induced or persistent nystagmus is usually pathological. Table 13-3 summarizes normal eye movements and impairments.

The vestibular system includes the labyrinths and their mechanoreceptors, the vestibulocochlear nerve (cranial nerve VIII), the vestibular nuclei in the brainstem, central projections to the cerebellum and vestibular cortex, and the long tracts of nerves arising from the vestibular nuclei that influence motor neuron pools in the spinal cord.

The central components of the vestibular system receive information from the peripheral components. Input arriving via cranial nerve VIII to the vestibular nuclei in the brainstem is combined with information from the cerebellum to coordinate head and eye movements and control equilibrium. The central components of the vestibular system also send information to the reticular formation, which facilitates arousal and motor responses. These connections result in increased extensor tone and postural responses, activation of cervical musculature for head position, and eye reflex reactions.

The vestibular system is one of the nervous system's most important tools for controlling posture. It has four primary roles: (1) sensing and perceiving self-motion, (2) orienting to vertical, (3) controlling the **center of mass,** and (4) stabilizing the head.[14] In perceiving self-motion, the vestibular system can help differentiate self-motion from environmental motion[11] and thus compensate for misinformation from another sense. For example, if the eyes see movement in the environment, but the labyrinths register no concurrent head movement, the brain can

TABLE 13-3	Normal Eye Movements	
Type	**Description**	**Impairments that Increase Risk of Loss of Balance or Falls**
Conjugate	Eyes move at the same time to follow object moving across visual field	Paresis/paralysis of extraocular eye muscles of one eye, diplopia
Convergence	Eyes move toward each other to follow object approaching face head-on	Paresis/paralysis of extraocular eye muscles, diplopia
Smooth pursuit	Eyes move to follow image whether head or image is moving, or both	Impaired tracking resulting from acute vestibular lesions, coordination deficits resulting from cerebellar lesions
Saccades	Quick recovery phase to resume smooth pursuit after eyes slip off an image during head or image movement, or both; function of the VOR	Slowed movement resulting from CNS disorders, such as MS or PD, or deficits, either peripheral or central
Nystagmus	Multiple slow movements of eyes interspersed rhythmically by quick recovery phases; normal if noted at ends of ranges of eye movements and after spinning (for a few seconds)	Inability to fix gaze normally, resulting from uncompensated peripheral or central vestibular deficits; vertical or oblique nystagmus may result from CNS disorders

VOR, Vestibulo-ocular reflex; *CNS*, central nervous system; *MS*, multiple sclerosis; *PD*, Parkinson's disease.

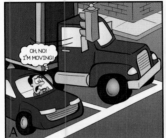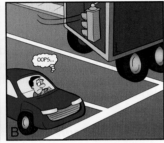

FIG. 13-2 As you sit in your car at a stop sign, the truck next to you starts to move forward. Visual information suggests you are moving backward and you slam on your brakes and brace **(A).** An instant later, information from the labyrinths lets you know you really are not moving and you relax **(B).**

abort any postural adjustments triggered by visual information initially intended to react to body movement (Fig. 13-2). By sensing, integrating, and producing motor responses, the vestibular system can orient the head and body to vertical and activate antigravity muscles and **automatic postural responses** to control the stability of the head and the body's center of mass (COM). Vestibular disorders cause **vertigo,** which is a sensation of the person or the room spinning, resulting in reduced balance when the person moves his or her head.[15]

Information about muscle length, stretch, tension, and contraction and about pain, temperature, pressure, and joint position is provided by somatosensory receptors located in joints, ligaments, muscles, and the skin. This information allows individuals to know where they are in space and to glean information from their environment needed for postural control.[16] Receptors, particularly in the feet, ankles, knees, hips, back, and neck, provide information needed for static and dynamic balance control. Disease or trauma can impair peripheral sensory receptor and sensory nerve function, causing data to be inaccurate or absent and the person to have poor balance because

they do not have information about where they are in space.

Central Sensory Impairments. Sensory information from the periphery, including vision, the vestibular system, and somatosensation, is integrated in the central nervous system (CNS).[5] This is needed because information from a single system does not distinguish specific movements and positions. For example, information from the somatosensory system alone cannot discriminate between a tilting body and a tilting support surface, and input from the visual or vestibular system alone cannot distinguish movement of the body from movement in the surrounding environment.[4] If this central processing is impaired, a person will have difficulty with certain balance tasks. For example, if one cannot integrate information from the right and left sides of the body, one may have difficulty maintaining balance when turning or performing other asymmetrical movements.

Central processing is particularly important when there are sensory conflicts within or between sensory systems. Conflict can occur within a system if there is disproportional information from the two sides. For example, if there is damage to the vestibular system on one side, then symmetrical head movements may be interpreted as turning, triggering inappropriate postural adjustments that could cause a loss of balance. In this case, to compensate, the central processing system must relearn what sensory input to expect with various head movements.[17] When there is conflict between systems, the central processing system must select which input(s) to use to drive motor responses or reactions. If one system provides inaccurate or conflicting information while the other two systems concur, then the concurrent systems will be relied on. However, if more than one sensory system provides inadequate or inaccurate information, or if sensory conflict is not resolved quickly, selection of an appropriate motor response will be difficult and decreased or poorly controlled movement, unsteadiness, **dizziness,** or falls may result.

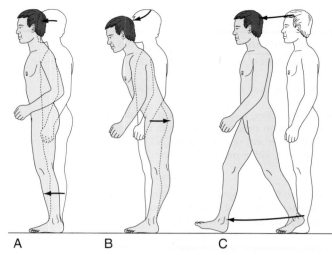

FIG. 13-3 Strategies used to maintain balance. **A,** Ankle strategy. **B,** Hip strategy. **C,** Change-in-support strategy.

Certain common environments or activities, such as descending stairs, walking in busy traffic or on escalators, walking on uneven ground, moving in dimly lit or overly bright areas, and making quick movements or turns, can also create sensory conflict. These environments are particularly challenging for individuals with limited or inaccurate sensory input from one or more systems.

CNS disease, such as stroke, multiple sclerosis (MS), cerebral palsy, or brain tumors, as well as trauma, can adversely affect central sensory processing, particularly if there is parietal lobe involvement.[11,14] This is because the parietal lobes process complex sensory and perceptual information, especially information related to somatosensation, spatial relations, body schema, and motor learning.

Peripheral Motor Impairments. The peripheral motor system executes all of the movements required for postural control. Strategies utilized for postural control are specific to the demands of the task. Although most people also have upper extremity reactions when balance is disturbed,[18] the most studied of the postural strategies for responding to balance perturbations include variations of three basic lower extremity strategies: The ankle, hip, and stepping (change-in-support) strategies (Fig. 13-3).[18] These basic strategies may be used to prevent falls during a wide range of tasks.[19]

The **ankle strategy** primarily controls body sway during stance. It starts with early activation of the ankle dorsiflexor or plantarflexor muscles followed by recruitment of hip and then trunk musculature to create small shifts in the alignment of the COM over the BOS. When someone uses an ankle strategy in quiet standing, the upper and lower body sway together in the same direction, with the body moving as a single entity over the ankle joints. The ankle musculature can generate relatively small forces to control sway through a small range of motion (ROM) at a slow speed.

When the COG moves more quickly over the BOS, moves unexpectedly laterally, or sways more than a very small amount, a **hip strategy** is used to control balance.

A hip strategy involves activation of large hip and trunk muscles first, including the hip abductors, followed by ankle muscle activation. When a patient uses a hip strategy in standing, the upper body and lower body move in opposite directions to maintain balance. If the COG suddenly shifts forward, the upper trunk will move rapidly backward and the pelvis will move forward; the arms may also flail before balance is regained.

The **stepping strategy** initiates establishment of a new BOS when the boundaries of stability are exceeded or even approached.[18] Boundaries of stability vary among individuals: A person with reduced boundaries will use a stepping strategy in response to smaller movement of the COG than a person with normal boundaries. When using a stepping strategy, the individual takes a step to avoid a fall.

The various strategies have several requirements to function well. The ankle strategy requires good ankle ROM in midrange, adequate plantar and dorsiflexor strength, intact sensation in the feet and ankles, and a broad, firm surface of support. Hip strategies require adequate hip strength and ROM along with somatosensation about the hips and trunk. Lateral hip strategies specifically require hip abductor and adductor muscles. Stepping strategies require adequate lower body strength for weight bearing on the stepping leg and adequate ROM at the ankles, knees, and hips. Central processing speed and the ability to initiate and coordinate the timing of movements are also critical.

⊚ *Clinical Pearl*

Muscle weakness, skeletal asymmetry, or joint dysfunction can impair balance and increase the risk of falling.

Central Motor Impairments. The CNS directs the execution of postural control and movement through the motor nerves and muscles. The central motor systems refine reflexive movements and initiate and coordinate voluntary movement needed for balance. They determine reaction time and movement speed and also coordinate and inhibit movement patterns. Motor planning provides timing, sequencing, and force modulation, as well as limb, joint, and muscle selection, for an activity.[4] Disorders that affect areas of the CNS that control motor output, primarily the motor cortex, the basal ganglia, and the cerebellum, can cause difficulties with motor control and thus impair static, anticipatory, adaptive, and reactive postural control and balance.[4,20]

Cognitive Impairments. Once learned, postural control functions automatically, without much conscious thought. However, cognition, attention, and memory still play important roles in balance. Attention is needed for the individual to collect information about the immediate environment. Attention deficits may limit anticipatory control by decreasing awareness of hazards. Cognitive problems, including poor judgment, distractibility, and limited multitasking skills, also increase fall risk. Cognitive problems also limit an individual's ability to learn or relearn balance skills.

Clinical Pearl

Individuals who have had a stroke, head injury, multifocal cerebral infarcts, tumors, or dementia may have significant changes in cognition that can increase their risk of falling.

IMPACT OF POOR BALANCE AND LIMITED POSTURAL CONTROL ON GAIT

Although much of the research on balance has evaluated standing balance, the same principles apply to gait. Walking involves moving toward the boundaries of stability with each step and then catching oneself with a stepping strategy. Individuals with a history of falls have more and faster sway during the stance phase of gait than those who have not fallen[10]; they also have slower motor responses and altered motor organization during gait. Several changes that coincide with advanced aging, including multisystem degeneration and musculoskeletal and neuromuscular changes, can result in responses to postural perturbations like those seen in individuals who fall. Individuals with balance disorders and the elderly often walk more slowly to improve accuracy during gait and use hip rather than ankle strategies when stance is perturbed. Without a functioning ankle strategy, the amount and direction of sway during standing can also affect progression through the stance phase of gait. Central sensory, central motor, and cognitive impairments can slow planning and execution of postural control during gait and impair problem solving when gait is challenged. With poor balance, gait speed is reduced, time in unilateral stance is decreased, initiation of swing phase of gait is delayed, step length is shortened, and toe clearance is reduced during the swing phase of gait.[3]

Clinical Pearl

Many older adults use hip strategies rather than ankle strategies, and walk more slowly, to improve accuracy during gait.

NEUROLOGICAL DISORDERS THAT AFFECT BALANCE

Many neurological disorders adversely affect balance. The problems can be compounded in older adults in whom the remaining systems typically available to compensate for specific deficits may also have problems. This section addresses specific effects on balance of PD, cerebellar degeneration, stroke, MS, vestibular disorders and multisensory **disequilibrium** resulting from peripheral neuropathy, diabetes, or other systemic illness (Fig. 13-4).

PD is a progressive disease of gradual onset caused by disruption of the dopamine pathways in the substantia nigra (see Chapter 17). Tremor, rigidity, flexed or forward posture, slowing of movements, or bradykinesia, all seen with PD, prolong reaction times and diminish balance strategies and fall prevention options. PD often causes unsteadiness and increased postural sway because of slowed response times when turning, negotiating stairs, experiencing perturbations, or completing transitional movements. Loss of balance and falling are common in patients with PD, especially falling backward.[21-23]

Cerebellar degeneration may occur in chronic alcoholics and in patients with certain metabolic, degenerative, or inherited disorders.[24] Ataxia, a muscular incoordination seen especially with voluntary movement, and dysmetria are frequently seen in patients with cerebellar lesions or degeneration. Ataxia and dysmetria decrease the effectiveness of balance strategies and impair occulomotor control, increasing the risk of falls.

After a stroke or head trauma (see Chapter 16), people often have problems with balance and falls.[25-27] This can be due to paresis, sensory loss, visual field defects, or impaired spatial perception. Additionally, brainstem lesions that affect the vestibular nuclei can cause vertigo, disequilibrium, and incoordination; basal ganglia lesions can cause slowed or involuntary movement; and cerebellar lesions can cause ataxia.

MS, primarily a demyelinating disorder of the CNS (see Chapter 17), affects balance by impairing function associated with multiple locations of the brain and spinal cord.[28] Symptoms depend on the locations of the lesions and may include vertigo, nystagmus, and imbalance with disruption of central vestibular pathways or interruption of vestibular integration. Optic neuritis may result in blurred vision and inaccurate visual input. Motor and cerebellar pathway disruption lead to weakness, incoordination, and poor motor control. If MS affects the posterior columns of the spinal cord, the resulting changes in somatosensory input will also alter postural control.

Multisensory disequilibrium refers to combined dysfunction of the vestibular, visual, and somatosensory systems. Diabetes can cause vestibulopathy, retinopathy, and peripheral neuropathy resulting in changes in all three sensory systems. Aging may also result in impairment of all three sensory systems along with the motor systems critical to postural control.[29] Common symptoms of multisensory disequilibrium include imbalance when walking, especially in dim lighting or on uneven surfaces, sensory complaints such as numbness and tingling in the lower extremities and feet, poor proprioception, poor use of the vestibular system, and poor vision.

TYPICAL EXAMINATION FINDINGS

PATIENT HISTORY

The patient history for a patient at risk for loss of balance and falling generally includes the following:
- Fall history, including number, time, and circumstances of any falls
- The type and overall number of medications
- A number of targeted standardized self-report questionnaires concerning balance and fall history
- Complaints of imbalance, dizziness, vertigo, **oscillopsia,** nausea and/or vomiting, diminished strength, sensation changes (diminished or paresthesia), hearing loss, tinnitus, or vision changes, including precipitating events, rate of onset, duration, termination, and easing or aggravating conditions

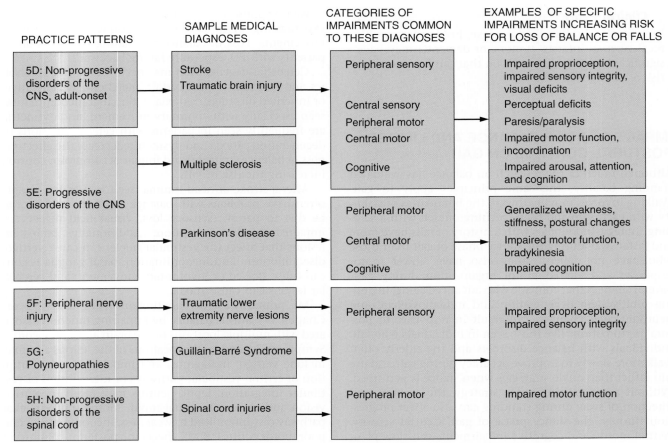

FIG. 13-4 Effects of common neuromuscular disorders on balance and falling. *CNS*, Central nervous system.

TESTS AND MEASURES

The patient history for a patient at risk for loss of balance and falling generally includes information about the following areas:

- Musculoskeletal
  - Standing posture
  - Joint ROM
  - Muscle strength
- Neuromuscular
  - Arousal and cognition
  - Cranial nerve function, particularly as it relates to the vestibular nerve; may include the Hallpike-Dix and head thrust tests
  - Cerebellar screening and equilibrium testing
  - Specific tests of sensory integration or sensory organization
  - Peripheral nerve integrity
  - Motor function—control and learning

INTERVENTION

Current theories underlying interventions for balance and fall prevention focus on the individual, the task, the environment, and their interactions.[10] In general, improving individual capabilities, manipulating the task and/or the environment, and progressing tasks from lower to higher demands can improve balance and reduce fall risk. However, the same interventions are not indicated for all patients with balance deficits.[30-32]

FLEXIBILITY EXERCISES

Flexibility exercises can increase ROM in patients with limited ROM and consequent poor balance.[33,34] Patients with balance problems and increased fall risk often have tight trunk flexors, hip flexors, and ankle plantarflexors that may be lengthened by spinal extension, hip extension in a prone position, and heel cord stretching, respectively. Decreased tightness in these muscle groups should improve balance, although few studies have specifically evaluated the effects of flexibility exercises on balance.

STRENGTH TRAINING

Studies have found that strength affects balance and that strengthening exercises, even when they do not produce measurable changes in strength, can improve balance or reduce fall risk, particularly in older adults.[35-37] Strengthening functional groups of muscles together may more effectively improve balance than strengthening specific muscles in isolation. In a group of frail healthy older adults (75 to 88 years of age), Brown et al found no correlation between the strength of individual muscles and balance but a fair correlation between the strength of functional muscle groups combined (e.g., hip extensors, knee extensors, and plantarflexors together) and balance.[35]

Although many studies report strength changes as a result of strength training (see Chapter 5), some specifically relate changes to improved balance or reduced fall risk.

Strengthening exercises for patients with poor balance and increased fall risk usually focus on the lower extremities, particularly the ankle and hip muscles, and include task specific activities such as weight shifting, step-up or step-over-objects exercises, and single-leg or tandem standing activities. Standing activities on uneven surfaces can also be used to activate and strengthen the ankle muscles (dorsiflexors and plantarflexors). Continuing exercises to increase endurance, as well as strength, should include monitoring the vital signs and perceived exertion of the patient or client. (See Chapter 5 for other types of strengthening exercises and Chapters 22 and 23 for approaches to patient monitoring.)

SENSORY TRAINING OR RETRAINING

Sensory training is intended to optimize the function of the visual, vestibular, and proprioceptive sensory systems to enhance delivery of information to the CNS where it can be integrated and processed, and then used to control balance. Although sensory training and retraining typically augment other types of balance training included in multidimensional or multifactorial training,[3,30,31,38] sensory training can prove effective when combined with limited numbers of other interventions.

Training differs depending on whether the sensory systems are functioning poorly or not at all. Poorly functioning sensory systems can be trained to assist with balance by "forcing" them to be more active. To force any one system to function better, one should minimize or provide confounding input from the other systems. Thus, to improve visual system balance functions, such as VOR and gaze stabilization, somatosensory and vestibular input should be confounded. This can be achieved by having the patient stand on a soft or moving surface or by having the patient move the head. To force use of an underused proprioceptive or vestibular system, the patient could close the eyes. To specifically force use of proprioceptive systems, the patient could stand on a firm surface while both visual information and vestibular information are removed by having the patient close the eyes or read while moving the head. To force use of the vestibular system, visual and proprioceptive information can be minimized or confounded by having the patient close the eyes or read while standing on a compliant surface.

Another common method of sensory training or retraining is to enhance the feedback provided via one sensory system until the patient learns to associate the sensation from the other systems with balance in a particular activity. For example, to enhance visual feedback, patients could watch a computer screen that indicates how much sway is occurring as measured by the change in pressure of the patients' feet on a force platform. After sufficient training, patients are expected to be able to perform the newly learned tasks without the external feedback. Visual feedback has not been shown to be more effective than other types of feedback. Compensatory strategies can be used when a system does not and cannot be trained to function. Research suggests reducing the height of shelving when patients cannot control their increased postural sway when their heads are tilted back.[9] Adding high contrast and vertical visual cues can optimize a patient's ability to maintain stability in a particular environment.[9] Compensatory strategies may also involve using environmental assistance such as lights, reflective tape at the edge of surface changes, timing of activities, shopping carts, or canes. Visually fixating on an object 20 to 30 feet ahead can improve balance in persons with vestibular problems or poor functioning of the VOR. When walking, as the person passes the object, he or she should pick a new point for visual fixation. This strategy helps to stabilize the head and reduce dizziness.

PERCEPTUAL TRAINING

Perceptual training for patients with balance problems focuses on integrating all sensory information relevant to certain environmental conditions, particularly vertical orientation relative to gravity and surface orientation relative to the BOS. Patients who lack perception of the vertical or of the surface generally need to retrain their automatic postural responses to use all available sensory information.

Individuals at risk for falls often have lost their internal sense of true vertical and may have additional trouble controlling movement at or around the midline of the body. Activities in midline that require movement in vertical directions, or activities that move in, out of, and back into a full upright position can promote greater facility with these functions. Progressive use of developmental postures can grade the BOS and height of the COG for the patient as activities progress through more challenging tasks. Exercises could include moving the body's COG in various directions and then returning to midline. Further progression could incorporate factors such as having the body on a firm surface with the eyes open and then closed, the body on a compliant surface with the eyes open and then closed, stationary and then dynamic movements, and movements with and without manipulation of something in the hands while performing a balance task.[39] The goal is to develop an accurate internal representation of true vertical and midline that is not dependent on vision or verbal cues.

Tips for Finding Vertical
- Complete a postural assessment using a plumb line or computerized equipment to determine the COG.
- Increase sensory awareness using the following verbal cues:
  - Sit or stand tall.
  - Are your ears directly above your shoulders?
  - Is your nose in line with your belly button?
  - Is there equal weight on your feet? (Two side-by-side bathroom scales can confirm this.)
- Increase sensory awareness using the following visual cues:
  - Use a door jam for a vertical reference.
  - Use a mirror and look for a vertical stripe or button placket on a shirt.
  - Use visual feedback on computerized equipment.
- Hold center and move limbs; start with arms, progress to one leg at a time.
- Hold steady with perturbation.
- Move away from vertical, then back with eyes closed. Open eyes to see if vertical was attained.

Similar progressions can help improve perception of the surface on which the BOS rests. Surface orientation exercises focus on activities performed on several gradations of firm to compliant and dynamic surfaces. The use of mats, wobble boards, Swiss balls, and variations can progress activities so that patients must use available sensory information to attain and retain balance on the progressively more challenging surfaces. Visual information can be minimized by closing the eyes or distracting vision, while vestibular information can be confounded by patients moving their head or by the clinician creating movement of the environment. For advanced activities, challenges may be combined.

POSTURAL AWARENESS TRAINING

Training a patient to be aware of posture could incorporate some of the sensory or perceptual training suggestions discussed previously but could also include COG training and postural strategy training, which focus on attaining and regaining an upright posture.

COG training requires a progressively smaller BOS for succeeding trials of activities that shift the COG progressively closer to the edge and then outside of the BOS. One study that used this approach with subjects 60 years or older who scored less than 45 on the Berg Balance Scale (BBS) and received treatment for 45 minutes twice a week for 6 weeks, found that both the experimental and the "current practice" group, who received transfer, bed mobility, and gait training, improved in BBS scores, number of falls, and a Falls Handicap Inventory (FHI). However, only COG training produced significant improvements in walking speed and quality-of-life scores.[40]

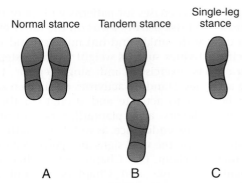

FIG. 13-5 Stances with smaller bases of support. **A,** Normal stance. **B,** Tandem stance. **C,** Single-leg stance. *Redrawn from Hasson S:* Clinical exercise physiology, *St. Louis, 1994, Mosby.*

Tips for COG Training
- Shift weight over the BOS, circumscribing the **cone of stability.** Sequence weight shifts from easier-to-harder directions as follows:
  - Forward-backward
  - Lateral
  - Forward diagonal
  - Backward diagonal
- Progress weight-shifting activities from head movements only, to trunk and limb movements that have a greater effect on the COG.
- Progress weight-shifting activities to performing them over a smaller BOS (Fig. 13-5) as follows:
  - Normal stance
  - Tandem stance
  - Single-leg stance
- Progress weight-shifting activities to performing them on more compliant surfaces.

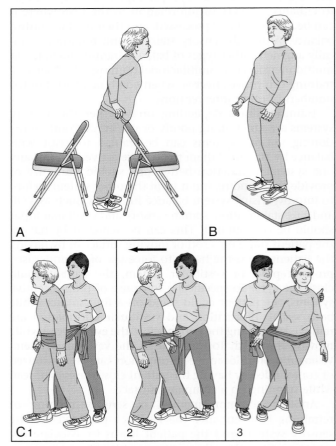

FIG. 13-6 Postural strategy training. **A,** Using ankle strategy. **B,** Using hip strategy. **C,** Using stepping strategies: (1) forward, (2) backward, and (3) sideways.

Postural strategy training involves selecting postural tasks that require each type of strategy (ankle, hip, or stepping strategies; Fig. 13-6) and then practicing the task first in a protected environment and then in progressively more challenging environments or at faster speeds.[10] Postural strategy training is designed to help clients select and implement, efficiently and effectively, the most appropriate strategy to prevent falls. By varying the task, support surface, BOS, and the intensity of a perturbation, one can promote selection of certain strategies. For example, standing quietly on a firm, broad surface promotes the use of ankle strategies to control postural sway. A narrow or unsteady surface will tend to trigger hip strategies while large perturbations that move the COG outside the BOS or cause fear of falling will trigger a stepping strategy. Careful guarding during practice sessions is particularly critical for individuals with a higher fall risk or limited mobility. Because older adults tend to require multiple steps to recover from loss of balance and have particular difficulty with lateral instability even with anterior-posterior displacement,[18] practice of lateral weight transfer, rapid foot movement, and cross-over steps may be particularly helpful in this population.

Tips for Postural Strategy Training
- Closely guard patients.
- Determine that joint ROM allows the requested movement.
- Start with voluntarily controlled strategies, then request a specific action within the patient's ability.
- Progress to involuntary strategies, and then to rapid automatic responses. Stay within the patient's ability.
- Start with easier directions (usually forward), progress to more difficult ones. The easier-to-harder sequence is usually anterior, posterior, side to side, then diagonal.

TASK-SPECIFIC TRAINING: LOCOMOTION

Locomotion, particularly gait, generally requires an advanced level of postural control. Balance during gait can be made more challenging by increasing its speed, number of stops and starts, variation of surfaces, and closing the eyes. A treadmill can be used to alter gait velocity and adding head and eye movements can increase the challenge of this controlled activity. Further challenges include walking around stationary and then moving obstacles; being in quiet or more distracting environments, such as grocery stores or malls; carrying objects; and performing dual tasks such as walking and talking.

Assistive devices (see Chapter 33) are prescribed for use during gait to compensate for certain types of balance problems. Although assistive devices may improve balance by increasing the BOS, they can increase fall risk in some circumstances because they can inhibit stepping strategies, particularly laterally.[41] Research has evaluated the effects of ambulation aids on balance and weight-bearing patterns on several populations of patients, including those with stroke, PD, and lower extremity amputation.

VESTIBULAR REHABILITATION

Vestibular rehabilitation is widely used in the management of patients with disequilibrium, dizziness, a history of loss of balance or falls, and gait instability caused by peripheral or central vestibular dysfunction.[42] Vestibular rehabilitation has been shown by a number of studies to help patients with peripheral and central vestibular disorders, although outcomes are better for patients with peripheral disorders.[42-45]

Dysfunction resulting from vestibular loss may resolve through spontaneous cellular recovery, vestibular adaptation, compensation, habituation, or canalith repositioning. Vestibular rehabilitation may incorporate all of these except spontaneous cellular recovery.

Adaptation exercises are designed to help the nervous system adapt to a change in or loss of vestibular input. In essence, the brain must relearn which vestibular signal patterns from the two sides indicate movement of the head in which directions. This learning requires practice of moving the head, which is often avoided because moving the head initially provokes dizziness. To improve patient adherence, adaptation exercises should start with minimal stimuli and gradually be made more challenging. An adaptation response can be triggered by as small a stimulus as a retinal slip, the movement of a visual image across the retina.[11] This can be progressed by varying visual input and/or head and body movement and continually reorienting to one's head position in space. Adaptation exercises can incorporate movements called X 1 (times one) and X 2 (times two) viewing. X 1 viewing involves keeping the eyes fixed on a stationary visual target while the subject moves the head back and forth, and up and down (Fig. 13-7, *A*). X 2 viewing involves maintaining visual fixation on a visual target when the head and target move in the same or opposite directions (Fig. 13-7, *B*). These exercises can be performed sitting, standing, or walking and may involve horizontal or

X 1 Viewing

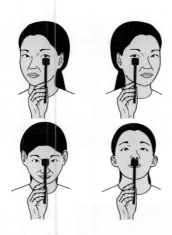

Eyes fixed on target, head moves and target stays stationary. Head may move side to side or up and down.

A

X 2 Viewing

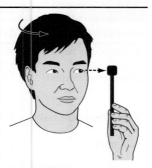

Eyes fixed on target, head moves same direction as moving target.

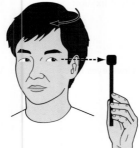

Eyes fixed on target, head moves opposite direction as moving target.

B

FIG. 13-7 **A,** X 1 viewing. **B,** X 2 viewing.

vertical movements progressing from small to large and from slower to faster.[11]

When the vestibular system is not working well, balance can require compensation with increased use of the other sensory systems, either vision or somatosensation or both, as discussed in the section on sensory training. Compensation specifically directed toward dysfunction of the VOR includes use of a number of possible strategies (Table 13-4).

Gaze stabilization exercises can be used to help patients learn to keep an image on the fovea during head movements. These exercises are designed to decrease eye saccades during head movement and to compensate by moving the eyes either before or after the head moves. Different patients will prefer different strategies, so it is best to provide situations and gaze stabilization exercises and let patients choose their own strategy.[11,46] Gaze stabilization strategies are appropriate for both training and

compensation. They can be used if the VOR is unlikely to return, as with bilateral vestibular loss, as well as in the initial stages of an acute unilateral lesion when a patient is too symptomatic to tolerate adaptation exercises. Exercises may start with X 1 viewing (see Fig. 13-7, *A*) for less than a minute, with the client sitting and the visual target placed on a plain background. Exercises can be progressed by increasing the distance between targets or the complexity of targets. Only a few patients with bilateral vestibular loss may eventually tolerate X 2 viewing.

Habituation exercises involve repeated exposure to a symptom-causing stimulus or movement to reduce the pathological response to that movement. These exercises can help with balance in patients with vestibular hypofunction or benign paroxysmal positional vertigo (BPPV). In contrast to adaptation exercises that use mostly head and eye movements to learn what altered signals mean, habituation generally focuses on whole body movements and repeats these until the patient no longer reacts adversely to the stimuli. The patient is provided with a list of functional motions to rate according to which motions trigger symptoms: none, some, or a lot.[7,11] The clinician picks a few of the motions that trigger moderate symptoms. The patient then repeats these motions with the goal of eventually generalizing the lack of symptoms to all functional motions.

TABLE 13-4	Compensatory Strategies for Vestibulo-Ocular Reflex Dysfunction	
Alternative Strategy	**Technique**
Cervico-ocular reflex	Very slow head movements, may allow eyes to compensate.
Saccade modification	Using saccades as a compensatory strategy, move the eyes then the head between two targets.
Create predictable tasks	Central preprogramming is possible if it is a predictable task.
Visual tracking	Use visual tracking to maintain gaze stability during head movement.
Visual fixation	While walking, patient fixates on object 20-30 feet away. Once past the object, the patient picks another object and continues to maintain visual fixation.
Move eyes first	When turning, teach the patient to move the eyes first, focus on an object, then turn the head, and then the body, all in the target direction.
Stop	When dizziness starts or imbalance begins, stop and focus on an object. Let symptoms pass before moving.

TABLE 13-5	Components of Multidimensional Balance Training
Exercise and Progression	**Activities**
Balance Exercises • Sitting • Standing • Walking	• Balance recovery • Using sensory information for postural orientation (center alignment) • Anticipatory postural adjustment activities • Integration of sensory and motor strategies for posture and balance control • Functional activities
Mobility Retraining • Unperturbed gait • Perturbed gait • Transfers • Stair climbing	• Various light conditions • With and without distractions • Variety of surfaces • With and without head movements • With and without cognitive tasks
Specific Exercises as Determined by the Therapist Based on Impairment	
Weakness	Strengthening
Fatigue	Endurance training
Stretching	Limited ROM

MULTIDIMENSIONAL OR MULTIFACTORIAL TRAINING

Multiple risk factors and multiple problems contribute to most individuals' falls. Therefore it can be important to target interventions toward multiple factors simultaneously. Multifactorial interventions normally include gait training, strengthening programs, balance training, training in appropriate assistive device use, review of health management (monitoring blood pressure, numbers and types of medications, vision correction, and assessment of dementia) and environmental assessment or modification, including a home safety evaluation and patient and/or caregiver education regarding fall risk.[47] Programs are targeted to the specific areas identified in the examination. Several studies have shown that falls can be prevented through appropriately targeted examination and implementation of multidimensional interventions.[30,31,34,48] These interventions have been tested in individual and group settings, with community-dwelling elderly, homebound elderly, and nursing home residents, and in acute care settings. Most of the studies report similar components to their interventions (Table 13-5).

PATIENT- OR CLIENT-RELATED INSTRUCTION: EDUCATION AND SAFETY

Even if patients have the potential for improving their postural control over time, the risk for falls may be so great that compensatory strategies will be required. Patients should be taught to stop, hold onto a stable surface, and refocus if they feel dizzy or unbalanced. When turning, they should move their eyes first, focus, and then turn their head and body to help minimize dizziness.

All individuals should be taught to identify safety hazards at home and in the community; for people with poor balance, hazards might include poor lighting, uneven surfaces, and visually conflicting environments. Compensation for such hazards might include using night lights, carrying pocket flashlights, securing throw rugs, and safely using extension cords. A home safety checklist should be used to assess environmental hazards and help educate the patient, client, care-provider, and/or family. Safety checklists typically include external factors that impact fall risk but should review internal factors to heighten awareness of risks.

Clinical Pearl
Night lights, or a pocket flashlight, can help prevent falls in the home at night.

INJURY PREVENTION OR REDUCTION

A primary focus of fall prevention and balance intervention is to reduce or prevent injury from falls. The previously mentioned interventions—strengthening, ROM, general conditioning, use of assistive devices, sensory and multisensory training, vestibular rehabilitation, and patient education, as well as environmental modification—can all be used to reduce or prevent injury from falls. Research regarding the effect of external hip protectors on reducing injuries from falls is equivocal, with some studies suggesting that these are helpful and others reporting no benefit. The most important considerations in making home modifications to reduce falls are modifications of surfaces, lighting, obstacles, and activity in the home. Adding grab bars and other safety devices to bathrooms may help reduce the risk of falls.[48] However, some evidence suggests that changing a familiar environment may increase the risk of falls for the elderly, particularly if they are used to using furniture in its current location for maintaining balance.

ONGOING ASSESSMENT TOOLS

A number of functional assessment tools are used by the physical therapist as part of the initial examination to help identify functional abilities and limitations. These tools also may be used by the physical therapist assistant to provide ongoing assessment of a patient with impaired balance and increased fall risk. Functional tools are particularly helpful because most falls occur during functional activities. These tools can provide quantitative measures of patient progress and the effectiveness of interventions and can help guide ongoing intervention.

Tinetti's Performance-Oriented Mobility Assessment (POMA)[49] is a balance test developed specifically for older adults that has since been used with a number of other populations.[50,51] The instrument has a 7-item gait subscale and a 9-item balance subscale. Each item can receive 1 to 2 criterion-referenced points. Scores from the balance and gait subscales total 28 in normally functioning adults. A score of 19 or less indicates a high risk for falling; a score of 19 to 24 points indicates a moderate risk. Balance activities assessed include sitting, rising from sitting, standing with eyes open or closed, nudge test, tandem stance, single limb stance, reaching, bending, and turning 360 degrees.

The Dynamic Gait Index (DGI)[10] was developed to assess walking under various dynamic conditions. It consists of eight walking tasks that patients would likely perform on a daily basis. These tasks are (1) walking on a level surface, (2) capacity for changing gait speed, (3 and 4) ability to walk and turn the head in horizontal and vertical directions, (5) balance for rapid directional changes, (6 and 7) capacity for stepping over and around an obstacle, and (8) stair performance. Each item is scored 0 to 3; lower scores indicate greater impairment. A score of 19 or less correlates with a history of more falls.[31,52]

The Timed Up and Go (TUG) test[53,54] combines several common functions that patients are likely to perform many times each day. For this test the subject rises from a standard chair, walks 3.0 m (10 feet) at a comfortable pace to a mark placed on the floor, turns around, walks back to the starting point, and sits back down in the chair. The score is the number of seconds the subject takes to complete the test. People who take 20 seconds or less to complete the test remain functionally independent. People who take longer than 20 seconds to complete the test are considered at high risk for falling[54] and people who take more than 30 seconds will need assistance with activities of daily living (ADLs).

The Berg Balance Scale (BBS) was developed to assess balance and fall risk in elderly adults. Its 14 items test various sitting and standing balance activities that are scored on a 0 to 4 scale.[55] A score of 4 is given if the client is fully able to perform the activity and a score of 0 indicates inability to perform any aspect of the item. Total scores below 45 out of the maximum 56 indicate impaired balance and greater risk for falls.

The Functional Reach test provides a quick clinical assessment of **anticipatory postural control** in the anterior direction.[56] A yardstick is taped to the wall at shoulder height. The patient stands with the tested shoulder next to the wall, then, without touching the wall or using any other support, reaches forward as far as possible along the wall without moving the feet or losing balance (Fig. 13-8). Most people can reach more than 10 inches. A reach of 6 inches or less indicates limited functional balance.

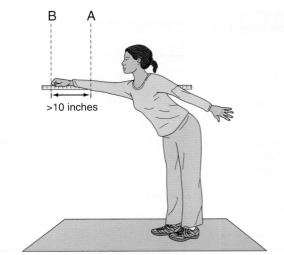

FIG. 13-8 The Functional Reach test. **A,** Starting position. **B,** Normal functional reach of more than 10 inches.

The Physical Performance Test (PPT) is a simple clinical test that takes about 10 to 15 minutes to complete.[57] In the 7-item version, patients write a sentence, simulate eating, put a jacket on and take it off, lift a book, turn 360 degrees in standing, pick up a penny from the floor, and walk 50 feet. The 9-item version also scores the time it takes to climb a flight of stairs and the number of flights (up to 4) the patient is able to climb. Each item has 5 levels of performance, scored 0 to 4, based on completion of the task and the time taken. Higher scores equal higher level of performance. Patients admitted to a geriatric rehabilitation unit were more than 3 times as likely to fall during hospitalization if they had PPT scores below 14/28.[58]

CASE STUDY 13-1

BALANCE

Patient History

FA is an 84-year-old woman who was independent in all ADLs, including driving, until 3 days ago when she fell and fractured her left humerus and broke her glasses. She underwent open reduction internal fixation (ORIF) of the left humerus, and the fracture is stable. She has a history of hearing loss and recent cataract surgery. Her confidence in her balance has been decreasing. She reports having most problems on uneven surfaces and in dark areas. She also notes problems with balance in the shower when she tips her head back and closes her eyes to wash her hair. Until this most recent fall, she has stayed active, walking once every day for 30 minutes, going out with friends, and gardening. She generally ambulated without an assistive device but used a cane for walks around the block.

Tests and Measures—Significant Findings
Musculoskeletal

- Slight forward head and kyphosis. Center of gravity was relatively forward.

- Range of motion (excluding left upper extremity) was within normal limits with the exception of bilateral ankle passive dorsiflexion limited to –10 degrees.
- Muscle strength in lower extremities by manual muscle testing (MMT): 4+/5, with the following exceptions: 4–/5 peroneals, dorsiflexors, hip abductors, and hip flexors.

Function
- Unable to stand on one leg; requires moderate assistance to get up from floor.
- Functional assessment tests: Tinetti's POMA: 18/28, DGI: 18/24, TUG: 12 seconds, functional reach: 4 inches.
- Gait is cautious, unsteady, with short steps, and forward lean. Ambulates 60 feet before losing balance and/or needing a rest. Cannot turn head and maintain path.

Diagnosis
Preferred practice patterns: 4G: Impaired joint mobility, muscle performance, and range of motion associated with fracture; 5A: Primary prevention/risk reduction for loss of balance and falling.

Interventions
- Lower extremity strengthening, plantarflexor stretching.
- Weight shifting exercises; ankle, hip, and stepping strategy practice.
- Dynamic gait activities: Obstacle course, gait training with head turns, curb training.
- Vestibular activities: Uneven surfaces, dark environment, gaze stability exercises.

Role of the Physical Therapist Assistant
- Describe what is indicated by each of FA's functional assessment test scores.
- What do her functional reach limitations tell you about her balance?
- Describe some of the specific dynamic gait activities that would be helpful for this patient.
- Why is lower extremity strengthening important for this patient?
- What would you do to increase FA's confidence in her balance?

Additional Information
For the full version of this case study, including detailed examination results, interventions, and outcomes, see the Evolve site that accompanies this book. Full case studies for a patient with a history of multiple falls and for a patient with vertigo caused by canalithiasis also appear on the Evolve site.

CHAPTER SUMMARY
This chapter discusses the pathology, intervention, and ongoing assessment for patients with impaired balance and increased fall risk. Poor balance can result in reduced activity and falls. Reduced activity has many secondary sequelae, including reduced participation and reduced fitness. Falls can result in fractures, particularly for those with fragile bones. Impaired balance may have many causes, including cognitive, vision, vestibular, sensory, or motor dysfunction. Interventions can help improve balance and decrease fall risk. Procedural interventions that can improve balance include exercises that address musculoskeletal impairments found in the examination and specific balance exercises and mobility retraining. Education in safety and injury prevention can also be helpful for patients in this practice pattern. Evidence demonstrates that rehabilitation intervention can reduce the risk of loss of balance and falls, particularly in the elderly, and thus reduce injury risk and increase participation in activities.

ADDITIONAL RESOURCES

Useful Forms
Berg Balance Scales (BBS)
Dynamic Gait Index (DGI)
Performance-Oriented Mobility Assessment (POMA)
Physical Performance Test (PPT)

GLOSSARY

Ankle strategy: A coordinated small amplitude motor sequence used to maintain balance, particularly when standing with feet about hip-width apart.

Anticipatory postural control: Motor activity that occurs before a planned movement to maintain balance when a shift in the center of mass is anticipated.

Automatic postural responses: Motor responses that maintain or restore balance when unexpected events or environmental demands occur; also known as *reactive postural responses.*

Balance: Process by which one controls the body's center of mass with respect to the BOS, whether the body is stationary or moving.

Base of support (BOS): The area defined by the outer boundaries of one's contact with external supportive surfaces; the foundation over which the center of mass moves during balance activities.

Center of mass (COM): The central point of the object or body given the current location and mass of all parts of the object or body; sometimes known as center of gravity (COG).

Cone of stability: Approximate shape of the area around a standing body, with the small end of the cone around the BOS, within which stability may be maintained without changing the base of support.

Disequilibrium: Unsteadiness, clumsiness in upright movement, increased postural sway.

Dizziness: A lay term that may include giddiness, swimming sensation, sensation of whirling or reeling, faintness, lightheadedness, or vertigo.

Hip strategy: A moderate amplitude coordinated motor sequence used to maintain balance, particularly when the standing base of support is small or sway is perceived to be too far for an ankle strategy to correct.

Oscillopsia: The illusion of visual motion.

Perturbations: Disturbances, either internal or external, to a system, as in disturbances to balance.

Postural control: Effective and efficient management of the body while holding still or moving in a particular environment.

Reactive postural responses: Motor activity used to maintain or restore balance when unexpected events or environmental demands occur; also known as *automatic postural responses.*

Somatosensation: Sensory input from the body from cutaneous and internal exteroceptive and proprioceptive receptors.

Stepping strategy: Coordinated motor sequence that may be large in amplitude used to restore balance when the COM is displaced beyond stability limits over the current base of support.

Vertigo: The illusion of movement of self or the environment.

Vestibular system: The anatomical components and physiological functions that allow sensation of head movement and head position relative to gravity and that initiate some of the body's response to head movement and position.

Vestibulo-ocular reflex (VOR): A sensorimotor connection that links the sensation of head movement (or stability) to eye movement so that functional vision is less interrupted by head position or movement.

Chapter 14

Impaired Neuromotor Development

Debra Clayton-Krasinski, Susan Klepper

OBJECTIVES

After reading this chapter, the reader will be able to:
1. Define impaired neuromotor development.
2. Discuss the core concepts of development and principles of motor development.
3. Identify tests and measures.
4. Differentiate between typical and atypical motor development and milestones.

INTRODUCTION

Children are different than adults. The clinician working with pediatric patients must be aware of the many unique characteristics of children to appropriately manage their care. Three important attributes that differentiate children from adults are rapid growth and maturation of multiple organ systems, rapid accession of **developmental milestones,** and an ever-increasing range of functional capacities. Appreciation of normal growth and **development** is needed to understand what are normal, normal variants, and deviations from normal. Knowledge of growth and development provides the fundamental theoretical basis for rehabilitation examination, evaluation, and intervention for pediatric patients. Age-specific variations from normal remain some of the best early indicators of childhood disorders, particularly neuromotor disorders, and provide the basis for patient evaluation and for planning of therapeutic intervention.

This chapter includes an overview of typical development and sequential acquisition of important functional skills. Salient developmental concepts, principles of motor development, and a model for the examination and evaluation of body structure and function, activities, and participation are also presented. Specific standardized pediatric tests are also discussed. The next chapter, Chapter 15, applies the information from this chapter to guide intervention for pediatric patients with specific conditions.

DEVELOPMENT TERMINOLOGY

Development is the process of change in behavior or capacity that relates to the age of the individual.[1] Neuromotor development is development in the domains of physical or motor behaviors. Thus **impaired neuromotor development** infers the opposite of "normal or typical" and denotes a problem with the acquisition of motor skills and/or the occurrence of atypical movements. Impaired neuromotor development is generally caused by central and/or peripheral nervous system damage or dysfunction. However, the focus on nervous system damage or dysfunction as the cause for impaired neuromotor development does not clearly express the dynamic interplay between the complex and diverse systems responsible for development. Neuromotor damage can profoundly affect the development of musculoskeletal, cardiopulmonary, and other systems, which may in turn affect neuromotor development. Additionally, development emerges from an interplay between the child, his or her tasks, and the environment in which the tasks are being performed.[2]

Clinical Pearl

Impaired neuromotor development refers to abnormal or impaired development of physical or motor behaviors that are generally caused by central and/or peripheral nervous system damage or dysfunction.

CORE DEVELOPMENTAL CONCEPTS

Human development refers to changes that occur over the entire spectrum of a person's life, from conception to death. Development is generally divided into age-related segments (Table 14-1).[3] Adolescence is described by changes in physical growth and sexual maturation rather than by age alone. Tanner's classic scales describe five stages of physical development in adolescence.[4] In girls,

TABLE 14-1	Pediatric Developmental Periods	
Developmental Period	**Stage**	**Time Frame**
Prenatal: Conception to birth	Embryonic	First 8 weeks
	Middle fetal	9 to 24 weeks
	Late fetal	25 weeks to birth (38-40 weeks)
Infancy: Birth to 2 years	Neonate	Birth to 1 month
	Infancy	1 month to 1 year
	Late infancy	1-2 years
Childhood:	Early childhood/toddler/preschool	2-5 years
Ages 2-10 years, girls	Middle childhood/elementary school age	6-10 years, girls
Ages 1-12 years, boys		6-12 years, boys
Adolescence:	Early adolescence (prepubescence): Tanner stage 1	10-13 years, girls
Ages 10-18, girls	Middle adolescence (pubescence): Tanner stage 3	10.5-14 years, boys
Ages 12-20, boys	Late adolescence (postpubescence): Tanner stage 5	11.8-14 years, girls
		12.8-15 years, boys
		14-17 years, girls
		14.8-16 years, boys

From Valadian I, Porter D: *Physical growth and development: From conception to maturity,* Boston, 1977, Little, Brown; Solorio MR, Wyatt-Henriques L: Health care of the adolescent. In David AK, Johnson TA, Phillips M, et al (eds): *Family medicine: Principles of practice,* ed 6, New York, 2003, Springer-Verlag; STAT!Online Electronic Medical Library, http://online.statref.com/document.aspx?fxid=32&docid=113; posted 8/26/2003; date accessed 3/18/2004.

Tanner's stages are based on breast size and pubic hair distribution. In boys, Tanner's stages are based on penis and scrotum size and shape and pubic hair development.

◎ *Clinical Pearl*

Human development refers to the changes that occur over the entire range of a person's life. Development is generally divided into age-related segments from conception to death.

The Committee on Integrating the Science of Early Childhood Development[5] (CISECD) generated a 10-item list of core concepts that structure the overall understanding of the nature of early development (Box 14-1). (The CISECD is a multidisciplinary committee charged to stay up-to-date on the scientific literature and knowledge about early development and discuss the implications of this knowledge for early childhood policy, practice, professional development, and research. The comprehensive findings are a highly recommended source for pediatric specialists.[6]) The core concepts particularly relevant to neuromotor development are summarized next.

Development Is Multidimensional. Human development is complex and can be divided into four dimensions: Physical, cognitive, emotional, and social (Box 14-2). Although each dimension concentrates on a particular aspect of development, all of them are closely intertwined. For example, mobility can be thought of as only encompassing the physical dimension when one looks at activities such as rolling, crawling, creeping, or walking. However, mobility may also involve other dimensions. For example, walking across a busy intersection requires the interaction of cognitive and physical, as well as possibly social, skills for the child to decide when, where, and how to proceed so that the task is safely executed.

Development Is Influenced by Heredity and Environment. Both nature (heredity, genetic endowment) and nurture (environment, personal life experiences) influence development.[5] Some aspects of development seem to be influenced more by heredity, particularly growth parameters such as body size, whereas other aspects of development seem more influenced by environment. Environmental influences that can impact development include illness, poverty, lack of opportunity or experience, and poor nutrition. The nature and quality of life experiences continuously and dynamically interact with genetic predispositions to shape individual development.

Development Reflects Individual Differences. The timing and rates of development of many factors, including height, weight, and physical abilities, vary among children, making it difficult to distinguish normal variations from maturational **delays** and transient disorders from persistent activity limitations.[5] There are many possible causes for individual differences in development, including cultural differences in child-rearing beliefs and practices, environmental factors that affect the opportunity to practice movements and skills, and gender. Although rates of development vary from child to child, there is a range of normal progression and timing for development, and a number of **norm-referenced tests** try to take into account this variability while also identifying delays in development, activity limitations, and participation restrictions. For example, the Denver Developmental Screening Test II illustrates typical variability for all test items graphically with a bar spanning the ages at which a percentage of the standardization sample passes that item. Thus the test item "walks well," which is defined as the child has good balance, rarely falls, and does not tip from side to side, has the ages at which 25%, 50%, 75%, and 90% of children can perform this task (11.1, 12.3, 13.6, and 14.9 months, respectively) on the graph (Fig. 14-1).

Developmental Influences Are Reciprocal. Researchers have traditionally emphasized the influence of adults and the environment on a child's development.[3]

BOX 14-1   **Ten Core Concepts of Early Development**

1. Human development is shaped by a dynamic and continuous interaction between biology and experience.
2. Culture influences every aspect of development and is reflected in child-rearing beliefs and practices designed to promote healthy adaptation.
3. The growth of self-regulation is a cornerstone of early childhood development that cuts across all domains of behavior.
4. Children are active participants in their own development, reflecting the intrinsic human drive to explore and master one's environment.
5. Human relationships are the building blocks of healthy development.
6. The broad range of individual differences among young children often makes it difficult to distinguish normal variations and maturational delays from transient disorders and persistent impairments.

7. The development of children unfolds along individual pathways whose trajectories are characterized by continuities and discontinuities, as well as by a series of significant transitions.
8. Human development is shaped by the ongoing interplay among sources of vulnerability and sources of resilience.
9. The timing of early experiences can matter, but more often than not the developing child remains vulnerable to risks and open to protective influences throughout the early years of life and into adulthood.
10. The course of development can be altered in early childhood by effective interventions that change the balance between risk and protection, thereby shifting the odds in favor of more adaptive outcomes.

From Committee on Integrating the Science of Early Childhood Development: Ten core concepts of development. In Shonkoff JP, Phillips DA (eds): *From neurons to neighborhoods: The science of early childhood development,* Washington, DC, 2000, National Academy Press.

BOX 14-2   **Dimensions of Human Development**

Physical	Cognitive	Emotional	Social
• Physical body growth	• Intellectual processing	• Attachment	• Family
• Skeletal	• Thinking	• Trust	• Socialization
• Muscle	• Learning	• Security	• Relationships
• Cardiopulmonary	• Memory	• Love	• Peers
• Nervous system	• Problem solving	• Affection	• Family members
• Sensory system	• Language	• Affect	• Work
• Motor development	• Communication	• Emotions	• Play
• Mobility	• Reasoning	• Feelings	• Social norms
• Postural control		• Temperament	• Cultural norms
• Reach, grasp, manipulation		• Motivation	
• Reproduction		• Interest	
• Vision		• Desire	
• Hearing			
• Endocrine			

However, recent emphasis has shifted to include the influence of the child on its own development. Children are active participants in their own development as a result of the intrinsic human drive to explore and master the environment.[3] Human development is shaped by the ongoing interplay of all participants. The CISECD categorically concludes that children's early development is influenced most significantly by the health and well being of their parents.[5] Children thrive in relationships that provide love, stability, responsive interaction, and encouragement of exploration and learning. Reciprocal influence can be seen when a child who exhibits shy, passive, and cautious characteristics when exploring a playground may be protected by the concerned caregiver. The child's behavior triggers a reactive restriction in exploration and experimentation in a novel environment. Additionally, early experiences influence the development of the brain: The brain itself is molded through experience.[6,7]

Culture Influences Development. Culture exerts a profound effect on human development.[3,6] Values, aspirations, expectations, and practices shape developmental experiences. Culture affects parents and influences how disability and illness are perceived. The influence of culture on development can interfere with interpretation of standardized developmental tests because most of these are based on middle-class, European-American norms and

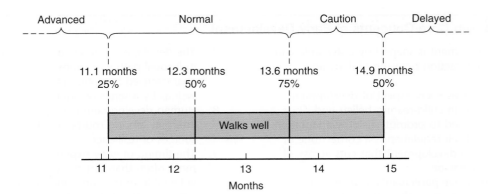

FIG. 14-1 "Walks well" test item of the Denver Developmental Screening Test II. *Modified from Frankenburg WK, Dodds J, Archer P, et al: Denver II training manual, Denver, 1992, Denver Developmental Materials.*

reflect their values. A straightforward example is the use of utensils for eating. Developmental tests value the use of the spoon, fork, and knife rather than the use of chopsticks or the fingers for eating.

PRINCIPLES OF MOTOR DEVELOPMENT

Observing movement and remembering the progression of milestones becomes easier when general principles of motor development are applied.

Movements Progress from Generalized to Specific. One of the first principles to keep in mind is that movements develop from generalized, with a whole limb moving together, to specific, with delicate specific movements of each individual part.

Movement Is an Interplay Between Stability and Mobility. In the 1960s, Margaret Rood, a physical therapist, proposed a four-stage sequence of motor development: Mobility, followed by stability, followed by combined mobility and stability in a weight-bearing position, followed by skill (Fig. 14-2).[8] Mobility encompasses the range and speed of movements that translate a body part in space and is characterized by the development of antigravity movement. Stability is the ability to maintain weight-bearing postures against gravity. Combined mobility and stability in a weight-bearing position is when there is a proximal movement on a fixed distal extremity. An example of this is when a child is in the quadruped position, the extremities are "fixed," and the trunk rocks forward and backward over the supporting extremities. Combined mobility and stability in a weight-bearing position is analogous to the term "closed chain." Skill refers to combined mobility and stability in a non–weight-bearing position. An extremity is free from the supporting surface (lower extremity is lifted from the floor), and movements are superimposed on a

stable proximal part (trunk holds lifted lower extremity). Examples of this pattern are reaching in sitting, creeping, cruising, and walking. Skill is analogous to the term "open chain." Rood's sequence seems rudimentary by today's developmental knowledge base and is not well studied, yet it provides a simple and straightforward method to categorize movement: Can the child move into a position (get to sitting), can the child hold the position (maintain sitting for a period of time), can the child move in the position with extremity support (move forward and backward, turn the head from side to side), and can the child move in the position without extremity support (sit without arm support, sit and reach for a toy)?

There Is More than One Right Way to Move. In studying the descriptions of important milestones and scrutinizing the criteria for passing standardized motor tests, one could think that there is only one typical way a specific movement is or should be performed. Take, for example, "sitting without arm support." The criteria could outline the proper posture, weight-bearing position, and position of the upper and lower extremities for this activity within a specified age range. But children can sit without arm support in many different ways, including with the lower extremities crossed, side-sitting to either side, long-sitting, or W-sitting, each of which would alter the criteria. Clinically, when planning an intervention program, it is important to encourage a repertoire of movement choices for a single motor task.

Movement Is the Product of Multiple Developing Elements. Movement arises from a confluence of interdependent processes and from constraints in the person and within the environment.[7] Multiple elements developing together, potentially at different rates, promote movement. These include the following:

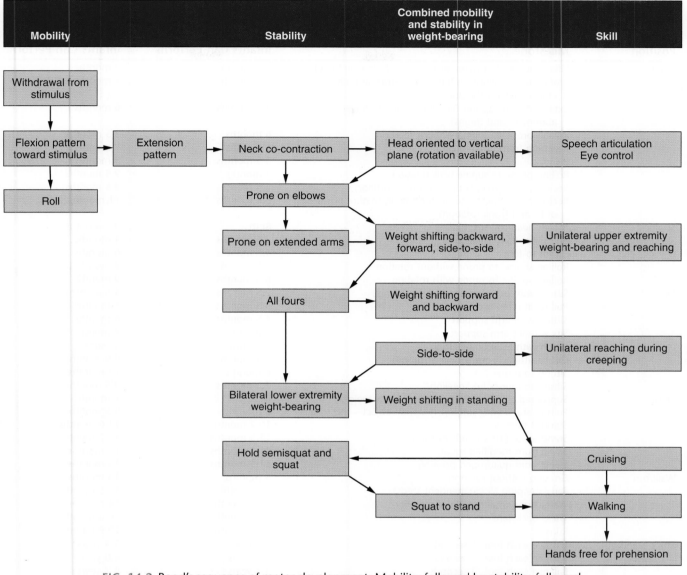

Mobility	Stability	Combined mobility and stability in weight-bearing	Skill

FIG. 14-2 Rood's sequence of motor development: Mobility, followed by stability, followed by combined mobility and stability in a weight-bearing position, followed by skill. *Redrawn from Case-Smith J (ed): Occupational therapy for children, ed 4, St. Louis, 2001, Mosby.*

- Sensation: The senses of touch, vision, hearing, and smell obtain information about the environment and receptors within muscles, skin, joints, and the vestibular system to detect body position, force, and movement.
- Biomechanics of skeletal muscles, including movement production, force production, and endurance.
- Energy, including cardiopulmonary parameters.
- Motivation.
- Cognition.
- Anthropometric measures, including height, weight, height-to-weight ratio, and head circumference.
- Perception: Coordinating movements with concurrent perceptual information.
- Central and peripheral nervous system processing.

Each of these is essential for typical movement.

Clinical Pearl

It is important to understand normal motor development and remember the sequence of motor milestones.

ACQUISITION OF MOTOR MILESTONES

A milestone is a significant point in development or a significant functional ability achieved during the development process. A developmental progression can be described for individual motor components, including postural reflexes, postural control, mobility function, reach, grasp, and manipulation. Age-related norms for important motor milestones are summarized in Table 14-2.

TABLE 14-2 Motor Developmental Milestones*

Position	Milestone	Age When 50% of Infants Can Perform	Age When 90% of Infants Can Perform
Prone	Lifts head to 45° (asymmetrically, holds momentarily)	0.5 months	2 months
	Prone prop, (weight on hands, forearms, and chest; elbows behind shoulders)	1.5 months	3 months
	Extended arm support (weight on hands, lower abdomen, and thighs)	4.5 months	6 months
	Rolling prone to supine without rotation	6 months	8.5 months
	Reaching from forearm support	5 months	7 months
	Pivoting	5.5 months	8 months
	Rolling prone to supine with rotation	7 months	9.5 months
	Reciprocal crawling (stomach touching floor)	7.5 months	9.5 months
	Reciprocal creeping (stomach off floor, mature posture of LE and trunk rotation)	8.5 months	11 months
Supine	Moves head toward midline	Birth	0.5 months
	Brings hands to midline	2.5 months	4 months
	Hands to feet	4.5 months	6 months
	Rolling supine to prone without rotation	5.5 months	9 months
	Rolling supine to prone with rotation	6.5 months	9 months
Sit	Sitting with propped arms (momentarily)	2.5 months	4.5 months
	Pull to sit (chin tuck)	3.5 months	5 months
	Sitting with arm support	4.5 months	6 months
	Sits without arm support	6 months	8 months
	Reach with rotation in sitting	7 months	8 months
	Get to sitting (from supine or prone)	8.4 months	9.9 months
	Sitting to prone	8 months	12 months
	Sitting to four-point kneeling	7.5 months	9.5 months
Stand	Supported standing (intermittently bears weight)	Birth	1 months
	Pulls to stand with support (external object—crib, chair)	8 months	9.5 months
	Stand 2 seconds	10.2 months	11.6 months
	Stand alone (10 seconds or more)	11.5 months	13.7 months
	Stand from modified squat	11.5 months	14 months
	Stand from quadruped position	11.5 months	15 months
Walk/run	Cruising without rotation	9 months	13 months
	Early stepping (5 independent steps)	11 months	13.5 months
	Walks alone (main mode of mobility)	11.5 months	14 months
	Walks backward	13.8 months	16.6 months
	Runs	15.8 months	19.9 months
Static standing balance	Balance each foot: 1 second	2.5 years	3.4 years
	Balance each foot: 2 seconds	3.1 years	4.0 years
	Balance each foot: 3 seconds	3.3 years	4.7 years
	Balance each foot: 4 seconds	4.0 years	5.1 years
	Balance each foot: 5 seconds	4.3 years	5.4 years
Curbs/stairs	Walk up steps	16.6 months	21.6 months
	Up/down curbs	1.5-2.0 years	2.0-2.5 years
	Climbs in/out of bed (using arms)	1.5-2.0 years	2.0-2.5 years
	Walks up full flight of stairs no difficulty	2.0-2.5 years	3.0-3.5 years
	Walks down full flight of stairs no difficulty	2.0-2.5 years	3.0-3.5 years
	Steps in/out of tub	2.5-3.0 years	4.0-4.5 years
Kick	Kick ball forward	18.3 months	23.2 months
	Coordinated kick (backward and forward LE motion)	—	4 years
	Runs forward, kicks ball	—	6 years
Jump/hop/skip	Gallops: Leading with one foot	—	6-7 years
	Jumps up (both feet off floor)	23.8 months	2.4 years
	Broad jump (approximately 8 inches)	2.7 years	3.2 years
	Hops (on 1 foot, 2 or more times in a row)	3.5 years	4.2 years
	Jump rope (3 consecutive times)	—	5-6 years

Data from Piper MC, Darrah J: *Motor assessment of the developing infant,* Philadelphia, 1994, WB Saunders; Frankenburg WK, Dodds J, Archer P, et al: *Denver II training manual,* Denver, 1992, Denver Developmental Materials; PEDI Research Group: *Pediatric Evaluation of Disability Inventory (PEDI) development, standardization and administration manual,* Boston, 1992, PEDI Research Group; Brigance AH: *Brigance Inventory of Early Development-II,* North Billerica, MA, 2004, Curriculum Associates.

LE, Lower extremity.

*Norms should be used as guidelines only. Clinically significant variations in rates of development exist between subgroups because of variables such as race, sex, maternal education, and place of residence.

The acquisition of motor milestones emphasizes the attainment of specific motor skills such as an infant learning to roll, sit, creep, and walk. Over time, the emphasis on milestones is translated into addressing a child's ability to function within their environment. **Functional activities** include age-expected day-to-day functional skills the children can perform within their natural environments of home, school, and community.[9] Functional activities allow the child to access their environment and independently meet their own needs. Some functional activities common to all children include independence in self-care, mobility, and social function.[10] Specific examples of functional activities include basic activities of daily living (BADLs), such as feeding, dressing, and grooming, and instrumental activities of daily living (IADLs), such as play skills and school performance. It is important for a child to perform essential functional activities as safely and independently as possible.[10]

TYPICAL EXAMINATION FINDINGS

The examination of a child deepens the understanding of the individual's competencies and resources for the purpose of intervention planning.[11] An examination confirms the presence and extent of an impairment, determines activity limitation or participation restriction in neuromotor development, determines appropriate remediation (intervention planning), and monitors the child's neuromotor progress.

Information obtained from a variety of sources and by a variety of methods can expand the understanding of the child's optimal and typical performance. Sources of information can include parents; caregivers; school personnel, including teachers and assistants; day care providers; and health care professionals.

PATIENT HISTORY

The patient history for a child with impaired neuromotor development is obtained by reviewing medical and educational records and interviewing the child, parents, caregivers, and/or teachers. The clinician should establish a working alliance with the parents and listen to their views of the child's strengths and challenges and understand their concerns.[11] The parents can generally provide information on personal and environmental contextual factors, including a developmental and medical history,

environmental demands, and formal and informal support structures.

TESTS AND MEASURES

Standardized Tests of Participation and Activity. A number of **standardized tests** can be used to examine a child's activity and participation developmental status. These tests assess different levels of the International Classification of Functioning, Disability and Health (ICF) model, use a variety of examination approaches, appraise different neuromotor components, and produce a variety of outcome scores and descriptions to aid in interpretation of the child's performance. There is no single "best" test.

Pediatric Evaluation of Disability Index. The Pediatric Evaluation of Disability Index (PEDI), introduced in 1992, is a statistically sophisticated, innovative, comprehensive, and norm-referenced diagnostic test.[10] The test focuses on what a child can accomplish and excludes information on how the child accomplishes the task. It also relies on information gathered from the child's caregiver rather than on direct observation of the child. The PEDI is intended to (1) detect if a functional deficit or delay exists, and if so, (2) determine the extent and content area of the delay or deficit, and (3) monitor individual progress and assess outcomes for program evaluation. The test can be administered to children ranging in age from 6 months to 7.5 years of age and to older children whose functional abilities fall within those expected for this age range. The major attribute measured is the ability of the child to perform daily activities independently and safely within the environment.

The PEDI measures (1) capacity, rated on the Functional Skills Scales, (2) performance, rated on the Caregiver Assistance Scale, and (3) environmental alterations and equipment used by the child in routine daily functional activities, rated on the Modifications Scale (Table 14-3). The PEDI manual contains a wealth of information that can augment the interpretation of a child's performance.

> ◎ *Clinical Pearl*
>
> The PEDI focuses on what tasks the child can achieve and not on how the child accomplishes the tasks. The test is generally administered to children aged 6 months to 7.5 years.

TABLE 14-3	Rating Criteria for the Pediatric Evaluation of Disability Index (PEDI): Self-Care, Mobility, Social Function		
Part I: Functional Skills (197 Discrete Items of Functional Skills)	**Part II: Caregiver Assistance (20 Functional Activities)**	**Part III: Modifications (20 Complex Functional Activities)**	
0 = Unable, or limited, in capability to perform item in most situations. 1 = Capable of performing item in most situations, or item has been previously mastered and functional skills have progressed beyond this level.	5 = Independent 4 = Supervise/prompt/monitor 3 = Minimal assistance 2 = Moderate assistance 1 = Maximal assistance 0 = Total assistance	N = No modifications C = Child-oriented (nonspecialized) R = Rehabilitation equipment E = Extensive modifications	

From PEDI Research Group: *Pediatric Evaluation of Disability Inventory (PEDI) development, standardization and administration manual,* Boston, 1992, PEDI Research Group.

School Function Assessment. The School Function Assessment (SFA), introduced in 1998, offers a seminal, comprehensive, and sophisticated method for examining a child within the context of the school environment.[12] One major contribution of the SFA is its extensive analysis of the physical requirements needed to participate effectively in an educational program. The SFA is intended for children in kindergarten through sixth grade.

The SFA consists of three scales: Participation, Task Supports, and Activity Performance. The SFA is completed by an individual or group of individuals who are familiar with the student's typical performance, have observed the student in a variety of school contexts on multiple occasions, and know the type and level of supports typically provided to the student. The SFA is similar to the PEDI in that items are rated on what the child can do and not on how the child performs the task. Ratings reflect the student's participation, need for supports, and activity performance compared to typical students in the same grade as the assessed child. Scores are graphically displayed on the SFA Summary Score Form. Item maps can also be generated to assist the examiner in identifying the child's strengths and limitations and to note any unusual or unexpected performance.

> ### Clinical Pearl
>
> The SFA is used in the school environment for children in kindergarten through sixth grade and consist of three parts: participation, task supports, and activity performance.

Alberta Infant Motor Scale. The Alberta Infant Motor Scale (AIMS), introduced in 1992, is an instrument designed to evaluate the motor development of infants between birth and 18 months of age. The AIMS provides a model for examining the sequence of motor maturation in infants. The test highlights what the child can do and notes any deviations from the normal pattern of motor maturation. The two primary uses of the AIMS are to (1) identify infants with immature, delayed, or abnormal patterns of motor development and (2) evaluate motor development over time.

The AIMS contains 58 items divided into four subscales: Prone (21 items), supine (9 items), sit (12 items), and stand (16 items). Each item is accompanied by a photograph(s), caricature sketch, normative graph showing the age at which 50% and 90% of infants are credited for the item, and a qualitative description of the weight-bearing, posture, and antigravity movements the infant must exhibit to receive credit (Fig. 14-3). This test is quick and

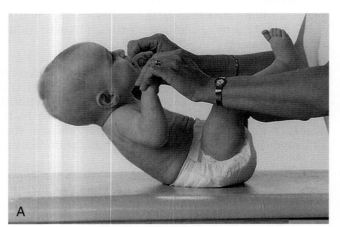

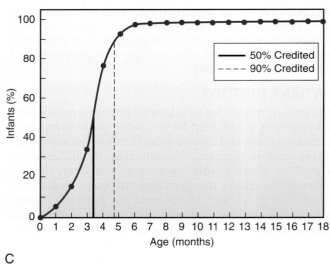

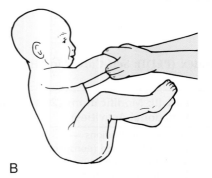

FIG. 14-3 "Pull to sit" item from the Alberta Infant Motor Scale (AIMS). **A,** Photo. **B,** Caricature sketch. **C,** Normative graph showing the age at which 50% and 90% of infants are credited for the item. **A** *from Martin S:* Neurologic interventions for physical therapy, *ed 2, St. Louis, 2007, Saunders;* **B** *and* **C** *redrawn from Piper MC, Darrah J:* Motor assessment of the developing infant, *Philadelphia, 1994, Saunders.*

easy to administer. The least and most mature item in the infant's skill repertoire is noted for each of the four positions (Fig. 14-4). The AIMS allows the child's performance to be classified as normal, suspect, or abnormal.

◎ *Clinical Pearl*

The AIMS is used to examine the motor development of children from birth to 18 months of age.

Peabody Developmental Motor Scales-2. Folio and Fewell published the original Peabody Developmental

Motor Scales (PDMS) in 1983 to provide physical education instructors with a way to assess and program motor patterns and skills within the physical education segment of a school program for children up to 6 years old. The second edition (PDMS-2) was revised and restandardized in 2000.

The PDMS-2 includes a gross motor scale and a fine motor scale. The purpose of the PDMS-2 is fivefold: (1) to estimate motor competence relative to the child's peers, (2) to compare gross and fine motor skills to determine if there is disparity in motor abilities, (3) to assess qualitative

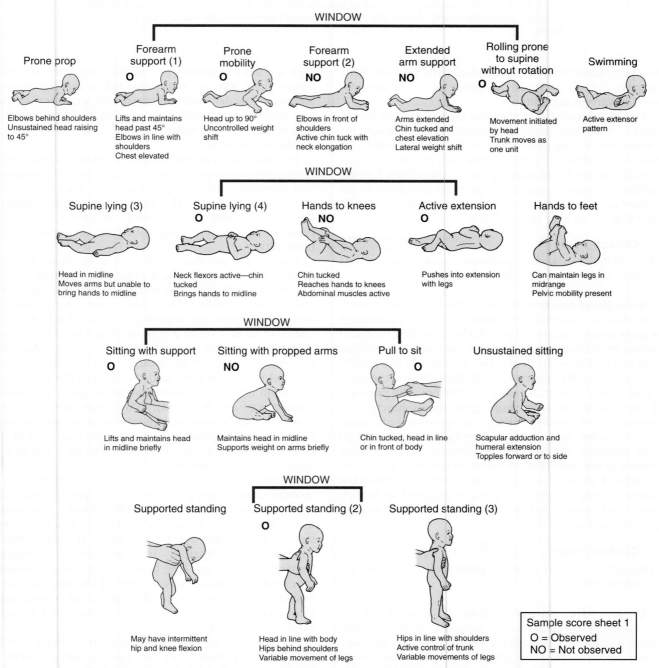

FIG. 14-4 Sample items from the AIMS score sheet. The least mature and most mature observed item is identified. The items between these two observed items are considered the motor window. *From Piper MC, Darrah J: Motor assessment of the developing infant, Philadelphia, 1994, Saunders.*

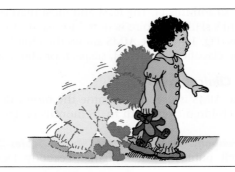

Item 36:	Standing and Moving Balance
Age:	13 Months
Position:	Standing
Stimulus:	Toy
Procedure:	Place the child in a standing position. Place a toy on the floor 2 ft. in front of the child. Say, "Get the toy and bring it to me."
Criteria:	2 Child picks up toy, returns to standing, and takes 3 steps without losing balance.
	1 Child picks up toy, returns to standing, and takes 1 or 2 steps before losing balance.
	0 Child remains stationary or loses balance when picking up toy.

FIG. 14-5 Item 36, standing and moving balance from the Peabody Developmental Motor Scales-2. *From Folio MR, Fewell RR:* PDMS-2 examiner's manual, *ed 2, Austin, 2000, Pro-Ed.*

and quantitative aspects of individual skills, (4) to evaluate progress, and (5) to study the nature of motor development in various populations.

The test manual describes the administration procedures for each item, provides an illustration of the activity, and lists the scoring criteria (Fig. 14-5). The type of instruction, demonstration, verbal instruction, or both, are specifically outlined and vary by item. The PDMS-2 yields multiple standard scores: The child's fine and gross motor performance can be classified as below average (80-89), poor (70-79), or very poor (35-69).

> ### Clinical Pearl
>
> The PDMS-2 assesses qualitative and quantitative aspects of gross and fine motor development.

Gross Motor Function Measure. The Gross Motor Function Measure (GMFM), introduced in 1993, is a measure of gross motor function. The GMFM is the first validated evaluative measure of gross motor function for children with cerebral palsy (CP). The two versions of the GMFM are the original 88-item measure (GMFM-88) and the more recent (2002) 66-item measure (GMFM-66). The purposes of the GMFM are to measure gross motor function in children with CP and to evaluate the magnitude of change in gross motor function over time or after treatment in these children. The test can be administered to children ranging in age from birth to 5 years of age and can be used for older children whose functional abilities fall within the norms for this age range. The test is designed so that all items can be completed by a 5-year-old child with normal gross motor function.

> ### Clinical Pearl
>
> The GMFM is used to assess gross motor function in children with CP.

Criterion-Referenced Scales. An array of curriculum-based, interdisciplinary, informal, criterion-referenced instruments is available for therapists to examine motor performance. These scales often have a checklist of milestones in several developmental areas and are intended for administration by multiple examiners to provide a comprehensive description of a child's relative strengths and limitations. An age is assigned at which the average typical child can successfully perform the item. Unfortunately, these tests are often misused in that age equivalents are generated, and children receive a motor diagnosis and referral for rehabilitation services based on information without proven norms.

Musculoskeletal

Posture and Postural Control. Postural control is fundamental to movement and is essential for the emergence and refinement of motor milestones.[13] Postural control allows an individual to (1) maintain a position (stability), (2) move into and out of positions (mobility), (3) recover from instability, and (4) anticipate and prepare for instability.

Postural control shows a distinct, continuous developmental progression and is a critical component of skill acquisition.[13] At birth, an infant's movement repertoire and control is limited. Over time, head control emerges, motor milestones are acquired, and the child gains the ability to sit and stand independently. The development of postural control appears to follow a cephalocaudal sequence starting with the head. Infants have limited head postural control at birth and do not develop good head control in response to positional perturbation until about 2 months of age (Fig. 14-6).[14] Over time, sensory inputs about the body's position with respect to the environment are integrated to produce motor actions that control the body's position. Vision seems to be the first step that is mapped to head control.

Infants begin to sit independently at about 6 to 8 months of age when they can control spontaneous body sway sufficiently to stay upright. Directionally appropriate motor responses to sitting platform perturbations develop slowly. Two-month-old infants show no directionally appropriate responses; 3- to 4-month-olds coordinate responses in the neck 40% to 60% of the time; 5-month-olds coordinate trunk muscles 40% of the time; and by 8 months of age, neck and trunk responses are coordinated into effective patterns for controlling forward and backward sway (Fig. 14-7).[15]

Infants begin to stand independently at about 9 to 11 months of age when they can control many degrees of freedom over a small base of support (Fig. 14-8). As with sitting, directionally appropriate motor responses to platform perturbations when standing develop gradually. In response to a backward fall, 2- to 6-month-olds show no

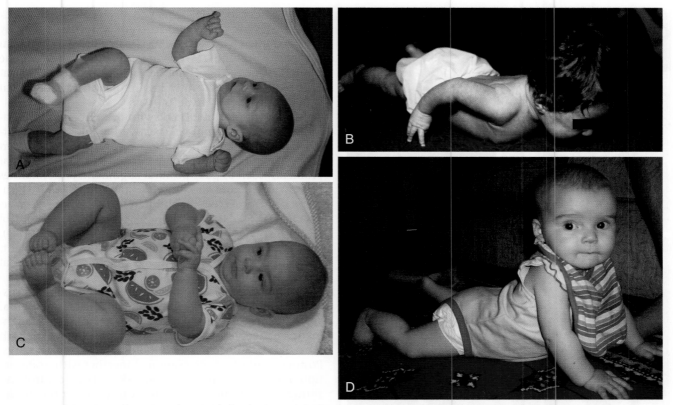

FIG. 14-6 Head control development. **A,** Supine, a newborn infant tends to keep her head rotated to one side. **B,** Prone, a 2-month-old infant can lift his head momentarily just high enough to clear his airway. **C,** Supine, a 4-month-old infant can maintain his head in midline. **D,** Prone, a 5-month-old can raise and maintain her head upright.

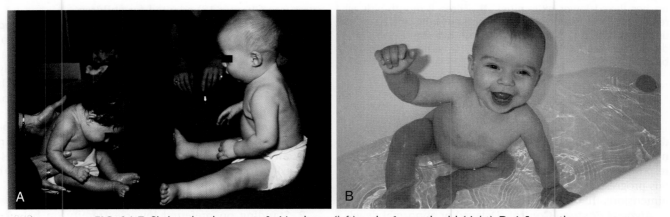

FIG. 14-7 Sitting development. **A,** Newborn *(left)* and a 6-month-old *(right).* **B,** A 5-month-old requires one hand support when reaching forward on a slippery surface.

directionally appropriate responses, 7- to 9-month-olds begin to show directional responses at the ankle, and 9- to 11-month-olds show a complete postural standing synergy pattern, with responses at the ankle, thigh, and trunk in a distal to proximal sequence.[16,17] Visual maps to muscles controlling standing posture occur at approximately 5 to 6 months of age, followed by somatosensory maps at around 8 to 9 months of age.[18] A stepping strategy emerges at around 12 to 15 months of age as an adaptation to

maintain standing in response to a perturbation. Hip strategies with minimal abdominal activity develop in new walkers with 3 to 6 months of walking experience, and a consistent hip strategy with active abdominal activity develops by 7 to 10 years of age.[19]

Studies of postural adjustments to reactive perturbations show that 1½- to 3-year-olds produce well-organized muscle responses but with larger amplitudes and longer latencies and durations than adults.[20] Postural control

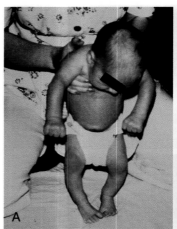
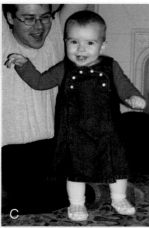
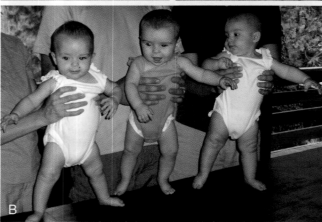

FIG. 14-8 Standing development. **A,** Newborn requires total support to stand; she bears some body weight intermittently on her flexed lower extremities. **B,** Three 8-month-olds all require support to stand, bear full body weight, and have an upright trunk and head. **C,** 12-month-old stands independently but cannot take a step forward without losing her balance.

develops gradually over time, and although progression is not linear, by the age of 7 to 10 years, reactive postural responses are similar to those of an adult. The discontinuous progression may be the result of the changes in body dimensions that occur in a growing child.

Atypical Postural Control. Delayed or abnormal development of postural control limits a child's ability to develop age-appropriate motor skills, including independent mobility and manipulation skills.[13] A wide range of problems can contribute to poor postural control, including insults to the motor or sensory components of the central and peripheral nervous system involved in postural control. Problems with sequencing, timely activation, and scaling of postural responses and poor adaptation of motor responses to task conditions are associated with motor coordination disturbances.[13] Abnormal sequencing of muscle recruitment in response to perturbations occurs in children with spastic hemiplegic and spastic diplegic CP.[21] Children with spastic diplegia tend to recruit muscles in a proximal to distal sequence, beginning at the neck and progressing downward in contrast to neurologically intact children who recruit muscles in a distal to proximal sequence, beginning with the muscles closest to the support surface. This abnormal pattern of muscle activation produces significantly less torque and larger lateral shifts of the body's center of mass.[21]

Spasticity is also associated with delayed muscle activation, inappropriate muscle coactivation and poor recruitment and regulation of motor neuron firing in children with CP and Down syndrome. Secondary musculoskeletal problems, such as poor postural alignment, abnormalities of muscle structure and function, and decreased strength, commonly observed in children with central nervous system (CNS) damage can also limit postural control responses.[13] Additionally, solid ankle-foot orthoses (AFO), used to control the position and motion of the ankle joint, limit the use of ankle strategies and distal-to-proximal response sequencing.[22]

Examination of Postural Control. Examination of postural control requires testing musculoskeletal and neural systems. Musculoskeletal constraints, poor postural alignment, changes in muscle structure, function, and strength must also be integrated with motor and sensory findings. Postural control can be examined together with examination of milestones and functional skills. Head control and sitting and standing milestones can be described under steady-state, anticipatory, and reactive conditions. There are few tests to assess functional balance in typical children and there are even fewer for children with neuromuscular impairments.[23] Common measures of postural control are tests of **reflexes** and **reactions,** balance as a component of a multidimensional test, and adult measures (see Chapter 13) adapted for children.

Adult Postural Control Tests and Measures Adapted For Children. Three adult measures of postural control have been used in the pediatric population: the Clinical Test for Sensory Interaction and Balance (CTSIB), fondly referred to as the "foam and dome"; the Functional Reach test; and the Berg Balance Scale (BBS) (see Chapter 13 for descriptions of these tests).

Postural Control as One Component in a Multidimensional Test. Postural control, which is called balance in this circumstance, is a component of the Bruininks-Oseretsky Test of Motor Proficiency (BOT).[24] The BOT balance subscale contains the following eight items:

1. Standing on preferred lower extremity on floor.
2. Standing on preferred lower extremity on balance beam.
3. Standing on preferred lower extremity on balance beam, eyes closed.
4. Walking forward on walking line.
5. Walking forward on balance beam.
6. Walking forward heel-to-toe on walking line.
7. Walking forward heel-to-toe on balance beam.
8. Stepping over response speed stick on balance beam.

Each task is administered and scored using specified criteria. Scoring criteria include amount of time (items 1 to 3), number of steps (items 4 to 7), or ability to perform, fail, or pass (item 8). The balance subtest score can be compared to an age-matched standardization sample.

A wide range of problems can contribute to poor postural control in children, including insults to the motor or sensory components of the central and peripheral nervous systems.

Anthropometric Characteristics

Range of Motion. Because of the uterine molding of the fetus, especially during the last weeks of gestation, the neonate has a strong flexion bias and torsional deviations of the lower limbs. In the typically developing infant, these resolve over time as routine handling, gravity, and muscle action elongate the shortened flexor muscles and activate the extensor muscles of the trunk and lower limbs.[25] Joint range of motion (ROM) changes significantly from birth through the growing years.

The basic shape of the skeleton and individual bones remains the same throughout life; however, bones increase in length, width, and girth because of postnatal skeletal modeling of the cartilage models. Intermittent compressive forces within a physiological range, the result of normal muscle pull and loading during weight bearing, stimulate longitudinal bone growth. The degree of modeling is greatest in young bone because it is highly compliant and responsive to dynamic strain from mechanical forces.

The shape and joint angles of the knees also change throughout childhood. The knee joint in the newborn has a mean of 16 degrees of tibiofemoral varum,[26] and this gradually decreases to approximately 0 degrees by the first or second year of life, then progresses to a valgus angle that peaks at approximately 11 degrees between the ages of 3 and 5 years. The mature angle of 5 to 7 degrees valgus is achieved between the ages of 6 and 12 years. There are slight gender differences by approximately age 15.

Atypical neuromuscular activity during the years of musculoskeletal growth can result in modeling errors that can cause joint dysfunction and disability. For example, in children with CP the configuration of the acetabulum often remains immature and the infantile femoral anteversion and neck to shaft angle fail to resolve, increasing the risk for hip subluxation or dislocation. Most newborns undergo screening for hip instability by a pediatrician.

Lower limb rotational deformities are also common in children with neuromuscular disorders and often present as an "in-toeing" or "out-toeing" gait. These conditions may result from persistent torsional deformities in the lower limbs, abnormal muscle activity, or habitual sitting and sleeping postures. For example, sitting in the reversed tailor or W position, with the feet internally rotated and beneath the buttocks encourages medial rotation contracture of the hips, medial tibial torsion, and adduction of the forefoot.[27,28] These complex conditions require careful and systematic examination to pinpoint the location and cause of the problem.

Muscle Performance. Many factors contribute to the development of strength during childhood and adolescence, including gender, age, body size and type, muscle cross-sectional area, and fiber type proportions. Strength increases throughout childhood, and gains in strength generally parallel the typical growth curves for height and weight. There are gender differences in strength in children as young as 3 years of age that continue throughout development.[29] Strength increases linearly in boys until puberty, at which time strength increases sharply, probably a result of the influence of androgenic hormones. Smaller increases in strength continue through the adolescent years. In contrast, in girls the curve either plateaus or continues to increase linearly at puberty.

Muscle size accounts for much of the age and gender differences in strength during childhood and adolescence. Changes in muscle function follow increases in muscle size, but qualitative improvements also result from neural changes, including myelination, increased coordination of muscle synergists and antagonists, and improvements in motor unit recruitment.[30]

Abnormalities in muscle structure or function may have a number of causes, including defects in neuromuscular development during gestation and deficits in blood supply, nutrition, or innervation after birth. Muscle function may also be affected by disease, immobilization, disuse, and postural imbalances.

Measuring Muscle Strength in Children. Measurement of muscle strength in children with neuromotor disorders helps to identify deficits that may contribute to activity restrictions. Observation of antigravity movements can be used to determine functional strength in infants and very young children. Fig. 14-9 shows tests for assessing strength of the neck extensor muscles in an infant.

In older children, manual muscle testing (MMT) is usually used to test strength in the clinic (see Chapter 5). Instruments for measuring strength, including handheld or isokinetic dynamometers, provide reliable results in most children. Field tests that measure relative strength, using the body as resistance, are commonly used in schools. In typically developing children, height, weight, percentage of body fat, and gender impact performance on field tests of upper body strength, including the pull-up, modified pull-up, flexed arm hang, and push-up. Most health-related fitness tests provide age- and gender-based criterion-referenced standards to determine if a child's test scores are consistent with good health.

Neuromuscular

Reflex Integrity. Traditionally, developmental reflexes are examined as part of the assessment of postural control. Developmental reflexes consist of attitudinal reflexes, righting reactions, and balance and protective reactions.[31] A developmental reflex is a stereotyped response to a specific stimulus and is categorized as primitive or reactive. A primitive reflex appears during fetal development or at birth and is difficult to elicit after approximately 6 months of age in children with typical development. A reactive reflex appears in infancy or childhood and persists throughout life. Developmental reflexes are evaluated in terms of when they appear and disappear in relation to typically developing children. For example, the reaction "forward protective extension" should appear at 6 months of age and persist thereafter. It would therefore be considered normal if this response was absent at 4 months of age but abnormal or delayed if still absent at 12 months. However, since the reported norms for age of onset for

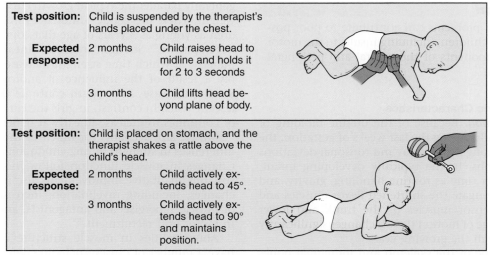

Test position:	Child is suspended by the therapist's hands placed under the chest.	
Expected response:	2 months	Child raises head to midline and holds it for 2 to 3 seconds
	3 months	Child lifts head beyond plane of body.
Test position:	Child is placed on stomach, and the therapist shakes a rattle above the child's head.	
Expected response:	2 months	Child actively extends head to 45°.
	3 months	Child actively extends head to 90° and maintains position.

FIG. 14-9 Assessing neck extensor strength in an infant. *Redrawn from Connelly B: Testing in infants and children. In Hislop H, Montgomery J (eds):* Daniels and Worthingham's muscle testing, *ed 6, Philadelphia, 1995, Saunders.*

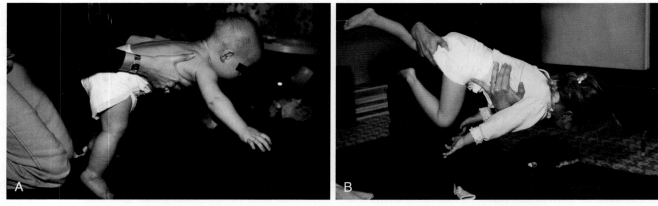

FIG. 14-10 Forward upper extremity protective extension. **A,** Normal response by an 8-month-old with arms outstretched to protect the body. **B,** Absent response in a 3-year-old child with athetoid cerebral palsy.

developmental reflexes are broad and variable, they must be used judiciously in assigning a label of normal or abnormal.[32]

Examination of developmental reflexes also provides a standardized format for observing symmetry, comparing upper and lower body responses, responses of the head and trunk, and association of the intensity of the stimulus to the size of the response and can also be useful in young infants in whom the expected movement repertoire is limited. Table 14-4 outlines reported developmental reflexes, and Figs. 14-10, 14-11, and 14-12 show responses of forward upper extremity protective extension, asymmetrical tonic neck reflex, and Landau righting reaction, respectively.

Motor Function—Control and Learning. Muscle tone abnormalities are common in children with impaired neuromotor development and range from hypertonicity,

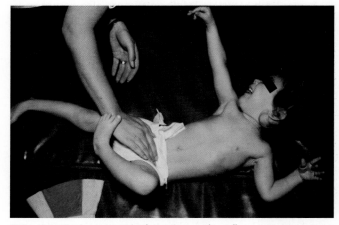

FIG. 14-11 Asymmetrical tonic neck reflex response in a 3-year-old child with athetoid cerebral palsy.

TABLE 14-4	Selected Developmental Reflexes and Reactions		

Time Course	Position	Test Procedure	Response
ATTITUDINAL REFLEXES			
Asymmetrical Tonic Neck			
Birth to 6 months	Supine	Rotate head, actively or passively, to one side.	"Bow and arrow position." UE and LE extension on "chin side." UE and LE flexion on "skull" side.
Symmetrical Tonic Neck			
4/6 months to 8/12 months	Prone, overlap	1. Flex the head. 2. Extend the head.	1. UE flexion and LE extension. 2. UE extension and LE flexion.
Tonic Labyrinthine			
Birth to 6 months	1. Prone 2. Supine	1. Position in prone. 2. Position in supine.	1. Increased flexion of all limbs. 2. Increased extension of all limbs.
RIGHTING REACTIONS			
Optical Righting			
Birth-Persists	Body held vertical in space	Tilt body: Forward. Backward. Left. Right.	Head orients to vertical position. Head extension. Head flexion. Head laterally flexes right. Head laterally extends left.
Labyrinthine Righting			
Birth-Persists	Body held vertical in space	Obscure vision, tilt body: Forward. Backward. Left. Right.	Head orients to vertical position. Head extension. Head flexion. Head laterally flexes right. Head laterally flexes left.
Body-on-Head Righting			
Birth/2 months to 5 years	Prone	Place prone.	Head extends and rotates to one side.
Neck-on-Body Righting			
Neonatal: 34 weeks' gestation to 2 months	Supine	Rotate head passively to one side.	Body rotates as a whole (log rolls, no rotation) to align body with head.
Mature: 4/6 months to 5 years	Supine	Rotate head passively to one side.	Body rotates with rotation to align body with head.
Body-on-Body Righting			
Neonatal: 34 weeks' gestation to 4/5 months	Supine	Flex and rotate LE across body.	Neonatal: Body rotates as a whole (log rolls, no rotation) to align body with head.
Mature: 4/6 months to 5 years	Supine	Flex and rotate LE across body.	Mature: Body rotates with rotation to align body with head.
Landau Righting			
3 months to 12/24 months	Prone	Hold in horizontal suspension.	Head, limbs, and trunk extend.
BALANCE AND PROTECTIVE RESPONSES			
Protective Extension: UE			
Forward: 6 months-Persists	1. Support body in space	Plunge body downward.	UEs extend, abduct to support and protect the body from falling: Forward.
Left/right side: 7 months-Persists	2. Sitting	Push sideways.	To the left and right side.
Backward: 9/10 months-Persists	3. Sitting	Push backward.	Backward.
Tilting Reactions			
Prone: 5 months-Persists	Prone	Place on tilt board in one of the four positions, then tilt board.	Preserve the equilibrium of the body under conditions of instability.
Supine: 7/8 months-Persists	Supine		
Sit: 7/8 months-Persists	Sit		Head rotates, trunk curvature,
Stand: 12/21 months-Persists	Stand		extension and abduction of limbs toward upward side of board.

Data from Barnes MR, Crutchfield CA, Heriza CB: *The neurophysiological basis of patient treatment,* Morgantown, WV, 1978, Stokesville.
UE, Upper extremity; *LE,* lower extremity.

spasticity, and rigidity to hypotonicity, hypotonia, and flaccidity. Tone abnormalities are associated with a wide variety of conditions including Down syndrome, Prader-Willi syndrome, and cognitive impairments such as mental retardation. Abnormalities in tone are consistent and predictive findings in young children at risk for CP and are hallmarks of children described as having CP.[33,34] Spasticity is the most common impairment in children with CP and is associated with limited selective motor control, abnormal and limited movement synergies, limited active ROM, and abnormal timing of muscle activation and postural responses.[35] Hypotonicity in infants may also herald a neuromuscular condition. The tonal pattern can gradually change over time from low tone to high tone. Muscle tone normally changes in the premature infant during the first year of life.[36]

It is important to examine how a child moves to guide rehabilitation evaluation and interventions. The quality of a child's movement is emphasized by the

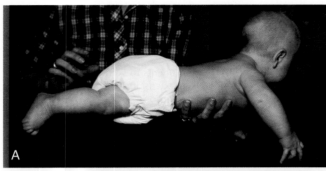

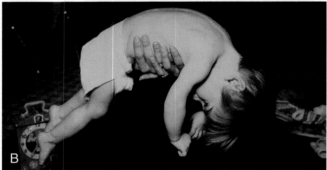

FIG. 14-12 Landau righting reaction. **A,** Normal response by 6-month-old (head, trunk, and limbs extending). **B,** Absent response in a 1-year-old child with spastic diplegic cerebral palsy.

neurodevelopment treatment (NDT) approach introduced by Berta Bobath and Dr. Karel Bobath in the early 1940s and remains important today. Unfortunately, there is no consensus on what movement components should be observed and analyzed to assess movement quality. This is further complicated by the fact that typical movements change with age; infant movement is not as smooth and coordinated as that of an adult. Movements performed with age-appropriate quality are thought to be the most efficient and least likely to be associated with future secondary complications.[37]

There is no well-accepted procedure for examining movement quality. Movement quality is generally documented with a detailed, narrative description.

Cardiovascular/Pulmonary. A basic examination of vital functions and exercise performance are essential components of the assessment of a child with impaired neuromotor development. The examination should include measurements of heart rate (HR), respiratory rate (RR), and blood pressure (BP) (see Chapter 22). Periodic examination of the child's aerobic fitness and energy expenditure during exercise is useful for planning and monitoring the effects of interventions.

Studies indicate that children with CP[38] and muscular dystrophy[39] have reduced aerobic capacity and use a higher percentage of their available aerobic function during routine activities, resulting in poor mechanical efficiency. Multiple factors may be involved, including abnormalities in structures (heart, lung, and muscle tissue) or physiological function, resulting in poor delivery or uptake of oxygen by tissues, as well as increased energy use for maintaining postural stability as a result of impaired muscle tone or motor control. Exercise tolerance may also be limited by poor muscle endurance in children with neuromuscular impairments. Table 14-5 illustrates a physical fitness profile for a 10-year-old girl with CP, using standards for the general population and specific standards for children with CP.

TABLE 14-5	Sample Physical Fitness Test Profile for a 10-Year-Old Girl with Cerebral Palsy			
Attribute	Test Item	Unit of Measure	Score	Health Fitness Standards*
Aerobic function	9MRWT	Yards	900 yards	1,480 yards
Body composition	Sum of triceps and subscapular skinfold thickness	Millimeters (mm)	36 mm	18-41 mm
	BMI	Weight (kg)/height (m²)	26	16.6-23.5
Muscle strength	Upper body: Modified pull-up	Number of pull-ups performed correctly	2	4 (minimal standard)
	Trunk: Curl-up	Number of curl-ups performed correctly	8	13 (preferred standard)
	Lower body: 40-meter walk	Time in seconds	90 seconds	60 seconds
		HR (bpm): Score as pass/fail	HR: 150 bpm	HR <125 bpm
Flexibility	Back-saver sit and reach	Inches	5 inches	9 inches
	Shoulder stretch	Inches (score as pass/fail)	Fingertips meet behind back	Fingertips meet behind back

*Standards from *Physical best: The AAHPERD guide to physical fitness education and assessment,* Reston, VA, 1990, AAHPERD; Winnick J, Short F: *The Brockport physical fitness test manual,* Champaign, IL, 1999, Human Kinetics. General standards are shown for all measures except the 40-meter walk, for which specific standards for a child with cerebral palsy are shown.
9MRWT, 9-Minute run-walk test; *HR,* heart rate; *bpm,* beats per minute; *BMI,* body mass index.

CHAPTER SUMMARY

Children with impaired neuromotor development frequently exhibit participation restrictions, activity limitations, and **primary** and/or **secondary impairments** in one or more of the musculoskeletal, neuromuscular, cardiovascular/pulmonary, and integumentary systems. This chapter reviews typical and atypical neuromotor development and referenced standardized tests and measures of development.

ADDITIONAL RESOURCES

For links to these and additional web-based resources, see the Evolve site.

National Institute of Neurological Disorders and Stroke (NINDS)
Children's Hemiplegia and Stroke Association (CHASA)
National Down Syndrome Society

Useful Forms

Pediatric Evaluation of Disability Inventory (PEDI)
Alberta Infant Motor Scale (AIMS)
School Function Assessment (SFA)
Peabody Developmental Motor Scales-2 (PDMS-2)
Gross Motor Function Measure (GMFM, GMFM-66, GMFM-88)

GLOSSARY

Body mass index: A person's weight (kg) divided by his or her height squared (meters^2). An estimate of body composition.

Delay: A significant lag in achieving age-appropriate developmental milestones. Delay can occur in one or more dimensions, including physical, cognitive, emotional, and social.

Development: Changes that occur over a person's life from conception to death.

Developmental milestones: Skills, abilities, or physical attributes specific to age.

Functional activities: Age-expected day-to-day skills performed within an individual's natural environments of home, school, and/or community.

Impaired neuromotor development: A delay in the acquisition of motor skills, and/or the occurrence of atypical movements

Norm-referenced test: A type of test that ranks an individual numerically and compares their score with a set of external standards. These tests allow comparison of an individual's performance to test scores from a defined population.

Primary impairments: Direct effects of the disease or pathology on the body's particular structures and function. Examples of primary impairments in children with CP include insufficient muscle force generation, spasticity, and hyperactive reflexes.

Reaction: Stereotyped response to specific stimuli.

Reflex: An involuntary response to a stimulus applied to the periphery and transmitted to the brain or spinal cord.

Secondary impairments: Changes in body structures and functions that are indirect consequences of the primary impairments. For example, decreased aerobic capacity may occur in children with CP as a consequence of a sedentary lifestyle as a result of the primary impairments of spasticity, muscle weakness, and joint stiffness.

Standardized test: Uniform testing procedure.

Chapter 15

Pediatric Nonprogressive Central Nervous System Disorders

Debra Clayton-Krasinski, Linda Fieback

OBJECTIVES

After reading this chapter, the reader will be able to:
1. Explain the pathology and natural history of cerebral palsy and describe how cerebral palsy influences typical development and motor control.
2. Describe the essential musculoskeletal, neuromuscular, cardiovascular/pulmonary, and integumentary clinical manifestations in children with cerebral palsy that impact a child's motor performance.
3. Understand interventions selected for pediatric clients with cerebral palsy and indicate how the treatment outcomes

address specific impairments, functional limitations, and/or disability.
4. Explain the pathology and natural history of one type of open spinal dysraphism, myelomeningocele, and describe how myelomeningocele influences typical development and motor control.
5. Describe the essential musculoskeletal, neuromuscular, cardiovascular/pulmonary, and integumentary clinical manifestations in children with myelomeningocele that impact a child's motor performance.
6. Understand interventions selected for pediatric clients with myelomeningocele and indicate how the treatment outcomes address specific impairments, functional limitations, and/or disability.

*P*ediatric nonprogressive central nervous system (CNS) disorders include a range of conditions such as cerebral palsy, Down syndrome, open and closed spinal dysraphism, meningitis, and traumatic brain injury. Each condition results in a unique combination of disability, functional limitations, and impairments that may be ameliorated by rehabilitation. The *Guide to Physical Therapy Practice* (the *Guide*)[1] preferred practice pattern 5C: Impaired motor function and sensory integrity associated with nonprogressive disorders of the central nervous system—congenital origin or acquired in infancy or childhood outlines the generally accepted elements of physical therapy management for this group of conditions.

This chapter focuses on the two most common pediatric nonprogressive CNS disorders encountered by rehabilitation clinicians: cerebral palsy and myelomeningocele. Myelomeningocele is a type of spinal dysraphism. Spinal dysraphism is also known as spina bifida. Cerebral palsy is the term used to describe postural and movement abnormalities caused by damage to the brain before, at, or close to the time of birth. Cerebral palsy is the most common form of chronic motor disability in children.[2,3] Patients with cerebral palsy present with a spectrum of delayed motor development and impaired motor function. Myelomeningocele is a neural tube defect in which the vertebrae are incomplete and the spinal cord and meninges protrude from the back. Myelomeningocele is the most severe form of spinal dysraphism. It causes paralysis and produces secondary complications involving multiple body systems.[4] This chapter focuses on the pathology of and interventions for children with cerebral palsy and myelomeningocele, applying the concepts for patient examination presented in Chapter 14.

CEREBRAL PALSY

PATHOLOGY

Cerebral palsy (CP) is not one single disease but rather a clinically defined complex of static, nonprogressive posture and movement abnormalities caused by damage to the developing brain before, during, or soon after birth.[5,6] Although the clinical manifestations of CP often change over time, these changes are not due to additional brain damage. CP is cerebral in origin and is associated with lifelong chronic motor impairments. The prevalence of CP is estimated at approximately 2 to 3 per 1,000 live births.[7] Although motor dysfunction is the hallmark of CP, CP is also associated with other disabilities, including mental retardation or learning disabilities (50% to 75%), speech and language disorders (65%), hearing impairments (25%), epilepsy (25% to 35%), and visual disorders (25%).

> ◎ *Clinical Pearl*
>
> Cerebral palsy is a static, nonprogressive deficiency of motor control caused by damage to the developing brain before, during, and/or soon after birth.

RISK FACTORS

Although CP has a wide range of causes, all are thought to be related to aberrations in brain maturation or to brain injury. Risk factors for CP are often broadly categorized according to the timing of the insult as prenatal (antepartum), perinatal (intrapartum), or postnatal. In the past, isolated perinatal events or difficulties during labor or delivery were thought to be the most common cause of brain injury.[8] However, recent findings indicate that children with CP often have abnormalities long before birth that make them less able to tolerate stresses that then occur during delivery.[9]

Premature Birth and Low Birth Weight. Evidence shows that the risk of CP is greater with premature birth (<37 weeks) and **low birth weight** (<2,500 gm). However, although full-term and near-term infants are at relatively low risk for CP, because they constitute the majority of live births, they still represent approximately half of all births of children with CP.[2]

Perinatal Stroke. Stroke before birth or within the first month after birth is associated with an increased risk of CP.

Maternal Infection. Intrauterine infection, whether established during or before pregnancy, is associated with an increased risk of CP. Certain nonuterine maternal infections, particularly toxoplasmosis, rubella, cytomegalovirus, herpes simplex virus, and syphilis, also increase the risk of CP and premature birth.

Multiple Births. The incidence of CP is higher among twins and triplets than among singletons. The increased risk associated with multiple gestation appears to be chiefly related to the higher rate of premature delivery. In

vitro fertilization (IVF) and other embryo implantation procedures are associated with a higher frequency of multiple births and CP. These risks are largely attributed to the high incidence of twin pregnancies, low birth weight, and prematurity.[10]

Birth Asphyxia. Birth asphyxia caused by alterations in the delivery of blood and oxygen to the fetus may also increase the risk for CP. There is a narrow margin between the levels of hypoxia that cause no damage and those that result in CP or perinatal death; of the infants who survive a hypoxic event, only a few develop CP. There is also no consistent association between the magnitude of the hypoxia and the degree of neurological damage. Multiple innovations and substantial research have been directed at preventing CP caused by intrapartum hypoxia, but none have been successful. The prevalence of CP has not decreased even with increased cesarean section operations and fetal monitoring aimed at detecting adverse events during labor.

Postnatal Risk Factors. The postnatal period refers to the first few hours or days after birth to the first few years of life.[11] Approximately 16% of children with CP acquire it postnatally.[12] Children who acquired CP postnatally are more likely to be black and male than children with congenital CP. Acquired CP can result from brain infections; head injuries caused by falls, motor vehicle accidents, or child abuse; or from near-drowning. The risk of neurological injury to infants and children has been reduced through a range of interventions, including the requirement in many areas for proper use of helmets and car seats for infants and older children.[2]

> ◎ *Clinical Pearl*
>
> Risk factors for CP include premature birth and low birth weight, perinatal stroke, maternal infection, multiple births, birth asphyxia, postnatal infection, or trauma.

CLASSIFICATION

CP is generally classified by severity (Gross Motor Disability Classification System [GMDCS] and/or mild, moderate, or severe), clinical type (spastic, dyskinetic, ataxic, or hypotonic), and topographical distribution of movement impairment (hemiplegia, diplegia, or quadriplegia).[13] A complete diagnosis includes findings in each domain to best describe the individual's condition. For example, a diagnosis could be recorded as level V (severe), spastic (type) diplegic (topographical distribution) CP.

SEVERITY

The severity of impairments caused by CP may be described as mild, moderate, or severe; however, these terms are generally poorly defined, with no universally agreed on meaning, and are based primarily on the individual examiner's prior experience.

The **Gross Motor Function Classification System (GMFCS)** for CP is a new system for categorizing the severity of CP and has clearly established itself as the principal classification system of functional ability for children with CP.[14] It is used across the spectrum of health professions and throughout the world. The GMFCS has been shown to be a valid and reliable measure when used by various professionals for children 2 to 12 years of age.

The GMFCS includes the following five levels of severity:
- Level I: Walks without restrictions; limitations in more advanced gross motor skills.
- Level II: Walks without assistive devices; limitations walking outdoors and in the community.
- Level III: Walks with assistive mobility devices; limitations walking outdoors and in the community.
- Level IV: Self-mobility with limitations; children are transported or use power mobility outdoors and in the community.
- Level V: Self-mobility is severely limited even with the use of assistive technology.

Each level has a different description for four separate age groups: 1 to 2 years, 2 to 4 years, 4 to 6 years, and 6 to 12 years of age.

CLINICAL TYPE

Spastic Cerebral Palsy. The hallmark of spastic CP is hypertonicity. Muscles are perceived as excessively stiff, especially during movement.[3] Children with spastic CP have upper motor neuron signs, including hypertonicity, hyperreflexia, clonus, and positive Babinski reflex; abnormal posturing of the extremities (abnormal flexor or extensor synergy patterns); and limited selective control and abnormal timing of muscle activation. Spastic CP is the most common type of CP and accounts for about 75% of all children with CP.[13]

> ◎ *Clinical Pearl*
>
> Spastic CP is the most common type of CP and is characterized by increased muscle tone, abnormal motor control, and abnormal posturing of the extremities.

Dyskinetic Cerebral Palsy. The hallmark of **dyskinetic CP** is impaired volitional activity with uncontrolled and purposeless movements that affect the entire body. Dyskinesias associated with this type of CP include athetosis, rigidity, and tremor. Athetosis refers to involuntary slow, irregular, writhing movements of the extremities, face, neck, and trunk.[15] Athetosis can impair postural control, increase latency of movement onset, and cause oral-motor dysfunction leading to dysphagia and dysarthria. Athetosis occurs in about 20% of all people with CP and is the most common type of dyskinesia.[13] Rigidity, an uncommon manifestation of CP, involves constant resistance throughout a movement in both agonist and antagonist muscles. CP can also rarely present with tremor (a rhythmic involuntary small amplitude motion).

Ataxic Cerebral Palsy. The hallmarks of ataxic CP are dysfunction in coordination, gait, and rapid distal movements of the extremities.[15] Ataxic CP is primarily a disorder of postural control and timing of coordinated movement.[13] Ataxia results from damage to the cerebellum and is characterized by dysarthria, dysmetria, and dysdiadochokinesia. Ataxia is also usually associated with hypotonia.

Hypotonic Cerebral Palsy. Diminished resting muscle tone is the hallmark of hypotonic CP. Children with hypotonic CP present with excessive joint range of motion (ROM), postural instability, and a decreased ability to generate voluntary muscle force.[16] Hypotonia is often seen temporarily during development and can be the precursor to either spasticity or athetosis.

Mixed Cerebral Palsy. It is not unusual for a child to have signs of more than one of the previously described types of CP. The most common mixed type of CP is spastic with athetoid but other combinations can also occur.

TOPOGRAPHIC DISTRIBUTION

Spastic CP can be classified as hemiplegia, diplegia, or quadriplegia according to the area of the body affected.

Spastic hemiplegia chiefly involves one side of the body. A typical clinical presentation for spastic hemiplegia includes atypical posturing, such as upper extremity forearm pronation; elbow, wrist, and finger flexion; lower extremity hip internal rotation, adduction, and flexion; knee flexion; and ankle plantarflexion (Fig. 15-1).

Spastic diplegia involves the entire body but with the lower extremities more involved than the upper extremities. Children with spastic diplegia are frequently born prematurely. Children with spastic diplegia often have trunk weakness and varying degrees of mobility and posture difficulties. Children with severe mobility restrictions may require a wheelchair, and those with moderate mobility difficulties may require assistive devices such as a walker or quad canes. Children with mild mobility difficulties require no assistance but may have difficulties performing more advanced gross motor skills such as running, jumping, and skipping. Standing and walking gait in severely and moderately involved children is frequently "crouched" and characterized by flexion,

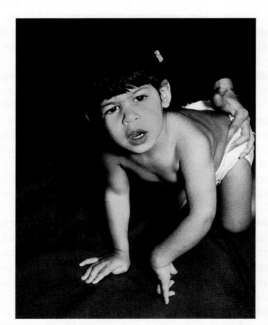

FIG. 15-1 A child with left-sided spastic hemiplegic cerebral palsy. Note the left forearm pronation; elbow, wrist, and finger flexion; and hip adduction and flexion.

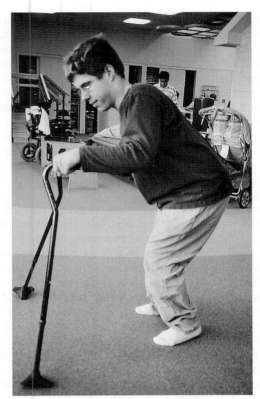

FIG. 15-2 A young man with spastic diplegic cerebral palsy. Note crouched stance with flexion, adduction, and internal rotation of the hips; flexion of the knees; and equinus feet.

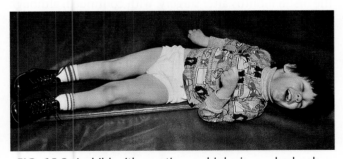

FIG. 15-3 A child with spastic quadriplegic cerebral palsy.

adduction, and internal rotation of the hips, flexion of the knees, and equinus feet (Fig. 15-2). Upper extremity impairments can result in difficulties with fine motor tasks and cause difficulty with school work such as handwriting.

Spastic quadriplegia involves the entire body with all four extremities relatively equally involved (Fig. 15-3). Children with spastic quadriplegia tend to have more severe impairments than children with hemiplegia and diplegia. They are likely to have swallowing and respiratory difficulties, drooling, and dysarthric speech. Hip subluxation or dislocation, contractures, and scoliosis can all occur in this population.

TYPICAL EXAMINATION FINDINGS

Chapter 14 includes detailed examination procedures for patients with CP.

EVALUATION, DIAGNOSIS, AND PROGNOSIS

Most children with CP, even those with severe disabilities, survive well into adulthood. However, respiratory problems, especially aspiration pneumonia, remain the leading cause of death. The future level of disability in a person with CP is largely predicted by the initial severity of gross motor disability as defined by the GMFCS. Although those with more severe impairments may need more caregiver assistance and have more restrictions in participation, assistive devices can promote higher achievement and performance, as well as lighten the burden of care.

Children with CP may ambulate independently or with support at a young age but often lose this ability by the time they reach adulthood because of the increased challenge of a larger body. Access to rehabilitation services generally also decreases once individuals with CP reach adulthood despite increased frequency and severity of deformities. Deformities are often the result of abnormal biomechanical forces and immobility that lead to excessive physical stress and strain, as well as overuse.

MEDICAL AND SURGICAL INTERVENTION FOR CHILDREN WITH CEREBRAL PALSY

A range of medical and surgical interventions available to help improve function in children with CP is discussed briefly in this section. Rehabilitation interventions for children with CP are discussed later in this chapter together with interventions for children with myelomeningocele (MM).

MEDICAL MANAGEMENT

A few oral medications can be used to reduce spasticity in children and adults. The most common is **baclofen** (Lioresal). Other oral options for spasticity management are tizanidine (Zanaflex) and diazepam (Valium). These medications are variably effective and often cause sedation.

Baclofen can also be administered by continuous intrathecal infusion (CIBI). With CIBI, baclofen is delivered in small, controlled doses from a pump to the spinal fluid via a catheter inserted into the intrathecal space at L1-L2 and threaded up to as high as T6 (Fig. 15-4). The primary indication for CIBI is spasticity severe enough to impair motor function and self-care that is not well managed with alternative therapies, including oral medication and physical therapy.[17] CIBI has the advantage of localizing the effects of the drug but is associated with infection at the site of pump implantation.

Botulinum toxin (BT), botulinum toxin type A (Botox), or botulinum toxin type B (Myobloc) can also be used to reduce muscle tone and spasticity and thereby increase ROM and improve function in children with CP. BT paralyzes muscles by inhibiting the release of acetylcholine at the neuromuscular junction.[18,19] In patients with CP, BT is injected into selected muscle groups to produce a dose-dependent reduction in muscular activity. The effects of BT take about 3 to 7 days to reach their

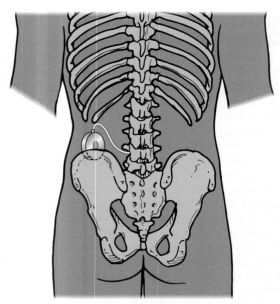

FIG. 15-4 Baclofen administration by continuous intrathecal infusion.

maximum and last about 12 to 16 weeks, during which time physical therapy, orthoses, and orthopedic surgery may be helpful. Fixed contractures can be addressed by combining BT with serial casting.

The usefulness of pharmacological intervention to manage spasticity in children with CP remains controversial because reducing spasticity does not necessarily improve function, and in some children, spasticity may actually allow for certain functional abilities. Reducing spasticity in the limbs generally improves function, but reduction of spasticity in the trunk is usually counterproductive.

◎ *Clinical Pearl*

A variety of medications, delivered orally, intrathecally, or by injection, can be used to reduce spasticity, but the functional benefits of these interventions may be limited by sedation or reduced motor control.

SURGICAL MANAGEMENT

Surgical interventions, as opposed to pharmacological interventions, generally cause permanent, irreversible changes in spasticity. **Selective dorsal rhizotomy (SDR),** in which selective sensory nerve roots in the lumbar and sacral region are transected, can reduce lower extremity spasticity. This intervention results in decreased spasticity and temporary or permanent muscle weakness. SDR was popular during the mid-1980s but has fallen from favor with the advent of a greater selection of reversible pharmacological interventions. An intense therapy program focusing on improving lower extremity antigravity strength and motor function typically follows this type of surgery.

Orthopedic surgery can alter bony mechanical alignment and deformities, control effects of spasticity on individual joints, correct dislocation or contraction, or control scoliosis for the purpose of maximizing function in patients with CP. Typical orthopedic procedures in children with CP include correction of bony abnormalities such as excessive femoral anteversion or tibial torsion or hip subluxation or dislocation. Surgery may also be used to release, lengthen, or transfer muscles. A muscle lengthening procedure may also reduce spasticity by placing the joint in a more effective position for muscle activation or by altering the balance of muscle forces at a joint. Single operative procedures were once common, but recently, single-event multilevel surgery correcting all existing soft tissue and bony deformities at the same time has gained popularity. For example, a 10-year-old child with spastic diplegic CP may undergo a bilateral femoral derotation osteotomy and distal hamstring lengthening, left psoas intramuscular lengthening, and left gastrocnemius slide all at one time. This type of procedure offers the advantages of lower incidence of recurrence of deformities than with single operative procedures and improvements in ambulatory status and joint ROM at the cost of longer operating times and more intraoperative blood loss. Postoperatively, the limb is generally immobilized with a cast for 3 to 6 weeks, after which an orthosis may be used. Postoperative rehabilitation generally includes passive ROM (PROM) and active ROM (AROM), strengthening, functional training, and gait training, depending on the examination findings at the time. Gross motor function tends to deteriorate immediately after surgery because of weakness in the released muscle, decreased physical fitness, and immobility, and functional abilities may take months to recover. Improvements are generally fastest in the first 6 months after surgery, with continued, although slower, improvements reported to occur up to 12 months after muscle release surgery. The effectiveness of orthopedic surgery in children with CP remains controversial. Outcome measures generally assess more for correction of the deformity than for improvement of function.

SPINAL DYSRAPHISM

PATHOLOGY

Spinal dysraphisms (Greek = bad + suture), also known generically as **spina bifida,** are congenital malformations of the spine and spinal cord, including anomalies of the skin, muscles, vertebrae, meninges, and nervous tissue. Dysraphism occurs within the first 2 months of gestation if the spine fails to fuse as the result of a disturbance in embryonic development. It is the most frequent permanently disabling neural tube defect with a prevalence of approximately 70,000 in the United States in 2001. During 1996-2001 the incidence of spinal dysraphisms decreased by 24%, largely as a result of increased maternal prenatal intake of folic acid.

Spinal dysraphisms usually involve the lumbosacral spine, although lesions can occur in the cervical and thoracic regions. Spinal dysraphisms are categorized as either **open spinal dysraphisms (OSD)** or **closed spinal dysraphisms (CSD)** (Fig. 15-5). In OSD, the nervous tissue and/or meninges are exposed through a congenital bony defect. In CSD, neural tissue is covered by skin, although cutaneous stigmata, such as a hairy nevus, capil-

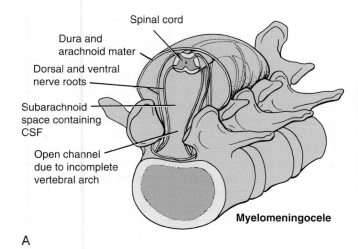

A

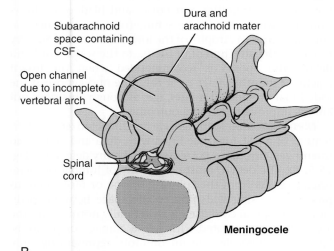

B

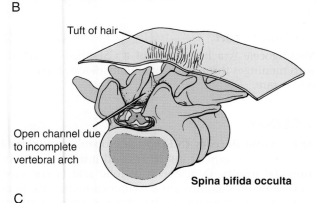

C

FIG. 15-5 Spinal dysraphisms. **A,** Myelomeningocele: An open spinal dysraphism with a cyst-like pouch containing spinal cord (myelo-) and meninges. **B,** Meningocele: A closed spinal dysraphism with a cyst-like pouch lined with meninges. **C,** Spina bifida occulta: A closed spinal dysraphism with posterior spinal bony defect and a hairy tuft on the skin. *From Larsen W:* Human embryology, *ed 3, Philadelphia, 2001, Churchill Livingstone.*

lary hemangioma, dimples, dystrophy, and subcutaneous masses, indicate the presence of dysraphism in as many as 50% of cases.[20] CSDs are more common than OSDs.

OPEN SPINAL DYSRAPHISMS

There are four types of OSDs: **Myelomeningocele (MM),** myeloschisis, hemimyelomeningocele, and hemimyelocele.[21] MM is the most common, accounting for more than 98% of all OSDs. OSDs are typically located at the lumbar or lumbosacral level. OSDs can be detected during pregnancy by maternal serum biochemical tests and ultrasound assessments.

Myelomeningocele. MM is an OSD that occurs when a segment of the spinal cord and meninges protrudes through a bony defect in the midline of the back and is exposed to the environment (see Fig. 15-5, *A*). MM occurs in 0.6 per 1,000 live births and is slightly more frequent in females than in males.[21] The incidence of MM in infants has been reduced in western countries by maternal folic acid supplementation before and during pregnancy and by parents choosing to terminate a pregnancy if MM is diagnosed prenatally.[21,22] Should MM be diagnosed prenatally and the parents elect to complete the pregnancy, delivery by cesarean section is recommended to reduce the risk of injury to the exposed neural tissue.

Shortly after birth, the open area of the back is surgically repaired to avoid ulceration and infection of the exposed tissue. Closure of the dural defect can change cerebrospinal fluid (CSF) dynamics, resulting in insufficient drainage and hydrocephalus. Hydrocephalus occurs in 70% to 90% of children with MM and may occur prenatally or 48 to 72 hours after surgical repair of the spinal malformation. Hydrocephalus may be treated by ventriculoperitoneal (VP) shunting. Intrauterine repair of MM has been performed since 1994.[23] It has been suggested that the fetal surgery is associated with a reduction in hindbrain herniation and a decrease in the need for VP shunting for hydrocephalus during the first year of life.[22] Hydromyelia, an increase in fluid in the dilated central canal of the spinal cord, may also occur in as many as 80% of infants who have surgery for MM and is a leading cause of neurological deterioration.[21] Children may have intellectual and psychological disturbances as the result of brain damage caused by hydrocephalus.

Findings on examination of children with MM may include sensorimotor deficits of the lower extremities, bowel and bladder incontinence, and hindbrain dysfunction. Children with MM differ from children with spinal cord injury in that they often have impairments of both the spinal cord and the brain. Each child has a different spectrum and severity of impairments, functional limitations, and disability. Some children will be nearly normal, whereas others will be severely involved with complete lower extremity paralysis and very impaired cognition.

> ◎ *Clinical Pearl*
>
> Myelomeningocele is an open spinal dysraphism that occurs when a segment of the spinal cord and meninges protrudes through a bony defect in the back and is exposed to the environment.

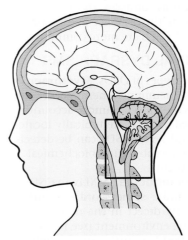

FIG. 15-6 Chiari II malformation. Note the downward displacement of the cerebellum through the foramen magnum.

Chiari II Malformation. All people with an OSD also have a **Chiari II malformation.** This malformation is an anomaly of the hindbrain characterized by: (1) downward displacement of the cerebellum through the foramen magnum; (2) resulting changes in the fourth ventricle; (3) downward displacement of the brainstem with potential for altered pressures on the lower cranial nerves; and (4) a smaller, tighter posterior fossa and a somewhat larger foramen magnum than is usual (Fig. 15-6).[24,25] The severity of the Chiari II malformation can range from a nearly normal-sized posterior fossa to a severe abnormality that can produce life-threatening symptoms such as respiratory failure as a result of brainstem dysfunction. The most common early symptom of this malformation is respiratory stridor, especially with inspiration, occurring within 1 to 2 weeks of birth. Stridor is a high-pitched, noisy respiration associated with obstruction commonly of the trachea or larynx. The stridor usually disappears spontaneously within a few days but may persist until up to 3 months of age. Stridor caused by lower brainstem dysfunction is associated with difficulties swallowing and intermittent apnea (cessation of breathing). In these cases, serious consideration is given to decompression of the hindbrain by surgical removal of the posterior arch of the upper spine.

CLOSED SPINAL DYSRAPHISMS

Many spinal dysraphisms are CSDs. Some CSDs, such as tethered cord syndrome (TCS), are not clinically evident at birth; however, cutaneous stigmata, such as an area of abnormal hair growth over the thoracic or lumbar spine, often indicate the presence of an underlying spinal malformation[26] (see Fig. 15-5, *C*). A subcutaneous mass in the lumbar or lumbosacral region can also be associated with two common malformations: lipomyeloschisis and lipomyelomeningocele. Meningocele and terminal myelocystocele are two other rare forms of CSD.

Lipomyeloschisis and Lipomyelomeningocele. Lipomyeloschisis and lipomyelomeningocele are forms of CSD that occur in conjunction with lipomas (subcutaneous fat masses) in the lumbosacral region. With lipomyeloschisis the lipoma is inside the spinal canal, whereas with lipomyelomeningocele the lipoma is outside the spinal canal inside a meningeal outpouching. The lipoma grows through the vertebral defect and attaches to an elongated and tethered spinal cord and often disturbs the formation of neural elements by adhesion or pressure. Lipomas with dural defects account for 87.4% of all CSDs. More than 90% of infants with these disorders will have an obvious soft tissue swelling over the spine in the lumbosacral region, and most will develop neurological symptoms within the first few months to years of life. Neurological symptoms are caused by tethering of the spinal cord, especially during growth spurts, and compression that results from progressive deposition of fat, especially during periods of rapid weight gain. Clinical manifestations include deformity and weakness of one or both lower extremities and bowel and bladder dysfunction. The weakness may be symmetrical or asymmetrical and may result in atrophy of the lower extremities. Surgery to release the attachment of the fat to the spinal cord and debulk the lipoma is recommended when the infant reaches 2 months of age or at the time of diagnosis if the individual presents at a later age, although this does not always improve functional outcome.

Meningocele. Meningocele is characterized by herniation of a CSF-filled sac lined with dura and arachnoid (meninges) through a posterior spinal bony defect (see Fig. 15-5, *B*). The deficit, most commonly of lumbar or sacral origin, results from the splitting of one or more spinous processes causing widening of the space between pedicles.[27] The spinal cord itself is structurally normal, and the lesion is not associated with nerve damage or paralysis. Spinal meningoceles are uncommon, representing only 2.4% of all CSDs.

> ### Clinical Pearl
>
> Meningocele is a herniation of a CSF-filled sac lined with meninges through a spinal bony defect. Meningocele is rare.

ETIOLOGY

Neural tube defects (NTDs) are probably caused by a combination of genetic influences and intrauterine environmental insults. Deficiencies in folic acid (a common water-soluble B vitamin) are a well-documented cause of NTDs, and supplemental folate before conception has been shown to reduce the recurrence rate of NTDs. A number of medications, as well as alcohol, are known to increase the risk of NTDs in humans.

PRENATAL TESTING AND PREVENTION

It is estimated that 50% to 70% of spinal dysraphisms can be prevented if a woman consumes sufficient folic acid (400 μg daily) before conception and throughout the first trimester of pregnancy.[28] Therefore the United States Public Health Service recommends that all women of reproductive age consume 400 μg of folic acid daily. Additionally, a healthy diet rich in folic acid that emphasizes fresh fruits, green leafy vegetables (spinach, broccoli, and asparagus), orange juice, enriched whole grain foods, and fortified cereals is recommended. In January 1998, all enriched cereal grain products were fortified with folic acid by mandate of the Food and Drug Administration (FDA).[29] After folic acid fortification, spinal dysraphism incidence decreased by 24% and anencephaly incidence decreased by 21%.[23]

Early intrauterine detection of spinal dysraphism followed by pregnancy termination is the only other option for preventing the birth of children with spinal dysraphisms. The majority of NTDs occur in families with no prior history of birth defects, thus screening tests are used to identify individuals at sufficient risk to warrant further evaluation. A blood test can be performed between 15 to 22 weeks of pregnancy to check for abnormalities common with NTDs.[30] If an elevated serum level is detected, the fetus is then evaluated for NTDs by targeted ultrasound. OSDs, anencephaly, and other cranial defects are usually readily visualized. When the diagnosis by ultrasound is uncertain, amniocentesis is performed and the amniotic fluid is tested. CSDs cannot be detected by maternal serum or amniotic fluid tests.

TYPICAL EXAMINATION FINDINGS

PATIENT HISTORY

Children with MM present with a broad spectrum of impairments, functional limitations, and disabilities. The nonprogressive spinal cord injury preferred practice pattern 5H of the *Guide*[1] can serve as a template for physical therapy practice for children with MM (see Chapter 20). However, children with MM differ substantially from children with spinal cord injury because of the potential multifocal involvement of the CNS, including not only the spinal cord but also the brain and the brainstem. The complex and challenging problems of MM require a multidisciplinary team approach and age-specific, life-long medical and rehabilitation management. The impairments in individuals with MM include paralysis, musculoskeletal deformities, sensory deficits, cranial nerve deficits, cognitive and language dysfunction, visuoperceptual deficits, seizures, neurogenic bowel and bladder, osteoporosis, obesity, and skin breakdown. Ongoing, objective monitoring is essential for proper medical management as the degree of impairment may increase over time.

TESTS AND MEASURES
Musculoskeletal

Posture. Spinal and lower extremity deformities and joint contractures frequently occur in individuals with MM.[4] A combination of hip flexion, adduction, and internal rotation contractures leading to hip subluxation or dislocation is common. Many of the musculoskeletal deformities are present at birth and are exacerbated by the effects of gravity as the child grows.[31] Musculoskeletal deformities observed in MM may result from an imbalance between muscle groups; the effect of stress, posture, and gravity; lack of mobility; and coexisting congenital malformations.

Patients with MM commonly have musculoskeletal deformities in all lower extremity joints and the spine.

These deformities can affect activities, especially in sitting and standing, and can alter postural control mechanisms. Foot deformities occur in 60% to 90% of children with low level MM,[32] and 41% of children with L4-L5 spinal lesions have calcaneus deformities. This is caused by strong ankle dorsiflexion from the anterior tibialis and toe extensors with weak or absent plantarflexion resulting from denervation of the toe flexors and the gastrocnemius/soleus group. Surgically transferring the tibialis anterior muscle to the calcaneus can improve this deformity, with the best outcomes occurring if the surgery is performed when the child is 4 to 7 years of age.[25] Lower sacral lesions can result in cavus foot deformities. When the deformity is mild, orthotic shoe inserts may assist with balance and comfort; however, for more severe cases, metatarsal osteotomies or triple arthrodesis of the hindfoot may be required.

Knee contractures, in both flexion and extension, are also common in this population and are seen with all levels of cord involvement. Knee flexion contractures occur in children who primarily use a wheelchair for mobility. Knee extension contractures occur after periods of immobilization in bed necessitated by pressure ulcers or surgical procedures. Up to a quarter of young to middle-aged adults with MM report chronic knee pain or have instability.[25]

Hip dislocations are seen in about a quarter to a third of individuals with thoracic to L2 level lesions, in up to half of those with L4 level lesions, and infrequently with lower lesions. It is uncommon for hips that are stable through the first decade of life to subsequently dislocate. Hip dislocations do not usually cause pain or interfere with seating, and surgical hip reduction is not a requirement for ambulation in children with MM.[25] Surgical management of hip dislocations differs among surgeons and medical centers and may be based on whether the dislocation is unilateral or bilateral, where the spinal lesion is located, and the strength of the quadriceps muscles. Potential adverse outcomes from such surgeries include postoperative contractures (stiff hip) that can affect seating, wound complications, and redislocation.

The spinal deformities most frequently associated with MM are scoliosis, kyphosis, and lordosis (Fig. 15-7) (see Chapter 4). The obvious malformation of vertebrae at the site of the lesion, hemivertebrae, and their corresponding ribs contribute to spinal instability. A lumbar kyphosis may also be present as a result of the original deformity.[31] Scoliosis may be present at birth as a result of the vertebral abnormalities or may be acquired later because of muscle imbalance. Progressive scoliosis is one of the most severe complications of MM.[31] Scoliosis frequently occurs in children with higher spinal lesions, and curves tend to progress with age.[4] Excessive lordosis or lordoscoliosis is common in the adolescent and is associated with hip flexion deformities and a large spinal defect. Spinal orthoses, a custom molded thoracolumbosacral orthosis (TLSO) or total contact body jacket, may support the spine during growth or after surgical spinal procedures (see Chapter 34).

An uncorrected postural deformity can cause joint contractures and deformities, muscle weakness, poor joint alignment, and musculoskeletal pain, ultimately leading

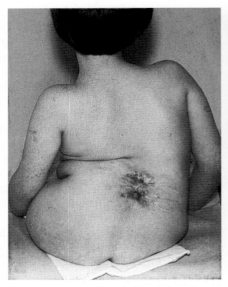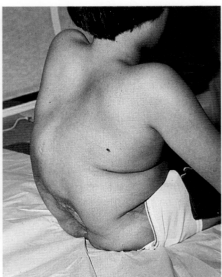

FIG. 15-7 Musculoskeletal deformities in patients with myelomeningocele. Note scoliosis and kyphosis. *From Hinderer KA, Hinderer SR, Shurtleff DB: Myelodysplasia. In Campbell S, Vander Linden D, Palisano RJ (eds): Physical therapy for children, ed 3, St. Louis, 2006, Saunders.*

to functional limitations.[4] Additionally, musculoskeletal deformities can adversely affect positioning, body image, sitting and standing weight bearing, activities of daily living (ADLs), energy expenditure, and mobility throughout the lifespan.[4]

Management of musculoskeletal deformities associated with MM requires good coordination between all members of the rehabilitation team, including the physical therapist (PT) and physical therapist assistant (PTA), occupational therapist (OT), orthotist, and orthopedic surgeon. Interventions are directed at decreasing the impact of congenital malformations, when possible, and preventing the development of secondary deformities. A regular, diligent program combines positioning and handling, PROM exercises, stretching, adaptive functional training, and parent education and instruction in following through with these activities when away from therapy. Older children with MM must collaborate in and become responsible for their own care once they understand the program.

Clinical Pearl

An uncorrected postural deformity can cause joint contractures, weakness, poor joint alignment, and pain, ultimately leading to functional limitations.

Anthropometric Characteristics

Osteoporosis. Osteoporosis can occur in children with MM. Paralysis, disuse, immobility, and decreased loading of long bones of the lower extremities contribute to decreased bone mineral density and increased risk of osteoporotic fractures. Fractures can occur after minor, painless trauma (as a result of sensory deficit); postsurgical immobilization; or prolonged bed rest for skin breakdown.[31] There is often redness and swelling around the fracture site, but the child will not complain of pain because of a lack of sensation. A passive weight-bearing standing program does not seem to decrease the risk of fractures in

children with MM, probably because maintenance of bone density depends on torque generated from volitional muscle activity.[4,32] Nonetheless, upright positioning and mobility is important, and restricting physical activity for fear of a fracture is not indicated.[4]

Obesity. About two-thirds of children with MM are significantly overweight.[33] Children with MM, especially those with higher level lesions (thoracic to L2), are at increased risk for obesity because of decreased physical activity and decreased lower extremity muscle mass. To help control body weight the clinician can help the child find age-appropriate physical activities that they can perform and enjoy. A physical fitness program tailored to the needs of the individual child can be developed and implemented at home and/or at school.

Muscle Performance. The most obvious impairment of MM is paralysis of the lower extremities, paraplegia, that results from the spinal cord malformation.[4] Upper extremity weakness can also occur with lesions in the cervical spine. Patients with complete cord transections have normal function down to a specific spinal level, below which there is flaccid paralysis, loss of sensation, and absent reflexes. Incomplete lesions present with mixed upper and lower motor findings, spasticity, and flaccidity. Skip lesions manifest either with isolated muscle function below the last functional level or with inadequate muscle strength of muscle groups that have innervation higher than the lowest functioning group. Children with MM may also present with asymmetrical signs (right side differing from the left side) and with both upper and lower motor neuron findings that change over time. They may also have discordant motor and sensory levels.[31] The International Myelodysplasia Study Group (IMSG) provides criteria for assigning motor levels from manual muscle test results.[34] The motor level is the lowest intact functional neuromuscular segment, with segments below this level not being intact. Table 15-1 shows the motor levels and

TABLE 15-1	Motor Levels and Commonly Associated Muscle Dysfunctions in Children with Myelomeningocele			

Motor Level	Muscle Function	Musculoskeletal Deformities	Mobility Options	Equipment Needs
T10	*Function:* Neck, upper extremity, shoulder girdle, upper trunk musculature *Absent or weak (>grade 3):* Weak lower trunk musculature No volitional lower extremity movements	Kyphoscoliosis; congenital hip subluxation or dislocation, often bilateral; hip abduction and external rotation contractures; club feet	Exercise ambulation Household (short distances) ambulation in young children Wheeled mobility for functional household and community	Parapodium, THKAO, TLSO, night splints
T12	*Function:* Some pelvic control in supine and sitting (abdominals or paraspinal muscles) *Absent or weak (>grade 3):* Hip hiking (quadratus lumborum, grade 2)			
L2	*Function as above plus:* Hip hiking Hip flexion (iliopsoas, sartorius, grade 3 or better) Hip adduction (grade 3 or better)	Congenital hip subluxation or dislocation (L1, L2), scoliosis, calcaneus-valgus, hip flexion contracture	Exercise ambulation Household (short distances) ambulation in young children Wheeled mobility for functional household and community	Parapodium, THKAO, RGO, KAFO, upper extremity support (crutches, walker)
L3	*Function as above plus:* Strong hip flexion and adduction Some knee extension (quadriceps; grade 3 or better)	Congenital hip subluxation or dislocation (L1, L2), scoliosis, calcaneus-valgus, hip flexion contracture	Household and community (short distance) ambulation Wheeled mobility for community	RGO or HKAFOs, upper extremity support (forearm crutches)
L4	*Function as above plus:* Stronger knee extension (medial hamstrings; grade 3 or better) Some ankle dorsiflexion and inversion (tibialis anterior; grade 3 or better) Weak peroneus tertius	Calcaneal foot deformities, ankle-knee valgus deformities	Household and community ambulation Wheeled mobility for distance, sports, etc	Standard or ground reaction force (AFO) or KAFOs RGO Upper extremity support (crutches)
L5	*Function as above plus:* Stronger dorsiflexion with inversion Stronger knee flexion (lateral hamstring; grade 3 or better) Plus one of the following: • Stronger plantarflexion with inversion (peroneus tertius; grade 4 or better) • Tibialis posterior (grade 3 or better) • Weak hip extension and abduction (gluteus minimus; grade 2)	Calcaneal foot deformities, hindfoot valgus, late hip dislocation, lumbar lordosis	Household and community ambulation Wheeled mobility for distance, sports, etc	Standard or ground reaction force AFO Bilateral upper extremity support
S1	*Function as above plus:* At least 2 of the following: • Improved hip stability • Gastrocnemius/soleus (grade 2 or better) • Gluteus medius (grade 3 or better) • Gluteus maximus (grade 2 or better)	Calcaneal varus	Community ambulation	AFO, SMO, or shoe insert for proper foot alignment and/or medial/lateral ankle stability
S2	*Function as above plus:* Gastrocnemius/soleus (grade 3 or better) Gluteus medius and maximus (grade 4 or better)	Toe-clawing	Community ambulation	AFO, SMO, or shoe insert for proper foot alignment and/or medial/lateral ankle stability
S2-S3	All muscles grade 5 except for one or two groups with grade 4	None	Community ambulation	AFO, SMO, or shoe insert for proper foot alignment and/or medial/lateral ankle stability

THKAO, Thoracic hip-knee-ankle-foot orthoses; *TLSO,* thoracolumbosacral body orthoses; *KAFO,* knee-ankle-foot orthoses; *AFO,* ankle-foot orthoses; *SMO,* supramalleolar orthoses; *RGO,* reciprocating gait orthoses; *HKAFO,* hip-knee-ankle-foot orthoses.

commonly associated muscle dysfunctions observed in children with MM.

Muscle strength is tested to determine the extent of paralysis; however, the testing method varies according to the child's age and cognitive ability. Detailed muscle testing should be performed every 6 months to 1 year and before and after any surgical procedure.[31]

Neuromuscular

Arousal, Attention, and Cognition. Specific and general learning problems and mental retardation are commonly associated with MM. These have a range of causes, including complications of untimely treatment of hydrocephalus, cerebral infection from an infected shunt, and prenatal hydrocephalus.[35,36] Approximately three-quarters of children with MM without hydrocephalus or with uncomplicated hydrocephalus have intelligence within the normal range.[37] Children who have had significant CNS infections tend to have lower intelligence than those who have not and intelligence tends to be higher in children with lumbar and sacral level lesions than in children with higher level lesions.[38] However, children with normal intelligence with MM still tend to have learning problems and poor academic achievement that are thought to result from deficits in perceptual skills, organizational abilities, attention, sequencing, reasoning, speed of motor response, memory, and hand function.[31,39,40]

Language dysfunction observed in children with MM and hydrocephalus is characterized by a high frequency of irrelevant content and excessive chatter.[4,41] In addition, some children with MM have speech deficits and/or hearing loss.

Sensory Integrity. MM causes sensory deficits, as well as paralysis. Although sensory levels often do not coincide with motor levels, findings from sensory and motor testing can help to establish the spinal lesion level.[42] Different sensory modalities (light touch, pain, proprioception, kinesthetic, vibration, and thermal) are tested and recorded on a dermatome chart indicating areas of absent and altered sensitivity.

Educating the family and individual with MM about the sensory deficit is an important component of management. Insensitive areas require vigilant attention and protection from skin breakdown, abrasions, and burns. Most children with spina bifida experience some form of skin breakdown before they reach adulthood.[43] Persons with insensitivity may develop skin problems from sitting because they do not shift their weight, change their position, or relieve pressure.[42] Skin breakdown commonly occurs over bony prominences such as the greater trochanter, ischii, sacrum, or heels. Bowel and bladder deficits contribute to skin maceration in the diaper area. Skin abrasions of the knees and feet can occur as the child moves by crawling or creeping. Proper shoe and orthotic fit is also essential to avoid pressure sores and abrasions. Bath water temperature must always be tested before placing the child in the tub. Serious burns can and do occur because of the inability to sense temperature. Pressure relief and skin inspection should be taught early on, so they are incorporated into the daily routine.[4]

Clinical Pearl

The family and the individual with myelomeningocele should be taught to protect areas with reduced sensation from skin breakdown, abrasions, and burns.

Motor Function—Control and Learning. The bladder, urinary outlet, and rectum are innervated by spinal segments S2-S4. Because these nerves leave the spinal cord in the lower sacrum, bowel and bladder dysfunction occurs in most children with MM and fewer than 5% develop voluntary urinary and anal sphincter control.[44] Even children with sacral level lesions with normal leg movement often have bowel and bladder problems.[45] Children with MM have problems with both storing urine and emptying the bladder, resulting in incontinence.[46] Incomplete emptying of the bladder may predispose the child to urinary tract infections and kidney damage; therefore regular urological evaluations are necessary throughout life. Urological management objectives are prevention of kidney damage and socially acceptable control of incontinence.[31] Bladder training programs include regularly scheduled clean intermittent catheterization. Children who are 6 to 8 years of age can usually master the catheterization technique.

Neurogenic bowel dysfunction is closely associated with neurogenic bladder dysfunction. Bowel problems are related to uncoordinated propulsive action of the intestines, an ineffective anal sphincter, and a lack of rectal sensation.[45] The anal sphincter can be flaccid, hypotonic, or spastic, causing different types of dysfunction during defecation. The lack of anorectal sensation prevents the individual from receiving sensory information of an imminent bowel movement and frequently results in bowel incontinence.[4] Constipation and impaction are also common and may be interspersed with periods of overflow diarrhea. Bowel training programs can be highly successful and bowel continence should be a goal for the preschool or early elementary school-aged child with MM.[25]

Rehabilitation management to facilitate bowel continence may include abdominal strengthening and wheelchair push-ups to assist bowel motility; education about skin inspection; ADL functional training for bathing, dressing, and toileting; recommendations for adaptive equipment, including wheelchair cushions and bathroom modifications; and functional transfer training.

Function

Gait, Locomotion, and Balance. Mobility achievement by children with MM has received much attention in the literature, with most of the focus on bipedal ambulation. In this population, mobility must be expanded from the concept of walking to include any efficient and effective means of moving about that enables the individual to easily traverse and explore the environment and independently pursue an education, vocation, or avocation.[47] Endurance, efficiency, effectiveness, safety, degree of independence, and accessibility can all be monitored for the different types of mobility, including bed mobility, floor mobility, wheelchair mobility, ambulation, and transfers.[4] Mobility options must be examined throughout the lifespan as body proportions and environmental demands change. Selecting appropriate ambulation aids and orthoses at any time is an important role of the rehabilitation clinician (see Chapters 33 and 34).

The prognosis for walking in an individual with MM depends on the extent and location of paralysis and associated muscle weakness, as well as other factors that include the degree and extent of medical complications and the level of cognitive, executive, hand, visuospatial, and emotional functioning.[31,48] The higher the spinal lesion level, the greater the muscle weakness, and thus the more ambulation is compromised. Most children with MM learn to belly crawl as their first means of mobility. Children with strong hip flexors and some knee movements may assume the quadruped position. Children with sacral lesions generally learn to walk by 2 or 3 years of age with or without orthoses. Children with midlumbar (L3) paralysis often require upper extremity support and orthoses. Children with thoracic or high lumbar paralysis may stand upright and walk for exercise with extensive support of the hips, knees, and ankles (parapodium, reciprocal gait orthosis [RGO]). The wheelchair will supplement and often become the primary means of mobility by early adolescence in children with lumbar level lesions because it is quick and energy efficient. Children with a 24-month developmental level can learn to operate a motorized wheelchair.

Energy expenditure is also an important determinant of ambulation status in children with MM. Children with MM fatigue sooner than children without disability because of the high energy demand of their walking pattern. This high-energy cost becomes more apparent and limiting as individuals are required to travel longer distances.[31] To adapt to this high-energy demand, individuals with MM may reduce their walking speed,[49] walk shorter distances, and pause more frequently during ambulation.[50] The ability to walk may regress during growth as a result of changes in body proportion or the development of musculoskeletal deformities or obesity.

◎ *Clinical Pearl*

Mobility for children with spinal dysraphism includes any efficient and effective means of moving about that enables the individual to easily traverse and explore the environment and independently pursue an education, vocation, or avocation.

Self-Care and Home Management. Children with MM have delayed gross and fine motor skills and functional limitations in ADLs.[51,52] Significant delays occur before achievement of sitting and standing. Motor delays are likely influenced by many factors, including level and extent of the spinal lesion, brain involvement, musculoskeletal deformities, cognitive delay, habilitation training, parental expectation, and ability to practice. Children with MM are typically able to perform ADLs as they acquire the necessary motor skills. Uncoordinated and immature hand function, decreased performance speed, and deficits in visual-perceptual and visual-motor skills are thought to explain why activities primarily involving the

upper extremities, such as washing the face and hands, are also delayed in children with MM as compared with age-matched typical norms.

Work, Community, and Leisure Integration. The goal of habilitation for individuals with MM is a satisfying, self-directed lifestyle with active community involvement. At least 75% of children born with MM can be expected to reach their early adult years. However, many have medical complications. Today's challenge is to establish a network of care throughout the lifespan for people with spinal dysraphisms because many of these individuals are now surviving longer and experiencing pain, loss of function, and loss of independence beginning in the their mid-twenties. People with MM are increasingly being employed in many areas of industry and commerce. In most instances, the choice of occupation is influenced by the degree of disability in adulthood. At present there are agencies, statutes, and attitudes that try to ensure that people with disabilities who desire to work are given equal opportunity to find employment

EVALUATION, DIAGNOSIS, AND PROGNOSIS

The evaluation process allows the therapist to determine (1) what specific problems are evident on the participation, activity, and impairment level and which of those are priorities; (2) which constraints from the child, task, and environment hinder the child's performance; and (3) what risk factors can be addressed to reduce the risk of secondary impairments in the future. According to the *Guide*,[1] children with CP and MM fall into one of two preferred practice patterns: 5B: Impaired neuromotor development or 5C: Impaired motor function and sensory integrity associated with nonprogressive disorders of the CNS—congenital origin or acquired in infancy or childhood.

REHABILITATION INTERVENTION FOR CHILDREN WITH CEREBRAL PALSY AND MYELOMENINGOCELE

Rehabilitation interventions for children with CP and MM are selected based on findings from the examination and the clinician's evaluation. Pediatric neuromotor rehabilitation intervention programs require consideration of the multiple systems (musculoskeletal, neuromotor, cardiovascular/pulmonary, and integumentary) that may be affected, the developmental progression of motor skill acquisition, and the levels of outcome (impairments, functional limitations, and disability) to be addressed. Because children with nonprogressive CNS disorders have many and varied clinical manifestations the intervention program generally requires dynamic multidisciplinary collaboration.[53]

A physical rehabilitation intervention program aimed at optimizing independence in all aspects of the client's life through improving motor performance is based on the principles of motor learning and motor control, task analysis, knowledge of typical and atypical motor development, knowledge of therapeutic exercise such as strength training, and development across domains. Individuals with functional limitations related to CP or MM require rehabilitative services throughout life. Their problems and goals and thus the indicated interventions will change over time. Successful intervention requires the therapist to know and understand the complexity and multifaceted nature of the diagnosis and the specific deficits and goals of the individual patient. The intervention program must often focus on several disparate but related system outcomes; be relevant across different venues (home, school, and community); be tailored to the patient's age, cognitive, physical, and emotional level; and complement the family social and cultural structure. An array of activity-focused and impairment-focused intervention approaches are incorporated to promote independence.

The level of the lesion in children with MM and the severity and clinical type of CP influences selection of interventions related to achieving motor milestone and ambulation goals and consideration of mobility alternatives, assistive devices, and orthoses. Although there are common goals and intervention strategies for any stage of life, the therapist will need to adapt different age-appropriate strategies and focus and redirect attention so the individual can be independent, efficient, and effective in an ever-widening range of environments. Before beginning any treatment session, keep in mind that how the child is handled today may impact his or her long-term outcome and ability to participate in long-term life roles. This is especially true for a growing and developing child. Table 15-2 outlines the major components of an intervention program for children with MM across the lifespan. Treatment in the hospital, outpatient clinic, home, school, and day care center may be necessary to achieve the most effective, well-integrated, and well-adapted intervention.

GENERAL INTERVENTION PRINCIPLES

Consider All Domains of Development. Motor skills are not acquired in a vacuum. Their development depends on the development of cognitive, emotional, and social skills. Movement promotes cognitive and perceptual development; likewise, cognition and perception promote movement development.[54] Therefore all developmental domains are considered when designing an intervention program for a child with CP or MM. Goals, play activities, and toys should be at the child's cognitive level, regardless of the child's chronological age and level of motor development. For example, a 15-year-old with level I spastic diplegic CP (mild motor involvement) but with a severe cognitive impairment may require toys intended for infants, whereas a 15-year-old with level IV spastic diplegia but with age-appropriate cognitive skills may be interested in adaptive sports.

Goal-Directed, Functional, and Meaningful Interventions. Habilitation interventions include tasks that are purposeful, relevant, developmentally appropriate, active, voluntarily regulated, goal directed, and meaningful to the child.[55-57] Intervention goals will be part of the child's day-to-day life, and achievement of the goals should make a difference in the lives of the child and family. A child's age, gender, extent and type of impairments, cultural background, cognitive level, and interests are all considered when establishing goals.

Encourage Practice. In general, the more one practices the more one learns; therefore activities should be repeated many times in each treatment session and throughout each day.[58] Each practice attempt is an opportunity to optimize the child's motor learning and motor performance.[57] Practice also increases efficiency, stability, and flexibility of performance.[13] Repetition of movements may also promote muscle strengthening, generation of an effective movement strategy through trial and error, testing of the limits of balance, and learning ways to manage reactive forces generated for stability and mobility.[54]

HEALTH PROMOTION AND PREVENTION OF SECONDARY COMPLICATIONS

A goal for habilitation of children is to promote the attainment and long-term maintenance of functional goals and community participation. Life-long, early-onset chronic disabilities cause not only primary impairments but also secondary conditions that develop with age. Secondary conditions develop for a variety of reasons, including (1) overuse of an already weakened neuromuscular system; (2) underuse or misuse because of poor movement quality, immobility, or deconditioning; (3) poor lifestyle behaviors such as lack of exercise and/or poor nutrition; and (4) environmental and attitudinal barriers that may limit access to preventive services and opportunities for social participation and health-promoting activities.[59] A child who acquires movement of poor quality may develop compensatory patterns that over time lead to musculoskeletal deformities (e.g., scoliosis), skin breakdown, joint pain, and osteoporosis. Intervention strategies must weigh the inherent trade-offs between facilitating function despite poor movement quality and restricting function with a goal of higher movement quality.[60] Neither of these is ideal nor is it currently possible to totally resolve the neuromuscular impairments that contribute to atypical movement quality.

It is suggested that individuals with neuromuscular impairments maintain higher levels of physical fitness than the general population to offset the decline in function associated with the disorder in addition to the changes related to typical aging.[61] The *Guide* emphasizes the importance of primary prevention and risk reduction strategies within a complete physical therapy intervention program.[1] Promotion of physical fitness and life-long habits of physical activity can enhance health and prevent diseases in adulthood.[62] Physical fitness programs for children with neuromuscular disorders should include activities that promote cardiorespiratory endurance, muscular strength and endurance, flexibility, and ideal body composition. The principles of an effective conditioning program, including specificity of training, intensity, frequency, and duration, should be incorporated in an intervention program for children with neuromuscular disorders.

TABLE 15-2	Relationship of Intervention to Impairments and Goals for Children with Myelomeningocele Across the Lifespan	
Impairment	**Goal**	**Intervention**
INFANCY		
Paralysis or decreased muscle strength	• Increase strength in innervated muscles	• Facilitate movement • Educate parents about possible movements
Absent or decreased sensation	• Establish areas of sensory loss to pain	• Educate parents on areas of absent sensation and avoidance of injury (test bath water before placing infant in tub; avoid placing infant close to hot surfaces such as radiators or fireplace); need for foot and knee protection during developmental tasks (crawling, walking) • Educate parents in skin inspection • Assist parents in following physician instructions
Musculoskeletal deformities (hip dislocation, foot deformities)	• Note muscle imbalance	• Positioning (double diapering for dislocated hips) • Serial casting, positioning splints for foot deformities
Delayed fine and gross motor development	• Achieve age-appropriate motor abilities (head and trunk control; upright posture—sit, stand; early mobility—roll, pivot, crawl)	• Facilitate age-appropriate motor skills (positions, guided movement, mobile surfaces, and reach and move for toys) • Educate parents to handle and interact with infant
Delayed ADL skills	• Achieve independence in age-appropriate ADL abilities	• Facilitate age-appropriate ADL skills • Educate parents in importance of developing independence
TODDLER AND PRESCHOOL		
Paralysis or decreased muscle strength	• Increase and maintain strength in innervated muscles	• Facilitate movement in different positions and on mobile surfaces (push a toy, pull a toy) • Functional electrical stimulation • Biofeedback
Decreased ROM	• Increase and maintain age-appropriate ROM	• Continue stretching program • Positioning
Absent or decreased sensation	• Determine stability of sensory findings	• Instruct child on skin safety and skin inspection • Teach child pressure relief techniques (sitting push-ups) • Order needed equipment (cushions) as per PT instructions • Instruct in joint protection techniques • Assist parents and child in following physician instructions
Musculoskeletal deformities		• Positioning, stretching
Delayed fine and gross motor development	• Achieve age-appropriate motor abilities (independent sitting, transitions, creeping, kneeling, standing)	• Continue to facilitate age-appropriate motor skills • Promote balance and trunk control, upright posture, and pull to stand
Delayed mobility	• Independent, effective short-distance and household ambulation	• Ambulation training • Wheelchair training for children 2 years of age and older (sitting balance, arm strengthening, transfer training, wheelchair propulsion, electrical switch operation, safety, and environmental exploration)
Delayed ADL skills	• Reassess ADL ability level (use fork and knife; drink from cup; wash hands; brush hair; remove shirt, socks, and shoes; put on shirt) • Facilitate age-appropriate ADL skills (donning and doffing orthoses, eating, dressing, and bathing) • Achieve efficient and effective independence in age-appropriate ADL abilities	• Continue to educate parents and child on importance of promoting independence
Decreased environmental exploration	• Promote independent exploration within the child's environments	
SCHOOL-AGE		
Paralysis, decreased muscle strength; loss of sensation; decreased ROM	• Continue to monitor for signs of progressive neurological dysfunction (result of tethered cord, shunt malfunction)	• Continue stretching and strengthening program (include low back extensor, hip flexor, hamstring, and shoulder girdle musculature) • Reinforce skin inspection, pressure relief strategies • Proper positioning in class (flat feet, seat and desk height fit child's body proportions, and tilted desk top) • Joint protection techniques

Continued

TABLE 15-2	Relationship of Intervention to Impairments and Goals for Children with Myelomeningocele Across the Lifespan—cont'd

Impairment	Goal	Intervention
Delayed mobility for longer distances	• Independent, effective short-distance and household ambulation • Independent, effective, and efficient long-distance and community mobility • Examine energy expenditure (keep up with peers with energy left to attend classroom activities)	• Ambulation and wheelchair training; managing streets, sidewalks, crosswalks, parking lots, playgrounds, all surfaces, and doorways; maneuvering in tight places, elevators, elevations, and public transportation
Decreased socialization and peer interaction	• Examine barriers to socialization at home, school, and community environments (stores, shopping malls, libraries, restaurants, theaters, sports arenas, public transportation, physician's offices, or religious institutions)	• Consultation with classroom/PE teacher (play, recreation, and PE class) • Full participation in PE classes, field trips, and sport activities • Modify task, equipment, or environment for full independent participation • Encourage participation in age-appropriate community activities (scouts, school clubs, or sports)
Delayed ADL skills	• Achieve efficient, effective independence in age-appropriate ADL abilities	• Educate parents and child on normative data for ADL skills • Promote positive parental expectations of independence
Decreased endurance	• Maintain and improve endurance, aerobic capacity, cardiovascular fitness, coordination, and weight control	• Promote a physical fitness program (low impact aerobic, strengthening, or flexibility) • Promote recreational activities (swimming, cycling, or rowing)
ADOLESCENCE TO ADULTHOOD		
Delayed mobility for long distances within the community	• Independent, effective, efficient, and safe long-distance and community mobility	
Delayed ADL skills	• Achieve efficient and effective independence in age-appropriate ADL abilities	• Prepare for mobility and motor skills necessary in different environments (higher education, employment, and independent living)
Regression of motor skills and mobility	• Continue to monitor for signs of progressive neurological dysfunction (result of tethered cord, shunt malfunction) • Achieve independent basic and community mobility	• Review all therapeutic programs (strength, ROM, and motor skill) • Promote sitting and standing postural control • Instruct in advanced community skills
Immobilization due to secondary complications (orthopedic surgeries, fractures, or decubitus)	• Prevent secondary complication (obesity, hypertension, osteoporosis, urinary tract infections, or skin wounds)	• Educate on prevention of secondary complications (skin protection pressure relief, exercise benefits) • Achieve highest level of independence • Promote recreational activities • Educate on maintenance of adaptive equipment • Instruct in physical fitness program • Promote recreational activities
Degenerative joint changes (especially weight-bearing joints) and overuse syndrome	• Prevent further degenerative joint changes	• ROM and strength training • Stretching (two joint muscles, hip and knee flexors; trunk musculature) • Educate and train in proper body mechanics (lift and carry groceries, laundry, or books)

ADL, Activities of daily living; *PE,* physical education; *ROM,* range of motion.

Clinical Pearl

Individuals with neuromuscular impairments should maintain a high level of physical fitness to offset the decline in function associated with the disorder, in addition to the changes related to typical aging.

FOCUSED INTERVENTIONS

The overall goal is for the child to participate in a variety of venues (e.g., home, school, or playground) using their upper extremities freely while engaging in body transport or movement with a stable posture and paying attention to the environment. The intervention program addresses goals that can be maintained over the lifetime of the client. Box 15-1 outlines areas of focus for an intervention program with life-long benefits.

Interventions for children with neuromuscular disorders may be activity-focused and/or impairment-focused. **Activity-focused interventions** involve structured practice and repetition of functional actions. **Impairment-focused interventions** address impairments in

BOX 15-1	Characteristics of an Intervention Program That Produces Life-Long Results

- Promotes engagement in life-long fitness activities, including exercise, proper nutrition and hydration, weight control, stress management, and energy conservation for meaningful pursuits.
- Promotes the individual's ability to take personal responsibility for personal health, to be knowledgeable about their own condition, and to be assertive in addressing needs: Is the individual encouraged to speak, or otherwise communicate for himself or herself?
- Program supports the child's motivation to persist in attaining difficult goals, despite failure along the way.
- Program develops the individual's perception of self-control and successful accomplishment of personally meaningful goals that are likely to foster self-esteem.
- Program uses activities that over the short and long term are not likely to lead to chronic musculoskeletal problems and excess fatigue to the detriment of engagement in meaningful activities.
- Program fosters prevention of increasing impairment rather than promoting function at all costs.

Adapted from Campbell SK: *Phys Occup Ther Ped* 17(1):10-15, 1997.

BOX 15-2	General Guidelines for Applying a Task-Oriented Approach to Clinical Practice

- Identify important, meaningful tasks that the child has difficulty performing.
- Select tasks that are the focus of intervention reasonably within the child's capabilities.
- Observe the child perform the task in the environment in which it is naturally performed, when possible, and document current level of abilities.
- Analyze the requirements and characteristics of the task.
- Analyze the demands and characteristics of the environment in which the task is performed. Consider physical characteristics, regulatory conditions, and the sociocultural context.
- Examine and evaluate the child's performance on the task and determine what the child is able to do, what the child is unable to do, task and environmental constraints that interfere with successful performance, and task and environmental factors that support the success of the performance.
- Identify possible intervention strategies directed toward reducing the constraints considering the influence of the musculoskeletal, neuromuscular, cardiovascular or pulmonary, and integumentary systems; possible modifications of the task and environment; type of feedback; and practice schedule.
- Allow the child to practice the task under the specific conditions, provide feedback, and document performance level.

Adapted from Kaplan M, Bedell G: Motor skill acquisition frame of reference. In Kramer P, Hinojosa J (eds): *Frames of reference for pediatric occupational therapy*, ed 2, New York, 1999, Lippincott Williams & Wilkins.

body structure and functions. Activity-focused interventions are system-based and include the task-oriented approach and constraint-induced movement therapy. An activity-focused intervention often adapts the physical environment by using therapeutic equipment, such as balls and bolsters, and adaptive equipment, such as seating and mobility aids. Impairment-focused interventions include neurodevelopmental treatment, strength training, electrotherapeutic modalities, biofeedback, and aerobic conditioning.

Passive impairment-focused interventions are aimed at reducing primary or secondary musculoskeletal impairments. Passive impairment-focused interventions include manual therapy techniques, therapeutic electrical stimulation administered while the child sleeps, positioning equipment (stander, long-sitter, orthoses, splints, and casts), and therapeutic exercises such as ROM and flexibility procedures not administered in the context of a purposeful task.

Activity-Focused Interventions

Task-Oriented Approach. There is no single, generally accepted task approach for children with CP or MM; rather, therapists individually combine concepts of motor learning, motor control, motor development, and learning theory to best suit the individual child. The concepts emphasized are the therapeutic use of purposeful, functional skills; active role of the learner; role of feedback in learning; type and amount of practice and experimentation; promotion of flexible strategies through variation of practice; and the transfer of learning from one skill to another and among different environments (Box 15-2).

Activity-based interventions focus on outcomes that allow the child to increase function and/or participation at home, school, or in the community. Components that limit achievement of these goals, including impairments such as decreased strength and ROM, are then assessed. Activity-focused interventions involve practice of actions that produce results related to overall goals rather than on patterns or quality of movement. The intervention is planned according to motor learning guidelines, taking into consideration the strengths and learning needs of the child. Impairment-level interventions are integrated with activity-focused interventions so that impairments that critically limit performance are addressed within the context of active practice.

In general, studies have shown that children who participate in task-oriented therapy do improve in their ability to perform functional skills; however, there is insufficient data from well-controlled trials to definitively

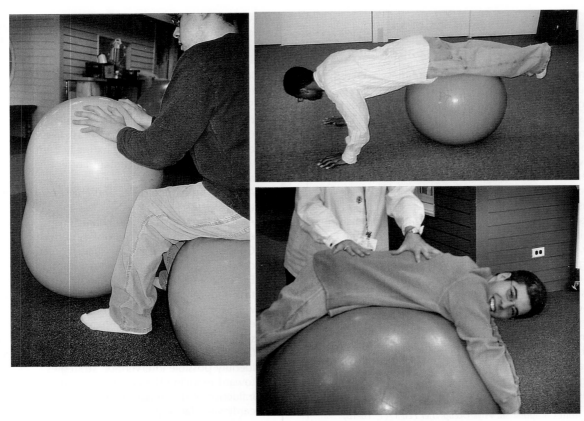

FIG. 15-8 Interventions using balls of various shapes and sizes.

conclude that this type of intervention is superior to others or exceeds the effects of time and maturation alone.

Therapeutic Equipment. The clinician may use various equipment, such as mats, benches, bolsters, balls, "eggs" (egg-shaped balls), and "peanuts" (peanut-shaped balls) (Fig. 15-8), to alter the physical environment during practice to support the performance of motor skills such as rolling from prone to supine, moving from prone to sitting, or moving from half-kneeling to standing.[63] Equipment can allow the therapist to control the degree and direction of movement within the context of the environment, introduce instability to the movement, and control the degree to which a movement is assisted by or performed against gravity.[64]

Assistive Mobility Devices. The success of activity-based interventions often depends on the use of appropriate assistive devices to help the child with functional, energy-efficient mobility (bed, floor, wheelchair, ambulation, and transfers). These devices include walkers, crutches, canes, wheelchairs, bicycles, and tricycles (see Chapter 33). Once the child is identified as needing an assistive device, the therapist must decide which devices provide the appropriate support, minimize secondary complications such as overuse syndromes, support energy efficient mobility for needed distances, and are useful in the child's home, school, outdoor, and community settings. Changes in body proportions and environmental demands necessitate reevaluating mobility options across the lifespan.[4]

Less restrictive devices, such as canes or crutches, have the advantage of allowing children to negotiate smaller spaces. Their weight and height will affect how much support they give, upper extremity orientation, and the child's center of gravity. Support may be reduced gradually from Lofstrand crutches, quad canes, tripod canes, or offset handle straight canes to encourage more weight bearing through the lower extremities as the child develops better control (Fig. 15-9).

Tricycles and bicycles can be a fun adjunct to any intervention program and provide a means of mobility for children who cannot walk. The cycle should be evaluated for fit and alignment. The ease with which the cycle can be pedaled, as well as the effort it takes to move the wheels, should be considered in cycle selection. Cycling promotes weight shift through the pelvis, lower extremity dissociation, upright posture with bilateral hand use, and an age-appropriate means of negotiating the environment and provides an opportunity to socialize with peers.

Mobility methods vary by age, severity of involvement, and environmental setting. Children are more dependent on adult assistance for mobility when outdoors and in the community than at home. Mobility in all settings, physical and social features of the environment, and the physical abilities of the caretaker are considered when selecting mobility methods for a child.

Constraint-Induced Movement Therapy. **Constraint-induced movement therapy (CIMT)** is an approach to therapy that was developed for adults with

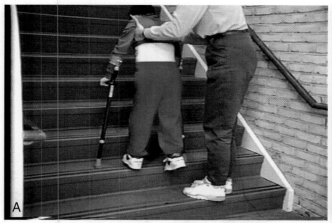
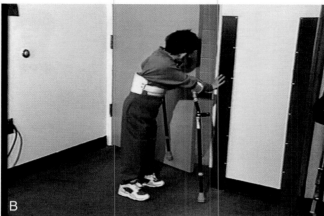

FIG. 15-9 Child with T12 myelomeningocele using Lofstrand crutches during functional mobility tasks. **A,** Ascending stairs. **B,** Opening a door.

hemiparesis caused by stroke (see Chapter 16 for details of this approach). This intervention approach can also be used for children with CP. CIMT involves immobilizing the individual's less impaired upper extremity and having them perform interesting and useful activities that provided immediate, frequent, and repetitive rewards. For a child, these activities may include reaching, grasping, holding, or manipulating an object; weight bearing on the arm; making hand gestures; and performing functional tasks such as dressing, eating, bathing, and grooming. Over time, the task demands are increased by requiring greater precision, strength, fluency, automaticity, and/or functional versatility.

Clinical Pearl

Activity-focused interventions emphasize the therapeutic use of purposeful, functional skills and transferring the use of skills between tasks and environments.

Impairment-Focused Interventions

Neurodevelopmental Treatment. **Neurodevelopmental treatment (NDT)** is an approach used in the treatment of neuromuscular disorders. It has been, and remains, one of the most popular approaches for management of children and adults with neuromotor disabilities (see Chapter 16). NDT was developed and first introduced in the early 1940s by Berta Bobath and Dr. Karel Bobath. This approach has changed over time and continues to change as theories of motor control, motor learning, and developmental theory evolve. NDT uses a developmental framework that necessitates a comprehensive knowledge of both typical and atypical development and components of movement and postural control.

To apply an NDT approach to treating a child with CP, the therapist must first describe the child's functional skills and analyze the quality of movement used to accomplish these skills. A central assumption of NDT is that abnormal movement patterns may be changed by altering sensory input to the CNS.[65] One technique used for altering sensory input is termed *handling* and is also known as *guided movement*. This consists of the clinician applying graded sensory input to specific areas on the child's body

---

BOX 15-3	General Principles for Applying the Neurodevelopmental Approach to Clinical Practice

- Guide the child's movement to experience a variety of motor patterns in a variety of positions with structured repetition. Guided movement is active; the child initiates and follows through with the movement.
- Assist the child in developing improved alignment, anticipatory postural control, selective control, strength, endurance, and variety in response options.
- Inhibit unwanted compensatory patterns that lead to secondary impairments or deformities that can lead to decreased functional performance.
- Reduce guidance as the child is able to move more effectively to advance the child's independent function.
- Provide interesting play activities and tasks that support meaningful practice and build strength and endurance.
- Provide carryover through independent and supervised practice in multiple settings.

Adapted from Howle JM: *Neuro-developmental treatment approach: Theoretical foundations and principles of clinical practice,* Laguna Beach, CA, 2003, Neuro-Developmental Treatment Association.

(known as *key points of control*) to elicit and facilitate specific motor responses.[65] The key point of control may be proximal (shoulder girdle, trunk, or pelvis) or distal (hands or feet). Handling is thought to facilitate appropriate motor responses that can be incorporated by the child into functional activities. Box 15-3 lists general principles for applying the NDT approach to clinical practice. Clinicians learn NDT through practice under the supervision of an experienced therapist and through specialized training programs (ranging from a 2-day to an 8-week course that leads to NDT certification).

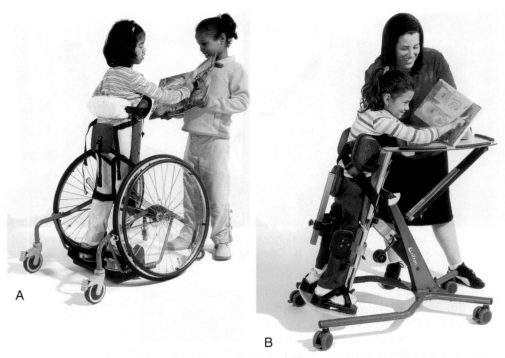

FIG. 15-10 Adaptive equipment used by children with neuromotor conditions. **A,** Mobile standing system. **B,** Prone stander with a table attachment. *Images courtesy Rifton.*

The effectiveness of NDT in the management of CP has been evaluated in many studies. There is consistent but scanty evidence that NDT immediately improves dynamic ROM. Although the evidence was deemed credible, the strength of evidence is impaired by (1) relatively small sample sizes; (2) considerable heterogeneity in the type and severity of CP, associated disabilities, and age at treatment; (3) questionable measures in terms of validity and sensitivity to detect changes; and (4) variability in therapy over time and among therapists.

Strength Training. Strength training can be a valuable component of an intervention program for a child with CP and MM. Despite variability in subject characteristics and program parameters, the literature reviewed indicated that strength training can increase strength and improve activity in children and young adults with CP without adverse effects. In addition, strengthening does not increase (or possibly even reduces) spasticity and also leads to increased ROM, especially in the lower extremities. Further studies are needed to evaluate the effects of strength training on mobility, function, and the ability of children with CP to participate in society.

Strength training can also help children with MM. Strengthening exercises are indicated for innervated but weak functioning muscles. The level of the lesion dictates the specific muscle groups that can be strengthened. Muscles that are important for postural control, ADL, mobility, or balance of muscle forces around joints should be emphasized.[4] Upper extremity strengthening is important for performing transfers, wheelchair propulsion, and using assistive mobility devices. Trunk strengthening is important for static, anticipatory, and reactive postural control in sitting and standing. Lower extremity strength-

ening is crucial for ambulation, improving gait, and possibly reducing the need for assistive devices and orthoses.[4]

Electrical Stimulation. Electrical stimulation at a sensory or motor level has been used to increase muscle strength and function in children with CP and MM. Neuromuscular electrical stimulation (NMES) is the transcutaneous application of an electrical current to elicit repetitive muscle contractions by stimulating motor nerves. Functional electrical stimulation (FES) is the use of such electrically stimulated muscle contractions during functional activities. In contrast, threshold electrical stimulation (TES), also called *therapeutic electrical stimulation,* involves stimulating only sensory nerves but applying the stimulation at home for many hours each night while the child is asleep. It has been suggested that all of these forms of electrical stimulation can enlarge atrophic muscles and secondarily improve motor function.

Adaptive Devices. Adaptive equipment is commonly used to correct positioning, achieve mobility and promote performance of tasks and movements, support weak or ineffective joints or muscles, and facilitate ADLs in individuals with neuromuscular disorders.[1,66] Examples include special chairs, adaptations to chairs, seating devices, wheelchair lapboards, standing frames (supine and prone), and adapted tricycles (Fig. 15-10). There are a myriad of commercially produced and custom-fabricated options available, and new devices are constantly being developed. The best device for a given individual offers support while having the least risk of causing complications. There are few clear scientific objective guidelines on which to base decisions regarding selecting equipment to address a particular issue.[66]

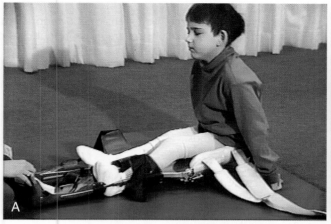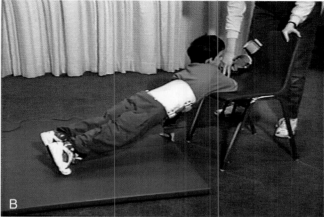

FIG. 15-11 Child with T12 myelomeningocele. **A,** Donning a reciprocating trunk-hip-knee-ankle-foot orthosis (THKAFO). **B,** Transfer from floor to standing while wearing a reciprocating THKAFO.

Appropriate positioning of children with CP and MM promotes function and participation within the environment; improves head control; permits greater control of upper extremity use; improves ability to perform ADLs, such as eating and dressing; improves postural alignment; manages pressure and thereby reduces the risk of developing pressure ulcers; and can increase ROM and decrease fatigue.[67] Positioning devices include recumbent systems that provide support in supine, prone, or sidelying positions and upright positioning systems that support the child in either a sitting or standing position. Recumbent systems are often used with children with severe impairments and functional limitations as a means of alternative positioning throughout the day. A sidelyer, for example, promotes neutral sidelying, elongation on the weight-bearing side, dissociation of the lower extremities, and midline hand use.

Upright seating systems can adapt a high chair, classroom chair, wheelchair, and/or stroller. The seating system includes an array of devices such as seat and back cushions and head, trunk, knee, foot, and arm supports (chest straps, shoulder harness, armrests, lap tray, knee guides, abductor wedge, and footrests). Any child who requires a seating system must be evaluated carefully as the incorrect orientation of even one strap can adversely affect the child's overall alignment and function. Seating systems should provide support while allowing function.

Upright standing systems usually have table or tray attachments that allow the child to play while standing. Standing can help elongate knee, hip flexor, and plantarflexor muscles; maintain or improve bone mineral density; encourage neutral and symmetrical lower extremity weight bearing; and facilitate development of hip, knee, and ankle joint muscles.[68] Children should be encouraged to experience upright weight bearing as close to the typical age of standing as possible if they can accept weight through their feet and have sufficient head and trunk control to be aligned correctly.

Orthoses. Orthoses are external appliances worn to correct extremity alignment, achieve mobility, promote performance of tasks and movements, and support weak or ineffective joints or muscles.[1] Lower limb orthoses range from shoe modifications to trunk-hip-knee-ankle-foot orthoses (THKAFOs; Fig. 15-11).[69] Chapter 34 contains detailed information on the selection, fitting, and use of upper and lower extremity and trunk orthoses. In children with MM, lower limb orthosis selection is based on multiple factors, including motor level, motivation, learning capacity, desire for movement, and other patient goals. Lower limb orthoses range from supramalleolar foot orthoses for S1 motor level, knee-ankle-foot orthoses (KAFOs) for L3-L4 motor level, to THKAFOs for thoracic to L1 motor level. If a child is able to pull to stand with support at the ankles, a parapodium is sometimes recommended at around 12 to 15 months of age.[70] This standing device supports the child upright on a base, allowing the child to develop pre-orthosis skills while the hands remain free. In children with CP, lower extremity orthoses may promote neutral foot alignment to allow muscles to work more effectively and efficiently and reduce the degrees of freedom the individual must control.

Clinical Pearl

Impairment-focused interventions focus on improving the quality of movement to achieve functional goals.

CASE STUDY 15-1

CEREBRAL PALSY

Patient History

TQ is a 15-year-old boy with a medical diagnosis of spastic diplegic CP. He was born prematurely at 32 weeks of gestation with a birth weight of 2 lb 15 oz. He was enrolled in an outpatient-center–based rehabilitation program at 1 year of age. This case will follow him from 1 through 15 years of age.

Diagnosis

Preferred practice pattern 5C: Impaired motor function and sensory integrity associated with nonprogressive disorders of the central nervous system—congenital origin or acquired in infancy or childhood.

Tests and Measures—Significant Findings at 1 Year of Age

Musculoskeletal
- Posterior pelvic tilt and kyphotic spine in sitting.
- Reduced bilateral PROM for straight leg raising, ankle dorsiflexion, and hip extension.

Neuromuscular
- Clonus at both ankles, left greater than right, and a positive Babinski sign bilaterally.
- Upper extremity protective extension is present anteriorly and sideways (left and right) but is absent posteriorly.
- Spasticity and increased muscle stiffness are present in both lower extremities, left greater than right, distal greater than proximal, and extensor greater than flexor.

Function
- TQ can roll from prone to supine and back without rotation and can sit independently with bilateral upper extremity support. He cannot bear weight on his lower extremities.

Interventions
- Functional activities include rolling with rotation, independent sitting with functional reaching, and bimanual hand skills for play, standing, getting to standing from the floor with upper extremity assistance, and cruising.
- TQ will be placed in a prone stander for 30 minutes per day.
- A nighttime stretching program, using an A-frame and bilateral solid ankle orthoses (SAOs) should be implemented for 2 to 3 hours per night.
- SAOs to be used during the day at school to assist with upright control at the ankle joint.

Role of the Physical Therapist Assistant
- What do the bilateral clonus and positive Babinski sign indicate?
- Write a paragraph for the caregivers of this patient explaining how to properly use the A-frame and SAOs.
- Describe three specific play activities that would help this patient's sitting skills to allow bimanual hand skill development in sitting.

Patient History at 4 Years of Age

TQ underwent bilateral hamstring lengthening and percutaneous adductor release at 30 months of age to address bilateral contractures. He continues his nighttime stretching program using the A-frame along with bilateral SAOs.

Tests and Measures—Significant Findings

Musculoskeletal
- Good sitting posture, kyphotic spine and posterior pelvic tilt in sitting resolved.
- PROM within normal limits (WNL).
- Lower extremity strength graded at 3 to 4/5 in all lower extremity muscles.

Neuromuscular
- Upper extremity protective extension posteriorly and equilibrium responses in sitting are now present. Standing responses are emerging.
- Tone is significantly reduced in all lower extremity muscles.

Cardiovascular/Pulmonary
- TQ can ambulate for short periods of time requiring frequent rest periods.

Function
- TQ can come to standing from the floor through half-kneeling with upper extremity support.
- Beginning to throw, catch, and kick a ball and play on playground equipment.

Interventions
- Functional activities include transitions, walking on level and nonlevel surfaces, community ambulation with increased speed and longer distances, and ascending and descending stairs and curbs.
- An adapted tricycle program (30 minutes per day at home) and a pool therapy program (3 times per week for 30 minutes) to improve endurance and lower extremity strengthening.
- Articulating ankle-foot orthoses (AFOs) to be used outside of therapy. Supramalleolar orthoses are to be used during therapy to control pronation and supination with hip extension and upright control.

Role of the Physical Therapist Assistant
- How will you engage TQ in the recommended activities at the age of 4?
- What sort of adaptations will be needed to allow TQ to use a tricycle safely? And to use the pool safely?
- Why are different orthoses used in therapy and at home?

Patient History at 9 Years of Age

TQ had two rounds of botulinum toxin injections bilaterally in the gastrocnemius soleus muscle group to reduce spasticity, eliminate clonus during heel strike, and promote a heel-toe gait pattern. The most recent injections were given 3 weeks before this examination.

Tests and Measures—Significant Findings

Musculoskeletal
- ROM is WNL except for excessive knee extension. Gastrocnemius soleus muscle group weakness is evident after botulinum toxin injections.

Neuromuscular
- Tone is significantly reduced in the injected muscle groups. TQ reports feeling "loose" and being able to "move more freely" when performing functional skills.

Cardiovascular/Pulmonary
- TQ can ambulate all day at a speed comparable to his able-bodied peers. Distance is no longer a limiting factor.

Function

- TQ ambulates with knee recurvatum, greater on the left than on the right, and a lateral thrust of the tibia to advance the tibia over the foot during midstance.
- He reports feeling stiff at the end of the school day.

Interventions

- Lower extremity strengthening through functional activities.
- The genu recurvatum is addressed with articulating AFOs and strengthening.

Role of the Physical Therapist Assistant

- What would help with this patient's end-of-day stiffness?
- Name three play activities that could be used as a home exercise program to strengthen the lower extremity.
- Why is persistent genu recurvatum of concern in this patient?

Patient History at 15 Years of Age

TQ is currently a sophomore in high school and attends regular classes.

Tests and Measures—Significant Findings

Cardiovascular/Pulmonary

- Ambulatory endurance and speed is similar to his peers.
- Endurance and speed on a bicycle is below age-norms but is steadily improving.

Function

- TQ ambulates all day without an assistive or orthotic device.
- He is very active in scouting and recently completed a 17-mile hike. He proudly reported that he did not finish in last place.

Interventions

- Fitness is promoted with treadmill training (20 minutes), aiming for speed and distance age-norms, and riding a stationary bicycle at school for 15 to 20 minutes.
- TQ is interested in learning to dance and do yoga and in participating in sport activities, specifically hiking, river rafting, and basketball. When working on these activities, weight shifting, hip stability, and active isolated muscle control of lower extremities are emphasized.

Role of the Physical Therapy Assistant

- How could TQ's interests be worked into his therapy program?
- What aspects of this patient's care will continue in the long term?
- Are there any activities that should be limited because of TQ's condition?

Additional Information

For the full version of this case study, including detailed examination results, interventions, and outcomes, see the Evolve site that accompanies this book.

CASE STUDY 15-2

MYELOMENINGOCELE

Patient History at 6 Months of Age

JM is a 6-month-old boy with a diagnosis of MM at T12. He was born 1 month premature and his MM was repaired at birth. He also has a Chiari II malformation with hydrocephalus and was born with a right subluxed hip and bilateral equinovalgus with calcaneus deformities.

Diagnosis

Preferred practice pattern 5C: Impaired motor function and sensory integrity associated with nonprogressive disorders of the central nervous system.

Tests and Measures—Significant Findings

Musculoskeletal

- Lower extremities tend to be in a "windswept" (hip flexion and adduction) position to the right.
- Minor limitations in hip abduction and external rotation ROM.
- Significantly reduced ankle plantarflexion ROM as a result of his bilateral foot deformity.

Neuromuscular

- Flaccid paralysis and sensory loss at T12 and below, with slightly more motor and sensory function on the right than on the left side.

Function

- JM can prop himself on flexed arms in the prone position and commando crawl. He cannot sit independently.

Interventions

- Lower extremity stretching.
- SAOs during the day to maintain lower extremity ROM. An A-frame with SAOs is used for nighttime positioning.
- Activities to promote independent sitting balance with the trunk over the pelvis and activation of innervated abdominal muscles.
- A parapodium will be introduced around 8 to 10 months of age to promote static standing, as well as beginning ambulation skills.

Role of the Physical Therapist Assistant

- Describe three activity-based exercises that would help promote sitting balance and be appropriate for JM's age and ability levels.
- Create a document which explains to JM's caregivers how to use the A-frame and SAOs.
- Demonstrate how you would stretch JM's lower extremities.

Patient History at 5 to 6 Years of Age

- JM underwent a right iliopsoas and percutaneous adductor longus tenotomy, varus osteotomy, and acetabular shelf procedure at 18 months of age.

Tests and Measures—Significant Findings

Musculoskeletal

- Upper extremity mobility and strength are within normal limits for age.
- Lower extremity ROM is WNL, except for the bilateral calcaneal deformity.

Neuromuscular

- Righting and equilibrium responses are intact for his upper extremities and trunk above the T12 level.
- Upper extremity protective extension responses are intact in all directions.

Integumentary

- Skin is currently intact, but there is a scar on his right knee from a pressure ulcer that developed during his hospitalization at 18 months of age.

Function

- JM can roll, sit independently with arms free, transition from the floor to sitting, and maintain tall kneeling with upper extremity support.
- He ambulates using reciprocating gait orthoses and Lofstrand crutches.
- He can don and doff his orthoses independently and can lock his orthoses and come to standing independently.

Interventions

- Lightweight Lofstrand crutches for ambulation.
- Functional exercises to practice ascending and descending stairs and curbs.
- Daily ROM and strengthening exercises of the intact muscles during practice of functional skills.
- Massage to keep scar tissue mobile. Training in skin inspection and monitoring.

Role of the Physical Therapist Assistant

- What play activities could also serve as ROM and/or strengthening exercises for JM?
- How can JM avoid developing pressure ulcers in the future?
- Which muscles/muscle groups will JM need to keep strong to allow him to ambulate? Describe three strengthening exercises for these muscles.

Patient History at 14 to 15 Years of Age

- As a teenager, JM has had poor compliance with wearing orthoses.

Tests and Measures—Significant Findings

Musculoskeletal

- Lower extremity malalignment is developing due to lack of orthosis use, uneven muscle innervation, and prolonged effects of gravity.
- Tibial valgum on the left, and bilateral knee and hip flexion contractures.

Function

- JM continues to use lightweight Lofstrand crutches for mobility, but he no longer wears any type of orthosis.

Interventions

- Mobility is augmented with a wheelchair.
- Exercises to maintain integrity of the shoulder girdle, ensure that full mobility and strength are maintained, and optimize trunk and lower extremity alignment and mobility.
- Endurance and strength training to help JM participate in competitive wheelchair racing.
- Soft tissue mobilization.
- Adaptations to extracurricular activities (such as scouting) to allow for full participation.

Role of the Physical Therapist Assistant

- What could you do to encourage JM to use his orthoses as prescribed?
- What exercises would help JM train for participation in wheelchair racing? Begin by finding an organization in your community that offers this type of program to learn more about what is physically involved in this sport.
- List two possible adaptations JM might need to use when participating in a scouting event such as camping.

Additional Information

For the full version of this case study, including detailed examination results, interventions, and outcomes, see the Evolve site that accompanies this book.

CHAPTER SUMMARY

This chapter addresses the management of children with nonprogressive CNS disorders. Cerebral palsy and myelomeningocele are presented to illustrate how their pathology and natural history are linked to the clinical judgments regarding rehabilitation interventions aimed at improving motor performance and promoting the attainment and maintenance of functional goals and community participation. The evidence supporting or refuting clinical interventions is reviewed. Further studies are needed to evaluate the plethora of therapeutic approaches addressing multiple neuromuscular conditions across the lifespan. To paraphrase the Committee on Integrating the Science of Early Childhood Development,[71] "successful interventions are determined by sound strategies, acceptability to the child and caregivers, and quality implementation."

ADDITIONAL RESOURCES

For links to these and additional web-based resources, see the Evolve site.

Campbell SK: *Decision making in pediatric neurologic physical therapy,* New York, 1999, Churchill Livingstone.

Campbell SK, Vander Linden DW, Palisano RJ (eds): *Physical therapy for children,* ed 2, Philadelphia, 2000, Saunders.

Effgen SK (ed): *Meeting the physical therapy needs of children,* Philadelphia, 2005, FA Davis.

Long T, Cintas H: *Handbook of pediatric physical therapy,* Baltimore, 1995, Williams & Wilkins.

Shumway-Cook A, Woollacott MH: *Motor control: Theory and practical applications,* ed 2, New York, 2001, Lippincott Williams & Wilkins.

Spina Bifida Association of America

United Cerebral Palsy (UCP)

Useful Forms

Gross Motor Function Classification System (GMFCS) for Cerebral Palsy

GLOSSARY

Activity-focused intervention: Plan of care that incorporates structured practice and repetition of functional activities and emphasizes a child's ability to learn motor tasks to increase independence and participation in daily responsibilities.

Baclofen: Pharmacological agent, administered either orally or intrathecally, to reduce spasticity.

Botulinum toxin: A toxin that paralyzes muscles by interfering with transmission at the neuromuscular junction. Botulinum toxin can be administered by injection into selected muscles to temporarily reduce muscle tone and spasticity and thereby promote increased ROM and improved function in children with neuromuscular disorders.

Cerebral palsy (CP): A symptom complex of static, nonprogressive posture and movement abnormalities caused by damage to the developing CNS in which motor impairment occurs before, during, and/or soon after birth.

Chiari II malformation: Anomaly of the hindbrain associated with open spinal dysraphism.

Closed spinal dysraphism (CSD): Congenital malformation of the spine and spinal cord where the neural tissue is covered by skin, although cutaneous stigmata, such as hairy nevus, capillary hemangioma, dimples, and subcutaneous masses, may exist.

Constraint-induced movement therapy (CIMT): A task-oriented intervention involving restraining the nonparetic upper extremity in conjunction with highly intensive, repetitive, and structured functional activities for the hemiparetic upper extremity.

Dyskinetic CP: A type of CP characterized by impaired volitional activity (athetosis, rigidity, and tremor) with uncontrolled and purposeless movements affecting the entire body.

Gross Motor Function Classification System (GMFCS): An ordinal, five-level system for categorizing the severity of CP based on self-initiated movement, need for assistive technology, and movement quality at a given age.

Impairment-focused intervention: A plan of care that addresses impairments in body structure and functions.

Low birth weight: A baby who weighs less than 2,500 gm (5 lb, 7½ oz) at birth.

Myelomeningocele (MM): An OSD that occurs when a segment of the spinal cord and meninges protrudes through a bony defect in the midline of the back and is exposed to the environment.

Neural tube defect (NTD): Incomplete development of the brain, spinal cord, and/or meninges as a result of errors or disturbances in any of the embryogenic processes.

Neurodevelopmental treatment (NDT): Impairment-focused intervention that uses a developmental framework emphasizing a child's ability to learn functional skills and typical movement patterns.

Open spinal dysraphism (OSD): Congenital malformation of the spine and spinal cord in which nervous tissue and/or meninges are exposed to the environment through a congenital bony defect of the vertebrae.

Selective dorsal rhizotomy (SDR): Neurosurgical intervention in which selective sensory nerve roots in the lumbar and sacral region are transected to reduce spasticity.

Spastic diplegia: A clinical type of CP characterized by paresis and hypertonicity of the entire body, with the legs being more involved than the arms.

Spastic hemiplegia: A clinical type of CP characterized by paresis and hypertonicity on one side of the body, including the arm, trunk, and leg.

Spastic quadriplegia: A clinical type of CP characterized by paresis and hypertonicity of the entire body with all four extremities relatively equally involved.

Spina bifida: Generic term used to describe spinal dysraphism.

Spinal dysraphism: Congenital malformations of the spine and spinal cord, including anomalies of the skin, muscles, vertebrae, meninges, and nervous tissue.

Chapter 16

Adult Nonprogressive Central Nervous System Disorders

Lisa L. Dutton

OBJECTIVES

After completing this chapter, the reader will be able to:
1. Describe and differentiate between different types of adult nonprogressive central nervous system disorders.
2. Understand the tests and measures used in the examination of adults with nonprogressive central nervous system disorders.
3. Discuss the theoretical principles underlying neurodevelopmental treatment, proprioceptive neuromuscular facilitation, and task-oriented approaches to rehabilitation intervention.
4. Apply interventions to address common impairments, functional limitations, and disabilities observed in individuals included in this practice pattern.
5. Apply knowledge of patient/client management for the individual who has sustained a stroke or traumatic brain injury to case studies.

This chapter addresses the rehabilitation of adults with impaired motor function and sensory integrity associated with nonprogressive central nervous system (CNS) disorders. The most common of these disorders are cerebrovascular accident (stroke) and traumatic brain injury. Patients with nonprogressive CNS disorders may exhibit a range of impairments, functional limitations, and disabilities that include the following:

- Altered cognition and behavior
- Impaired motor control and performance, including weakness, abnormal tone, abnormal reflexes, and altered movement patterns
- Disturbances in postural control and balance
- Decreased endurance
- Impaired sensory and perceptual integrity, including altered proprioception, vision, and unilateral neglect
- Decreased ability to perform functional activities such as bed mobility, transfers, and ambulation
- Decreased ability to function in work or home environments and fulfill social roles

In addition to the influence of varied pathology, all of these impairments, functional limitations, and disabilities are uniquely expressed in each patient based on the impact of individual and environmental factors. Individual factors include demographics, culture, lifestyles, psychological traits, and social support. Environmental factors are composed of influences such as social, political, and economic structures; the physical environment; available medical and/or rehabilitation care; and societal views of disability.[1]

Using the frameworks provided by Nagi's disablement model[2] and the *Guide to Physical Therapist Practice,*[1] this chapter discusses pathologies commonly linked with preferred practice pattern 5D: Impaired motor function and sensory integrity associated with nonprogressive disorders of the central nervous system—acquired in adolescence or adulthood. This is followed by consideration of appropriate examination procedures, including tests and measures for impairments and functional limitations often observed in patients with nonprogressive CNS disorders. A variety of intervention approaches for these patients is then discussed. All of these are considered within the context of "the conscientious, explicit, and judicious use of current best evidence in making decisions about the care of individual patients."[3]

PATHOLOGY

CEREBROVASCULAR ACCIDENT

Stroke or cerebrovascular accident (CVA) has been defined as an "acute neurologic dysfunction of vascular origin ... with symptoms and signs corresponding to the involvement of focal areas of the brain."[4] As the third leading cause of death and the number one cause of serious disability in the United States (US), stroke poses a significant public health concern.[5] Strokes are typically classified as occlusive or hemorrhagic. Occlusive strokes are associated with a restriction in blood flow to the brain that results in ischemia. Occlusive strokes account for 80% of all CVAs[6] and may be thrombotic or embolic in origin. A thrombotic stroke is caused by the development of a blood clot or thrombus in a vessel in the brain. An embolic stroke is caused by material from another area of the body moving to a blood vessel in the brain and occluding it. Emboli that go to the brain are typically blood clots that detach from blood vessels, or from within the heart, that travel through the bloodstream to suddenly occlude a cerebral artery.[7] Emboli may also be composed of other materials such as fat, which occurs occasionally after fractures of long bones, or necrotic material, which can occur with infection of the heart valves (endocarditis).

The clinical syndromes associated with occlusive strokes vary according to the cerebral artery involved (Fig. 16-1). For example, occlusion of the middle cerebral artery, the most common site of stroke,[8] typically results in contralateral paralysis and sensory deficits in the face and upper extremities that are greater than in the lower extremities, as well as motor speech impairment and aphasia if the dominant hemisphere is involved. When the anterior cerebral artery is occluded, contralateral paralysis and sensory loss are generally greater in the lower extremity than the upper extremity. In addition, ischemia in the frontal lobe may cause declarative memory loss and behavioral impairments. When the posterior cerebral artery is involved, homonymous hemianopsia (a loss of vision in the half of the visual field contralateral to the lesion), cortical blindness, and memory deficit can ensue. In addition, with loss of blood supply to the thalamus, patients often develop choreoathetosis, spontaneous pain and dysesthesias, sensory loss, and intention tremor.

◎ *Clinical Pearl*

Middle cerebral artery occlusion is the most common cause of stroke.

Hemorrhagic strokes, which are those associated with the rupture of a blood vessel, account for approximately 20% of strokes.[6] They are often associated with hypertension or vascular malformations such as cerebral aneurysms and arteriovenous malformations (AVM). With this type of stroke, brain tissue death occurs because of ischemia and mechanical and chemical injury associated with the release of blood into the extravascular space. The mortality rates for hemorrhagic stroke are much higher than for occlusive strokes.[9] Eighty percent of hypertensive hemorrhages involve the cerebral hemispheres, they are often large, and common sites of involvement include the basal ganglia, thalamus, cerebellum, and the pons.[10] Subarachnoid hemorrhages are often seen in normotensive individuals, with 85% arising from congenital berry aneurysms, and they frequently occur in the circle of Willis. The clinical syndromes associated with hemorrhagic stroke tend to be more varied because they are related to the size and extent of damage associated with the bleed. Cases can

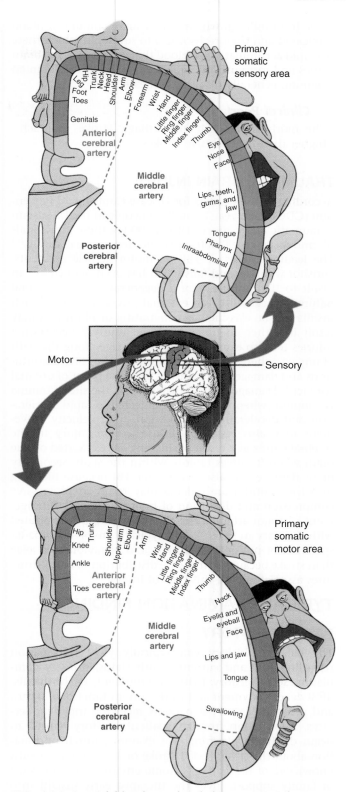

FIG. 16-1 Arterial blood supply of the motor and sensory cortex. *Adapted from Thibodeau GA, Patton KT: Anatomy and physiology, ed 6, St. Louis, 2006, Mosby.*

range from mild, in which only a small amount of blood is released and then reabsorbed, to severe, in which there is a rapid accumulation of blood that compresses the brain tissues and can push the brainstem through the foramen magnum, generally resulting in death.

◎ *Clinical Pearl*

The mortality rate for hemorrhagic strokes is much higher than for occlusive strokes.

TRAUMATIC BRAIN INJURY

According to the Centers for Disease Control and Prevention (CDC), each year 1.5 million people in the US sustain a traumatic brain injury (TBI); 50,000 of these individuals die and 80,000 to 90,000 experience long-term disability.[11] The leading causes of TBI are motor vehicle accidents, gunshot wounds, and falls.[12] TBI has been defined as "an insult to the brain, not of a degenerative or congenital nature, but caused by an external physical force."[13] Such insults can be classified as penetrating or blunt and may result in either an open or closed injury.[14] Penetrating injuries tend to cause more focal damage along the path of impact, whereas blunt injuries can cause cortical contusions and damage in areas away from the point of original contact.[15] Damage in areas distant from the site of trauma is common when the brain is subjected to rapid acceleration and deceleration. In addition, high velocity movement may also result in diffuse axonal injury in the cerebral cortex as a result of shearing forces exerted on the brain when it moves rapidly within the skull. Secondary brain damage can also occur after TBI because bleeding into the cranium and edema may result in progressive compression and distortion of brain tissue and impingement of major arteries. The clinical syndromes associated with TBI vary in severity and typically involve a broader spectrum of physical, cognitive, and behavioral sequelae than stroke because of the wide distribution of brain structures associated with this type of injury.

TYPICAL EXAMINATION FINDINGS

PATIENT HISTORY

The patient's history will typically yield information regarding past and current health status, primary complaints, social history, living environment, health habits, lifestyle, employment and work, current functional status, and personal goals. For patients receiving inpatient services, information from the patient's history is used to begin discharge planning. For example, initial information about the severity of a stroke or TBI, combined with knowledge of the patient's home environment and level of family support, gives the therapist early insight into potential needs for equipment and support services on discharge.

TESTS AND MEASURES

Musculoskeletal. Strength can be assessed as reliably through isometric, isokinetic, and functional measures in individuals with neurologic dysfunction as in those with musculoskeletal dysfunction[16-18] (see Chapter 5).

TABLE 16-1	Classification of Neglect
Classification	**Definition**
Sensory neglect	Decreased awareness of sensory stimulation on the involved side of the body. Can include decreased awareness of auditory, visual, or somatosensory input.
Motor neglect	Decreased ability to generate a movement response despite awareness of stimuli. May be observed throughout the body, including the eyes, head, neck, trunk, and limbs.
Representational neglect	Failure to construct one side of a visual memory or image. May be observed when a patient is asked to describe a familiar place from a particular orientation (e.g., if asked to describe the front of his/her home only one side is described, but if the orientation is changed by having the patient imagine he/she is facing a different direction, then the previously omitted side of the image is included).
Personal neglect	Decreased awareness of the limb or side of the body opposite the brain lesion.
Spatial neglect	Decreased awareness of space on the side of the body opposite the brain lesion.

From Schmidt RA: *Motor control and learning: A behavioral emphasis,* Champaign, IL, 1982, Human Kinetics.

Neuromuscular

Arousal, Attention, and Cognition. One frequently used measure of arousal, particularly in the case of individuals with TBI, is the Glasgow Coma Scale (GCS) (see Chapter 21).[19] This scale was designed to provide a measure of altered consciousness through assessment of eye opening, best motor response, and a verbal score. The GCS score within the first 24 hours after injury has also been used as an indicator of severity and a predictor of outcome after TBI.

One commonly observed attentional deficit after stroke is unilateral spatial neglect. Individuals with this behavioral syndrome fail to "report or respond to people or objects presented to the side opposite a brain lesion."[20] This lack of response cannot be attributed to sensory or motor deficits.[21] Some researchers have reported the incidence of unilateral neglect after stroke to be as high as 82% for strokes in the right hemisphere and 65% for strokes in the left hemisphere.[22] Understanding the type of neglect allows the therapist to more appropriately structure patient intervention. Types of neglect are more specifically described in Table 16-1.[23-25]

Cognition includes **skills** such as the ability to discriminate between relevant and irrelevant information, understanding and retention, and the ability to appropriately apply knowledge.[26] Deficits in cognitive function are a significant cause of disability after TBI and stroke and can decrease a patient's capacity to complete routine daily tasks and impair the ability to respond to new or challenging situations.

The most common screening test used for cognition is the Mini-Mental State Examination (MMSE).[27] This test

TABLE 16-2	Rancho Los Amigos Levels of Cognitive Functioning	
Level	**Response**	**Characteristics**
I	No response	Unresponsive to any stimulus.
II	Generalized response	Limited, inconsistent, nonpurposeful responses, often to pain only.
III	Localized response	Purposeful responses. May follow simply commands. May focus on presented object.
IV	Confused, agitated	Heightened state of activity. Confusion, disorientation. Aggressive behavior. Unable to do self-care. Unaware of present events. Agitation appears related to internal confusion.
V	Confused, inappropriate	Nonagitated. Appears alert. Responds to commands. Distractable. Does not concentrate on task. Agitated responses to external stimuli. Verbally inappropriate. Does not learn new information.
VI	Confused, appropriate	Goal-directed behavior, needs cueing. Can relearn old skills as ADLs. Severe memory problems. Some awareness of self and others.
VII	Automatic, appropriate	Appears appropriate. Oriented. Frequently robot-like in daily routine. Minimal or absent confusion. Shallow recall. Increased awareness of self, interaction in environment. Lacks insight into condition. Decreased judgment and problem solving. Lacks realistic planning for future.
VIII	Purposeful, appropriate	Alert, oriented. Recalls and integrates past events. Learns new activities and can continue without supervision. Independent in home and living skills. Defects in stress tolerance, judgment, abstract reasoning persist. May function at reduced levels in society.

From Hagan C, Malkmus D, Durham P: Levels of cognitive functions. In *Rehabilitation of the head injured adult: Comprehensive physical management,* Downey, CA, 1979, Professional Staff Association of Rancho Los Amigos Hospital.
ADLs, Activities of daily living.

addresses orientation to time and place, registration of words, attention, calculation, recall, language, and visual construction. Although designed for patients with dementia, it has been shown to be a valid and reliable tool in a range of populations, including patients with stroke.[27-29]

A second test of cognition that is recommended by the Agency for Health Care Policy and Research (AHCPR) in their clinical practice guideline for stroke[5] is the Neurobehavioral Cognitive Status Examination (NCSE).[30] This examination addresses ten domains: Orientation, attention, comprehension, naming, construction, memory, calculation, similarities, judgment, and repetition. The test starts with a difficult item in each domain as an initial screen. If a patient fails this screening item, he or she completes additional items, progressing from easy to more difficult, to identify the extent of his or her deficit. If a patient passes the screening item, he or she is considered to have no deficit in that domain. The NCSE has been validated in samples of neurosurgical patients,[31] patients with TBI,[32,33] and patients with stroke.[34] In addition, the NCSE was found to be more sensitive than the MMSE at detecting cognitive dysfunction in a sample of 30 neurosurgical patients.[35]

Finally, while the GCS is primarily used as an acute measure of arousal, the Rancho Los Amigos Levels of Cognitive Functioning Scale (LCFS) is the most commonly used measure of arousal and cognitive functioning in the TBI population (Table 16-2).[36] This scale classifies individuals recovering from TBI into one of eight possible categories. These categories range from no response to purposeful and appropriate responses. Although commonly used as a means of quantifying improvement in individuals with TBI, no literature supports the validity or reliability of this tool.

Sensory Integrity. Patients within the adult nonprogressive CNS disorder practice pattern typically present with sensory and in some cases, perceptual deficits. Sensory deficits can include impairments in discriminative touch, proprioception, and sensation of pain and temperature (see Chapter 18 for further details of tests and measures of sensation). The ability to discriminate light touch can be grossly assessed with the patient's eyes closed by asking her to indicate whether she feels the stimulus. Proprioception, including joint position and joint motion, can be assessed with the patient's eyes closed by asking the patient to indicate the position of a limb or the direction of movement.[37]

Spasticity and Muscle Tone. **Spasticity** is characterized by a velocity-dependent increase in tonic stretch reflexes accompanied by exaggerated tendon jerks.[38] **Muscle tone** has been defined as resistance to passive stretch,[39] and increased muscle tone in individuals with neuromuscular disorders can be related to both changes in the intrinsic properties of muscle, tendon, and connective tissue, as well as hyperactive stretch reflexes. The most commonly used clinical measure of muscle tone is the Modified Ashworth Scale (Table 16-3).[40] This 6-point scale grades muscle tone based on resistance to passive movement. Specifically, the test is conducted by passively moving the muscle or muscle group under consideration through its full range of motion (ROM).

Coordination. Nonequilibrium coordination tests are typically used to assess motor performance deficits related to cerebellar dysfunction. For example, they may be used to identify impairments such as **dysdiadochokinesia, dysmetria,** or **dyssynergia.**[41] Common coordination tests include examination of alternating finger to nose movement, rapid finger opposition, pronation/supination, tapping of the hand or foot, and moving the heel up and down the shin.

Movement Patterns. Abnormal movement patterns, or synergies, have been described after CNS disorders such as stroke or TBI.[41,42] Abnormal synergies are stereotyped patterns of movement that limit an individual's ability to dissociate movement at one joint from movement at another and generate a variety of movement patterns in response to task demands.[43] For example, when asked to raise his arm, the patient with an abnormal flexor synergy in the upper extremity may be unable to flex his shoulder without shoulder elevation, shoulder abduction, and elbow flexion accompanying the movement. The full **abnormal synergy** patterns for the upper and lower extremity are shown in Fig. 16-2.

Cardiovascular/Pulmonary. Tests and measures commonly associated with the assessment of aerobic capacity and endurance in adults with nonprogressive CNS disorders include measures such as heart rate, blood pressure, and respiratory rate at rest and during and after functional activities and exercise, as well as standardized tests such as the 6-minute walk test (6MWT). The 6MWT measures the distance that an individual can walk in 6 minutes[44] and is considered a submaximal test of aerobic capacity.[45]

Function

Balance. Balance is a multidimensional construct that has been described as including the ability to maintain one's position in space, stabilize in anticipation of voluntary movement, and respond to external perturbations.[46,47] In addition, one's ability to demonstrate symmetry or equal weight distribution in sitting or standing is also often included as an important aspect of balance.[48-50] A variety of tests and measures (see Chapter 13) has been developed to examine one or more of these components. These include scales such as the Berg Balance Scale (BBS), Tinetti's Performance-Oriented Mobility Assessment (POMA), Timed Up and Go, and Functional Reach Test (see Fig. 13-8). Of these, the BBS addresses all three components of balance: Maintenance of position, postural adjustment to voluntary movement, and reaction to external disturbances. In addition, it has well-established validity and reliability in the elderly.[46,51]

Gait. For adults with neuromuscular disorders, one of the most clinically practical measures of gait ability is gait speed. This measure has been shown to be valid, reliable, and sensitive to change in a wide range of populations.[52-58] Measures of gait speed are only appropriate for individuals who are able to ambulate without significant manual assistance. In addition to measures of gait speed, it is also important to consider the patient's ability to negotiate different types of surfaces and obstacles.

Self-Care and Home-Management. A number of global measures of function can be used for adults with nonprogressive CNS disorders. These measures include the Functional Independence Measure (FIM) and the Barthel Index. The FIM is probably the most widely used outcome measure for individuals with neuromuscular disorders, particularly for those receiving inpatient rehabilitation services. The FIM measures function in the areas of self-care, sphincter control, mobility, locomotion, communication, and social cognition and is reported to be valid, reliable, and generally sensitive to change for most individuals, including those with stroke and TBI, with the exception of those functioning at the lowest and highest

TABLE 16-3	Modified Ashworth Scale

Muscle Tone Grade	Definition
0	No increase in muscle tone.
1	Slight increase in muscle tone, manifested by a slight catch and release or by minimal resistance at the end of the ROM when the affected part(s) is moved in flexion or extension.
1+	Slight increase in muscle tone, manifested by a catch, followed by minimal resistance throughout the remainder (less than half) of the ROM.
2	More marked increase in muscle tone through most of the ROM, but affected part(s) easily moved.
3	Considerable increase in muscle tone, passive movement difficult.
4	Affected part(s) rigid in flexion or extension.

From Bohannon RW, Smith MB: *Phys Ther* 67:206-207, 1987.
ROM, Range of motion.

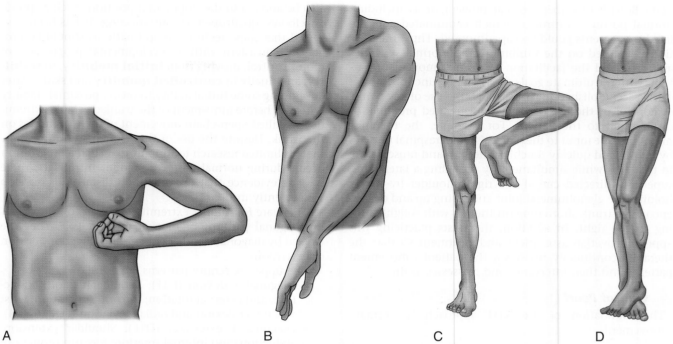

FIG. 16-2 Abnormal synergy patterns for the upper and lower extremities. **A,** UE flexion—shoulder abduction, elbow flexion, forearm supination, wrist and finger flexion; **B,** UE extension—shoulder adduction, elbow extension, forearm pronation, wrist and finger extension; **C,** LE flexion—hip abduction, hip and knee flexion, ankle dorsiflexion; **D,** LE extension—hip adduction, hip and knee extension, ankle plantarflexion.

A B C D

levels.[59,60] This measure is a good predictor of level of disability and discharge status in patients who have sustained strokes.[61] A FIM score of 80 or above is associated with discharge to home.[62,63]

The Barthel Index is primarily intended for patients after stroke. This index assesses activities in two major categories: Personal care and mobility. The personal care items include tasks such as drinking from a cup, dressing, grooming, bathing, and bowel and bladder continence. The mobility items include wheelchair maneuvering, walking, stairs, and transfers.

INTERVENTION

There are a variety of approaches to intervention for adults with nonprogressive CNS disorders. These approaches can be classified according to the motor control theories that support them. The more traditional neurofacilitation techniques, such as proprioceptive neuromuscular facilitation (PNF) and neurodevelopmental treatment (NDT), have historically been associated with the reflex and hierarchical models of motor control.[39] In these models, sensory input is used to influence motor output and the CNS is considered to be organized hierarchically, beginning with the spinal level as the lowest level of integration and extending upward to the prepontine, midbrain, and cortical levels, respectively. It should be noted that NDT in particular has begun to move away from its historical theoretical base to incorporate tenets of the systems model into its underlying assumptions.[64] The emphasis of intervention in these approaches is on facilitation of normal movement patterns while inhibiting abnormal synergies,

and motor recovery is assumed to follow a predictable sequence.[39,65] In contrast, the task-oriented approaches[43,66,67] are supported by the systems theory of motor control. The theoretical basis for these approaches was originally proposed by Nicoli Bernstein and suggests that movement emerges as the result of the interaction of multiple systems.[68] Furthermore, this theory posits that in the case of motor control, these systems are organized around the goal of accomplishing a particular motor task as opposed to the generation of a selected movement pattern.[39,65] Also associated with the task-oriented approaches are more recently introduced interventions such as constraint-induced movement therapy (CIMT) and body weight–supported (BWS) ambulation (see later).

Although few studies evaluate their effectiveness, PNF and NDT continue to be widely used approaches in clinical practice and therefore are discussed in the next section. In contrast, more recent task-oriented approaches, such as BWS gait training and CIMT, are less commonly used in clinical practice but have been more extensively studied. These approaches have good scientific evidence demonstrating efficacy and are also described later.

NEURODEVELOPMENTAL TREATMENT

The NDT approach was originally developed by Berta Bobath and Dr. Karel Bobath in the early 1940s.[42] The Bobaths described their approach as "not a method but a living concept ... a management."[69] As such, the approach has changed and adapted over the years to accommodate emerging knowledge in neuroscience.[70] A key element of this approach is its foundation in normal movement.[42,71]

Berta Bobath described normal movement as including normal postural control on which coordinated and isolated movements could be superimposed. Thus intervention is focused on the inhibition of abnormal synergies and tone and the facilitation of normal movement patterns with the ultimate goal of optimizing function.[42,64,71,72] This is accomplished in part through the use of key points of control or the use of therapist-generated proximal or distal input to the patient. For example, the therapist might provide input to the patient's left paraspinal muscles by lightly and quickly touching the skin and musculature in that area while simultaneously providing a lateral and superiorly directed cue at the right shoulder by gently holding the glenohumeral joint and lifting up and over to encourage trunk shortening on the left with weight shifting to the right. In addition, therapists practicing this approach overlap assessment and treatment so that the therapist continually reassesses the patient's movement patterns and then intervenes and reassesses again.

◎ *Clinical Pearl*

The foundation of the NDT approach is normal movement.

Aside from the possible immediate effects related to NDT facilitation, there is limited evidence to suggest that NDT is superior to other neurorehabilitation approaches as measured by short- or long-term outcomes.

PROPRIOCEPTIVE NEUROMUSCULAR FACILITATION

PNF is based on concepts first introduced by Dr. Herman Kabat in the 1950s and later expanded on by Margaret Knott and Dorothy Voss. This intervention approach was described by Voss as including "methods of promoting or hastening the response of the neuromuscular mechanism through stimulation of proprioceptors."[73] PNF is carried out using defined combinations of movement that include diagonal and spiral components. The use of these movement combinations takes into consideration Dr. Kabat's observations that (1) normal coordinated activities are accomplished through complex movement patterns that do not occur in straight planes; (2) the stretch reflex is most effectively elicited when the extremity is elongated in a specific diagonal; and (3) the muscular response is more coordinated and forceful when resisted within a specific diagonal. In addition, PNF incorporates the use of a variety of sensory inputs, such as traction, approximation, resistance, quick stretch, verbal stimuli, and visual stimuli, to facilitate a desired motor response.[74] The goals of this facilitation may include either increased contraction or relaxation of various muscle groups.

◎ *Clinical Pearl*

PNF uses defined combinations of movement, including diagonal and spiral components, to increase contraction or relaxation of various muscle groups.

In PNF, specific diagonal patterns are applied to the trunk, pelvis, shoulder girdle, and extremities. They may also be applied to developmental positions such as prone on elbows, quadruped, or tall kneeling. It has been suggested that these techniques and patterns should be progressed consistent with a developmental progression of motor control, moving from **initial mobility,** to **stability,** and finally to **controlled mobility** and skill.[75] After developing some initial ability to move, proximal stability is needed before movement of the trunk on stable extremities or skilled open-chain movement of the extremities on the trunk. Despite the use of this sequencing in practice, there is limited research to support that such a progression occurs during normal motor development. In fact, there is some evidence that proximal and distal skills develop concurrently in infants.[76,77]

There are four upper extremity and four lower extremity diagonal patterns of motion used in PNF. They are labeled by diagonal number (1 or 2) and direction (flexion or extension).

The upper extremity patterns are as follows[74]:

- Diagonal 1 flexion (D1F): Shoulder flexion, adduction, and external rotation; forearm supination; wrist and finger flexion and radial deviation (Fig. 16-3, *A*).
- Diagonal 1 extension (D1E): Shoulder extension, abduction, and internal rotation; forearm pronation; wrist and finger extension and ulnar deviation (Fig. 16-3, *B*).
- Diagonal 2 flexion (D2F): Shoulder flexion, abduction, and external rotation; forearm supination; wrist and finger extension and radial deviation (Fig. 16-3, *C*).
- Diagonal 2 extension (D2E): Shoulder extension, adduction, and internal rotation; forearm pronation; wrist and finger flexion and ulnar deviation (Fig. 16-3, *D*).

The lower extremity patterns are as follows:

- Diagonal 1 flexion (D1F): Hip flexion, adduction and external rotation; ankle/foot dorsiflexion and inversion; toe extension (Fig. 16-4, *A*).
- Diagonal 1 extension (D1E): Hip extension, abduction, and internal rotation; ankle/foot plantarflexion and eversion; toe flexion (Fig. 16-4, *B*).
- Diagonal 2 flexion (D2F): Hip flexion, abduction, and internal rotation; ankle/foot dorsiflexion and eversion; toe extension (Fig. 16-4, *C*).
- Diagonal 2 extension (D2E): Hip extension, adduction, and external rotation; ankle/foot plantarflexion and inversion; toe flexion (Fig. 16-4, *D*).

When applying these diagonals specifically to the shoulder girdle or pelvis, there are generally two diagonals considered: Anterior-elevation/posterior-depression and posterior-elevation/anterior-depression, and intervention is generally conducted with the patient in sidelying (Fig. 16-5). In addition, the extremity, shoulder girdle, and pelvic diagonals can also be applied with the patient in various developmental postures. For example, in quadruped a patient could be asked to shift weight down and back to the right and up and forward to the left, thus incorporating pelvic, shoulder, and portions of the extremity diagonals.

A number of techniques associated with PNF are superimposed on these diagonals as applied to the extremities,

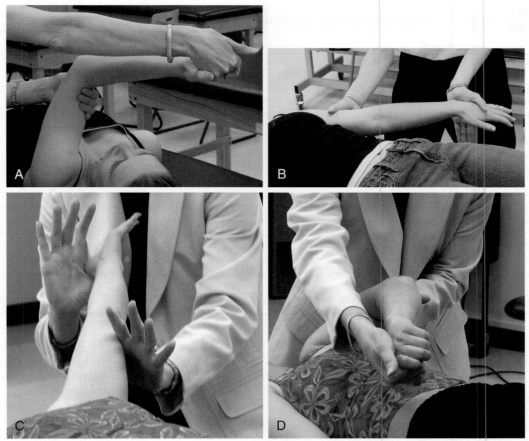

FIG. 16-3 Upper extremity diagonal patterns. **A,** Diagonal 1 flexion (D1F). **B,** Diagonal 1 extension (D1E). **C,** Diagonal 2 flexion (D2F). **D,** Diagonal 2 extension (D2E).

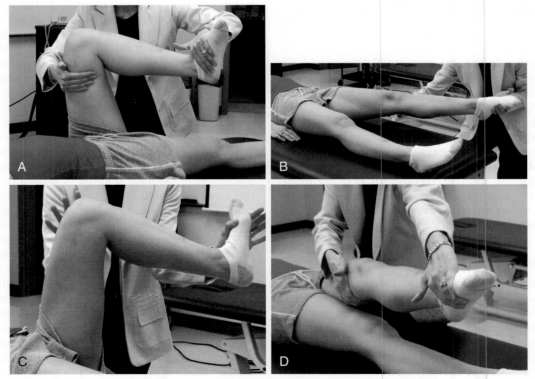

FIG. 16-4 Lower extremity diagonal patterns. **A,** Diagonal 1 flexion (D1F). **B,** Diagonal 1 extension (D1E). **C,** Diagonal 2 flexion (D2F). **D,** Diagonal 2 extension (D2E).

TABLE 16-4	Proprioceptive Neuromuscular Facilitation Techniques
Technique	**Method**
Hold-relax active motion	An isometric contraction in the shortened range of the diagonal, followed by passive movement into the lengthened range and then followed by active contraction into the shortened range.
Repeated contractions	Repeated use of the stretch reflex to initiate a contraction or reinforce and strengthen an existing contraction.
Rhythmic initiation	Progression of movement in diagonal from passive to active assistive to active to resisted.
Timing for emphasis	Maximal isometric resistance applied to stronger components of the diagonal to allow for facilitation or irradiation to weaker components.
Rhythmic rotation	Active or passive rotation around the longitudinal axis with the extremity positioned in the desired diagonal.
Alternating isometrics	Alternating isometric contractions of the agonist and antagonist.
Rhythmic stabilization	An extension of alternating isometrics in which the manual contacts are on opposite joint surfaces simultaneously.
Contract-relax	Movement into agonist pattern until a point of limitation, followed by isometric contraction of all components of the antagonist pattern except for the rotation component, which is allowed to contract isotonically; repeated with passive movement into any newly gained range after each trial.
Hold-relax	Isometric contraction of the agonist or antagonist musculature in the desired diagonal at the point of range limitation; repeated with passive movement into any newly gained range after each trial.
Slow reversals	Slow concentric contractions alternating between the agonist and antagonist muscle groups.
Slow reversal-hold	Slow concentric contractions alternating between the agonist and antagonist muscle groups with an isometric contraction applied at the end of each diagonal.
Agonist reversals	Isotonic contraction in the diagonal followed by an eccentric contraction of the same muscle groups.

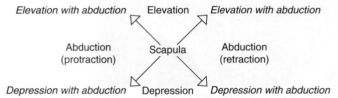

FIG. 16-5 Anterior-elevation/posterior-depression of the shoulder girdle. *From Waddington PJ: PNF head and neck, scapular, and trunk patterns. In Hollis M, Fletcher-Cook P: Practical exercise therapy, ed 4, Oxford, 1999, Blackwell Science.*

trunk, or in developmental postures. These techniques are based on neurophysiological evidence that sensory inputs can influence motor output[78,79] and are described in Table 16-4.[73,74]

For initial mobility, techniques such as **rhythmic initiation, repeated contractions,** and **timing for emphasis** are used. For stability, **rhythmic stabilization** and **alternating isometrics** are suggested. For controlled mobility and skill, therapists may utilize **hold-relax active motion, slow reversal-hold, slow reversals,** and **agonistic reversals. Hold-relax** and **contract-relax** are intended to improve ROM and flexibility.

TASK-ORIENTED APPROACHES

The task-oriented approaches are based on scientists' current understanding of how movement arises from the interaction between systems at the level of the individual, the environment, and the task. In addition, these approaches more fully incorporate emerging knowledge regarding neural plasticity and **motor learning** and take into consideration the implications of research in the areas of environmental and task analysis, feedback, and practice. Gentile's Taxonomy of Movement Tasks is

often used as the framework for environmental and task analysis for the purpose of guiding examination and intervention.[80] In this taxonomy, functional activities are evaluated based on the environmental context of the task and its functional role. Specifically, **regulatory conditions,** or those elements of the environment to which a task must conform, are conceptualized as being either stationary or in motion and presenting with or without intertrial variability. For example, if one were to practice a sit-to-stand transfer from a kitchen chair in the patient's home, the regulatory conditions (the chair) would be stationary and assuming that the person only practiced from one specific chair, present no intertrial variability. This is considered a closed task. On the other hand, if the patient were to practice sit-to-stand from a therapy ball, the regulatory conditions (the ball) would be in motion and that motion would be variable from trial to trial. This is considered an open task. This taxonomy is described in Table 16-5.

One can also analyze the function of the task. From this perspective, Gentile suggested considering whether the task required body stability or transport and whether the upper extremities were used primarily for stability or manipulation. In this case, if an individual was practicing sitting balance with the upper extremities providing support on the mat, the task would be stable with the upper extremities yoked into the postural system. If the person was ambulating while looking for a pencil in his or her pocket, the task would be more difficult and require both transport and manipulation. This taxonomy is provided in Table 16-6. From these two taxonomies, a full 16-cell taxonomy, combining both analysis of the environment and the task, can be created that allows one to structure interventions based on the inclusion of appropriately challenging activities. For example, a task such as ambulating through a busy shopping mall while carrying a wiggling baby would be at the highest level of the full

TABLE 16-5	**Environmental Context: Task Categories and Examples**	
Regulatory Conditions	**Intertrial Variability: Absent**	**Intertrial Variability: Present**
Stationary	Closed tasks: 　Climbing stairs at home 　Brushing teeth 　Unlocking the front door 　Stepping on the bathroom scale	Variable motionless tasks: 　Walking on different surfaces 　Climbing stairs of different heights 　Drinking from mugs, glasses, cups
Motion	Consistent motion tasks: 　Stepping onto an escalator 　Lifting luggage from an airport 　　conveyor 　Moving through a revolving door	Open tasks: 　Sitting in a moving automobile 　Catching a ball 　Walking down a crowded hallway 　Carrying a wiggling child

From Gentile A: Skill acquisition: Action, movement, and neuromotor processes. In Carr J, Shepherd R (eds): *Movement science: Foundations for physical therapy in rehabilitation,* ed 2, Gaithersburg, MD, 2000, Aspen.

TABLE 16-6	**Function of the Action: Task Categories and Examples**	
Body Orientation	**Manipulation: Absent**	**Manipulation: Present**
Stability	Body stability: 　Sit 　Stand 　Lean on table	Body stability plus manipulation: 　Hold object while standing 　Reach for glass while sitting 　Writing at a desk
Transport	Body transport: 　Run 　Walk 　Crawl	Body transport plus manipulation: 　Carry child while walking 　Run to catch a ball 　Drive an automobile

From Gentile A: Skill acquisition: Action, movement, and neuromotor processes. In Carr J, Shepherd R (eds): *Movement science: Foundations for physical therapy in rehabilitation,* ed 2, Gaithersburg, MD, 2000, Aspen.

taxonomy and includes regulatory conditions that are variable and in motion, as well as transport and upper extremity manipulation.

Feedback and its use to enhance motor learning, recovery, and control is also an important component of the task-oriented approaches. A variety of types of feedback are available to patients as they learn and refine motor skills. For example, patients have access to **intrinsic feedback** about both the outcome of a functional task, as well as the movement used to accomplish that outcome.[80] Intrinsic feedback includes any type of feedback that is naturally available to the individual such as somatosensory, proprioceptive, or visual input. External or **augmented feedback** related to **knowledge of results (KR)** or **knowledge of performance (KP)** is also often provided to patients by therapists with the goal of improving motor control. Examples of augmented feedback include verbal or tactile cues, and such feedback may be provided concurrently, immediately following, or be delayed in relation to the action.[81] The impact of augmented feedback on both the performance of motor skills and motor learning has been studied in individuals with and without neurological deficit. Motor learning has typically been defined as a process associated with practice that leads to a relatively permanent change in performance of motor skills.[82,83] As such, changes in performance observed immediately after a treatment session are not generally considered evidence of motor learning

unless these changes are retained over time. For example, if a patient moved from sit-to-stand asymmetrically and with assistance at the beginning of a treatment session and demonstrates the ability to move from sit-to-stand symmetrically and independently at the end of the session, this would be evidence of improved performance. If the patient continues to be able to demonstrate a symmetrical and independent sit-to-stand at the beginning of his or her next treatment session, this would be evidence of retention of that skill and thus motor learning.

In general, although more research has been conducted on the use of feedback in people without neurological conditions than in people with neurological impairments, the evidence suggests that the timing and frequency of feedback may significantly influence its effects on motor performance and learning. For individuals poststroke, explicit knowledge of the task goals before practice appears to most effectively improve implicit learning of motor skills.

◎ *Clinical Pearl*

Patients who have had a stroke learn skills best when they know the goals of the task.

One of the more promising task-oriented approaches for facilitating function of the hemiplegic upper extremity is CIMT (Fig. 16-6). In this approach, the nonparetic upper extremity is typically restrained for most of the patient's

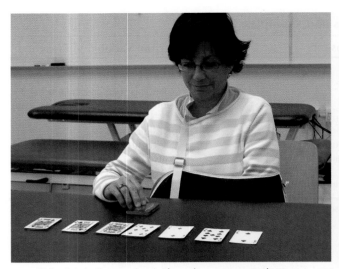

FIG. 16-6 Constraint-induced movement therapy.

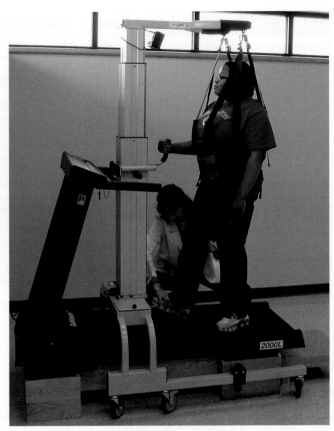

FIG. 16-7 Body weight–supported treadmill training.

waking hours, and the patient spends 6 hours per day for 2 weeks performing repetitive and structured functional activities that require use of the hemiparetic upper extremity.[84] An important component of CIMT is shaping. Shaping is an operant conditioning method in which the difficulty of the movement task is progressively increased, and individuals are given regular positive reinforcement and feedback regarding their performance. Positive results associated with CIMT have been documented in individuals with chronic stroke and have been shown to be sustained over time.[84-86]

It appears that CIMT may benefit some patients with neuromuscular disorders. In general, CIMT is most beneficial for subjects with intact cognition and moderate active movement in the involved upper extremity. In addition, there may be different effects for those with sensory disorders. In general, the intensity of training appears to be a key factor in this approach, with greater intensity (e.g., 6 hours per day) producing more substantial and clinically meaningful results.

Finally, another promising task-oriented approach to rehabilitation for individuals with nonprogressive neuromuscular disorders is treadmill training with partial body weight support. A growing body of evidence indicates that this intervention is an effective means of gait rehabilitation for individuals after a stroke (Fig. 16-7). Body weight–supported treadmill training (BWSTT) may improve functional gait and velocity, particularly for individuals who are either unable to walk or require maximal assistance of one or more individuals for ambulation (see Chapter 32). For this patient population, reported advantages of BWSTT include the ability to begin gait training earlier in the recovery process and its repetitive, task-specific nature.[87] Although no studies were identified that included individuals with TBI as subjects, given the effectiveness of this approach in patients with stroke and the similarities in impairments and functional limitations associated with both pathologies, this approach also holds promise for patients with TBI.

THERAPEUTIC EXERCISE

Aerobic and Endurance Conditioning/Reconditioning. Many of the impairments associated with stroke and TBI, such as abnormal motor control, reduced strength and power, impaired sensation, and hypertonicity or hypotonicity, may lead to inefficient motor control that results in increased energy expenditure during ambulation and other functional activities.[88,89] In addition, individuals with stroke are often physically deconditioned and have reduced aerobic capacity compared to age-matched controls.[90] As such, there is good evidence that individuals with nonprogressive CNS disorders may benefit from aerobic exercise and endurance training.

◎ *Clinical Pearl*

Many of the impairments associated with stroke and TBI result in increased energy expenditure during ambulation and functional activities.

A number of different aerobic exercise training regimens, particularly for individuals at least 6 months post-stroke, have been evaluated in the literature.[88,90-92] Positive effects have been reported for submaximal training programs involving 6 months of treadmill ambulation 2 to 3 times per week for 40-minute sessions.[88,91] Specifically, in these studies, individuals who exercised at 50% to 60% of their heart rate reserve significantly improved their fitness reserve or their percentage of peak oxygen consumption during submaximal exercise. These programs were conducted without BWS on the treadmill. Although treadmill training can be conducted with BWS, not surprisingly, oxygen uptake and heart rate measures have been found to be lower under these conditions.[92] It should be noted that almost 25% of the patients screened for this treadmill training study could not participate because of either co-morbidities or neurological deficits that prevented full weight-bearing treadmill walking.[88] It is possible that more individuals could have participated if some percentage of BWS had been allowed. While these studies provide preliminary support for the effectiveness of treadmill exercise training programs after stroke, they are all limited by small sample sizes, ranging from 9 to 23 subjects, and no meta-analyses of these studies have been published.

Balance, Coordination, and Agility Training. Individuals with diagnoses of stroke or TBI often present with perceptual, sensory, and motor impairments that impact balance and coordination. In addition, balance status has been associated with length of stay and other rehabilitation outcome measures.[93] As such, significant attention is often given to addressing these functional limitations and interventions to improve balance or postural control may take various approaches. Interventions can be designed to improve postural control in either sitting or standing, and they may be focused on symmetry, stability, anticipatory, or reactionary control.

Postural Symmetry. From an NDT perspective, postural symmetry, or the ability to evenly bear weight in sitting or standing, is a key indicator of improved motor control.[42,72] A symmetrical base of support allows individuals to appropriately prepare for movement and provides a foundation for normal equilibrium reactions, as well as other functional activities. For example, by establishing equal weight bearing with a neutral pelvis in sitting, a patient with a stroke or TBI can better activate his or her trunk musculature to move from a sitting position to standing.

In preparation for sitting, therapists using an NDT approach should first work to establish symmetrical alignment and a neutral pelvis. This would include even weight bearing on the ischial tuberosities, lower extremities, and feet.[71] In addition, the shoulders and head should be positioned symmetrically and there should be no rotation in the trunk. From this position, the therapist can facilitate anterior and posterior tilts of the pelvis, as well as lateral weight shifting. To facilitate an anterior pelvic tilt, while sitting in front of the patient, the therapist's hands are positioned around the patient's trunk to the back, aiming down and in. The hands then give a cue forward and up and the fifth digit can be used to cue the abdominal musculature (Fig. 16-8). For a posterior pelvic tilt, similar hand holds are used, but the fifth digit is used to cue the patient's trunk down and back.

From a PNF perspective, to achieve good sitting balance and symmetry, repeated contractions or resistance in a diagonal through the anterior superior iliac spines can be used to facilitate an anterior pelvic tilt. Once a neutral pelvic position is achieved, rhythmic stabilization or

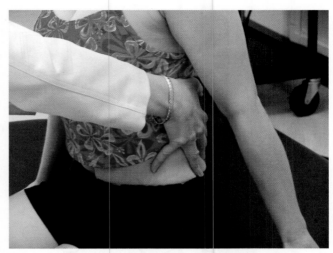

FIG. 16-8 Neurodevelopmental treatment facilitation of sitting posture.

alternating isometrics can be applied to the trunk to promote a stable posture.

In standing, postural symmetry can be encouraged through NDT techniques by facilitating alignment of the trunk and lower extremities. Important key points of control to achieve this alignment include the trunk, pelvis, and knees. As with sitting, PNF stability techniques, such as rhythmic stabilization and alternating isometrics, can be superimposed at the shoulders or pelvis to encourage symmetry and stability in standing. As discussed earlier, there is limited evidence to support the effectiveness of these approaches to postural control.

Another approach to retraining symmetry is through the use of postural biofeedback. For this method, patients typically sit or stand on a force platform and perform activities with or without visual and auditory feedback regarding the symmetry of their position. This training can also involve weight shifting either laterally or in an anterior/posterior direction. In this case, the patient may be provided with visual feedback about the position of his center of mass (Fig. 16-9). There is evidence that this intervention approach is more effective than others in improving stance symmetry.

Dynamic Balance/Stability. After symmetry has been established, NDT theory suggests that the therapist begin to work on dynamic postural control. Activities that may be incorporated at this stage include facilitated weight shifting that is progressed to stepping forward and back with the nonparetic leg and weight shifting in a stride position (Fig. 16-10). This can then be progressed to include lifting and stepping with the paretic lower extremity. NDT facilitation is structured based on the needs of the patient and possible hand placements to facilitate dynamic postural control, including bilateral control at the pelvis, control at the pelvis on the nonparetic side, control at the paretic shoulder or upper extremity, control at the nonparetic shoulder with support for the involved upper extremity, and control from the side at the paretic pelvis and knee.

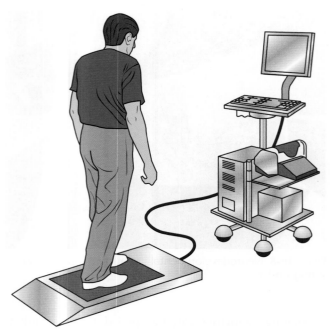

FIG. 16-9 Force-plate biofeedback training for postural symmetry.

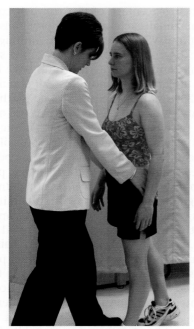

FIG. 16-11 Application of slow reversals to weight shifting in standing.

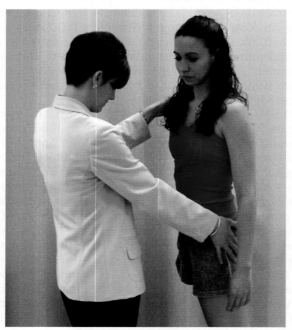

FIG. 16-10 Neurodevelopmental treatment facilitation of weight shifting in standing.

From a PNF perspective, the recommended activities to facilitate dynamic postural control are similar to those that would be used with an NDT approach, but the facilitation techniques differ. For example, the therapist working from this perspective might start by applying rhythmic initiation and repeated contraction to weight shifting in stride to assist with initiation of movement. This can be progressed to the application of slow reversals and agonistic reversals (Fig. 16-11). From this point, the patient can begin to work on pre-gait activities such as repeated stepping with one lower extremity. This is typically facilitated by providing approximation through the stance leg at midstance and applying repeated contractions down and back through the anterior superior iliac spine during swing.

From a task-oriented perspective, dynamic postural control in sitting and standing is addressed through specific tasks designed to facilitate lateral and anterior/posterior control. For example, patients may be asked to reach for objects in different directions or catch objects while sitting or standing on different surfaces.[66] The principles of feedback and practice previously discussed would be superimposed on these activities.

Flexibility. Bobath suggested that reducing spasticity is a key step in moving patients with CNS disorders toward increased flexibility and more normal motor control.[42] Specific techniques that may assist with this include gentle stretching of spastic muscles and approximation of proximal joint structures.

When severe, splints or casts may be recommended to reduce spasticity and increase joint ROM. These are most commonly applied to the ankle, knee, or elbow. It has been proposed that casts are effective because they provide prolonged stretch, warmth, and pressure.[94-96]

The two most common PNF techniques that address flexibility in patients with neuromuscular disorders are hold-relax and contract-relax. The evidence related to these techniques has been previously discussed and supports their use over passive stretching for the improvement of flexibility in individuals without neuromuscular disorders.

The task-oriented approaches recognize the importance and impact of impairments in flexibility on motor control and function.[66,67] In addition to standard stretching and joint mobilization, therapists employing this approach use functional activities to improve flexibility and ROM. For example, sit-to-stand activities can be structured to use more dorsiflexion range based on foot placement and surface height. Similarly, reaching activities can be structured so that they demand more hip or knee extension.

Gait and Locomotion Training. From an NDT perspective, gait rehabilitation involves both pre-gait and gait activities. Pre-gait activities related to dynamic postural control were addressed previously and are believed to provide a foundation for gait activities.[72] Direct gait training activities may include facilitation through the use of key points of control at the shoulders, trunk, hip, knee, ankle, or foot, depending on the gait deviations observed. The objective is to facilitate biomechanical alignment and muscle activation that is as close to normal as possible.

With PNF, gait is typically facilitated by applying approximation through the weight-bearing limb and repeated contractions to the pelvis during swing phase. As with the NDT approach, pre-gait activities typically precede facilitation of gait.

Strength, Power, and Endurance Training. A positive relationship between hip flexor, knee flexor, and ankle plantarflexor torque on both the paretic and nonparetic side and speed of gait and stair climbing has been documented for individuals with stroke.[97] Knee extension force has also been correlated to sit-to-stand ability for patients with a variety of diagnoses receiving inpatient rehabilitation.[98] Furthermore, a number of studies indicate that strength training benefits individuals with nonprogressive CNS disorders and that this training does not adversely affect muscle tone or spasticity.

Proponents of the NDT approach only address strength as it relates to normal movement patterns and functional activities because they are concerned that the effort associated with resisted strength training may worsen hypertonicity and thereby interfere with normal movement.[71] One NDT method used to improve lower extremity strength is the facilitation of bridging (Fig. 16-12). For this activity, the therapist uses key points of control on both thighs or at the pelvis to assist the patient to bridge. Bridging can be progressed to single leg bridging and single leg bridging with the leg over the edge of the mat and

supported on a stool or step. A proposed advantage of this activity is that it facilitates hip extension strength with knee and ankle flexion and therefore does not encourage an abnormal synergy pattern.

A number of PNF techniques are designed to increase strength through the use of manual resistance. Strength training in the extremity diagonals using rhythmic initiation, slow reversal-hold, and slow reversals are suggested for individuals after stroke or TBI.[74] In addition, these techniques can be applied to the pelvis, shoulder girdle, and trunk and in a variety of positions such as prone on elbows, quadruped, kneeling, or half-kneeling. Although limited evidence exists, it is suggested that this approach can improve strength, ROM, and motor control.[73]

The task-oriented approaches include a number of strategies designed to strengthen muscles in patients with hemiparesis. For example, patients may be asked to step up and down from surfaces of different heights and in different directions, raise and lower the foot while standing on steps of different heights, or complete other activities requiring single leg stance on the hemiplegic extremity.

FUNCTIONAL TRAINING IN SELF-CARE AND HOME MANAGEMENT

Functional training can include a variety of activities such as bed mobility, transfers and activities of daily living (ADLs). When facilitating rolling using NDT principles, the therapist is encouraged to pay close attention to the positioning of the involved upper extremity, particularly if it is flaccid, to ensure that the scapula maintains a protracted position and that the extremity is protected. The patient can also be taught to use the nonparetic extremity to support the paretic lower extremity during rolling to facilitate this motion. When training the patient to move from sidelying on the hemiparetic side to sitting upright, it is suggested that the therapist facilitate lateral trunk flexion on the paretic side and weight shift through the pelvis on the nonparetic side. In addition, the therapist may support the hemiparetic scapular region and incorporate weight bearing through the hemiparetic arm. This can assist with muscle activation, reduce tone, and increase stability in the involved extremity. In transfers, the goal is to facilitate symmetrical, normal movement during the activity. Special attention is given to trunk activation, symmetrical lower extremity weight bearing, and activation of the involved extremity. The therapist can use key points of control at the trunk or lower extremity or both. If the involved upper extremity is flaccid, it should be supported on the patient's knee or by the therapist to avoid shoulder or upper extremity injury.

With a PNF approach, rolling can be encouraged with techniques that promote either mass or reciprocal trunk patterns. With mass rolling patterns, the upper and lower trunk move simultaneously to complete the roll. To facilitate mass flexion or extension, techniques, such as rhythmic initiation, slow reversals, and agonistic reversals of the pelvis and shoulder, can be used. For example, in sidelying, mass flexion can be facilitated through simultaneous resistance of anterior depression at the shoulder

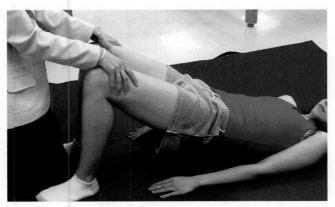

FIG. 16-12 Neurodevelopmental treatment facilitation of bridging with key points of control on the distal femurs.

girdle and anterior elevation at the pelvis. Reciprocal trunk patterns in rolling occur when the roll is initiated by either the upper or lower trunk. This can be facilitated in sidelying by applying rhythmic initiation to anterior elevation at the shoulder girdle with posterior depression at the pelvis. This can be followed by rhythmic initiation to posterior depression at the shoulder and anterior elevation at the pelvis. The verbal cue, "twist," can be used to assist the patient with this activity.

In the task-oriented approach, functional activities are facilitated through the therapist's design of the task, structure of the environment, feedback, and practice. For example, the therapist can structure transfers from sitting to standing to incorporate different seat heights or surfaces. A higher seat height makes the task easier because the patient does not need to raise his or her center of gravity as far. This activity can be progressed by reducing the seat height or by asking the patient to perform an upper extremity task, such as picking up a glass, while moving from sitting to standing. Feedback can also be provided in summary form after three to five trials. In addition, the therapist should withhold feedback for a short period to allow the patient to reflect on his or her performance and engage him or her in active problem solving. Rolling can also incorporate functional reaching activities. For example, the patient could be asked to reach for items located in a variety of spatial positions at the bedside.

CASE STUDY 16-1

STROKE

Patient History

Three weeks ago, MF, a 72-year-old man, was diagnosed with a stroke caused by a left anterior cerebral artery occlusion and was admitted to the hospital. Since that time, he has progressed well, with improvements in right upper and lower extremity motor control and functional status. MF's past medical history includes hypertension. He was recently discharged home with his wife and has been referred for outpatient services.

Tests and Measures—Significant Findings
Musculoskeletal
- MF has 3/5 strength throughout the right lower extremity. Other strength is 5/5.

Neuromuscular
- Proprioception decreased at right ankle.
- Decreased selective motor control at the hip, knee, and ankle.

Function
- MF can stand for less than 1 minute without support. He has increased postural sway when standing.
- Gait deviations include decreased right hip extension in terminal stance, right knee hyperextension in midstance, and decreased right ankle push-off.

- MF can ambulate with minimal to moderate assist and use of cane for 50 ft.

Diagnosis
Preferred practice pattern 5D: Impaired motor function and sensory integrity associated with nonprogressive disorders of the central nervous system—acquired in adolescence or adulthood.

Interventions
- PNF beginning with slow reversals of the right lower extremity in the D1F/D1E diagonal.
- Task-oriented activities: standing with his right lower extremity on steps of varying heights and raising and lowering his left heel from the ground in a controlled manner.
- Static standing activities and activities during which he must reach outside of his base of control. Treadmill ambulation to improve gait and increase strength and endurance.

Role of the Physical Therapist Assistant
- Would you expect this patient to have speech or visual loss as a result of his stroke? Why?
- Describe three standing activities that could be done with this patient to improve balance and strength.
- Write two home exercises for this patient that he can do safely by himself to improve his gait pattern.

Additional Information
For the full version of this case study, including detailed examination results, interventions, and outcomes, see the Evolve site that accompanies this book. Full case studies for a patient undergoing rehabilitation after TBI and for another patient undergoing rehabilitation after stroke also appear on the Evolve site.

CHAPTER SUMMARY

This chapter addresses the management of adult patients with impaired motor function and sensory integrity secondary to nonprogressive CNS disorders. Common pathologies related to this practice pattern, as well as tests and measures for aerobic capacity and endurance; arousal, attention, and cognition; gait, locomotion, and balance; motor function; muscle performance; self-care and home management; and sensory integrity, were introduced. Evaluation, diagnosis, and prognosis were then discussed along with research related to outcomes for these patient populations. Finally, interventions associated with NDT, PNF, and task-oriented approaches were discussed, and the evidence available to support or refute these interventions was presented. The chapter concludes with case study examples of the application of the above information related to the rehabilitation of individuals with nonprogressive CNS disorders.

ADDITIONAL RESOURCES

For links to these and additional web-based resources, see the Evolve site.

Adler SS, Beckers D, Buck M: *PNF in practice: An illustrated guide*, Berlin, 1993, Springer-Verlag.

Bobath B: *Adult hemiplegia: Evaluation and treatment,* ed 3, Oxford, 1990, Heinemann Medical Books.

Carr J, Shepherd R: *Neurological rehabilitation: Optimizing motor performance,* Oxford, 1998, Butterworth Heinemann.

Carr J, Shepherd R: *Stroke rehabilitation: Guidelines for exercise and training to optimize motor skill,* Edinburgh, 2003, Butterworth Heinemann.

Davies PM: *Steps to follow: A guide to the treatment of adult hemiplegia,* New York, 1984, Springer-Verlag.

Davies PM: *Right in the middle: Selective trunk activity in the treatment of adult hemiplegia,* New York, 1990, Springer-Verlag.

Howle JM: *Neuro-developmental treatment approach: Theoretical foundations and principles of clinical practice,* Laguna Beach, CA, 2002, NDTA.

Voss DE, Ionta MK, Myers BJ: *Proprioceptive neuromuscular facilitation: Patterns and techniques,* ed 3, Philadelphia, 1985, JB Lippincott.

American Heart Association

Brain Injury Association of America

National Resource Center on Traumatic Brain Injury

GLOSSARY

Abnormal synergy: Stereotyped patterns of movement that cannot be changed or adapted in response to task or environmental demands.

Agonistic reversals: Isotonic contraction in the diagonal, followed by an eccentric contraction of the same muscle groups.

Alternating isometrics: Alternating isometric contractions of the agonist and antagonist.

Augmented feedback: External feedback provided to the patient by the therapist; examples include verbal, visual, or tactile cues.

Contract-relax: Movement into agonist pattern until point of limitation followed by isometric contraction of all components of the antagonist pattern except for the rotation component, which is allowed to contract isotonically; repeated with passive movement into any newly gained range after each trial.

Controlled mobility: Ability to alter a position or move in a weight-bearing position while maintaining postural stability.

Dysdiadochokinesia: Impaired ability to perform rapidly alternating movements.

Dysmetria: Impaired ability to judge the distance or range of a movement.

Dyssynergia: Impaired interjoint coordination.

Hold-relax: Isometric contraction of the agonist or antagonist musculature in the desired diagonal at the point of range limitation; this is repeated with passive movement into any newly gained range after each trial.

Hold-relax active motion: An isometric contraction in the shortened range of the diagonal, passive movement into the lengthened range, followed by active contraction into the shortened range.

Initial mobility: Discrete movements that are not well controlled; postural or antigravity control is lacking.

Intrinsic feedback: Any type of feedback that is naturally available to the individual such as somatosensory, proprioceptive, or visual input.

Knowledge of performance (KP): Augmented feedback on the individual's movement performance.

Knowledge of results (KR): Verbal, terminal, augmented feedback on the outcome of a motor task.

Motor learning: Process associated with practice that leads to a relatively permanent change in one's ability to produce skilled movement.

Muscle tone: Resistance to passive stretch.

Regulatory conditions: Elements of the environment to which a task must conform.

Repeated contractions: Repeated use of the stretch reflex to initiate a contraction or reinforce and strengthen an existing contraction.

Rhythmic initiation: Progression of movement in diagonal from passive to active assistive to active to resisted.

Rhythmic stabilization: An extension of alternating isometrics in which the manual contacts are on opposite joint surfaces simultaneously.

Skill: Highly coordinated movement that allows for adaptability to meet the demands of the individual and the environment.

Slow reversals: Slow concentric contractions alternating between the agonist and antagonist muscle groups.

Slow reversal-hold: Slow concentric contractions alternating between the agonist and antagonist muscle groups with an isometric contraction applied at the end of each diagonal.

Spasticity: A motor disorder characterized by a velocity-dependent increase in tonic stretch reflexes accompanied by exaggerated tendon jerks.

Stability: Ability to maintain a steady position in a weight-bearing, antigravity posture.

Timing for emphasis: Maximal isometric resistance applied to stronger components of the diagonal to allow for facilitation or irradiation to weaker components.

Chapter 17

Progressive Central Nervous System Disorders

Lori Quinn, Vanina Dal Bello-Haas

OBJECTIVES

After reading this chapter, the reader will be able to:
1. Describe and differentiate different types of adult progressive central nervous system disorders, including Alzheimer's disease, amyotrophic lateral sclerosis, Huntington's disease, multiple sclerosis, and Parkinson's disease.
2. Describe the underlying pathology and common presentation of impairments and functional limitations for adults with progressive central nervous system disorders.
3. Discuss factors that may affect the intervention of an individual with an adult progressive central nervous system disorder.
4. Identify and provide a rationale for rehabilitation interventions for adults with progressive central nervous system disorders.

This chapter concerns the pathology, examination, and treatment of patients with progressive central nervous system (CNS) disorders that result in impaired motor function and sensory integrity. These include such commonly known diseases as Alzheimer's disease, Parkinson's disease, and multiple sclerosis, as well as a range of other disabling disorders, such as amyotrophic lateral sclerosis, Huntington's disease, cerebellar disorders (including cerebellar **ataxia**), and progressive muscular **atrophy.** Other disorders that have progressive effects on the CNS include acquired immune deficiency syndrome (AIDS), basal ganglia disease, idiopathic progressive cortical disease, neoplasms, primary lateral palsy, and progressive muscular atrophy.

PATHOLOGY

ALZHEIMER'S DISEASE

Dementia is an acquired syndrome of progressive deterioration in global intellectual abilities that interferes with the person's usual occupational and social performance, excluding impairments in consciousness. Alzheimer's disease (AD) accounts for 45% to 75% of patients with dementia,[1,2] and it has been estimated that prevalence rates double every 4.5 years until at least age 90.[3]

The pathological hallmark of AD is the development of neurofibrillary tangles within neurons and plaques (deposits of amyloid matter).[4,5] The density of the filaments within neurons in the brain is directly related to the severity of dementia. The ultimate effect of these tangles is compromise of microtubular function and eventual destruction of the neuron.[5-7] Plaques seem to form as a result of disordered processing of beta-amyloid and its precursors, and it is thought that inflammation around plaques destroys neighboring neurons.

Synaptic degeneration and neuronal death in the cortex and limbic brain regions (limbic cortex, anterior and medial nuclei of the thalamus, hippocampus, amygdala, and basal forebrain) result in cognitive and behavioral abnormalities (Fig. 17-1). AD is manifested by impairments in memory and one or more of the following: Aphasia, apraxia, agnosia, or disturbances in executive abilities such as abstracting, organizing, planning, and sequencing.[8] In addition to memory loss, individuals with AD may have dramatic personality changes, disorientation, declining physical coordination, and an inability to care for themselves.[9] In the final stages of the disease, patients are bedridden, lose urinary bladder and bowel control, and are completely dependent on the care of

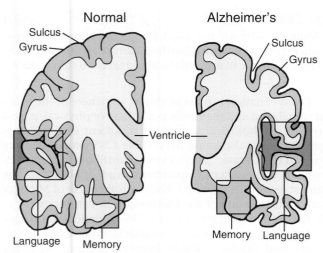

FIG. 17-1 Typical changes in the brain with Alzheimer's disease. Note that there is loss of cortex, particularly in the areas controlling memory and language; widening of the sulci; and enlargement of the ventricles.

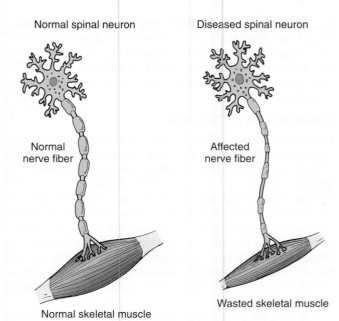

FIG. 17-2 Motor nerve degeneration and its effect on the muscle fibers it innervates.

others. Death is usually due to pneumonia or urinary tract infection. Studies have found survival after a diagnosis of AD depends on age at diagnosis. Median survival was almost 9 years for persons diagnosed at age 65, whereas survival was approximately 3 years for persons diagnosed at age 90.[10]

> ### ⊚ *Clinical Pearl*
>
> As Alzheimer's disease progresses to the final stages, patients will be completely dependent on others for care and will often die from pneumonia or urinary tract infection.

AMYOTROPHIC LATERAL SCLEROSIS

Amyotrophic lateral sclerosis (ALS), commonly known as Lou Gehrig's disease, is the most common and devastatingly fatal **motor neuron disease** among adults. The prevalence of ALS is 5 to 7 per 100,000 in the United States, and the disease affects men slightly more than women. The average age of onset is 58 years, with a range of 40 to 70 years.[11-14]

ALS is characterized by degeneration and loss of upper motor neurons in the cortex; brainstem nuclei for cranial nerves (CNs) V, VII, IX, X, and XII; and anterior horn cells (lower motor neurons) in the spinal cord. As motor neurons degenerate, they can no longer control the muscle fibers they innervate (Fig. 17-2). Healthy, intact surrounding axons sprout and reinnervate the partially denervated muscle,[15] thereby preserving strength and function early in the disease. This reinnervation can compensate for the progressive degeneration until about 50% of motor units are lost.[16,17] With disease progression reinnervation can no longer compensate for the degeneration,[18] resulting in a combination of upper motor neuron and lower motor neuron signs and symptoms. These include weakness,

muscle atrophy, hyperreflexia or areflexia, and muscle **fasciculations.**

The most frequently presenting symptom, occurring in more than 70% of patients with ALS, is focal weakness beginning in the leg, arm, or bulbar muscles.[19] Patients gradually become weaker all over, eventually having difficulty breathing because of diaphragmatic weakness. Most patients remain relatively intact cognitively, although speech production becomes difficult and alternative communication methods are required. Although disease progression varies between individuals, death usually results from respiratory failure, and the 50% survival after the first symptom appears is about 3 years, unless mechanical ventilation is used to sustain breathing.[20]

HUNTINGTON'S DISEASE

Huntington's disease (HD) is a fatal, autosomal dominant hereditary disorder affecting 5 to 10 per 100,000 people.[21] The disease has an insidious onset, generally manifests when the patient is in the mid-thirties to mid-forties, and causes cognitive and emotional disturbances, in addition to problems with voluntary and involuntary movement.[22] The disease typically progresses over 15 to 20 years, although progression is faster in individuals with an earlier age of onset.[22]

Chorea, abnormal extraocular movements, hypertonic reflexes, and abnormal rapid alternating movements are the most consistent early manifestations of HD.[23] As the disease progresses, other functionally limiting motor symptoms, such as dystonia,[24] athetosis, **akinesia,** and **bradykinesia,** develop.[21,25,23] In addition to motor problems, depression, cognitive decline, and personality changes occur, progressing from deficits in executive function, short-term memory, and visuospatial functioning in the early stage of the disease to dementia in the later stages.[23,25] Cognitive impairments and depression are associated with more rapid functional decline.[26,27] The most common cause of death is respiratory complications.[28]

PARKINSON'S DISEASE

Parkinson's disease (PD) is an idiopathic, hypokinetic movement disorder of the basal ganglia. It affects men slightly more often than women, and approximately 1.5 million Americans are currently diagnosed with the disease. The typical age of onset is 60; however, 15% of those diagnosed are under age 50. The risk of PD increases with age. In certain cases, there is a strong genetic predisposition, but PD is not an inherited disease. Although the cause of PD is unknown, researchers believe that several factors may be involved, including accelerated aging, exposure to environmental toxins, and free radical oxidative damage.[29,30]

The primary pathology in PD is degeneration of neurons that produce dopamine and degeneration primarily within the substantia nigra. Symptoms do not generally appear until approximately 80% of dopaminergic cells in the substantia nigra are lost. First symptoms typically include resting tremor, bradykinesia, **rigidity**, and impaired balance or postural control. Disease progression is quite variable: Some patients are able to live for many years with PD, whereas others decline rapidly. Medication can control symptoms for many years by increasing levels of dopamine in the brain. As the disease progresses, medications are less effective and produce more side effects, particularly bradykinesia and rigidity as they wear off, and **dyskinesias** at peak dose. Many patients also experience varying degrees of dementia. In the end stages of the disease, patients are generally totally dependent for physical care and have problems communicating. The cause of death is typically respiratory failure.

> ### ◎ *Clinical Pearl*
> Parkinson's disease is not an inherited disease, although in certain cases, there is a strong genetic predisposition.

MULTIPLE SCLEROSIS

Multiple sclerosis (MS) is a demyelinating disease of the CNS.[31] The typical age of onset of symptoms is between 20 to 50 years of age, and the disease affects women almost 3 times more often than men. The prevalence of the disease in the United States is 1 in 700. Although the exact cause of MS is unknown, studies suggest that genetics may play a role; however, MS is not a directly inherited disease.[32,33] MS has been found to occur more frequently in people with northern European ancestry and those who live in areas of the world far from the equator. The proposed pathogenic mechanisms for the onset for MS include (1) an autoimmune response causing a widespread attack on the neural tissue, (2) a slow-acting or latent viral infection that triggers an immune response, or (3) environmental factors.[33]

> ### ◎ *Clinical Pearl*
> Multiple sclerosis has been found to occur more frequently in people with northern European ancestry and those who live in areas of the world far from the equator.

Demyelination can occur almost anywhere in the brain or spinal cord and manifests as a variety of physical, cognitive, or psychological impairments. Recent evidence suggests MS may also cause irreversible CNS axonal damage early in the disease,[34] and this may contribute to the development of persistent impairments and disability in the later stages of the disease.[35] The clinical course of MS typically falls into one of the following four categories:

1. Relapsing-remitting (85% to 90% of patients): Characterized by episodes of acute attacks followed by recovery and disease stability between relapses. Recovery after a relapse may be full but is usually characterized by some residual deficits. Over time, the degree of disability increases.
2. Primary progressive (10%): Characterized by steady progression of the disease and continuous worsening over time. There may be occasional plateaus and temporary minor improvements in impairments and functional limitations.
3. Secondary progressive (40% to 50% of people with relapsing-remitting develop this form within 10 years of initial diagnosis): Characterized by relapsing-remitting disease for a period of time followed by progressive disease with or without occasional minor relapses, remission, or plateau.
4. Progressive relapsing (rare): Characterized by progressive disease from the onset, with periods of acute relapses, with or without recovery; between relapses there is progressive worsening of the disease.[36]

In newly diagnosed cases of MS, most experience a relapsing-remitting course, with relapses occurring usually a little less than once a year.[37,38] A typical relapse increases in severity over a few weeks, begins to remit after 4 weeks, and resolves over 2 to 3 months.[36] In the early stages, clinical recovery is virtually complete, although persistent structural and conduction abnormalities can be detected. Although the course of the disease is variable, after a number of years, neurological impairments begin to accumulate after each relapse.[36] After 10 years, 40% to 50% of patients with a relapsing-remitting disease will develop a progressive course in which there is a continuous accrual of impairments and functional limitations, with or without relapses.[36] Approximately 50% of patients are unable to work 5 years after disease onset,[39] and approximately 50% of patients require an assistive device or wheelchair within 15 years of diagnosis.[40] Respiratory complications are the most common cause of death in patients with MS.[41]

STAGES OF PROGRESSIVE CENTRAL NERVOUS SYSTEM DISORDERS

A commonality among progressive CNS disorders is their progressive and deteriorating trajectory. Although the course of some diseases (such as MS) can be altered or slowed by disease-modifying agents (typically medications), there is currently no cure for any of the progressive CNS disorders discussed in this chapter.

Most progressive CNS diseases can be viewed in three functional stages: Early, middle, and late. In the early stage of the disorder, the pathology manifests as a variety of signs and symptoms recognized by the individual as abnormal. At this stage, resultant impairments may or may not cause minor functional limitations, and the individual's ability to perform typical roles is usually not affected. In the middle stage of the progressive CNS disorder, an individual experiences increasing signs and symptoms and develops an increasing number of impairments or more severe impairments. The individual is minimally to moderately functionally limited and experiences disabilities. In the late stage, progression of the disease leads to numerous and increasingly more severe impairments. The individual becomes increasingly more limited functionally because of the lack of voluntary motor control and numerous disabilities ensue. The individual becomes dependent in essentially all aspects of mobility and self-care, and depending on the disease process, speech, swallowing, pulmonary, bowel, bladder, and cognitive function may also be significantly compromised, if not already affected.[42] Table 17-1 summarizes the pathology, common impairments, and disabilities of the progressive CNS disorders discussed in this chapter.

> ◎ *Clinical Pearl*
>
> There is no cure for the progressive CNS disorders discussed in this chapter, although the course of the specific disease can often be altered or slowed, typically with medications.

TYPICAL EXAMINATION FINDINGS

Progressive CNS disorders can affect many regions of the CNS at any one time and in various combinations for some diseases. Impairments may occur as (1) a direct result of the CNS pathology (primary impairment), (2) a sequela to the primary pathology (secondary impairment), (3) a result of preexisting pathology (co-morbid condition), and (4) as a result of habits independent of a specific disease process (disuse and abuse). Most individuals who have been diagnosed with a progressive CNS disorder will have a complex array of examination findings. Even patients with the same diagnosis can present with a significantly different presentation of symptoms. Reexamination at regular intervals is necessary to determine the extent and rate of progression of the disorder and the effectiveness of interventions; however, it may be difficult to differentiate between the progressive course of the disorder and ineffectiveness of the interventions.

PATIENT HISTORY

In patients with a progressive CNS disorder, the patient history should identify what is most important, relevant, and valued by the individual and may give a sense of the rate of progression. There may be many immediate and future potential impairments, as well as functional limitations, as the disease progresses. Identifying the spouse, caregiver, and/or family members will be important because their participation is frequently crucial to the viability and success of any intervention program.

TESTS AND MEASURES

Typically, the examination of a patient with progressive CNS disorders includes the following information.

Musculoskeletal

Posture. Progressive CNS disorders often affect posture. For example, PD causes forward tilt of the trunk, rigidity and trembling of the head, reduced arm swing, rigidity and trembling of the extremities, and shuffling gait with short steps (Fig. 17-3).

Range of Motion and Muscle Length. Functional range of motion (ROM), active ROM (AROM), active-assisted ROM (AAROM), passive ROM (PROM), muscle length, and soft tissue flexibility and extensibility are usually examined in patients with progressive CNS disorders because they are at risk for loss of ROM. **Hypertonicity,** specifically rigidity (seen in PD) and hyperreflexia (seen in ALS, MS, and HD), can result in muscle shortening over time. Risk of contractures is one of the key reasons why one tries to control **spasticity** and rigidity in patients.

TABLE 17-1	Summary of Progressive Central Nervous System Disorders	
Disorders	**Pathology**	**Common Impairments And Disabilities**
Alzheimer's disease	Synaptic degeneration and neuronal death in the cortex and limbic regions of the brain	Memory loss, disorientation, aphasia, decreased abstracting, sequencing, organizing, and planning
Amyotrophic lateral sclerosis	Degeneration and loss of UMN and LMN LMN degeneration in the anterior horn cells UMN degeneration in the cranial nerves	Weakness, muscle atrophy, hyperreflexia, areflexia, muscle fasciculations, and diaphragmatic weakness
Huntington's disease	Degeneration of the caudate nucleus, putamen, frontal cortex, globus pallidus, and thalamus	Chorea, abnormal extraocular movements, dystonia, hypertonic reflexes, depression, and cognitive decline
Parkinson's disease	Degeneration of neurons that produce dopamine and degeneration within the substantia nigra	Tremor, bradykinesia, rigidity, impaired balance, and postural control
Multiple sclerosis	Demyelination of the CNS	Unilateral muscle weakness, fatigue, gait and balance impairment, visual impairment, pain, and spasticity

UMN, Upper motor neuron; *LMN,* lower motor neuron; *CNS,* central nervous system.

Muscle Performance. Any patient with a progressive CNS disorder is at risk for strength deficits because of lack of activity and subsequent muscle disuse. Therefore, at a minimum, therapists perform a screening examination of the strength of the upper extremities, lower extremities, and the trunk musculature, using manual muscle tests (MMT) or functional tests. Functional testing, such as checking if a person can get out of a chair or reach for an object, may be more appropriate in patients with significant cognitive impairments (e.g., patients with AD or PD-related dementia) because these patients may have difficulty following the commands for MMT.

Neuromuscular

Arousal, Attention, and Cognition. Examination of cognition, communication, language, and learning style is performed in patients with progressive CNS disorders associated with significant impairments in cognition and behavior such as AD and HD and the later stages of MS and PD.

Pain. Pain is common in individuals with ALS, MS, and PD. In addition to pain caused by direct effects of progressive CNS disorders, individuals with any of these disorders may develop pain as a result of indirect (e.g., decreased ROM or contractures secondary to muscle weakness, spasticity, or rigidity) or composite impairments (e.g., joint malalignment secondary to spasticity). Thus pain is generally examined in patients with progressive CNS disorders who report pain in the patient history (see Chapter 22).

Cranial Nerve Integrity. Many patients with progressive CNS disorders have impairments in CN integrity, particularly in the nerves that control eye movements and the bulbar muscles. Eye movements are examined by having the patient look in different directions. Bulbar function is assessed through evaluation of speech and swallowing.

Impairments in Motor Control and Motor Learning. Motor control and motor learning abilities are examined in individuals with progressive CNS disorders because deficits in these areas can significantly impact functional abilities (Table 17-2).

Motor learning is typically examined by observing the ability of a patient to learn a new skill (acquisition), the ability to retain that skill (retention), and the ability to transfer the skill to a similar (but slightly different) task (transfer).

Cardiovascular and Pulmonary.

A variety of ventilatory impairments may be seen in patients with progressive CNS disorders, and the incidence and severity of these impairments vary. In all patients with progressive CNS

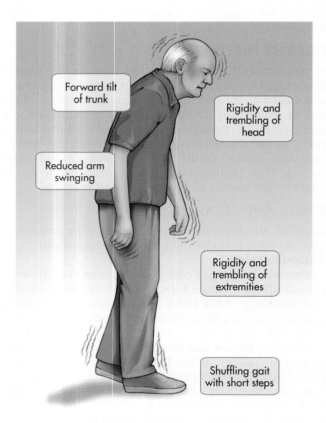

Forward tilt of trunk

Rigidity and trembling of head

Reduced arm swinging

Rigidity and trembling of extremities

Shuffling gait with short steps

FIG. 17-3 Typical posture of a person with Parkinson's disease. *From Thibodeau GA, Patton KT: The human body in health & disease, ed 4, St. Louis, 2002, Mosby.*

TABLE 17-2	**Common Motor Impairments in Patients with Progressive CNS Disorders**
Motor Impairment: Description	**Typically Seen in:**
Akinesia: Impaired initiation of movement	PD, HD
Bradykinesia, **hypokinesia:** Slowness of movements, reduced movement speed and amplitude	PD, HD
Chorea: Involuntary writhing movements of varying amplitude of almost any part of the body	HD
Dysdiadochokinesia: Inability to alternately contract and relax agonist and antagonist muscles or muscle groups	MS, HD, PD
Dyskinesia: Involuntary movements of the face, trunk, or limbs	Treated PD
Dysmetria: Inability to control the direction and amplitude of muscle force during a purposeful movement	MS, HD, PD
Dystonia: Involuntary, sustained contractions of the muscles of the head, limbs, or trunk, producing abnormal postures	PD, HD
Freezing: Sudden inability to move during the execution of a motor sequence	PD
Rigidity: Excessive muscle activity in all directions	PD
Spasticity: Velocity-dependent increased resistance to passive stretch of a muscle	ALS, HD, MS
Tremor: Involuntary, rhythmic contractions of opposing muscles, producing the appearance of trembling. May be present at rest (resting tremor), during specific postures (postural tremor), or during a voluntary movement (intention tremor)	PD

Adapted from Nolan MF: *Introduction to the neurologic examination,* Philadelphia, 1994, FA Davis and Morris ME: *Phys Ther* 80(6):578-597, 2000.
PD, Parkinson's disease; *HD,* Huntington's disease; *ALS,* amyotrophic lateral sclerosis; *MS,* multiple sclerosis.

disorders, respiratory and ventilation impairments may lead to atelectasis, pneumonia, and ventilatory failure. Respiratory complications are a major cause of morbidity and mortality in many patients with these disorders.[43-45]

Individuals with a gradual progression of respiratory muscle weakness may not complain of respiratory symptoms because they tend to decrease their overall level of physical activity caused by concomitant muscle weakness in the extremities. As weakness progresses, truncated speech, **orthopnea** (shortness of breath when lying supine), **dyspnea** at rest, paradoxical breathing, accessory muscle use, and a weak cough occur. If an individual does not receive ventilatory support, eventually carbon dioxide (CO_2) retention will lead to acidosis, coma, respiratory failure, and death.[45]

Integumentary. Examination of integumentary integrity in patients with progressive CNS disorders focuses on the skin. In general, skin breakdown tends to develop in individuals with conditions that impair sensation, such as MS, and in those who become incontinent. Contact points between the patient's skin and any devices and the patient's bed should be examined, especially when the patient's mobility becomes increasingly dependent. In patients with HD, bruising and skin abrasions on the feet, shins, forearms, and elbows can occur because of frequent choreiform movements.

Function

Gait, Locomotion, Balance, and Postural Control. Problems with gait and balance are common in patients with progressive CNS disorders. Gait or balance impairments are often one of first signs in individuals with these types of disorders.

Gait abnormalities,[46,47] impaired tandem gait,[48] postural instability,[47,49,50] decreased gait speed,[47,51-55] decreased stride length,[56] decreased step length,[57] increased cadence,[51] and stride length variability[50,56] are described in all types of dementia. The annual incidence of falls in persons with dementia is twice the rate in cognitively normal elderly.[58-60] In ALS, ambulation difficulties and impaired postural control and balance are caused by muscle weakness and/or spasticity. Almost 50% of people with ALS are reported to fall.[61] In HD, ambulation is characterized by a wide-based staggering gait, sometimes in a zigzag pattern of progression, with the arms fixed. Early in the progression of HD, chorea, weakness of specific muscle groups (often the upper back and trunk), and mild cognitive and visuospatial impairments may all contribute to balance problems, difficulty walking, and falls. Patients may lose their balance when turning quickly, especially while carrying a load, changing directions suddenly, or wearing unsupportive footwear.[62]

Akinesia (lack of movement), bradykinesia (slowed speed and amplitude of movement), rigidity (resistance to passive movement), dyskinesia (extraneous movement), and postural instability are associated with the balance and gait impairments seen in individuals with PD.[63] Preambulation is marked by a lack of normal preparatory trunk and extremity movements. Patients may have difficulty transferring their weight from one foot to the other to initiate gait ("ignition disorder"). In most patients, ambulation is initially characterized by a shortened stride, with intact cadence,[64-66] producing short shuffling steps with a narrowed base of support.

Patients with MS usually have gait problems because of proprioceptive loss, lower extremity weakness, or spasticity. Common impairments include weakness of the hip flexor muscles, resulting in difficulty lifting the lower extremity; weakness of the hip abductors, resulting in a Trendelenburg gait pattern; and weakness of the dorsiflexors and evertors of the foot, resulting in foot drop. Patients with spasticity (usually increased extensor tone) will ambulate stiffly and will drag the toes and circumduct the hip during swing phase.

Orthotic, Protective, and Supportive Devices. Most individuals with a progressive CNS disorder have primary or secondary impairments in muscle strength or secondary impairments in joint integrity. Devices and equipment that enhance function or performance may be prescribed by the physical therapist (see Chapter 34).

For example, in individuals with ALS and MS, foot drop is common and an ankle-foot orthosis (AFO) may be prescribed to increase safety during gait. Individuals with HD with dystonic posturing may benefit from a shoe insert to control the position of the foot during ambulation. Individuals with ALS often develop cervical extensor muscle weakness, making it difficult to keep the head up for prolonged periods or with unexpected movements. To address this, a soft, foam neck collar may help initially when weakness is mild, and a semirigid collar may help when weakness becomes more severe. Protective devices, such as helmets or elbow and knee protectors, may be prescribed for individuals at risk of falling or for individuals with HD who are prone to injuries because of chorea. Not surprisingly, it is often difficult to persuade an individual to wear a protective device.

Environmental Barriers at Home and Work. The patient's home and work environments are often examined for current and potential barriers, including access and safety issues.

Self-Care and Home Management. Loss of independence in activities of daily living (ADLs) and instrumental ADLs (IADLs) can be the result of physical and/or cognitive impairments. Physical impairments, such as weakness, decreased ROM, spasticity, or impaired coordination and balance, can limit independence or impair performance of ADLs. Cognitive impairments, resulting from dementia, can also significantly impact functional abilities. This decline in functional abilities, which is inevitable for patients with progressive CNS disorders, is one of the most troubling aspects of dementia for patients[67] and their caregivers.[68] Early in the dementing process, the loss of ability to function may cause the patient to feel useless, dependent, and burdensome.[67] For families of persons with more advanced stages of dementia, such as seen in AD, HD, and PD, the major problems of care include impairments of communication, eating, bathing, and wandering.[69] Incontinence is also a significant problem that causes stress for the patient and caregiver.

Work, Community, and Leisure Integration. The physical therapist will evaluate a patient's ability to work and be involved in their community and leisure activities because these are very important for patients with progressive CNS disorders. These disorders often cause progressive loss of independence and reduced involvement in activities that are central to a fulfilling life.

Psychosocial Function. Depression and anxiety are common in individuals with neurodegenerative disorders,[70,71] thus screening is important and referral to a psychologist or psychiatrist for further evaluation may be warranted.

EVALUATION, DIAGNOSIS, AND PROGNOSIS

According to the *Guide to Physical Therapy Practice*,[72] the preferred practice pattern for patients with progressive CNS disorders is 5E: Impaired motor function and sensory integrity associated with progressive disorders of the central nervous system. With progressive CNS disorders, progression of pathology, impairments, functional limitations, and disabilities is inevitable. It is imperative that clinicians understand the nature and progression of the disease and the stage of the disease to not only address an individual's immediate problems but also to plan ahead for future problems.

Adults with progressive CNS disorders will have a number of different abnormal examination findings that will vary considerably in severity and in their impact on prognosis. Many factors can affect a patient's functional prognosis.

INTERVENTION

Interventions for individuals with progressive CNS disorders are influenced by numerous factors, including the examination findings, the patient's goals, financial and human resources, the nature and course of the disease, individual variability throughout the disease course, age at disease onset, disease stage, and the availability of disease-modifying agents.

Therapeutic management for individuals with a neurodegenerative disease will typically occur along a care continuum. The care continuum suggests the disease process has a trajectory that varies and changes over time, as a result of progression and deterioration. Along the continuum, resultant impairments, functional limitations, and disabilities are managed through interventions tailored to the stage of the disease and grounded in evidence-based research whenever possible. Even though the course of the disease itself cannot be altered, appropriate rehabilitation can help an individual maintain his or her independence and function for as long as possible, within the context of his or her goals and resources, throughout the stages of the disease and in different health care settings (acute care, rehabilitation, outpatient, long-term care, home care, and hospice settings).

◎ *Clinical Pearl*

Tailoring interventions along the continuum is important as the patient's needs will change over time.

AEROBIC EXERCISE

An aerobic exercise program may be indicated to address deconditioning, decreased endurance, or fatigue for patients with progressive CNS disorders. The physical therapist will design the aerobic exercise program considering frequency, duration, intensity, and mode of exercise. Despite a clearly stated plan, careful monitoring may be necessary to ensure the safety of patients with progressive CNS disorders. For example, HD, MS, AD, and PD can all cause autonomic dysfunction, resulting in orthostatic hypotension, excessive sweating, heat intolerance, and abnormal cardiovascular responses.[73-77] Vital signs; symptoms of exertion, such as dyspnea, excessive fatigue, pallor, and dizziness; and signs and symptoms specific to the disorder will be monitored and documented, at rest, and during and after exercise. The Borg Rating of Perceived Exertion (RPE) Scale (see Chapter 23) can also be used to objectively record perceived exertion.

Amyotrophic Lateral Sclerosis. When implementing an exercise program for patients with ALS, there is the possibility of overwork damage or overuse fatigue. Patients should be advised not to carry out any activities to the point of extreme fatigue and should keep track of symptoms of overuse, such as the inability to perform daily activities after exercise because of exhaustion or pain, increased fasciculations, or muscle cramping.

Parkinson's Disease. While several studies have investigated the benefits of general exercise in patients with PD (see section on Strength Training later in this chapter), the few studies that have specifically assessed the benefits of aerobic conditioning in PD found that this intervention increased cardiorespiratory fitness and habitual activity level, stabilized functional ability, and marginally improved mood.

Multiple Sclerosis. In patients with MS, Uthoff's phenomenon, an adverse reaction to external heat or increased body temperature, can occur with exercise, resulting in extreme fatigue and worsening of symptoms. An ear thermometer can be used to monitor temperature before, during, and after exercise in patients with MS. Precooling with cold water immersion,[78] cooling garments (Fig. 17-4),[79] or ice packs or by the patient consuming iced drinks or having the patient exercise in an air-conditioned room can prevent excessive gains in core temperature with physical work and may allow heat-sensitive individuals with MS to perform aerobic exercise without adverse effects.

The few studies examining the effects of aerobic exercise in patients with MS found that this intervention improved aerobic capacity, strength, body composition, cholesterol, mood, and quality of life.

Alzheimer's Disease and Huntington's Disease. There is limited information evaluating the effects of aerobic training in patients with AD or HD; however, several studies report that general exercise is beneficial in these populations.

BALANCE, COORDINATION, AND AGILITY TRAINING

Balance training activities in general are progressed from a wide to narrower base of support, from static to dynamic activities, from a low to a high center of gravity, and with increasing degrees of freedom that must be controlled (see Chapter 13). When restoration is not possible,

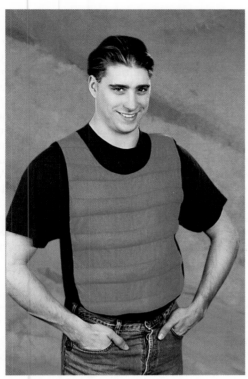

FIG. 17-4 Patient using a cooling vest. *Image of Miracool Cooling Vest courtesy OccuNomix International.*

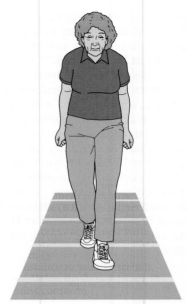

FIG. 17-5 Visual cueing for a patient with Parkinson's disease.

compensatory interventions may be needed to address sensory, visual, vestibular, and motor impairments and promote balance safety. Modifications of the home, work, and community environments and recommendations for assistive and adaptive devices may also be required for balance safety.

Huntington's Disease. For patients with HD, strategies found to be useful in individuals with PD described in the next section, such as attentional strategies and avoiding dual-task performance, may be useful.[80] Balance retraining, strengthening of the postural muscles to enhance postural stability, and increasing the base of support of footwear is recommended in the early stage of HD.[81] As the disease progresses, compensatory strategies, such as teaching the patient the Touch-Turn-Sit maneuver are implemented. The Touch-Turn-Sit maneuver involves instructing the patient to touch the chair initially and then turn before sitting down (i.e., a sensory cue attentional strategy). Assistive devices (walker with wheels is preferred) and safety equipment, such as a helmet or elbow and knee protectors, may be recommended. Because cognitive impairments also increase in number and severity as the disease progresses, additional compensatory strategies, such as providing cues, teaching skills using one-step commands, and providing treatment in a quiet, nondistracting environment should also be incorporated into treatment.[81]

Parkinson's Disease. Because balance is often affected in the early stages of PD, balance training will typically begin early.[82] This training usually takes place in the environment where the individual's problems are the worst. Patients with PD have difficulty maintaining stability when they do not have sufficient time to prepare for threats to balance. They are taught to deliberately prepare in advance for forthcoming threats to balance, or to focus their attention on maintaining balance before a task in which equilibrium is challenged.[83] This strategy may allow patients to use intact frontal cortical systems to regulate stability to substitute for impaired basal ganglia mechanisms.[83] Training the patient to step in response to perturbations, with an emphasis on speed and accuracy of the stepping strategy, is also recommended.[84] Balance training may also be enhanced through the use of auditory and visual cueing (Fig. 17-5) (see section on Gait and Locomotion Training for more details).[85]

Dancing, particularly ballroom dancing, and karate, both of which incorporate changes in direction, rhythmical movement, rotation, balance, and coordination, may be useful in addressing several impairments.[86,87] To address the inability to attend to more than one task at a time, patients can be taught to break down complex activities into simple tasks and to focus their attention on performing each task separately, and to practice performing two activities at the same time under various practice and context conditions.

Multiple Sclerosis. In MS, sensory and vestibular disorders, ataxia, dysmetria, muscle weakness, spasticity, and tremor may cause balance impairments and incoordination. Interventions will typically focus first on the cause of these specific problems and then on improving postural stability and accuracy of upper and lower extremity movements through balance and coordination training during functional activities. For example, if the patient has weak trunk muscles, strengthening exercises usually are prescribed to increase strength and stability before coordination and balance problems are addressed.

Light weights (cuff weights, weight belt, or weighted jacket) and weighted ambulation devices, which provide proprioceptive loading and can stabilize movements, are sometimes used clinically to control the incoordination of ataxic and dysmetric movements in patients with MS. However, research studies have not consistently found these interventions to be beneficial.[88-91]Frenkel's exercises are a series of exercises that emphasize normal daily activities, increase in difficulty, and are performed in four positions: Lying, sitting, standing, and walking[92] (Box 17-1). These exercises have also been suggested as an intervention for MS-related ataxia and dysmetria, although there are no published studies examining the effects of these exercises in people with MS. Incoordination caused by poor proximal joint control may be addressed by proprioceptive neuromuscular facilitation (PNF) techniques, including rhythmic stabilization, alternating isometrics and slow reversal hold, and by activities that emphasize weight-bearing activities through proximal joints (e.g., 4-point kneeling).

STRENGTH TRAINING

Alzheimer's Disease. Dementia is commonly associated with reduced activity, which is thought to contribute to weakness, gait abnormalities, and falls. Therefore exercise programs are often prescribed to minimize the functional impact of any type of dementia, including AD.

Amyotrophic Lateral Sclerosis. The benefit of muscle strength training in patients with ALS is controversial and there is a concern that strength training may cause muscle damage in these patients. However, one randomized controlled trial found that patients with ALS can derive short-term benefits from 3 months of individualized, moderate intensity, endurance type exercises for the trunk and limbs.[93]

Huntington's Disease. Relatively few studies have examined the effects of any type of physical therapy for

---

BOX 17-1   Frenkel's Exercises

Exercises While Lying

Starting position: Lie on bed or couch with a smooth surface so your feet may be moved easily. Your head should be raised on a pillow so that you can watch every movement.

1. Bend one leg at the hip and knee, sliding your heel along the bed. Straighten the hip and knee to return to the starting position. Repeat with the other leg.
2. Bend one leg at the hip and knee as in #1. Then slide the same leg out to the side, leaving your heel on the bed. Slide your leg back to the center and straighten your hip and knee to return to the starting position. Repeat with the other leg.
3. Bend one leg at the hip and knee with the heel raised from the bed. Straighten your leg to return to the starting position. Repeat with the other leg.
4. Bend and straighten one leg at the hip and knee sliding your heel along the bed stopping at any point of command. Repeat with the other leg.
5. Bend the hip and knee of one leg and place the heel on the opposite knee. Then slide your heel down the shin to the ankle and back up to the knee. Return to starting position and repeat with the other leg.
6. Bend both hips and knees sliding heels on the bed, keeping your ankles together. Straighten both legs to return to starting position.
7. Bend one leg at the hip and knee while straightening the other in a bicycling motion.

Exercises While Sitting

Starting position: Sit on a chair with feet flat on the floor.

1. Mark time, raising just the heel. Then, mark time lifting the entire foot and placing the foot firmly on the floor on a traced foot print.

2. Make two cross-marks on the floor with chalk. Alternately glide the foot over the marked cross: forward, backward, left and right.
3. Rise from the chair and sit again to a counted cadence. At one, bend knees and draw feet under the chair; at two, bend trunk forward; at three, rise by straightening the hips and knees and then the trunk. Reverse the process to sit down.

Exercises While Standing and Walking

Starting position: Stand erect with feet 4-6 inches apart.

1. Walk sideways, beginning with half steps to the right. Perform this exercise in a counted cadence: At one, shift the weight to the left foot; at two, place the right foot 12 inches to the right; at three, shift the weight to the right foot; at four, bring the left foot over to the right foot. Repeat exercise with half steps to the left. The size of the step taken to right or left may be varied.
2. Walk forward between two parallel lines 14 inches apart, placing the right foot just inside the right line and the left foot just inside the left line. Emphasize correct placement. Rest after 10 steps.
3. Walk forward, placing each foot on a footprint traced on the floor. Footprints should be parallel and 2 inches from a center line. Practice with quarter steps, half steps, three-quarter steps, and full steps.
4. Turn to the right in a counted cadence. At one, raise the right toe and rotate the right foot outward, pivoting on the heel; at two, raise the left heel and pivot the left leg inward on the toes; at three, complete the full turn, and then repeat to the left.
5. Walk up and down the stairs one step at a time. Place the right foot on one step and bring the left up beside it. Later, practice walking up the stairs, placing one foot on each step. At first use the railing, then as balance improves, do not use the railing.

people with HD. However, preliminary evidence supports the use of physical therapy interventions, in particular exercise involving strengthening and balance training, to improve function in patients with HD.

Parkinson's Disease. Strength training has been found to be particularly beneficial for patients with PD. A study with 14 patients with mild-to-moderate PD and 6 age-matched controls, found that 8 weeks of resistance training twice a week focusing on lower extremity strengthening produced significant increases in strength in both groups and improved stride length, walking velocity, and postural angles in the patients with PD.[94] Intensive exercise training over 14 weeks was also found to improve motor disability, mood, and well-being in patients with mild-to-moderate PD.[95]

Strengthening exercises can also improve impairments in areas other than strength, flexibility, and coordination.

Multiple Sclerosis. Several studies show that strengthening exercises and general physical therapy interventions help patients with varying stages of MS.[96-101] It appears that resistance training of the lower extremities at submaximal levels (e.g., 5% to 50% of maximum voluntary contraction) is safe for patients with MS, as long as fatigue is appropriately monitored. Although research suggests that strengthening improves various impairments, such as strength[97,99] and fatigue,[101] and functional abilities, such as walking,[96,98] in patients with MS, improvements in disability have only been demonstrated when strengthening exercises are components of a more comprehensive rehabilitation program.[102,103]

Aquatic exercise, in which patients perform strengthening and endurance exercises in a pool, has been found to improve lower extremity fatigue and strength[104] and health-related quality of life in patients with MS.[105] Ideally, aquatic exercise should be performed in cooler water (less than 85° F). Several studies have also demonstrated that respiratory muscle training produces significant improvements in measures of respiratory function (maximal expiratory pressure or maximal inspiratory pressure) in individuals in the middle and late stages of MS.[106-108]

> ◎ *Clinical Pearl*
>
> Strength training has generally been shown to be effective for most progressive CNS disorders, at least in the short term.

GAIT AND LOCOMOTION TRAINING

Gait impairments are common in individuals with progressive CNS disorders, and many patients hope that physical therapy interventions will improve their walking ability (speed, coordination, balance, and safety) or allow them to continue walking for as long as possible. Gait training will typically focus on ameliorating or compensating for impairments that most contribute to functional gait limitations to help patients reach their ambulation goals.

Patients with progressive CNS disorders can benefit from task-specific gait training, including extended practice of walking. In addition, for best results, since the practice environment can influence carryover, walking practice should occur in an environment that is similar to the patient's current life situation (e.g., including obstacles or timing constraints). For patients with cognitive impairments, practice with much contextual interference (random practice) and extensive verbal feedback should be avoided because this may interfere with task performance.

Parameters and characteristics of gait (speed, stride length, step width, episodes of **freezing**) during forward, backward, and sideward walking are be examined and documented, as well as overall stability, safety, and endurance. Gait and walking ability is analyzed in a variety of contexts and during complex, functional walking tasks,[109,110] including during performance of dual tasks, such as walking and talking[111] or walking while performing a cognitive task.[112] Energy expenditure, alignment, fit, practicality, and safety and ease of orthotic and assistive devices used during gait are examined and documented. Postural orientation, postural stability, reactive control, anticipatory control, and adaptive postural control will be assessed. Any falls and related injuries that have occurred are documented.

Treadmill Training. Within the past 10 years, many studies have examined the effects of treadmill gait training in patients with CNS disorders. This work began primarily in patients with stroke and spinal cord injury but is now continuing in patients with PD and MS. Research suggests that body weight–supported treadmill training, as well as regular unsupported treadmill training, increases gait speed and step length.

SENSORY CUEING

Sensory cueing involves the use of augmented sensory information, typically in the form of external visual,[113] auditory, or manual cueing, to improve task performance. Visual or auditory sensory cueing is commonly used in patients with PD to facilitate movement and overcome episodes of freezing and akinesia during gait. This approach is thought to work by using frontal pathways that respond to visual or auditory input to bypass damaged basal ganglia structures that are usually involved in self-initiating movement.[114] Use of visual cues, such as brightly colored objects or lines at consistent intervals along a walkway, during a walking task has been shown to improve walking performance (stride length and step length) in patients with PD[65,66,113,114] (see Fig. 17-5). Auditory cues, such as a series of tones or a metronome, to which a patient can entrain the tempo of their walking have also been found to improve gait cadence,[115-117] velocity, and stride length[115,116] in patients with PD. Synchronizing gait to rhythmic beats has also been shown to help modulate gait speed in people with HD.[118]

RELAXATION

Although there are no published studies examining the effects of relaxation on spasticity and rigidity, clinical observations demonstrate that slow, rhythmic rotational movements through small ranges of movement can temporarily reduce hypertonicity. For example, lower trunk rotation in hook or sidelying can decrease tone in patients with ALS or MS with increased lower extremity extensor muscle tone.

PNF, especially the technique of contract-relax, and biofeedback may also promote relaxation. In addition, a generalized decrease in muscle tone and overall increased well-being may be achieved through cognitive relaxation techniques such as Jacobsen's progressive relaxation exercises.[119] Because stress can induce fatigue and anxiety, effective recognition and management of stress are also important in an overall rehabilitation program.

FUNCTIONAL AND TASK-SPECIFIC TRAINING

Functional training is often essential for patients with progressive CNS disorders. Functional training refers to strategies to improve the ability to perform daily functional tasks, such as dressing, bathing, and climbing stairs, as well as training in the use of devices and equipment, and in injury prevention or reduction. Task-specific training, such as working on the speed of reaching, may be particularly helpful for patients with movement disorders, such as those caused by PD, because motor disturbances are typically context-dependent and occur during complex, well-learned tasks such as walking and reaching.[82,120] A task-based model of intervention can enhance skill learning through identification of tasks to be learned, followed by appropriately sequenced practice of these tasks within a structured environment and with augmented information before, during, and after task performance.[121,122]

APPLICATION OF ASSISTIVE DEVICES AND EQUIPMENT

Patients with progressive CNS disorders frequently benefit from use of assistive and adaptive devices. Some equipment, such as a cane or a walker, is usually quickly and readily available, although customized equipment, such as a customized wheelchair, may take many months to be made, by which time a patient's needs may have changed. The physical therapist should be available to reevaluate if a patient's physical needs or cognitive ability have changed.

At some point during the disease course, most patients with progressive CNS disorders require some sort of assistive or adaptive device (see Chapter 33) to maintain or assist with function. In fact, many patients require several different types of devices over the course of their disease. For example, a patient with HD may initially walk independently but soon may need a straight cane for help with balance. Later on, a rolling walker may be prescribed, and later still, as the disease progresses, a customized wheelchair is likely to be required. Because of the expense of adaptive equipment, clinicians must consider not only the current needs of a patient but also his or her needs as the disease progresses. In addition, one should keep in mind the cognitive skills needed to use a device when considering a device for a patient with a dementing disorder, such as AD, and in the later stages of HD, PD, and often MS.

INTEGUMENTARY REPAIR AND PROTECTIVE TECHNIQUES

Integumentary protection is indicated for patients who have very limited ability to move, which is common in the late stages of most progressive CNS disorders, and for patients who have an increased risk of bruising and fractures because of involuntary movements, such as those with HD. Patients may benefit from pressure relief interventions, including positioning, turning, and appropriate support surfaces (see Chapter 28) and if mobile, from protective padding on the elbows, forearms, knees, and shins. For added safety in the ambulatory patient with poor movement control, a helmet, hip protectors, and other body padding may be used to prevent more serious injuries such as a fracture or head injury.

CASE STUDY 17-1

EARLY-MIDDLE STAGE MULTIPLE SCLEROSIS

Patient History

RC is a 45-year-old woman who was diagnosed with MS 5 years ago. She has had 3 relapses over the last 5 years. During each episode, her legs became weak and she had visual problems. After each episode, she recovered most but not all of her strength. Her most recent episode was 2 months before this evaluation. RC requires assistance for heavy lifting and activities that require her to walk for extended distances (>¼ mile). She is independent with all ADLs, but it takes her longer to get dressed and finish her grooming routine because of fatigue and leg weakness (approximately 30 minutes after showering). She had enjoyed playing tennis and running until about 1 year ago, when she found these activities too difficult because of balance problems. RC requested physical therapy to address her worsening balance difficulties, weakness, and fatigue.

Tests and Measures—Significant Findings
Musculoskeletal

- Passive ROM: Hip abduction left 0-35 degrees, right 0-40 degrees; ankle dorsiflexion left 0 degrees, right 0-5 degrees; all others within normal limits (WNL).
- Strength: Significant manual muscle test results:

	Left	Right
Hip flexion	4/5	4/5
Hip extension	4/5	4/5
Hip abduction	4/5	4/5
Hip adduction	3/5	3/5
Knee extension	3/5	4/5
Knee flexion	4/5	4/5
Ankle dorsiflexion	2/5	3/5
Ankle plantarflexion	3/5	4/5

Neuromuscular

- RC reports problems with short-term memory (e.g., what she ate for breakfast) but not with long-term memory.

- Patient reports **diplopia,** particularly when looking at close objects.
- Moderate spasticity in both lower extremities in the hamstrings, adductors, and calf muscles.

Sensory Integrity
- Impaired sensation to light touch and pinprick below the knees bilaterally.
- Proprioception impaired in both ankles and knees.

Cardiovascular/Pulmonary
- 6-Minute Walk Test (6MWT): Distance walked: 850 ft. Surface: Outdoor/level/pavement. Borg RPE during the test: 5 (RC was requested to report when fatigue level was greater than 6 at any point during the test, and a rest was taken. RC took 3 rests during the entire test).
- Fatigue: RC reported fatigue as averaging 3/7 on the Fatigue Severity Scale (scale 1-7, 7 = highest severity).

Function
- RC can ascend and descend the 12 stairs she has at home with a step-over-step gait, while holding the railing, in 16 seconds.
- Gait: RC has a slight steppage gait on the left, likely to compensate for the profound left DF weakness. She also has a wide-based gait and decreased arm swing.
- Balance: RC can sit erect for 10 minutes without upper extremity support but could not do this for longer because of fatigue. RC can stand independently for up to 5 minutes, limited by fatigue.
- Patient has difficulty with all of the following tasks: Standing with eyes closed, turning 360 degrees, placing an alternate foot on a step, standing in tandem, and standing on one foot.
- She dresses and bathes independently, but it takes at least 15 minutes to get dressed and although she has not fallen, she is worried about falling while in the shower.

Diagnosis
Preferred practice pattern 5E: Impaired motor function and sensory integrity associated with progressive disorders of the central nervous system.

Interventions
- Instruction in energy conservation techniques and fatigue management.
- Balance training.
- Strengthening exercises.
- Cardiovascular training.
- AFO for the left ankle to compensate for ankle dorsiflexion weakness and improve foot clearance during ambulation and prevent steppage gait.
- Gait training with a straight cane for long distance ambulation.
- Recommendations for safety measures to be taken in the home.
- Instruction in an ongoing daily exercise routine.

Role of the Physical Therapist Assistant
- Why are the manual muscle test results significant?
- Define **nystagmus.**

- What additional safety measures are important in this patient's home?
- Describe three balance training activities, three strengthening exercises, and a cardiovascular training activity suitable for the patient.

Additional Information
For the full version of this case study, including detailed examination results, interventions, and outcomes, see the Evolve site that accompanies this book. A full case study for a patient with Huntington's disease midstage and a patient with middle-late stage Parkinson's disease also appears on the Evolve site.

CHAPTER SUMMARY
Patients with progressive CNS disorders present with a variety of impairments and functional limitations. There is currently no cure for any of the disorders presented here, although for some there are medications that alter symptoms or the course of the disease. All of these disorders progress over time, ultimately leading to disability and change in a patient's quality of life. All of these disorders involve the neurological system, often causing an array of cognitive and emotional changes that can compound the devastating effects on the motor and sensory systems.

Therapists should keep in mind that these disorders do progress and that the interventions need to progress accordingly. Appropriate rehabilitation intervention can improve quality of life, functional abilities, and possibly, disease progression. While we wait for a cure, therapists can help patients maintain functional independence and optimize quality of life.

ADDITIONAL RESOURCES
For links to these and additional web-based resources, see the Evolve site.
Alzheimer's Association
American Parkinson's Disease Association
Amyotrophic Lateral Sclerosis Association

GLOSSARY
Akinesia: Lack of movement.
Ataxia: Uncoordinated movement.
Atrophy: Wasting or loss of muscle tissue resulting from disease or lack of use.
Bradykinesia: Slowed speed and amplitude of movement.
Clonus: Alternate muscular contraction and relaxation in rapid succession.
Diplopia: Double vision.
Dyskinesia: Extraneous movement.
Dyspnea: Shortness of breath.
Fasciculations: Involuntary contraction, or twitching, of groups of muscle fibers.
Freezing: A sudden transient inability to move.
Hypertonicity: Increase in muscle tone.
Hypokinesia: Abnormally decreased motor function or activity.
Motor neuron disease: A heterogeneous spectrum of inherited and sporadic clinical disorders of the upper motor neurons, lower motor neurons, or both.
Nystagmus: Rapid involuntary oscillations of the eye.
Orthopnea: Shortness of breath in supine.
Rigidity: Non-velocity–dependent resistance to passive movement.
Spasticity: Velocity-dependent resistance to passive movement.

Chapter 18

Peripheral Nerve Injuries

Ginny Gibson

OBJECTIVES

After reading this chapter, the reader will be able to:
1. Describe the mechanisms of and classification systems for peripheral nerve injuries and their relevance to functional outcomes.
2. Describe the etiology and resultant clinical picture of common peripheral nerve injuries.
3. Explain the physiological processes after nerve injury and repair.
4. Summarize current approaches to surgical and medical management of peripheral nerve injuries.
5. Explain the relevance and general methods of electromyography and nerve conduction testing.
6. Be familiar with typical examination findings specific to the client with peripheral nerve pathology.
7. Describe rehabilitation interventions for patients with traumatic peripheral nerve injury, nerve compression, and nerve entrapment.

Depending on the nature and extent of peripheral nerve pathology, individuals with peripheral nerve injury* experience various degrees of recovery and with more advanced or severe injury, often do not return to their prior functional status. Appropriate interventions can reduce the extent of long-term dysfunction. This chapter describes the nature of peripheral nerve injury, reviews the examination, and describes interventions shown to be effective in the rehabilitation of individuals with peripheral nerve injuries.

OVERVIEW OF THE PERIPHERAL NERVOUS SYSTEM

The nervous system is typically divided into central and peripheral components. Central components include nerves that are wholly contained within the brain and spinal cord. Peripheral components include nerves that originate in the brain or spinal cord and end peripherally, as well as cranial and spinal nerves. The **peripheral nervous system (PNS)** includes motor, sensory, sympathetic, and parasympathetic **neurons,** with most nerves containing a mixture of these types of neurons. **Efferent** pathways (those that send messages from the center to the periphery) include somatic motor nerves that innervate skeletal muscles and the **autonomic nervous system (ANS)** with sympathetic and parasympathetic divisions that regulate smooth muscle, cardiac muscle, and glandular activity (Fig. 18-1). **Afferent** pathways (those that send messages from the periphery toward the center) transmit a range of sensory modalities including touch, position, vibration, and pain.[1,2]

Motor nerves originate in the anterior horn of the spinal cord, and sensory nerves originate in the dorsal root

---

*For clarity, this chapter will use the term *injury* to refer to all insults to peripheral nerves.

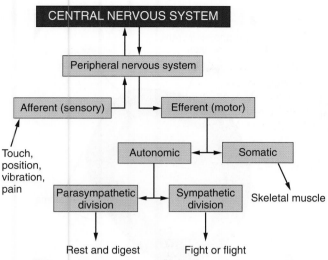

FIG. 18-1 The nervous system, including divisions of the peripheral nervous system.

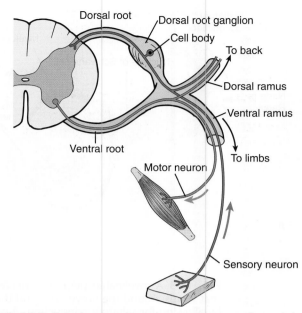

FIG. 18-2 Spinal nerves contain motor nerves that originate in the anterior horn of the spinal cord and sensory nerves that originate in the dorsal horn of the spinal cord.

ganglia. Sympathetic nerves originate in the lateral horn of the thoracic spinal cord and continue in sympathetic ganglia. Parasympathetic nerves originate from the brain and lateral grey matter of the sacral spinal cord and continue in the parasympathetic ganglia. Motor neurons of **cranial nerves** extend from the brainstem, and sensory neurons of cranial nerves have their cell bodies in cranial nerve ganglia. Motor and sensory cranial nerves serve structures in the head and neck, with the exception of the vagus nerve, which also continues to the chest and abdomen. Spinal nerves, of which there are 31 pairs, extend from their cell bodies and provide sensory and motor functions to all of the body, except the head.[1,2]

Spinal nerves, with their contributory dorsal and ventral roots, exit the intervertebral foramen and divide into dorsal and ventral rami (Fig. 18-2). With the exception of the thoracic region, the ventral rami combine to form the cervical, brachial, and lumbosacral **plexuses.**[1,2] This chapter discusses the examination and management of clients with nerve damage distal to these plexuses, as well as injuries to cranial nerves.

◎ *Clinical Pearl*

The peripheral nervous system (PNS) includes motor, sensory, sympathetic, and parasympathetic nerves.

ANATOMY OF A PERIPHERAL NERVE

Neural tissue includes excitable neurons (nerve cells) that propagate electrical impulses and **glia** cells that facilitate impulse conduction and support and protect the neurons.[1] All neurons have a cell body that contains a nucleus and organelles (mitochondria, rough endoplasmic reticulum, ribosomes, and Golgi apparatus). Almost all of a neuron's proteins, enzymes, and organelles are synthesized in the cell body. Most neurons have **dendrites,** an **axon,** and terminal branches. Dendrites are branching and tapering extensions of the axon that receive signals from other neurons, which the axon then carries to the cell body.

Signals are then carried away from the cell body toward terminal branches, where electrical and chemical signals are transmitted to other nerves or end-organs.

In the PNS, axons are wrapped in **myelin** from **Schwann cells.** A single Schwann cell wraps around an axon in a spiral fashion with small gaps, known as **nodes of Ranvier,** approximately 1 mm apart. The segments of axon between the nodes of Ranvier are called the *internodes* (Fig. 18-3). The myelin sheath accelerates the propagation of signals along the axon because impulses can jump from node to node rather than traversing the entire length of the nerve. This is known as *saltatory conduction.* Unmyelinated neurons conduct more slowly because they do not have a myelin sheath, although there are some Schwann cells within bundles of unmyelinated neurons.

A nerve consists of multiple neurons. Each neuron is surrounded by a semipermeable membrane called the **plasmalemma.** Groups of neurons are arranged in bundles, called **fascicles,** and groups of fascicles make up a nerve. Along a nerve, the thickness and presence of connective tissue layers vary. Where nerves cross over joints there is more connective tissue. Nerves may be more prone to injury at locations where the layers are thinner or absent.[3]

BLOOD SUPPLY OF PERIPHERAL NERVES

Peripheral nerves require oxygen to maintain the energy levels needed for axonal transport and cell viability. Nerves receive oxygen via extraneural and intraneural blood vessels. Peripheral nerves are immunologically isolated from the rest of the body by a blood-nerve barrier, comprised of tightly packed endothelial cells of the endoneurium and the internal layers of the perineurium. Injury to a nerve and the blood-nerve barrier may result

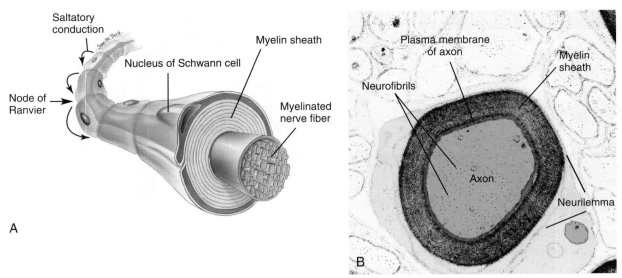

FIG. 18-3 A myelinated peripheral nerve. Note that the Schwann cell forms the myelin that wraps around the nerve axon and that the myelin promotes faster nerve transmission by allowing for saltatory conduction. *A courtesy Brenda Russell, PhD, University of Illinois at Chicago; B from Thibodeau GA, Patton KT:* Anatomy and physiology, *ed 6, St. Louis, 2006, Mosby.*

in exposure of the nerve and trigger an immunological response.

PERIPHERAL NERVE FUNCTION AND CLASSIFICATION

Peripheral nerves connect distally to end-organs that are sensory receptors, muscles, or glands. Sensory end-organs include mechanoreceptors, thermoreceptors, nociceptors, chemoreceptors, photoreceptors, and free nerve endings. In the somatic motor system, a single alpha motor neuron and all of the muscle fibers it innervates are known as a **motor unit.** A single motor unit, when stimulated sufficiently, will cause all of the muscle fibers it innervates to contract. Within the ANS, efferent pathways signal glands, including sweat glands, to secrete.[1,2] Peripheral nerves can be classified by axon diameter or by speed of conduction.

PHYSIOLOGY OF THE PERIPHERAL NERVOUS SYSTEM

AXONAL TRANSPORT

Neurotransmitters, proteins, and organelles are transported along axons using a system of microtubules and neurofibrils. Anterograde flow provides transport away from the cell body and occurs either quickly or slowly. Neurotransmitters and structures necessary to replenish the plasmalemma are transported quickly, whereas proteins and organelles needed for new axoplasm or to replenish axoplasm in regenerating neurons or mature neurons are transported more slowly. Retrograde flow, toward the cell body, occurs at a constant slow rate and returns organelles to the cell body for disposal and carries nerve growth factor toward the cell body. Both anterograde flow and

retrograde flow require an energy source that is compromised if circulation is disrupted.[4]

ION CHANNELS AND NERVE CONDUCTION

Two ions, potassium (K^+) and sodium (Na^+), are primarily responsible for nerve conduction. At rest, there is more sodium outside and more potassium inside a neuron. These concentrations are maintained by chemical and electrical gradients together with the sodium-potassium adenosinetriphosphatase (ATPase) pumps that pump three sodium ions out of the cell for every two potassium ions they pump into the cell. At rest, a neuron is more negatively charged inside than outside.

When the nerve is stimulated sufficiently, sodium ions enter the neuron, depolarizing it. This depolarization is quickly followed by potassium rushing out, causing repolarization. This sequence of depolarization and repolarization is known as an **action potential** (Fig. 18-4, *A*). The action potential will then be propagated along the nerve until it reaches the end of the nerve (Fig. 18-4, *B*).

A **synapse** is the meeting point of the axon terminal of one neuron (the presynaptic neuron) and a dendritic ending or cell body of another neuron (the postsynaptic neuron). The presynaptic axon terminal has vesicles containing a neurotransmitter that is released into the synaptic cleft, the space between the presynaptic and postsynaptic nerve, in response to an electrical signal (Fig. 18-5). The neurotransmitter then binds to postsynaptic receptors, causing the postsynaptic nerve to become excited (i.e., less negative), if more sodium ions enter the neuron, or inhibited (i.e., more negative), if chloride ions enter the neuron.[1,2] Each neuron can receive inputs from many other neurons and with a sufficient dominance of depolarizing inputs, an action potential will start in the postsynaptic neuron and propagate along the length of this nerve.

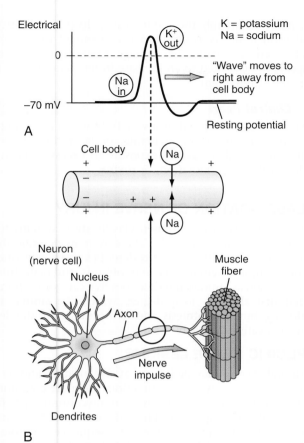

FIG. 18-4 An action potential propagating along a nerve. *Copyright Royal Society of Chemistry, 2006.*

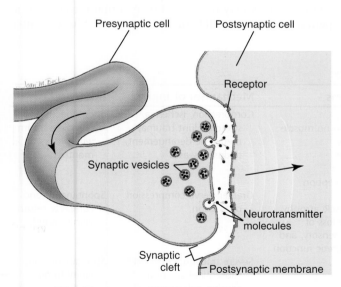

FIG. 18-5 Synaptic transmission. *From Thibodeau GA, Patton KT: Anatomy and physiology, ed 6, St. Louis, 2006, Mosby.*

EFFECTS OF MOVEMENT ON PERIPHERAL NERVES

Movement and positioning of the limbs, head, neck, or trunk can cause nerves to slide, become elongated, or recoil.[5-7] The tissues around peripheral nerves, including bone, cartilage, muscle, tendon, vessels, and fascia, form tunnels or passageways of various sizes through which the nerves pass. These tunnels may apply pressure to the nerves when the nerves move. Movement at one joint may require the nerve to lengthen at that joint and can pull on the nerve where it crosses other joints.[7] When a nerve is elongated, it gets narrower,[8] intraneural pressure increases,[8-10] blood flow decreases,[11,12] and strain increases.[7,13] Strain on the median and ulnar nerves has also been shown to increase more with movement (activity) than with maintained postures that impose incremental strain.[6]

NERVE PATHOLOGY

Nerve pathology can be localized or diffuse and may be caused by acute or cumulative trauma. An isolated nerve lesion is termed a **mononeuropathy,** and a condition with asymmetrical lesions of multiple nerves is termed **mononeuropathy multiplex.** Symmetrical diffuse nerve dysfunction is termed **polyneuropathy.** Polyneuropathy generally presents initially with symmetrical distal symptoms and is most often caused by a disease process rather than trauma (see Chapter 19).

MECHANISMS OF NERVE INJURY

How a nerve is injured influences the acute and long-term consequences of the injury and the selection of medical, surgical, and rehabilitation interventions. Nerves may be injured by excessive stretch or compression, inadequate blood supply, or exposure to excessive electric energy, radiation, or toxins. Inadequate blood supply is a feature of most mechanically induced nerve injury. Regardless of the mechanism of injury, the clinical findings of pain, paresthesia, and motor impairment are similar for most nerve injuries.

Nerves may be injured by a single application of high force traction or by repeated application of lower levels of traction that would not cause injury if they occurred only once.[14] Acute traction injuries are associated with fractures, either directly or secondary to reduction or fixation; joint dislocation; extreme limb or body segment positioning, as might occur during positioning for surgical access; and pulling on a limb segment, as seen in obstetrical brachial plexus injury. Traction injuries have also been reported during and subsequent to limb-lengthening procedures.[15] Traction that stretches the nerve a small amount may only impair circulation within the nerve. But a greater stretch can cause structural failure and complete conduction block and affect sensory and motor function.

Nerves may be compressed by a variety of mechanisms. Edema from acute and chronic inflammation,[16] inflammatory diseases, increased compartmental pressures, space-occupying lesions, contact against bones, and entrapment within soft tissues, as well as iatrogenic causes, such as tourniquet[17] and blood pressure cuff application, are all associated with compression neuropathies.[18,19]

The force (measured in mm Hg) and duration of compression applied to a nerve affects the nature and degree of nerve damage. Acute and localized compression generally causes less severe injury than chronic and diffuse compression.[20] Experimental studies of controlled vibration and studies with workers using vibrating tools have also found that vibration can damage myelin and cause nerve fibrosis.[21,22] Vibration-induced nerve injury is common in workers using heavy machinery such as jackhammers.[23] Nerve **ischemia** may also be caused by vascular occlusion[24] and other vascular disorders.

When a nerve is subjected to accidental injection, it may be damaged by the physical trauma of the needle and by exposure to the drug or agent. Accidental injection injuries occur most often during medication delivery,[25,26] with the sciatic nerve being the nerve most frequently injured by injection.[27] Needle-stick injuries to nerves during acupuncture are rare but have also been reported.[28] Injection of a nerve usually causes severe, radiating pain.

Nerve lacerations can occur as result of contact with a sharp object, such as a piece of glass, metal, knife, razor blade, or scalpel, or from contact with a blunt object, such as components of power tools or other machinery, and gunshot wounds. Sharp injuries may occur intraoperatively.[29] Blunt objects generally produce jagged, shredded injuries with ill-defined edges, whereas sharp objects produce injuries with a well-defined edge. Gunshot wounds may injure a nerve directly or secondarily as the result of shock, blast, or cavitation effects.[30,31]

Nerves may also be damaged by heat, either through direct exposure or by exposure to electrical current or radiation. Nerve tissue has the lowest electrical impedance of any body tissue, therefore electrical currents tend to travel along neurovascular bundles. Most neurovascular bundles run deep to the muscles they innervate, thus tissues lying close to this pathway may also be damaged. An electrical current can injure nerves directly by heating them and causing coagulation necrosis or by damaging the nerve cell membrane and increasing its permeability.[32] Radiation injury is associated with treatment for cancer, and when it occurs, the damage to irradiated nerves appears to be related to an increase in temperature and is generally permanent.[33]

> ◎ **Clinical Pearl**
>
> Nerves may be injured in a variety of ways, including traction, compression, ischemia, or laceration. They may also be damaged by exposure to excessive heat, electrical energy, radiation, or toxins.

CLASSIFICATION OF NERVE INJURY

Several authors have proposed classification systems for nerve injury (Table 18-1).[34-37] These systems describe the extent of nerve injury. Seddon describes three categories of nerve injury: Neurapraxia, axonotmesis, and neurotmesis,[34,36] whereas Sunderland describes five categories, numbered first through fifth degree, which are similar to Seddon's, but axonotmesis and neurotmesis are divided into two categories each.[35]

SPECIFIC NERVE LESIONS

Although nerves may be injured at any location and by a variety of mechanisms, certain lesions are more common. The following section discusses the more common specific peripheral nerve injuries and includes examples of unique mechanisms of injury. This section is sequenced anatomically, starting cranially and proximally and moving caudally and distally.

Nerve Lesions Affecting the Head and Neck. Cranial nerves may be injured by external forces, such as penetration from bullets or needles, or by blunt trauma,

TABLE 18-1	Classification of Peripheral Nerve Injury				
Seddon	**Sunderland**	**Injury**	**Symptoms**	**Mechanism of Injury**	**Recovery**
Neurapraxia	First degree	Structure of nerve intact, focal demyelination, localized area of conduction block	Pain Minimal to no muscle atrophy Numbness Diminished proprioception	Compression, ischemia, stretch, blunt trauma, metabolic derangement, toxins, diseases	Spontaneous and complete return within days to months
	Second degree	Interruption of axons, epineurium, perineurium, and endoneurium intact	Pain Some muscle atrophy Complete loss of motor, sensory, and sympathetic function	Greater nerve compression or traction	Spontaneous and complete return within months
Axonotmesis	Third degree	Disruption of axons, injury to funiculi		Severe traction, crush with subsequent scarring causing entrapment	Spontaneous but faulty to no recovery
	Fourth degree	Disruption of perineurium	No pain Muscle atrophy Complete loss of motor, sensory, and sympathetic function	No conduction because of scar	Incomplete spontaneous recovery, surgery likely required for repair or grafting
Neurotmesis	Fifth degree	Complete transection of nerve		Complete laceration	No spontaneous recovery without surgical intervention

causing fractures.[38] Injury may also occur from compression by edema, tumors, and entrapment. For example, pituitary tumors often compress the optic nerves[38]; the trigeminal nerve may be injured in association with mandibular or maxillary fractures,[38] mandibular surgery,[39] or dental work[40,41]; and the facial nerve may be injured in association with mandibular condyle,[42] laterobasal fractures,[38] and parotidectomy.[43] Bell's palsy, the acute onset of idiopathic facial nerve palsy, may occur subsequent to a viral infection[44] or may have a vascular cause.[38] Glossopharyngeal, vagus, and hypoglossal nerve injuries have been reported after subluxation of the cervical spine in subjects with rheumatoid arthritis.[45,46] Spinal accessory nerve injuries may occur during lymph node biopsy,[47-49] and the hypoglossal nerve may be injured by intubation.

Nerve Lesions Affecting the Upper Extremity. Brachial plexus injuries can be caused by blunt trauma from falls and lacerations from penetrating injuries, as well as compression and traction. In a report of 100 consecutive cases of subjects undergoing surgical repair of brachial plexus injuries, most injuries included trauma (motorcycle accidents, gunshot wounds, and penetrating wounds) and nine were iatrogenic. Positioning the shoulder in hyperabduction for surgical procedures, such as mammoplasty, can also be associated with brachial plexus traction injuries.

Obstetrical brachial plexus palsy (OBPP) is a brachial plexus injury in the newborn. OBPP is associated with increased birth weight, operative vaginal delivery,[50] advanced maternal age, and maternal diabetes.[51] Most infants with OBPP have complete neurological recovery.[52] Predictors of optimal recovery include intact active elbow flexion by 3 months of age, C7 involvement, and high birth weight.[53] Children with OBPP may develop secondary deformities around the shoulder because of muscle imbalance, which progress with suboptimal neural recovery.[54]

There are many injuries that may occur more distally in the upper extremity. Nerve injuries beyond the cords of the brachial plexus are summarized in Tables 18-2 and 18-3.

Nerve Lesions Affecting the Lower Extremity. Peripheral nerve injuries of the lower extremities in women are often associated with labor and delivery and pelvic surgery. In a study of 6,057 women after childbirth, 55 reported a new onset of nerve injury.[56] Cardosi, Cox, and Hoffman described a 1.9% incidence of postoperative neuropathy involving (in order of decreasing frequency) the obturator, ilioinguinal/hypogastric, genitofemoral, femoral, or lumbosacral nerves in a group of women who underwent pelvic surgery.[57] Although rare, compression of the femoral nerve was reported in three cases to be associated with entrapment at the iliopectineal arch.[58] Traumatic femoral nerve injuries may occur as a result of displaced acetabular fractures,[59] total hip arthroplasty,[60-62] and anterior dislocation of the femur.[63] Iatrogenic injuries are associated with inguinal hernia repair, arterial bypass, appendectomy,[64] and hysterectomy.[65,66] Sciatic nerve lesions can occur after a blunt force to the buttock region[67] or accidental injection[27] and as an iatrogenic consequence of hip arthroplasty.[61,68] Other nerve injuries that occur

TABLE 18-2	Etiology of Upper Extremity Nerve Lesions
Nerve	**Mechanism of Injury**
Axillary	Anterior shoulder dislocation, trauma during anterior shoulder stabilization procedures, fracture of the humeral neck
Musculocutaneous	Clavicular fracture
Radial nerve	Humeral fractures, compression in the radial tunnel
Median nerve	Entrapment in pronator teres, compression in the carpal tunnel
Ulnar	Cross-pinning after supracondylar fractures, entrapment in the cubital tunnel, entrapment in Guyon's canal

Data from Kline DG, Kim DH: *J Neurosurg* 99(4):630-636, 2003; Bartosh RA, Dugdale TW, Nielsen R: *Am J Sports Med* 20(3):356-359, 1992; Ring D, Chin K, Jupiter JB: *J Hand Surg* 29(1):144-147, 2004; Portilla Molina AE, Bour C, Oberlin C, et al: *Int Orthop* 22:102-106, 1998; Johnson RK, Spinner M, Shrewsbury MM: *J Hand Surg* 4A(1):48-51, 1979; Skaggs DL, Hale JM, Bassett J, et al: *J Bone Joint Surg Am* 83(5):735-740, 2003; Taniguchi Y, Matsuzaki K, Tamaki T: *J Shoulder Elbow Surg* 9(2):160-162, 2000.

more distally in the lower extremity are summarized in Tables 18-4 and 18-5.

NERVE DEGENERATION AND REGENERATION

Nerve recovery after complete nerve transection (neurotmesis) occurs if there is no damage to the cell body (Fig. 18-6). This process involves changes in the proximal and distal axon segments, as well as the nerve cell body. After neurotmesis, nonviable tissue must be removed and then the nerve must regenerate. First, within hours of the injury, chromatolysis, with breakdown of rough endoplasmic reticulum, occurs in the injured part of the nerve. The proximal axon degenerates from the site of injury up to at least the closest node of Ranvier. Following this degeneration, protein production accelerates to provide materials for nerve regeneration. These new proteins are transported to the stump of the proximal axon where they are assembled within approximately 24 hours from the initial injury. While more proteins are being made for nerve repair, the production of proteins for neurotransmission and the proliferation of Schwann cells decrease.[69] Axonal sprouting then occurs from the stump, just distal to the last intact node of Ranvier. Each axon forms up to 15 sprouts, collectively called a *growth cone*. These sprouts migrate, directed in part by signals received by projections of the basement membrane of the axon called *filopodia*. The filopodia are sensitive to growth factors, such as nerve growth factor (NGF), that act as targets, attracting regenerating axons.

◎ *Clinical Pearl*

A nerve cannot recover if the cell body is damaged.

Because the organelles required for protein synthesis are only located in the cell body, when a nerve is

TABLE 18-3	Major Nerve Injuries of the Upper Extremity	

Nerve	Muscles	Clinical Signs
Dorsal scapular	Rhomboid major Rhomboid minor	Weakened scapular adduction.
Suprascapular	Supraspinatus Infraspinatus	Weakened shoulder abduction and external rotation.
Subscapular	Subscapularis Teres major	Weakened shoulder medial rotation.
Long thoracic	Serratus anterior	Weakened scapular abduction and upward rotation, incomplete shoulder elevation through flexion and abduction, scapular winging.
Thoracodorsal	Latissimus dorsi	Diminished ability to depress scapula against resistance.
Lateral pectoral	Pectoralis major	Weakened shoulder flexion, medial rotation, and horizontal adduction.
Medial pectoral	Pectoralis major (PMa) and pectoralis minor (PMi)	PMa: Weakened shoulder flexion, medial rotation, and horizontal adduction. PMi: Weakened scapular downward rotation.
Axillary	Deltoid Teres minor	Weakened shoulder abduction, flexion, and/or extension, shoulder impingement.
Musculocutaneous	Coracobrachialis Biceps Brachialis	Significantly diminished elbow flexion. Requires abduction of shoulder to flex the elbow via brachioradialis.
Radial	Triceps Anconeus Brachioradialis Extensor carpi radialis longus Extensor carpi radialis brevis	Supination diminished, loss of wrist and MCP extension.
Posterior interosseus	Supinator Extensor digitorum communis Extensor digiti minimi Extensor carpi ulnaris Abductor pollicis longus Extensor pollicis brevis Extensor pollicis longus Extensor indicis proprius	Full-wrist extension but weak, weak ulnar deviation, unable to extend MCP joints.
Median	Pronator teres Flexor carpi radialis Palmaris longus Flexor digitorum superficialis Flexor pollicis brevis (superficial head) Opponens pollicis Lumbricales (1 and 2)	High (above or near elbow): Weakened pronation; weakened wrist flexion; loss of digital flexion of IF, MF; weakened flexion of RF and MF; weakened thumb MCP flexion, loss of thumb opposition, and palmar abduction. Benedictine hand: clawing of the index and middle finger.
Anterior interosseus	Flexor pollicis longus Flexor digitorum profundus (1 and 2) Pronator quadratus Abductor pollicis brevis	Weakened forearm pronation; weakened flexion of IF, MF; loss of thumb palmar abduction. Unable to make the "O" sign with thumb and index finger.
Ulnar	Flexor carpi ulnaris Flexor digitorum profundus (3 and 4) Palmaris brevis	High (at or above elbow): Weakened wrist flexion and ulnar deviation, loss of DIP flexion RF, SF; loss of MCP flexion SF; weakened MCP flexion RF; loss or significantly diminished IP extension IF, MF, RF, and SF; loss of lateral pinch; loss of SF opposition to thumb. Froment's paper sign: In presence of ulnar nerve palsy, client will flex the thumb IP joint instead of contracting the adductor pollicis muscle when asked to hold paper between the pads of the thumb and index finger. Jeanne's sign: The client may hyperextend the MCP joint in the above task. Egawa's sign: Client cannot radially and ulnarly abduct the MF.
Deep branch	Abductor digiti minimi Flexor digiti minimi Opponens digiti minimi Lumbricales (3 and 4) Palmar interosseus Dorsal interosseus Adductor pollicis	Weakened MCP flexion SF; loss or significantly diminished IP extension IF, MF, RF, and SF; loss of lateral pinch; loss of SF opposition to thumb. Froment's sign, Jeanne's sign, Egawa's sign, clawing of RF and SF.

MCP, Metacarpophalangeal; *IF,* index finger; *MF,* middle finger; *RF,* ring finger; *SF,* small finger; *DIP,* distal interphalangeal; *IP,* interphalangeal.

TABLE 18-4	Common Causes of Lower Extremity Nerve Lesions
Nerve	**Cause**
Peroneal	Fractures of the femur, tibia, and fibula; knee dislocation; leg crossing; positioning in persons who are mobility impaired or comatose; and positioning during surgical procedures
Deep peroneal	Compression beneath fibular fibrous arch in the anterior tarsal tunnel, from constricting shoe laces and in the presence of pes cavus
Superficial peroneal nerve	Inversion sprain
Tibial	Compression because of entrapment in the tarsal tunnel or in the popliteal fossa
Sural	Lateral malleolus fracture, calcaneus fracture, small saphenous vein stripping

Data from Mont MA, Dellon AL, Chen F, et al: *J Bone Joint Surg Am* 78:863, 1996; Goitz RJ, Tomaino MM: *Am J Orthop* 32(1):14-16, 2003; Fabre T, Piton C, Andre D, et al: *J Bone Joint Surg Am* 80(1):47-54, 1998; Johnston EC, Howell SJ: *Foot Ankle Int* 20(9):576-582, 1999; Mastaglia FL: *Muscle Nerve* 23(12):1883-1886, 2000; Seror P: *Am J Phys Med Rehabil* 81(11):876-880, 2002.

transected, the proteins needed for its maintenance and repair can only reach the proximal nerve segment. Therefore the distal nerve segment degenerates. This type of degeneration is known as **Wallerian degeneration** and involves disintegration of the axoplasm and axolemma over the course of 1 to 12 weeks and degradation of the surrounding myelin. The remnants of these materials are cleared from the area by macrophages. Residual Schwann cells in the area of the distal portion of the injured nerve, responding to the Wallerian degeneration, stimulate the production of high levels of NGF for up to 2 weeks after nerve injury.[70] Although NGF promotes nerve regeneration, it has also been implicated in the development of **neuromas** and neuropathic pain after nerve injury.

After repair of a transected nerve, the rate of regeneration is at the most 10 mm per day. However, regeneration rates differ among fibers, depending on their type and location (Table 18-6). Small fibers regenerate more quickly than larger diameter fibers. Therefore C fibers carrying information about dull, aching pain and temperature will regenerate more quickly than A-beta and A-delta fibers that carry information about discriminative touch, proprioception, and sharp pain.

Surgical repair of transected nerves does not ensure full functional return. Nerve cell viability, rate of recovery, and axonal direction all affect the degree of nerve regeneration and the viability of end-organs.[71] Additionally,

TABLE 18-5	Signs and Symptoms of Lower Extremity Nerve Injuries		
Nerve	**Muscle(s)**	**Clinical Signs**	**Sensory Loss**
Superior gluteal	Tensor fascia lata	Trendelenburg gait	None
Sciatic	Abductor magnus Semimembranosus Biceps femoris	High steppage gait, inability to stand on heel or toes	Posterior thigh and calf Entire foot with exception of medial malleolus and medial aspect
• Common peroneal			
Superficial	Peroneus longus Peroneus brevis	Foot drop, inability to evert the foot	Lateral aspect of calf Dorsum of foot
Deep	Tibialis anterior Extensor digitorum longus Extensor hallucis longus Peroneus tertius Extensor digitorum brevis Extensor hallucis brevis	Foot drop	First web space of toes
• Tibial	Gastrocnemius Soleus Tibialis posterior Flexor digitorum longus Flexor hallucis longus Intrinsics on plantar foot	Inability to plantarflex the ankle and invert the foot Toe flexion, abduction, and adduction lost	Plantar aspect of foot and toes except medial border
Femoral	Pectineus Sartorius Rectus femoris Vastus medialis Vastus intermedius Vastus lateralis	Falling because of an unstable knee and difficulty with stair climbing	Medial distal thigh Medial aspect calf and foot
Obturator	Adductor brevis Adductor magnus Adductor longus Gracilis	Weak thigh adduction	Medial aspect of thigh

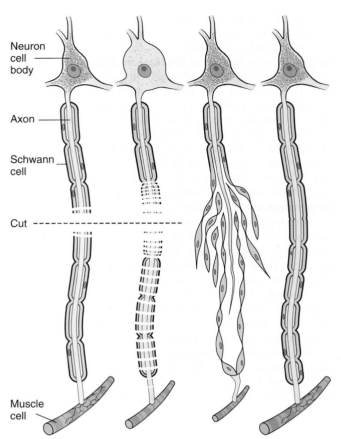

Neuron
cell
body

Axon

Schwann
cell

Cut ------------------------

Muscle
cell

FIG. 18-6 Nerve degeneration and regeneration after complete nerve transection. *From Damjanov I: Pathology for the health professions, ed 3, St Louis, 2006, Saunders.*

TABLE 18-6	Rate of Nerve Regeneration by Region
Location	**Rate of Regeneration (mm/day)**
Upper arm	2.5-8.5
Proximal forearm	2-6
Wrist	1-2
Hand	1-1.5
Upper leg	2
Lower leg	1.5
Ankle	1

neuroma development and neuropathic pain can contribute to poor functional outcomes despite optimal surgical repair and subsequent regeneration.

FUNCTIONAL RECOVERY FROM PERIPHERAL NERVE INJURY

For a peripheral nerve to successfully regenerate, four criteria must be met: Survival of the cell body; absence of barriers, such as scar or bone that would prevent axonal sprouting; accurate growth toward appropriate end-organs;

and accommodation of the **central nervous system (CNS)** to reorganize mixed afferent signals.[72] In addition, functional recovery from peripheral nerve injury may be affected by the age and cognitive capacity of the patient, the circumstances or nature of the nerve injury, and the subsequent repair.[73]

Children tend to have better functional outcomes from peripheral nerve injury than adults.[74-76] Proposed reasons for this include that the nerves have less distance to cover to reach their end-organ[74] and that children have more cerebral plasticity[77,78] and better nerve regeneration.[79] The latter theory, however, is controversial with studies showing both better[74] and similar nerve regeneration in adults and children.[80,81]

Patients with traumatic peripheral neuropathies have worse outcomes than patients with peripheral neuropathies from nontraumatic causes.[82] Functional outcomes after crush injuries are better than those after transection followed by repair or nerve grafting.[83] Nerves repaired sooner fare better, with less cell death, than those repaired later.[84] Generally, the more proximal a nerve injury is the poorer the outcome because of the length of nerve that needs to regrow for reinnervation.

TYPICAL EXAMINATION FINDINGS

PATIENT HISTORY

Information obtained from the medical record and patient interview includes the patient's name, gender, race/ethnicity, and primary language. Gender appears to be a risk factor for certain peripheral nerve injuries. For example, carpal tunnel syndrome (CTS) seems to be more common in women,[85] whereas cubital tunnel syndrome affects more men.[86] In the presence of OBPP, a developmental and birth history should be obtained.

Specific aspects of the patient history to be emphasized for patients with peripheral nerve pathology include employment status and sports activities. Since entrapment mononeuropathy may be caused by specific activities, the clinician will ask the patient about the nature of their activities at work, school, and home. Particular attention will be paid to repetitive activities and positions or activities in which compression may be placed on a nerve by an external object. For example, suprascapular nerve entrapment has been reported to occur in video cameramen as a result of compression of the nerve by the weight of the camera on the shoulder.[87] Although work activities may affect the risk for nerve injury, there is evidence that other factors, such as body mass index, age, and anatomical variation, may play a greater role for industrial workers with abnormal nerve function.[88] Sports-related injuries, whether as employment or leisure activity, are commonly reported. Examples include suprascapular and dorsal scapular nerve injury in volleyball players[89] and cubital tunnel syndrome in throwing athletes.[90,91]

The medical chart will be reviewed for results of radiographs, computed tomography (CT), magnetic resonance imaging (MRI), nerve conduction studies (NCS), and diagnostic nerve blocks. Radiographic studies, particularly CT and MRI, may reveal presence of a soft tissue mass along nerves causing compression. Diagnostic nerve blocks and nerve conduction studies aid in localizing sources of noxious stimuli and pathways for transmission of noxious stimuli. Further discussion of nerve conduction studies follow later in this chapter.

The client's understanding of the current problem and reason for referral to rehabilitation therapy are recorded. The physical therapist will record the response to other therapies, including past and present, to help determine prognosis. The mechanism of injury and date of injury or onset of symptoms are also crucial for diagnostic and prognostic determination. Since more proximal injuries have less favorable outcome, recording the level of injury is also essential.

SYSTEMS REVIEW

The systems review is used to target areas requiring further examination and to define areas that may cause complications or indicate a need for precautions during the examination and intervention processes. Chapter 1 includes details of the systems review.

TESTS AND MEASURES

There is no single test shown to accurately assess the presence and status of nerve pathology, thus a battery of tests will often be used to examine subjects with suspected nerve lesions.

Musculoskeletal

Posture. Posture may play a role in the development or exacerbation of symptoms associated with peripheral nerve entrapment or compression (see Chapter 4).

Anthropometric Characteristics.

Edema. Peripheral nerve injury may be associated with edema, heat, and redness when there is inflammation present and with edema, coolness, and pallor when active motion is significantly impaired. Limb volume can be estimated by water displacement using commercially available hand volumeters or by circumferential measurements. Hand volumeters have been found to be accurate. Circumferential measurements and volumetry have both been found to have high interrater and test-retest reliability. When estimating hand or foot volume with a tape measure, the figure-of-eight method has been found to be most reliable.[92-95]

There are no standards for these measurements, but comparison with the uninvolved limb and over time can be used to evaluate for abnormalities and changes. Note that it is not uncommon for the dominant hand to be larger than the nondominant hand.

Range of Motion and Muscle Length. Joint contractures and muscle shortening frequently occur after peripheral nerve injury as a result of unbalanced forces around a joint. For example, 52% of a sample of patients with cubital tunnel syndrome were found to have elbow flexion contractures.[96] Therefore both active range of motion (AROM) and passive ROM (PROM), as well as muscle length, should be examined in patients with peripheral nerve injuries. These measurements will be performed for all areas that the involved nerve crosses.

Muscle Performance. Muscle strength testing is essential for patients with peripheral nerve injuries because a peripheral motor nerve injury will produce specific weakness in the muscles innervated by that nerve. Muscles will be tested individually rather than with others performing similar movements because muscles performing similar movements may have different innervations. Muscle weakness that results from peripheral nerve injury is examined using manual muscle tests (MMT). Prolonged weakness as a result of motor nerve injury may also be detectable by observation of muscle atrophy and loss of muscle bulk. Although changes in girth measurements over time have been shown to correlate with other measures of strength, the poor specificity of this method limits its utility (see Chapter 5).[97]

The British Medical Research Council (BMRC) scale, that was later modified by Dellon (Table 18-7), is often used for grading motor and sensory function after peripheral nerve injury.[98] This scale grades motor function based on the strength of proximal and peripheral muscles innervated by the nerve in question. This scale is helpful for localizing and determining the severity of peripheral nerve injuries and in evaluating recovery. A modified BMRC scale appropriate for use in children is also available.

Neuromuscular

Pain. Peripheral nerve injury is often associated with changes in sensation. Although decreased sensation,

TABLE 18-7	British Medical Research Council (BMRC) Scale of Nerve Function		
Motor Function		**Sensory Function**	
M0	No contraction	S0	Absence of sensibility in the autonomous area
M1	Perceptible contraction in proximal muscles	S1	Recovery of deep cutaneous pain in the autonomous area
M2	Perceptible contraction in proximal and distal muscles	S1+	Recovery of superficial pain in the autonomous area
M3	Contraction of proximal and distal muscles with sufficient power to allow movement against resistance	S2	Return of some degree of superficial cutaneous pain and some tactile sensibility in the autonomous area
		S2+	S2 but with an overresponse
M4	Return of function as in stage 3 but synergistic and independent movements possible	S3	Return of superficial cutaneous pain and tactile sensitivity throughout the autonomous area, with disappearance over response, static 2-point discrimination >15 mm
		S3+	S3, with localization and recovery of 2-point discrimination at 7-15 mm in the autonomous area
M5	Complete recovery	S4	Complete recovery with static 2-point discrimination at ≤6 mm

Modified from Dellon A, Curtis R, Edgerton M: *Plast Reconstr Surg* 53:297-305, 1974.

causing numbness and tingling, is most common, burning, shooting, and sharp electrical-type pains are also often associated with peripheral nerve injuries. In addition, tingling or paresthesias may also be described by the patient as pain.[99] The nature of the pain may help to distinguish nerve-related pain from pain of musculoskeletal origin. Pain associated with peripheral nerve injury may indicate normal nerve regeneration but is thought more often to be a result of irritation of small diameter nociceptive A-delta and C fibers.

Pain may also be caused by neuromas, which are benign tumors made up largely of nerve cells and nerve fibers, that often occur after peripheral nerve injury. Neuromas are thought to be formed when nerve regeneration is blocked by scar tissue, preventing further regeneration. Movement of adjacent tissues or direct application of pressure on neuromas often causes pain by stimulating the nerve enclosed by the neuroma. Standard pain assessment measures (see Chapter 22) may be used to measure pain in clients with peripheral nerve injury and should be reexamined at each therapy encounter.

Cranial and Peripheral Nerve Integrity

Electrophysiological Testing. Electrodiagnostic studies are generally considered the gold standard for evaluating peripheral nerve integrity. NCS and electromyography (EMG) will provide information on the nature, severity, and location of peripheral nerve injury by sending pulses of electricity down the nerve. These tests are usually conducted by a physician (neurologist or physiatrist) but may also be performed by therapists with specific advanced training and necessary certification.

Provocative Tests to Detect Nerve Injury. Clinicians often subject nerves to compression or traction in an attempt to detect nerve injury or dysfunction. Production of symptoms by these provocative testing maneuvers is thought to indicate nerve injury. Compression can be applied manually or with a device, and tension is generally applied by placing the client in positions that are thought to put the nerve on stretch and would not elicit symptoms in normal subjects. This latter type of maneuver is referred to as a *neural tension test*.

Tinel's Test. Tinel's test is used to detect Tinel's sign, which is a hyperirritability or response to mechanical inputs such as tapping, and is thought to indicate nerve injury. Tinel's test is performed by tapping on the skin directly over the nerve in question. Production of distal pain or tingling may indicate a nerve injury at the location of tapping.

Phalen's Test. Phalen's test is used in the evaluation of suspected CTS. The client is asked to flex both wrists for 1 minute. Any numbness or tingling in the median nerve distribution during the 1-minute period is considered a positive test.

Neural Tension Tests. Neural tension tests can be performed on the upper and the lower extremities. Neural tension tests for the lower extremities include the straight leg raise (SLR) test, the slump test, and the prone knee bend test. The SLR and slump test primarily apply tension to the sciatic nerve, whereas the prone knee bend test primarily applies tension to the femoral nerve (see Chapter 8). A number of neural tension tests, collectively known as *upper limb neural tension tests* (ULNTTs), have been described for the upper extremities. The different ULNTTs attempt to selectively apply most tension to the brachial plexus or to the median, radial, or ulnar nerve. Although ULNTTs have been found to be reliable in symptomatic and asymptomatic individuals, ULNTTs can also produce symptoms or less than full ROM in many asymptomatic people without nerve pathology.[100]

Reflex Integrity. Deep tendon reflex (DTR) testing can help establish the presence of nerve pathology even in the absence of other clinical findings and is performed by tapping on tendons with a reflex hammer. With peripheral nerve injury, the DTRs will be hyporeactive. Although widely used as part of the clinical examination, some limitations of this test include variability in force during the tapping procedure, subjectivity in qualifying the response, and the fact that different responses can be produced by exerting different amounts of force.

Sensory Integrity. Testing of sensibility is an essential component of the examination of individuals with peripheral nerve injury and can help localize a nerve lesion, and facilitate diagnosis, prognosis, and selection of interventions including patients' educational needs. Sensory test selection should be based on the expected progression of sensory return:

Pain and temperature
↓
Sharp, pressure
↓
Moving 2-point discrimination
↓
Static 2-point discrimination

Sensory Testing. Sensory testing is most commonly performed with hand-held tools. Consequently, some variables cannot be fully controlled, including the amount of force used when applying the testing instrument, the amount of vibration caused by shaking of the clinician's hand, the amount of time the device touches the client's skin, and the speed at which the device is applied to the skin.[101]

For sensory testing, the examiner should ensure a mutually agreeable communication system, establish patient understanding of the testing procedure, and maximize patient comfort. Additionally, for all cutaneous sensory testing, vision should be occluded, and after orientation to testing procedures, distracting noise and activities in the testing environment should be minimized. Comfort may improve accuracy as the client will be less likely to reposition, thus minimizing extraneous proprioceptive inputs. The body part to be tested should rest on a supportive surface to minimize extraneous movement and stretching of tissues.[102]

Vibratory sensation is the first sensory function affected by peripheral nerve compression.[103-105] Vibratory sensation can be tested with a hand-held tuning fork. Sensation of cutaneous pressure is best tested with nylon monofilaments. These have high sensitivity and reliability but low specificity for perception of touch.[106] Monofilaments are made of a single nylon thread attached to a plastic, hand-held rod. Monofilaments come in different thicknesses and stiffness (denoted by different colors in Table

TABLE 18-8	Interpretation of Monofilament Test Findings	
Filament	Interpretation	Color
1.65-2.83	Normal	Green
3.22-3.61	Diminished light touch	Blue
3.84-4.31	Diminished protective sensation	Purple
4.56-6.65	Loss of protective sensation	Red
≥6.65	Untestable	Red striped

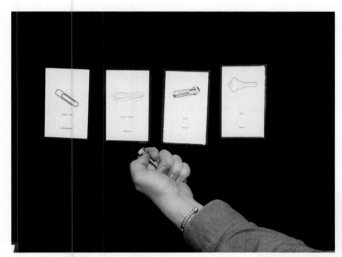

FIG. 18-7 Items from the Moberg pick-up test for tactile gnosis.

18-8), corresponding to the amount of force required to bend them. The end of the thread is pressed against the area being tested until it bends, and the subject is asked to note if they did or did not feel pressure from the thread.

Tactile Gnosis Testing. Patients with peripheral nerve injuries affecting sensation in the hand may have difficulty with tactile gnosis, which is the ability of the hand to perform complex functions by feel. A number of tests have been devised and evaluated for assessment and measurement of tactile gnosis. These include the Moberg pick-up test (Fig. 18-7) and the shape and texture identification (STI) test.

Function. Compression neuropathy may be associated with activities that involve repetitive movements or vibration. However, since this is not a universal association, the majority of people with CTS or ulnar entrapment do not perform jobs that involve repetition,[107,108] and most people with repetitive strain injuries do not have compression neuropathy,[109] it should not be assumed that a patient's nerve injury is related to their occupation.

EVALUATION, DIAGNOSIS, AND PROGNOSIS

Most clients who fall into the *Guide for Physical Therapist Practice*[110] preferred practice pattern 5F: Impaired peripheral nerve integrity and muscle performance associated with peripheral nerve injury will have the following types

of abnormal examination findings: Loss of or diminished strength, loss of or diminished ROM, impaired sensation, and hyporeactive stretch reflexes. In addition, integumentary integrity may be secondarily compromised. The following section describes rehabilitation interventions that have been shown to optimize outcomes for patients with peripheral nerve injury.

INTERVENTION

Clients with peripheral nerve injuries are referred for rehabilitation before and after surgical interventions and when surgery is not anticipated. After peripheral nerve injury, interventions will progress from those that focus on protection and immobilization to those that focus on restoring physical and functional abilities as the nerve recovers. These interventions will be modified according to findings on the examination, the level and mechanism of injury, and any associated injuries.

PATIENT EDUCATION

Clients with absent or impaired protective sensation should be instructed in measures to protect skin integrity. For patients with upper extremity involvement, this should include abstaining from holding cigarettes or cooking at a stovetop. For those with lower extremity involvement, this should include wearing shoes whenever walking. All patients with sensory impairment should be especially vigilant during activity involving use of sharp objects such as nail clippers, and patients who require splinting should regularly inspect under the splint for areas of pressure, rashes, and signs of maceration.

Personal and ergonomic factors may increase the risk for nerve compression or entrapment. Since smoking and obesity increase the risk for CTS, wellness programs that promote smoking cessation and weight reduction may reduce the incidence or severity of CTS.[111]

THERAPEUTIC EXERCISE

Although muscle strengthening exercises will not increase strength in patients with complete motor **denervation,** strengthening exercises can be effective with partial innervation and during reinnervation. Strengthening exercises may be started as soon as the patient can perform active muscle contraction (see Chapter 5). The use of electrical stimulation for strengthening denervated muscles is discussed in detail in the section on Electrotherapeutic Modalities.

JOINT RANGE OF MOTION AND MUSCLE STRETCHING

Once immobilization for acute nerve injury is no longer necessary, joint ROM and muscle stretching may be needed to regain ROM and soft tissue length lost because of immobilization. After surgical nerve repair, soft tissue lengthening should be performed with caution, particularly if the nerve was repaired under tension or with a graft. Muscle stretching is recommended when nerve compression or entrapment is caused by muscle shortening, as with cubital tunnel syndrome caused by tightness of the flexor carpi ulnaris or piriformis syndrome caused by a tight piriformis muscle compressing the sciatic nerve.

Muscle stretching is also recommended when motor nerve injury causes weakness of one muscle and consequent shortening of its antagonist.

SENSORY RETRAINING

Sensory desensitization and reeducation programs are generally performed together or in sequence in patients with sensory nerve injuries that cause reduced sensation or pain. These interventions are intended to reduce hyperesthesia and promote reorganization of cortical representation of the involved limb.

Desensitization. Desensitization programs consist of graded introduction of stimuli with a specific progression of textures, from less irritating to more irritating sensory stimuli. Treatment recommendations suggest anywhere from 10 to 30 minute sessions, 2 to 4 times a day. Media commonly used for desensitization programs are shown in Fig. 18-8.

Sensory Reeducation. After nerve injury, even with optimal surgical repair, cell death and axonal misdirection can result in poor sensory localization and poor functional outcome.[83,112] The initial nerve injury, as well as axonal misdirection during regeneration, can alter sensory representation because of cortical reorganization.[113,114] The degree of cortical reorganization varies according to the nature of the injury. Crush injuries, in which the basement membranes remain relatively intact, cause less axonal misdirection[83] and therefore little cortical reorganization after recovery.[115] In contrast, after complete nerve lacerations and repair, there is much distortion of somatosensory cortical maps, causing previously well-defined areas to become diffuse[114] and adjacent areas to expand.[116]

Sensory reeducation may improve functional outcome after nerve injury by facilitating more appropriate cortical reorganization. There is some suggestion that training should also occur bilaterally[117] because tactile sensory inputs to one side can activate the ipsilateral, as well as the contralateral, cerebral hemisphere.[118] Sensory reeducation is recommended as a component of the treatment of patients with sensory loss after peripheral nerve injury. Sensory reeducation programs generally include introduction and identification of increasingly complex tactile inputs with and without vision occluded. Stimulation should be focused on the area with reduced sensation, and correct performance should be consistently and strongly reinforced.

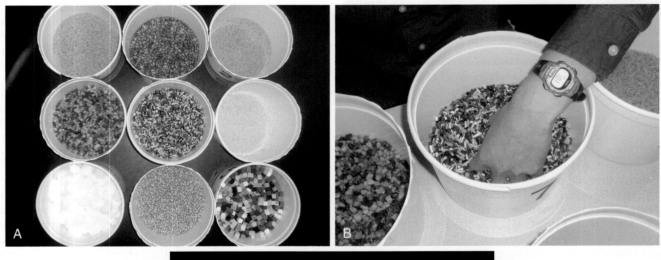

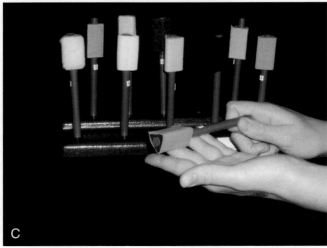

FIG. 18-8 Media for graded desensitization. **A** and **B**, Containers of loose materials. **C**, Tactile sticks.

MANUAL THERAPY TECHNIQUES

Nerve gliding techniques are commonly employed after nerve injury or repair with the goal of mobilizing nerves from sites of compression or entrapment after a period of immobilization.[119] These techniques are often applied by therapists but, because the techniques are complex and require ongoing patient evaluation and technique modification, they are rarely applied by therapist assistants.

PRESCRIPTION, APPLICATION, AND FABRICATION OF DEVICES AND EQUIPMENT

Splinting and Orthotics. Orthotics may be used to protect repaired nerves or insensate areas, rest limb segments to assist in resolving inflammation, promote function, or prevent deformity after nerve injury. Fig. 18-9 shows examples of functional splints for the upper extremity.

Assistive Devices. Patients with peripheral nerve injuries may need assistive devices for a short period of time while waiting for reinnervation or reconstructive surgery, such as a nerve or tendon transfer, or for the long term, if motor reinnervation does not occur (see Chapter 33).

ELECTROTHERAPEUTIC MODALITIES

In patients with peripheral nerve injuries, electrical stimulation (ES) may be used to stimulate contraction of denervated muscle, to facilitate muscle contraction in weakened reinnervated muscle, and for pain management. Although research on the use of ES to denervated muscle has had mixed outcomes, some clinicians use ES to try to preserve muscle function and reduce the rate of atrophy and fibrosis in denervated muscle. Such stimulation is generally provided via surface electrodes using direct current stimulation. Some studies suggest that iontophoresis with a corticosteroid may help patients with inflammatory nerve

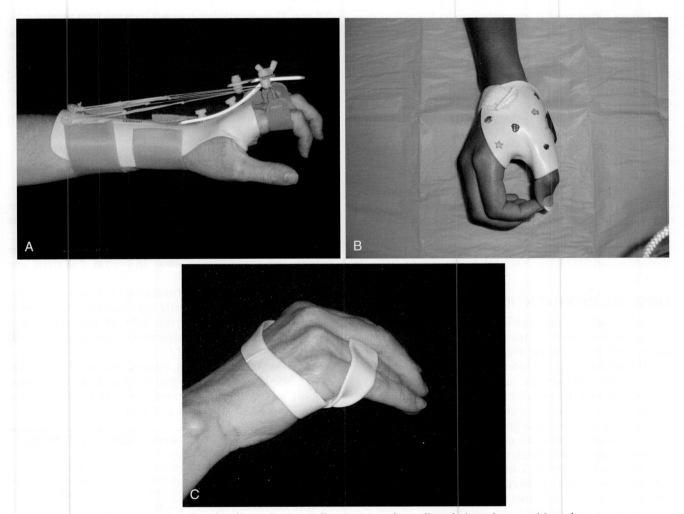

FIG. 18-9 Functional splints. **A,** A median nerve palsy splint designed to position the thumb to allow opposition. **B,** A radial nerve palsy splint designed to assist wrist and finger extension. **C,** An ulnar nerve palsy splint designed to prevent hyperextension of the MCP joints and allow the long finger extensors to extend the fingers when the intrinsic muscles are not able to contract. All of these splints are intended to be used during functional activities.

injuries. However, since iontophoresis can cause skin burns where the electrodes are placed, these electrodes should not be placed on skin with reduced sensation.

PHYSICAL AND MECHANICAL MODALITIES

Heat. Heat is not commonly used for treatment of patients with nerve injury because it can increase inflammation during the acute recovery phase. However, heat may be used in the later rehabilitation of patients with peripheral nerve injury to facilitate stretching muscles that have shortened as a result of weakness or denervation of the antagonist and for pain management.

Cold. Cryotherapy may occasionally be used to control inflammation and edema after trauma that includes damage to peripheral nerves, surgical nerve repair, or decompression,[120] or when soft tissue inflammation causes nerve compression.

Ultrasound. Pulsed ultrasound may promote recovery from nerve injury by nonthermal mechanisms. Furthermore, unlike continuous ultrasound, which increases tissue temperature and may adversely affect nerve latencies, pulsed ultrasound at intensities up to 1.0 W/cm^2 has been found to improve comfort and function and not adversely affect nerve conduction.[121]

Hydrotherapy. Despite a dearth of evidence, contrast baths, which involve immersing a limb segment in alternating cold and hot water, are often used clinically in patients with edema from any cause, including peripheral nerve injury.[122,123] It is proposed that the alternating cooling and heating will cause alternating vasoconstriction and vasodilation, respectively, to pump fluid out of an edematous area.

Laser Light Therapy. Laser light therapy, also known as *low level laser therapy* (LLLT), is thought to promote nerve recovery by enhancing energy production, reducing inflammation,[124,125] and promoting formation of new blood vessels[126] and proliferation of fibroblasts.[127] LLLT was first cleared for clinical use by the Food and Drug Administration (FDA) in 2002 for treatment of patients with CTS.

SURGICAL INTERVENTION

Although rehabilitation clinicians do not perform surgery, they are often involved in the care of patients with nerve injuries that are surgically treated. Several factors determine the need for surgical interventions, including nature of the injury, whether the injury produces a closed or open wound, and the amount of time between injury and presentation. For severe nerve transections that present early, surgical nerve repair is generally indicated. If a nerve injury is associated with an open wound, the wound is generally surgically explored, whereas closed wounds are often observed for up to 3 months and only surgically explored if evidence of nerve regeneration is lacking. Surgery is also often indicated when pressure on a chronically compressed nerve produces symptoms.

The primary options for surgical nerve repair are end-to-end coaptation and nerve graft (autograft, allograft). End-to-end coaptation, after partial or complete nerve transection, involves suturing the epineurium of the separated nerve endings together (known as *epineurial repair*)

or suturing individual fascicles or groups of fascicle endings together (known as *fascicular repair*). Individual fascicle repair is uncommon because the many sutures required can cause excessive scarring.

If there is a gap between the nerve endings because the proximal and distal nerve segments have retracted or a portion of the nerve was so damaged it needed to be excised, then a repair by end-to-end coaptation, which would require bringing the proximal and distal nerve stumps together, would place excessive tension on the nerve. In this circumstance, a nerve graft may be used. A conduit may also be placed around a nerve lesion or an area of nerve repair to reduce adhesion of the nerve to surrounding tissues and to direct nerve growth.

CASE STUDY 18-1

TRANSECTION OF THE ULNAR NERVE

Patient History

TR is a 31-year-old, left-handed construction worker who fell through glass and sustained a puncture wound to the left cubital tunnel, resulting in transection of the ulnar nerve. Two weeks ago he underwent an ulnar nerve repair without anterior transposition on the day of injury and was placed in a long-arm, above-elbow cast postoperatively. The patient is now completing 100% of bilateral activities of daily living (ADL) tasks with his nondominant right hand.

Tests and Measures—Significant Findings
Musculoskeletal

- Volumetric testing of TR's hand revealed moderate edema in the left hand with displacement of 37 cc more water than the right.
- Circumferential measures of the elbow taken in line with the elbow crease were 26 cm on the right and 32 cm on the left.
- PROM testing of the left shoulder and elbow was deferred to avoid placing the recently repaired ulnar nerve under tension. Left wrist PROM was full with the exception of wrist extension (0 to 60 degrees compared with 0 to 80 degrees on the right).
- AROM of both shoulders, elbows, and wrist joints was measured. The proximal and distal joint to each tested joint was positioned to avoid placing tension on the ulnar nerve. Results were as follows:

Joint motion	Right AROM	Left AROM
Shoulder flexion	0-180°	0-120°
Shoulder hyperextension	0-60°	0-40°
Shoulder abduction	0-180°	0-150°
Elbow flexion	0-140°	15-60°
Wrist extension	0-80°	0-20°
Wrist flexion	0-75°	0-40°
Wrist ulnar deviation	0-40°	0-25°
MCP abduction index	0-25°	0-10°
Middle (radial/ulnar)	0-15°, 0-15°	0-5°, 0°
Ring	0-20°	0°
Small	0-35°	20°

MCP flexion*		
Ring	0-90°	15°
Small	0-90°	20°
PIP flexion*		
Ring	0-110°	15-90°
Small	0-110°	20-90°
DIP flexion*		
Ring	0-70°	0°
Small	0-70°	0°

*Composite MCP, PIP, and DIP passive flexion is full, indicating adequate length of the extensor digitorum communis.

- MMT revealed weakness of the muscles innervated by the ulnar nerve with flattening of the hypothenar eminence.
- Left-hand grip strength measures were approximately 44% of the right (nondominant hand). Left 2-point pinch strength average was 86% of the right, left three-point pinch strength average was 66% of the right, and left lateral pinch strength average was 27% of the right. On testing lateral pinch strength, Froment's sign was noted.

Neuromuscular
- TR reported pain about the elbow at a level of 5/10 with activity and 2/10 at rest.
- There was a positive Tinel's sign at the left inferior cubital tunnel with pain radiating proximally and distally.
- Semmes-Weinstein monofilament testing showed absent sensation (6.65 monofilament) along the ulnar nerve distribution.

Diagnosis
Preferred practice pattern 5F: Impaired peripheral nerve integrity and muscle performance associated with peripheral nerve injury.

Intervention
Integumentary
- TR was instructed in measures to protect skin integrity.
- A light compressive garment was provided to minimize edema. The patient was instructed to elevate the left arm while sleeping to minimize accumulation of fluids in the distal extremity.

Musculoskeletal
- Muscle stretching and passive joint ROM exercises were incorporated.
- The patient was instructed on how to avoid overstretching the ulnar nerve.
- Active contraction of uninvolved muscles of the left upper extremity was initiated to maintain ROM throughout the limb. A resistive exercise program is to be initiated when innervation to the flexor carpi ulnaris is evident.

Neuromuscular
- TR will incorporate ulnar nerve gliding techniques by the fifth postoperative week with full flexion of the elbow avoided until the sixth postoperative week.

- A sensory reeducation program will be initiated when TR begins to perceive moving touch along the volar surface of the small and ring fingers.

Splinting and Orthotics
- A thermoplastic anterior elbow splint was fabricated to maintain the elbow in almost full extension.
- On reinnervation of the flexor digitorum profundus, a splint will be fabricated to block the MCP joint of the ring and small finger in flexion.

Modalities
- Pulsed ultrasound was used initially. On reinnervation of muscles supplied by the ulnar nerve, ES will be used.

Role of the Physical Therapist Assistant
- Create a diagram showing the basic distribution of the ulnar nerve.
- Describe two possible sensory reeducation activities for this patient.
- Create a patient handout which outlines skin protection guidelines, edema reduction measures, and positioning suggestions to avoid overstretching the ulnar nerve.
- Describe the difference between nerve gliding and stretching. What would you expect the patient to feel during these interventions and how would your manual technique differ?

Additional Information
For the full version of this case study, including detailed examination results, interventions, and outcomes, see the Evolve site that accompanies this book. A full case study for a patient with carpal tunnel syndrome also appears on the Evolve site.

CHAPTER SUMMARY

This chapter describes the typical examination findings and interventions for patients with peripheral nerve injuries. Motor function, sensation, and sympathetic function are likely to be compromised, requiring examination of muscle strength, length, and balance, as well as quantitative and qualitative measurement of sensory functions, and examination of skin integrity. Intervention for patients with nerve injury may be brief, and the goals of treatment aimed toward relieving the causative factors, or long term, while waiting for reinnervation of motor and sensory end-organs. In the latter case, treatment emphasis may shift to prevention of associated deformities and skin injuries, as well as facilitation of functional independence. Treatment may include patient education, edema management, muscle strengthening and lengthening, desensitization, sensory reeducation, ES, ultrasound, splinting, and training with assistive devices.

ADDITIONAL RESOURCES

For links to these and additional web-based resources, see the Evolve site.

Dyck PJ, Thomas PK: *Peripheral neuropathy*, ed 4, Philadelphia, 2005, Saunders.

Senneff JA: *Numb toes and aching soles: Coping with peripheral neuropathy,* San Antonio, 1999, Medpress.
Senneff JA: *Numb toes and other woes: More on peripheral neuropathy,* San Antonio, 2001, Medpress.
The Neuropathy Association
National Institute of Neurological Disorders and Stroke

GLOSSARY

Action potential: The change in electrical potential of a nerve when it is stimulated.

Afferent: Carrying impulses toward a center, as in nerves transmitting impulses toward the CNS.

Autonomic nervous system (ANS): Efferent pathways that include the sympathetic and parasympathetic divisions, which regulate smooth muscle, cardiac muscle, and glandular activity.

Axon: A projection or outgrowth of a nerve cell that conducts impulses away from the cell body.

Central nervous system (CNS): Nerves that are wholly contained within the brain and spinal cord.

Cranial nerves: Twelve pairs of nerves that have their origin in the brain.

Dendrite: Branching and tapering extensions of the axon that receive signals from other neurons.

Denervation: Loss of nerve supply.

Efferent: Carrying impulses away from a center, as in nerves transmitting impulses away from the CNS.

Fascicle: A bundle of fibers, as in a nerve fiber tract.

Glia: Cells and fibers that form the supporting elements of the nervous system.

Ischemia: Local deficiency of blood supply can be caused by mechanical obstruction of the circulation.

Mononeuropathy: An isolated nerve lesion.

Mononeuropathy multiplex: Asymmetrical lesions of multiple nerves.

Motor unit: A single alpha motor neuron and all the muscle fibers it innervates.

Myelin: Lipids and proteins that form a sheath around certain nerves.

Neuroma: Abnormal growth of nerve cells.

Neurons: Nerve cells.

Neurotransmitter: A chemical agent released by a presynaptic cell that stimulates or inhibits the postsynaptic cell.

Nodes of Ranvier: A short interval in the myelin sheath of a nerve.

Peripheral nervous system (PNS): Nerves that may originate in the brain or spinal cord but end peripherally and include cranial and spinal nerves.

Plasmalemma: Plasma membrane.

Plexus: A network of nerves, or blood or lymphatic vessels.

Polyneuropathy: Symmetrical diffuse nerve dysfunction.

Schwann cells: Any of the cells that cover the nerve fibers in the PNS and form the myelin sheath.

Synapse: The meeting point of the axon terminal of one neuron and a dendritic ending or cell body of another neuron or cell.

Wallerian degeneration: The degenerative changes of an axon and its myelin sheath distal to a focal lesion.

Polyneuropathies

Mohamed Ibrahim

OBJECTIVES

After reading this chapter, the reader will be able to:
1. Define different types of polyneuropathies.
2. Differentiate the motor and sensory dysfunctions commonly seen in patients with polyneuropathies.
3. Identify specialized equipment needs, assistive technology, and rehabilitation intervention considerations appropriate for patients with polyneuropathy.
4. Describe effective rehabilitation intervention programs for patients with polyneuropathies.

Polyneuropathies are peripheral neuropathies affecting multiple nerves. **Polyneuropathy** affects approximately 2,400 individuals per 100,000 (2.4%), and this prevalence increases with age to a maximum of 8,000 per 100,000 (8%).[1,2] Annually, **peripheral neuropathy** is newly diagnosed in 118 people per 100,000.[3,4]

It is important to distinguish among different kinds of peripheral nervous system (PNS) dysfunctions. Polyneuropathy generally refers to a bilateral symmetric disturbance of peripheral nerve function.[5] When the spinal nerve roots or the roots and the peripheral nerve trunks are involved these are termed *polyradiculopathy* and *poly-*

radiculoneuropathy, respectively. **Mononeuropathy** is a focal lesion of one peripheral nerve, and multiple mononeuropathy, or mononeuropathy mutiplex, is defined as multifocal isolated lesions of more than one peripheral nerve.[5] Neuropathies with different anatomical distributions have characteristic causes and primary underlying pathology (**demyelination** or axonal degeneration) and tend to affect sensory, motor, or a combination of both types of nerves (Fig. 19-1). These associations are summarized in Table 19-1. This chapter discusses pathology, examination, evaluation, and rehabilitation intervention for patients with impaired motor function and sensory integrity associated with acute and chronic polyneuropathies. The examination, evaluation, and rehabilitation intervention for patients with peripheral nerve injuries are covered in Chapter 18.

There are many types and causes of polyneuropathy. This chapter focuses on the types of polyneuropathy that occur most commonly in patients treated by rehabilitation clinicians in North America and Europe today.

> ### ◎ Clinical Pearl
>
> Polyneuropathy generally refers to a bilateral symmetrical disturbance of peripheral nerve function.

PATHOLOGY

ACQUIRED DEMYELINATING POLYNEUROPATHIES

Guillain-Barré Syndrome. **Guillain-Barré syndrome (GBS)*** is an inflammatory disorder of the peripheral nerves, with a number of variants. It generally

---

*American and British literature uses the term *Guillain-Barré syndrome* in all recent publications. However, the terms *acute inflammatory demyelinating polyneuropathy, acute infective polyneuritis, Guillain-Barré-Strohl syndrome, Landry-Guillain-Barré syndrome, idiopathic polyneuritis, postinfectious polyneuritis, acute toxic neuronitis, mononeuronitis, radiculoneuritis, polyradiculoneuritis, myeloradiculoneuritis, acute immune-mediated polyneuritis,* and *acute inflammatory polyneuropathy* are all also used to describe this syndrome.

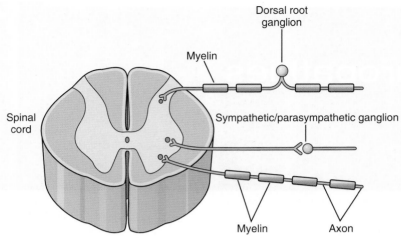

FIG. 19-1 Target areas for damage in polyneuropathies.

TABLE 19-1	Causes and Anatomical Distribution of Neuropathies					
Examples	Subtype	Predominantly Sensory	Mixed	Predominantly Motor	Axonal Degeneration	Demyelination
MONONEUROPATHY						
Entrapment neuropathies/ trauma		Yes		Yes		Yes
MULTIPLE MONONEUROPATHY						
Diabetic mononeuropathy		Yes	Yes	No		
Vasculitis		No	Yes	No		
AIDS		Yes		Yes	Yes (excluding acute)	No
Focal CIDP		Yes		Yes		
POLYNEUROPATHY						
Acquired demyelinating polyneuropathies	GBS (acute infective polyneuritis)	No	Yes	Yes	Yes	Yes
	CIDP					Yes
Neuropathies associated with systemic disorders	Diabetic neuropathies	Yes	Yes	No	Yes	Yes
	Nutritional deficiency (vitamins)	Yes	Yes		Yes	No
Hereditary and idiopathic peripheral neuropathy	Hereditary motor and sensory neuropathies (CMT)	Yes		Yes	Yes	Yes
Neuropathies associated with drugs, metals, and industrial agents	Neurotoxic drugs*	Yes	Yes	No	Yes (excluding acute)	No
	Alcoholic neuropathy	Yes		Yes	Yes	Yes
Neuropathies associated with infection	HIV	Yes		Yes	Yes (excluding acute)	No

*For example, cisplatin, nitrofurantoin, and vincristine.
AIDS, Acquired immunodeficiency syndrome; *CIDP,* chronic inflammatory demyelinating polyneuropathy; *GBS,* Guillain-Barré syndrome; *CMT,* Charcot-Marie-Tooth disease; *HIV,* human immunodeficiency virus.

presents with an acute ascending flaccid paralysis and areflexia. The Miller Fisher variant of GBS presents with ataxia, areflexia, and ophthalmoplegia without weakness.[6] This variant affects 3% to 5% of patients with GBS.[7]

Etiology and Pathogenesis. Although GBS often seems to be preceded by an acute bacterial or viral infection,[8-12] to date there is no evidence that GBS is communicable nor are there specific genetic factors that increase vulnerability to GBS.[13] Approximately two-thirds of the cases are

TABLE 19-2	Comparison of Guillain-Barré Syndrome (GBS) with Chronic Inflammatory Demyelinating Polyneuropathy (CIDP)	
Characteristic	**GBS**	**CIDP**
Duration to develop full clinical picture	<4 weeks	>8 weeks
Responds to corticosteroids	No	Yes
Respiratory muscle	Usually affected	Generally not affected
Prognosis	Better	Worse
Recovery	>80% recover in 6-8 months	>80% fail to have spontaneous recovery

preceded by an acute, influenza-like illness (presumed viral infection) or diarrhea (presumed bacterial infection) from which the patient has recovered by the time the neuropathy becomes symptomatic.[14]

In most cases, clinical, electrophysiological, and pathological findings indicate that GBS is an autoimmune disease directed against myelin, hence the name, **acute inflammatory demyelinating polyneuropathy (AIDP)**. However, there may also be some axonal damage.

Clinical Presentation. Despite the many variants of GBS, all present with acute or subacute peripheral nerve dysfunction and all take about 2 to 4 weeks to cause peak neurological deficits. All variants are commonly preceded by a trigger (e.g., upper respiratory tract infection, gastrointestinal infection), although this may be difficult to determine from the history. The neurological signs and symptoms partially or completely resolve over weeks to months, with the long-term prognosis depending on the site and extent of axonal injury. A good functional recovery is expected in most but not all cases, and this syndrome has a mortality of about 2% to 5%, generally from respiratory failure or infection.[15]

◎ *Clinical Pearl*

Many cases of Guillain-Barré syndrome (GBS) are preceded by an acute influenza-like illness or diarrhea that the patient recovers from before there are signs of neuropathy.

Chronic Inflammatory Demyelinating Polyradiculoneuropathy. **Chronic inflammatory demyelinating polyradiculoneuropathy (CIDP)** has a similar clinical presentation to GBS but with a slower onset and more chronic course. Patients with what appeared to be a chronic form of GBS have been described in the literature for many years, and their disorders were given a variety of names, including polyneuritis idiopathica, nonfamilial hypertrophic neuritis, relapsing or recurrent neuritis, idiopathic neuritis, or chronic GBS.[16,17]

Etiology and Pathogenesis. Although the pathogenesis of CIDP is not proven, most authors consider it to be an autoimmune disease directed against myelin.[18]

Clinical Presentation. CIDP generally presents with slowly progressive or relapsing motor and/or sensory symptoms in more than one limb, developing over at least 8 weeks.[16,19,20] There is symmetrical involvement of the proximal and distal muscles, with atrophy being less pronounced than the weakness. Although depressed or absent reflexes are found in all patients, these are generally

confined to the ankles. Eighty percent of patients also have sensory disturbances (numbness).[16,21]

Some patients with CIDP present atypically, with symptoms similar to lumbar stenosis or cauda equina syndrome, caused by inflammation and recurrent demyelination and remyelination of the hypertrophied lumbar nerve roots.[22-24] Other patients present primarily or only with sensory symptoms.[25]

CIDP and GBS are differentiated clinically by the criterion of how long it takes for maximum deficits to develop (Table 19-2). CIDP develops over more than 8 weeks, whereas GBS symptoms peak in less than 4 weeks. Another difference is that CIDP responds to corticosteroids, whereas GBS does not, and respiratory muscles are often involved in GBS but are not affected in CIDP. Finally, although prognosis for recovery from GBS is usually good, CIDP has a poor prognosis and most patients do not fully recover.

Although children are rarely affected by CIDP,[26] when affected, their disease course is generally similar to that of adults.[27] Compared to the clinical presentation in adults, children often have weakness and loss of reflexes and sensation and rarely have pain or cranial nerve involvement. Children generally have an abrupt onset of symptoms and present with gait abnormalities and other significant neurological dysfunctions. The initial response of children with CIDP to immune modulating therapy is often excellent.[26,28]

◎ *Clinical Pearl*

Chronic inflammatory demyelinating polyradiculoneuropathy (CIDP) and Guillain-Barré syndrome (GBS) are the result of an autoimmune attack against myelin.

NEUROPATHIES ASSOCIATED WITH SYSTEMIC DISORDERS

Diabetic Neuropathies. One of the most common complications of diabetes mellitus in the Western world is neuropathy. Because virtually every type of peripheral nerve fiber can be affected, including sensory, autonomic, and motor nerve fibers, **diabetic neuropathy** can have diverse presentations.[29] The term, *diabetic neuropathy*, includes all of these, and no single classification system identifies all subtypes.[30-32] Nonetheless, most diabetic neuropathies can be classified as focal or multifocal neuropathies or as polyneuropathies.

Etiology and Pathogenesis. Over the past 20 years, research has helped to clarify the pathogenesis of diabetic

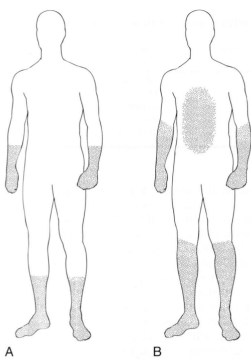

A   B

FIG. 19-2 Sensory loss in length-dependent polyneuropathy. **A,** Stocking-glove distribution. **B,** Truncal sensory loss occurs in advanced cases, usually when the limbs are affected up to the knees and elbows.

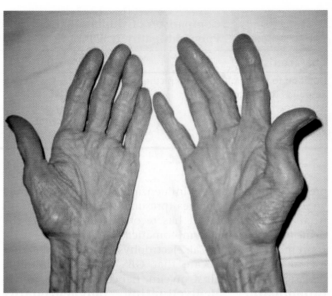

FIG. 19-3 Advanced case of diabetic neuropathy with thenar eminence muscle wasting bilaterally. *Courtesy Rehab R US Physical Therapy, Brooklyn, NY.*

neuropathy. However, how exactly diabetes results in nerve damage is controversial. One theory is that nerve damage is caused by altered sugar or fatty acid metabolism and the production of products that are toxic to nerves. Alternatively, the nerves may be damaged by poor blood flow as a result of the damage diabetes causes to the microvascular circulation.

Clinical Presentation. Diabetic neuropathy most commonly presents with distal symmetrical sensorimotor signs and symptoms. Typically, the distribution follows a length-dependent pattern, with the most distal extremities (the toes) being involved first, followed by the feet, and spreading up the legs in a stocking distribution.[30] The neuropathy may then advance to involve the fingers, spreading up to the hands and forearms in a glove distribution.[33,34] Later still, the trunk may be affected in an anterior wedge-shaped pattern (Fig. 19-2).[30,35] There are usually sensory changes and mild weakness of the ankle dorsiflexor and toe extensor muscles, accompanied by electromyographic (EMG) evidence of denervation.[30,32] Distal muscle weakness and atrophy can be profound in advanced cases (Fig. 19-3). Positive symptoms, such as paresthesias, burning, tingling, aching, cold sensation, lancinating (sharp) pain, or pain produced by normal touch **(allodynia)** or by a change in temperature, are often reported.[34,36] When there is pain, it is often worse at night.[30] Negative signs and symptoms, such as sensory loss, depression or absence of ankle jerks, and loss of vibratory sensation, are also often present, but these may not be reported by patients unless they are asked about them directly.[34,36]

Foot ulcers are common late complications in people with diabetic neuropathy. Foot ulcers are usually caused by sensory loss and vascular insufficiency and often result in amputations in patients with diabetes (see Chapter 30 for further information on neuropathic ulcers).

Charcot arthropathy, also known as neuropathic arthropathy, also occurs in some people with diabetic neuropathy. This condition involves damage to the joints of the foot and foot deformity. Charcot arthropathy usually occurs about 8 to 10 years after the onset of sensory loss from peripheral diabetic neuropathy. It is caused by lack of pain sensation and proprioception that results in unnoticed injuries to joints in the foot. Repeated small injuries, such as strains and fractures, tend to occur as the joint becomes more unstable until finally the joints are permanently destroyed and the foot becomes deformed.

The autonomic nerve involvement that commonly accompanies diabetic sensorimotor polyneuropathy may also cause postural hypotension, impotence (erectile dysfunction, initially with preserved ejaculation and orgasm), bladder atony, gastroparesis and nocturnal diarrhea, postprandial sweating, and diminished distal limb sweating.[32]

◎ **Clinical Pearl**

Diabetic neuropathy can cause sensory loss in the toes, feet, and legs in a stocking distribution. As it progresses, it may affect the hands and forearms in a glove distribution.

HEREDITARY MOTOR AND SENSORY NEUROPATHIES

Charcot-Marie-Tooth Disease. Charcot-Marie-Tooth disease (CMT), also called *hereditary motor and* *sensory neuropathy,* is a clinically and genetically heterogeneous group of inherited peripheral nerve disorders that can affect the sensory and/or motor nerves. It usually presents with distal weakness and sensory loss. Symptoms typically start in the patients' teens or twenties and progress gradually over their lifetimes.

Etiology and Pathogenesis. CMT is caused by mutations in genes that produce proteins involved in the structure and function of either the peripheral nerve axons or the myelin sheath.

Clinical Presentation. CMT neuropathy affects both motor and sensory nerve fibers. Therefore patients with CMT typically present with distal muscle weakness or atrophy, structural foot abnormalities, soft tissue complications (e.g., calluses, ulcers), and EMG abnormalities. Furthermore, absent or diminished deep tendon reflexes and impaired sensation are also present to varying degrees in certain forms of CMT.[37] Findings are similar among affected family members.[38]

Generally, distal muscle weakness (dorsiflexors and evertors) results in foot drop and a steppage gait with frequent tripping or falls. Pes cavus and hammertoes, which are also common, are caused by weakness in the intrinsic foot muscles and the unequal action of the long toe flexors and extensors.[38] Typically, few patients seek help, suggesting that they experience few symptoms, that they are accustomed to their symptoms and manage well functionally, or that they believe that no help is available.[38]

CMT symptoms usually present in the second or third decade of life, ranging from infancy to mid-adulthood, depending on the CMT subtype.[39,40] Symptoms usually progress gradually and vary in severity. Some may have such mild symptoms that they do not notice, while others with a severe form of the disorder may be severely compromised because of respiratory muscle involvement.[39,40] CMT is rarely fatal, and most people who have the disease have a normal life expectancy.[41,39]

> ### ◎ Clinical Pearl
>
> Charcot-Marie-Tooth disease (CMT) usually presents with distal weakness or atrophy of the lower extremities that result in foot drop and a steppage gait.

TOXIC NEUROPATHIES

Alcoholic Neuropathy. Neuropathy as a complication of excessive alcohol consumption was first reported over 200 years ago.[42,43] Controversy still exists as to whether **alcoholic neuropathy** is a direct toxic effect of alcohol or is caused by the secondary nutritional deficiencies that are common in alcoholics.[43-45] This debate persists in part because the clinical presentation of alcoholic neuropathy is similar to that of neuropathy caused by certain nutritional deficiencies such as thiamine deficiency.[44] In addition, because alcohol provides so many calories, many alcoholics have little other nutritional intake and are therefore often relatively malnourished.[46] Furthermore, alcohol may interfere with gastrointestinal absorption of nutrients, exaggerating malnutrition.[46]

Current evidence, however, gives greatest support to the hypothesis that alcoholic neuropathy is primarily a result of the toxic effects of alcohol. This is supported by the finding that neuropathy develops in alcoholics who are not malnourished and that nutritional supplementation alone does not alter the course of neuropathy in these patients.[44,47,48] Alcoholic neuropathy presents with a gradual decrease in sensory and motor peripheral nerve function in patients who chronically consume excessive amounts of alcohol.

Etiology and Pathogenesis. Although the precise pathogenesis and pathophysiology of alcoholic neuropathy remain unclear, it is known that alcoholic neuropathy causes axonal involvement of both myelinated and unmyelinated peripheral nerve fibers and can cause segmental demyelination.[44,45,49]

Clinical Presentation. Ethanol alcohol consumption of 100 gm per day for 3 years has been suggested as the minimum amount likely to cause alcoholic neuropathy.[43,46] Generally, alcoholic neuropathy presents initially with distal sensory or sensorimotor findings, including symmetrical distal loss of all sensory modalities (light touch, pin prick, vibration, and temperature), foot and calf pain, and diminished ankle reflexes.[50-52] The sensory loss is in a stocking-glove distribution (see Fig. 19-2). Almost 50% of patients with alcoholic neuropathy have muscle weakness, progressing to foot drop, gait disturbances, and wrist drop, depending on the severity of the disease.[46] Generally, weakness is more pronounced in the lower extremities than in the upper extremities.[46,44]

Alcoholic neuropathy is usually associated with a number of other medical conditions, including liver cirrhosis, gastrointestinal bleeding, Wernicke-Korsakoff syndrome (a memory disorder caused by thiamine deficiency), alcoholic cerebellar degeneration, and alcoholic dementia. However, many patients seek medical assistance for pain from neuropathy rather than for symptoms associated with these conditions.

TYPICAL EXAMINATION FINDINGS

The physical therapist will perform a thorough examination to establish a diagnosis and prognosis (including plan of care) and select interventions for patients with suspected polyneuropathy.[53]

PATIENT HISTORY

Patients with polyneuropathy generally present with complaints of motor or sensory disturbance, or both. When there are motor disturbances the patient may report muscle incoordination, distal weakness (causing frequent tripping and difficult walking on uneven surfaces), or proximal weakness (causing difficulty with getting out of a chair and with going up and down stairs). Sensory presentations include feelings of tingling, burning, stabbing, throbbing, clumsiness, cold, hot, wooden, and/or dead.

The progression of symptoms may indicate their likely cause. However, some patients with polyneuropathy present with an unclear history, particularly if the symptoms developed very gradually, as in many inherited neuropathies.[54] Such patients may have had subtle symptoms

TABLE 19-3   Typical Examination Findings and Likely Diagnosis in Patients with Polyneuropathy

Impairments	Functional Limitations	Pathology/Medical Diagnosis
LOWER LIMB		
Distal muscle weakness	Frequent tripping/difficulty walking	Distal denervation
Foot drop	High-steppage gait	GBS
Proximal muscle weakness	Difficulty getting up from deep chair/stairs and rising from squatting position	CMT (hereditary)
Pes cavus and hammertoes	Difficulty walking	Distal denervation
Loss of hair extending up to the midcalf	None	Length-dependent neuropathies
Thin and dry skin	None	Length-dependent neuropathies
Ulceration	None	Hereditary sensory neuropathy or diabetic neuropathy
UPPER LIMB		
Proximal muscle weakness	Difficulty reaching overhead, shaving, combing hair	CMT disease (hereditary)
Distal muscle weakness	Difficulty opening doors, buttoning, and manipulating small objects, etc	Distal denervation
Repeated trauma to joint, pathological fracture, and osteomyelitis	Loss of pain sensation	Neuropathic joint, Charcot joint
TRUNK		
Scoliosis–kyphoscoliosis	Difficulty breathing	Denervation of paraspinal muscle

GBS, Guillain-Barré syndrome; *CMT*, Charcot-Marie-Tooth disease.

since childhood that presented as poor performance in sports, frequent falls, or frequent ankle sprains and only now have developed severe enough symptoms to seek medical advice or intervention. In contrast, other causes of polyneuropathy, such as GBS, produce symptoms that develop rapidly, over a few days to up to 4 weeks[55]; whereas symptoms of CIDP develop over more than 8 weeks and alcoholic or diabetic neuropathy symptoms generally develop over years.[56]

The family history can help distinguish different types of polyneuropathy because some types, particularly CMT, are inherited. The clinician will often ask about similar symptoms in immediate and more distant family members, including children, parents, siblings, aunts, uncles, cousins, and grandparents. Questions about family members will also include information about the use of assistive devices, functional limitations, and any complaints similar to those of the patient.

A social and occupational history can help identify risk factors for certain types of polyneuropathies. Welders, printers, and manufacturers of batteries are often exposed to lead and are therefore at risk for neuropathy from lead toxicity.[57,58] Patients with a history of drug or alcohol abuse are at increased risk for alcoholic neuropathy,[43,45] and HIV-related neuropathies are more common among intravenous drug users and men who have sex with men.[59]

The patient's past medical history can also be revealing and should focus on surgeries, illnesses, and medications. Recent surgeries or illness, as explained earlier, can precipitate GBS. Side effects of medication can lead to toxic neuropathy. A history of multiple nerve entrapment is usually associated with hereditary neuropathies.

TESTS AND MEASURES
Musculoskeletal

Anthropometric Characteristics. Certain skeletal deformities, masses, and atrophy are associated with certain polyneuropathies (Table 19-3). Pes cavus, with or without hammer toes, is common in CMT neuropathies.

Muscle Performance. Muscle strength will be tested by manual muscle testing in patients with polyneuropathy. Polyneuropathies have characteristic presentations, distributions, and courses of muscle weakness. For most polyneuropathies, weakness progresses from distal to proximal, starting with the intrinsic foot muscles; followed by the extensor digitorum brevis, anterior tibialis, posterior tibialis; and finally the lower parts of the thigh muscles (Fig. 19-4, *A*). This sequence causes a steppage gait early on, secondary to bilateral foot drop, and later as atrophy develops, a physical appearance resembling an inverted champagne bottle (Fig. 19-4, *B*).

Neuromuscular

Cranial Nerve Integrity. Cranial nerve (CN) function distinguishes among different types of polyneuropathy and is therefore an important part of the examination.

Reflex Integrity. The distribution of changes in muscle stretch reflexes can help distinguish between polyneuropathy and mononeuropathy.

Sensory Integrity. Abnormal or absent sensation is common in patients with polyneuropathies.

Cardiovascular/Pulmonary.
Breathing may be impaired in any polyneuropathy that affects the motor nerves to the diaphragm or trunk muscles. This is of particular concern in GBS in which involvement of the trunk or diaphragm may be severe and comes on rapidly, necessitating intubation and ventilator-assisted breathing in some patients.[60]

Integumentary

Integumentary Integrity. Clinicians should inspect the skin for trophic changes, skin discoloration, sweat pattern abnormalities, and ulceration, particularly on the feet. Foot ulcers are common in patients with diabetic polyneuropathies, as well as in those with other sensory and autonomic neuropathies[61] (see Chapter 30).

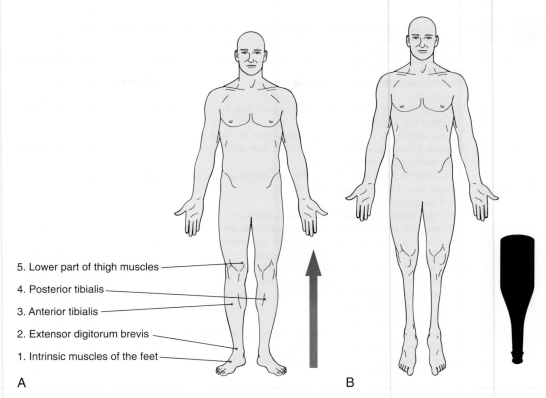

5. Lower part of thigh muscles
4. Posterior tibialis
3. Anterior tibialis
2. Extensor digitorum brevis
1. Intrinsic muscles of the feet

A   B

FIG. 19-4 **A,** Progression of most polyneuropathies from distal to proximal, starting with weakness of the intrinsic foot muscles, followed by the extensor digitorum brevis, anterior tibialis, posterior tibialis, and finally the lower parts of the thigh muscles. **B,** Inverted champagne bottle appearance of lower extremities in Charcot-Marie-Tooth disease. *Redrawn from Feldman EL, Stevens MJ, et al: A practical two-step quantitative clinical and electrophysiological assessment for the diagnosis and staging of diabetic neuropathy,* Diabetes Care *17:1281-1289, 1994.*

Trophic changes, such as hair loss in the lower leg, occur in length-dependent polyneuropathies, such as alcoholic or other toxic neuropathies, secondary to denervation of hair follicles. Furthermore, autonomic denervation of sweat glands can cause the skin to become thin and dry.

Electrodiagnostic Testing. EMG and nerve conduction studies (NCS) are among the most informative, widely available, and reliable medical tests for examination of patients with peripheral neuropathy.[62-64] Electrodiagnostic testing is generally performed by a physician (usually a neurologist or a physiatrist) but may be performed by suitably trained and qualified physical therapists. These studies help identify the type of fibers involved (motor, sensory, or both), the underlying pathophysiology (axonal damage versus demyelination), and the pattern of involvement (symmetrical, asymmetrical, or multifocal).[62,64] NCS can identify 80% of patients with diabetic neuropathy and 80% to 100% of patients with GBS.

EVALUATION, DIAGNOSIS, AND PROGNOSIS

Most patients who fall into the *Guide to Physical Therapy Practice*[56] preferred practice pattern 5G: Impaired motor function and sensory integrity associated with acute or chronic polyneuropathy will typically have the following abnormal examination findings: Muscle weakness in one or more extremities; diminished or lost deep tendon reflexes; and abnormal tone, strength, and sensation.

INTERVENTION

This section includes discussion of evidence-based interventions for patients with polyneuropathies. These include patient education and exercise, physical modalities, electrical stimulation (ES), and the use of orthoses and other durable medical equipment.

PATIENT AND FAMILY EDUCATION

Patient and family education regarding the progression and course of recovery and the need for compliance with instructions can impact the success of rehabilitation.[65] Compliance with instruction and recommendations for home activities, including exercise, can be influenced by variables related to the patient, the disease, the interventions, and interactions between the patient and the practitioner.[66,67]

EXERCISE

Studies indicate that various types of exercise, including progressive strengthening, balance, moderate resistance and higher resistance dynamic exercise, result in

TABLE 19-4	Published Exercise Guidelines for Patients with Peripheral Neuropathy	
Conditions	**Recommendations**	**Source**
Neuromuscular diseases	Adopt an active lifestyle. Moderate-intensity (defined by frequency, load, and duration) resistive strengthening exercise programs. Moderate aerobic exercise training program may be recommended without concern for any deleterious effect. Reduce fatigue by using brief work-rest-interval training programs.	Fowler[76]
Neuromuscular diseases	Resistance exercise with a relatively slow rate of progression may be beneficial if the degree of weakness is not severe. High-intensity resistance exercise has no advantage over more moderate program.	Kilmer[75]
Neuromuscular diseases	Aerobic conditioning is encouraged. Avoid eccentric exercise. Brace the joints with inadequate muscle support. Start exercise at a low level and progress gradually. Begin strength training with 20% of the maximum weight the patient can lift. Do 8-15 repetitions of each resisted exercise. Patients with severely affected muscles, with less than 10% of the normal strength, are unlikely to benefit from exercising these muscles. Patients with rapidly progressive disease will not benefit from strength or endurance exercise.	Forrest[68]
Guillain-Barré syndrome	Assess overwork weakness. Submaximal strength training. Aerobic training using Borg rating of perceived exertion (RPE). Recruit/train fast-twitch muscle fibers. Intense eccentric contractions should be avoided. Practice functional activities.	Bassile[73]

improvements in impairments and functional abilities in patients with polyneuropathies. To avoid overwork, exercise should be adjusted so that it does not produce delayed-onset muscle soreness or postexercise soreness that worsens rather than improves over time.[68,69] It has also been suggested that eccentric exercise be avoided since this type of activity causes more muscle damage and postexercise soreness than isometric and concentric contractions in healthy persons.[70-72]

The Borg rating of perceived exertion (RPE) may also be used to guide the cardiovascular intensity of exercise in patients with polyneuropathies (see Chapter 23).[68,73,74] It is suggested that to increase their cardiovascular endurance, patients with neuromuscular diseases, including those with polyneuropathy, start their exercise at very light intensity and gradually increase to the level of somewhat difficult.[68] Further guidelines and recommendations for exercise in patients with peripheral nerve and neuromuscular diseases are summarized in Table 19-4.[68,73,75,76]

PHYSICAL MODALITIES

Although heat and cold are of limited benefit in patients with polyneuropathy,[77] if patients have other indications for such interventions, it is essential that their ability to sense temperature be carefully examined because the absence of such sensation increases the risk for burns. The application of deep or superficial heating agents is contraindicated in patients with impaired or absent temperature sensation. The patient should be able to distinguish between very cold, cold, room temperature, warm, and hot for the application of heat to be safe.[78]

ELECTRICAL STIMULATION

ES can be used in patients with various types of polyneuropathy to produce contractions in denervated muscles and, at a sensory or motor level, to control pain. However, research on the effects of ES in denervated muscle has produced conflicting results with some showing prevention or retardation of muscle atrophy and others reporting that this intervention is ineffective or even detrimental. No studies have demonstrated that ES enhances reinnervation and some animal studies have found that ES is associated with inhibition of axonal sprouting to denervated muscle fibers. In contrast, most studies have found that sensory level ES does help to control pain in patients with peripheral neuropathy. This effect depends on transcutaneous electrical nerve stimulation (TENS) preferentially stimulating A-beta myelinated sensory fibers while avoiding stimulation of C and A-delta fibers and therefore is most likely to be effective in patients with neuropathic pain but intact touch sensation.

ORTHOSES

An orthosis is an externally applied device intended to correct and/or prevent deformity and improve function[79] (see Chapter 34). When using orthoses in patients with polyneuropathy and impaired sensation, particular attention should be paid to distributing pressure evenly over a large area and frequently inspecting the skin for early signs of breakdown.[77] The most commonly used lower extremity orthosis in patients with polyneuropathy is the total contact cast used in patients with neuropathic ulcers.[80] This device is designed to redistribute pressure on the foot, minimize shearing force, and protect wounds from contamination and infection.[65,81,82] In addition, ankle-foot orthoses (AFOs) may also be used to prevent plantar-flexion contractures and assist with gait in patients with polyneuropathies that cause ankle dorsiflexor weakness.

CASE STUDY 19-1

DIABETIC POLYNEUROPATHY

Patient History

AM, a 76-year-old retired college professor, complained of progressive lower extremity pain over a number of years. She was diagnosed with non–insulin-dependent diabetes mellitus 18 years ago, noted numbness and tingling in her feet for the first time 7 years ago, and first noticed pain 4 years ago. The pain has become progressively worse and more constant. The patient described it as a burning ache with her "feet on fire" that was exacerbated by walking. AM reported two falls within the last 6 months. She was diagnosed by her physician as having diabetic polyneu-ropathy, and in addition to interventions to optimize blood sugar control, she was referred to physical therapy to address her pain, weakness, balance deficits, and fall risk.

Tests and Measures—Significant Findings
Musculoskeletal
- Muscle strength was graded as 4+/5 in the upper extremities and 4–/5 in the lower extremities.

Neuromuscular
- Pain severity at rest was 8/10.
- Vibration and pin-prick sensation absent from midleg distally. She had pain when a cotton ball was stroked gently across the skin of her feet.
- Unable to feel the 10 gm (5.07 Semmes-Weinstein) nylon monofilament from the midleg distally.

Function
- Functional reach test: 5 inches.
- Berg Balance Scale score: 41/56.
- Timed up and go test score: 22 seconds.

Diagnosis
Preferred practice pattern 5G: Impaired motor function and sensory integrity associated with acute or chronic polyneuropathies.

Interventions
- TENS, with a pulse duration of less than 150 μs, a frequency of 80 pulses per second, and a current amplitude that will produce a comfortable tingling sensation to be used at home.
- Neuromuscular reeducation and balance exercise to be performed 3 times a week.
- Instruction on ways to improve safety at home.

Role of the Physical Therapist Assistant
- What symptom is being treated with TENS? How long is the effect expected to last?

- Write instructions for how AM can improve her safety at home and include at least three recommendations.
- Describe three balance exercises appropriate for AM to perform in the clinic and three balance exercises appropriate for her to perform at home.

Additional Information
For the full version of this case study, including detailed examination results, interventions, and outcomes, see the Evolve site that accompanies this book.

CHAPTER SUMMARY

Polyneuropathies are conditions that affect the function of multiple peripheral nerves. Polyneuropathies have a wide range of etiologies and presentations that impact patient function and the selection of the ideal plan of care and interventions. Most polyneuropathies are associated with reduced sensation and strength, particularly in the distal extremities. There is some evidence that rehabilitation intervention, including patient and family education, exercise, physical modalities, ES, and orthotics, may reduce impairments and functional limitations in patients with polyneuropathies.

ADDITIONAL RESOURCES

For links to these and additional web-based resources, see the Evolve site.

Ahroni JH: *101 Foot care tips for people with diabetes,* Alexandria, VA, 2000, American Diabetes Association.

Brown WF, Bolton CF, Aminoff MJ: *Neuromuscular function and disease: Basic, clinical, and electrodiagnostic aspects,* Philadelphia, 2002, Saunders.

Dyck PJ: *Peripheral neuropathy,* Philadelphia, 1993, Saunders.

Ouvrier RA, McLeod JG, Pollard JD: *Peripheral neuropathy in childhood,* New York, 1990, Raven Press.

Senneff JA: *Numb toes and aching soles: Coping with peripheral neuropathy,* San Antonio, 1999, MedPress.

Staal A, Van Gijn J, Spaans F: *Mononeuropathies: Examination, diagnosis and treatment,* Philadelphia, 1999, Saunders.

Weiner WJ, Goetz CG: *Neurology for the non-neurologist,* Philadelphia, 1999, Lippincott Williams & Wilkins.

Neuromuscular Disease Center

GBS/CIDP Syndrome Foundation International

CIDP International Organization

GLOSSARY

Acute inflammatory demyelinating polyneuropathy (AIDP): An autoimmune disease directed against myelin. Most common variant of GBS.

Alcoholic neuropathy: Decreased nerve functioning caused by damage from excessive drinking of alcohol.

Allodynia: The sensation of pain in response to sensory stimulation that is usually not painful.

Charcot-Marie-Tooth disease (CMT): A group of inherited, slowly progressive disorders that result from progressive damage to nerves. Symptoms include numbness and muscle atrophy that first occur in the feet and legs and then in the hands and arms.

Chronic inflammatory demyelinating polyradiculoneuropathy (CIDP): An autoimmune disease directed against myelin or Schwann cell antigens that causes slowly progressive or relapsing motor and/or sensory symptoms in more than one limb, developing over at least 8 weeks.

Demyelination: Loss of myelin.

Diabetic neuropathy: A common complication of diabetes mellitus in which nerves are damaged as a result of hyperglycemia (high blood sugar levels).

Guillain-Barré syndrome (GBS): An autoimmune disease directed against myelin that causes progressive muscle weakness or paralysis over a few days, which often starts a few days after resolution of an infectious illness.

Mononeuropathy: Dysfunction of a single nerve or nerve group.

Peripheral neuropathy: Dysfunction of the peripheral nerves.

Polyneuropathy: Generally, a bilateral symmetrical disturbance of peripheral nerve function.

Chapter 20

Nonprogressive Spinal Cord Disorders

Lynda L. Spangler

OBJECTIVES

After reading this chapter, the reader will be able to:
1. Describe the most common types of spinal cord injuries and their primary sequelae.
2. Understand tests and measures for an individual with spinal cord injuries.
5. Execute and modify within the plan of care selected interventions for individuals with spinal cord injuries.
6. Recognize the impact of spinal cord injuries on physical, emotional, social, and psychological health.
7. Participate with the physical therapist in decision making for equipment selection and home program for individuals with spinal cord injuries.

Injuries and illnesses that affect the spinal cord are devastating for the individual involved and for those who surround them. A fleeting moment can mark the difference between being independently mobile and being dependent on personal determination, mechanical equipment, and other people for all daily activities. The occurrence of **spinal cord injury (SCI)** is statistically low compared to many other diagnoses, but the personal and financial expense is high.

There are approximately 247,000 people in the United States (US) today living with SCI, and approximately 11,000 people in the US, equivalent to 40 per million, are newly diagnosed with SCI each year.[1,2] This group includes people of all age groups and ethnicities. Trauma is the most common cause of SCI, although most of the information applies similarly to SCIs of nontraumatic origin.

Data concerning the traumatic spinal cord–injured population in the US is gathered by the National Spinal Cord Injury Database (NSCID) and processed at the National Spinal Cord Injury Statistical Center (NSCISC). The following data are based on figures from current and past reports of the NSCID and NSCISC.[1,2]

Motor vehicle accidents (MVAs) account for the largest percentage of SCIs (about half). Other causes of SCI include falls, violent acts (stab and gunshot wounds), and sports injuries. The proportion of injuries represented by each of these groups is shown in Fig. 20-1. Although the incidence of SCI as a result of these primary causes has remained fairly constant over the last 30 years, there are some noteworthy changes in overall distribution. The proportion of injuries as a result of sports has decreased, presumably because of better training techniques and emergency care and improvements in protective equipment. With the aging of the US population in general, the percentage of SCI attributed to falls has increased. Below the age of 45, the leading cause of SCI is MVAs, but after age 45, falls become the leading mechanism of injury. Acts of violence have declined from a peak of 21% in 1990-1992 but remain disproportionately higher among African-Americans and Hispanics compared to other racial groups.

PATHOLOGY

The neurological deficits associated with SCI occur when sufficient force is exerted on the spinal cord to cause nerve damage. The forces may be direct, as when an object like a bullet or a bone fragment directly enters the spinal canal and severs some or all of the nerves of the spinal cord. More often forces are indirect, with the spinal cord remaining physically contiguous, but the neural components being adversely affected by secondary damage that impacts the site of injury and the surrounding tissues.

The mechanism of injury dictates the initial type of mechanical damage to the spine, the spinal cord, and surrounding structures. Flexion (or hyperflexion) injuries (Fig. 20-2, *A*) occur when forces cause anterior movement of one segment of the spine on another (e.g., forward contact of a lower part of the body with an immovable object, causing extreme flexion in higher segments) and can result in posterior ligament disruption, posterior intervertebral disk herniation or tear, and vertebral body fracture and/or dislocation.[3-5] Extension (or hyperextension) injuries (Fig. 20-2, *B*) occur when forces are directed toward the posterior surface of the body (e.g., backward contact of the lower part of the body with an immovable object) and may result in tearing of the anterior longitudinal ligament, tear or anterior herniation of the intervertebral disk, and fractures of the posterior spine elements with compression and/or subluxation. Flexion and extension injuries are most likely to occur where the spine is the most flexible and has the greatest bending moment. In the cervical spine the greatest flexion moment occurs at C5-6 and the greatest extension moment occurs at C4-5, making these the segments most vulnerable to flexion and extension injuries, respectively.[5]

Axial loading (vertebral compression) with sufficient vertical force, from the cranial or caudal end or both, can cause one or more vertebral bodies to burst.[4,6] A burst fracture produces bone fragments that scatter and cause damage to surrounding tissues, often including the spinal cord (Fig. 20-2, *C*). Rotational injury occurs when one segment of the body is forcefully twisted longitudinally on another segment that is either stable or moving in the opposite direction.[3] The opposing movements create a rotational force that can have a variety of results, including stretching and tearing of neural tissue, ligament tears, and vertebral fractures (Fig. 20-2, *D*).

The primary damage to the spinal cord is classified as a concussion if there is injury as a result of violent movement or a blunt blow that results in temporary loss of function.[4] In contrast, a contusion is when the surface of the spinal cord and its coverings remain intact, but there is loss of neural tissue (grey and/or white matter) in the central portion of the cord. The injury is considered a laceration or maceration if the glia is disrupted and there is possible direct disruption of the spinal cord tissue.

Secondary damage to the spinal cord is damage that occurs after the primary structural damage and that extends beyond the area of initial trauma.[6,7] Secondary damage occurs at the site of the primary lesion and over time may spread as far as four spinal segments above and/or below the initial lesion.[4,5,7] Initially, there is necrotic destruction of axons where they were damaged by the trauma. This is followed by a progression of tissue injury that is only partially understood but is most likely related in part to vascular and immune system responses.

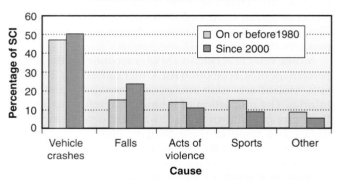

ETIOLOGY OF SPINAL CORD INJURY

FIG. 20-1 Causes of spinal cord injury. *Data from the National Spinal Cord Injury Database.*

◎ *Clinical Pearl*

Spinal cord injuries (SCIs) are classified as primary (injury to the cord as a direct consequence of some force or trauma) or secondary (injury to the cord that occurs over time after the initial trauma).

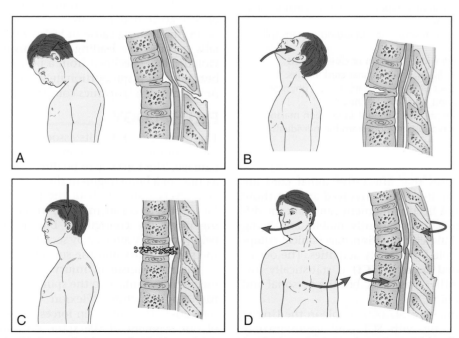

FIG. 20-2 Mechanisms of spinal cord injury. **A,** Flexion. **B,** Extension. **C,** Axial loading. **D,** Rotation.

Changes in blood flow because of ischemia and/or hemorrhage contribute to local nerve cell destruction. At the site of injury, intraparenchymal hemorrhage contributes to early tissue damage because of shear stress on vessels located centrally in the grey matter and in a margin of the surrounding white matter.[7] The vessels in the periphery of the spinal cord are relatively spared from this early damage, owing to the greater compliance (and thus reduced shearing force) of the white matter. The microvascular damage to the grey matter results in diminished blood flow to the spinal cord and impairment of autoregulation. Ischemic damage in this region can also occur as a result of vasogenic edema (secondary to breakdown of the blood–spinal cord barrier), by direct compression by surrounding tissues, or as the result of local vasospasm.

It appears that immune cells trigger posttraumatic inflammatory responses that contribute to the acute and chronic secondary pathogenesis of SCI.[4,7-10] Hemorrhage and disruption of the blood–spinal cord barrier allows inflammatory cells to infiltrate the injured area of the spinal cord, beginning at the first hour after injury and continuing over a period of weeks. These cells are associated with neuronal death and demyelination and other changes in the white matter, including Wallerian degeneration. Further detrimental effects can also be attributed to changes in ion levels and free radical production in the spinal cord.

Some aspects of the immune response may promote recovery from SCI.[4,7] Beneficial immune responses may include scavenging of cellular debris and release of nerve growth factors. These and other actions can have a neuroprotective function and may enhance neural regeneration.

Clinical Pearl

The inflammatory response to spinal cord injury (SCI) can exacerbate the injury but may also promote recovery.

Despite the predominance of destructive forces, some nerve tissue in the spinal cord may be spared, particularly in the peripheral regions. The amount of the nerve preservation, combined with appropriate early medical intervention to minimize primary and secondary damage, will dictate the degree of motor and sensory function preserved at and below the level of injury.

Since traumatic physical impact is the primary cause of SCI, it is not surprising that many other injuries can be associated with SCI. For all persons enrolled in the NSCID between 1985 and 1995, 29% had fractures and 29% had loss of consciousness. Traumatic pneumothorax or hemothorax occurred in 18% of cases. Traumatic brain injury severe enough to impair cognitive or emotional functioning was also reported in 11.5% of the SCI population.

Although trauma is the cause of most SCIs, there are other pathologies that can cause spinal cord damage. Nontraumatic causes include any injury or disease process that results in damage to the neural components of the spinal cord such as transverse myelitis and multiple sclerosis.[11] The cord may also be damaged by compressive forces from tumors, spinal degeneration, or intervertebral disk distention. Vascular events can also cause ischemia or hemorrhage in the spinal cord or spinal column. Congenital malformation of the spine or spinal canal, such as spina bifida (see Chapter 15) or severe scoliosis (see Chapter 4), may also result in spinal cord damage.

An incomplete SCI is one with partial preservation of sensory and/or motor function below the **neurological level** that also includes some function of the lowest sacral segment. A complete injury is defined as one that causes absence of all sensory and motor function below the neurological level, including the lowest sacral segment. **Zone of partial preservation (ZPP)** is a term associated with complete injuries and refers to the dermatomes and myotomes caudal to the neurological level in which some modalities of function remain. Although these definitions are recognized for research and documented classification, in the clinical setting an individual with any sparing of function below the neurological level of injury is frequently considered to have an incomplete SCI, whereas an individual without detectable sparing is often considered to have a complete SCI, regardless of sacral segment function.

SCI is termed **tetraplegia** (or **quadriplegia**) if the impairment or loss of motor and/or sensory function is a result of damage of the neural elements in the cervical segments of the spinal cord. Tetraplegia results in impairments involving the upper extremities (UEs), as well as more caudal functions. **Paraplegia** is loss of function as a result of injury to the thoracic, lumbar, or sacral segments, sparing UE function but causing impairments in the trunk, pelvis, and lower extremities (LEs), depending on the level of the lesion.

An injury to the spinal cord above the cauda equina (approximately the L1-2 intervertebral space in adults) will preserve the sacral reflex arc but damage upper motor neurons (UMNs) and lower motor neurons (LMNs).[5,12] This type of injury is characterized by motor weakness or paralysis, hypertonia, co-contraction, and hyperreflexia below the level of the lesion. SCI to regions caudal to the beginning of the cauda equina will damage only LMNs, resulting in destruction of the sacral reflex arc and loss of reflexes, muscle atrophy, flaccid paralysis, and fibrillations below the injury level.

SPINAL SHOCK

A major contributing factor to complications during the acute phase of SCI is a phenomenon called **spinal shock** (also known as *areflexia*). Spinal shock is characterized by a total loss of sensory, motor, and autonomic control below the level of the lesion. It occurs immediately at the time of injury and can last for days to weeks after the injury.[4,5] During this period, there is flaccid paralysis of all musculature below the level of the lesion, including the smooth muscles of the visceral systems.

Where UMNs are affected, resolution of spinal shock is signified by the return of deep tendon reflexes (DTRs) and the onset of **spasticity** in skeletal and visceral muscles. Where only lower motor neurons are affected, skeletal muscle and visceral muscles remain flaccid after the resolution of spinal shock.

Because of spinal shock, many individuals with SCI have low tone and good flexibility below their injury level early on, during the acute management phase, but may develop potentially limiting hypertonicity, spasticity, and contractures as their rehabilitation progresses and the spinal shock resolves (see later discussion of spasticity).

AUTONOMIC DYSREFLEXIA

Autonomic dysreflexia (AD), also known as *autonomic hyperreflexia,* is a serious, life-threatening emergency caused by uncontrolled episodes of hypertension that can occur in individuals with SCI at or above the T6 level. AD occurs after the period of spinal shock, as reflexes and autonomic responses return. A survey of the model SCI systems (1996-1998) found that 7.9% of patients experienced AD during rehabilitation.[13] In patients with complete tetraplegia, the incidence was as high as 29%. Because of the frequency and the danger of AD, it is extremely important for therapists dealing with individuals with SCI to be able to recognize the symptoms of AD and to respond appropriately when AD occurs.

AD is the result of an uncontrolled autonomic response to a noxious stimulus from either an external or internal (visceral) source. The most common causes for AD are bladder or bowel distention, although there are other causes, such as a blocked catheter, bowel impaction, or urinary tract infection.[4,14] A noxious stimulus normally causes a sympathetic response that results in vasoconstriction and an increase in blood pressure (BP). In an individual without SCI, the body compensates for this phenomenon with inhibitory impulses that cause vasodilation and a normalization of BP. SCI prevents activation of the body's normal compensation mechanism below the level of injury and results in steadily escalating blood pressure. If not treated immediately, the rising BP may damage the brain by causing subarachnoid hemorrhage or seizure, may damage the kidneys or eyes by causing local hemorrhage, or may damage the heart by causing a myocardial infarction.[15,16]

◎ *Clinical Pearl*

Autonomic dysreflexia (AD) is an uncontrolled life-threatening autonomic response that can occur in individuals with spinal cord injury (SCI) at or above the T6 level. AD is usually caused by a noxious stimulus, most commonly bowel or bladder distention.

Symptoms of AD reflect the pathological sympathetic response and high BP (elevation of systolic BP by 20 to 40 mm Hg or more above the patient's baseline). Initial flushing of the skin above the injury level and sweating followed by the fairly rapid onset of a severe, pounding headache; possible blurred vision; and worsened sweating with chills or goose bumps (in the absence of fever).[15,16] There may be a period of cardiac arrhythmias and bradycardia as the body attempts to compensate for the elevated BP. The individual may also experience an unexplained feeling of apprehension or anxiety. All members of the treatment team (especially the individual with SCI and his or her family) must be taught to recognize these symptoms and to respond to AD as a medical emergency.

Interventions by therapists and other medical personnel should include an immediate check for obvious sources of noxious stimuli (e.g., kinked urinary catheter, distended bladder, tight or twisted clothing, positioning resulting in abdominal compression) and removal of the stimulus if possible.[16] If the person is prone or supine, they should be brought into a sitting position to reduce intracranial pressure. BP and heart rate should be monitored immediately and frequently. Caregivers should also notify the individual's nurse and/or physician and prepare to activate the emergency medical system if removing the most obvious stimuli does not result in immediate resolution of signs and symptoms. It may be necessary to administer BP-reducing medications until the noxious stimulus can be identified and resolved. After an episode of AD, symptoms and BP should be monitored for at least 2 hours to check for and prevent recurrence.

◎ *Clinical Pearl*

All members of the treatment team (including the client and his or her family and caregivers) must be able to recognize the symptoms of autonomic dysreflexia (AD) and know how to respond to them.

PRESSURE ULCERS

Pressure ulcers (also known as *decubitus ulcers* or *pressure sores*) are one of the most frequent problems after SCI and are a major cause of hospital readmission. Pressure ulcers are characterized by ischemic ulceration of soft tissue as a result of unrelieved pressure and shearing forces. (See Chapter 28 for more information on pressure ulcers.)

Sixty percent to 80% of individuals with SCI will develop a pressure ulcer at some time during their lifetime, and 30% will have more than one ulcer.[17,18] Many individuals (approximately 30%) will develop their first pressure ulcer during their initial hospital stay after injury, and the trend continues over a lifetime, with surveys of SCI populations showing that in a given postinjury year, approximately 20% or more individuals have a pressure ulcer.[19] In the US alone, the Centers for Disease Control and Prevention (CDC) estimates the annual cost of treating SCI-related pressure ulcers at $1.2 billion.[21] These direct medical costs are compounded by the economic, vocational, social, and psychological costs to the individual who requires an extended period of wound care.

Risk factors for pressure ulcer development include sensory loss, prolonged pressure, immobility, shearing forces, skin maceration, and inadequate nutrition. These factors may be compounded by substance abuse, obesity, smoking, poor hygiene, psychosocial stressors, and noncompliance with preventive behaviors (e.g., proper bed positioning).[5,19,20] Although any area of bony prominence is at risk for ulcer development, during acute care, the sacrum, heels, and scapulae are particularly susceptible because of prolonged supine positioning. As an individual begins to spend more time out of bed in a wheelchair, the ischia are at greater risk.

Prevention of pressure ulcers involves multiple members of the health care team. Table 20-1 includes some of the steps that should be taken to reduce pressure ulcer risk. If

TABLE 20-1	Pressure Ulcer Prevention
Prevention Technique	**Suggested Strategies**
Proper positioning in bed and in wheelchair	Good postures and positions with bony prominences protected and pressure distributed equally over large surface areas. Use pressure distribution equipment such as wheelchair cushions, custom mattresses, and alternating-pressure mattress pads.
Frequent changes in position	Every 2 hours when in bed. Every 15-20 minutes when seated.
Keep skin clean and dry	Good bowel and bladder care with immediate cleansing after episodes of incontinence. Thoroughly cleanse and dry skin at least once daily. Inspect skin for areas of redness in morning and evening. Use recommended commercial skin care products.
Nutrition	Diet with adequate calories, protein, vitamins, and minerals. Sufficient water intake. Limit alcohol.
Clothing	Avoid clothes that are either too tight or too loose fitting. Avoid clothes with thick seams, buttons, or zippers in areas of pressure.
Activity	Regular cardiovascular exercise. Gradual build-up of skin tolerance for new activities, equipment, and positions. Avoid movements that rub, drag, or scratch the skin.

a pressure ulcer develops, immediate intervention includes getting and keeping the area clean and avoiding as much as possible any position that puts pressure on the affected area.[18] Additional physical therapy wound care interventions may be utilized during the recovery process. Physical therapy may also play a role in helping modify mobility and positioning to help protect the skin during a period of wound healing.

TYPICAL EXAMINATION FINDINGS

PATIENT HISTORY

Patient history obtained from the medical record and the patient interview is used to help guide the testing and measurement portion of the examination.[21] This portion of the examination includes the medical and surgical history related to the SCI (e.g., mechanism of injury, fractures, stabilization surgeries) and alerts the clinician to precautions that may need to be observed. The records are reviewed for background information, including but not limited to patient demographics (e.g., age, sex), previous medical conditions and interventions, developmental history, and family history. Specifics related to the current injury include medical conditions directly and indirectly related to the SCI, medications, and clinical laboratory and other diagnostic tests.

The patient and family interview gathers information that allows the therapist to develop an idea of the patient's lifestyle before the SCI. Information obtained during the interview includes living environment, prior functional level, educational level, school and/or employment situation, social habits, previous health habits, recreational/hobby interests, general personality characteristics, and life goals.[21] This information will guide evaluation, interventions, and discharge planning. Patients will often be assessed for understanding of their current condition and the associated medical prognoses. The final piece of the patient interview is discussion of the patient's goals and expected outcomes for his or her rehabilitation and the role that he or she expects therapy to play in their recovery.[11]

SYSTEMS REVIEW

The systems review is used to target areas requiring further examination and to define areas that may cause complications or indicate a need for precautions during the examination and intervention processes. Chapter 1 includes details of the systems review.

Physical therapists (PTs) can make better clinical decisions regarding patient care if they understand the global influence of SCI on multiple body functions. During the systems review, it is important to recognize how changes in system functions may affect the individual's participation in the rehabilitation process. The following describes the impact the SCI can have on multiple body systems.

Musculoskeletal. Major changes in bone metabolism that start within a few days after SCI result in steady decreases in bone mineral density (BMD). This bone loss leads to osteoporosis, with resulting increased risk of fractures. The exact mechanism of this phenomenon is unknown, but it may be related to neurological, circulatory system, and/or hormonal changes, combined with the effects of immobility after injury.[4,22,23]

Neurogenic **heterotopic ossification (HO)** is defined as abnormal bone growth within the extraarticular soft tissues. Progressive HO can result in severe restriction of muscle and joint movement. Although the exact pathophysiology of HO is not well understood, it is generally accepted that microtrauma and mechanical stress to the musculotendinous apparatus induces ossification directly by releasing osteoblast-stimulating factors or indirectly by instituting a local inflammatory response.[24,25]

Interventions for HO involve prophylactic medications and gentle mobilization of muscles and joints.[11] Cautious passive range of motion (ROM) and joint mobilization exercises to prevent tissue shortening should be initiated as soon as the patient is stable and should be performed consistently during rehabilitation.[24,25] Delaying the onset of ROM activities increases the risk that tissue shortened by periods of immobility will be traumatized by later ROM activities and that aggressive ROM exercises begun at this later point may actually contribute to microtrauma and the formation of HO. In severe cases of HO, surgery may be indicated to remove the excess bone and try to regain joint movement required for functional mobility.

⊚ *Clinical Pearl*

Heterotopic ossification (HO), which is abnormal bone growth in soft tissues surrounding paralyzed joints, can result in severe restriction of muscle and joint motion and is likely caused by microtrauma and mechanical stress to the soft tissue surrounding the joint.

Cardiovascular/Pulmonary

Respiratory Considerations. Individuals with spinal cord compromise are at risk for developing respiratory complications. Pneumonia is the leading cause of death for all persons with SCI, and pulmonary embolism (PE) is the second leading cause of death within the first year after injury.[26]

For individuals with tetraplegia, the work of breathing is increased because of a number of factors, including inspiratory muscle paresis or paralysis, decreased chest wall mobility, expiratory muscle paresis or paralysis, altered position of the diaphragm, postural changes, and decreased functional mobility.[27] Complete spinal cord lesions at or above C3 result in complete paralysis of the diaphragm and require immediate resuscitation and life-long mechanical ventilator support to sustain life. Mechanical ventilation may also be required on a temporary or long-term basis for individuals with acute ascending edema in a lower cervical SCI, for patients with preexisting pulmonary disease, or for patients with direct trauma to the lungs or abdomen. For individuals with lower cervical or high thoracic SCI, injury may result in complete or partial paralysis of the diaphragm, intercostal, and abdominal muscles. They may have a weak cough and lack the ability to clear secretions, increasing the risk for pulmonary infections.

Within several months after injury, as strength and mobility increase, vital capacity should improve for patients with an intact diaphragm. Vital capacity may also be helped by providing support for the abdominal wall with an external device (e.g., an abdominal binder), or by the development of mild trunk spasticity.[27] However, severe thoracic spasticity may decrease chest wall compliance and increase the work of breathing (see Chapter 26).

Cardiovascular. Three major acute cardiovascular conditions are associated with SCI. Autonomic dysreflexia and PE have been discussed previously. Deep vein thrombosis (DVT) is the third complication that is of particular concern, especially during early postinjury management.

Factors contributing to DVT in the SCI population include decreased or absent muscle function, prolonged periods of decreased functional mobility, and loss of sympathetic innervation. These combine to cause vasodilation and pooling of blood in the venous system.[5,28] Failure to recognize and treat DVT can result in PE and death. Clinical signs of DVT may include swelling, localized warmth or redness of the affected extremity, pain in the calf with muscle stretch (if sensation is present), and fever.[3] Because clinical signs have poor sensitivity and specificity for DVT, medical screening tests may be indicated for patients with SCI.[5] Active DVT is managed with anticoagulation medications and occasionally with surgical placement of a vascular filter.

⊚ *Clinical Pearl*

Because of reduced lower extremity muscle contractions, people with SCI are at risk for deep vein thrombosis (DVT). Signs of DVT include swelling, redness, or warmth of the affected area.

Gastrointestinal. At the time of SCI, although gastrointestinal (GI) complications are less common and less severe than many other deficits, ileus (profoundly decreased bowel motility) and GI hemorrhage can occur in the early stages.

SCI can also disrupt the normal motility and evacuation of the colon. AD associated with bowel distention is therefore not uncommon. Patients with alterations in bowel function secondary to SCI are described as having a neurogenic bowel.[29,30] The primary intervention used to control neurogenic bowel dysfunction is a regular bowel program that is initiated during acute hospitalization.[30] The program always includes diet and fluid management and regularly scheduled bowel elimination. Elimination may be assisted or controlled with chemical or mechanical stimulation, positioning, medications, or elimination devices. The goal of the bowel program is to prevent impaction or unplanned bowel movements. The bowel program must be continued throughout the individual's life or until neurological recovery improves volitional bowel function.[5]

Genitourinary

Bladder Management. Establishing a consistent and effective method of emptying the bladder is one of the first routines that needs to be developed after SCI. Failure to regularly and completely drain the bladder can result in urinary tract infection (the most common complication among SCI survivors). The primary intervention for bladder management in the acute stages of SCI (during the period of spinal shock) is catheterization (either indwelling or intermittent).

Sexual Function. Questions about sexual function will likely arise for both male and female SCI patients during the rehabilitation process. Because sexuality is a sensitive issue, patients may approach the subject with any member of the treatment team with whom they feel a level of confidence and trust, including their PT assistant (PTA). For this reason, it is important for therapists to have at least a basic knowledge of how SCI affects sexual function and available referral and reference information to direct questions beyond the therapist's knowledge. All patients should be encouraged to seek medical and counseling advice to deal constructively with concerns about sexuality and sexual function.

Male Sexual Function. Male sexual function after SCI is altered based on the level of injury. Sensory function is often absent or impaired after injury, resulting in absent or changed responses to tactile stimuli below the injury level. Erectile function may be altered at two levels. Psychogenic erections (erections resulting from sensory input that produce erotic emotions) are mediated at the T10 to T12 spinal levels. SCI at or above this level results in loss of psychogenic erection, whereas injury below this level or incomplete injury may result in preservation of this function.

While some erectile ability is often preserved, the quality and duration of the erection may or may not be sufficient for intercourse. The patient should also understand that even with erection sufficient for sexual activity, as many as 90% of men with SCI are not able to ejaculate during intercourse.[31] Poor ejaculatory function combined with poor sperm motility and concentration results in very low fertility rates for men with SCI.[32,33] Because of this, a man with a SCI may need medical intervention to father children.

Female Sexual Function. The impact on sexual function for women with SCI is significantly less than for their male counterparts. Sensory loss may alter the experience and a patient may experience reduced or absent vaginal lubrication because sexual response cannot get from the brain to the sacral region (similar to the effects on the psychogenic erection response in the male). Sensory loss may alter the experience of orgasm after SCI.

Pregnancy is possible for women with any level of spinal injury. Because of this, women with SCI need to consider the same issues related to contraception as women without SCI. If a woman with SCI chooses to become pregnant, there are several factors that put her in a higher risk pregnancy category: Pressure of the fetus, complicating bowel and bladder programs; weight gain, affecting mobility skills and increasing pressure ulcer risk; increased risk for urinary tract infections; changes in patterns of spasticity; decreased respiratory capacity from pressure of the fetus on the diaphragm; cardiovascular changes; and alterations in normal feeling of and response to contractions during labor.[34,35] AD also occurs more often during all stages of pregnancy, particularly during labor. Despite these complicating factors (most of which are to a lesser extent issues for able-bodied women during pregnancy), women with SCI can safely give birth to children with the guidance of a physiatrist and obstetrician who are familiar with the special needs of women with SCI.

TESTS AND MEASURES

Musculoskeletal

Posture. Observation of sitting posture focuses on the ability to remain upright against gravity, symmetry, scapular position, use of UEs to assist with and maintain posture, and position of lower trunk and pelvis.

Anthropometric Characteristics. General body composition and proportion are noted. An individual who is very thin or who has lost a large amount of weight during acute care may have more prominent bony prominences, with increased susceptibility to pressure ulcers.

Range of Motion. Range of all motions available at all joints is noted but may be complicated by medical precautions, presence of spinal stabilization devices or orthoses, or by the patient's inability to tolerate some standard testing positions.

Muscle Performance. Manual muscle testing (MMT) is performed for all muscle groups[5,21] (see Chapter 5).

Joint Integrity and Mobility. Joint integrity and mobility are frequently assessed during the ROM examination, using palpation and observation during active, active assistive, and passive movement. Because of the increased demand for UE weight bearing during mobility for SCI patients, the integrity of the scapulothoracic, shoulder, elbow, and wrist joints are of particular concern in this population.

Neuromuscular

Cognition. A basic cognitive screen, such as the Mini-Mental State Examination (MMSE), is often administered to determine the patient's potential for participation in rehabilitation.[36]

Pain. The incidence of pain after SCI varies greatly, but pain can significantly impact the rehabilitation process, functional mobility, quality of life, and the psychological well-being of many people with SCI. The presence, intensity, and location of pain will be noted at the time of examination and needs to be reexamined at each therapy encounter. Pain may be measured with a variety of standard pain scales, indices, and questionnaires as described in Chapter 22.

Reflex Integrity. Reflexes are tested using a tap of a reflex hammer on the tendon of a relaxed muscle.

Sensory Integrity. Testing of light touch, pain (sharp/dull), discriminative touch, temperature sensation, proprioception, and kinesthesia will be noted in the examination.

Motor Function—Control and Learning. Motor control varies, depending on the type of injury and the resulting loss or preservation of motor function. Complete SCI causes total loss of voluntary movement below the level of injury but spasticity, which produces an involuntary increase in muscle tone, can still occur and may interfere, or be used to assist, with motor control and mobility skills. In incomplete injuries, there will be some overlap of voluntary control and spasticity across spinal levels, making the resultant motor function more difficult to predict.

The pathological synergy patterns and spasticity frequently associated with other nonprogressive UMN central nervous system disorders, such as stroke[12,37,38] (as described in Chapter 16), differ somewhat from the abnormal movement patterns commonly seen in SCI. Spasticity in SCI is caused by changes in neural control and in the muscles themselves.[12,39,40] This combination of changes can result in weakness, impaired coordination, changes in posture, and involuntary movements.[5,41]

The incidence of spasticity in SCI is difficult to ascertain because there is no universally agreed on way to measure spasticity in this population. If spasticity is severe and uncontrolled, it may contribute to muscle and joint contractures, interfere with activities of daily living (ADLs) and mobility skills, prevent proper positioning, impair hygiene, increase the risk for pressure ulcers, interfere with sleep, create pain, and cause other disruptions to quality of life.[5,11,42-45] The presence and severity of spasticity may be influenced by the individual's physiological state[43] and be increased by physiological stressors[5,44] such as urinary tract infection, fever, menstruation, bowel or bladder distention, mechanical shortening/contractures of muscles, changes in environmental temperature, presence of pressure ulcers, tight clothing, and emotional stress.

Cardiovascular/Pulmonary

Circulation. Persons with high level SCI are particularly prone to orthostatic hypotension because of decreased venous return, decreased cardiac output, and pooling of blood in dependent body parts.[5] Therefore careful initial measurement and ongoing observation of blood pressure is required in this population. As noted previously, AD is a dangerous consequence of SCI that results in circulatory changes and requires frequent BP monitoring. (See Chapter 22 for further information on blood pressure measurement and AD.)

Ventilation and Respiration/Gas Exchange. The examination of respiratory function may include measurement of oxygen saturation, respiratory muscle strength (diaphragm, abdominals, pectorals, serratus, scalenes, sternocleidomastoid, and latissimus), respiratory capacities, respiratory rate, and chest expansion.[5,14] Oxygen saturation may be measured with a pulse oximeter. Vital capacity and inspiratory and expiratory reserve volumes may be measured using a spirometer.[5,46]

Respiratory pattern (especially the presence of **paradoxical breathing**), chest shape and symmetry, ability to cough, and duration of phonation (length of vocalization and syllables per breath) are noted and recorded. Auscultation (use of a stethoscope) may be performed to determine the types and location of breath sounds. The use of respiratory assistive devices like ventilators or positive pressure ventilatory support should also be noted, along with the settings and critical values that have been determined for the patient.[5,47]

Aerobic Capacity and Endurance. The examination of endurance and aerobic capacity in individuals with SCI will be performed by using tests that do not require the ability to ambulate (the skill most often used to judge cardiovascular fitness in able-bodied individuals). One of the most frequently used alternatives for research and training is performance on arm ergometry tests.[48-50] Heart rate, power output, and oxygen uptake ($\dot{V}o_2$) may all be measured with continuous or interval arm ergometry. For individuals without a normal heart rate response to exercise because of sympathetic system alterations, ratings of perceived exertion (e.g., the Borg Rating of Perceived Exertion [RPE] scale[51]) may be used to determine exercise intensity[48] (see Chapter 23).

Function

Basic Mobility and Self-Care. The examination generally includes the following functions: Rolling in bed to both sides, rolling from supine to prone and returning to supine, moving supine to/from long sitting, transitioning from supine to/from sitting at edge of bed, and transferring from bed or mat to/from a wheelchair. Additional ADL and instrumental ADL (IADL) skills may be examined and recorded using any of a number of functional mobility scales based on the patient's level of function.

Locomotion and Gait. For most acute patients with SCI the primary means of locomotion is by wheelchair. Initial examination of wheelchair mobility includes observing the individual's ability to manage wheelchair parts (e.g., wheel locks, foot rests) and to propel the chair on level surfaces. For higher level tetraplegic patients, the skills required for managing the control mechanism of a power wheelchair may need to be tested. The patient should be tested on his or her ability to perform an effective pressure-relief technique when seated in the wheelchair.

More extensive tests have been developed to measure additional dimensions of wheelchair propulsion such as endurance, speed, and exertion. For example, the Wheelchair Circuit was specifically developed to assess manual wheelchair mobility in persons with SCI.

Standard gait assessment tools (see Chapter 32) and functional measures, such as the Functional Independence Measure (FIM) and the Modified Barthel Index (MBI), may be used to assist with gait examination and determination of level of independence with gait skills in individuals with SCI who can ambulate. Two scales have recently been developed to assist with the standardized description of gait in patients with SCI. The Spinal Cord Injury Functional Ambulation Inventory (SCI-FAI) is an observational gait assessment instrument with three domains: Gait parameters, assistive device use, and a walking mobility score (based on typical walking practices and timed test).[52] The Walking Index for Spinal Cord Injury (WISCI)[53,54] is a scale that incorporates gradations of functional limitation (based on physical assistance and assistive devices required) for walking 10 m.

EVALUATION, DIAGNOSIS, AND PROGNOSIS

Evaluation of SCI usually includes grading the degree of impairment using the American Spinal Injury Association (ASIA) Impairment Scale[55] (Fig. 20-3). The ASIA Impairment Scale is scored from A, which is more impaired, to E, which is normal sensory and motor function. A number of clinical syndromes associated with incomplete SCI result in typical patterns of impairment (Table 20-2).[3,5,12,55] Recognizing these syndromes can help predict functional limitations and can assist with treatment planning.

INTERVENTION

Because of the global effects of SCI, case management needs to be team-based and include interventions for multiple musculoskeletal and neuromuscular systems. The rehabilitation team may include nursing, medicine (specifically physicians with specialization in physical medicine and rehabilitation), occupational therapy, physical therapy, speech and language therapy, psychology, social work, and recreation therapy. Other medical specialists and allied health practitioners may be involved, depending on the exact nature of the patient's needs. The remainder of this chapter addresses basic intervention options in the acute and rehabilitation phases of recovery

ASIA IMPAIRMENT SCALE

☐ **A = Complete:** No motor or sensory function is preserved in sacral segments S4–S5.

☐ **B = Incomplete:** Sensory but not motor function is preserved below the neurological level, including sacral segments S4–S5.

☐ **C = Incomplete:** Motor function is preserved below the neurological level, and more than half the key muscles below the neurological level have muscle grade less than 3.

☐ **D = Incomplete:** Motor function is preserved below the neurological level, and at least half the key muscles below the neurological level have muscle grade of 3 or more.

☐ **E = Normal:** Motor and sensory function are normal.

CLINICAL SYNDROMES

☐ Central cord
☐ Brown-Séquard
☐ Anterior cord
☐ Conus medullaris
☐ Cauda equina

FIG. 20-3 American Spinal Injury Association Examination Form. *Courtesy American Spinal Injury Association, Atlanta, GA.*

from SCI. Because of the infinite combinations of motor and sensory loss and preservation after injury, no single intervention plan can be applied to the majority of patients with SCI. The following suggestions will be modified according to the results of a thorough examination and evaluation process.

THE ACUTE PHASE

Early intervention in the acute stage of recovery from SCI focuses on prevention of secondary complications from immobility and beginning the transition to upright postures. Emphasis is placed on passive and active assistive exercise, positioning to prevent skin breakdown and preserve ROM, and on maintaining or restoring as much respiratory function as possible.

Patient-Related Instruction. Education of the patient and any identified caregivers must begin at the time of onset of therapy services. The patient must learn to direct the assistance he or she needs to control their physical care, their comfort, and their psychosocial needs. In particular, physical therapy instruction in the acute setting will include instruction in bed positioning, skin inspection and pressure ulcer risk factors, respiratory exercises, and assisted ROM exercises. Instructions should be provided and learning assessed for accuracy, since an error in understanding could lead to submaximal care and possible complications in recovery. Once the patient is stable, he or she should also begin to be educated about the long-term rehabilitation process.

Therapeutic Exercise. Passive ROM (PROM) exercises are used to minimize shortening of muscles and articular structures. Traditional ROM exercises are provided to all limbs, trunk, and cervical region as allowed by immobilization devices and by medical restrictions to movement. ROM exercises are begun as soon as the patient is medically stable and cleared for activity. Because of the possible risk of increased incidence of HO development associated with delayed-onset of ROM activities, early

TABLE 20-2	Spinal Cord Injury Syndromes	
Name of Syndrome	**Pattern of Neurological Injury**	**Associated Impairments**
Central cord syndrome	Injury to the central portion of the cord, with sparing of peripheral areas. Occurs almost exclusively in the cervical region.	Sparing of sacral sensation. Weakness more severe in the UEs with lesser impairment or preservation of function in the LEs.
Brown-Séquard syndrome	Anterior-to-posterior hemisection of the spinal cord or other injury resulting in unilateral cord damage.	Ipsilateral proprioceptive and motor loss and contralateral loss of sensitivity to light touch, pressure, pain, and temperature.
Anterior cord syndrome	Destruction of the anterior portions of the white and grey matter of the cord, with preservation of posterior components.	Complete loss of motor function and some loss of light touch and temperature sensation. Sparing of proprioception and discriminative touch.
Posterior cord syndrome	Destruction of the posterior portions of the cord, with relative preservation of anterior components.	Severe impairment of proprioception, discrimination, and vibration. Motor function minimally affected or preserved.
Cauda equina syndrome	Damage to the lumbar or sacral nerve roots caudal to the level of spinal cord termination.	Sensory loss and flaccid paralysis of LE muscles, bladder, and bowels.

UEs, Upper extremities; *LEs,* Lower extremities.

intervention is stressed. A standard ROM protocol usually includes twice daily exercises of all joints through full available ROM for 5 to 10 repetitions.[5,11]

Some extra precautions must be taken when performing ROM exercise with an individual with SCI because of the future ROM required for mobility and the hypotonicity present during early recovery:

1. Extreme or forceful ROM is avoided because of the risk of soft tissue trauma and possible predisposition to HO.
2. Straight leg raises and combined hip and knee flexion may be limited in acute phases, particularly after lower thoracic or lumbar surgery, because of the possible stretch on dural tissue and lumbar structures.
3. Combined movements of the wrist and fingers are rarely applied in the same directions (e.g., wrist flexion combined with finger flexion or wrist extension with finger extension) to avoid overstretching the long finger flexor or extensor tendons. The natural passive movement of the fingers into flexion with wrist extension will be used by many patients to perform grasp functions (called **tenodesis grip**), so preservation of some tightness in the long finger flexors in combination with wrist extension must be preserved. Concomitantly, extensor length must be preserved to allow the passive opening of the tenodesis grip when the wrist is flexed. The exception to this rule occurs if the patient is developing severe spasticity, at which time prolonged stretching or splinting may be required to prevent contractures of the involved muscle groups.
4. Because of the need for strength and mobility in the shoulders and scapulae for all future mobility skills, these areas must be addressed along with distal extremity motions.
5. During the areflexive period of spinal shock, care should be taken to fully support the limbs during ROM to prevent trauma to intermediate joints.

While ROM is initially a passive activity performed by the therapist or trained caregiver, as patient progress allows, these exercises are advanced to active assistive or active exercise, and the patient is instructed in how to perform self-ROM exercises for maintaining flexibility.

◎ Clinical Pearl

Range of motion (ROM) exercises should be initiated early: Observe spinal precautions, do not force movement, and do not overstretch muscles.

Positioning. Because of the prolonged period of time most acute SCI patients spend in bed, it is very important that correct positioning be used to reduce the risk of pressure ulcers, maintain postural and skeletal alignment, and reduce the secondary effects of spasticity. A pressure-relief bed, mattress, or mattress overlay should always be used in addition to constant monitoring of positioning and skin condition. Turning between positions is generally performed every 2 hours.

When the patient is supine, the following postures are recommended:

Body Area	Anatomical Point	Position
LEs	Hips	In extension and slightly abducted, with neutral rotation.
	Knees	In extension but supported and not hyperextended.
	Ankles	In dorsiflexion, generally with the use of an orthotic device.
	Toes	Extended.
UEs (for patients with tetraplegia)	Shoulders	In adduction, slight flexion, neutral rotation.
	Elbows	In extension, especially in the presence of biceps function without opposing triceps function. Air splints or other orthotic devices may be used to maintain elbow extension in the case of biceps spasticity.
	Wrists	In extension of approximately 30 to 45 degrees. A schedule of intermittent splinting may be used to facilitate proper wrist position.
	Fingers	In slight flexion.

Patients are rarely positioned in direct sidelying because of the pressure this places on the bony prominences at the shoulder and hip. Instead, they are positioned slightly away from sidelying in the supine direction. In this position, the hips and knees are slightly flexed and the upper leg is slightly posterior to the lower, with padding provided between the limbs (especially at the knees and ankles). The lower side shoulder is flexed to about 90 degrees and is slightly protracted, the elbow extended, and the forearm supinated and supported on a pillow. The upper arm is supported on a pillow in shoulder flexion and elbow extension.

Prone positioning is an excellent option for prolonged stretching of hip and knee flexors and is an especially good position for patients with a good prognosis for recovery of ambulation. The presence of medical devices (e.g., tracheotomy or feeding tube) may complicate but does not preclude the use of the prone position in early intervention. The presence of a Halo brace is not necessarily a contraindication for prone lying, but many patients with a Halo have to be slowly introduced to time spent prone secondary to the initial helpless feeling of lying face down and because the feeling of compression on the chest may create a perceived change in respiratory function. In fact, prone positioning improves oxygenation and may increase circulation to dependent lung regions.[56] Even if a patient with a Halo does not tolerate prolonged prone positioning, he or she should still be turned to prone for a few minutes daily to allow skin inspection and cleaning under the posterior portion of the Halo vest and to help with respiratory secretion mobilization.

As the patient's condition stabilizes, he or she may be progressed to upright sitting. An abdominal binder and LE ace wrapping are used for vascular support, and the individual is gradually raised into a sitting position in bed or in a reclining wheelchair with elevating leg rests, while BP and heart rate are monitored and the patient is observed for signs of light-headedness or dizziness. When the patient can tolerate sitting in this position for extended periods (15 to 30 minutes), the patient can be progressed to sitting with the LEs in a dependent position.

Airway Clearance. Many individuals with SCI, especially at the cervical level, require mechanical ventilation during their acute management. Patients with complete injuries above C4 will require life-long full or partial ventilatory support. Physical therapy interventions during acute patient management will include techniques for improving respiratory muscle strength and endurance and improving airway clearance and for minimizing the respiratory complications of prolonged immobilization. Treatment should be closely coordinated with other members of the treatment team, including nursing, respiratory therapy, speech therapy, and occupational therapy.

Interventions chosen are based on the results of the pulmonary examination and evaluation. If airway secretions are present or suspected, interventions may include positioning for postural drainage, percussion, and vibration (see Chapter 24). These interventions are applied to lung areas involved (as noted on radiograph or with auscultation), and the treatment time is determined by the changes in airway clearance. Treatments may take 20 to 30 minutes and are continued as long as there are productive secretions (with induced cough or suctioning) and breath sounds are improving.[47] A change in breath sounds from diminished or absent before treatment to crackles, rhonchi (coarse rattling sound somewhat like snoring, usually caused by secretion in bronchial airways), or vesicular during and after treatment indicates effective secretion mobilization. Periodic suctioning and/or assisted coughing may be used to clear the mobilized secretions. A pneumatic vest that supplies mechanical vibration to the entire chest wall may also be used to mobilize secretions. Once a patient is more active and can mobilize secretion with coughing, passive airway clearance techniques may be discontinued.

An abdominal binder to support breathing may be used once the patient is performing some spontaneous breathing. The binder is applied in the area 2 to 3 inches below the xiphoid process and extending slightly below the anterior superior iliac spine (ASIS).[47] Binders placed too high may impair inspiration, and binders that extend too low may cause skin breakdown. Although the use of abdominal binders to support respiration is controversial, there is evidence that binders can help some individuals.[57,58] Vital capacity, respiratory rate, breathing pattern, and oxygen saturation may be monitored in supine and in sitting with and without the binder to determine if the binder is helping a specific individual.

To support weaning from mechanical ventilation, respiratory muscle training may be performed with inspiratory muscle training devices and/or with abdominal weight training.[5,47] Manual cues and facilitation may be used to target specific muscles and excursions during exercise. The duration and resistance of training is progressed slowly to prevent respiratory muscle fatigue. As respiratory endurance improves, interventions for mobility may be added during the periods when the patient is off the ventilator. During the weaning process, continuous positive airway pressure (CPAP) may be used to assist breathing when the patient is off mechanical ventilation.

Patients with higher cervical SCI may be taught a technique called *glossopharyngeal breathing* (GPB), which uses the upper accessory muscles (innervated by the cranial nerves) to expand the oral cavity to draw air into the mouth and create a negative inspiratory pressure to facilitate inspiration. The air is then "pushed" into the lungs by pulling the chin and tongue back toward the neck, creating a positive pressure in the mouth. This air "gulping" or "stroke" is repeated multiple ($\approx$3 to 12) times per breath.[59] Some patients who would otherwise be ventilator-dependent can use GPB to allow extended time off the ventilator. For others, it serves as an emergency procedure to sustain breathing for short periods in the case of temporary failure of mechanical ventilatory support.

As the patient becomes more medically stable and physically active during rehabilitation, a number of respiratory interventions may be added to those begun during the acute phase. Initial emphasis is on improving active mobilization and expectoration of secretions. Expectoration is addressed by techniques designed to improve the ability to cough. Intervention may involve manual assistive cough techniques, including but not limited to "quad cough" (forceful expiration assist provided via a Heimlich-type or abdominal thrust maneuver), costophrenic assist, anterior chest compressions, or trunk counter-rotation.[5,11,59] Patients may learn to do self-assisted versions of the quad cough by using techniques like positioning their hands under the rib cage and using biceps to pull up and in, or by timing a forward trunk lean with the expulsion phase of coughing. Individuals with sufficient balance and inspiratory lung volume may also learn to use an independent airway clearance strategy called *active cycle of breathing* (ACB) followed by a forced expiratory technique (FET)[59,60] (see Chapter 24).

Once the individual is upright, obtaining proper postural alignment will assist with facilitation of respiratory muscles. Alignment should include slight shoulder retraction (opening of the anterior chest wall), shoulder neutral or external rotation, thoracic spine extension, and pelvic positioning that avoids excessive posterior tilt. This alignment facilitates recruitment of primary and accessory breathing muscles and prevents the development of secondary postures (e.g., kyphosis) that may impair respiratory capacity.[5,59]

Pairing respiratory efforts with complementary movements and cues can help to maximize both the breathing effort and the mobility skills.[5,59] If a task involves trunk extension (e.g., overhead reaching, UE proprioceptive neuromuscular facilitation [PNF] flexion patterns, rolling sidelying to supine), it may be paired with inspiration (expansion of thoracic cage). Conversely, movements involving thoracic flexion and compression (forward lean or reach, rolling supine to sidelying with head and upper trunk flexion pattern, PNF extension patterns) should be paired with expiratory efforts. Concentric trunk and extremity movements can be paired with concentric respiratory movements and eccentric with eccentric. Manual cues and verbal cues can also be used to facilitate the appropriate combination of movements, with strong cues associated with concentric (inspiratory or expiratory) breathing efforts and slower, softer cues associated with eccentric (expiratory) breathing efforts. By combining the appropriate cues and movements, the efficiency of both mobility and breathing are increased and the benefits of interventions for training mobility skills are compounded.

The endurance and power of the respiratory system can be augmented with training of the respiratory musculature. The length and control of expiratory efforts can be practiced with common activities like singing, humming, or blowing through a straw or blow toy. Incentive spirometers with target ranges can be used for repetitive breathing exercise. Utilizing ventilatory muscle training (VMT) devices strengthens breathing by adding resistance to respiratory muscle contractions. Most VMT training programs are used during the rehabilitation phase for 15 to 20 minutes, 2 times per day, 5 to 7 days per week for approximately 6 weeks. Studies have shown improvement in inspiratory muscle strength and endurance and subjective reports of decreased breathing effort with the use of VMT training.[61,62]

Pain Management. Interventions for pain management vary with the type of pain. Although any structure above or below the injury level may be affected, nociceptive pain is often musculoskeletal in nature and frequently occurs above the level of injury secondary to the increased stresses of weight bearing and mobility placed on the UEs.[63] The shoulder is the most common site of pain above the level of injury. Nociceptive pain symptoms are addressed with similar regimens to those used for able-bodied populations, including the use of analgesic and antiinflammatory medications, rest, lifestyle modifications, therapeutic modalities, and exercise.[63,64] Additional interventions for people with SCI may involve ergonomic assessment and modification of wheelchair seating and propulsion technique.[65,66] No controlled study evidence was found for SCI patients related to the efficacy of various interventions for nociceptive pain. In a self-report study of pain management in 120 individuals with SCI, 40 had tried physical therapy and 50% of them rated it as making pain "considerably better" or "disappear."[67]

Neuropathic pain is more difficult to classify and treat, particularly if it occurs below the injury level. Treatment options for this type of pain are similar to those used in other patients with chronic pain and may include medication (e.g., opioids, antidepressants, anticonvulsants, and antispasticity agents), psychosocial support, cognitive-behavioral therapy, and surgical intervention.[64,66,67] Spinal

cord stimulation and drug infusions are additional possibilities.[68]

THE REHABILITATION PHASE

During the rehabilitation phase of recovery, interventions focus on training mobility skills and providing education in self-care to the individual with SCI. This phase will at a minimum include training in pressure relief techniques, bed mobility skills, transfer training, wheelchair mobility skills, respiratory care, and gait training (when appropriate). Training for each of these tasks may be accompanied by specific exercises to increase the strength, flexibility, or control components necessary to increase task performance and efficiency. Information in this section of the chapter is categorized according to task and includes descriptions of techniques that may be used for achieving and improving task performance.

Patient-Related Instruction

Pressure Relief in Sitting. Patients with SCI are at an increased risk for developing pressure ulcers during their initial episode of care after injury. It is therefore imperative that pressure relief techniques are taught as soon as possible after injury and frequently reinforced throughout the rehabilitation process. The patient must understand the importance of these skills, and all team members must cue and reinforce their performance.

When seated, tissue around the ischial tuberosities is at greatest risk for breakdown. If the patient has a kyphotic posture with a posterior pelvic tilt, the area over the sacrum is also at increased risk.[69,70] Recommendations about how long and often pressure should be relieved over the bony prominences to reduce ulcer risk vary greatly.[11,17,18] Most sources agree that pressure relief should initially be performed for 15 seconds or more, at least every 15 to 30 minutes. However, recent evidence suggests that this may not be sufficient for reoxygenation of compressed tissue. Based on monitoring of transcutaneous oxygen levels during pressure relief, studies have concluded that most subjects tested required 1.5 to 2 minutes of pressure relief to restore oxygen equivalent to baseline unloaded levels.[71,72]

For patients with tetraplegia at or above the C4 level, pressure relief is performed by an assistant or a powered system tilting or reclining the wheelchair (Fig. 20-4). An assistant can tilt the wheelchair by sitting behind the wheelchair, grasping its push handles, and tilting the chair back onto its rear wheels until the chair is tilted at least 65 degrees (the back of the chair may be resting on the assistant's knees).[73] Some wheelchairs have a mechanism that allows the back of the wheelchair to be reclined separately from the seating surface. With this type of mechanism, the chair back should be reclined as far back as comfortably possible (120 to 150 degrees)[74] and the legs elevated. Further weight shifting can be accomplished by partially rolling the individual to each side once in the supine position. A disadvantage of reclining the patient is that this involves changing the patient's position relative to the chair. The patient then needs to be repositioned when the chair is returned to the upright position after the pressure relief, and this can trigger spasticity. It is also important to realize that some angles of recline that reduce ischial pressure can increase surface shear force and thus risk tissue breakdown.[74]

For patients with SCI at the C5-6 level with good head and neck control and some UE function (not including triceps), several techniques may be used to assist with pressure relief in a manual wheelchair. The individual may lean forward with the chest moving toward the thighs (Fig. 20-5, *A*). Henderson et al found this technique to be more effective in reducing pressure over the ischial tuberosities than tilting the chair back by 35 or 65 degrees.[73] The most difficult part of this technique is learning to recover from the forward position without triceps function. Patients can be taught to use their anterior shoulder muscles to push up to sitting, or to throw one arm back

and "hook" the back of the chair or push handle to pull themselves back to an upright position. Another technique is to lean sideways in the wheelchair as far as possible, using the opposite arm (i.e., left arm for right lean) to hook the wheelchair back or push handle (with the forearm for individuals with C5 function and with wrist extension for individuals with C6 function) to control the lean and to recover from the lean (Fig. 20-5, *B*). This technique must then be repeated to the opposite side for bilateral pressure relief.

For individuals with functional use of the triceps, pressure relief may be performed using the push-up technique (Fig. 20-5, *C*). This involves placing the hands on the wheelchair tires or arm rests and lifting the body off of the seat with a push-up motion. Some individuals without triceps function may be able to perform a version of this skill, if their seating configuration allows them to position the UEs in way that passively locks the elbow into extension while the shoulder depressors are used to create the lifting force. The disadvantage of the push-up technique is that it contributes further to the overuse of the shoulders and wrist already inherent in wheelchair mobility.[75] It is also extremely difficult for someone to maintain the push-up position long enough to allow sufficient tissue perfusion (1.5 to 2 minutes).

In addition to regular pressure relief techniques, it is essential that every individual with SCI use a seat cushion designed to distribute pressure when sitting in the wheelchair or on any surface for an extended period of time. Wheelchair cushions are available in four basic types, each with advantages and disadvantages. Cushions that use air for support consistently reduce pressure over bony prominences[76,77] and are generally lightweight, but they require regular maintenance and provide a less stable surface for performing mobility skills. Gel cushions require minimal maintenance and are generally easier to move on and off

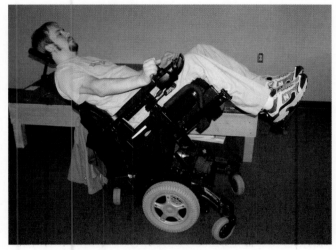

FIG. 20-4 Passive pressure relief using a tilt-in-space wheelchair.

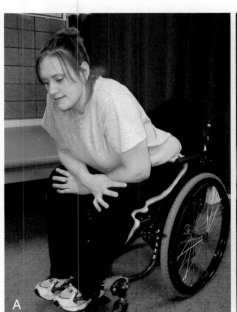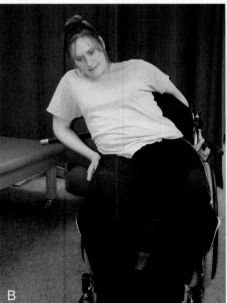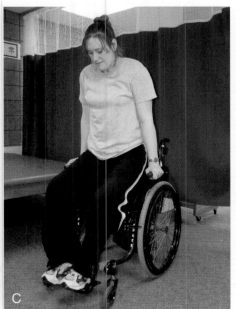

FIG. 20-5 Active pressure relief techniques. **A,** Forward lean. **B,** Side lean. **C,** Push-up.

of but can be heavy and trap moisture. Foam cushions come in a large variety of shapes and various combinations of foam density and material. The effectiveness of the pressure relief and the longevity of the material vary greatly between types of foam, and careful assessment is needed to match the fit, the mobility needs, and the pressure distribution requirements of the individual to the characteristics of the cushion. Other cushions are made from any of a number of synthetic materials in a variety of configurations (e.g., honeycomb construction), with variable attributes related to pressure distribution, positioning, and mobility skills.

◎ *Clinical Pearl*

A variety of pressure-reducing seat cushions are available. These provide differing degrees of pressure reduction and vary in longevity. Cushions require regular maintenance and inspection.

Gait and Locomotion Training

Wheelchair Mobility. Training individuals with any level of SCI to use a wheelchair is essential for independent daily mobility. After an initial period of skill and endurance training, an individual should be able to propel his or her wheelchair throughout an average day at the community level without creating muscle soreness or fatigue. The level of SCI will dictate the skills required and the type of wheelchair needed to meet this goal.

Individuals with SCI at C4 or above will use a power wheelchair for mobility. Power chairs may be controlled by any of a number of control mechanisms that are matched to the patient's mobility. Small movements of the head, chin, lips, breath, or shoulders can be used to control the chair and to control power pressure relief options. A variety of hand and arm mounting systems enable individuals to drive a wheelchair with limited UE motion. Portable ventilators can be mounted on power wheelchairs to allow ventilator-dependent individuals to be mobile at the household and community levels. Initial practice with powered mobility should be done in an open area with the wheelchair controls adjusted to a slow speed. As the individual's skills progress, he or she should be instructed in using the chair on uneven terrain, around obstacles, in public places, and on elevators. The power chair user must be able to direct the management and maintenance of all parts of his or her wheelchair, including the mechanism that disengages the drive mechanism and allows the wheelchair to be pushed by an assistant in case of mechanical failure.

SCI at the midcervical level (C5-6) results in motor control that allows limited manual wheelchair propulsion. Specially designed push rims on the wheelchair give patients projections or tacky surfaces that can be used to "grip" the rim in the absence of finger function. For these individuals, the wheelchair push stroke involves planting the hands on the rims behind the hips and pulling with the biceps to start the propelling motion, following through with a squeeze motion of the anterior shoulder and chest muscles to complete the push stroke. The wheelchair should be adjusted to allow maximum maneuverability, while at the same time having stable seat and back support sufficient to allow maximum push stroke efficiency without compensatory postural changes.[78,79] While most individuals with this level of SCI can be independent on smooth level surfaces with manual wheelchair propulsion, community level mobility often requires the use of a power-assist manual wheelchair or a power wheelchair.

Most individuals with complete SCI at or below C7 will use a manual wheelchair for mobility. The push stroke for these individuals involves grasping the push rim behind the hips (with modifications to the rim as needed with cervical injuries), pushing forward on the rims, allowing the hands to drop down and then extending the shoulders during the recovery phase, and then gripping the rims again. In this way the push stroke becomes a circular motion rather than a back and forth "sawing" type of motion.

After mastering the basic push stroke required for propulsion on a level surface, manual wheelchair users should be instructed in a variety of additional skills that they can then adapt to their daily needs. The ability to open and close doors, operate an elevator, and perform ADL tasks from the seated position should all be taught during the patient's rehabilitation. The "wheelie" skill should also be introduced (Fig. 20-6) to allow for balance during steep descents, to unload the front of the wheelchair to improve mobility over rough surfaces, and as a component of the skill of ascending curbs. The wheelie position is achieved by giving a firm forward push on the hand rims from a position just behind the hips, while at the same time leaning the head and shoulders back. This results in the front castors of the chair coming off the floor and all of the weight being transferred to the rear wheels. With practice, most individuals can learn to maintain the chair in a balanced position with weight on the rear wheels

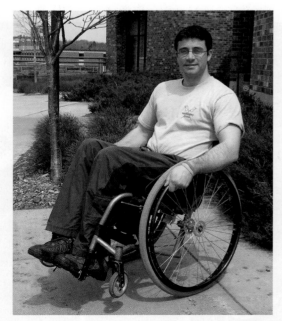

FIG. 20-6 Patient with complete T10 paraplegia balancing in the wheelie position.

only. When training a patient in this skill, the therapist must maintain a firm grip on the wheelchair push handles or on a safety strap looped around the rear of the wheelchair frame. This allows the therapist to help the patient get tilted far enough back to find the balanced position, while also preventing the patient from losing their balance backward.

Patients should be taught to protect themselves in the case of a fall. If falling backward, the individual should lean forward with their head turned (to avoid having their legs fall directly into their face) and try to grasp the front of the wheelchair frame. At no time should they try to reach back and catch themselves to prevent a fall; this puts the UE at high risk for shoulder injury or dislocation.

Ascending and descending curbs are skills that require repeated practice to master. A low curb can be ascended using a wheelie to lift the front wheels up over the curb, pushing the chair forward until the rear wheels are against the curb, leaning the trunk as far forward as possible, and then pulling up and pushing forward on the hand rims. This technique requires good UE and grip strength. A low curb may be descended by backing down the curb with the rear wheels while leaning as far forward as possible over the front of the chair. Once the back of the chair is on the lower surfaces, the front end is moved off the curb by turning to the side or by using a wheelie to lift the front end and pulling back away from the curb. A more efficient technique for ascending curbs is to have the chair rolling forward throughout the ascent so that the forward momentum of the moving chair provides most of the force needed to get up the curb (Fig. 20-7). This involves approaching the curb with the chair rolling at a steady, moderate speed; just as the footplate is about to reach the curb the front end is lifted with a wheelie, and as soon as the front of the chair clears the curb, the upper body is thrown forward (lean or fall, depending on trunk control) while the arms continue the push stroke. Descending the curb is

performed similarly by approaching the curb rolling and performing a small wheelie at the edge of the curb to hold up the front end of the chair as the rear wheels descend the curb, thus allowing the rear wheels to land on the lower surface either slightly before or at the same time as the front castors. Note that both of these skills require a good sense of timing, motor coordination, and a fair command of the wheelie skill. Patients should be assisted to allow success during early practice and should be closely guarded to prevent injury as they progress with their training.

In addition to learning wheelchair mobility skills, the individual must also be comfortable with the mechanics of the wheelchair: Managing leg rests and arm rests (required for transfers), using the wheel locks, making the chair compact for travel (this may involve folding the chair and/or removing the wheels), making mechanical adjustments to alter the performance of the chair (e.g., camber, seat to back angle), and performing basic maintenance.

Gait. Traditionally, gait training for individuals with SCI focused on using orthotics and assistive devices to allow individuals to bear weight on their LEs and achieve upright positioning and a limited measure of functional mobility in standing. While this approach maintains some utility and is discussed later in this section, more recent investigation has led to a shift in intervention paradigm that seeks to better exploit the spinal neural circuitry. Treatment programs consistent with this paradigm include various forms of "locomotor training," which are sometimes combined with additional modalities (e.g., functional electrical stimulation [FES], drug therapies) and other traditional therapy interventions.

Locomotor Training. Locomotor training takes advantage of neural networks in the spinal cord called **central pattern generators (CPGs)** that can produce rhythmic neural activity without supraspinal and proprioceptive input. CPGs may provide basic motor patterns, with the higher centers and sensory inputs initiating and modifying

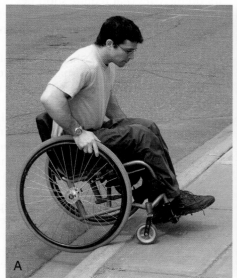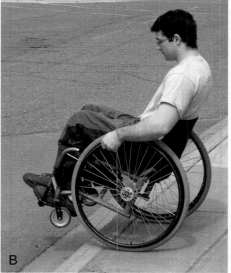

FIG. 20-7 Patient with complete T10 paraplegia ascending and descending a curb.

these patterns. The presence of CPGs contributing to a variety of movements is well established in a number of vertebrates other than humans, and evidence from these animals suggests that repetitive motor training may provide sufficient input to modify or enhance CPG motor output.[80-84] While the presence and exact function of CPGs in humans is more controversial, studies have shown that individuals with complete and incomplete SCI can produce locomotor-type movements and EMG patterns when LE stepping movements are assisted externally to provide appropriate sensory cues to the spinal cord.[85-87]

The evidence supporting the existence of human CPGs has led to the development of a number of interventions aimed at using these neural pathways to produce locomotor movement in patients with SCI. This is generally done by suspending the individual above a treadmill with a harness connected to a device that allows a portion of the person's body weight to be lifted off of their feet. As the treadmill starts to move, the LEs are passively moved or electrically stimulated to produce a stepping pattern that is as kinematically correct as possible. Over time, the repetitive stepping practice results in greater spontaneous stepping and the amount of body weight suspended and the amount of assistance provided are decreased as tolerated. The goal of this intervention is to maximize the use-dependent plasticity of the spinal neural networks to increase the effectiveness of ambulation. There are many studies and treatment protocols in this area, some of which demonstrate positive outcomes. In addition to the physical and functional benefits, locomotor training has been associated with psychological gains, including increased confidence, self-esteem, hope, and quality of life in patients with SCI.

Gait Training with Bilateral Knee-Ankle-Foot Orthosis. In patients with complete SCI or incomplete SCI without functional ambulation skill, interventions may include bracing accompanied by instruction in alternative gait patterns. The most commonly taught pattern is a 2-point swing-through pattern with the use of forearm crutches and bilateral knee-ankle-foot orthoses (KAFOs) with the knee joints locked in extension and the ankles locked in slight dorsiflexion. To utilize this technique effectively, individuals must have normal UE function with excellent strength and endurance and preferably some preservation of active trunk control (T8 and below). They must also have full passive hip extension, ankle dorsiflexion, and lumbar extension ROM.

The most efficient KAFO gait sequence is as follows (Fig. 20-8):

1. Momentary balance is achieved by extending the hips and trunk with weight shifted forward over the ball of the foot and arms extended with the crutch tips behind the position of the feet. In this position the locked ankle of the brace is providing the forward stability.
2. Both crutches are lifted and extended forward simultaneously, and weight is transferred to the crutches in a forward falling motion.
3. Full weight is then borne on the UEs while both legs are lifted and simultaneously swung through to a point in front of the crutch tips.

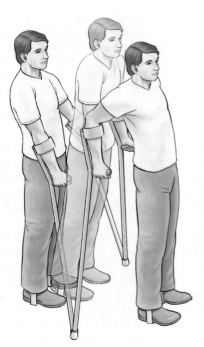

FIG. 20-8 Gait with bilateral knee-ankle-foot orthoses.

4. A forceful push on the crutches is used at the same time the trunk is extended to push the hips forward into extension and achieve the balance position noted in item 1.

Repetition of this momentary balance followed by forward "fall" creates the gait sequence. Although this sequence can be mastered by some individuals, the energy demand is so high, the burden on the UE joints so great, and the risk of loss of balance so significant that most people choose to use a wheelchair as their primary means of locomotion. Mobility with the KAFOs is then reserved for spaces that are too small to accommodate a wheelchair (e.g., bus or plane aisles), for short distance mobility, or for doing ADLs that require short periods of standing (e.g., reaching objects from overhead cabinets).

Functional Training in Self-Care and Home Management

Mobility Skills. The limited use of multiple muscle groups after SCI requires that the patient use alternative methods for performing mobility skills. Unlike many other physical therapy applications in which the patient is trying to return to a previously known movement pattern, many patients with SCI will need to learn new and different ways of performing everyday movements. For many individuals with SCI the rehabilitation process will involve the slow and difficult process of learning to use the UEs to compensate for absent or weak LE movement. The PT performs a key role in helping the individual to discover the most effective and efficient means of mobility according to their particular pattern of movement preservation.

What follows is a description of several functional postures that are key to mobility and ADLs, with training techniques that can be used to increase control within the

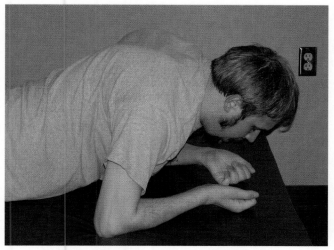

FIG. 20-9 Individual with complete C5 tetraplegia in the prone-on-elbows position. Note the scapular winging indicating poor innervation of the serratus anterior muscles and the wide base of support used for lateral stability.

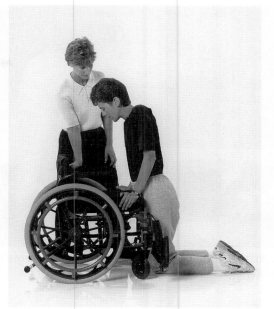

FIG. 20-10 Tall-kneeling position. *From Martin ST, Kessler M: Neurological interventions for physical therapy, ed 2, Edinburgh, 2006, Saunders.*

postures and techniques that can be taught to help with transitions between these functional postures.

Basic Postures

Prone on Elbows. The prone-on-elbows posture is useful for bed positioning, rolling, and progressing to sitting positions. This position also relieves pressure from posterior structures after periods of sitting or lying supine and stretches anterior hip muscles at the hips and trunk that can easily become shortened with prolonged sitting. The prone-on-elbows position is a very stable position with a large base of support that is used extensively during the rehabilitation process to improve all levels of motor control (mobility, stability, controlled mobility, and skill) in partial weight bearing at the shoulder in preparation for full UE weight-bearing activities like transfers. One precaution to consider for this position is whether the individual has sufficient lordosis to comfortably achieve the position. This position should be avoided in individuals with extremely unstable shoulder joints that may be traumatized by even partial weight bearing.

Push-ups in the prone-on-elbows position (Fig. 20-9) emphasize strengthening of the serratus anterior and anterior shoulder muscles and eccentric control of scapular musculature. These are vital points of control for progressing independence with functional mobility. Individuals with weak or absent (above C6 level) serratus anterior function will have marked winging of the scapulae during prone-on-elbows push-ups.

Progression through the stages of motor control in the prone-on-elbows position may be facilitated with combinations of various activities, including:

1. Mobility—Assuming the prone-on-elbows position from sidelying or prone, push-ups.
2. Stability—Weight bearing in the position, manually applied joint approximation, alternating isometrics in multiple directions, and rhythmic stabilization.
3. Controlled mobility—Controlled anterior-posterior and side-to-side weight shifts, push-ups (on elbows or

onto hands), unilaterally supporting on one arm while unweighting and/or reaching with the other (static dynamic movement).
4. Skill—"Walking" on the elbows side to side and forward and back (commando type movements).

Supine on Elbows. The supine-on-elbows position is primarily used to increase flexibility and mobility at the shoulder and in preparation for moving from supine to long sitting. Similar to the prone-on-elbows position to enhance motor control, activities like weight shifting, stability activities, and side-to-side movements may be practiced in this position. The process of assuming the supine-on-elbows position is described in the section on transitioning from supine to long sit.

Quadruped and Tall Kneeling. The quadruped and tall-kneeling positions function as progressions from the positions noted previously. In most cases, patients in the tall-kneeling position will use UE support on a table or bolster to assist in maintaining upright trunk posture (Fig. 20-10).

For individuals with tetraplegia and high paraplegia, these positions are useful for practicing motor control in partial weight bearing through the entire UE with the elbow maintained in extension. Individuals without triceps control will need the therapist's assistance to keep the elbows extended when in the quadruped or tall-kneeling position. A therapy ball or large bolster may also be placed under the trunk to give support during quadruped activities. Tall kneeling is used most often with individuals who have partial preservation of trunk function and who can use their UEs to control movement through a support surface.

Individuals with complete lower paraplegia or with incomplete injuries at any level may be put in these postures to challenge trunk, pelvic, and LE control in preparation for activities requiring upright balance and control in

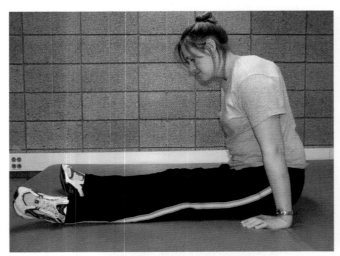

FIG. 20-11 Individual with incomplete C7 tetraplegia in the long-sitting position with head forward for balance.

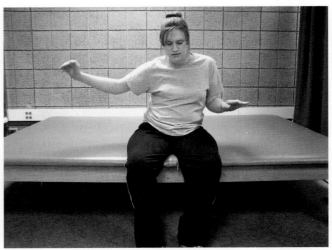

FIG. 20-12 Individual with a C7 incomplete spinal cord injury using her head and arms to compensate for limited balance during static short sitting without upper extremity support. Note the scoliotic collapse of her trunk.

sitting and standing. The quadruped position may be assumed from prone on elbows or from side sitting; both provide a significant challenge at the mobility level of motor control. The kneeling position is assumed from quadruped, generally using UEs for assist. Once in kneeling the individual is encouraged to find a balance position with hips and trunk extended and weight bearing on arms minimized. Once either of these positions is achieved, isometric and dynamic activities can be added to challenge the individual's skills at progressive levels of motor control.

Long Sitting. Long sitting is the primary position used during dressing and other ADLs, especially for individuals without trunk or full UE control (Fig. 20-11). Long sitting is also a stable position for practicing and progressing associated skills. Stability is provided by the large base of support and by the taut hamstring muscles holding the pelvis in a stable midway position. It is important that hamstring length is not too short, which would pull the pelvis into a posterior pelvic tilt, nor too long, which would allow the pelvis to fall into an anterior tilt. Either of these would be less stable than a midway position. Ideally, hamstring length should allow approximately 100 degrees of passive straight leg raise.

Activities in long sitting would be similar to those practiced in the prone-on-elbows position. Push-ups in this position help with strength and allow practice in preparation for mastering transfer skills. This position also allows practice of static and dynamic balance activities with bilateral or unilateral UE support, or without arm support. The patient should learn to transition from a supported position with the hands in front of the hips, to a position with the hands behind the hips with the upper body supported on the extended arms. This transition requires the ability to maintain balance briefly without UE support. For individuals with trunk muscle innervation, long sitting is a good position to begin trunk strengthening and practice of static and dynamic control.

Short Sitting. The ability to maintain balance and move in the short-sit position is crucial for independence with transfers, mat or bed mobility, and some ADLs and to have the arms free for functional activities. Most patients with SCI at or below the C5 level can find a position in short sitting where they can maintain static balance without UE support and have some degree of dynamic balance in this position with UE weight bearing. It is important during sitting activities that the feet are supported with hips and knees near 90-degree angles to allow partial weight to be borne on the feet to stabilize the lower body. It is also essential for patients with cervical injuries that the hands are positioned with fingers flexed when weight bearing on the UEs in sitting to avoid overstretching the long finger flexors and weakening the possible tenodesis grip.

The amount of preservation of active movement will determine what postures and compensatory balance strategies must be used to function in the short-sitting position. Patients with low thoracic injury levels should be able to achieve a fairly upright static posture with little or no posterior pelvic tilt. Dynamic movements will be possible in a small "cone of stability," with movements of the head, shoulder, and arms used to create and control weight shifting. Moving much beyond the base of support will require support on at least one UE. Patients with high thoracic or lower cervical injuries will most often maintain static balance with a combination of posterior pelvic tilt, trunk flexion, and forward head position. In this position, they may be able to unload one or both UEs for brief periods of time with compensatory movements of head and UEs (Fig. 20-12), but their stability remains poor and almost any dynamic movement in the seated position will require use of one or both UEs for weight bearing to increase the base of support.

As with long sitting, patients should learn to transition from a forward-propped position (hands in front of hips), to a backward-lean position (hands and shoulders behind hips) in short sitting. To maintain elbow extension in these weight-bearing positions, individuals without triceps function will need to mechanically lock the elbows by positioning the extremity in shoulder external rotation with the hand in a fixed position distally. This posture moves the elbow joint in front of the line of force through the UE and passively maintains the elbow in extension. During a forward lean with hands fixed, the anterior deltoid and the clavicular head of the pectoralis major can also be used to draw the humerus into adduction, thus creating a push-up motion that moves the extremity toward extension at the elbow.

The same sequence of activities used in the prone-on-elbows position to move through the stages of motor control may be used in the short-sitting position. It is particularly important that the patient master a push-up from the short-sitting position sufficient to clear the buttocks from the seating surface as this is required for scooting and transfer activities. This skill is performed by locking the elbows in extension, using the fixed shoulders and scapulae as a fulcrum, then leaning the head forward and lifting the trunk and pelvis, using scapular depressors (lower trapezius muscles among others) and any available trunk musculature. The mechanics of this motion are contrary to the "normal" use of the scapular depressors in which the pelvis and trunk are fixed and concentric contraction draws the scapulae down relative to the trunk. In this case, the scapulae are fixed and concentric contraction of the depressors draws the trunk and pelvis upward relative to the scapulae.[88] Mastery of this skill requires much practice as it requires high levels of strength, endurance, and motor control.

Transitioning Between Positions

Rolling. Rolling is taught early in rehabilitation because it is essential for many ADLs (e.g., dressing), for independence in bed mobility and bed positioning, and is a building block for other mobility skills (e.g., moving from supine to sitting). Initial training for rolling is performed on a treatment mat, but the patient must be able to perform this skill on a bed for it to be functional. Whenever possible, rolling is taught without the use of assistive devices such as bed rails, webbing loops, or an over-bed trapeze. However, some individuals with complete cervical injuries may need assistive devices to perform this skill independently.

Moving from supine to sidelying requires a coordinated sequence of movements. Most people will use slight variations of the following (Fig. 20-13):

1. The arms are extended over the chest as far as possible. For individuals without triceps, the hands may be pressed together or the arms lowered slightly toward the hips to allow gravity to help maintain as much elbow extension as possible.
2. Both arms are rocked from side to side in a symmetrical pattern to generate momentum.
3. Flexion and rotation of the head are combined with the arm motion to help move the upper body in the desired direction.
4. Once momentum is gained with the rocking motions of the arm and head, a single forceful rock is used to start the turn, followed by reaching as far as possible with the upper arm, protracting the

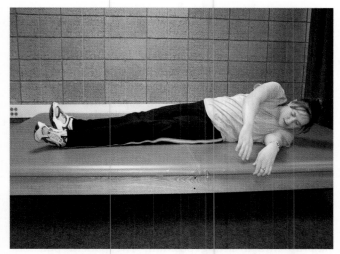

FIG. 20-13 Individual with a C7 incomplete spinal cord injury rolling from supine to sidelying using her head and upper extremity reach to turn her upper body.

shoulder, elongating the trunk, and turning the head to rotate the upper body toward prone.
5. The lower body passively follows the upper body into the rotated position.
6. The patient returns to supine by reaching back with the upper arm and turning the head in the desired direction of movement, thus rotating the upper trunk toward supine. Horizontal abduction of the lower shoulder can assist this motion. Once the upper body has rolled past midline, the lower body will follow because of gravity. If needed, the UEs and head can be rocked or forcefully "thrown" in the direction of movement to further turn the upper body to help complete the lower body roll.

During early training, rolling can be made easier in several ways. The roll may be started from a partially turned position rather than from full supine. The LEs may be crossed passively before starting the roll to partially tilt the pelvis and help move the lower body. For individuals without triceps function, air splints may be used to maintain elbow extension and increase the lever arm of the UE rocking motion. With elbows extended, weights may be added at the wrist to increase the momentum of the rocking motion. The entire mat table may be propped up on one side to tilt the table in the desired direction to allow gravity to further assist with the roll. The therapist may also provide help with the reaching motion in step 4 or help the pelvis to turn to complete the roll. These same techniques may be reversed to further challenge the skill after it has been mastered: Tilting the mat table so the roll is performed uphill, partially flexing the UEs to shorten the lever arm of the rocking motion, providing some manual resistance to the roll at the shoulders or pelvis.

Suggested exercises that may be used to practice components of this activity include bilateral symmetrical UE PNF patterns, incorporating inspiration and expiration with the rhythmic rocking and reaching motions, and strengthening exercises for the serratus anterior and pectoral muscles to facilitate the reach and trunk elongation required to complete the roll.

Supine to Long Sitting Transition. Being able to come to a sitting position from supine assists with ADLs, bed mobility, and preparation for transfers. Several techniques may be used to achieve this skill, depending on the functional muscle groups available. The selected techniques will depend most on whether the triceps muscles and the abdominal muscles are functioning.

Individuals without good triceps or abdominal muscle function generally use their biceps and assistive devices to move from supine to sitting. Bed rails of various heights and sizes can be used to provide leverage for maneuvering. Some individuals may use a series of webbing loops attached to the foot of the bed (a webbing "ladder") to pull up into a sitting position. The patient puts one forearm through a loop of the ladder, contracts the biceps to partially raise the body, then puts the other arm through the next loop, and pulls further forward. This is repeated, using successive loops, until the body is in the upright long-sitting position.

A technique commonly used for moving from supine to long sitting consists of rolling to the side and then "walking" the upper trunk around on the elbows until the sitting position is achieved. Again, each individual will vary the technique slightly, but the primary steps are as follows (Fig. 20-14):

1. Roll toward prone as described (Fig. 20-14, *A*).
2. Move from sidelying or three-quarters prone to partial prone lying on elbows. This is a difficult maneuver that usually combines shoulder abduction and depression of the lower arm with horizontal adduction of the upper arm to lever into the on-elbows position (Fig. 20-14, *B*). Functional use of triceps enables a push-up motion onto elbows or directly onto the hands with the elbows extended (note: the hands are positioned with fingers flexed when weight bearing on the UEs in sitting to avoid overstretching the long finger flexors and weakening the possible tenodesis grip).
3. The upper body is "walked" on elbows toward the legs. As the legs are approached, it may be possible to use the upper arm to pull on the hips or legs to bring the upper body further toward the legs (Fig. 20-14, *C*).
4. Transition from on-elbows position to on-hands position. Without triceps, this involves a push-up motion using pectoral muscles proximally with hands fixed distally (Fig. 20-14, *D*), or "hooking" the legs with the upper arm, pulling with biceps sufficiently to unload the lower arm, which is then quickly repositioned in the extended position. With triceps, this maneuver can be achieved with a traditional push-up maneuver.
5. The upper body is then walked around, alternately weight bearing on extended UEs until a balanced long-sitting position is achieved (Fig. 20-14, *E* and *F*).

For individuals with paraplegia or lower cervical tetraplegia, alternative techniques for coming to long sitting are also possible. One possible sequence is as follows (Fig. 20-15):

1. In supine, the hands are caught under the hips and elbow flexion and neck flexion are used to pull up into a position of supine on elbows (Fig. 20-15, *A1*). Alternately, the move is begun from sidelying, with the upper arm rapidly extended at the shoulder with the elbow flexed as the body rolls toward supine to "catch" the weight on that elbow (Fig. 20-15, *A2*). Head lean and rocking of the shoulders are then used to shift the weight onto one elbow while the other shoulder is extended and the flexed elbow is positioned for weight bearing (Fig. 20-15, *B*).
2. Body weight is shifted to one elbow with head and upper body lean while the other arm is fully extended at the shoulder (with the momentum of the shoulder movement used to create elbow extension in the absence of strong triceps), and the hand is then planted on the mat with elbow extended. This requires good strength and flexibility of the shoulder girdle (Fig. 20-15, *C*).
3. Weight is then shifted onto the arm in extension with a combined rocking and leaning motion until the original support arm is unweighted and can also be reached back into the extended position (Fig. 20-15, *D*)
4. From the position of supporting on extended arms, the upper body is moved forward by leaning the head forward, alternate side shifting, and slow forward movements of the hands until a balanced long-sitting position is achieved (Fig. 20-15, *E*).

This technique may also be used by some higher level tetraplegics with exceptional balance and proximal UE control.

For patients with at least partial control of the abdominal muscles, a head and trunk curl motion can be used to initiate coming to sitting and then augmented as needed by pushing up with the UEs. With fully intact abdominal muscles, patients with lower paraplegia may be able to perform a traditional sit-up, although they may need to use their UEs for assistance because the LE muscles will not be able to stabilize the pelvis.

Exercises that may be used to practice components of this activity include PNF mobility and controlled mobility techniques while in supine on elbows, partially prone on elbows, or in long sitting with weight on extended arms; static and dynamic balance activities in long sitting; biceps curls in the supine position; and push-ups and partial push-ups in prone, long sitting, or short sitting.

Transitioning from Short Sitting to Long Sitting to Supine. When transferring from a wheelchair to lying down, the individual generally goes from sitting in the wheelchair to short sitting on another surface, then getting the legs on to the new surface and ultimately moving into a supine position. These transitions require good balance and coordination, as well as sufficient hamstring length. LE and/or trunk spasticity can interfere with these transitions.

Individuals with midcervical tetraplegia can use the following steps to bring their legs up onto the bed, moving from short sitting to long sitting. In this example the individual is turned to his or her right (Fig. 20-16):

1. In the short-sitting position, scoot as far back as possible on the seating surface (at least until the

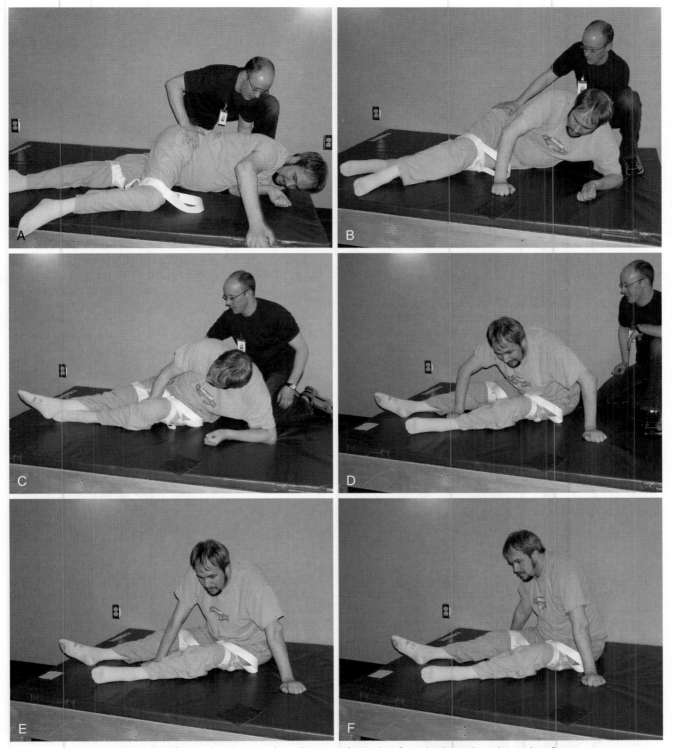

FIG. 20-14 Individual with complete C5 tetraplegia (no functioning triceps) moving from supine to long sitting using the sidelying "walk-around" technique.

popliteal fossa contacts the edge) and partially turn the upper body toward the end of the bed where the feet will ultimately be positioned.

2. Support on the lead (right) arm while using the trailing (left) arm to begin lifting the right leg onto the mat (Fig. 20-16, *A*). For individuals without grasp function, the wrist or the forearm is hooked under the leg to lift it, or the leg is lifted with a webbing

leg loop secured around the distal thigh (an example of a leg loop is shown in Fig. 20-14). At this point, it may be necessary to drop onto the elbow of the lead arm to gain enough stability and leverage to lift the weight of the leg (Fig. 20-16, *B*).

3. Once the lead leg is securely on the mat, the body may be scooted sideways, further onto the mat, using a partial long-sit push-up technique or if

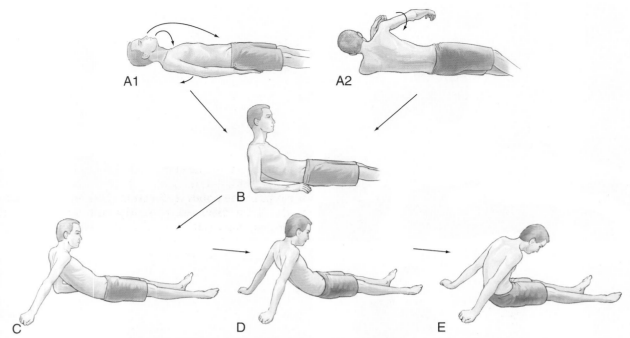

FIG. 20-15 Moving from supine to long sitting using a supine on elbows technique; for individuals with paraplegia or lower cervical tetraplegia.

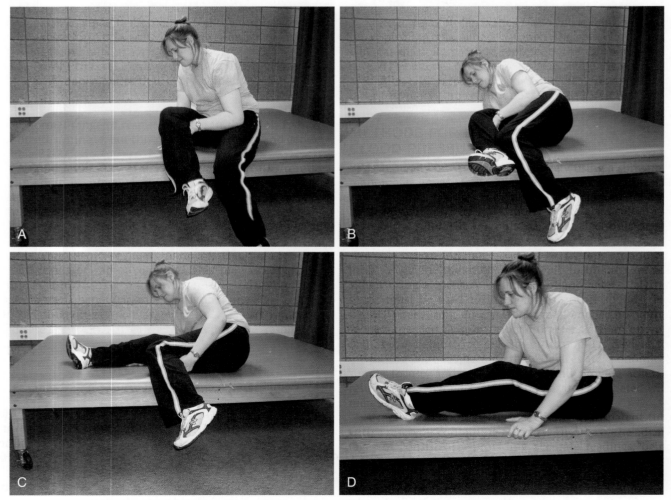

FIG. 20-16 Individual with incomplete C7 tetraplegia moving from short sitting to long sitting.

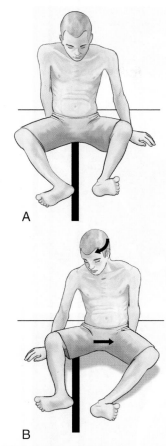

A

B

FIG. 20-17 Seated scooting. Note the use of the head-hips relationship.

propped on elbow in step 2, by pulling the body on the elbows in commando fashion.

4. The second leg is then lifted onto the mat using a similar technique as the first, the legs are then straightened into extension, and balance achieved in long sitting (Fig. 20-16, *C* and *D*).

5. Any of the supine to long-sitting techniques described earlier can be reversed to complete the transition to supine (lean to side and "walk" around on elbows, extend arms behind body, and flex elbows into supine-on-elbows position).

Seated Scooting. The ability to move from side to side in the seated position improves functional capabilities in transfers and bed mobility. Scooting can be performed with similar techniques in the long-sitting and the short-sitting position (Fig. 20-17):

1. Weight is supported on extended UEs with one arm positioned next to the body, and the arm on the lead side (desired direction of movement) abducted to place the hand a small distance from the hip.

2. A push-up is performed with the head lowered and leaned forward as described in the short-sitting section above (Fig. 20-17, *A*).

3. Once the hips are off the mat the head is rotated to the side away from the desired direction of move-

ment, and the hips are twisted in the desired direction (Fig. 20-17, *B*).

4. The hips are then lowered to the mat and the arms repositioned to attain a balanced position.

5. Weight bearing is shifted to the lead arm, and the following arm is used to pull the legs toward the lead arm and back into alignment with the pelvis. Patients without good grip may use webbing leg loops to help control the LEs.

During these actions, the head is always moving in the opposite direction from the hips around a pivot point at the shoulders; the head is lowered and brought forward to raise the hips, and the head is moved to the side to move the hips in the opposite direction. This principle is known as the **head-hips relationship** and is frequently used during mobility skills involving UE weight bearing.

Transfers. Transitioning from one surface to another (e.g., from a wheelchair to bed) requires combinations of the mobility, balance, and motor control developed in the postures and movement sequences described previously. The basic sequence of the transfer is similar in most circumstances, although the individual's pattern of motor preservation, body proportions, endurance, and personal preferences will determine the exact technique used for various transfer situations. In all situations, the following general guidelines should be observed during transfers:

1. The buttocks should be lifted and not dragged between surfaces. If the individual cannot do this alone, manual assistance should be provided and/or a sliding board or similar device should be used to minimize shear forces during scooting.

2. The environment should be arranged before transferring to allow the most level, controlled transfer possible.

3. Use of momentum for movement should be minimized, with emphasis placed on slow, controlled movements.

4. Early in transfer training, just enough assistance and instruction should be provided to allow for successful performance of the skill. It is important that the individual accomplish the task as independently as possible so that they gain a sense of independence and control.

The transfer is generally begun by positioning the transfer surfaces. When transferring from the wheelchair, the chair is generally positioned at a 30- to 45-degree angle to the mat table (or other surface). This allows the patient to stay in front of the wheelchair wheel during the transfer. The feet are then positioned in preparation for the transfer; with rigid frame chairs, one or both feet may be left on the foot plate and turned slightly in the direction of the transfer; with folding frame chairs, the footrests are usually removed and the feet placed flat on the floor, and for individuals with poor balance control the feet may be lifted onto the mat to put the individual in a more stable long-sit position before beginning the scooting portion of the transfer. The pelvis is then moved forward slightly in the chair to bring the hips closer to the transfer surface, to move the hips anterior to the wheelchair wheel, and to put some weight through the LEs (Fig. 20-18, *A*).

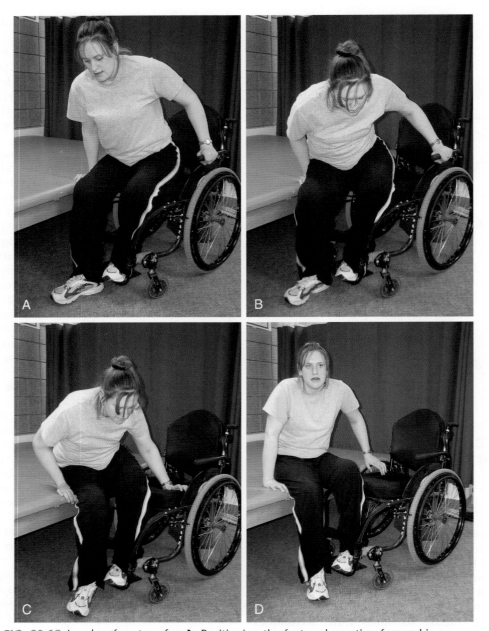

FIG. 20-18 Level surface transfer. **A,** Positioning the feet and scooting forward in preparation for the transfer. **B,** Leaning forward and lifting the hips during initial scooting. **C,** Repositioning the hands and trunk for the next scoot. **D,** Hips securely on the transfer surface and balance regained. Note that the feet have not yet been repositioned after the transfer.

Tetraplegic patients often achieve this forward scooting by twisting the head and upper body with one arm hooked around the push handle of the wheelchair and then repeating this technique on the other side.

If a sliding board is required (generally for individuals with midcervical SCI without triceps or during initial training for patients with lower level injuries), the board is placed under the midthigh of the lead leg and angled toward the ischial tuberosity on the opposite side. The individual then leans the head forward, performs a push-up, lifts the hips, and pivots the head away from the transfer surface, thus using the head-hips relationship to swing the hips toward the transfer surface (Fig. 20-18, *B*). The hips are lowered, balance is regained, and hands repositioned (Fig. 20-18, *C*), and then the sequence is repeated until the hips are securely positioned on the transfer surface (Fig. 20-18, *D*). The legs may be repositioned after each scoot, if needed for balance, or they may be left to trail the body and repositioned after the final sitting position is achieved. Variations on this basic technique are used for transfers to a bathtub bench, toilet, car, or any other relatively level surface.

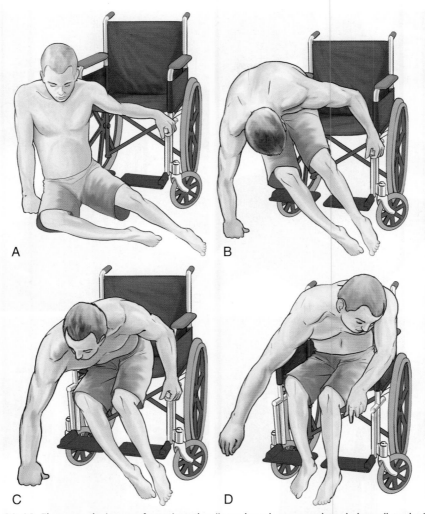

FIG. 20-19 Floor to chair transfer using the "one hand up, one hand down" technique.

Patients with high cervical level injuries will be physically dependent for transfers but should become independent in directing the required assistance before they are discharged from rehabilitation. A mechanical lift can be used to transfer a patient in the hospital or in the modified home setting. A mechanical lift, although cumbersome at times, reduces the long-term strain on caregivers who have to repeatedly lift and move an individual. When a mechanical lift is impractical, a pivot transfer with a sliding board and assistance by one or two people is generally used. Note that it is still important that the person being transferred has his or her feet on the floor, if possible, to allow partial weight bearing through the legs (which are braced by the assistant's legs) and reduce the lift required during the transfer. The head-hips relationship should also be employed; the individual being transferred has his or her head and upper trunk turning away from the transfer surface and hips moving toward the transfer surface. In this case, the weight-bearing pivot point for the head-hips relationship is the feet of the individual being transferred. Care must be taken to avoid pulling on the UEs during assisted transfers to avoid straining unstable shoulder joints.

Transferring from the floor into the wheelchair is an advanced skill that is mastered only after the individual has mastered level surface transfers and developed considerable strength, flexibility, and coordination. Variations on a few basic techniques are used to accomplish this skill. The first technique begins with the individual positioned next to and approximately parallel to the front edge of the wheelchair. The lead hand is placed on the wheelchair seat, and the other hand is placed next to the hip (Fig. 20-19, *A*). The legs may be flexed up and held in place by leaning into them with the head and shoulders, or they may be left straight during the transfer. The individual then leans the head as far forward as possible and pushes with the arms to raise their hips to the edge of the wheelchair seat (Fig. 20-19, *B* and *C*). Once the lead hip is securely on the seat, a series of small lifts and scoots may be used to bring both hips firmly onto the seating surface. The trunk is brought into the upright position by pushing up with the arms on the front of the wheelchair frame or seat (Fig. 20-19, *D*). This skill can be made easier by removing the wheelchair cushion from the chair (effectively reducing the height required with the lift) and using it under the hips on the floor (effectively raising the floor

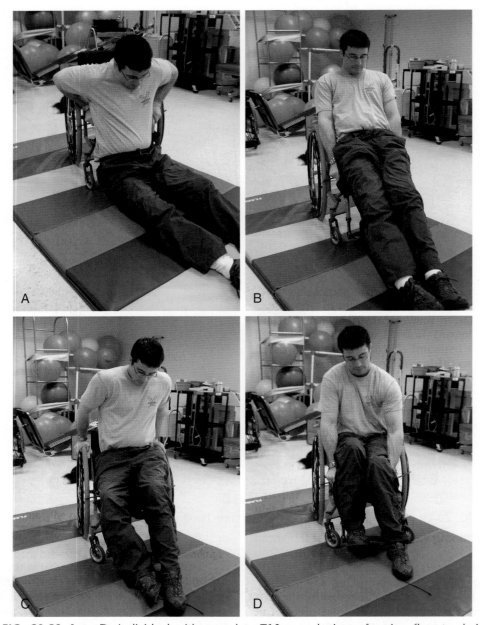

FIG. 20-20 **A** to **D,** Individual with complete T10 paraplegia performing floor-to-chair transfer using the back push-up technique. Note spasticity producing extension of the trunk and lower extremities in **B.**

surface and further reducing the lift required). The skill may also be trained or simplified by using intermediate height surfaces to break up the task.

Another technique for moving from the floor to a chair is to use a front push-up from an intermediate quadruped position. The knees are positioned by the front of the wheelchair and the individual pulls himself or herself up on the chair until his or her weight is distributed on the knees on the floor and on the chest resting on the seat of the chair. A push-up is then performed with the hands on the wheelchair seat until the hips clear the edge of the chair. The individual then twists and pivots the trunk to move the lead hip onto the seating surface. The hands are then repositioned, and additional push-ups are performed

to bring the hips fully into the seated position. Because of the large twisting motion required by this technique, it is most effectively used by an individual with some degree of active trunk control.

Another option is to use a back push-up (Fig. 20-20). The individual begins in sitting with his or her back to the chair seat and reaches back and up with both arms until the hands are on the top of the wheelchair frame or the front edge of the seat. A push-up is then performed to lift the body into the chair. This technique requires a lot of strength in a mechanically disadvantageous position of extreme shoulder extension and elevation.

Although some individuals with SCI will master independent floor transfers, all patients with SCI should be independent in directing others to safely and effectively move them from the floor to a chair. This should be practiced in the rehabilitation setting so that when the individual either intentionally or accidentally finds themselves on the floor or ground, they are not intimidated by the circumstances and can be in control of safely returning to the wheelchair.

Functional Training in Leisure Integration or Reintegration. Advances in wheelchair and other adaptive device technology have made many leisure and recreational opportunities open to individuals with SCI. Sports like tennis, basketball, and quad rugby draw many participants and have competitions at every level from local to international. Recreational activities like snow skiing and water skiing may also be enjoyed by individuals with all levels of mobility. Specific competitions and team events have been developed for individuals using power wheelchair mobility. Therapists can assist in preparation for these activities by providing assessment for adaptive devices, training in activity-specific mobility skills, strength building and conditioning, and education about injury prevention and management. Referral should also be made to school, community, state, and national programs that can provide information and assistance that allow individuals to pursue areas of interest.

CASE STUDY 20-1

COMPLETE SPINAL CORD INJURY AT T10

Patient History

JD is a 20-year-old student who was involved in an MVA 22 days ago. He was admitted to the trauma center with a fracture and complete SCI at the level of T10. He sustained fractures of his ninth, tenth, and eleventh ribs on the right. He was initially immobilized in a thoracolumbosacral orthosis (TLSO) of a plastic body-jacket style. He underwent spinal stabilization surgery. His hospital stay was complicated by pneumonia with decreased secretion clearance. Acute therapies involved ROM, positioning in bed and transitioning to sitting, patient and family education, and active breathing exercises. JD was unable to tolerate assisted coughing or manual facilitation for respiration because of pain from soft tissue bruising and rib fractures. JD used the TLSO at all times when out of bed and no brace when in bed per his physician's instructions. After 3 weeks in the hospital, the pneumonia was resolving and JD was considered medically stable and appropriate for further rehabilitation in an inpatient rehabilitation center.

Tests and Measures—Significant Findings
Musculoskeletal
- Active ROM in both UEs was grossly within normal limits. LE PROM was within normal limits except dorsiflexion was not measured in the end-range of hip flexion and straight leg raise was not tested because of JD's recent spine surgery.
- Strength throughout both UEs was greater than or equal to 4/5 on MMT. JD had no active movement or visible

contractions in either LE (0/5). LEs are hypotonic throughout.

Neuromuscular
- JD reported some back pain around the surgical site. Rib pain was present at all times (2/10 at rest) and increased with deep breathing, moving, and donning the TLSO (8/10 at worst). Oral medications were being used for pain, with pain remaining less than or equal to 3/10 during mobility with the medications.

Cardiovascular/Pulmonary
- JD was short of breath during wheelchair propulsion and practice of mobility skills.
- JD's vital capacity was 40% lower than normal for a person of his age and height.

Function
- JD could propel his wheelchair independently on smooth, level surfaces for 50 feet. Sitting at the edge of a treatment mat, JD could maintain his balance statically with bilateral UE support with stand-by assistance. He was unable to maintain sitting balance without using his UEs, and he had poor dynamic balance.
- He had been using an overhead trapeze for mobility in bed but was trying to wean off of this device. The bed JD was using had a pressure-relieving overlay.
- He used a long-handled reacher and a leg loop for ADL skills and an incentive spirometer to encourage deep breathing.
- JD required maximal assistance from one person and a sliding board to transfer between level surfaces. He required moderate assistance from one person for all bed mobility.
- JD was dependent for all ADLs except feeding himself independently after he, his food, and utensils had been set-up.
- JD was incontinent of bowel and bladder. His indwelling catheter had been removed, and he was started on an intermittent catheterization program that he was learning to perform himself. He was on an every-other-day bowel elimination program.

Diagnosis
Preferred practice pattern 5H: Impaired motor function, peripheral nerve integrity, and sensory integrity associated with nonprogressive disorders of the spinal cord.

Interventions
- Skin care training, including pressure relief techniques, bed and wheelchair positioning, and skin protection during mobility skills. Instruction to turn every 2 hours in bed and to perform a pressure relief technique for 2 out of every 15 minutes of sitting.
- Respiratory training (incentive spirometry, ventilatory muscle training). Breathing techniques education and practice, cardiovascular conditioning, and positioning for postural drainage.
- Mobility skills training in the use of his wheelchair, mobility in bed, training in sitting balance, and transfer training. Training should include level and uneven

surfaces and on ramps and stairs (with assistance as needed).
- Training for ADL and IADL skills required in dressing, bathing, and toileting and utilizing adapted equipment and performing household and community level tasks.
- Flexibility exercises and training in self-ROM activities for the LEs. In addition, muscle strength and endurance training should be performed with an emphasis on the shoulder and scapular muscles utilized during mobility skills.
- Gait training is initiated with standing in a standing frame for building tolerance to being in an upright position and to maintain ROM. Gait training should also include body weight–supported locomotor training.
- Integration to community through introduction to wheelchair level sport and recreation activities as part of functional training. JD will be referred to a community organization that provides sport and recreational opportunities for individuals with disabilities.

Role of the Physical Therapist Assistant
- Describe some of the skin care techniques this patient should practice. Why are they important?
- Describe three interventions to improve this patient's aerobic capacity. What are the goals of gait training for this patient?
- List four organizations in your community that would benefit JD.
- Describe three of the transfer techniques JD will need to be independent in by the end of his inpatient rehabilitation stay.

Additional Information

For the full version of this case study, including detailed examination results, interventions, and outcomes, see the Evolve site that accompanies this book. A full case for a patient with **anterior cord syndrome** also appears on the Evolve site.

CHAPTER SUMMARY

SCI alters the function of multiple body systems, including the GI, skeletal, respiratory, cardiovascular, genitourinary, integumentary, musculoskeletal, and neuromuscular systems. Many of these changes require ongoing medical management and changes in an individual's ADLs. Some of the possible systemic effects of SCI, such as pressure ulcers or AD, are potentially life threatening. A careful plan of care developed and administered by a multidisciplinary team of rehabilitation professionals is necessary to manage the acute needs of the SCI patient and provide a rehabilitation process that will prepare the individual to lead a healthy and fulfilling life after injury.

ADDITIONAL RESOURCES

For links to these and additional web-based resources, see the Evolve site.

ASIA Standard Neurological Classification of Spinal Cord Injury Form
American Spinal Injury Association (ASIA)
Paralyzed Veterans of America
Spinal Cord Injury Information Network

GLOSSARY

Anterior cord syndrome: Destruction of the anterior portion of the spinal cord that results in a pattern of impairments characterized by complete loss of motor function and some loss of light touch and temperature sensation, with sparing of proprioception and discriminative touch.

Autonomic dysreflexia (AD): A serious, life-threatening emergency condition that is the result of an uncontrolled autonomic response to a noxious stimulus from either an external or an internal (visceral) source.

Brown-Séquard syndrome: Damage to one-half of the spinal cord, resulting in a pattern of impairments characterized by ipsilateral proprioceptive and motor loss and contralateral loss of pain and temperature sensation.

Cauda equina syndrome: Damage to the lumbar or sacral nerve roots, resulting in sensory loss and flaccid paralysis below the injury level.

Central cord syndrome: Injury to the central portion of the spinal cord, resulting in a pattern of impairments characterized by weakness more severe in UEs than in LEs, with sparing of sacral sensation.

Central pattern generators (CPGs): Neural circuits within the spinal cord that can produce rhythmic neural activity without supraspinal and proprioceptive input.

Head-hips relationship: Descriptive term describing a mechanical principle used during mobility skills; with UE weight bearing, the shoulders act as a fulcrum, and the head and hips move in opposite directions around this point.

Heterotopic ossification (HO): Abnormal bone growth within the extraarticular soft tissues that can result in severe restriction of muscle and joint movement.

Neurological level: The most caudal segment of the spinal cord with normal sensory and motor function on both sides of the body.

Paradoxical breathing: An abnormal breathing pattern common in tetraplegia and occurring occasionally in high paraplegia, in which the abdomen rises and the chest is pulled in on inspiration and the abdomen falls and the chest expands on expiration.

Paraplegia: Loss of function in the thoracic, lumbar, or sacral segments of the spinal cord, resulting in sparing of UE function but possible impairments in the trunk, pelvis, and LEs, depending on the segment of the lesion.

Pressure ulcer: A common complication of SCI characterized by ischemic ulceration of soft tissue as a result of unrelieved pressure and shearing forces.

Quadriplegia: SCI affecting all four extremities; synonym for tetraplegia.

Spasticity: A disorder that can occur below the level of SCI characterized by velocity-dependent hypertonia, resulting from a combination of multiple changes in neural control and muscle properties.

Spinal cord injury (SCI): Damage to the neurological components of the spinal cord as the result of primary or secondary effects of disease or trauma.

Spinal shock: A temporary condition that occurs after acute SCI, characterized by a total loss of sensory, motor, and autonomic control below the level of the lesion.

Tenodesis grip: Use of the passive properties of the long finger flexors to perform grasp functions. With the finger flexors slightly tight, the motion of wrist extension is used to pull the fingers toward the palm in a grasping motion.

Tetraplegia: Loss of function because of damage of the neural elements in the cervical segments of the spinal cord, resulting in impairment or loss of motor and/or sensory function involving the upper extremities, as well as more caudal functions.

Zone of partial preservation (ZPP): Those dermatomes and myotomes caudal to the neurological level that remain partially innervated (in the absence of sacral function) in complete SCI.

Chapter 21

Disorders of Consciousness: Coma, Vegetative State, and Minimally Conscious State

Susan Grieve

OBJECTIVES

After reading this chapter, the reader will be able to:
1. Define and understand the uses of the terms coma, vegetative state, and minimally conscious state.
2. Identify and distinguish between the clinical criteria and characteristics of coma, vegetative state, and minimally conscious state.
3. Understand the pathology causing altered or impaired consciousness.
4. Understand the prognostic indicators for coma, vegetative state, and minimally conscious state and how they affect selection of rehabilitation interventions
5. Identify the clinician's role in educating family and other caregivers to perform passive range of motion, positioning, and skin integrity checks in people with low levels of consciousness.

Over the past two decades, advances in medical technology have reduced mortality from severe medical disease and brain injuries significantly, allowing many people to survive despite being in severely impaired states of **consciousness.** It is predicted that 30% to 40% of survivors of brain injury and approximately 80% of survivors of cardiac arrest will remain in a state of impaired consciousness after medical stabilization.[1,2] Although some of these people regain some degree of consciousness, many have severely limited neurological function and continue to have disorders of consciousness for prolonged periods and often for the rest of their lives. These patients are often admitted to rehabilitation facilities for management by a multidisciplinary rehabilitation team.

Clinical Pearl

Because of advances in medical technology, patients with severe medical disease or brain injuries survive despite severely impaired states of consciousness.

This chapter discusses pathology, typical examination findings, and intervention for patients with disorders of consciousness. For rehabilitation specialists, these disorders most commonly include **coma, vegetative state,** and **minimally conscious state,** resulting from trauma, tumor, stroke, cerebral anoxia, and/or metabolic dysfunction. Coma, vegetative state, and minimally conscious state may be permanent conditions or transient states from which patients may evolve or regress.

The *Guide to Physical Therapist Practice* (the *Guide*) classifies these patients under preferred practice pattern 5I: Impaired arousal, range of motion, and motor control associated with coma, near coma, or vegetative state.[3] The terminology used in this chapter is slightly different from that used in the *Guide* to be more consistent with most of the current literature on states of impaired consciousness. In this chapter, the terms *minimally conscious, coma,* and *vegetative state* are used, whereas the term *near coma* is not. The definitions and diagnostic criteria sections further discuss the use of these terms.

PATHOLOGY

Understanding the pathology of impaired consciousness first requires knowledge of intact or normal consciousness. Consciousness is studied by various disciplines, including neurophysiology, philosophy, psychology, and psychiatry. All agree that the essential components of normal or intact consciousness are arousal and awareness of self and the environment.[4] Arousal, the more primitive element of consciousness, is clinically intact if a person opens his or her eyes either spontaneously or in response to an external stimulus. Arousal requires a functioning ascending **reticular activating system** (ARAS). The ARAS is a diffuse network of nerves located in the upper two-thirds of the brainstem that connects to the thalamus and the cerebral cortex (Fig. 21-1). The ARAS may be activated by somatosensory stimuli, such as touch and sound, or by basic needs, such as hunger or thirst.

Awareness, the more complex component of consciousness, involves not only awareness of self but also awareness of the relationship of self to the environment. The combination of self-awareness and the awareness of one's relationship to the environment requires cerebral functioning and leads to conscious cognitive behavior. Awareness requires cerebral hemisphere function, whereas arousal does not. Arousal requires only a functioning upper brainstem. Arousal can occur without awareness, but awareness is not possible without arousal.

It may be helpful to think of arousal as the light switch and awareness as the light bulb (Fig. 21-2). For consciousness to be normal, a person must have a functioning ARAS in the brainstem (the light switch), functioning cerebral hemispheres (the light bulb), and functioning connections through the thalamus (wiring) to send information between the two. Injuries or medical conditions that affect any of these areas in the central nervous system (CNS) can impair or alter consciousness.

Clinical Pearl

Arousal is intact if a person opens his or her eyes either spontaneously or in response to an external stimulus. Awareness involves both awareness of self and awareness of one's relationship to the environment. Awareness requires brainstem and cerebral hemisphere function; arousal requires only brainstem function.

There are three mechanisms by which the cerebral hemispheres, thalamus, and/or the brainstem may be affected to alter consciousness. The first is a structural lesion caused by conditions such as stroke, tumor, abscess, or trauma. The second results from toxic or metabolic abnormalities, and the third results from diffuse brain insults such as anoxia.[5]

Alterations of consciousness from toxic causes may be a result of excessive intake of substances, such as alcohol or other psychoactive drugs, or a result of poor elimination or toxin production because of kidney or liver dysfunction. In addition, hypoglycemia or severe hyperglycemia may also impair consciousness. Toxic and metabolic abnormalities are the most common nontraumatic causes of impaired consciousness, accounting for 47% of emergency room presentations for "coma of unknown origin."[5] Of these, 55% are caused by alcohol or other drugs. When consciousness is impaired by toxic or metabolic causes, patients typically present clinically with somnolence or **delirium** preceding the state of coma. They generally do not have focal neurological signs such as localized motor or sensory abnormalities.

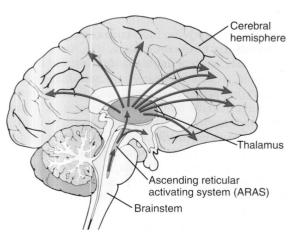

FIG. 21-1 Areas of the brain responsible for consciousness: The ascending reticular activating system in the brainstem and the cerebral hemispheres.

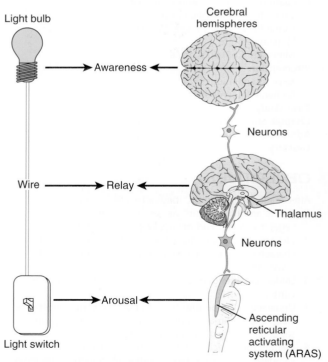

FIG. 21-2 Light bulb and light switch analogy for arousal as it relates to awareness.

Consciousness may also be impaired by diffuse brain damage as the result of subarachnoid hemorrhage, infection, cerebral anoxia secondary to cardiac arrest, or diffuse axonal injury secondary to trauma. Diffuse brain damage is the least common cause of impaired consciousness, accounting for only 4.5% of patients presenting with nontraumatic causes of coma.

After trauma, the two leading causes of coma are toxic/metabolic insults, primarily from drug overdose, and cardiac arrest, causing diffuse global ischemia. Some believe that with increased access to automated defibrillators in public places and a greater public interest in learning basic life support, more people may survive cardiac arrest after prolonged impairment of circulation to all areas, including the brain. This will consequently increase the incidence of "cardiac arrest coma."[2]

Many medical conditions can also cause impaired consciousness and unresponsiveness. Coma can be thought of as the final common pathway in many untreated disease states. The underlying cause of impaired consciousness may give an indication of patient prognosis and be used to guide rehabilitation interventions and family education.

CLINICAL DEFINITIONS AND CRITERIA FOR DIAGNOSIS OF DISORDERS OF CONSCIOUSNESS

One of the problems facing clinicians who care for patients with impaired consciousness is the lack of consistent nomenclature for defining disorders of consciousness. Understanding the criteria for each disorder and the differences among them allows allied health professionals involved in the rehabilitation of patients with impaired consciousness to most accurately determine an individual's expected functional outcome and amount of time needed to achieve that outcome.

COMA

Coma is the neurobehavioral diagnostic term for a patient in a state of "unarousable unawareness." This description was first used by Plum and Posner in their widely referenced text, *The Diagnosis of Stupor and Coma*, first published in 1966. The latest edition (third) published in 1982 expands the description of coma to "the total absence of awareness of self and environment even when the subject is externally stimulated."

> **Clinical Pearl**
>
> *Coma* is the term for a person in a state of unarousable unawareness.

VEGETATIVE STATE

Jennett and Plum first used "persistent vegetative state" in 1972 to label the population of patients who demonstrated "arousal in the absence of awareness."[6] Over the past 10 years, there has been a great deal of discussion and controversy in the medical community regarding the use of the term *persistent* in labeling patients in a vegetative state.[7-9] Many believe that use of the term *persistent* implies

that a patient in this state cannot make any improvements and that the modifier "persistent" adds nothing to the meaning of the diagnosis or prognosis of vegetative state.

Patients in the vegetative state have some activity in the ARAS but lack relay (thalamic) or cerebral function. The vegetative state is defined as a clinical condition of complete unawareness to the self and the environment accompanied by sleep-wake cycles with either complete or partial preservation of hypothalamic and brainstem autonomic functions.[10]

> **Clinical Pearl**
>
> *Vegetative state* is the term for a person who demonstrates arousal in the absence of awareness.

MINIMALLY CONSCIOUS STATE

The term *minimally conscious state* does not appear in the *Guide*[3] but is found in the literature concerning patients in low-level neurological states that cause impaired consciousness. The American Congress of Rehabilitation Medicine first used "minimally responsive state" in 1995 to describe patients who were no longer in a coma or vegetative state but who remained severely disabled. This diagnostic term was recently changed to "minimally conscious state" because patients in a vegetative state have reflex responses, so the term *minimally responsive* fails to clearly distinguish between vegetative state and minimally responsive state. The distinguishing feature between these states is the presence of some cognitive function in the latter state, which is therefore most clearly termed the *minimally conscious state*.[11]

Unlike the criteria for coma or vegetative state in which a patient must meet all of the criteria for a diagnosis, an individual is determined to be in a minimally conscious state if only one or more of the above criteria are met.

> **Clinical Pearl**
>
> *Minimally conscious state* is the term for a person no longer in a coma or vegetative state who remains severely disabled but has some cognitive function.

NEAR COMA

The preferred practice pattern 5I: Impaired arousal, range of motion, and motor control associated with coma, near coma, and vegetative state, included in the *Guide*,[3] includes the term *near coma*. This term appears in the Coma/Near Coma (CNC) scale, as described later, but is not used elsewhere in current literature. The definition of near coma according to the CNC scale is "consistently responsive to stimuli presented to two sensory modalities and/or inconsistently or partially responsive to simple commands."[12] Since the publication of this scale and the *Guide,* the term *near coma* has fallen out of favor. It appears that the diagnostic category "minimally conscious state" is now used to describe patients who were previously described as in near coma. Patients in a minimally conscious state are unconscious but occasionally show signs of consciousness such as tracking with their eyes, reaching for an object when asked, or grabbing for someone's hand. Since the term *near coma* is no longer in current usage in other literature, it is not used in this chapter and has been replaced with the term *minimally conscious state* where relevant.

Other terms used in the medical community to describe decreased levels of alertness but that have not been defined as diagnostic categories are **stupor, somnolent, obtunded,** and delirium.

DIFFERENTIAL DIAGNOSIS OF DISORDERS OF CONSCIOUSNESS

Correct diagnosis of a disorder of consciousness requires not only an understanding of the specific clinical features and behavioral characteristics of each but also an understanding of conditions that can mimic these states. One such condition is **locked-in syndrome.** This syndrome often results from a stroke at the base of the pons in the brainstem. Patients with this condition have a functioning ARAS, as well as normal thalamic and cortical connections, and therefore have intact normal consciousness; however, all motor pathways to the face, trunk, and limbs are lost. Thus these patients are awake and fully aware of their condition and environment but cannot move. Often the ability to blink and move the eyes vertically are spared and become the patient's only means of communicating. Patients with locked-in syndrome are frequently misdiagnosed as being in a persistent vegetative state.[13,14]

◎ *Clinical Pearl*

A person with locked-in syndrome has intact normal consciousness and is cognitively intact but cannot move their face, trunk, or limbs.

Brain death is another term sometimes confused with coma and vegetative state. For a patient to be brain dead, they must meet three neurological criteria: coma, absent brainstem reflexes, and apnea.[15] The concept of brain death was developed in the late 1950s and 1960s, with the advent of intensive care units (ICUs) and sophisticated ventilators that made it possible to maintain respiration in patients with severe irreversible brain injuries. The principal aim of the concept was to facilitate organ transplantation by providing justification for the removal of organs from individuals who were not dead by cardiopulmonary criteria.[16] Before the development of effective ventilators, these patients usually died within minutes because of the irreversible stoppage of respiration and heartbeat. Brain death is considered legally equivalent to death, and although cardiopulmonary function may occasionally be supported for prolonged periods, most patients lose cardiopulmonary function within a few days despite maximal support[17] and there are no documented cases of recovery of any degree of consciousness in patients who meet the criteria for brain death. Given their poor prognosis, patients who are brain dead are not candidates for rehabilitation. Box 21-1 summarizes the major clinical criteria for coma, vegetative state, minimally conscious state, locked-in-syndrome, and brain death.

◎ *Clinical Pearl*

A person who is brain dead is in a coma with absent brainstem reflexes and absence of spontaneous breathing. Brain death is the legal equivalent to death. A brain-dead patient's heart and breathing usually stop within minutes without the support of a ventilator.

BOX 21-1	Clinical Criteria for Coma, Vegetative State, Minimally Conscious State, Locked-In Syndrome, and Brain Death			
Coma	**Vegetative State**	**Minimally Conscious State**	**Locked-In Syndrome**	**Brain Death**
• Eyes do not open spontaneously or to external stimuli. • Does not follow commands. • Does not mouth or utter meaningful words. • Does not demonstrate intentional movement. • Cannot sustain visual pursuit. • Not under the influence of any paralytic agent.	• Eyes open spontaneously. • Sleep-wake cycles present. • No evidence of awareness of self or environment. • Inability to interact with others. • No language comprehension or expression. • No purposeful movement. • No visual pursuit. • Bowel/bladder incontinence. • Variably preserved cranial nerve and spinal reflexes.	• Follows simple commands. • Gestures or verbal yes/no responses. • Intelligible verbalization. • Purposeful behavior not a result of reflex activity. • Minimally conscious state if one or more criteria are met.	• Eyes open spontaneously or in response to external stimulation. • Unable to follow motor commands except eye blink or some vertical eye movement. • Caused by total paralysis below the level of the oculomotor nuclei in the brainstem. • Full awareness of self and the environment. • Able to communicate through eye movement.	• Coma. • Absent brainstem reflexes (pupillary response, corneal, oculocephalic, oculovestibular, and gag). • Apnea. • Completely unresponsive to external visual, auditory, and tactile stimuli. • Incapable of communication in any manner.

EXAMINATION

PATIENT HISTORY

A rehabilitation examination will begin with a thorough patient history. The history will usually focus on the etiology of the disorder, the patient's neurological condition (whether improving or deteriorating and over what timeframe), the nursing notes (information about the patient's current activity level, vital sign stability), and the patient's medications (looking particularly for those that may cause sedation or paralysis). Together, these four elements of the patient history influence the frequency, intensity, and types of rehabilitation interventions best suited for the patient.

SYSTEMS REVIEW

The systems review is used to target areas requiring further examination and to define areas that may cause complications or indicate a need for precautions during the examination and intervention processes. Chapter 1 includes details of the systems review.

Patients with a disorder of consciousness typically undergo a period of bed rest; therefore it is important for clinicians to understand the physiological effects of bed rest on body systems when performing the systems review.

Musculoskeletal. Bed rest has many effects on the musculoskeletal system. Strength loss is greatest during the first week of immobilization, with skeletal muscle strength decreasing by 1% to 1.5% per day with strict bed rest and by 1.3% to 5.5% with cast immobilization.[18] With bed rest, tendons and ligaments also lose strength internally and in their connections to muscle and bone. Bone loss occurs, with the ratio of bone formation to bone resorption decreasing because there is less stress placed on the bones in the gravity-eliminated position. As bed rest continues, bones become less dense and more prone to fracture. Trabecular bone, as found in the neck of the femur, is more susceptible to resorption than cortical bone. Joints also remodel in response to bed rest, with cartilage degenerating, synovium atrophying, and fibrofatty tissue infiltrates appearing.[18]

If the patient's condition is caused by trauma, the clinician should document any fracture sites and any physician-ordered precautions to movement.

◎ *Clinical Pearl*

Skeletal muscle strength decreases by 1% to 1.5% per day during the first week of bed rest and by 1.3% to 5.5% with cast immobilization.

Neuromuscular. The neuromuscular system is carefully examined in this patient group. Patients are observed for abnormal spontaneous or reflexive movement patterns that are common in patients with severe brain damage. A response of upper extremity flexion together with lower extremity extension is known as a *decorticate response*. A response of extension of both the upper and lower extremities is known as a *decerebrate response* and indicates more advanced motor dysfunction, generally caused by deep bilateral cerebral hemispheric lesions or compression of the brainstem. Fig. 21-3 illustrates **decorticate** and **decerebrate posturing.**

A grasp reflex in response to tactile stimulation of the palm is sometimes present, as is trismus or biting down spontaneously or in response to something placed in the mouth. These reflexes may be mistaken for purposeful movement, particularly by family and friends of the patient who may perceive them as a sign of "waking up" or as conscious attempts at hand holding or eating.

Spontaneous ocular movements are also common in patients with disorders of consciousness, specifically roving eye movements from side to side or up and down and blinking at rest or in response to light, sound, or threat. These eye movements do not indicate that the patient is moving toward a higher state of arousal or awareness, but consistent visual tracking is an early indicator of some awareness and resolution of the vegetative state.[10]

Cardiovascular/Pulmonary. Bed rest significantly affects the cardiovascular and pulmonary system. Signs of orthostatic intolerance begin within 3 to 4 days of complete bed rest.[19] Both the central and peripheral components of the system are affected. Centrally, as the heart muscle atrophies, stroke volume decreases and heart rate (HR) increases to maintain cardiac output. This substantially decreases an individual's capacity to respond to increases in physical demand, including changes in position from supine to sitting or standing, as well as exercise. Peripherally, within 3 to 4 weeks of bed rest, blood volume shifts to the thorax. Any change in position from supine causes the volume of blood in the thorax to decrease, decreasing venous return to the heart and reducing cardiac output. This reduction in cardiac output is counteracted by a surge in HR, sometimes by more than 35 beats per minute (bpm), when moving a patient from supine to standing.[20]

Integumentary. The initial examination of the integumentary system also involves systematic observation. The patient should be visually examined from head to toe for any areas of skin breakdown or potential skin

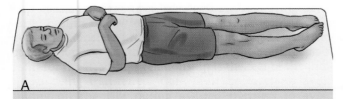
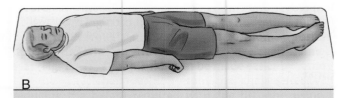

FIG. 21-3 **A,** Decorticate posture. **B,** Decerebrate posture. *From Cameron MH: Physical agents in rehabilitation, ed 3, St. Louis, 2009, Saunders.*

breakdown (see Chapter 28), changes in skin color, and location of dressings. These findings are recorded in the chart.

TESTS AND MEASURES

The final step in the examination of a patient with a disorder of consciousness is performance of specific tests and measures. Tests and measures are administered on initial patient contact and readministered at regular intervals to check for signs of changes in neurological status such as development of new purposeful movement. Initial examination by rehabilitation professionals of patients in a coma, vegetative state, or minimally conscious state commonly takes place in the ICU, where multiple monitoring lines, sedating drugs, and mechanical ventilatory support machines may complicate the examination. In this setting, rehabilitation professionals are most often asked to initiate interventions that assist in maintaining full extremity range of motion (ROM) and reduce the risk of contractures and pressure ulcers. As patients move from the ICU to step-down units and general medical floors, rehabilitation clinicians can examine patients more accurately and completely and adjust interventions accordingly.

Musculoskeletal

Range of Motion. Active ROM (AROM) and passive ROM (PROM) are measured with a goniometer.

Posture. The rehabilitation specialist may sit or stand a patient to see if this affects their level of arousal or awareness.

Neuromuscular

Arousal, Attention, and Cognition. Coma scales and cognitive function scales have been developed with the aim of achieving standardization in determining level of consciousness for clinical research, as well as for monitoring changes during acute illness, and serving as prognostic indicators.[21] Most coma and cognitive function scales are composite scales that include measures of motor function, level of disability, and levels of arousal, attention, and cognition.

The Glasgow Coma Scale (GCS), developed in 1974, is the scale most widely used in emergency departments, community hospitals, and research literature worldwide[22] (Table 21-1). Originally developed for use with patients after traumatic brain injury, this scale has also proven to be a reliable predictor of outcome for patients in coma with brain damage from nontraumatic causes.[23] The GCS shows high interrater and intrarater reliability when used by paramedics, physicians, and nurses.[24,25]

The GCS consists of three categories: Eye opening, best motor response, and best verbal response. Each category has a numerical scale assigned to specific responses. Scores for eye opening range from 1 to 4, for best motor response from 1 to 6, and for best verbal response 1 to 5. The totals for all categories are summed to give the final score. Total scores range from 3 to 15, with a score of 8 or less defining coma. A score of 9 to 11 indicates moderately severe brain injury, and a score of greater than or equal to 12 indicates minor injury.

The Rancho Los Amigos Levels of Cognitive Function Scale (LCFS) was developed in 1972 as a descriptive scale outlining the sequence of behavioral and cognitive recovery that typically takes place in patients after traumatic brain injury[26] (Table 21-2). The scale is frequently initially administered on admission to a trauma center and is readministered as the patient moves through acute, subacute, and inpatient rehabilitation. The scale does not require cooperation from the patient because a level is assigned based on observations of the patient's responses to external stimuli. The scale is recorded in roman numerals and consists of 8 levels ranging from I: No response to VIII: Purposeful, appropriate response. Patients can plateau at any level of the scale, which may indicate a temporary or permanent leveling off in the recovery process. The LCFS is not intended as a prognostic tool for patients with brain injury. The scale is intended only for patients with traumatic causes of brain injury and is primarily a means of standardizing communication between rehabilitation clinicians and between clinicians and patients' family members. Patients in a coma are assigned LCFS level I or II, and patients in a vegetative state or minimally conscious state are typically assigned level II or III. Levels III through VIII describe a patient exhibiting some degree of awareness or conscious behavior.

The CNC scale was developed to measure small clinical changes in patients with severe brain injuries who function at the very low levels characteristic of the vegetative state. The CNC scale is useful for recognizing patients in low-level neurological states most likely to respond to further rehabilitation. The CNC scale, as well as directions and tips for administering the scale, can be found at the Center for Outcome Measurement in Brain Injury (COMBI) web site (see Additional Resources). The CNC scale does not appear often in the literature concerning outcomes or treatment of patients with disorders of consciousness, and as discussed previously, the language of the scale used to label scoring levels does not correlate with the current

TABLE 21-1		The Glasgow Coma Scale (GCS)			
Eye Opening		**Best Motor Response**		**Best Verbal Response**	
Spontaneous	4	To verbal command	6	Oriented and converses	5
To speech	3	To painful stimulus	5	Disoriented and converses	4
To pain	2	Flexion withdrawal	4	Inappropriate words	3
No response	1	Flexion abnormal	3	Incomprehensible sounds	2
		Extension	2	No response	1
		No response	1		
E score		M score		V score	

Total score = E score + M score + V score.
Interpretation: ≤8 = Coma; ≥9 = Not in a coma; 9-11 = Moderate severity; ≥12 = Minor injury.

TABLE 21-2	Level of Cognitive Functioning Scale (LCFS)
Level	**Response**
Level I: No response	Patient does not respond to external stimuli and appears asleep.
Level II: Generalized response	Patient reacts to external stimuli in nonspecific, inconsistent, and nonpurposeful manner with stereotypic and limited responses.
Level III: Localized response	Patient responds specifically and inconsistently with delays to stimuli but may follow simple commands for motor action.
Level IV: Confused, agitated response	Patient exhibits bizarre, nonpurposeful, incoherent, or inappropriate behaviors; has no short-term recall; and attention is short and nonselective.
Level V: Confused, inappropriate, nonagitated response	Patient gives random, fragmented, and nonpurposeful responses to complex or unstructured stimuli. Simple commands are followed consistently, memory and selective attention are impaired, and new information is not retained.
Level VI: Confused, appropriate response	Patient gives context-appropriate, goal-directed responses, dependent on external input for direction. There is carry-over for relearned but not for new tasks, and recent memory problems persist.
Level VII: Automatic, appropriate response	Patient behaves appropriately in familiar settings, performs daily routines automatically, and shows carry-over for new learning at lower than normal rates. Patient initiates social interactions, but judgment remains impaired.
Level VIII: Purposeful, appropriate response	Patient oriented and responds to the environment but abstract reasoning abilities are decreased relative to premorbid levels.

Data from Hagan C, Malkmus D, Durham P: Levels of cognitive functions. In *Rehabilitation of the head injured adult: comprehensive physical management*, Downey, Calif, 1979, Professional Staff Association of Rancho Los Amigos Hospital.

language used in describing patients with disorders of consciousness.

Cranial Nerve Integrity. Rehabilitation clinicians do not usually perform tests of cranial nerve function or reflexes in this population, but an understanding of these tests and their results gives information regarding brainstem integrity and overall prognosis. As mentioned previously, the ARAS is located in the upper two-thirds of the brainstem, specifically the upper pons and midbrain, and is responsible for the arousal component of consciousness. Awareness and cognitive functioning are not possible without arousal, and this requires a functioning ARAS. The nuclei of the cranial nerves (CNs) are located throughout the brainstem, so tests of certain CN reflexes provide information about brainstem integrity. Generally, if cranial nerve reflexes are present, brainstem function is intact, but if the reflexes are absent, one cannot be sure that brainstem function is absent. Various illicit drugs, antibiotics, neuromuscular-blocking agents, and vestibular diseases can block CN reflexes.[5]

The CN reflexes commonly tested in this population are the pupillary light reflex (CN II and III), corneal reflex (CN V and VII), and/or the oculocephalic and oculovestibular reflexes (CN III, IV, VI, and VIII). Shining a bright light into each eye and looking for direct and consensual constriction of the pupil tests the pupillary reflex. The corneal reflex is tested by touching each cornea with a cotton swab, looking for the eyelids to shut (and/or upward deviation of the eyes, which is an ocular movement known as Bell's phenomenon). The oculocephalic reflex test, also known as the *doll's eye phenomenon,* is tested by rapidly moving the patient's head from one side to the other, then up and down, briefly holding the endpoints. The patient's eyes are watched for movement in the opposite direction to the movement of the head, indicating a positive test or intact reflex. The oculocephalic reflex test is not used if there is a concern that

the patient may have an unstable cervical spine, so that rapid movement of the head from side to side or up and down is contraindicated. The oculovestibular reflex test is often referred to as *caloric stimulation* and elicits the same but stronger response than the oculocephalic reflex. The integrity of the patient's tympanic membranes must be assessed before caloric stimulation is done, since the test involves introducing cold and warm water into the ears. To test this reflex, the patient's head is elevated 30 degrees from horizontal and a small amount of ice water is first used to irrigate each ear canal. The eyes of an unconscious patient should deviate toward the side of irrigation. Then, both ear canals are irrigated simultaneously with ice water, producing an upward deviation of both eyes and then with warm water to produce a downward deviation of the eyes.

Reflex Integrity. Abnormal deep tendon reflexes and tone abnormalities (see Chapters 16 and 17) are common in patients in a coma, vegetative state, or minimally conscious state.

Cardiovascular/Pulmonary. It is not uncommon for patients in a vegetative or minimally conscious state to have a fever, elevated systolic blood pressure (BP), and high HR during the acute phase of recovery.[27-29] Tests and measures for respiratory rate (RR), BP, temperature, HR, and oxygen saturation of patients in vegetative and minimally conscious states can be found in Chapter 22.

Integumentary. Patients with disorders of consciousness are at increased risk for pressure ulcers because of their impaired mobility, as well as impaired nutritional and respiratory status (see Chapter 28).

EVALUATION, DIAGNOSIS, AND PROGNOSIS

Prognosis for recovery from conditions causing disorders of consciousness vary greatly with age, underlying etiology of the low-level state, depth of unresponsiveness, length of unresponsiveness, and response to brainstem reflex testing. The state of complete unarousal and unresponsiveness characteristic of patients in a coma rarely continues beyond 14 days, with patients usually dying or becoming vegetative within that timeframe.[30-32]

COMA FROM TRAUMATIC CAUSES

The prognosis for traumatic coma differs from that for nontraumatic coma. In general, patients with coma resulting from trauma achieve better outcomes than patients in coma from nontraumatic causes.[33] Younger age and a higher GCS score 1 week after injury are the most reliable predictors of functional recovery at 6 months in patients with coma from trauma.

COMA FROM NONTRAUMATIC CAUSES

Prognosis after nontraumatic coma is most affected by coma etiology, depth of coma, duration of coma, and clinical signs. Coma induced by drug overdose has the best prognosis. Patients with coma caused by drug overdose often present as deeply comatose with depressed brainstem reflexes but high levels of motor activity, and all have the potential for a good prognosis. The probability of waking from coma within 2 weeks is 8 times better for drug-induced coma than for coma from other nontraumatic causes. Coma resulting from hypoxic/global ischemic etiologies has the next most favorable prognosis followed by ischemic stroke. Patients with hemorrhagic etiologies of coma have the worst prognosis for functional recovery.[32]

Depth of coma as measured by the GCS is also predictive of outcome in nontraumatic coma. Patients with higher scores 6 hours after the onset of coma have better outcomes. The longer a patient remains in a coma the worse his or her chance of a good outcome. If a comatose state lasts 3 days or longer, the chance for a good recovery is only 7% and drops to 2% by day 14. Absence of CN reflexes (corneal, pupillary light, oculocephalic, and oculovestibular) at 24 hours after onset of coma is also predictive of poor outcome.

VEGETATIVE STATE

In general, recovery of awareness is unlikely in people in a vegetative state 1 year after traumatic brain injury or 3 months after nontraumatic brain injury. The prognosis for functional recovery is slightly better if awareness returns by 6 months after traumatic injury and is generally slightly better for children than for adults.

MINIMALLY CONSCIOUS STATE

Because the term *minimally conscious state* is relatively new, there is limited information on the prognosis for patients in this state.[8] The Aspen Neurobehavioral Conference formally defined the term in 1997 and stated "there is as yet inadequate information in the research literature to corroborate the natural history and prognosis for patients in minimally conscious state."

INTERVENTION

There is little specific evidence and no evidence-based guidelines or standard treatment approaches for rehabilitation of patients with disorders of consciousness.[34,35]

Nonetheless, it is widely recommended that active rehabilitation should begin early.[32,36] Several reports have highlighted the generic benefits of early rehabilitation,[8,28,36,37] and most rehabilitation centers follow consensus-based guidelines for the care and treatment of patients with impaired consciousness.

The Aspen Neurobehavioral Conference recommends that treatment interventions focus on four areas: Augmenting communication, promoting meaningful behavioral responsiveness, preventing complications, and facilitating nursing care.[8] It has been suggested that for patients who lack awareness (coma and vegetative state), treatment should be focused on "maintaining or attaining physical health so that there is a useful body for the brain to control should recovery of awareness occur."[27]

The Aspen Neurobehavioral Conference proposes that treatment interventions be classified into two categories: Basic interventions, consisting of treatments that are vital to maintaining physical health, such as ROM, positioning protocols, and tone normalizing methods; and optional interventions, or those considered to be nonessential but appropriate on a case by case basis. Sensory stimulation programs and pharmacological trials are given as examples of optional interventions.[8] Casting of limbs with goals of improving ROM and decreasing hypertonia is also considered to be an optional intervention.

BASIC INTERVENTIONS

Range of Motion Exercises. Despite the lack of supporting research, it is thought that daily ROM exercises in bed-bound patients assist with maintaining joint ROM. These exercises are also thought to prevent contractures and reduce the risk of developing **heterotopic ossification,** both of which are common in patients with severe brain injuries.

As stated earlier, maintaining functional PROM in certain joints is key in assisting with the long-term care of these generally bed-bound patients because reduced ROM can cause difficulty with turning and positioning. Stretching increases the extensibility of soft tissues and is used widely to increase joint mobility. Prolonged stretching, for at least 20 minutes a day and for up to 12 hours a day, may be necessary.

Despite the lack of evidence supporting the use of passive stretching to minimize contracture and **spasticity** in patients, most agree that stretching should be used as an intervention until the results of further studies emerge.[38-40]

Positioning Protocols. Positioning protocols should be developed in conjunction with the nursing staff whose primary concerns are to avoid the development of pressure ulcers secondary to prolonged bed rest, to mobilize static lung secretions, and to prevent aspiration to reduce the risk of pneumonia. Aspiration pneumonia is common in patients with disorders of consciousness. This can be challenging as the semirecumbent position reduces aspiration risk but increases the risk for pressure ulcers. Correct wheelchair positioning may also help to temporarily normalize tone and reflexes. Furthermore, standing with the help of a tilt table can sometimes facilitate higher level behavioral responses.

Normalizing Tone. Tone abnormalities, particularly high tone, are common in patients with disorders of consciousness. High tone can lead to posturing, which can result in contracture formation and positioning difficulties.[29] A number of physical interventions, including electrical stimulation, vibration, altering body position, and prolonged muscle stretch (including splinting), are thought to decrease tone in hypertonic muscles. Several authors also advocate the use of sitting programs with patients in a vegetative state because clinical observation seems to suggest that proper sitting position can temporarily normalize tone.

OPTIONAL INTERVENTIONS

Sensory Stimulation. Sensory stimulation is the application of environmental stimuli by an external agent for the purpose of promoting arousal and behavioral responsiveness.[41] Formalized sensory stimulation programs as a treatment for patients in a coma or vegetative state became popular in the 1980s but have to some degree fallen out of favor because of the lack of scientific evidence proving or disproving their effectiveness. These programs vary in intensity and frequency of intervention, as well as targeted senses. At a minimum, most programs include stimulation of visual, auditory, olfactory, kinesthetic, and tactile senses.

Casting. The use of casts in management of tone in adults with impaired consciousness is controversial. Three goals are suggested for casting in these patients: Improved ROM, decreased spasticity, and improved function. A systematic review of the literature published in 2003 revealed that improved PROM is the only outcome supported by the current evidence and that there is insufficient evidence to support that casting decreases spasticity or improves function in brain-injured adults.[42]

CASE STUDY 21-1

METABOLIC COMA

Patient History

MM is a 38-year-old male who was found unconscious by a family member in his home 10 days ago. Medical work-up showed him to be in diabetic ketoacidosis with respiratory failure. He also had acute renal failure, left lung pneumonia, low BP, and hypoxia. On the tenth day of his hospitalization, he began moving his fingers and toes and was able to consistently squeeze the physician's hand on command. Hours after first being noticed to squeeze his hand on command, MM could open his eyes to voice command. He was extubated the following morning, and a physical therapy evaluation was initiated at the physician's request.

Tests and Measures—Significant Findings
Musculoskeletal

- Ankle dorsiflexion PROM was limited to neutral bilaterally, and MM complained of "tightness" in both calfs when passive stretch into dorsiflexion was applied.

Neuromuscular

- MM was alert and oriented to self and place but not time. He could remember events the day before his hospitalization but had no memory of the past 10 days.

Cardiovascular

- MM was assisted to sitting at the edge of the bed and immediately complained of feeling dizzy. Vital signs were measured as follows:
  - Sitting: HR 105 bpm, BP 95/60 mm Hg, RR 21 breaths/min, O_2 saturation 100%. MM's dizziness worsened over the next 20 to 30 seconds, and he was assisted back to supine and his symptoms resolved over the next minute.
- He was again assisted to sitting, and his vital signs measured again: HR 92 bpm, BP 105/65 mm Hg. Minor dizziness quickly resolved.
- MM was asked to stand at the bedside and required close contact guard assistance for balance. Vital signs were measured 1 minute after standing as follows: HR 80 bpm, BP 105/70 mm Hg.

Diagnosis

Preferred practice pattern 5I: Impaired arousal, range of motion, and motor control associated with coma, near coma, or vegetative state.

Interventions

- Calf stretching to increase PROM
- Practice of position changes, and progressively increased time in an upright position
- Progressive ambulation

Role of the Physical Therapist Assistant

- How would you stretch this patient's calf muscles?
- What do his changes in heart rate and blood pressure indicate?
- Name three places where heart rate can be measured.
- What will be the main focus of this patient's physical therapy sessions?

Additional Information

For the full version of this case study, including detailed examination results, interventions, and outcomes, see the Evolve site that accompanies this book.

CHAPTER SUMMARY

The past two decades have provided advances in medical technology that have caused the mortality from severe brain injuries to decrease significantly. Patients who previously would have died are living in a vegetative or minimally conscious state and are being evaluated for admission to rehabilitation facilities with greater frequency. Rehabilitation professionals working together as a multidisciplinary team must understand the prognostic indicators for this population to make the most appropriate and informed recommendations for rehabilitation.

The role of rehabilitation in the early stages of injury is to help prevent deterioration of the sensory motor system and to maintain physical health to reduce the risk of complications associated with prolonged bed rest. Clinicians also have the responsibility of monitoring changes in the behavior and function of these patients and understanding what these changes might indicate. It is imperative that all rehabilitation professionals understand the differences between specific definitions, clinical features, and prognostic indicators for this group of patients so appropriate decisions regarding care can be made.

There is a lack of evidence-based data concerning behavior measurement, rehabilitation interventions, and outcomes for patients in preferred practice pattern 5I. Quality research is needed in this area to develop rehabilitation programs consisting of interventions that have the potential to optimize recovery of awareness and function in these patients.

ADDITIONAL RESOURCES

For links to these and additional web-based resources, see the Evolve site.

Glasgow Coma Scale (GCS)

Rancho Los Amigos Levels of Cognitive Function Scale (LCFS)

Jennett B: *The vegetative state: Medical facts, ethical and legal dilemmas,* London, 2002, Cambridge University Press.

Plum F, Posner JB: *The diagnosis of stupor and coma,* ed 3, Philadelphia, 1982, FA Davis.

Young B, Ropper A, Bolton C: *Coma and impaired consciousness,* New York, 1998, McGraw Hill.

Brain Injury Association

Center for Outcome Measurement in Brain Injury (COMBI)

National Rehabilitation Information Center (NARIC)

GLOSSARY

Coma: A neurobehavioral diagnosis indicating the patient is unarousable and without sleep-wake cycles. The patient has no ability to interact with the environment. Eyes do not open spontaneously or to external stimulation, and the patient does not follow any commands.

Consciousness: The totality in psychology of sensations, perceptions, ideas, attitudes, and feelings of which an individual or a group is aware at any given time or within a given time span; waking life (as that to which one returns after sleep, trance, or fever) in which one's normal mental powers are present; the upper part of mental life of which the person is aware as contrasted with unconscious processes.

Decerebrate posturing: Extension of the elbow, internal rotation of the shoulders, and extension of the lower extremities. Usually occurs with lesions affecting the midbrain portion of the brainstem.

Decorticate posturing: Flexion of the upper extremities and extension of the lower extremities. Usually occurs with lesions affecting the corticospinal tracts. Usually more favorable than decerebrate posturing.

Delirium: An abnormal mental state characterized by disorientation, irritability, fear, visual hallucinations, and misperception of sensory stimuli. Delirium is characterized by rapid onset and rarely persists longer than 7 days. Delirium is common with toxic and metabolic disorders of the nervous system.

Heterotopic ossification: The appearance of ectopic bone in soft tissue usually in periarticular locations. Can present clinically with erythema, warmth, and edema and decreased ROM.

Locked-in-syndrome: A neurobehavioral diagnosis referring to patients who are alert, aware of the environment, and able to interact with it but who cannot move or speak. Communication is usually through limited eye movements (blinking or vertical movements). The syndrome is the result of a brainstem lesion usually involving the pons.

Minimally conscious state: A neurobehavioral diagnosis indicating severely altered consciousness in which minimal but definite behavioral evidence of self-awareness or environmental awareness is demonstrated. The patient's eyes open spontaneously or in response to stimulation; the patient follows commands inconsistently.

Obtunded: A decreased alertness and interest in the environment, slow response to stimuli, and increased sleep time with drowsiness characterizing awake time.

Reticular activating system: A part of the reticular formation that extends from the brainstem to the midbrain and thalamus with connections distributed throughout the cerebral cortex and that controls the degree of activity of the central nervous system (as in maintaining sleep and wakefulness and in making transitions between the two states).

Somnolent: Inclined to or heavy with sleep.

Spasticity: Velocity-dependent resistance to passive movement.

Stupor: A state of deep sleep from which a patient can be awoken with vigorous and repeated stimuli. Once the stimulation is stopped, the patient falls back into a state of unresponsiveness.

Vegetative state: A neurobehavioral diagnosis indicating complete loss of ability to interact with the environment but with intact sleep-wake cycles. The patient's eyes open spontaneously or in response to stimulation; the patient does not follow any commands.

Chapter 22

Vital Signs

Brian K. Peterson

OBJECTIVES

After reading this chapter, the reader will be able to:
1. Identify the vital signs.
2. Discuss the importance and physiological implications of each vital sign.
3. Describe and perform appropriate procedures to measure the vital signs, including pulse, respiratory rate, blood pressure, pain level, and oxygen saturation.
4. Identify normal ranges for the vital signs.
5. Know when to monitor vital signs during rehabilitation.

Vital signs are critical indicators of a person's health and current medical status. The body's cells and organs require a relatively constant internal environment to function and the vital signs reflect whether specific body systems (circulatory, pulmonary, neurological, and endocrine) are functioning appropriately.[1] Vital signs often provide the first indication of harmful physiological changes or disturbances in the body and may also be the first indication of a return to a more stable condition.[2]

There are four traditional vital signs (also known as cardinal signs): Temperature, **pulse**, respiratory rate, and blood pressure. Two additional measures, pain level and oxygen saturation, were more recently added to these. Pain level was added because many patients have pain, and pain is often why patients seek medical help. Thus pain can be an indicator of patient progress, status, and comfort.[1] Additionally, the level of oxygen saturation, as measured by pulse oximetry, provides information about the amount of oxygen a patient is carrying in their blood and can indicate changes in cardiac, circulatory, and pulmonary status.

Recording baseline measurements of vital signs during the initial patient contact is important for comparison with future measurements. Regular recording and documentation of vital signs may reveal sudden or gradually progressive changes that might not otherwise be observed. Accurate reliable measurements of the vital signs are needed to detect such changes. Knowledge of normal ranges of vital signs is also important for direction of interventions.

This chapter provides information about the vital signs of temperature, pulse, blood pressure, respiratory rate, pain level, and oxygen saturation. Included is information about the implications of the vital sign, measurement methods, normal ranges for each vital sign, and suggestions for when each should be measured during the management of patients involved in rehabilitation.

TEMPERATURE

IMPLICATIONS OF TEMPERATURE

Heat is produced by virtually every chemical reaction within the body, and core body temperature represents the balance between heat production and heat loss. Body temperature is tightly regulated within a narrow physiological range but may increase significantly in response to infection or increased physical activity. Many other factors, such as **ambient temperature,** circadian rhythm, neurological function, clothing, age, gender, menstrual cycle, pregnancy, emotion, and injury, influence core body temperature. Body temperature is regulated primarily by the hypothalamus, which acts like a thermostat, keeping core body temperature near a set point of approximately 37° C (98.6° F). The hypothalamus continuously monitors body temperature and directs the heat producing and heat loss mechanisms to keep the temperature near the set point.

Circulating blood in the body transfers heat by convection (the transfer of heat by mass flow of a liquid past a surface). The body adjusts its rate of heat transfer by **vasodilation** (an increase in the diameter of the blood vessels) and **vasoconstriction** (a decrease in the size of the blood vessels) in response to information processed in the hypothalamus regarding increasing or decreasing temperature. Temperature increases promote peripheral vasodilation and increased blood flow to the skin to help eliminate heat from the body and reduce the core temperature. Conversely, temperature decreases promote peripheral vasoconstriction to shunt blood to the core and preserve body heat.

If temperature regulation cannot keep up with environmental changes, core body temperature may shift too far down, resulting in **hypothermia** (too low a temperature) or up resulting in hyperthermia (too high a temperature). Hypothermia is defined as body temperature of 35° C (95° F) or lower. If unchecked, hypothermia causes a sequence of symptoms beginning with a sense of cold, progressing to shivering, vasoconstriction, muscle rigidity, decreased blood pressure, confusion, loss of reflexes, loss of spontaneous movement, coma, and death, usually by cardiac **arrhythmia**, when core temperature falls to 21.2° to 29.4° C (70° to 85° F).

> ◎ **Clinical Pearl**
>
> Hypothermia is defined as body temperature of 35° C (95° F) or lower.

METHODS FOR MEASURING TEMPERATURE

Body temperature may be measured with various types of thermometers and at various sites. Thermometer types include mercury-in-glass thermometers, electronic thermometers, **tympanic membrane** thermometers, and disposable/single-use thermometers. Sites for temperature measurement include oral, axillary, tympanic membrane, and rectal. The procedures for rectal temperature measurement and pulmonary artery catheter temperature monitoring are not described in this book because rehabilitation clinicians are unlikely to perform these procedures.

Types of Thermometers

Mercury-in-Glass Thermometer. Mercury-in-glass thermometers are discussed here briefly because they have been used extensively in the past. However, there is a growing trend nationally and internationally to phase out or ban the use of mercury thermometers and other equipment containing mercury, such as **sphygmomanometers,** because of the toxicity of mercury to the individual and the environment. Therefore, in clinical practice, electronic, tympanic membrane, and single-use thermometers will be encountered much more commonly than the mercury-in-glass thermometer.

Mercury-in-glass thermometers consist of a sealed glass tube calibrated in degrees Centigrade and/or degrees Fahrenheit, with a mercury-filled reservoir at one end. The mercury in the reservoir expands with increased temperature, climbing higher up the thermometer, and contracts and recedes as the temperature falls.

Tympanic Membrane Thermometers. Tympanic membrane thermometers use an **otoscope**-like probe that is inserted into the external auditory canal to detect and measure thermal infrared energy emitted from the tympanic membrane (Fig. 22-1). A scan button is pressed to start the measurement, and an audible signal indicates that the temperature is ready to be recorded from the digital display.

Tympanic thermometers are minimally invasive, record temperatures in approximately 3 seconds, register temperatures in the range of 25° to 43° C, have no direct

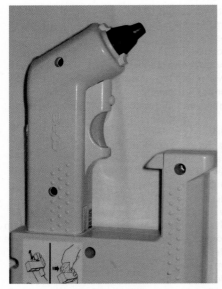

FIG. 22-1 A tympanic membrane thermometer resting in its storage base.

contact with mucous membranes, and work only if the disposable probe cover is in place.[3] The probe lens, however, can be easily damaged if not handled carefully. It is important to check the lens before each use and to replace its protective cover when not in use.[3] Operator handedness, patient position, and ear (right or left) does not produce clinically significant variability, but obstruction of the tympanic membrane by cerumen may lower tympanic measurements.[4]

Tympanic thermometers are accurate, easily usable clinically,[5] satisfactory for routine intermittent temperature measurement, and the most sensitive noninvasive devices for measuring body temperature above 37.5° C.

Inaccuracies in temperature measurement are more likely in children if the thermometer is calibrated for an adult, the incorrect size probe is used, or if the child is less than 1 year old, in whom even the smallest tip available is likely to fit poorly.[6,7] Additionally, inaccuracies may occur with incorrect positioning.[8]

◎ *Clinical Pearl*

Tympanic thermometers are accurate, easy to use, and ideal for measuring body temperature above 37.5° C.

Electronic Thermometers. Electronic thermometers detect temperature changes using a thermoresistive device in which the electrical resistance changes in response to changes in temperature (Fig. 22-2). This device may be a thermistor or a thermocouple and is incorporated into the tip of a probe. Thermistors are very small and therefore respond rapidly to changes in temperature.[9] The current flow from a thermistor is translated into a temperature reading that is displayed on a digital readout.

Electronic thermometers are relatively easy to use and portable. They can be used to measure oral, axillary, and rectal temperatures. Axillary temperature is measured in the same way as with a mercury-in-glass thermometer but using the electronic probe and waiting for the signal to indicate that the temperature is ready on the digital display. There are separate color-coded probes for oral and rectal measurements, and the disposable probe cover needs to be in place to operate, which helps reduce the risk of cross-contamination.[1,9] An audible signal indicates when the temperature on the digital display is ready to be recorded.

Disposable Single-Use Thermometers. Single-use thermometers usually consist of a plastic strip with a matrix of dots arranged to correspond with temperature registered in degrees Centigrade and/or Fahrenheit (Fig. 22-3). The dots contain two heat-sensitive chemicals that change color in response to temperature. This type of thermometer is usually calibrated to measure temperatures between 35.5° to 40.5° C (96.0° to 104° F) and takes 1 minute to measure an oral temperature and 3 minutes to measure an axillary or rectal temperature.[3,10]

Single-use thermometers have the advantages of being sterile when opened; unbreakable; easy to use; suitable for oral, axillary, and rectal temperature measurement; and possibly decreasing the risk of cross-infection.[3,10] The main disadvantages are that the chemicals within the dots may degenerate if stored above 35° C, costs may increase if repeated measurements are required, and as mentioned previously, they can only measure temperatures between 35.5° to 40.5° C.[3,10]

Single-use thermometers produce accurate, precise, and clinically valid temperature readings in adults and children with and without fever and are often recommended for clinical use because of their accuracy and efficiency.[11,12] They are also an appropriate choice when treating patients under isolation or with communicable diseases.

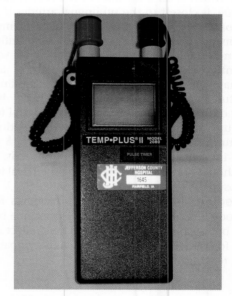

FIG. 22-2 An electronic thermometer.

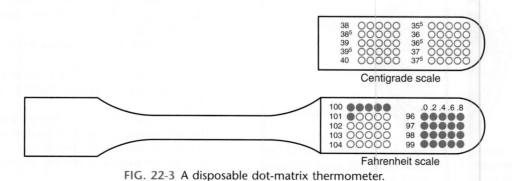

FIG. 22-3 A disposable dot-matrix thermometer.

Oral and axillary procedure and placement for using disposable thermometers is essentially the same as the mercury-in-glass thermometer. Remember to turn the dots inward when measuring at the axillary site.

Whatever type of thermometer used, correct and consistent procedure must be followed to ensure accuracy and reliability, and the same site and instrument should be used for repeated measurements to accurately reflect changes in body temperature over time.[3,13]

> ◎ **Clinical Pearl**
>
> Use the same correct procedure and the same instrument to accurately and reliably check for changes in body temperature over time.

Site of Temperature Measurement. Core body temperature may be estimated by measurement at oral, axillary, tympanic membrane, or rectal sites using the various types of thermometers as described. Site and instrument selection are determined partly by the patient's age, medical condition, comfort, ease of access to site, and instrument availability.

When taking a temperature orally, placing the thermometer in the **sublingual pocket** (Fig. 22-4) gives the most accurate estimate of core body temperature because this area, which is on both sides of the **frenulum** under the tongue, is closest to the sublingual arteries.[13-15]

Most of the problems with accuracy of oral temperature measurement result from environmental influences.[9] **Tachypnea** (rapid breathing) and drinking ice water can significantly reduce sublingual temperature, and hot drinks may increase oral temperatures.[16,17] Smoking before temperature measurement has little effect; however, smoking during measurement may increase oral temperature by up to 2° C.[18] Based on these observations, oral temperatures should not be taken for at least 15 minutes after the intake of cold drinks or even hot foods, and the patient should not smoke while having their oral temperature measured.

Procedure. The recommended procedures for measuring body temperature vary slightly from one source to another, but the procedures presented here reflect accepted practice for obtaining oral, axillary, and tympanic temperature readings.[1,19,20]

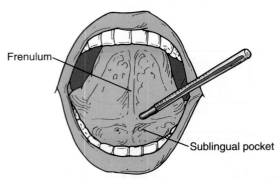

FIG. 22-4 The sublingual pocket area on either side of the frenulum underneath the tongue gives the most accurate estimate of core body temperature measured orally.

Oral Measurement with Mercury-in-Glass Thermometer

1. The patient should be resting comfortably, allowing easy access to the measurement site.
2. Don disposable gloves.
3. Grasp and hold the tip of the thermometer away from the reservoir. If color coded, the tip will be blue.
4. Read the level of mercury at eye level by rotating the thermometer until the scale is visible.
    A. If the temperature is above 35.5° C (96° F), shake the mercury below that level with a few quick flicks of the wrist.
    B. Be sure to stand clear of any objects you may hit with the thermometer and be sure to hold onto it securely.
5. Cover the end of the thermometer with a plastic sleeve if available.
6. Place the thermometer gently under the patient's tongue into the sublingual pocket (see Fig. 22-4).
7. Have the patient gently hold the thermometer with their lips. Instruct them to keep the thermometer still and in place and to not bite down.
8. The thermometer remains in place for 3 minutes.
9. Remove the thermometer gently, discard the plastic sleeve, and wipe away any remaining secretions with a clean tissue.
10. Read the thermometer at eye level and record the temperature.

Axillary Measurement with Mercury-in-Glass Thermometer

1. Prepare the thermometer as you would for steps 1 to 4 for measuring oral temperature.
2. Have the patient lie down supine if possible. Otherwise, they should sit comfortably.
3. Make sure the axilla is dry. Abduct the arm to expose the axilla. Place the thermometer tip at the center of the axilla then reposition the arm to the side of the patient with the forearm across the abdomen to hold the thermometer in place.
4. The thermometer remains in place for at least 3 minutes, but it may need to be left in place 6 to 9 minutes to reach a stable temperature.
5. Remove and discard the plastic cover and wipe off any remaining secretions with a clean tissue.
6. Read the thermometer at eye level and record the temperature.

Tympanic Membrane Thermometer

1. The patient should be in a comfortable position, either lying or sitting with the head turned away from the examiner.
2. Make a note if there is excess ear wax in the auditory canal.
3. Cover the sensor tip of the thermometer with the protective plastic sheath, making sure it locks in place.
4. Insert the tip into the auditory canal according to the manufacturer's positioning directions (Fig. 22-5). These may include the following:
    A. Pull the **pinna** of the ear up, out, and back for an adult.

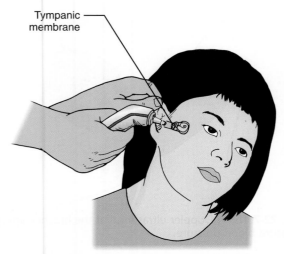

Tympanic membrane

FIG. 22-5 Position of tympanic membrane thermometer. One hand pulls pinna of the ear up, out, and back to help position the tip of the thermometer forward.

B. Move the tip in a figure-of-eight pattern to situate the tip of the probe.
C. Make sure the probe fits snugly and does not move.
D. Point the tip toward the nose.
5. Once the probe is properly placed, press the scan button and wait for an audible signal indicating that the temperature is ready to be read on the display.
6. Remove the tip from the ear and discard the plastic cover.
7. Record the temperature.

Electronic Thermometer
1. Don disposable gloves.
2. Make sure the oral/blue probe is attached and slide one of the plastic probe covers onto the probe until it locks.
3. Gently place the probe in the sublingual pocket (see Fig. 22-4) under the patient's tongue.
4. Instruct the patient to hold the probe in place with the lips closed until the signal is heard.
5. Read and record the temperature on the display.
6. Remove the probe and push the eject button to discard the plastic probe cover.

Measurement Time. Electronic and tympanic membrane thermometers make a sound to indicate when they have completed measuring the temperature. Most electronic thermometers register a temperature in less than a minute,[9] and tympanic membrane thermometers register temperature in about 3 seconds.[4] Disposable thermometers have measurement times of 1 minute for oral measurement and 3 minutes for axillary and rectal measurements.[10] Recommendations for how long to insert a mercury-in-glass thermometer vary from 3 to 10 minutes, with 3 minutes generally recommended for oral measurements and 5 minutes for axillary.[3,10,12,21]

NORMAL TEMPERATURE RANGES

Average normal temperatures are reported as 37° C (98.6° F) measured orally, 37.6° C (99.6° F) measured rectally, and 36.4° C (97.6° F) measured at the axilla.[3]

RELEVANCE OF TEMPERATURE MEASUREMENT TO REHABILITATION

Most outpatients will likely have a normal temperature, but occasionally a patient may not look well or may complain of fever or chills, at which time measuring their temperature would be indicated. If the patient has recently had surgery, check the incision site for heat, redness, swelling, drainage, and tenderness to evaluate for local infection. If the patient's temperature is abnormal, contact your supervising physical therapist and consider canceling the therapy session.

Inpatients are often admitted with an infection-related diagnosis. Review their temperature in the vital signs section of the chart to determine if it is nearing acceptable values. Patients with abnormal temperatures are likely to have reduced activity tolerance that will be more severe the greater the abnormality.

◎ *Clinical Pearl*

Patients with abnormal temperatures are likely to have reduced tolerance to activity.

PULSE

IMPLICATIONS OF PULSE MEASUREMENTS

A patient's peripheral pulse rate approximates their heart rate. The quality and regularity of the peripheral pulse may also give other information about cardiovascular function. The simplest and most common way of taking a pulse is by counting the number of beats felt in a specified amount of time at a location where a superficial artery can be palpated.

Blood ejected from the heart distends the arterial walls and rapidly travels in a pulsatile wave from the aorta to the arteries in the extremities. The beats produced by blood moving through the arteries with each heartbeat produces the palpable pulse. Palpating an artery that lies close to the surface of the body allows this wave to be felt. The number of times the heart beats in 1 minute is the pulse rate. An estimation of the pulse rate can be calculated if the pulse is counted for 15 seconds and then multiplied by 4 to derive the heart rate in beats per minute (bpm).

Pulse has characteristics of rhythm and strength, in addition to rate. Rhythm reflects the regularity of the heartbeat and strength reflects the volume of blood ejected. Documentation should include the heart rate, strength, and rhythm. For example, a pulse may be reported as 60 bpm, strong and regular, or as 70 bpm, weak and irregular.

The heart rhythm is generally noted as being regular when the beats occur at evenly spaced intervals, or irregular when the beats are unevenly spaced. Even though irregular heartbeats may be **benign**, they may indicate potentially life-threatening cardiac dysfunction and should be reported to the supervising physical therapist.

The pulse strength is generally noted as strong, bounding/full, or weak. A strong pulse is normal. It can be palpated easily with mild pressure of the fingers and is not easily obliterated. A bounding or full pulse is even more

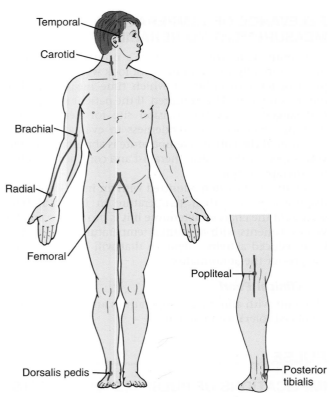

FIG. 22-6 Superficial locations where the peripheral pulses may be assessed.

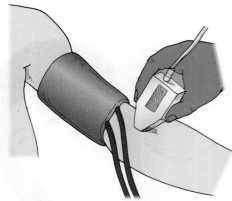

FIG. 22-7 Using Doppler ultrasound at the brachial artery to measure blood pressure.

pronounced and not easily obliterated with firm palpation. A weak pulse is one that is difficult to palpate and is easily obliterated with mild or light palpation. Weak pulses are also known as *feeble* or *thready* and may indicate a decreased stroke volume.

In addition to measuring the pulse to assess cardiac function, the quality of the pulse at peripheral sites can be used to assess local arterial perfusion. For example, a weak or absent femoral pulse can indicate that the lower extremity is not getting enough blood and a weak or absent pedal pulse can indicate that the foot is not getting enough blood.

METHODS FOR ASSESSING PULSE

The pulse may be assessed peripherally at sites where an artery is close to the skin (Fig. 22-6). The peripheral pulse most commonly assessed is the radial artery at the distal radial portion of the wrist because this site is easily accessible and the pulse is generally readily palpated here. Other sites that are easily palpated include the carotid artery at the neck; the brachial artery at the antecubital fossa or inner portion of the upper arm between the biceps and the triceps; the temporal artery on the head; and the dorsalis pedis, posterior tibial, femoral, and popliteal arteries on the lower extremities. These sites may be used if the radial pulse site is not accessible or if assessment of circulation in another part of the body is required.

Procedure. The recommended procedures for measuring the pulse vary slightly from one source to another, but the procedures presented here reflect accepted practice for measuring the radial pulse at the wrist.[1,2,19,20] Similar procedures should be used for measuring the pulse at the other peripheral sites.

1. The patient should rest for at least 5 minutes before the pulse is taken.
2. Explain to the patient what you are doing and why and how they can cooperate to get better results.
3. Position the patient comfortably, either sitting or supine, with the forearm supported and wrist slightly extended. If the patient is in bed, raise it to a height that allows easy access to the site chosen for measurement.
4. Press the flat part of the fingertips of your index, middle, and/or ring fingers in the shallow trough just medial to the radial border of the wrist and feel for a recurring pulsation. Do not use your thumb because it has its own pulse that may be mistaken for the patient's pulse.
5. Observe your watch or clock and count the number of pulsations that occur in 15 or 30 seconds and multiply by 4 or 2, respectively. If this is the first measurement or if the pulse is irregular, count for a full minute.
6. Record the pulse rate, rhythm, strength, and peripheral site used.
7. Report any anomalies.

If the pulse is too weak to be palpable at a peripheral site, if there is significant irregularity, or when measuring the heart rate in an infant, the **apical** heart rate may be measured by direct palpation or auscultation with a stethoscope over the apex of the heart. Alternatively, weak peripheral pulses that are difficult to palpate by hand may be detected and counted using a Doppler ultrasound (DUS) device (Fig. 22-7).

In addition to methods using palpation, auscultation, or DUS, there are a number of devices that monitor heart rate electronically. Some of these devices are available to the public for monitoring heart rate at rest and during activity at home, and some devices are intended for medical professionals to use in hospitals or clinics. The professional devices generally combine measurement of heart rate with measurement of other vital signs or cardiac performance parameters.

NORMAL RANGES

Normal resting pulse rate in adults ranges from 60 to 100 bpm.[30] **Tachycardia** or rapid pulse rate is defined as a pulse rate greater than 100 bpm at rest. Rapid and sustained tachycardia overworks the heart and can prevent adequate peripheral oxygenation by reducing cardiac output. When the heart rate increases, the heart has less time to fill with blood between contractions, resulting in less blood being ejected with each contraction.[20] **Bradycardia** or a slow pulse rate is defined as a heart rate of less than 60 bpm at rest.[2] Although bradycardia may be pathological, physical training with exercise commonly produces low resting heart rates in highly trained athletes that are not pathological.[22-24] The resting heart rate can be lower than 40 bpm in professional cyclists[25] and other endurance athletes. Although the exact mechanism of this training–induced resting bradycardia is not understood, it is likely due to both an increase in parasympathetic influence and a decrease in sympathetic influence.[26]

> ◎ *Clinical Pearl*
>
> Normal resting pulse rate in adults is between 60 and 100 bpm.

Although there is a normal range for the resting pulse rate, a number of factors, including age, time of day, gender, body build, activity, stress, body temperature, blood volume, and anemia, as well as various medications, may alter this rate. The heart rate is typically lower in the morning than in the evening.[20] After puberty, the pulse is generally about 7 to 8 beats slower in males than females.[2,19,20] Tall slender people usually have a slower heart rate than shorter heavier people.[2,20] Exercise increases heart rate during and shortly after the activity. However, regular aerobic exercise reduces the resting heart rate and causes it to rise more slowly with exertion. This causes both resting and exercise pulse to be lower than average in trained athletes.[19,20,22-24] In addition, physiological changes, such as sympathetic stimulation as a result of fear, anger, excitement, or pain, as well as increases in body temperature, dehydration, excessive blood loss, and anemia, will produce increases in the heart rate.[1,2,19,20] Furthermore, many drugs may increase or decrease the resting heart rate. For example, digitalis preparations and sedatives slow heart rate, whereas caffeine, nicotine, cocaine, thyroid replacement hormones, and epinephrine will all increase heart rate.[1,2,19,20]

Age consistently affects the resting heart rate, with the rate gradually decreasing from birth to adulthood to finally reach the average adult range of 60 to 100 bpm by adolescence[1,2,19,20] (Table 22-1).

RELEVANCE OF PULSE TO REHABILITATION

Pulse rate is often used as a measure of cardiac work when setting exercise intensity and goals in deconditioned patients and those undergoing cardiac rehabilitation (see Chapters 23 and 25). Slower heart rates indicate less cardiac work, and slower heart rates at the same overall workload indicate improvement in cardiac conditioning, as long as medications that influence heart rate have not

TABLE 22-1	Normal Pulse Rates at Various Ages	
Age	Approximate Range (bpm)	Approximate Average (bpm)
Newborn	100-180	140
1-12 months	80-140	120
1-2 years	70-130	110
3-6 years	75-120	100
7-12 years	75-110	95
Adolescence	60-100	80
Adulthood	60-100	80

Data from Perry AG, Potter PA: *Clinical nursing skills and techniques*, ed 5, St. Louis, 2002, Mosby; DeWit SC: *Rambo's nursing skills for clinical practice*, ed 4, Philadelphia, 1994, WB Saunders.
bpm, Beats per minute.

been changed. In general, conditioning exercise is prescribed based on a target heart rate that is related to the individual's resting heart rate and predicted maximum heart rate. Therapy should be stopped immediately and the physician contacted if a patient has an abnormal pulse along with symptoms of shortness of breath or lightheadedness because these may indicate life-threatening cardiac or pulmonary pathology.

> ◎ *Clinical Pearl*
>
> Aerobic exercise causes the pulse to go up during exercise. Consistent aerobic exercise causes the resting pulse rate to decrease.

RESPIRATORY RATE

IMPLICATIONS OF RESPIRATORY RATE MEASUREMENT

Breathing is the multistep physiological process that delivers oxygen to and removes carbon dioxide from the human body. Ventilation is made up of two phases. Inspiration (inhalation or breathing in) fills the lungs with air. Expiration (exhalation or breathing out) expels air from the lungs. The primary inspiratory muscles are the diaphragm and the external intercostals. Smaller accessory muscles, the scalenes, sternocleidomastoids, and pectorals, also aid inspiration during exertion or under certain pathological conditions.[27] Expiration is largely passive while at rest and during light activity and results from the relaxation of the inspiratory muscles and the recoil of the lungs through their natural elasticity. Respiratory rate is the number of breaths or the number of times a cycle of inspiration and expiration is completed in 1 minute.

> ◎ *Clinical Pearl*
>
> Respiratory rate is the number of breaths or the number of times a cycle of inspiration and expiration is completed in 1 minute.

METHODS FOR ASSESSING RESPIRATORY RATE

The clinician should try to assess the rate, regularity, and depth of breathing to determine if an adequate volume of air is being exchanged. Unusual sounds produced with respiration are noted because they may indicate additional pathology (see Chapters 24 and 26).

Procedure

1. The patient should be inactive for 5 minutes before testing.
2. Make sure the patient is comfortable in supine or a more upright sitting position and that the chest can be observed. If necessary, move blankets or bed linen for better viewing.
3. Since patients often voluntarily alter their breathing if they are aware that you are counting the respiratory rate, it is best to count when the patient is unaware that you are counting. It may be helpful to count respiratory rate while appearing to count pulse or while the patient is holding a thermometer in the mouth to measure temperature.
4. Count the number of times the chest rises and falls for a full minute if there appears to be anything unusual. Count for 30 seconds if breathing is noiseless and effortless, then multiply by two. If unable to observe the chest clearly, place a hand on the patient's upper abdomen to feel the inspiration and expiration cycle and count the number of times it rises and falls.
5. Record the respiratory rate, rhythm, and depth and any abnormalities that may be observed.

NORMAL RANGES

The normal range of respiratory rate in the adult is 14 to 20 breaths/minute, but this rate varies with age and gender (Table 22-2).

A rapid respiratory rate, faster than 20 breaths/minute in an adult, is known as *tachypnea,* and a slow respiratory rate, slower than 10 breaths/minute is known as *bradypnea.* Tachypnea commonly occurs during fever with the rate increasing by about 4 breaths/minute for each 0.5° C (1° F) increase in temperature.[2] Hyperventilation is when the rate and depth of breathing increase enough to lower blood levels of carbon dioxide. This may occur during periods of high anxiety, following severe exertion, or with fever and diabetic acidosis.[2] Bradypnea may be a result of sedating drugs such as morphine,[20] head injury, or increased intracranial pressure affecting the respiratory

center.[2] If an adult's respiratory rate falls below 10 respirations/minute and the depth is shallow, they may become apprehensive, restless, confused, dizzy, or less conscious because of inadequate delivery of oxygen to the brain.[2] Apnea is the absence of breathing and may occur for short periods or for periods that are long enough to be life-threatening. If prolonged, apnea can cause brain damage or lead to serious abnormal cardiac rhythms.[20]

BLOOD PRESSURE

Blood pressure (BP) is the pressure exerted by the blood on the arterial walls. It is determined by the contractile force exerted by the left ventricle of the heart, the amount of blood ejected with each heartbeat (i.e., the stroke volume), and the resistance of the blood vessels to flow. BP reflects the effectiveness of the heart's contraction, the adequacy of blood volume, and the presence of obstruction or interference to blood flow through the vessels.[2] Arterial BP changes cyclically with the heartbeat. The maximum arterial BP is known as the *systolic BP* and the minimum arterial BP is known as the *diastolic BP.*

> ### ◎ *Clinical Pearl*
> The maximum arterial blood pressure (BP) is known as the systolic BP, and the minimum arterial BP is known as the diastolic BP.

Systolic BP represents the peak ventricular contractile force pushing the blood through the vascular system, whereas diastolic pressure represents the minimum pressure in the arteries between heartbeats while the ventricles are refilling. BP is recorded as systolic/diastolic in millimeters of mercury (mm Hg), for example, 120/80 mm Hg.

METHODS FOR MEASURING BLOOD PRESSURE

BP is generally measured noninvasively using a sphygmomanometer and a stethoscope. A sphygmomanometer is a device that measures the pressure (the manometer) and an occlusive cuff. The manometer uses a glass column of mercury, a calibrated aneroid dial, or an electronic device to measure and display the pressure (Fig. 22-8). The occlusive cuff has an inflatable bladder that wraps around the limb to occlude the artery and a bulb to inflate the cuff. When using a mercury or aneroid manometer, a stethoscope must be used to listen for the heart sounds (Fig. 22-9). When using an electronic manometer, no stethoscope is needed. A sphygmomanometer with an aneroid dial and a stethoscope are the most popular devices for measuring BP today because these devices are economical, simple to use, and easy to handle and provide accurate results quickly while avoiding the hazards associated with mercury.

A mercury manometer is a calibrated transparent tube with a reservoir containing mercury. They have the advantages of consistently providing accurate readings, being easy to maintain, and not losing calibration.[28] The level of the top of the convex **meniscus** at the top of the column of mercury is used for readings. One must read the meniscus at about eye level or have it positioned in a

TABLE 22-2	Normal Respiratory Rate Ranges
Ranges	**Breaths/minute**
Newborn	30-60
Early childhood	20-40
Late childhood	15-28
Adolescence	18-22
Adult males	14-18
Adult females	16-20

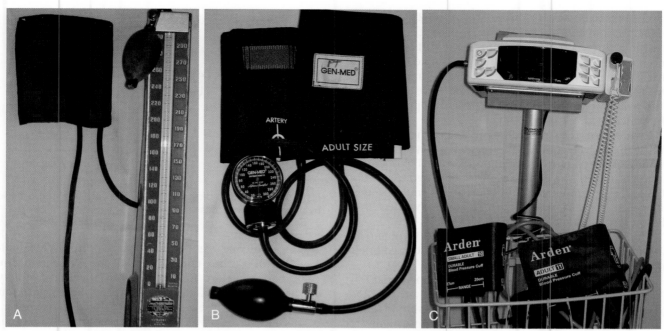

FIG. 22-8 Devices for measuring blood pressure. **A,** Mercury sphygmomanometer with arm cuff, inflation bulb, and manometer. **B,** Aneroid sphygmomanometer with arm cuff, inflation bulb, and manometer. **C,** Combination unit with electronic BP device, thermometer, and pulse oximeter.

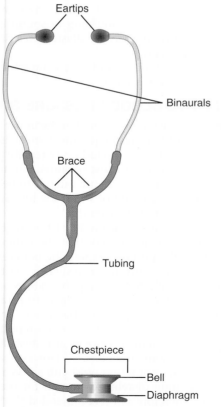

FIG. 22-9 Stethoscope and its parts.

direct line with the eye to avoid visual distortion that may skew the readings.

The aneroid manometer is made of a sealed canister with thin metal walls. One of the walls is flexible and moves with changes in pressure. This movement causes a needle on the calibrated dial to shift, indicating the pressure in mm Hg. Aneroid manometers are generally accurate, but their readings will vary with changes in outside temperature and they may be less accurate than mercury manometers if not calibrated regularly and handled gently.[29] Aneroid manometers should be recalibrated every 6-12 months or if their readings differ by more than 2 to 4 mm Hg from those taken with a mercury sphygmomanometer.[28] They tend to underread pressure when decalibrated.[28,29]

Electric sphygmomanometers use aneroid manometer technology and an electronic device to measure the maximum and minimum pressure after inflation of the cuff. This type of device displays diastolic and systolic BP on a digital display. These devices also require regular maintenance and accuracy checks.

BP cuffs range in size to fit different size limbs from the arm of a newborn, infant, child, small adult, or adult or large adult to the thigh. Small children require a narrower cuff with a shorter bladder, whereas muscular, large, or obese patients need a wider cuff with a longer bladder.[2] The bladder should be long enough to encircle at least 80% of the limb in the adult and the entire limb in the child.[28,30] Regular adult cuffs are generally 12 to

13 cm (4.8 to 5.2 inches) wide and 22 to 23 cm (8.5 to 9 inches) long.[1] The appropriately-sized cuff must be used to assure valid measurement. If the cuff is too small, too narrow, or too short, it will overestimate the BP, and if it is too large, it will to a lesser degree underestimate the BP.[28,31] Therefore clinicians should have several cuff sizes available to suit the typical patient population that they encounter.

Procedure. The procedures described here for measuring BP reflect commonly accepted practice.[28,30] Positioning of the patient and therapist is critical to obtaining accurate results. The clinician must be in a good position to view the manometer, and the patient must be positioned so that the results are not adversely affected by discomfort or undue exertion.

The upper arm is most commonly used to obtain BP, although other sites can be used and are discussed briefly after the following general description:

1. The patient should be seated comfortably for at least 5 minutes in a chair with their feet on the floor before measuring their BP. The patient should refrain from smoking, exercising, or ingesting caffeine for 30 minutes before the measurement is taken. The patient may be supine or standing if necessary. The surroundings should be quiet if possible.

2. The arm is supported at the level of the heart whether the patient is seated, supine, or standing. BP measures increase when the arm is below heart level and decrease when the arm is above heart level.[32-34] If measuring BP in a position other than sitting, note this position for consistency. The patient should not have to hold their arm at heart level actively or the isometric contraction involved may artificially increase the BP measurement. Crossing the legs should also be avoided as this has been found to elevate both systolic and diastolic pressures.[35]

3. Select the appropriately-sized cuff and position the manometer gauge so that the view is unobstructed, in line with the eyes, and the gauge indicates zero mm Hg while the cuff is deflated. The air bladder should be long enough to encircle at least 80% of the limb.

4. Expose the upper arm and apply the cuff directly on the skin. Clothing may prevent correct placement of the cuff and interfere with readings. Wrap the deflated cuff evenly around the upper arm so the center of the bladder is directly over the brachial artery in the antecubital fossa. Arrows on the cuff generally mark the area that should be over the brachial artery. The elbow should be slightly bent, and the lower border of the cuff should be placed approximately 1 inch above the antecubital fossa in adults (Fig. 22-10).

5. Place the earpieces of the stethoscope in your ears. The earpieces of the stethoscope should be pointing slightly forward in the direction of the ear canal to more clearly hear sounds. Make sure that the stethoscope tubing is hanging freely without rubbing or bumping anything that may interfere with the sounds to be auscultated. Place the diaphragm of the

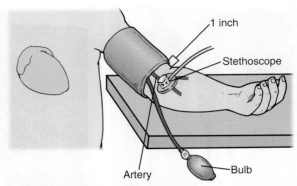

FIG. 22-10 Position of the arm with the cuff and stethoscope to measure blood pressure.

stethoscope over the brachial artery in the antecubital fossa firmly enough that all surface edges of the diaphragm are in contact with the skin. Rapidly inflate the cuff about 30 mm Hg above the point where the pulse was previously noted to disappear.

6. Gradually deflate the cuff at about 2 mm Hg per second while listening for the pulse with the stethoscope. The systolic BP is the number at which the pulse is first heard. The diastolic BP is the number at which the sound of the pulse is no longer heard. Once the diastolic BP is reached, the cuff can be deflated quickly all the way to zero. If readings are difficult to obtain, do not stop midway and try to reinflate to repeat the reading because this will produce unreliable results. Wait at least 2 minutes before repeating any measurement to confirm accuracy. If sounds are heard all the way down to zero, use the point where muffling of sound begins and record that number as the diastolic reading.

7. Remove the cuff.

8. Record your findings and note from which arm the measurement was taken.

ALTERNATIVE BLOOD PRESSURE SITES

Although BP is generally measured in the upper arm, thigh measurement of BP using the popliteal artery is indicated in certain circumstances, including when BP cannot be measured on either arm because of burns, trauma, or bilateral mastectomy; when BP in one thigh is to be compared with BP in the other thigh; or when the BP cuff available is too large for the upper extremity.[19]

The procedure for measuring BP at the thigh is similar to that used for the arm except that the patient must be lying down, ideally prone to expose the popliteal fossa, or if necessary, supine, with the knee slightly bent. The popliteal pulse is auscultated in the popliteal fossa.

Many wrist-cuff devices are available to measure BP in the forearm. They are appealing because of their convenience and portability, and a few studies report that they are comparable to standard upper arm auscultatory and electronic sphygmomanometers.[36,37] However, the majority of evidence has not found wrist-cuff sphygmomanometers to be accurate or reliable enough for practical use, and these are therefore not recommended.[28,38-41]

AGE-RELATED CONSIDERATIONS FOR BLOOD PRESSURE MEASUREMENT PROCEDURE

In infants, a pediatric stethoscope with a smaller diaphragm should be used for auscultation and the lower edge of the cuff can be placed closer to the antecubital fossa than in the adult because infants' arms are so much smaller. Arm and thigh pressure are essentially equivalent in children under 1 year of age, and therefore BP may be measured at the thigh if this is more convenient.[19]

In children, it is best to explain the steps and what it will feel like first and then demonstrate on a doll or stuffed animal if available. The bladder should be wide enough to cover about 40% of the arm and long enough to wrap around 80% to 100% of the arm's circumference. Ideally, BP measurements should be taken before uncomfortable procedures so that the measure is not artificially elevated. In children over 1 year of age, the thigh BP is about 10 mm Hg higher than the arm BP.

In the elderly, the cuff pressure should not remain high for any longer than necessary to minimize the risk of damaging fragile skin. Also, if the patient is taking any antihypertensive medication, one should note which one and when the last dose was taken.[42]

CONTRAINDICATIONS TO MEASURING BLOOD PRESSURE

BP should not be measured on the patient's arm if the patient has had breast or axilla surgery on that side, if the patient has an intravenous line or has had a recent blood transfusion on that limb, or if the patient has an arteriovenous fistula (for renal dialysis) in that limb. The thigh should not be used if there has been a recent surgery on that hip or lower extremity.

NORMAL RANGES

Normal BP in adults is less than 120/80 mm Hg. Hypertension is defined as a BP with either the systolic or the diastolic BP being at or above the cut-off of 140/90 mm Hg.

HYPERTENSION

The prevalence of hypertension, particularly systolic hypertension, increases with advancing age but multiple factors affect blood pressure (Table 22-3). Hypertension (systolic or diastolic) is an independent risk factor for all forms of cardiovascular disease, including heart attack, stroke, heart failure, peripheral vascular disease, and kidney failure.[28,30] The risk increases progressively as BP gets higher.

> ### ◎ *Clinical Pearl*
>
> Hypertension (elevated blood pressure) is a risk factor for heart attack, stroke, and kidney failure.

Cardiovascular disease risk is determined in part by BP but also by associated risk factors, including smoking, dyslipidemia, diabetes mellitus, age, gender, obesity, and family history. Prevention through risk factor modification is considered better than treatment. This mainly involves lifestyle changes such as decreasing caloric intake

TABLE 22-3	**Factors Affecting Blood Pressure**
Factor	**Impact**
Age	Systolic BP gradually increases through life.
	Diastolic BP increases until 50-60 years of age.
	Newborn mean systolic BP is 73 mm Hg.
	Ages 10-19 BP ranges from 124-136/77-84 mm Hg for boys and 124-127/63-74 mm Hg for girls.
	Geriatric adult BP commonly ranges from 140-160/90 mm Hg.
Gender	Women typically have lower BP than men until after menopause.
Exercise	Physical exertion increases BP acutely and decreases resting BP over time.
Position	BP can fall after a change of position from lying to sitting or sitting to standing (see section on Orthostatic Hypotension).
Medications/drugs	Many medications may increase or decrease BP.
	Antihypertensives, diuretics, beta-blockers, calcium channel blockers, vasodilators, ACE inhibitors, and narcotic medications all decrease BP.
	Stimulants, such as caffeine, generally increase BP.
Sympathetic nervous system stimulation	Stress, anxiety, fear, and pain increase BP.
Obesity	Obesity predisposes people to hypertension.
Diurnal variations	BP is usually lowest in the morning when metabolic rate is the lowest, rises throughout the day, and peaks in late afternoon when the person is mentally awake and physically active.
Fever/heat/cold	Increased metabolic rate associated with fever may elevate BP.
	External heat associated with vasodilation may decrease BP.
	Cold associated with vasoconstriction may increase BP.
Smoking	Smoking causes vasoconstriction, which increases peripheral resistance resulting in elevated BP.
	BP may remain elevated acutely for up to 15 minutes after smoking.[43]
Race/ethnicity	Typically, African-American men over 35 years of age have higher BP than European men of the same age.

BP, Blood pressure; *ACE,* angiotensin-converting enzyme.

to decrease body weight, moderating alcohol consumption, increasing exercise, stopping smoking, decreasing fat and salt intake, and decreasing stress. If and when these measures fail, then the physician may decide to prescribe medications.

HYPOTENSION

Hypotension is generally defined as a systolic BP of 90 mm Hg or lower, although in some adults such a low BP may be normal.[1] Signs and symptoms of clinically significant hypotension include tachycardia; dizziness; mental confusion; restlessness; cool, clammy, pale or **cyanotic** skin; and **syncope**.[19] Shock may be caused by a reduction in BP as a result of a wide range of causes, including hemorrhage, vomiting, diarrhea, burns, myocardial infarction, and overwhelming infection. Signs and symptoms of shock include hypotension, tachycardia, cold clammy skin, dizziness, blurred vision, and apprehension. The presence of low BP and any of these symptoms may indicate onset of shock or circulatory collapse and should be taken seriously, including ensuring immediate medical attention.

ORTHOSTATIC HYPOTENSION

Orthostatic hypotension, also known as *postural hypotension,* is a transient decrease in BP, occurring in response to a change in position, generally when moving from lying down to an upright position. It is typically defined by a decline of 20 mm Hg or more in systolic BP or a decline of 10 mm Hg or more in diastolic BP.[43,44] Orthostatic hypotension is common in patients when they first try to get up after a protracted period of bed rest.[45] When the patient stands, blood pools in the legs and trunk and causes venous return to transiently fall. This in turn decreases cardiac output and subsequently BP and cerebral perfusion.[44] Normally, autonomic reflexes quickly restore BP by causing vasoconstriction and a transient increase in heart rate to prevent dizziness or lightheadedness. However, if pooling is severe or if the autonomic response is delayed or inadequate, the patient will feel lightheaded and may faint.[44] Certain medications, including diuretics and beta-blockers, may promote or aggravate orthostatic hypotension.[43]

RELEVANCE OF BLOOD PRESSURE TO REHABILITATION

Physical therapists (PTs) and physical therapist assistants (PTAs) can participate in improving public health by providing education about exercise and other lifestyle-related interventions that help reduce resting BP and thus the community burden of hypertension and its sequelae. BP measures are used to indicate a patient's baseline hemodynamic status during rehabilitation and to guide the safety and vigor of activities during rehabilitation. Patients frequently perform exercises, such as treadmill walking, running, upper body ergometer pedaling, or cycling on a stationary bicycle, as a component of their physical therapy interventions. Although these exercises can be beneficial, they all place demands on the cardiovascular system and should be tailored to the individual needs and limitations of the patient.

Typically, systolic BP rises rapidly and diastolic pressure rises slightly during the first few minutes of aerobic exercise and then both level off.[46] With resistance training, systolic BP rises more dramatically. High-level resistance training can cause rises in systolic BP that can be harmful for individuals with preexisting hypertension or heart disease and therefore loads should be kept lower in such patients. Aerobic exercise performed with the arms produces a greater rise in systolic and diastolic BP than lower extremity exercise performed at the same intensity.[46] Therefore upper body ergometry should be avoided or used with caution and should generally be replaced with lower extremity exercise in those with increased cardiovascular risk. Although exercise causes an acute increase in BP, regular submaximal aerobic and resistance training does not cause long-term increases in resting BP but rather results in lowered BP for 2 to 3 hours after exercise, lowered resting BP, and less increase in BP during exercise.[46]

AUTONOMIC DYSREFLEXIA

The interruption of autonomic pathways by spinal cord injury (SCI) can cause dysfunction of the autonomic nervous system (see Chapter 20). SCI cranial to the sympathetic outflow may be complicated by a phenomenon known as *autonomic dysreflexia* (AD). Although AD is generally associated with injuries at or above the T6 level, there have been cases reported with SCI as low as the T8 and T10 level. AD occurs in between 19% and 70% of patients with SCI.

AD is an acute syndrome manifested by cardiovascular symptoms and characterized by a sudden increase in BP.[47] Along with paroxysmal hypertension, AD generally causes a throbbing headache, profuse sweating above the level of the spinal lesion, facial flushing, and tachycardia.[40-52] Headache is one of the most common symptoms of AD, occurring in approximately 50% of patients.[53] Less commonly, AD causes nasal congestion, piloerection, paresthesias, shivering, desire to void, anxiety, malaise, nausea, dullness in the head, or blurred vision.[48,50-52] Untreated, AD can cause seizures, strokes, cardiac arrhythmias, and death.[47,51-56]

The main objective sign of AD is a dramatic increase in systolic BP and diastolic BP,[48] which can reach as high as 250 to 300 mm Hg and 200 to 220 mm Hg, respectively.[53,57] Most authors consider a rise in systolic BP of 30 to 40 mm Hg or 20% of the baseline value to be diagnostic of AD when it occurs in conjunction with at least one of the following: Headache, flushing, piloerection, sweating, and chills.[48]

◎ *Clinical Pearl*

In general, in the right clinical setting, a rise in systolic BP of 30 to 40 mm Hg or 20% of the baseline value in conjunction with headache, flushing, piloerection, sweating, and/or chills is diagnostic of autonomic dysreflexia (AD).

The onset of AD is rapid and often dramatic,[48] and practically any cutaneous or visceral stimulus below the level of the spinal cord lesion can precipitate the AD reaction.[50] Common triggers for AD are distention or contraction of the hollow organs or activation of pain receptors. More than one stimulus occurring simultaneously may make the reaction more severe and easier to bring on.[48] Bowel and bladder distention are perhaps the most common causes of AD.[48] However, catheterization and manipulation of an indwelling catheter are also well-known precipitating factors.[58] Additional precipitating factors, although less common, are gastric ulcers,[59] gastroesophageal reflux,[60] skeletal fractures below the level of the spinal cord lesion,[61,62] pregnancy,[63,64] labor,[65] sexual activity,[48] surgery,[66] and numerous others.[67]

REHABILITATION AND AUTONOMIC DYSREFLEXIA

Because of its life-threatening potential, clinicians working with patients with SCIs must be familiar with and understand the signs and triggers for AD. Patients with SCI should be positioned carefully to avoid pain and undue pressure on the bladder or abdomen. One should keep in mind that aggressive stretching or range of motion (ROM) activities that stimulate nociceptors can trigger an AD reaction. In addition, urinary catheters should be checked for blockage, twisting of the tubing, or overfilling of the bag.

Clinical Pearl

Autonomic dysreflexia (AD) is a life-threatening medical emergency. Always alert appropriate personnel and inspect for any possible triggers.

An AD reaction should be treated as a medical emergency, and institutional policies for such situations should be followed. In addition, the patient should be kept as upright as possible and inspected for any possible triggers. Keep in mind that the trigger may be something as simple as tight clothing or sitting on a wrinkle in clothing. All potential triggers should be resolved as quickly as possible. For example, tight clothing should be loosened or removed and catheter tubing should be unkinked. The therapy session should be discontinued so that the patient is able to recover and stabilize.

PAIN*

IMPLICATIONS OF PAIN

Pain is an unpleasant sensory and emotional experience associated with actual or potential tissue damage or described in terms of such damage.[68] It is the most common symptom that brings patients to their health care practitioner, and patients' goals in rehabilitation frequently involve relieving pain. Measurement of pain helps evaluate the cause and source of symptoms, selection of interventions, and outcome assessment of the rehabilitation management.

---

*The information on measurement of pain in this chapter is adapted from Cameron MH: *Physical agents in rehabilitation,* ed 3, St. Louis, 2009, Saunders.

The case to consider pain as the fifth vital sign stems from attempts to overcome barriers to relieving pain,[69] goals to improve patient/practitioner communication,[70] and attempts to improve the overall quality of patient care.[71] Pain should be taken seriously and addressed even if the patient does not want to complain about it or if pain is an expected part of the patient's condition.[72]

Pain is not just the result of nociceptive signals reaching the brain but also encompasses an individual's experience of the sensation interwoven within their past and present experiences and emotions. Therefore, to be successful, pain management may need to address these issues, as well as the nociceptive aspect of pain.[73]

Pain measurement may include information about the nature, location, severity, and duration of the patient's experience of pain, as well as the degree to which the pain results in functional limitation or disability. Various methods and assessment tools have been developed to quantify and qualify both experimentally induced and clinical pain. These methods are based on patients rating their pain on visual analog or numeric scales or selecting words from a list to describe their present experience of pain. Different tools provide different amounts and types of information and require differing amounts of time and cognitive ability to complete.

Clinical Pearl

Pain is an unpleasant sensory and emotional experience associated with actual or potential tissue damage.

VISUAL ANALOG AND NUMERIC SCALES

The visual analog scale (VAS) and the numeric rating scale (NRS) assess pain severity by asking the patient to indicate the present level of pain on a drawn line or to rate the pain numerically on a scale of 1 to 10 or 1 to 100.[74] With the VAS, the patient marks a position on a horizontal or vertical line, where one end of the line represents no pain and the other end represents the most severe pain possible or the most severe pain the patient can imagine (Fig. 22-11). With the NRS, 0 is no pain and 10 or 100, depending on the scale used, is the most severe pain possible or the most severe pain the patient can imagine. The horizontal VAS has been validated and shown to be reliable.[75]

Scales similar to the VAS or NRS have been developed for use with individuals who have difficulty using these scales. For example, children who understand pictures but are too young to understand numeric representations of pain can use a scale with faces with different expressions to represent different experiences of pain (Fig. 22-12). The faces pain scale (FPS) is often used with children (3 to 12 years old) or individuals who are unable to communicate verbally.[76,77] This type of scale can also be used to assess pain in patients with limited comprehension because of language barriers or cognitive deficits. Pain scales are also available for rating pain in very young children and infants. These are based on describing the child's behavior, from inconsolable, constant crying to smiling.

These simple scales are frequently used to assess the severity of a patient's clinical pain because they are quick

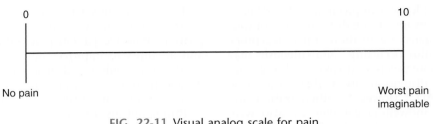

FIG. 22-11 Visual analog scale for pain.

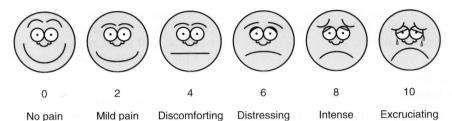

FIG. 22-12 Pain scale using graphic representations to assist small children or those with a language barrier. *Adapted from Wong DL, Hockenberry MJ, Perry SE, et al:* Maternal child nursing care, *ed 3, St. Louis, 2006, Mosby.*

and easy to administer, are easily understood, and provide readily quantifiable data.[74] VAS and NRS provide only a single measure of the patient's pain complaint and do not provide information about the patient's affective response to pain or the effect of the pain on his or her functional activity level. These types of measures are most useful in the clinical setting when a quick estimate of a patient's perceived progress or response to different activities or treatment interventions is desired.

SEMANTIC DIFFERENTIAL SCALES

Semantic differential scales consist of word lists and categories that represent various aspects of the patient's pain experience. The patient is asked to select words from these lists that best describe his or her present experience of pain. These types of scales are designed to collect a broad range of information about the patient's pain experience and to provide quantifiable data for intrasubject and intersubject comparisons. The semantic differential scale included in the McGill Pain Questionnaire, or variations of this scale, are commonly used to assess pain[78-80] (Fig. 22-13). This scale includes descriptors of sensory, affective, and evaluative aspects of the patient's pain and groups the words into various categories within each of these aspects. The categories include temporal, spatial, pressure, and thermal to describe the sensory aspects of the pain; fear, anxiety, and tension to describe the affective aspects of the pain; and the cognitive experience of the pain based on past experience and learned behaviors to describe the evaluative aspects of the pain. The patient circles the one word in each of the applicable categories that best describes the present pain.[78,80]

Semantic differential scales have a number of advantages and disadvantages compared with other types of pain measures. They allow assessment and quantification of various aspects of the pain's scope, quality, and intensity. Counting the total number of words chosen provides a quick gauge of the pain severity. A more sensitive assessment of pain severity can be obtained by adding the rank sums of all the words chosen to produce a pain-rating index. For greater specificity with regard to the most problematic area, an index for the three major categories of the questionnaire can also be calculated.[80] The primary disadvantages of this scale are that it is time consuming to administer and requires the patient to have an intact cognitive state and a high level of literacy. Given these advantages and limitations, the most appropriate use for this type of scale is when detailed information about a patient's pain is needed such as in a chronic pain treatment program or in clinical research.

OTHER MEASURES

Other measures or indicators of pain that may provide additional useful information about the individual's pain complaint and clinical condition include daily activity/pain logs indicating which activities ease or aggravate the pain, body diagrams on which the patient can indicate the location and nature of the pain (Fig. 22-14), and open-ended, structured interviews.[81]

In addition to the severity and nature of pain, pain can be described according to its presentation over time as constant or intermittent. Constant pain is pain that is present at all times. The person is never pain-free, although the severity of the pain may vary over time. Intermittent pain is pain that is not always present. The pain comes and goes, and the patient has some pain-free periods, although these may be brief. Chemically-induced pain associated with an inflammatory process is often constant. Mechanical pain, which is generally associated with positioning, malalignment, or pressure, is usually intermittent.

◎ *Clinical Pearl*

Chemically-induced pain associated with an inflammatory process is often constant. Mechanical pain, which is generally associated with positioning, malalignment, or pressure, is usually intermittent.

What does your pain feel like?

Some of the words below describe your *present* pain. Indicate which words describe it best. Leave out any word group that is not suitable. Use only a single word in each appropriate group—the one that applies *best*.

1	2	3	4
1 Flickering	1 Jumping	1 Pricking	1 Sharp
2 Quivering	2 Flashing	2 Boring	2 Cutting
3 Pulsing	3 Shooting	3 Drilling	3 Lacerating
4 Throbbing		4 Stabbing	
5 Beating		5 Lancinating	
6 Pounding			

5	6	7	8
1 Pinching	1 Tugging	1 Hot	1 Tingling
2 Pressing	2 Pulling	2 Burning	2 Itchy
3 Gnawing	3 Wrenching	3 Scalding	3 Smarting
4 Cramping		4 Searing	4 Stinging
5 Crushing			

9	10	11	12
1 Dull	1 Tender	1 Tiring	1 Sickening
2 Sore	2 Taut	2 Exhausting	2 Suffocating
3 Hurting	3 Rasping		
4 Aching	4 Splitting		
5 Heavy			

13	14	15	16
1 Fearful	1 Punishing	1 Wretched	1 Annoying
2 Frightful	2 Gruelling	2 Blinding	2 Troublesome
3 Terrifying	3 Cruel		3 Miserable
	4 Vicious		4 Intense
	5 Killing		5 Unbearable

17	18	19	20
1 Spreading	1 Tight	1 Cool	1 Nagging
2 Radiating	2 Numb	2 Cold	2 Nauseating
3 Penetrating	3 Drawing	3 Freezing	3 Agonizing
4 Piercing	4 Squeezing		4 Dreadful
	5 Tearing		5 Torturing

FIG. 22-13 Semantic differential scale from the McGill Pain Questionnaire. *From Melzack R: The McGill Pain Questionnaire: Major properties and scoring methods,* Pain *1:277-299, 1975.*

ARTERIAL OXYGEN SATURATION

IMPLICATIONS OF ARTERIAL OXYGEN SATURATION

As early as 1988, it was suggested that arterial oxygen saturation be considered a vital sign.[82] Arterial oxyhemoglobin saturation, more commonly known as *arterial oxygen saturation (Sao$_2$)*, is the degree to which hemoglobin in the blood is bound to oxygen. Each hemoglobin molecule has four oxygen-binding sites and is considered to be 100% saturated when all four sites are bound to oxygen. Oxygen saturation is generally measured by percentage saturation and may be as high as 100%. Values of 95% to 100% are considered normal, and pulse oximetry generally provides reliable measures of oxygen saturation in the range of 70% to 100%.[83]

Sao$_2$ may be measured by pulse oximetry or through an arterial blood gas (ABG) analysis from a sample of arterial blood. Oxygen saturation via pulse oximetry **(Spo$_2$)** is generally preferred because it is simple, painless, accurate, noninvasive, and provides instantaneous, continuous measures of oxygen saturation.[83] Pulse oximetry is used to monitor hypoxia in patients with moderate-to-severe pulmonary disease and also the effectiveness of oxygen supplementation in many patients.[82]

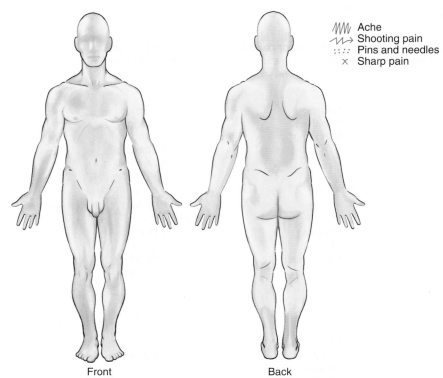

	Ache
	Shooting pain
	Pins and needles
✕	Sharp pain

Front   Back

FIG. 22-14 Body diagram to record pain symptoms.

HOW PULSE OXIMETRY WORKS

A pulse oximeter consists of a sensor connected to a micro-processor. Most sensors resemble a small clothespin or a flat patch. The clothespin type sensor is typically secured to a fingertip, and the patch sensor may be taped to the skin, wrapped around a digit, or wrapped about the foot of an infant or small child. The sensor has a light-emitting diode (LED) light source and a light detector or photode-tector positioned directly opposite the LED. The LED pro-duces alternating bursts of red and infrared light. Unoxygenated hemoglobin absorbs more of the red light, and oxygenated hemoglobin absorbs more of the infrared light. The photodetector measures how much of each type of light passes through the tissue and transmits this infor-mation to a microprocessor that calculates the SpO_2 from this data. Pulse oximeters only monitor light absorption that varies in a pulsatile manner and therefore only work if applied to an area with good arterial flow.[83] The device generally displays both SpO_2 and the pulse rate.

METHOD FOR MEASURING ARTERIAL OXYGEN SATURATION

Descriptions of the procedure for measuring SpO_2 vary slightly from one source to another. The procedure here reflects common accepted practice.[1,83] Before measuring an individual's arterial oxygen saturation you should, if possible, be aware of their hemoglobin level, previous baseline arterial oxygen saturation, and temperature. Additionally, check to see if the patient has a current or past history of using oxygen therapy.

Procedure

1. Explain what you are going to do, why, and how the patient can cooperate.
2. Wash your hands.
3. Provide for patient privacy, position patient com-fortably, and try to ensure that the patient is breathing regularly.
4. Choose the site for application of the sensor. The sensor should be applied to an area of high vascu-larity such as the finger-tip, toe, earlobe, pinna of the ear, or the bridge of the nose. It should have adequate perfusion, be as motionless as possible, and free of any substance that may interfere with the light transmission through the tissue.
5. Choose the appropriate sensor for the selected loca-tion. In infants, if finger or toe sensors of the appro-priate size are not available, then an adhesive type sensor may be used.
6. If using the finger, have the forearm supported and choose a finger without nail polish or artificial nails. If necessary, remove the polish or artificial nail. If that is not possible, use a toe or place the sensor sideways on the finger rather than over the nail bed.
7. Place the sensor on the patient. Let the patient know that it will not hurt and that they will feel only a little pressure. Make sure it is aligned cor-rectly. If pulse oximetry is to be continuous, be sure to move sensors secured by spring tension every 2 hours as a safety precaution.
8. Turn on the oximeter, and observe the pulse inten-sity display and listen for an audible beeping sound.

Correlate the oximeter pulse with a palpated pulse for accuracy.

9. Have the patient remain still, and inform them that an alarm will sound if the sensor falls off or if the patient displaces the sensor. If necessary, cover the sensor with a towel or washcloth to prevent bright ambient light from shining on the sensor, which may distort readings.

10. Leave the sensor in place until the oximeter reaches a stable value and the pulse display reaches full strength during each cardiac cycle. Read the SpO_2. If the SpO_2 is less than 95%, retake it or find an alternate site to retake the measurement unless the patient is known to have habitually low readings.

11. Document the SpO_2, pulse rate, sensor site, activity level, patient position, date, time, and, if the patient is on supplemental oxygen, the delivery rate and method of delivery. Discuss the findings with the physical therapist as needed.

FACTORS AFFECTING RELEVANCE AND ACCURACY OF PULSE OXIMETRY READINGS

A number of factors may affect the clinical relevance and accuracy of SpO_2 measurements taken using pulse oximetry. These include patient factors, such as hemoglobin level, carbon monoxide inhalation, and the type of hemoglobin, as well as factors during the test such as motion, ambient light, wearing nail polish, and mechanical problems with the device.

Hemoglobin Level. Arterial oxygen hemoglobin saturation must be interpreted in the context of the patient's complete clinical picture, particularly their hemoglobin level. Even though a patient may have a high level of saturation, oxygen delivery to the tissues will be poor if the hemoglobin level is low.[83] Normal hemoglobin levels typically range from about 12 to 16 gm/dL for women and 13 to 18 gm/dL for men. A reduction in oxygen-carrying capacity as occurs with low hemoglobin levels causes a reduction in the amount of oxygen delivered to the tissues and will produce the same symptoms as low SpO_2. Pulse oximetry can be used in patients with sickle cell anemia because even though SpO_2 is underestimated, the difference is not clinically significant.[84] Pulse oximetry can also be used in infants and neonates, who have fetal hemoglobin (HbF), because it provides accurate, reliable, and clinically acceptable estimates of arterial hemoglobin in this population.[85-87]

Carbon Monoxide Inhalation. Carboxyhemoglobin absorbs light similarly to oxyhemoglobin, and pulse oximeters cannot differentiate between hemoglobin saturated with carbon monoxide or oxygen. Therefore patients who have inhaled a significant amount of carbon monoxide may have pulse oximeter readings that give the false impression of being normal. If carbon monoxide poisoning is suspected, only an ABG test should be used to determine oxygen saturation.[83]

Low Perfusion States. Low perfusion states that weaken or eliminate peripheral pulses will decrease the precision of the pulse oximeter readings because the device must detect pulsatile flow to function.[83] Patients at risk for low perfusion are those with hypotension, peripheral vascular disease, peripheral vasoconstriction, peripheral edema, and hypothermia and those who are hypovolemic or in cardiac arrest.[1,83] These conditions can easily lead to unreliable readings. In patients who are cold but not hypothermic, it is recommended that more central sites, such as the forehead or earlobes, be used or peripheral sites be warmed, to avoid inaccuracies caused by distal peripheral vasoconstriction.[83]

Motion During the Test. A variety of errors can be produced by patient movement during the measurement of arterial blood saturation by pulse oximetry. These include reduced accuracy, loss of signal, false desaturation alarms, and missed hypoxic events.[88] Erratic movement, especially in small children and neonates, may partially dislodge the sensor, which in turn disrupts the light transmission through the tissue. Furthermore, rhythmic movements may make it difficult for the sensor to distinguish pulsatile flow, and other movements, such as shivering, exercise, and vibration, during transport may dislodge the sensor.[83] Therefore the patient should be as still as possible when measuring oxygen saturation. Newer devices, with different hardware and software designed to tolerate or compensate for movement, have been found to produce more reliable and accurate results than older units when patients are moving.[88-92]

Ambient Light. Ambient light can alter pulse oximeter readings if there is enough light of similar wavelengths to those produced by the sensor's LED. This may occur with fluorescent lighting but can be rectified by covering the sensor with an opaque towel.

Fingernail Polish. Fingernail polish, particularly dark polish, may interfere with pulse oximetry readings at the fingers or toes. Therefore, if the patient is wearing dark nail polish, either remove the polish from a finger or toe and use this digit or measure oxygen saturation at an alternate site. If necessary, the sensor may be placed sideways on the finger or toe.[83]

Mechanical Problems. Pulse oximeters like any other mechanical device need to be maintained and calibrated regularly. If inconsistencies are suspected in a unit, have it checked immediately and continue with a unit that is known to be in good working order.

Clinical Pearl

The accuracy of pulse oximetry may be hampered by carbon monoxide inhalation, the type of hemoglobin, motion, ambient light, wearing nail polish, and mechanical problems with the device.

NORMAL VALUES

Oxygen saturation values of 95% to 100% are generally considered normal. Values under 90% could quickly lead to a serious deterioration in status, and values under 70% are life-threatening.[19] Patients may deteriorate considerably before there is a dramatic change in oxygen saturation because, as discussed previously, the PaO_2 may fall from 100 mm Hg to 60 or 70 mm Hg before the oxygen saturation drops to 90%. Signs of deterioration include low BP, increased respiratory rate, and increased pulse rate.[83] Other signs of altered oxygen saturation that would indicate checking SpO_2 are altered respiratory rate; depth or rhythm; unusual breath sounds; cyanotic appearance of nail beds, lips, or mucous membranes; dusky skin; confusion; decreased level of consciousness; and dyspnea.[1,19]

CLINICAL APPLICATION

Pulse oximetry is a valuable tool to evaluate patients' exercise tolerance or progress in a rehabilitation program. Additionally, documentation of SpO_2 values with therapeutic intervention can lend support to the need for supplemental home oxygen therapy.

CHAPTER SUMMARY

Vital signs are indicators of a patient's general health. A history of recorded vital signs provides a view of a patient's health status over time and current measurements are valuable indicators of acute changes. The rehabilitation provider should be able to differentiate between normal and abnormal findings and have the proper skills and tools to gather and document vital sign measures. Accurate and reliable measures are needed for safe and effective patient management during therapeutic interventions.

GLOSSARY

Ambient temperature: The temperature in one's immediate location.

Apical: Of, at, or forming the apex of a structure.

Arrhythmia: Irregularity or loss of rhythm, especially of the heartbeat. Also known as dysrhythmia.

Benign: Not recurrent or progressive. The opposite of malignant.

Bradycardia: A slow heart rate usually less than 60 bpm.

Carboxyhemoglobin: Compound of hemoglobin and carbon monoxide formed in poisoning by carbon monoxide.

Cyanotic: Pertaining to the bluish, grayish, or dark purple discoloration of the skin, resulting from abnormal amounts of reduced hemoglobin in the blood.

Frenulum: Fold of mucous membrane that extends from the floor of the mouth to the inferior surface of the tongue along its midline.

Hypothermia: Having a body temperature below normal, usually considered 35° C (95° F) and below.

Meniscus: The curved upper surface of a liquid in a container. The surface is convex if the liquid does not wet the container and concave if it does.

Otoscope: A device for examination of the ear.

Pinna: The auricle or projected part of the exterior ear that collects and directs sound waves into the ear.

Pulse: The regular expansion felt over an artery as the wave of blood passes through the vessel in time with the heartbeat.

Sphygmomanometer: The instrument used to determine BP through the use of an arm cuff and an aneroid dial or a calibrated column of mercury.

SpO_2: Estimation of arterial blood saturation by pulse oximetry.

Sublingual pocket: The area to the back and underneath the tongue on either side of the frenulum.

Syncope: A transient loss of consciousness from inadequate blood flow to the brain. Also known as fainting or swooning.

Tachycardia: Abnormally rapid heart rate, usually considered over 100 bpm in adults at rest.

Tachypnea: Abnormally rapid respiration or rate of breathing.

Tympanic membrane: Eardrum. The membrane serving as the lateral wall of the tympanic cavity and separating it from the external acoustic meatus.

Vasoconstriction: Decrease in the caliber of a blood vessel.

Vasodilation: Increase in the caliber of a blood vessel.

Vital signs: The critical indicators of a person's health and current medical status (e.g., pulse, body temperature, respiration, BP, oxygen saturation, and perceived pain).

Chapter **23**

Deconditioning

Ahmed Samir Elokda, Kevin Helgeson

CHAPTER OUTLINE

OBJECTIVES

After reading this chapter, the reader will be able to:
1. Discuss the risk factors for pathologies associated with the consequences of deconditioning.
2. Use evidence-based interventions for patients with deconditioning.

Deconditioning is the decline of normal anatomical and physiological function caused by disease, aging, or inactivity.[1] **Deconditioning** can affect multiple body systems, and a decline in the function of any one system may affect the other systems. The cardiopulmonary system is most affected by deconditioning, and this secondarily has the greatest effect on the musculoskeletal system. Deconditioning of the cardiopulmonary system impairs the transport of blood and oxygen to the body's tissues, including the skeletal muscles that provide for mobility of the body. Musculoskeletal deconditioning leads to changes in muscle cellular metabolism, decreased capillarization, and decreased ability to work for long periods.[1]

Deconditioning can occur in many patients needing rehabilitation, ranging from high-level athletes who cannot perform sports-specific physical training because of injury to patients in the intensive care unit and less active elderly individuals.

Clinical Pearl

Many patients receiving physical therapy demonstrate deconditioning.

Patients with a high level of physical fitness will have a more rapid decline in physiological function with periods of extended immobility than patients with low levels of fitness.[2] Periods of immobility or decreased activity quickly result in a decline in maximum oxygen consumption rate, total blood volume, and stroke volume. These changes can be measured after as little as 2 weeks of inactivity.[1,2] Measures of pulmonary function, heart rate, and muscle metabolism decline more slowly, with measurable changes occurring after at least 30 days of inactivity.[1]

PATHOLOGY

The *Guide to Physical Therapist Practice* (the *Guide*) includes the preferred practice pattern 6B: Impaired aerobic capacity/endurance associated with deconditioning. This practice pattern describes physical therapy management for patients with deconditioning who develop impairments of decreased aerobic capacity and/or endurance. The functional limitations related to the **endurance impairment** are activities or tasks the patient cannot perform for long enough or with enough repetitions to be efficient or cannot carry out in a typically expected or competent manner. Patients classified in this preferred practice pattern have functional limitations primarily because of impaired endurance. Patients with conditions that best fit other practice patterns in the musculoskeletal, neuromuscular, or integumentary sections of the *Guide* may also have deconditioning and endurance impairments. Therefore the information presented in this chapter may serve as a useful reference for patients primarily categorized in other preferred practice patterns who develop problems related to deconditioning.

The musculoskeletal preferred practice pattern 4C: Impaired muscle performance (see Chapter 5) is closely related to deconditioning, since the loss of muscle endurance, the inability to perform repetitive work tasks, and decreased functional work capacity described in the inclusion criteria of this pattern may also be found in a patient fitting the deconditioning pattern. The impaired muscle performance pattern should be used for problems that primarily affect the musculoskeletal system in a specific region of the body, whereas the deconditioning pattern would be used for problems of a more global nature, affecting multiple systems.

PROCESSES THAT RESULT IN DECONDITIONING

The effects of detraining in athletic subjects and of bed rest in subjects without pathologies have been well studied.[1,2,4] The effects on the cardiopulmonary, musculoskeletal, and endocrine systems in these subjects serve as the basis for our understanding of the effects of deconditioning on patients with conditions that result in endurance impairments.

Maximum oxygen uptake ($\dot{V}o_{2max}$) rate is considered the best indicator of cardiopulmonary fitness.[5,6] $\dot{V}o_{2max}$ is the maximum amount of oxygen in milliliters (ml) that one can use in 1 minute (min) per kilogram (kg) of body weight. $\dot{V}o_{2max}$ is determined by measuring the amount of oxygen the body consumes during an activity such as walking, running, or bicycling with maximal effort. $\dot{V}o_{2max}$ in a healthy adult is usually in the range of 24 to 50 ml of oxygen/kg of body weight/min.[6] $\dot{V}o_{2max}$ has been shown to decline with inactivity, with the decline being fastest during the first month of inactivity but ongoing, albeit at a slower rate, for at least the next 2 months.[1,2] Changes in stroke volume, blood volume, heart rate, and ventilatory capacity all contribute to the decline in $\dot{V}o_{2max}$.

The oxygen consumption rate ($\dot{V}o_2$) at rest is about 3.5 ml/kg/min. Activities of daily living (ADLs), such as grooming, preparing a meal, and slow walking, require a $\dot{V}o_2$ of 7 to 10 ml/kg/min. The inability to tolerate activities that require a $\dot{V}o_2$ higher than 18 ml/kg/min has been used as a criterion for disability.[5] Activities, such as prolonged standing, walking at 3 miles per hour (mph), and climbing stairs, are examples of activities that could not be sustained by a person with a maximum $\dot{V}o_2$ of 18 ml/kg/min.[7]

Inactivity. Cardiac stroke volume declines by approximately 12% during the first 30 days of inactivity or bed rest.[2] This decrease is primarily a result of decreased filling of the left ventricle during diastole.[8] When the left ventricle is less full at the end of diastole, it has less blood available to pump out with each stroke and is able to exert less force because the ventricle is not optimally stretched. Associated with this decrease in stroke volume is a decline in blood volume and increase in heart rate at submaximal levels of activity.[1,9] The maximum ventilatory capacity of the lungs also declines, showing a 10% to 15% decline after 4 weeks of inactivity.[2]

Levels of mitochondrial enzymes and capillary density in muscles also decline with inactivity and inactivity causes muscle mass to decline, primarily because of atrophy of the lower extremity extensor muscles (see Chapter 5 for further information on the effects of inactivity on muscle performance). Inactivity and bed rest also affect anaerobic metabolism and neuroendocrine responses to exercise. Studies show that 3 days of bed rest result in

a decrease in insulin-mediated glucose uptake and diminished levels of cortisol and growth hormone.[10,11] Inactivity can also decrease leukocyte (white blood cell) counts, affecting the body's immune response and ability to fight infection.[12]

Aging. Aging is a gradual process that influences a person's function and endurance levels. Physical effects of aging include loss of bone mineralization, loss of muscle mass, reduction in mitochondrial enzymes, reduced pulmonary function, and vascular insufficiency.[13-15] All of these changes contribute to deconditioning of the aging adult. Each individual ages at a different rate as a result of the interaction of genetic predisposition, behaviors, ongoing and new disease processes, psychosocial factors, physical activity levels, and living environment. For healthy older adults, the rate of decline in physiological functional capacity is largely determined by the volume and intensity of exercise they maintain as they age.[16]

The effects of aging on endurance and functional activities have been extensively studied and reviewed.[13-15] Aging of the cardiovascular and musculoskeletal systems have the greatest influence on deconditioning. Aging is associated with reduced cardiac output during exercise and reduction in maximum cardiac output of about 1% per year.[16] Declining cardiac muscle function reduces both contraction force and conduction through the myocardium, resulting in a decreased stroke volume and heart rate response to exercise.[17]

Skeletal muscle atrophies with aging as a result of a decrease in the number of muscle fibers accompanied by an increase in connective and fatty tissues within the muscle.[18] The size of type II muscle fibers decreases with age, resulting in a greater percentage of type I fiber mass, particularly in the lower extremity muscles. These changes can cause muscle strength to decrease by up to 40% by the age of 80.[19] This decrease in strength can limit the amount of activity the aging adult can perform.

Obesity. Obesity can also contribute to deconditioning. A sedentary lifestyle and voluntary inactivity have been associated with rising obesity rates in the United States.[20-22] Obesity contributes to deconditioning by accelerating the progression of atherosclerosis, increasing the risk of type II diabetes and its pathological consequences, and reducing tolerance of activities that maintain physical fitness. Multiple physical and psychosocial factors influence the progression of obesity. Many of these factors also limit the performance of physical activities and thus the individual's ability to reverse obesity and deconditioning.

A patient with deconditioning may have multiple pathological conditions that contribute to their endurance impairment. The examination of the patient with deconditioning emphasizes the patient's tolerance of endurance activities and the factors that could motivate the patient to increase their activity level.

TYPICAL EXAMINATION FINDINGS

PATIENT HISTORY

The history will include information about the patient's general health (physical, psychological, and social functions), current level of activity, and any related symptoms, such as fatigue, dyspnea, or angina, during activities.

A patient's history of exercise participation and activities and possibly history of participation in recreational or competitive sporting activities will help the therapist select the types of interventions that will most likely result in the patient beginning and maintaining an exercise program. The patient's social history and habits, living environment, employment, and exercise habits and history will be assessed because these may all influence exercise participation and continuation.

An exercise program is a voluntary behavior that requires a certain level of physical exertion and period of time to complete and maintain.[6] **Patient motivation** has been shown to be the single most important factor for continuing an exercise program.[23-25] It therefore needs to be determined if the patient is ready to change his or her behavior to start and maintain an exercise program, and the program should be specific to the patient's background, current needs, and developmental status.[26]

> ◎ **Clinical Pearl**
>
> Patient motivation is critical in the success of a patient's exercise program.

SYSTEMS REVIEW

Because many of the tests of endurance require ambulation, the patient's gait will be briefly examined before beginning these tests. The patient's overall stability and safety with walking activities should be evaluated, and any significant gait deviations will be noted (see Chapter 32). The effect of fatigue on gait stability and safety will be monitored during the endurance tests.

TESTS AND MEASURES

Patients with deconditioning may have a range of other problems requiring measurement of musculoskeletal, neuromuscular, cardiorespiratory, and/or integumentary function. However, since deconditioning is primarily a condition of altered cardiorespiratory function, tests and measures will focus on this area. The tests and measures described cover areas of greatest importance for deconditioned patients.

Musculoskeletal. The patient with deconditioning may be examined with tests and measures of posture, range of motion (ROM), and muscle performance.

Body composition will be measured in the deconditioned patient because this can affect tolerance of certain types of exercise programs. **Body mass index (BMI)** is the most commonly used general indicator of body composition (Fig. 23-1). BMI is equal to a person's weight in kilograms (kg) divided by their height in meters (m) squared (kg/m^2).[27]

More accurate but more cumbersome measures of body composition and body fat percentage are achieved through underwater weighing, skinfold measurements, or through bioelectrical impedance analysis (BIA).[27] Using body fat percentage, obesity is generally regarded as greater than 30% for adult men and greater than 40% for adult women.

Minimal or essential body fat percentages are 5% for men and 10% for women.[27]

Neuromuscular

Arousal, Attention, and Cognition (Fatigue). A report of fatigue during the patient history may be an indication of deconditioning, and fatigue that is not the result of deconditioning may also severely limit activity participation by a deconditioned patient.

> ◎ **Clinical Pearl**
>
> A patient may report fatigue before other overt signs of deconditioning are exhibited.

Pain. A patient with deconditioning may have episodic or chronic pain that should be assessed and monitored. Measurement of pain intensity by a pain scale, words, or pictures can be performed during an exercise program (see Chapter 22).

Cardiovascular/Pulmonary. Examination of a patient with deconditioning will focus on assessment of cardiopulmonary function. Measurements of the vital signs of heart rate, blood pressure (BP), and respiratory rate (see Chapter 22) provide basic information about the patient's cardiopulmonary function and readiness for active exercise and serve as a baseline for responses to exercise.[28] Findings of an abnormal heart rate or BP will affect the intensity of exercise chosen for the patient and may require referring the patient to the supervising physical therapist and possibly another health care provider.

Ventilation and Respiration/Gas Exchange. Patients who report discomfort with breathing during activities should rate their dyspnea before and during exercise. The Borg CR10 scale (see Box 24-1), which was designed to measure intensities of perceptions of any sensation on a 0 to 10 scale, is often used for subjective rating of dyspnea (Table 23-1).

Aerobic Capacity and Endurance. As noted previously, the measure that most accurately reflects an individual's cardiorespiratory functional fitness is their maximum oxygen uptake $\dot{V}O_{2max}$.[6,29] A patient with a $\dot{V}O_{2max}$ less than 60% of the average $\dot{V}O_{2max}$ for individuals of the same age and gender is considered to have impaired aerobic capacity or endurance.[30]

Although maximum aerobic testing is the gold standard for assessing maximum aerobic capacity, this type of testing requires the patient to reach a state of $\dot{V}O_{2max}$ that may put the patient at risk, cause excessive fatigue, or not be achievable because of fatigue or limitations from other impairments. Clinicians assessing the aerobic capacity of patients with deconditioning therefore generally use submaximum aerobic testing to estimate the patient's $\dot{V}O_{2max}$.[6,31,32] Tests for estimating $\dot{V}O_{2max}$ primarily use changes in the patient's heart rate with increasing workloads to determine the cardiorespiratory response to aerobic demand. Because heart rate has a linear relationship with oxygen uptake, heart rate can be used to estimate a person's oxygen uptake during the test and to estimate $\dot{V}O_{2max}$. Stationary bicycling and treadmill walking are the most common activities used to provide a workload when estimating $\dot{V}O_{2max}$. The **modified Bruce**

To determine BMI, locate the height of interest in the left-most column and read across the row for that height to the weight of interest. Follow the column of the weight up to the top row that lists the BMI. A BMI of 18.5 to 24.9 is the healthy-weight range, BMI of 25 to 29.9 is the overweight range, and BMI of 30 and above is in the obese range.

BMI	19	20	21	22	23	24	25	26	27	28	29	30	31	32	33	34	35
Height									**Weight in Pounds**								
4'10"	91	96	100	105	110	115	119	124	129	134	138	143	148	153	158	162	167
4'11"	94	99	104	109	114	119	124	128	133	138	143	148	153	158	163	168	173
5'	97	102	107	112	118	123	128	133	138	143	148	153	158	163	158	174	179
5'1"	100	106	111	116	122	127	132	137	143	148	153	158	164	169	174	180	185
5'2"	104	109	115	120	126	131	136	142	147	153	158	164	169	175	180	186	191
5'3"	107	113	118	124	130	135	141	146	152	158	163	169	175	180	186	191	197
5'4"	110	116	122	128	134	140	145	151	157	163	169	174	180	186	192	197	204
5'5"	114	120	126	132	138	144	150	156	162	168	174	180	186	192	198	204	210
5'6"	118	124	130	136	142	148	155	161	167	173	179	186	192	198	204	210	216
5'7"	121	127	134	140	146	153	159	166	172	178	185	191	198	204	211	217	223
5'8"	125	131	138	144	151	158	164	171	177	184	190	197	203	210	216	223	230
5'9"	128	135	142	149	155	162	169	176	182	189	196	203	209	216	223	230	236
5'10"	132	139	146	153	160	167	174	181	188	195	202	209	216	222	229	236	243
5'11"	136	143	150	157	165	172	179	186	193	200	208	215	222	229	236	243	250
6'	140	147	154	162	169	177	184	191	199	206	213	221	228	235	242	250	258
6'1"	144	151	159	166	174	182	189	197	204	212	219	227	235	242	250	257	265
6'2"	148	155	163	171	179	186	194	202	210	218	225	233	241	249	256	264	272
6'3"	152	160	168	176	184	192	200	208	216	224	232	240	248	256	264	272	279
	Healthy Weight						**Overweight**					**Obese**					

From U.S. Department of Health and Human Services, U.S. Department of Agriculture: *Dietary guidelines for Americans 2005,* ed 6, Washington, DC, 2005, Authors. Accessible at *www.healthierus.gov/dietaryguidelines.*
   Source: National Institutes of Health, National Heart, Lung, and Blood Institute: *Evidence report of clinical guidelines on the identification, evaluation, and treatment of overweight and obesity in adults,* Bethesda, Md, 1998, Author.

FIG. 23-1 Body mass index is body weight in kilograms divided by height in meters squared (kg/m^2).

TABLE 23-1	Perceived Breathlessness Scale*
0	Nothing at all
0.5	Very, very slight (just noticeable)
1	Very slight
2	Slight
3	Moderate
4	Somewhat severe
5	Severe
6	Can't talk because of breathlessness
7	Very severe (gasping, all focus is on breathing)
8	
9	Very, very severe
10	Maximum

*Based on the Borg CR10 scale; see Box 24-1.

protocol is the treadmill exercise progression protocol usually used in clinical settings for estimating $V_{O_{2max}}$ in patients with low functional capacity.[29,31,32] The Astrand/Rhyming and YMCA protocols are alternative reliable methods for estimating $V_{O_{2max}}$ using a bicycle ergometer rather than a treadmill. The patient's heart rate, BP, and lung sounds are monitored before, during, and after the exercise test. The test is usually terminated when the patient reports exhaustion or when the heart rate reaches 85% of the person's age-predicted maximum.

Walking tests for distances or time may also be used when a stationary bicycle and treadmill are not available or appropriate. A self-paced walking test for a set distance can also be used as a baseline measurement of conditioning for patients who cannot maintain a consistent walking speed on a treadmill or pedaling speed on a stationary bicycle. The distance walked in a 2- or 6-minute test can be used for indoor settings with a measured walking course.[33] The self-paced walking tests do not require the patient to maintain a steady workload during the test and should not be used to estimate $\dot{V}O_{2max}$.[34]

Function. Patients with deconditioning are often limited in their self-care and home management abilities. The patient's ability to perform ADLs and work can be assessed by interview or by use of a number of functional abilities tools including the Barthel Index, Lower Extremity Functional Scale (LEFS), and Functional Independence Measure (FIM).

INTERVENTION

Interventions for a patient with deconditioning should focus on improving functional abilities, especially those related to ADLs and activities of independent living. Aerobic exercise and weight-training programs have been shown to most effectively improve aerobic capacity[35-37] and thus directly enhance the deconditioned patient's ability to use aerobic metabolism at rest and during activity. In addition to aerobic exercise, interventions for deconditioning should include communication, education, and coordination with the individual's other medical treatments.

COMMUNICATION

For a patient with severe deconditioning in an acute or long-term care setting, communication of which and how much activity a patient can perform safely can guide other health care providers and the patient's family members to avoid encouraging the patient to overexert or underexert. Activities should not be unnecessarily limited nor should too much assistance be given. Activities should also be paced to allow optimal function through the course of the day. It is also important to communicate the nature of a patient's signs of fatigue to avoid overexertion. Coordination of the patient's medical treatment and rehabilitation sessions should limit his or her overall fatigue and improve performance during therapeutic and functional activities.[35]

In an outpatient setting, communication with the patient, the patient's family, and caregivers should convey expectations of the patient's activities during rehabilitation sessions and during their daily activities. The patient and family should see their daily activities as part of the rehabilitation program. The family will need to learn to assist at an appropriate level so that the patient can increase his or her independence.

EDUCATION

The patient and family should receive education about the benefits of increased physical activity. Understanding the physiological and psychological benefits of exercise will help reinforce the patient's goals for treatment and assist the patient in adhering to the exercise program. The patient should also be educated to differentiate signs of normal physiological responses to exercise, such as increased respiratory and heart rate, from signs of fatigue that require rest.

The patient should understand that periods of rest during the day are important for pacing their activities and limiting fatigue. The patient should also use rest periods to prepare for potentially fatiguing activities, such as family functions or visits to medical professionals.[35] The patient and family should also be educated regarding safety issues. The patient and family should have a list of phone numbers to call, including their Emergency Medical System (911), in case problems or an emergency situation arise.

MOTIVATION

Because a patient's motivation has been shown to be the most important determinant of maintaining an exercise program,[23-25] the therapist should employ interventions to improve the patient's motivation and confidence to optimize the likelihood that they will maintain an exercise program. The therapist should discuss with the patient his or her beliefs about exercise and address issues about how the patient will maintain his or her exercise program. The discussion should include the patient's history of exercise and physical activities to help the therapist understand the types of activities and programs that have been successful and to avoid activities that the patient does not believe will be effective.[6,38]

> ◎ *Clinical Pearl*
> An individualized approach to a patient's aerobic program will improve success.

AEROBIC EXERCISE

The foundation of therapeutic exercise programs for patients with deconditioning is aerobic activity.[39-41] Aerobic activities should be prescribed with a specified level of intensity, duration, and frequency as developed by the physical therapist. The patient may initially be limited in the mode or type of aerobic activities he or she can perform, but as the patient progresses, the mode of exercise should be based on the patient's goals and individual preference.

Acute Care Inpatient Setting. For a patient in the acute care inpatient setting, the primary goal of an exercise program is to improve the patient's functional abilities to prepare for discharge home or to another health care facility. The exercise program will have other benefits, but because of the short duration of most inpatient hospital stays, the primary goal is to decrease fatigue with functional activities. The inpatient exercise program can also be the first stage of a more comprehensive, long-term exercise program that changes physiological function, improves endurance, and prepares the patient to return to his or her societal roles.[37]

For the patient with severe deconditioning, periods of sitting upright in bed or in a chair may be the first step of the conditioning exercise program. The patient may then be progressed to periods of standing and walking for short distances (less than 50 feet). Walking distance may be limited by fatigue or by monitoring or treatment equipment in a hospital room. Upper extremity active ROM exercises in a sitting or standing position can also be used to increase cardiovascular demand and thus improve function and endurance.[35,37]

◎ *Clinical Pearl*

Basic bed mobility and gait may be conditioning for very deconditioned patients.

The ambulatory patient may initially use walking as the primary mode of exercise, with walking distance and speed used to progress exercise intensity and monitor exercise tolerance. Patients who report fatigue with walking may be able to walk further if they take short rest periods, either in standing or sitting, between walking bouts. A walking exercise program can be progressed by increasing the total walking time, speed, or distance and/ or by reducing the frequency and duration of rest periods. The patient's heart rate, respiratory rate, dyspnea rating, and **rate of perceived exertion (RPE)** (see Box 23-1 and the section on Exercise Intensity) should be monitored during the exercise session to determine the intensity of walking activities.[37] The patient's BP, heart rhythm, and oxygen saturation levels (see Chapter 22) should be monitored before, during, and after these periods of walking to assess the patient's cardiorespiratory tolerance of the exercise session.

General guidelines for stopping an exercise session are as follows:

- Heart rate: A drop below the resting rate or an increase of more than 20 to 30 beats per minute (bpm) above the resting rate.
- Systolic blood pressure: A drop of more than 10 mm Hg below the resting rate.
- Oxygen saturation level: Below 90%.[42]
- Symptoms: Angina, significantly increased dyspnea.[6,35]

Depending on their length of stay, prior level of conditioning, and level of deconditioning at the initiation of exercise, a patient in an inpatient setting may progress to tolerate longer periods of exercise and other modes and forms of exercise. A stationary bicycle or arm ergometer can be transported to the patient's room or floor for more prolonged endurance exercises. The patient's pedaling speed or work level can then be used to progress and monitor the intensity of this exercise. Patients may also be able to use the long corridor and stairs of a hospital or rehabilitation center to increase their walking endurance. Upper extremity ROM exercises using light resistance with sets of 12 to 15 repetitions are also recommended.[5,35]

Outpatient Setting. A patient in the outpatient setting will generally have time for and tolerate a more comprehensive and long-term exercise program than the patient in the inpatient setting. The exercise program can be designed to improve performance of the patient's functional, vocational, and recreational activities, maintain and improve overall fitness, and often reduce the risk of recurrence of their disease processes.[35,41] Exercise appropriate at this stage should also improve physiological parameters.

The exercise prescription should be based on objective measures of physiological function, on what is attainable

for the patient based on their general health and medical history, and on evidence of the effectiveness of exercise. To reduce deconditioning, an exercise prescription should primarily involve activities to improve aerobic function, but some patients will also need activities to improve their strength and flexibility.

In the outpatient setting, whether in a clinic or health club, the patient will likely have a range of exercise modes and equipment available for their aerobic exercise program. Equipment selected should be safe and comfortable for the patient to use. The treadmill is the most commonly used equipment for endurance exercise because it allows one to easily change the speed of movement and the slope of incline. The patient should use a speed and incline that allows safe walking with good balance and efficient lower and upper extremity movement. Other equipment that allows movements similar to walking are the elliptical trainer and cross-country gliders, although these may require more balance and coordination, so patients should be closely monitored as they learn to use this equipment. Patients with poor balance may be safer using a stationary bicycle, although they may need assistance getting on and off the bicycle.

The exercise program for a patient with deconditioning needs to be individualized based on the patient's current medical condition and fitness level and available equipment or exercise settings. The exercises should be continually assessed and modified according to the patient's response. The exercises are usually defined by the parameters of exercise intensity, duration, and frequency.

The exercise session should include warm-up and cooldown periods, during which the activity level is slowly increased to and then later decreased from the prescribed levels. The warm-up period reduces the risk of cardiac arrhythmias and ischemia and improves muscle performance.[36,43,44] The warm-up period may include static stretching of large muscle groups and should also involve moving these muscle groups to prepare them and the cardiovascular system for the exercise session. The patient should be closely monitored during the cool-down period because adverse cardiac events are thought to occur most often during this period.[6] The cool-down period should be long enough to allow the heart rate and BP to return toward resting levels.

Exercise Intensity. The intensity of exercise after the warm-up period should be determined primarily by the physiological response of the patient. The American College of Sports Medicine (ACSM) recommends beginning the exercise program for unfit individuals at 55% to 65% of the estimated maximum heart rate or at 40% to 50% of the **heart rate reserve (HRR)**.[41,45] Measures of exercise intensity based on the patient's heart rate rather than oxygen consumption are generally used because heart rate can easily be monitored during an exercise session.

When using a percentage of the maximum heart rate to prescribe exercise intensity, maximum heart rate is generally estimated to be 220 minus the patient's age.[41] Thus a patient's initial exercise goal would be between $0.55 \times (220 -$ patient's age) and $0.65 \times (220 -$ patient's age). This method may be inaccurate in deconditioned patients because their maximum heart rate may actually be lower than the estimated 220 − age.[36] The HRR method (also known as the **Karvonen method**) is therefore the preferred method for exercise prescription for deconditioned patients.[41] HRR is equal to the maximum heart rate minus the resting heart rate. To calculate the target heart rate using the Karvonen method, use the following formula:

$$([\text{maximum heart rate} - \text{resting heart rate}] \times \text{goal percentage of HRR}) + \text{resting heart rate}$$

For this method, maximum heart rate is ideally the symptom-limited maximum heart rate as determined by a graded exercise test, although when this is not available, 220 minus the patient's age may be used as an estimate. For example, for a 50-year-old patient with a resting heart rate of 80 bpm whose target heart rate is 50% of HRR, the target heart rate would be: ([220 − 50 − 80] × 0.50) + 80 = 125 bpm.[41] This compares with a target heart rate of 94 to 111 based on 55% to 65% of the age-predicted maximum heart rate alone.

Using either method for estimating target heart rate, the clinician should keep in mind that this is only an estimate of the appropriate work level for the patient. During each exercise session the intensity of the exercise should be slowly progressed toward this level while monitoring the patient's tolerance of the activity by his or her respiratory effort and rate and fatigue level. A patient who cannot tolerate exercise at the calculated level should have the target level decreased or the mode of the exercise changed to better match their current fitness level.[35,36] As the patient progresses with their exercise program the intensity level can be gradually increased toward the maximum recommended levels of 90% of maximum heart rate or 85% of HRR.[36]

Another common method for monitoring exercise intensity during exercise uses the patient's own perception of their level of exertion. The RPE scale, as proposed by Borg, rates a patient's exertion using words such as "light" or "hard" with corresponding numbers 6 to 20 to describe the patient's workload (Box 23-1).[44,46] The RPE scale correlates well with other physiological measures of exertion and can be used reliably by patients, with instruction.[47] The RPE scale can be used with heart rate to monitor exercise intensity. An RPE level of 10 to 12 would be appropriate for deconditioned patients beginning an exercise program.[36] A patient's perceived exertion will change with different modes of exercise, and the prescribed level of exertion would need to be adjusted for each mode of exercise.[35,36] When patients are ready to perform an independent exercise program, they may use the RPE scale to maintain a specified level of intensity.[36]

A **metabolic equivalent (MET)** is another commonly used and convenient measure of activity intensity that can be used for exercise monitoring and prescription. One MET is equivalent to the energy used at rest, which is equivalent to approximately 3.5 ml of oxygen/kg/min.[6] The ACSM's *Guidelines for Exercise Testing and Prescription* include tables of MET ranges for ADLs and recreational activities (Table 23-2).[6] These tables can help the therapist direct the deconditioned patient to an appropriate level of activity.

BOX 23-1 Borg RPE Scale

6	No exertion at all
7	
8	Extremely light
9	Very light
10	
11	Light
12	
13	Somewhat hard
14	
15	Hard (heavy)
16	
17	Very hard
18	
19	Extremely hard
20	Maximal exertion

Borg-RPE-Scale®
©Gunnar Borg 1970, 1985, 1998
Instructions for the Borg-RPE-Scale®:
During the work we want you to rate your perception of exertion, i.e., how heavy and strenuous the exercise feels to you and how tired you are. The perception of exertion is mainly felt as strain and fatigue in your muscles and as breathlessness or aches in the chest.

Use this scale from 6 to 20, where 6 means "No exertion at all" and 20 means "Maximal exertion."

9 Very light. As for a healthy person taking a short walk at his or her own pace.
13 Somewhat hard. It still feels OK to continue.
15 It is hard and tiring, but continuing is not terribly difficult.
17 Very hard. It is very strenuous. You can still go on, but you really have to push yourself and you are very tired.
19 An extremely strenuous level. For most people this is the most strenuous exercise they have ever experienced.

Try to appraise your feeling of exertion and fatigue as spontaneously and as honestly as possible, without thinking about what the actual physical load is. Try not to underestimate, nor to overestimate. It is your own feeling of effort and exertion that is important, not how it compares to other people's. Look at the scale and the expressions and then give a number. You can equally well use even as odd numbers.

Any questions?
"Borg's RPE Scale," Borg G, 1994.

Exercise Duration and Frequency. The total volume of training depends on the exercise intensity and duration.[77,90] To maximize the benefits of an exercise program the exercise intensity should be progressed toward a target level, as previously described, and the duration of activities should be adjusted to the patient's tolerance. The optimal intensity and duration of exercise to improve and maintain aerobic fitness is controversial.

TABLE 23-2	Metabolic Equivalent (MET) Ranges for Various Activities	
Activity		**METs**
Bowling		2-4
Billiards		2.5
Shuffleboard		2-3
Music playing		2-3
Fishing: Standing from a bank		2-4
Canoeing: Two person		3-5
Golf: Power cart		2-3
Golf: Walking with pull cart		5
Dancing		3-8
Table tennis		3-5
Bicycling at 10mph		7

From Franklin BA (ed): *ACSM's guidelines for exercise testing and prescription*, ed 6, Baltimore, 2000, Lippincott Williams & Wilkins.

Initially, a patient may tolerate only 5-minute or shorter bouts of exercise with rest periods in between. The patient can then be progressed by increasing the duration of the bouts and decreasing the duration of rest periods by a few minutes each session.[36,39] A deconditioned patient should ideally maintain a low-to-moderate intensity of exercise for 20 to 60 minutes to gain physiological benefits of aerobic training.[41] As the duration of the exercise is increased, the intensity may need to be temporarily decreased, based on the patient's tolerance for the longer duration. These parameters may also affect adherence to the exercise program.[41,48]

The ACSM recommends two to five exercise sessions per week for improving aerobic capacity in deconditioned patients.[77] However, patients with severe deconditioning may initially do better with brief, daily sessions of exercise and functional activities.[32,37] As patients increase their tolerance for longer durations and intensity of exercise and activities, the frequency of exercise sessions can be adjusted to maximize performance and allow for longer durations of recovery, as demonstrated in the case study at the end of this chapter.[36,41]

WEIGHT TRAINING

Patients with deconditioning may also benefit from an exercise program that includes resistive weight training. A resistive weight training program will improve muscle strength impairments and may improve associated functional limitations.[25] Some patients prefer resistive weight training to aerobic exercise because of their perceived need to improve strength-related activities.[49]

CIRCUIT WEIGHT TRAINING

Patients with deconditioning may also benefit from weight training using a **circuit weight training (CWT)** program.[36,37,41] CWT is defined as the performance of 10 to 15 repetitions using 40% to 60% of one repetition maximum (1 RM) in a continuous fashion and moving from one exercise station or machine to another with short rest periods between stations. The circuit should contain 5 to 15 different exercise stations, each used 2 to 3 times per session, and sessions should be done 3 to 5 times per week.[50] The continuous activity of performing moderate resistance exercise and moving quickly from station to station is proposed to engage aerobic metabolism.[51] However, although CWT in healthy, untrained males has been shown to increase strength by 20% to 40% after 8 to 20 weeks of training,[50-52] it has been found to improve aerobic capacity only by 5% to 10%.[50,53]

CASE STUDY 23-1

CHRONIC OBSTRUCTIVE PULMONARY DISEASE WITH EMPHYSEMA

Patient History

TD is a 76-year-old man with a history of chronic obstructive pulmonary disease (COPD) with emphysema. He uses oxygen therapy primarily at night and a nebulized bronchodilator twice per day. He was referred to physical therapy by his pulmonologist because of decreased endurance and decreased ability to perform basic ADLs. He lives alone, and his activities have decreased over the past 3 months primarily because of his son moving out of town and the colder winter weather. TD is concerned that he will be unable to maintain his independent living status. A consultation with the referring pulmonologist reveals that this patient's pulmonary function only decreased slightly in the past 3 months.

Tests and Measures—Significant Findings
Musculoskeletal

- TD has a cachetic appearance, with a barrel chest and hypertrophy of the accessory respiratory muscles. He is 5 foot 9 inches tall and weighs 132 lb.
- Limited passive hip extension ROM bilaterally as a result of limited extensibility of the hip flexor muscles.

Cardiovascular/Pulmonary

- Vital signs at rest: BP 128/86, heart rate 82 bpm, respiratory rate 18 breaths/min, oxygen saturation 92%.
- Dyspnea rating at rest 4/10.
- Auscultation of the lungs finds reduced breath sounds in the middle and lower lobes on the right and lower lobe on the left.
- TD completed a 6-minute self-paced walk test without the use of oxygen. He walked 210 m with two short standing rest periods. At the end of the test, his oxygen saturation was 88% with a dyspnea rating of 8/10. He used pursed lip breathing during the last 4 minutes of the test. His vital signs at the end of the test were BP 140/104 mm Hg, heart rate 112 bpm, respiratory rate 24 breaths/min. His vital signs and dyspnea rating returned to resting levels within 10 minutes of sitting rest.
- A test of upper extremity endurance was performed by having the patient stand and hold a dowel with his arms elevated to 90 degrees. After 80 seconds, he reported more shortness of breath and requested to stop the test. Dyspnea rating at the end of the test was 7/10.

Diagnosis

Preferred practice pattern 6B: Impaired aerobic capacity/endurance associated with deconditioning.

Interventions

- Daily home walking program
- Home program of upper extremity exercises.

Role of the Physical Therapist Assistant

- Why are upper extremity exercises important for this patient?
- Calculate this patient's BMI. Is it high? Or is it low?
- Provide written instructions for this patient's home walking and upper extremity exercise program.
- How could this patient monitor and set the intensity of his exercises?
- How will you monitor his progress in the clinic?
- What community resources would benefit this patient?

Additional Information

For the full version of this case study, including detailed examination results, interventions, and outcomes, see the Evolve site that accompanies this book. A full case study for a patient with fatigue and weight gain and a patient with deconditioning after surgery also appears on the Evolve site.

CHAPTER SUMMARY

Deconditioning is the decline of normal anatomical and physiological function caused by disease, aging, or inactivity. Deconditioning primarily affects the cardiopulmonary system and its ability to supply the musculoskeletal system with oxygen for aerobic metabolism. This can result in impaired endurance and reduced ability to perform normal activities long enough or with enough repetitions to complete desired activities or tasks. The interaction of disease, aging, and decreased activities can result in deconditioning and impaired endurance and functional limitations.

Interventions for a patient with deconditioning should focus on improving their functional abilities, especially those related to ADLs and activities of independent living. Interventions to reverse the effects of deconditioning and to improve endurance and functional abilities primarily involve aerobic exercise. Because exercise programs for a patient with deconditioning need to be consistently followed for multiple weeks and months, an individualized exercise prescription should be fashioned for each patient to optimize the physiological effects of the exercise and to enhance the patient's motivation to continue with the exercise program. An individualized exercise program will include the type of activity, the intensity level and how the intensity will be monitored, the duration of the activity, and how often the activity will be performed daily or on a weekly basis. The exercise program should be reevaluated on a consistent basis to assess for progression toward the treatment goals and to adjust the exercise parameters.

ADDITIONAL RESOURCES

For links to these and additional web-based resources, see the Evolve site.

Barthel Index

Lower Extremity Functional Scale

Franklin BA: Abnormal cardiorespiratory responses to acute aerobic exercise. In *ACSM's resource manual for guidelines for exercise testing and prescription,* ed 4, Baltimore, 2001, American College of Sports Medicine.

Franklin BA (ed): *ACSM's guidelines for exercise testing and prescription,* ed 6, Baltimore, 2000, Lippincott, Williams & Wilkins.

Noonan V, Dean E: Submaximal exercise testing: Clinical application and interpretation, *Phys Ther* 80(8):782-807, 2000.

Williams MA (ed): *Guidelines for cardiac rehabilitation and secondary prevention programs,* ed 4, Champaign, Ill, 2004, Human Kinetics.

American Heart Association

American Association of Cardiovascular and Pulmonary Rehabilitation

American College of Sports Medicine

GLOSSARY

Body mass index (BMI): A general indicator of body composition calculated as weight in kilograms divided by height in meters squared (kg/m^2).

Circuit weight training (CWT): The performance of exercises with 10 to 15 repetitions using 40% to 60% of 1 RM in a continuous fashion, moving from one exercise station or machine to another with short rest periods between stations.

Deconditioning: The decline of normal anatomical and physiological function caused by disease, aging, or inactivity.

Endurance impairment: The primary impairment for individuals with deconditioning that can be measured by whole body activities or with repeated movements of an extremity.

Heart rate reserve (HRR): Estimated maximum heart rate minus the resting heart rate. This can be used to determine aerobic exercise intensity.

Karvonen method: Formula for determining target heart rate using the heart rate reserve: ([maximum heart rate − resting heart rate] × goal percent of HRR) + resting heart rate.

Maximum oxygen uptake (Vo_{2max}): The maximum amount of oxygen consumption of the body during activity. This is the best indicator of cardiopulmonary fitness.

Metabolic equivalent (MET): One MET is the rate of energy consumption at rest, which is approximately 3.5 ml of oxygen/kg/min. The MET is a convenient measure of intensity for prescribing activity levels.

Modified Bruce protocol: A protocol for exercise testing commonly used in clinical settings for estimating Vo_{2max} in patients with low functional capacity.

Patient motivation: A patient's internal state that activates their behavior and gives it direction. Motivation is the single most important factor for determining if a patient will maintain an exercise program.

Rating of perceived exertion (RPE): A common method for monitoring exercise intensity during exercise, using the patient's own perception of his or her level of exertion.

Chapter 24

Airway Clearance Dysfunction

Jan Stephen Tecklin

OBJECTIVES

After reading this chapter, the reader will be able to:
1. Identify four common causes of airway clearance dysfunction.
2. Describe associations between specific pathological findings and airway clearance techniques.
3. Understand the results of valid and reliable tests that guide selection of airway clearance techniques for a particular patient.
4. Execute safe and effective interventions for improving airway clearance.
5. Identify when airway clearance techniques should be taught to a patient's family members.

Airway clearance dysfunction is a problem common to individuals with a wide variety of medical and surgical diagnoses. Airway clearance dysfunction implies an inability to adequately clear the airways of obstructing material, such as mucus, secretions, fluid, cellular debris, or inflammatory exudate, or other items, such as aspirated foreign objects. Many immediate and potentially adverse outcomes may result from an inability to clear the airways, including airway obstruction, inflammation, infection, **atelectasis,** abnormal ventilation/perfusion relationships, and deterioration of arterial blood gas (ABG) values. Airway obstruction occurs in many groups of individuals and is a defining feature of chronic obstructive pulmonary disease (COPD) in adults and of cystic fibrosis (CF) in children, adolescents, and adults.

PATHOLOGY

Airway clearance dysfunction occurs in many diseases and conditions. In reviewing the codes from the *International Classification of Diseases—Ninth revision* (ICD9)[1] that are listed in the *Guide to Physical Therapist Practice*[2] for preferred practice pattern 6C: Impaired ventilation, respiration/gas exchange, and **aerobic capacity**/endurance associated with airway clearance dysfunction, it appears that patients in three large diagnostic groups are at risk for airway clearance dysfunction. One group includes patients with disorders caused by chronic inhalation of particulate matter, including organic (generally tobacco smoke) and inorganic dusts; another group of patients have infectious disorders; and the third large group is associated with operative procedures, including cardiovascular and orthopedic procedures and organ transplantation. In addition, the nature of the pathological process in CF, which leads to tenacious and voluminous bronchial secretions, inevitably produces airway clearance problems.

TYPICAL EXAMINATION FINDINGS

PATIENT HISTORY

The patient history will include questions about the following areas:
- Employment/work, including exposure to fumes, dusts, gases, or other particulate matter.
- Living environment, including space and resources for necessary respiratory support items.
- General health status, including mental health status (e.g., depression).
- Social/health habits, including smoking history, fitness level, and exercise habits.
- Medical/surgical history, including recent hospitalizations or illnesses.
- Current condition/chief complaint, including current airway clearance or exercise regimens and the patient's and family's expectations.
- Functional status/activity level, including independence level at home and with activities of daily living (ADLs).

- Medications, including the use of aerosolized **bronchodilator** and **mucolytic** medications.
- Available records should also be reviewed, including pulmonary function test results and ABG.

SYSTEMS REVIEW

The systems review is used to target areas requiring further examination and to define areas that may cause complications or indicate a need for precautions during the examination and intervention processes. Chapter 1 includes details of the systems review.

TESTS AND MEASURES

Musculoskeletal

Posture. Posture is commonly altered by chronic lung disease, particularly when hyperinflation is present for a long period of time.[3] An examination of postural alignment is therefore generally performed on any patient with chronic lung disease (see Chapter 4).[4] Increased anteroposterior (AP) diameter of the thorax is common. With hyperinflation the **thoracic index** (ratio of the AP diameter to the transverse diameter of the thorax) is often increased from the normal 1:2 to more than 2:1. This is termed a *barrel chest.*[5] The muscle shortening and increase in thoracic index associated with hyperinflation are generally accompanied by an increase in thoracic kyphosis and reduced thoracic excursion and spinal flexibility.

Range of Motion. Because of the degree of chronic inactivity and lack of mobility in many individuals with chronic lung disease, range of motion (ROM) of major joints is often reduced. Shoulder girdle and thoracic spine ROM are measured to assure that chest expansion is not impeded by soft tissue tightness or lack of joint mobility.

> ### ◎ Clinical Pearl
>
> People with chronic lung disease are commonly not able to be very active and spend a great amount of time seated. This can result in reduced lower extremity range of motion (ROM).

Muscle Performance. Individuals with COPD often have muscle weakness in their extremities, shoulder girdle, neck, and chest that limits physical activity.[6] Studies indicate that chronic lung disease results in muscle weakness and that oxidative stress reduces muscle endurance in individuals with COPD.[7] Peripheral muscle strength deficits in this population lead to exercise limitation and intolerance.[8-10] Strong abdominal muscles and expiratory muscles of the thorax are needed for effective coughing.

Neuromuscular. Chest wall pain resulting from musculoskeletal problems is common in patients with airway clearance difficulties. This pain is usually nonsegmental, localized to the anterior chest, and aggravated by deep breathing and has a palpable source. Chest wall pain is also usually unrelated to exercise. In contrast, chest pain caused by cardiac ischemia (angina pectoris) is typically a viselike, crushing midline pain that radiates to the jaw and arm and is aggravated by exercise. Thoracic nerve root inflammation can also cause chest pain, but this will follow a dermatomal distribution. A pain scale (see Chapter 22) is used to determine the level of pain.

Cardiovascular/Pulmonary

Ventilation and Respiration/Gas Exchange. Two important indicators of potential problems with respiration include the rate of perceived exertion (RPE) and the level of **dyspnea.** The Borg RPE scale has a range of scores from 6 to 20 (see Box 23-1). A score of 6 indicates no exertion at all and 20 indicates very, very hard exertion. The Borg category ratio 10 (CR10) scale, developed after the Borg RPE scale, measures intensities of perceptions of any sensation (e.g., breathlessness/dyspnea, pain, fatigue, loudness, taste, and chest pain/angina). The Borg CR10 scale (Box 24-1) has a range from 0 to 10, with 0 equating to none and 10 indicating extremely strong or maximal perception. For patients with cardiovascular or pulmonary dysfunction, the RPE scale is generally used for perceived exertion and the CR10 scale is used for perceived breathlessness/dyspnea. Alternatively, a visual analog scale (VAS) can be used to quantify dyspnea. A 10-cm horizontal line is presented with end points of "not breathless at all" to "worst breathlessness I can imagine." The patient indicates his or her level of breathlessness on the line.

Many of the findings associated with impaired ventilation and gas exchange have a direct bearing on procedural intervention selection. These findings are best gathered through the tools of a traditional chest examination, which include inspection, **auscultation,** palpation, and percussion.

Inspection. The inspection phase of the chest examination involves looking at the patient, specifically seeking signs of problems with breathing. Inspection first focuses on the patient's general appearance, noting body type as normal, obese, or cachectic, and then examines posture, taking particular note of any spinal misalignment or unusual postures including kyphosis, scoliosis, and forward bend, or professorial posture (Fig. 24-1). Signs of respiratory distress and oxygen desaturation, including flaring of the nares and cyanosis of the mucous membranes, are noted.[11]

Congenital defects, such as pectus carinatum (pigeon breast) and pectus excavatum (funnel chest or hollow chest) and the rib angles and intercostal spaces, are also noted.

> ### ◎ Clinical Pearl
>
> The first sign of respiratory distress with inadequate oxygenation is cyanosis or a bluish tinge to the lips and nail beds.

The respiratory rate, including the ratio of inspiratory and expiratory time (the I:E ratio), is assessed. Normally, expiration lasts twice as long as inspiration, giving an I:E ratio of 1:2. In obstructive lung disease, expiration is prolonged, commonly producing I:E ratios of 1:4 or 1:5.

Assessment of the sounds associated with breathing is made, including **stridor, stertor,** expiratory grunting, and gurgling. The pattern of breathing, including rate, depth, and regularity of the ventilatory cycle, is assessed. Some commonly encountered breathing patterns appear in Table 24-1.

BOX 24-1 Borg CR10 Scale

Instruction. Use this rating scale to report how strong your perception is. It can be exertion, pain, or something else. Ten (10) or "Extremely strong"—"Maximal" is a very important intensity level. It serves as a reference point on the scale. This is the most intense perception or feeling (e.g., of exertion) you have ever had. It is, however, possible to experience or imagine something even more intense. That is why we've placed "Absolute maximum" outside and further down on the scale without any corresponding number, just a dot "•". If your experience is stronger than "10," you can use a larger number.

First look at the verbal expressions. Start with them and then the numbers. If your experience or feeling is "Very weak," you should say "1"; if it is "Moderate," say "3." Note that "Moderate" is "3" and thus weaker than "Medium," "Mean," or "Middle." If the experience is "Strong" or "Heavy" (it feels "Difficult") say "5." Note that "Strong" is about 50 percent, or about half, of "Maximal." If your perception is "Very strong" ("Very intense") choose a number from 6 to 8, depending upon how intense it is. Feel free to use half-numbers like "1.5" or "3.5," or decimals like "0.3," "0.8," or "2.3." It is very important that you report what you actually experience or feel, not what you think you should report. Be as spontaneous and honest as possible and try to avoid under- or over-estimating. Look at the verbal descriptors and then choose a number.

When rating perceived exertion give a number that corresponds to your feeling of exertion, that is, how hard and strenuous you perceive the work to be and how tired you are. The perception of exertion is mainly felt as strain and fatigue in your muscles and as breathlessness or aches in the chest. It is important that you only think about what you feel, and not about what the actual load is.

Any questions?

0	Nothing at all	
0.3		
0.5	Extremely weak	Just noticeable
0.7		
1	Very weak	
1.5		
2	Weak	Light
2.5		
3	Moderate	
4		
5	Strong	Heavy
6		
7	Very strong	
8		
9		
10	Extremely strong	"Maximal"
11		
⚡		
•	Absolute maximum	Highest possible

The Borg CR10 Scale
©Gunnar Borg 1982, 1998.

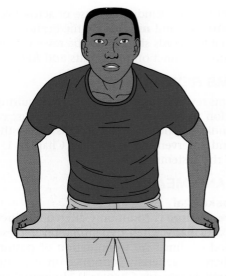

FIG. 24-1 Forward-bend or professorial posture.

The symmetry and synchrony of breathing is noted. The chronically hyperinflated thorax and flattened diaphragm, often seen with severe COPD, can result in a simultaneous in-drawing of the lower ribs and expansion of the upper ribs during inspiration.[12] Speech, breath, cough, and sputum are also assessed. Shortness of breath that causes frequent interruptions in speech is known as *dyspnea of phonation*. This is often quantified by the number of words that can be spoken between sequential breaths, for example, "three-word dyspnea" or "four-word dyspnea."

If a patient complains of coughing, the clinician next identifies characteristics of the cough, including whether it is persistent, paroxysmal, or occasional; dry or productive; and the circumstances associated with the onset or cessation of coughing. Patients with COPD often cough with poor inspiratory effort and negligible abdominal muscle compression, making the cough ineffective for airway clearance. Patients with COPD also often have much paroxysmal coughing that can be very fatiguing because it is so frequent and ineffective.

Quantity, color, and consistency of sputum are also assessed. Examination of the abdomen for factors that may affect diaphragmatic function, including morbid obesity, previous and recent abdominal surgeries, or insertion of a feeding tube, should be described.

Auscultation. Auscultation provides information about which parts of the lungs are being ventilated during breathing and about the location and presence of secretions in the lungs. During chest auscultation, the patient breathes in and out deeply with the mouth open.

Breath sounds are generated by the vibration and turbulence of airflow into and out of the airways and lung tissue during inspiration and expiration. Normal breath sounds can be divided into four specific types: Tracheal, bronchial, bronchovesicular, and vesicular. Each of these is considered normal when heard over a specific region of the thorax. However, when heard in a different region, these sounds are considered abnormal. In contrast,

TABLE 24-1	Breathing Patterns Commonly Found in the Examination of Patients with Airway Clearance Problems

Pattern of Breathing	Description
Apnea	Absence of ventilation
Fish-mouth	Apnea with concomitant mouth opening and closing; associated with neck extension and bradypnea
Eupnea	Normal rate, normal depth, regular rhythm
Bradypnea	Slow rate, shallow or normal depth, regular rhythm; associated with drug overdose
Tachypnea	Fast rate, shallow depth, regular rhythm; associated with restrictive lung disease
Hyperpnea	Normal rate, increased depth, regular rhythm
Cheyne-Stokes respiration (periodic)	Increasing then decreasing depth, periods of apnea interspersed with somewhat regular rhythm; associated with critically ill patients
Biot's respiration (cluster)	Slow rate, shallow depth, apneic periods, irregular rhythm; associated with CNS disorders such as meningitis
Apneustic	Slow rate, deep inspiration followed by apnea, irregular rhythm; associated with brainstem disorders
Prolonged expiration	Fast inspiration, slow and prolonged expiration yet normal rate, depth, regular rhythm; associated with obstructive lung disease
Orthopnea	Difficulty breathing in postures other than erect
Hyperventilation	Fast rate, increased depth, regular rhythm; results in decreased arterial carbon dioxide, tension; called *Kussmaul breathing* in metabolic acidosis; also associated with CNS disorders such as encephalitis
Psychogenic dyspnea	Normal rate, regular intervals of sighing; associated with anxiety
Dyspnea	Rapid rate, shallow depth, regular rhythm; associated with accessory muscle activity
Doorstop	Normal rate and rhythm; characterized by abrupt cessation of inspiration when restriction is encountered; associated with pleurisy

From Irwin S, Tecklin JS: *Cardiopulmonary physical therapy: A guide to practice*, ed 4, St. Louis, 1995, Mosby.
CNS, Central nervous system.

adventitious breath sounds including **crackles,** previously called *rales,* and **wheezes,** previously called *rhonchi,* are always abnormal. Crackles are nonmusical sounds that may be mimicked by rolling several strands of hair near your ear or by listening to a bowl of cereal that crackles when the milk is added. Wheezes are continuous and musical sounds that sound like whistling or growling. Other adventitious sounds that may be detected during auscultation of the lungs include rubs and crunches. Rubs are coarse, grating, leathery sounds. Crunches are crackling sounds heard over the pericardium during systole and suggest the presence of air in the mediastinum.

Palpation. The sternocleidomastoid and scalene muscle groups are the primary accessory muscles of inspiration.[13] Normally, accessory muscles are inactive during quiet breathing. Palpation of increased accessory muscle activity during inspiration indicates that the work of breathing is increased. Patients with airway clearance dysfunction who have chronic lung disease often habitually and unnecessarily use their accessory muscles. Intervention, including instruction in diaphragmatic breathing, may be directed at reducing accessory muscle use to conserve energy.

Steps for Palpating the Activity of Accessory Muscles of Breathing

1. Position the patient with his or her back toward you.
2. Place your thumbs over the spinous processes so that your fingers reach around to the anterolateral aspect of the neck.
3. Feel for activity and movement of scalene and sternocleidomastoid muscles (Fig. 24-2).
4. Feel during at least two respiratory cycles.

In addition, movement of the diaphragm can be palpated as shown in Fig. 24-3. Normal motion of the diaphragm produces equal upward motion of the costal margins. Inward motion of the costal margins during inspiration is associated with a flattened diaphragm that commonly occurs in individuals with chronic airway clearance dysfunction and COPD.[14] Flattening of the diaphragm caused by severe hyperinflation may reduce the ability of the diaphragm to contract because it alters the length-tension relationship of the muscle fibers.[14]

Percussion. Percussion is performed to check for changes in lung density. Percussion is performed by tapping the finger of one hand against the middle finger of the other hand placed on the chest wall. The sound produced by the tapping is affected by the density of the underlying tissue, with denser tissue (poorly inflated lung or other solid tissue) sounding flat or dull and less dense tissue (hyperinflated lung) sounding hyperresonant or tympanic. When examining lung density by percussion, the therapist may identify one of three sounds or notes: Normal, dull, or tympanic. A normal note is produced when percussion is performed over the thorax adjacent to resonant lung of normal density. A dull note is soft, brief, high-pitched, and thudlike and is heard over the thorax with lung of increased density because it is less air-filled. A tympanic note is loud, lengthy, low pitched, and hollow

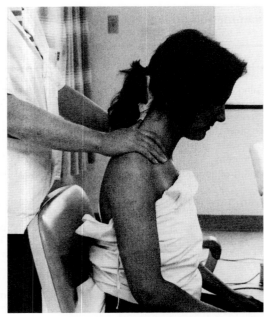

FIG. 24-2 Palpation of scalene muscle activity. *From Irwin S, Tecklin JS:* Cardiopulmonary physical therapy: A guide to practice, *ed 4, St. Louis, 1995, Mosby.*

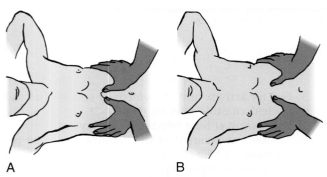

A   B

FIG. 24-3 Palpation of diaphragmatic motion. **A,** At rest. **B,** At the end of a normal inspiration. *A from Cherniack RM, Cherniack L, Naimark A:* Respiration in health and disease, *ed 2, Philadelphia, 1972, WB Saunders; B from Irwin S, Tecklin JS:* Cardiopulmonary physical therapy: A guide to practice, *ed 4, St. Louis, 1995, Mosby.*

and is heard over the thorax in areas of excessive air such as hyperinflated lung.

Aerobic Capacity and Endurance. Aerobic capacity and endurance may be tested in a variety of ways, ranging from simply noting symptomatic responses to a standard exercise challenge to technically sophisticated invasive aerobic testing in an exercise laboratory. Exercise testing to determine aerobic capacity typically involves progressive or incremental increases in exercise intensity while walking on a treadmill or riding a bicycle ergometer, as described in Chapter 23.

Function. Individuals with respiratory difficulty leading to airway clearance dysfunction often use supplemental oxygen devices, including metal oxygen cylinders of various sizes, liquid oxygen systems, oxygen concentration devices, and oxygen from wall-mounted oxygen sources in hospitals and nursing homes (as described in Chapter 26). Oxygen may be delivered from these sources by nasal cannula or mask.

INTERVENTION

COORDINATION, COMMUNICATION, AND DOCUMENTATION

Coordination, communication, and documentation are interventions used for all patients and are particularly important for this preferred practice pattern because patients with impaired airway clearance generally need intervention by many different types of health care professionals. Patients may need various types of equipment, help at home, or placement in some type of assisted living situation and often require ongoing case management. In addition, collaboration with various agencies, such as home care practitioners, equipment providers, and third party payers, is often necessary to ensure continuation of care across varied settings. Complex cases often include an interdisciplinary effort that requires communication across and between disciplines, with occasional referral to other professionals not involved with the team.

PATIENT/CLIENT-RELATED INSTRUCTION

Education and training about the lung disease underlying the airway clearance dysfunction is critically important for self-efficacy in patients in this preferred practice pattern.[15] The American Thoracic Society cites education as one of the four major components of any pulmonary rehabilitation program and includes the items in the following list as important parts of the educational component[16]:

1. Structure and function of the lung
2. Information regarding their specific disease
3. Instruction and participation in correct inhaler technique
4. Airway clearance techniques
5. Breathing, relaxation, and panic control techniques
6. Respiratory muscle training
7. Exercise principles
8. ADLs and instrumental ADLs (IADLs)
9. Nutrition interventions and considerations
10. Medications—their effects and side effects
11. Psychosocial interventions and means of coping with stress, anxiety, and depression
12. Avoidance of environmental irritants
13. Smoking cessation
14. Oxygen rationale and proper use of oxygen-delivery devices
15. Travel and leisure activities
16. Sexuality
17. End-of-life issues and planning for those with progressive diseases

Individualized teaching or a series of short, interactive lectures are commonly employed. DVDs, CDs, and various web sites covering specific topics can also be used. The ultimate goal for patient-related instruction in individuals with airway clearance dysfunction is to provide basic knowledge about their disease, its medical management, and daily techniques and activities to enhance their quality of life while recognizing the limitations imposed by the disease process.

AIRWAY CLEARANCE TECHNIQUES

Airway clearance techniques include a range of therapeutic interventions intended to clear the airways of secretions and other debris in individuals with pulmonary disease or respiratory impairment or those who are at risk for developing those conditions. The interventions include various physical maneuvers, manual procedures, breathing techniques, use of equipment, and instruction. A physical therapist or physical therapist assistant, a respiratory therapist, a nurse, or other health care worker, a family member, or the patient may apply airway clearance techniques to maintain patent airways and thereby reduce or eliminate airway obstruction, enhance ventilation, and reduce the likelihood of new or continuing infection of the respiratory tract.

Airway clearance, in one of its many forms, is universally employed for patients with almost all types of pediatric and adult lung diseases. There are many approaches and techniques used to remove secretions and other debris from the patient's airway. This section presents the more commonly used and evidence-based approaches and techniques for airway clearance.

Breathing Strategies for Airway Clearance

Forced Expiratory Technique. The forced expiratory technique (FET) employs a forced expiration or huff after a medium-sized breath.[17] The patient is instructed to take a medium breath (to midlung volume) then tighten the abdominal muscles firmly while huffing (expiring forcibly but with an opened glottis), without contracting the throat muscles. The "huff" should be maintained long enough to mobilize and remove distal bronchial secretions without stimulating a spasmodic cough. The important part of FET is the period (15 to 30 seconds) of relaxation with gentle diaphragmatic breathing after 1 or 2 huffs. This helps relax the airways as secretions continue to be mobilized during deep breathing. Once secretions are felt in the larger, uppermost airways, a huff or double cough should remove them.

Active Cycle of Breathing Technique. Active cycle of breathing technique (ACBT) uses several individual breathing strategies in sequential combination to accomplish the goals of mobilizing and evacuating bronchial secretions. A suggested sequence for ACBT is as follows:

- Breath control, another name for diaphragmatic breathing, is performed for 15 to 30 seconds in a quiet, relaxed manner.
- Several attempts at thoracic expansion are performed. (There is divergence of opinion regarding the necessity of having the patient assume one of the many postural drainage positions during this phase. Some might also suggest using the manual techniques of percussion or vibration during the expiratory phase of breathing.)
- Breath control is repeated for 15 to 30 seconds.
- Thoracic expansion is repeated.

This alternating cycle of breath control and thoracic expansion may continue until the patient feels ready to expectorate the built-up secretions. A medium-sized breath followed by tightening the abdominal muscles firmly while huffing (expiring forcibly but with an opened glottis) without contracting the throat muscles, or coughing, is then performed to help evacuate the accumulated secretions. The sequence of breath control and expansion is then repeated.

Autogenic Drainage. Autogenic drainage (AD) can also be used by the patient for airway clearance.[18] AD is performed in a sitting position and requires the patient to know when bronchial secretions are present in the smaller, medium, or larger airways. The patient then learns to breathe at low, medium, and high lung volumes to mobilize secretions in those airways.

Sequence of Autogenic Drainage

1. The patient sits upright with a minimum of distractions in the room.
2. After a brief period of diaphragmatic breathing, the patient exhales to a low lung volume and breathes at a normal **tidal volume** at that low lung volume. This is the "unsticking phase" of AD.
3. As the patient becomes aware of secretions in those smaller airways, breathing becomes a bit deeper and moves into midlung volume. This is the "collecting phase" in which secretions are mobilized proximally into the midsized airways.
4. At this point, breathing becomes deeper at normal to high lung volumes. The patient is asked to suppress coughing until it cannot be avoided. This "evacuation phase" enables secretions to accumulate in central airways and be evacuated by huffing or a cough, using minimal effort.

Proponents of AD believe it can be applied in all types of obstructive lung disease and for postoperative treatment and can be taught to children as young as 5 to 6 years of age. Intensive training in the technique is necessary before it can be used effectively. AD and ACBT are similarly effective at improving ventilation, removing secretions, and enhancing pulmonary function.

Coughing and Huffing. Coughing and huffing is an effective means of removing secretions and is critically important for the individual with airway clearance dysfunction. Coughing may be reflexive or voluntary. A reflexive cough has four phases: Irritation, inspiration, compression, and expulsion, whereas a voluntary cough has only the latter three phases. To be effective for airway clearance, either type of cough must generate enough force to clear secretions from the larger airways.[19]

Huffing is a popular airway clearance technique consisting of a single large inspiration followed by short expiratory efforts interrupted by pauses. The glottis remains open during huffing to reduce the potential for adverse effects from coughing. Huffing has been recommended in lieu of coughing because it is thought to reduce the physical work of the activity, but research has not shown huffing to be any more energy efficient than coughing.[20] If these techniques fail to clear the airway, endotracheal suctioning may be necessary, but where possible, coughing or huffing are preferred because suctioning can injure the tracheal epithelium and may cause sudden **hypoxemia** or cardiac arrhythmias.[21,22]

Proper cough technique, which facilitates airway clearance, requires that the patient sequentially (1) inspires to or near a maximum inspiration; (2) closes the glottis; (3) "bears down" by tightening the abdominal, perineal, gluteal, and shoulder depressor muscles to increase intrathoracic and intraabdominal pressures; and (4) suddenly opens the glottis to enable the pressurized inspired air to suddenly escape to provide the expulsive force. The patient should cough no more than two times during each expulsive, expiratory phase—a "double cough." To continue beyond this "double cough" usually produces little added benefit. Proper cough technique after surgery may also require incisional splinting. Splinting an abdominal or thoracic incision is commonly performed by having the patient hold a small pillow firmly against the incision while attempting to cough or using the hands to approximate the edges of the incision while attempting to cough. There is no scientific evidence that this type of splinting improves cough, but there is a great deal of anecdotal commentary on the usefulness of the techniques. Following are techniques that can be used to improve cough:

1. Positioning—sitting in the forward leaning posture with the neck flexed, the arms supported, and the feet firmly planted on the floor—promotes effective coughing (Fig. 24-4).
2. Tracheal stimulation—pressure or vibration applied to the extrathoracic trachea—may elicit a reflex cough.

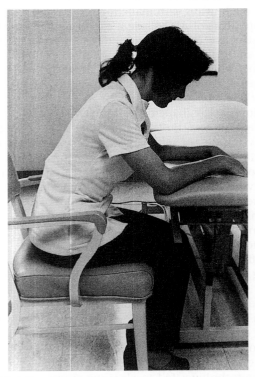

FIG. 24-4 Recommended position for effective coughing. *From Irwin S, Tecklin JS:* Cardiopulmonary physical therapy: A guide to practice, *ed 4, St. Louis, 1995, Mosby.*

3. Pressure applied to the midrectus abdominis area after inspiration may improve cough effectiveness if the pressure is suddenly released.
4. Pressure applied along the lower costal borders during exhalation may improve the effectiveness of an impaired cough.

◎ *Clinical Pearl*

Patients with trunk paralysis or weakness may require manual compression by the clinician along the lower costal borders and diaphragm during exhalation to make a cough effective.

Manual and Mechanical Techniques

Postural Drainage with Chest Percussion, Vibration, and Shaking. This group of techniques is often referred to as "chest physiotherapy," "chest physical therapy," "postural drainage," or "bronchial drainage" and represents the classic and traditional approach to airway clearance that has been used for many decades. Although the evidence for superiority of this technique over other more modern approaches is lacking, a number of studies have found it to be as effective as some of the newer equipment-intensive approaches to airway clearance described, including high-frequency chest compression,[23] intrapulmonary percussive ventilation (IPV),[24] and treatment with Flutter devices.[25] Furthermore, the experience of several generations of committed physicians, PTs, respiratory therapists, and nurses has borne out the ongoing utility of this approach to airway clearance. In addition, the face validity of airway clearance for properly selected patients is undeniable. As a result, most patients with chronic and acute respiratory problems that produce voluminous secretions are currently treated with some airway clearance technique, whether it be manual or mechanical.

Positioning. Before manual or mechanical approaches are used to loosen and mobilize secretions, it is generally recommended that the patient be positioned to optimally drain a particular lung segment or lobe. This requires that the area to be drained is uppermost, with the bronchus from the area in as close to a vertical position as possible or reasonable. Some refer to this notion as the "ketchup bottle theory." To get ketchup from the bottle, it must be turned upside down (and shaken).[26] Fig. 24-5 shows positions for postural drainage of different parts of the lungs.

These positions may need to be modified under certain conditions. Typically, the modification consists of reducing the angle for head-down positions for the middle lobe, lingula, and lower lobes. With severe dyspnea or gastroesophageal reflux and with increased intracranial pressure, all positions for the middle lobe, lingula, and lower lobes should be performed with the patient flat with no decline. Recent research indicates that in infants with CF, the head-down tipped position should be avoided for the first year of life because this position stimulates gastroesophageal reflux that can adversely affect lung tissue.[27]

Percussion and Vibration. Often referred to as "manual techniques" of airway clearance, percussion and vibration of the thorax are performed to loosen accumulated

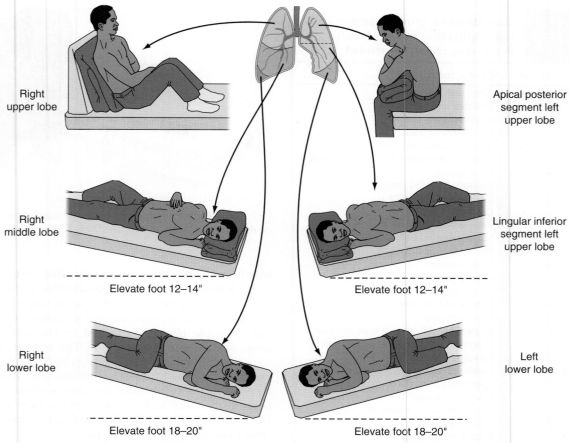

Right
upper lobe

Apical posterior
segment left
upper lobe

Right
middle lobe

Elevate foot 12–14"

Lingular inferior
segment left
upper lobe

Elevate foot 12–14"

Right
lower lobe

Elevate foot 18–20"

Left
lower lobe

Elevate foot 18–20"

FIG. 24-5 Positions for postural drainage of different parts of the lungs.

secretions. These techniques are intended to enhance movement of secretions to the more proximal airways during positioning for gravity-assisted postural drainage. Some clinicians also advocate "chest shaking," a more vigorous type of vibration. Percussion and vibration are usually performed in an area of the thorax corresponding to the lung segment being drained while the patient is positioned specifically to allow gravity to assist in secretion drainage.

Percussion, a massage stroke originally called "tapotement," involves rhythmically clapping with a cupped hand for 2 to 5 minutes over the appropriate area of thorax being drained by gravity (Fig. 24-6). Percussion may feel uncomfortable but should not be painful; a layer of clothing or towel may be employed to reduce any discomfort.

Vibration often follows percussion, although some advocate its use in lieu of percussion, particularly in postoperative treatment and in those for whom percussion should be done with caution (Table 24-2). Vibration involves placing one's hands on the area previously percussed (Fig. 24-7) and having the patient perform several deep breaths using sustained maximal inspiration as in the ACBT maneuver. During the expiratory phase, the therapist performs a fine, tremulous vibration to the chest wall. This may be repeated several times, although in individuals with copious secretions, the first vibratory

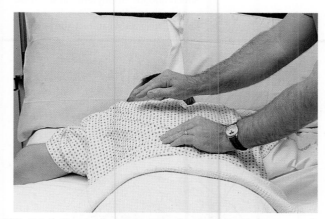

FIG. 24-6 Correct hand position for therapeutic chest percussion. *From Potter PA, Perry AG:* Fundamentals of nursing, *ed 7, St. Louis, 2009, Mosby.*

effort often stimulates coughing and evacuation of secretions and debris.

Clinical Pearl

Vibration of the thorax is best performed by a tight isometric contraction of both upper extremities without increased downward pressure on the chest.

TABLE 24-2	Conditions in Which Caution in the Application of Therapeutic Percussion Is Recommended
Type of Condition	**Characteristics**
Cardiovascular	Chest wall pain
	Unstable angina
	Hemodynamic lability
	Low platelet count
	Anticoagulation therapy
	Unstable or potentially lethal arrhythmias
Musculoskeletal	Osteoporosis
	Prolonged steroid therapy
	Costochondritis
	Osteomyelitis
	Osteogenesis imperfecta
	Spinal fusion
	Rib fracture or flail chest
Pulmonary	Bronchospasm
	Hemoptysis
	Severe dyspnea
	Untreated lung abscess
	Pneumothorax
	Immediately after chest tube removal
	Pneumonia or other infectious process
	Pulmonary embolus
Oncological	Cancer metastasis to the ribs or spine
	Carcinoma in the bronchus
	Resectable tumor
	Osteoporosis secondary to chemotherapeutic agents
Miscellaneous	Recent skin grafts
	Burns
	Open thoracic wounds
	Skin infection in the thoracic region
	Subcutaneous emphysema in the head or back regions
	Immediately after cataract surgery

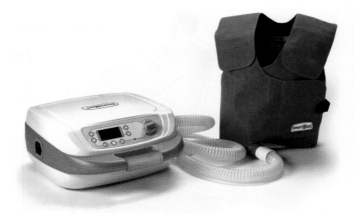

FIG. 24-8 High-frequency chest wall oscillation (HFCWO) device. *Courtesy Electromed, Inc, New Prague, MN.*

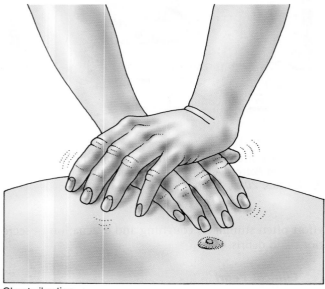

Chest vibration

FIG. 24-7 Correct hand position for chest vibration. *From Frownfelter D, Dean E: Cardiovascular and pulmonary physical therapy: Evidence and practice, ed 4, St. Louis, 2006, Mosby.*

Mechanical Devices for Airway Clearance

High-Frequency Chest Wall Oscillation. High-frequency chest wall oscillation (HFCWO) is provided by a device that uses an air compressor and a garment (a vest) that has inflatable bladders attached to the compressor by large, flexible tubing (Fig. 24-8). The compressor pumps bursts of air at varying frequencies (1 to 20 Hz) and varying pressures into the bladders within the vest. The bursts of air entering the vest bladder transmit oscillations or vibrations to the chest wall. Clinical studies have shown that HFCWO is as effective in the short term as manual bronchial drainage techniques.[23,28] HFCWO, which is typically used twice each day at several different frequencies for a total of 30 minutes per treatment, can be used concurrently with nebulized bronchodilators and mucolytics, whose deposition may be increased by the enhanced airflow generated by HFCWO.[29] Originally used for young adults with CF, HFCWO is now also used in other patients with a long-term need for airway clearance, such as those who have undergone heart/lung transplantation and those with respiratory pump dysfunction as a result of chronic neuromuscular disorders.

Positive Expiratory Pressure. Positive expiratory pressure (PEP) breathing employs another mechanical device for airway clearance dysfunction (Fig. 24-9). This device tries to maintain airway patency by applying positive pressure during expiration with the goal of dislodging and moving secretions proximally in the respiratory tract. PEP was originally provided via an anesthesia face mask, but a mouthpiece can also be used to deliver this treatment. As the patient exhales, the valve of the PEP device provides a positive pressure of 10 to 20 cm H_2O within the airways. This positive pressure stabilizes the small airways and prevents their collapse, which would otherwise trap the secretions distal to the point of collapse and interfere with evacuation of secretions by huffing or coughing. When using PEP, patients should take a large breath in and then breathe out slowly. While breathing out, the patient will experience positive pressure from the PEP device. Many PEP devices have an indicator that shows how much pressure is being exerted. Pressure of 10 to 20 cm H_2O should be maintained throughout the full expiration. This procedure is repeated for 10 to 20 breaths and is followed by

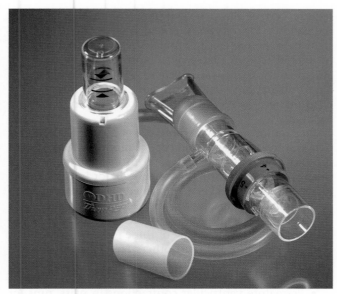

FIG. 24-9 A positive expiratory pressure (PEP) device. *Courtesy Smiths Medical, Rockland, MA.*

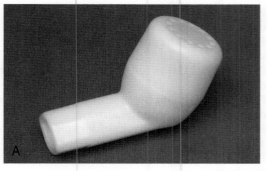

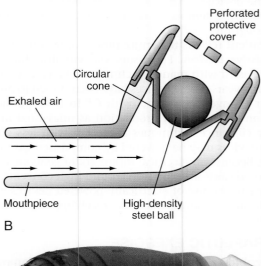

Perforated protective cover

Circular cone

Exhaled air

Mouthpiece

High-density steel ball

B

huffing or coughing to expel accumulated secretions. Some recommend performing the PEP maneuver while the patient is in bronchial drainage positions.

PEP has been shown to be more effective than bronchial drainage and vibratory PEP in patients with cystic fibrosis.[30,31] PEP is an effective, inexpensive, well-researched, and universally employed airway clearance device. It can be used effectively by people who can understand and follow the instructions. It is not particularly useful, however, for patients with significant neuromuscular weakness or dyscoordination who may not be able to achieve adequate flows to receive the benefits.

Use of a PEP Device

- Therapist washes hands and assembles the PEP device.
- Patient sits upright with elbows resting on a table.
- Patient completes a diaphragmatic breath with a larger than normal volume.
- Patient holds the inspiratory breath for 2 to 3 seconds.
- Patient exhales fully but not forced to functional residual capacity (FRC) through the device.
- The pressure manometer should read 10 to 20 cm H_2O pressure during exhalation.
- Therapist adjusts the orifice to result in an inspiratory-to-expiratory time ratio of 1:3.
- Patient performs 10 to 20 breaths.
- Follow with huffing or coughing.
- Repeat the cycle of 10 to 20 breaths at least 3 to 4 times.

Vibratory Positive Expiratory Pressure. Two vibratory positive expiratory pressure devices, the Flutter (Axcan-Pharma, Birmingham, AL) (Fig. 24-10, *A* and *B*) and the Acapella (Smiths Medical, Rockland, MA) (Fig. 24-10, *C*), are commonly employed. Each adds oscillation during the expiratory cycle of PEP breathing. The Flutter employs a pipelike device with a metal ball that is dislodged and reseated in its reservoir during expiratory effort. The

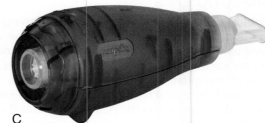

C

FIG. 24-10 **A** and **B**, The Flutter device. **C**, The Acapella airway clearance device. **A** and **B** courtesy Axcan Pharma, Birmingham, AL. **C** courtesy Smiths Medical, Rockland, MA.

dislodgment and reseating of the ball opens and closes the expiratory port, which in turn oscillates the expiratory airflow. The Acapella oscillates airflow using a magnet and a rocker with a metal pin. The variable distance between the pin and the magnet should be matched and set to the patient's needs to create the appropriate resistance and desired length of expiration. These devices have similar performance characteristics to each other, and the Flutter has been shown to have similar clinical efficacy to manual airway clearance techniques. The Acapella has the advantages of being less technique-dependent than the Flutter, it can be used at very low expiratory flows, and can generate PEP at any angle because it is not gravity dependent.

Suggested Sequence for Use of the Flutter and the Acapella

- Therapist washes hands and makes sure device is ready for use.
- Patient is seated with back and head erect.

- Patient places device in mouth and inhales more deeply than normal but not fully.
- Patient holds the inspiratory breath for 2 to 3 seconds.
- Patient now exhales fully but not forced through the device.
- Patient must hold cheeks firmly (not puffed out) to direct oscillation into the airways.
- Patient repeats each inspiratory/expiratory cycle 5 to 10 times and suppresses cough.
- Patient next takes 2 deep breaths in and out through the device.
- Patient attempts to remove sputum via huffing or coughing.
- Patient repeats the entire process 2 to 3 times.

Assistive Devices. Percussors and vibrators have been used to assist with manual techniques of airway clearance for many years. These devices have been shown to produce similar changes in patients with CF in both pulmonary function and secretion production as unassisted manual airway clearance techniques alone but with less effort.[32] These devices may be powered by compressed gas or electricity. Because an electrical motor could generate a spark that could cause an explosion around high concentrations of oxygen, the use of electrically-powered devices is contraindicated around patients receiving supplemental oxygen.

THERAPEUTIC EXERCISE

Aerobic Capacity/Endurance Conditioning or Reconditioning. Patients with pulmonary disease with associated inability to clear their airway often experience dyspnea on exertion that leads to abstaining from any activity that precipitates this unpleasant sensation. This continued avoidance of activity further decreases exercise tolerance and in turn lowers the patient's dyspnea threshold, thereby resulting in dyspnea with even minimal physical exertion such as produced by performing ADLs. Exercise is the most common and useful intervention to break this vicious cycle of deterioration. A cautionary note is that the work of breathing during physical activity in patients with airway clearance dysfunction and COPD may constitute a major portion of their oxygen consumption, which may reduce their ability to achieve the workload one might expect. Therefore the therapist must administer the exercise program judiciously and with close monitoring for signs of early fatigue that may include cyanosis and abnormal vital signs.

Rehabilitation interventions to improve aerobic capacity and exercise tolerance vary widely. They may be formal, based on a strictly derived exercise prescription, or informal, started from an arbitrary point and progressed according to a patient's symptoms and tolerance. They may require equipment, such as treadmills or bicycle ergometers, or merely require enough space to permit obstacle-free walking. Participants may have either subacute pulmonary disease or chronic pulmonary disease of varying severity, and the exercise regimen may begin in any setting from intensive care to home. Exercise may be administered while the patient breathes room air or supplemental oxygen. Completion of the programs may require several days, several months, or longer. Some indications for oxygen-supplemented exercise include right heart failure, cor pulmonale, resting partial pressure of arterial oxygen (PaO_2) of 50 mm Hg or less on room air, inability to tolerate exercise while breathing room air,[33] and oxygen saturation below 80% during physical exertion and while performing ADLs when breathing room air.[34]

Preparation for any aerobic exercise program requires determining the degree and type of monitoring needed to preserve the patient's safety. No formal guidelines that establish the monitoring requirements for informal exercise programs have been published; this determination must be made according to individual circumstances.

There are clear instances in which an exercise session should be terminated. Some of these reasons for termination are physiological, and others are symptom related. The exercise session should be terminated in the presence of the following:

- Premature ventricular contractions in pairs, runs, or increasing frequency
- New-onset atrial arrhythmias: Tachycardia, fibrillation, or flutter
- Heart block, second or third degree
- Angina
- ST-segment changes of greater than or equal to 2 mm in either direction
- Persistent heart rate or BP decline
- Elevation of diastolic pressure by more than 20 mm Hg above resting or to more than 100 mm Hg
- Dyspnea, nausea, fatigue, dizziness, headache, and blurred vision
- Intolerable musculoskeletal pain
- Heart rate greater than target rate
- Patient pallor or diaphoresis

Aerobic exercise training for patients with airway clearance dysfunction has been shown to produce benefits that include improved exercise tolerance, reduced dyspnea, and enhanced quality of life.[35-38]

Body Mechanics and Postural Stabilization Training. Body mechanics and postural stabilization training have two potential benefits for the patient with airway clearance dysfunction and COPD: Reducing general body work and diminishing the effects of dyspnea. Many anecdotal examples of dyspnea relief in the forward-flexed posture have precipitated research into proper positions for the patient with COPD. It is clear that the seated, forward-leaning posture is the preferred position to reduce dyspnea in patients with severe and moderate limitations of maximum inspiratory pressure associated with COPD. The forward-leaning posture produces a significant increase in maximum inspiratory pressures, thereby relieving the sensation of dyspnea.[39] In addition, this position may increase FRC in those with airflow limitations because the thorax approaches a similar position to prone in which FRC is increased.[40] In patients who are unable to tolerate functional walking because of either musculoskeletal stress or dyspnea, a high walker may be adapted to permit forward leaning, thereby reducing the work of breathing and the perception of dyspnea to permit the desired activity (Fig. 24-11).

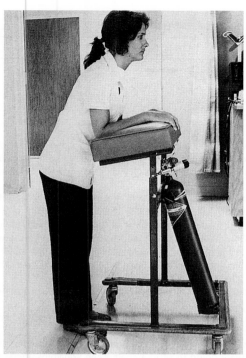

FIG. 24-11 A high walker to permit assumption of a forward-leaning posture in standing. *From Irwin S, Tecklin JS: Cardiopulmonary physical therapy: A guide to practice, ed 4, St. Louis, 1995, Mosby.*

ⓒ *Clinical Pearl*

The forward-leaning posture produces a significant increase in maximum inspiratory pressures, thereby relieving the sensation of dyspnea.[39]

Flexibility Exercises. Exercise to improve flexibility for the patient with airway clearance dysfunction and COPD may include stretching exercises to promote muscle lengthening, exercises to improve ROM, and mobilization exercises to improve joint function. There is little or no experimental evidence to support the use of flexibility exercises in this patient population. However, it seems intuitive that maintaining or improving thoracic and shoulder girdle flexibility would enhance respiratory effort by increasing thoracic compliance. A more flexible chest wall should require less muscular work to inflate the thorax. A similar benefit of increased thoracic compliance and reduced work of breathing may be implied for improving motion of a tight shoulder girdle in the patient with pulmonary disease. Many individuals with COPD have an increased AP thoracic diameter and a hyperinflated and often fixed thoracic cage, particularly during periods of dyspnea.[41] One suspects that using exercise to prevent or treat the fixed thoracic cage should be beneficial despite the dearth of evidence.

A series of flexibility exercises has been recommended as part of a traditional "warm-up" for a pulmonary rehabilitation session (Table 24-3). Although this program has not been formally evaluated from a scientific perspective, it serves as a model for a major long-established

pulmonary rehabilitation program.[42] These exercises may be used as a regular exercise routine to improve or maintain good thoracic and shoulder girdle motion.

Breathing Exercises. To increase **alveolar ventilation,** patients should be taught breathing exercises to influence the rate, depth, or distribution of ventilation or muscular activity associated with breathing. The breathing strategies commonly recommended to improve ventilation and oxygenation include diaphragmatic breathing, also referred to as *breathing control, pursed-lip breathing, segmental breathing, low-frequency breathing,* and *sustained maximal inspiration breathing exercises.* ACBT and AD are also breathing strategies, but they are used primarily with airway clearance and were discussed earlier in this chapter.

Diaphragmatic Breathing Exercises. The diaphragm is the principal muscle of inspiration. Historically, when muscles other than the diaphragm assumed a role in inspiration, therapeutic efforts were directed toward restoring a more normal, diaphragmatic pattern of breathing. The return to diaphragmatic breathing was thought to relieve dyspnea.

Diaphragmatic breathing exercises are intended to enhance diaphragmatic descent during inspiration and diaphragmatic ascent during expiration. Diaphragmatic descent is assisted by directing the patient to protract the abdomen gradually during inhalation. One assists diaphragmatic ascent by directing the patient to allow the abdomen to retract gradually during exhalation or by directing the patient to contract the abdominal muscles actively during exhalation. Although the exact techniques used to teach diaphragmatic breathing vary, in principle they are similar. They all recommend that the patient assume a comfortable position, usually one-half to three-quarters upright sitting, before beginning, and that the patient's hips and knees be flexed to relax the abdominal and hamstring muscles respectively. Diaphragmatic breathing exercises are then taught as follows:

1. Place the patient's dominant hand over the midrectus abdominis area.
2. Place the patient's nondominant hand on the midsternal area.
3. Direct the patient to inhale slowly through the nose.
4. Instruct the patient to watch the dominant hand as inspiration continues.
5. Encourage the patient to direct the air so that the dominant hand gradually rises as inspiration continues.
6. Caution the patient to avoid excessive movement under the nondominant hand.
7. Apply firm counterpressure over the patient's dominant hand just before directing the patient to inhale.
8. Instruct the patient to inhale as you lessen your counterpressure as inspiration continues.
9. Practice the exercise until the patient no longer requires manual assistance of the therapist to perform the exercise correctly.
10. Progress the level of difficulty by sequentially removing auditory, visual, and tactile cues. Then

TABLE 24-3	"Warm-up" Flexibility Exercises for Pulmonary Rehabilitation
Body Area	**Exercise**
Cervical	Look up/down (nod "yes"). Look left/right (shake "no"). Move left ear to left shoulder. Move right ear to right shoulder.
Shoulder and upper extremity	Shoulder circles forward and backward. Shoulder shrugs (up/relax). Shoulder blade squeeze: Rest your hands on your shoulders, touch your elbows together in front of your body, pull them apart, try to push them backward. Squeeze your shoulder blades together as you push back. Breathe IN as you push your elbows backward, and breathe OUT as you bring your elbows together in front. Front arm raises (shoulder flexion): Lift your arms overhead, lower them in front of you slowly, as if pushing against resistance. Breathe IN when lifting, and breathe OUT when lowering. Side-arm raises (abduction): Lift your arms out to the side and up overhead, lower them back to your sides slowly, as if pushing against resistance. Breathe IN as you lift, and breathe OUT as you lower. Arm circles forward: With your arms fully extended and raised to shoulder level, slowly make small circles with your arms, then reverse. (If the patient is extremely short of breath, he or she may lower the arms.)
Trunk	Trunk rotation (side-to-side twists): Start with your arms extended forward and slowly twist to the right and then to the left. Try not to move your hips. Sidebending (right and left): Reach one arm up over your head and lean to the opposite side, then reverse. Blow OUT as you bend, and breathe IN as you straighten.
Lower extremity	Wall slide: Stand with your hips and buttocks pressed as flat as you can against a wall. Shoulders should be relaxed. Slowly lower your body as if you were going to sit in a chair. Keep your hips above the level of your knees. Hold this position. Try to increase the holding time to at least 2 minutes. Hip flexion: Marching in place. Toe tapping. Gastrocnemius/soleus stretch: Stand facing a wall about a foot away and put your hands on the wall at about shoulder height. With knees extended, lean your body into the wall to put a stretch on your large calf muscles.
GENERAL INSTRUCTIONS	Begin with 3-5 repetitions of each exercise and then increase gradually to 7-10 repetitions. Once 10 repetitions of each can be done, a 1-lb weight may be added to the arm exercises. Perform pursed-lip breathing throughout the activity. Remember to have patients breathe IN through the nose and OUT through pursed lips, and remind patients to not hold their breath.

progress the exercise by practicing it in varied positions, including seated, standing, and walking.

The objectives and potential outcomes of diaphragmatic breathing exercises are summarized in Table 24-4.

Pursed-Lip Breathing Exercises. Pursed-lip breathing is another method, often associated with relaxation activities, suggested for improving ventilation and oxygenation and relieving respiratory symptoms in individuals with airway clearance dysfunction.[43] One method of pursed-lip breathing advocates passive expiration,[44] whereas the other recommends abdominal muscle contraction to prolong expiration.[45] Current use of the technique usually encourages passive rather than forced expiration. Pursed-lip breathing with passive expiration is performed as follows:

1. Position the patient comfortably.
2. Place your hand over the midrectus abdominis area to detect activity during expiration.
3. Direct the patient to inhale slowly.
4. Instruct the patient to purse the lips before exhalation.
5. Instruct the patient to relax the air out through the pursed lips and refrain from abdominal muscle contraction.

TABLE 24-4	Objectives and Potential Outcomes of Diaphragmatic Breathing Exercises
Therapeutic objectives	Alleviate dyspnea Reduce the work of breathing Reduce the incidence of postoperative pulmonary complication
Physiological objectives	Improve ventilation Improve oxygenation
Potential outcomes	Eliminate accessory muscle action Decrease respiratory rate Increase tidal ventilation Improve distribution of ventilation Decrease need for postoperative therapy

6. Direct the patient to stop exhaling when abdominal muscle activity is detected.
7. Progress the intensity of the exercise by substituting the patient's hand for yours, removing tactile cues, and having the patient perform the exercise while standing and exercising.

Clinical Pearl

Pursed-lip exhalation is a gentle exhalation like blowing out a candle. Forceful exhalation is avoided because it closes airways and increases the work of breathing.

Research has failed to fully explain the symptomatic benefits some patients ascribe to pursed-lip breathing. One theory is that pursed-lip breathing is effective because the slight resistance to expiration increases positive pressure within the airways and helps keep open the small bronchioles that otherwise collapse because of loss of support associated with lung tissue destruction. Alternatively, or additionally, pursed-lip breathing could be effective because it slows the respiratory rate. At the very least, pursed-lip breathing appears to reduce respiratory rate and increase tidal volume, thereby not compromising minute ventilation. It is recommended that clinicians continue to teach pursed-lip breathing exercises to patients complaining of dyspnea.

Segmental Breathing Exercises. Segmental breathing, also referred to as *localized expansion breathing,* is another type of exercise used to improve ventilation and oxygenation in individuals with airway clearance dysfunction. This exercise presumes that inspired air can be actively directed to a specific area of lung by emphasizing and increasing movement of the thorax overlying that lung area. This intervention has been recommended to prevent the accumulation of pleural fluid, to reduce the probability of atelectasis, to prevent the accumulation of tracheobronchial secretions, to decrease **paradoxical breathing,** to prevent the panic associated with uncontrolled breathing, and to improve chest wall mobility.[46] The attempt to preferentially enhance localized lung expansion uses manual counterpressure against the thorax to encourage the expansion of that specific area of thorax in the hopes of improving ventilation to a specific part of the lung. Segmental breathing exercises are performed as follows:

1. Identify the surface landmarks demarcating the affected area.
2. Place your hand or hands on the chest wall overlying the bronchopulmonary segment or segments requiring treatment (i.e., the areas of lung you hope to expand).
3. Apply firm pressure to that area at the end of the patient's expiratory maneuver. (Pressure should be equal and bilateral across a median sternotomy incision.)
4. Instruct the patient to inspire deeply through his or her mouth, attempting to direct the inspired air toward your hand, saying, "Breathe into my hand, or make my hand move as you breathe in."
5. Reduce hand pressure as the patient inspires. (At end inspiration, the instructor's hand should not be applying pressure to the chest.)
6. Instruct the patient to hold his or her breath for 2 to 3 seconds at the completion of inspiration.
7. Instruct the patient to exhale.
8. Repeat the sequence until the patient can execute the breathing maneuver correctly.
9. Progress the exercises by instructing the patient to use his or her own hands or a belt to execute the program independently.

There is a lack of persuasive evidence linking segmental breathing with other therapeutic effects. However, it is quite clear and demonstrable that improving local chest wall motion can improve breathing by converting intercostal muscle shortening into lung volume expansion.[47]

Sustained Maximal Breathing Exercises. Breathing exercises during which a maximal inspiration is sustained for about 3 seconds have also been associated with improved oxygenation.[48] Currently, sustained maximal inspiration is more commonly employed as part of the ACBT and is used in association with airway clearance techniques as described previously.

Relaxation Exercise Techniques. Relaxation exercise and training are currently used as adjunctive therapy for many different diseases; however, despite many anecdotal reports, there are little data to demonstrate discrete pulmonary benefits of relaxation.[49] Relaxation techniques coupled with breathing strategies and hypnosis have recently been shown to result in some symptomatic improvement in children with dyspnea.[50] Relaxation techniques are often administered to decrease unnecessary muscle contraction throughout the body and thereby reduce general body work. The traditional method or approach involves muscle contraction followed by relaxation, whereas a newer technique employs visual imagery to achieve the desired effects.

Strength, Power, and Endurance Training. Endurance training that focuses primarily on aerobic benefits has been used for decades in pulmonary rehabilitation programs. The issue of muscle strength and resistance exercise to improve strength and reduce related symptoms has only recently come to the fore as a means of improving physical functioning in patients with chronic airway clearance dysfunction. Recent work indicates that people with COPD have peripheral muscle weakness that is likely multifactorial in origin.[51] Among those factors are disuse atrophy, inadequate nutrition, long-term **hypercapnia** and hypoxemia, reduced anabolic steroid levels, and myopathy from continuous or periodic corticosteroid use. Muscle strength, particularly lower extremity strength, is reduced in individuals with COPD when compared to age-matched controls.[52] Although there is great patient-to-patient variability in this muscular dysfunction, research has demonstrated a 20% to 30% deficit in quadriceps strength in those with moderate-to-severe COPD. Muscle endurance is similarly decreased in this population. These deficits may limit exercise capacity and function in those with COPD.[6,53,54]

There is a growing body of evidence that strength training is beneficial and should become part of a comprehensive physical therapy program for patients with airway clearance dysfunction and COPD. The primary benefits of strength training in this population are improved muscle strength, endurance, function, and exercise tolerance and reduced dyspnea.[55-58] Although these benefits are reasonably well accepted, recent studies call into question the benefit of such exercises on a patient's quality of life.[59,60] Since the preponderance of

TABLE 24-5	Features of a Resistance Exercise Program for Patients with Airway Clearance Dysfunction
Frequency	Each major muscle group to be trained should be exercised 2-3 times per week. Specific suggestions will depend on where the program is carried out: At home, outpatient, inpatient, and other sites.
Intensity	Muscle load is typically and reasonably safely initiated with 50%-60% of the 1 repetition maximum (1 RM) established during the examination. Repetitions are typically 10 per muscle group at outset of program. One set of repetitions is a good starting point. A degree of success should be built into the prescription for the psychological benefits and to increase a likelihood of adherence. A rest period should provide time between the sets for recovery.
Mode	Various types of resistance devices may be employed—exercise tables, benches, pulleys, free weights, and so forth. Exercise should focus on the large muscle groups of the lower and upper extremities, as well as trunk musculature such as latissimus dorsi. To ensure continued interest and to vary the training stimulus, it is important to vary the types of exercise and consider including eccentric, concentric, isometric, isotonic, and isokinetic exercises.
Duration	ACSM recommends a 10-12 week duration followed by a period of active recovery using alternative forms of exercise.
Progression	Begin with lighter loads and increase number of repetitions and sets as the patient begins to demonstrate tolerance at each particular level of activity.

ACSM, American College of Sports Medicine.

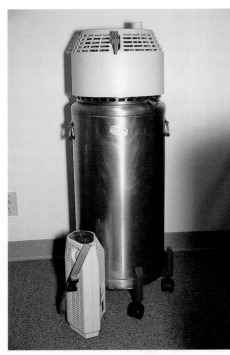

FIG. 24-12 Stationary and portable liquid oxygen units. *From Potter PA, Perry AG:* Fundamentals of nursing, *ed 6, St. Louis, 2005, Mosby.*

evidence indicates that strength training can improve impairments associated with quality of life, a comprehensive intervention plan for the patient with airway clearance dysfunction should include resistance training, as well as endurance training. Features of a resistance exercise program for patients with airway clearance dysfunction are described in Table 24-5.[61]

Functional Training in Self-Care and Home Management, Work, Community, and Leisure Integration/Reintegration. There is little direct evidence regarding functionally specific training programs and improvement in ADLs in patients with airway clearance dysfunction. However, it appears from recent data that whether the physical rehabilitation program focuses on endurance training using treadmill or bicycle ergometry or employs more traditional calisthenics, the intervention produces significant improvement in functional performance and overall health.[62]

Unlike patients with neuromuscular or musculoskeletal deficits who may need to learn new strategies and adapted tasks to regain functional independence, it appears that those with COPD need to gain control over their dyspnea and disease to use existing functional skills. These self-care skills have not been lost but have gone unused because of the physical and emotional impact of the severe dyspnea and resultant physical deconditioning that has accrued over months and years of disabling lung disease. Among the various functional tasks that may need to be relearned or adapted are the following:

- Bed mobility and transfers—use of transfer boards and overhead trapeze bars
- Self-care such as bathing, grooming, and dressing—raised toilet seat, long-handled brush, shower seat
- Household activities and related chores such as yard work—long-handled tools, rolling bench
- Activity adaptation to conserve energy—break complex or difficult tasks into component parts, motorized mobility device
- Injury prevention—use of grab-bars, walking aids

DEVICES AND EQUIPMENT

There are various oxygen sources and delivery devices available for use in the home, at work, or in the community. Oxygen may be supplied in gas cylinders of varying sizes. These cylinders must be replaced or refilled periodically to replenish the oxygen supply and most are large, bulky, and heavy. However, recent technology has made much smaller devices, such as liquid oxygen containers (Fig. 24-12) and oxygen concentrators, available. These devices can supply oxygen for up to several hours, depending on patient usage. Liquid oxygen systems have been available for use at home for many years. There is usually

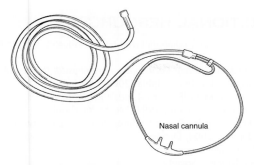

FIG. 24-13 Nasal cannula for oxygen delivery. *From Hillegass EA, Sadowsky HS: Essentials of cardiopulmonary physical therapy, ed 2, Philadelphia, 2001, Saunders.*

a large reservoir in the home from which a small, portable knapsack–size container may be filled for outside use. Oxygen concentrators, which have also been available for several years, are electrically powered and use a molecular sieve to separate oxygen from the ambient air and concentrate and store the oxygen. These devices are economical for use in the home and for activities immediately around the house, such as gardening, but are too large to take out into the community.

Oxygen must be delivered from its source to the patient via a device. Oxygen catheters may be inserted into the nasal passage or via a small surgical incision directly into the trachea, with a transtracheal device. Oxygen masks placed over the nose and mouth may also be used. These sometimes have a reservoir that enables high concentrations of oxygen to be provided. The most commonly used device is a nasal cannula that provides a small prong into each nostril for oxygen delivery (Fig. 24-13).

Mechanical ventilators are commonly used for patients with airway clearance disorders when acute or chronic respiratory failure occurs such as after acute disease processes, trauma, or surgery (see Chapter 26). Assistive devices, such as canes and walkers, are often indicated to assist with ambulation and enhance stability and safety.[2] When recommending such assistive devices for the patient with airway clearance dysfunction, the therapist must be aware that crutches, walkers, and similar devices tend to increase the oxygen requirement when compared to unassisted ambulation.[63] A cost-benefit decision about such devices must be made.[64] A wheeled walker can, however, be very helpful for individuals with chronic airway clearance dysfunction. The walker not only offers support and stabilization, but a walker with a basket or small platform can be used to carry a small oxygen delivery system during community activities. Motorized scooters are useful for community mobility outside the home for shopping, work, and recreational activities in individuals with significant airway clearance dysfunction. There are lift systems for automobile storage of the scooters to facilitate patient use. Motorized scooters and the appropriate lift devices are expensive but often make the difference between being housebound or active in the community.

CASE STUDY 24-1

CHRONIC BRONCHITIS

Patient History

NT is a 66-year-old woman with a history of chronic bronchitis. She was admitted to the hospital in acute respiratory distress and was diagnosed with bacterial pneumonia. Because NT previously participated in a pulmonary rehabilitation program, a physical therapy consultation was requested. She reported a 110 pack per year history of cigarette smoking. NT reported that it now exhausts her to prepare her meals and perform other IADLs. She is currently taking antibiotics for her infection, oral and inhaled bronchodilators, and oral and inhaled corticosteroids, and she is breathing supplemental oxygen at 2 L/min via nasal cannula.

Tests and Measures—Significant Findings

* Heart rate is 100 bpm, respiratory rate is 24 breaths/min with clear distress, BP is 130/85 mm Hg.

Musculoskeletal

* NT has forward head and shoulders and a significant thoracic kyphosis.

Cardiovascular/Pulmonary

* NT has minimal pedal edema.
* NT is in acute respiratory distress with tachypnea, flaring of the nares, use of accessory muscles of inspiration, and prolonged expiration with an I:E ratio of 1:4. She exhibits perioral cyanosis, digital clubbing, and a cough that produces thick, yellowish sputum without evidence of blood. Her thorax appears symmetrical.
* NT has minimal thoracic excursion with a very limited right hemithorax. Dullness to percussion is noted in the lower right posterior and lateral thorax.
* Distant breath sounds are heard throughout the lungs, except for bronchial and bronchovesicular sounds in the lower right posterior and lateral thorax. Coarse crackles and low-pitched wheezing are noted in that area on the right, along with some scattering of these sounds throughout the lung fields.
* NT is not able to complete a 6-minute walk test. She walked 100 feet in 2 minutes limited by severe fatigue (9/10 on the Borg CR10 scale).

Diagnosis

Preferred practice pattern 6C: Impaired ventilation, respiration/gas exchange, and aerobic capacity/endurance associated with airway clearance dysfunction.

Interventions

* Airway clearance techniques: NT was treated with bronchial drainage, percussion, and vibration during her hospital admission. She was instructed in proper use of autogenic drainage.

• Therapeutic exercise: Bedside cycle ergometry will be performed until the patient is able to travel to the physical therapy department where she will begin endurance walking on a motorized treadmill. She will continue treadmill exercise and free walking as part of her home program. Lower extremity strengthening exercises will be alternated each day with flexibility exercises. Relaxation exercises and diaphragmatic breathing will be done daily.

Role of the Physical Therapist Assistant

• Write a home program for this patient that includes one endurance exercise, one strengthening exercise, one flexibility exercise, and diaphragmatic breathing.
• What are the positions for postural drainage of the different parts of the lungs?
• Describe the sequence of autogenic drainage.
• Describe how you would instruct this patient to modify one of her household activities to conserve energy.

Additional Information

For the full version of this case study, including detailed examination results, interventions, and outcomes, see the Evolve site that accompanies this book.

CHAPTER SUMMARY

This chapter focuses on individuals with airway clearance dysfunction, particularly patients with COPD and CF. The principles and skills described are applicable to any patient with airway clearance dysfunction, including young adults with neurological trauma that has resulted in the inability to cough and clear secretions. Basic chest examination techniques—inspection, palpation, percussion, and auscultation—are described and are appropriate for any patient with respiratory or pulmonary disease. Interventions described include specific approaches to airway clearance and therapeutic exercise for strength, aerobic fitness, and breathing retraining.

ADDITIONAL RESOURCES

For links to these and additional web-based resources, see the Evolve site.

Irwin S, Tecklin JS (eds): *Cardiopulmonary physical therapy: A guide to practice,* ed 4, Philadelphia, 2004, Elsevier.

Burton GG, Hodgkin JE, Ward JJ (eds): *Respiratory care: A guide to practice,* ed 4, St. Louis, 1997, Mosby-Yearbook.

Wilkins RL, Stoller JK: *Egan's fundamentals of respiratory care,* ed 7, Philadelphia, 2004, Elsevier.

Borg CR10 scale
American Thoracic Society
American College of Chest Physicians
American Lung Association

GLOSSARY

Aerobic capacity: Another term for maximum oxygen uptake (Vo_{2max}). The highest amount of oxygen consumed during maximal exercise.

Alveolar ventilation: The volume of gas expired from the alveoli to the outside of the body per minute.

Atelectasis: Alveolar collapse because of poor lung expansion or complete obstruction of an airway.

Auscultation: Listening with a stethoscope.

Bronchodilator: Medication that reduces bronchial smooth muscle spasm and thereby causes an increase in caliber of a bronchial tube.

Crackles: Nonmusical sounds (previously called *rales*) that may be mimicked by rolling several strands of hair near your ear or by listening to a bowl of cereal that crackles when milk is added. Crackles may represent the sudden opening of previously closed airways. Expiratory crackles may indicate the presence of fluid in the large airways.

Dyspnea: Shortness of breath. A subjective difficulty or distress in breathing.

Hypercapnia: Increased carbon dioxide level in the arterial blood.

Hypoxemia: Low or insufficient oxygen in the arterial blood.

Mucolytic: A medication capable of dissolving or decreasing the viscosity of mucus.

Paradoxical breathing: Moving the belly in during inspiration and out during expiration.

Stertor: A snoring noise created when the tongue falls back into the lower palate.

Stridor: A crowing sound during inspiration.

Thoracic index: Ratio of the AP diameter to the transverse diameter of the thorax.

Tidal volume: The volume of air inspired or expired in a single breath during regular breathing.

Wheezes: Whistling sounds probably produced by air flowing at high velocities through narrowed airways.

Chapter 25

Congestive Heart Failure

Jennifer Dekerlegand

OBJECTIVES

After reading this chapter, the reader will be able to:
1. Define congestive heart failure and identify implications for rehabilitation interventions.
2. Understand the etiology and pathology of heart failure.
3. Describe classification systems for heart failure.
4. Identify typical examination procedures used to diagnose heart failure.
5. Provide effective rehabilitation interventions for patients with heart failure.
6. Modify a patient's program, as needed, based on the patient with heart failure's response to exercise.
7. Identify methods to measure outcomes of treatment of patients with heart failure, including exercise testing and self-report measures.

Heart failure affects 5 million people in the United States, with approximately 550,000 new cases being diagnosed each year.[1] According to the Centers for Medicare and Medicaid, **heart failure** is the most frequent Medicare diagnosis at hospital admission, and 250,000 deaths each year are caused by heart failure.[1] Whether a clinician works in an acute care hospital, an acute rehabilitation facility, an outpatient clinic, a long-term care facility, or in the home setting, they will certainly encounter patients with heart failure. Hallmarks of heart failure include decreased activity tolerance, decreased function, and edema. Patients with heart failure can benefit from the expertise of therapists to improve these deficits.

Heart failure is a progressive disease that results from the heart's gradual inability to pump enough blood to meet the body's demands. In the past, the term *congestive heart failure* was used to describe patients who presented with heart failure and the classic signs and symptoms of volume overload. However, we now realize that many patients with heart failure have reduced activity tolerance without evidence of fluid retention. Therefore, since the 1990s, heart failure has become the preferred term because it causes less confusion about the presenting signs and symptoms in these patients.

Heart failure research has generally focused on interventions aimed at reducing mortality and decreasing signs and symptoms in patients diagnosed with heart failure. There are also a few studies evaluating the effects of interventions intended to prevent or reduce the risk of heart failure. Based on these studies, the New York Heart Association, the American College of Cardiology (ACC), and the American Heart Association (AHA) have developed guidelines for classifying heart failure into one of four stages (Table 25-1) and recommend certain interventions for each of these stages.[2] This chapter presents and analyzes the evidence on rehabilitation examination, evaluation, and interventions for patients in all stages of heart failure.

PATHOLOGY

Heart failure is a clinical syndrome caused by a reduction in the heart's ability to fill with blood or eject blood to the rest of the body. There are many pathologies that can progress to heart failure. Structural causes of heart failure include disorders of the **myocardium,** pericardium, endocardium, or great vessels. Heart failure can also be caused by valvular disease, coronary artery disease (CAD), hypertension, **cardiomyopathy,** alcohol or drug abuse, and myocarditis.[2]

Hypertension causes heart failure because it leads to high peripheral arterial pressure and resistance, which increases the afterload on the heart, making it more difficult for the heart to eject blood. Cardiomyopathy of any type, restrictive, hypertrophic, or dilated, can also lead to

TABLE 25-1	New York Heart Association Classification of Heart Failure
NYHA class	**Description**
I	No symptoms with ordinary exertion
II	Symptoms with ordinary exertion
III	Symptoms with less than ordinary exertion
IV	Symptoms at rest

Data from The Criteria Committee of the New York Heart Association: *Nomenclature and criteria for the diagnosis of the heart and great vessels,* ed 6, Boston, 1964, Little Brown.

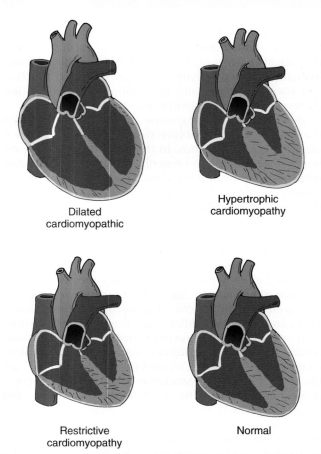

Dilated cardiomyopathic

Hypertrophic cardiomyopathy

Restrictive cardiomyopathy

Normal

FIG. 25-1 Types of cardiomyopathies and the normal heart.

heart failure. In **restrictive cardiomyopathy,** the walls of the ventricle become stiff. This stiffness prevents the heart from filling or ejecting blood adequately. **Hypertrophic cardiomyopathy** is characterized by thickening of the walls of the heart. The thickening reduces the size of the heart chambers and can also restrict the heart's ability to fill. **Dilated cardiomyopathy** is characterized by stretching and thinning of the heart muscle with consequent cardiac enlargement and increased filling but reduced ejection of blood. The various types of cardiomyopathy are depicted in Fig. 25-1.

CLASSIFICATION OF HEART FAILURE

Heart failure may be classified according to a variety of classification schemes. It is generally classified by whether it most affects systolic (ejection of blood from the heart) or diastolic (filling of the heart with blood) heart function. Systolic failure can be further divided according to its etiology as ischemic or nonischemic. Although the signs and symptoms of all types of heart failure may be similar, appropriate medical management can vary, depending on classification.[3]

Heart function is quantified either by **echocardiography** or by nuclear multiple-gated acquisition (MUGA) scanning, with the primary index generally being left ventricular **ejection fraction (EF)**.[4] The left ventricular EF is the percentage of the **end-diastolic volume** (i.e., the amount of blood in the left ventricle when it is full, at the end of **diastole**) pumped from the left ventricle with each heartbeat. A normal EF is between 55% and 65%. **Systolic dysfunction** is defined as an EF below 40%. In contrast, **diastolic dysfunction** is characterized by a normal EF with reduced filling.[4] Both systolic and diastolic heart failure can present with similar symptoms, including fatigue, **dyspnea**, and decreased exercise tolerance.

As noted, systolic dysfunction can be further categorized as ischemic or nonischemic. **Ischemic heart failure** is the breakdown of the heart muscle as the result of lack of blood flow to the coronary vessels and may occur with or without myocardial infarction. Approximately 50% to 70% of patients diagnosed with heart failure have ischemic systolic dysfunction.[5] Nonischemic heart failure is systolic heart failure that results from any process other than CAD. It can have many causes, including hypertension, alcohol abuse, valvular disease, and viral or other infectious diseases. Nonischemic systolic heart failure is also associated with pregnancy and certain medications or may be idiopathic. The prognosis for patients with ischemic heart failure is worse than for those with nonischemic failure, probably because more of these patients have other co-morbidities such as diabetes mellitus.[6]

From 20% to 70% of patients with heart failure have diastolic dysfunction, characterized by a normal left ventricular EF.[7-9] Patients with diastolic dysfunction are more often female, older, and obese and more likely to have high blood pressure (BP) and less likely to have CAD than patients with systolic heart failure.[9] With diastolic dysfunction, there is impaired filling of the left ventricle because of thickening, stiffening, and/or impaired relaxation of the walls of the heart. With aging, the heart's elasticity decreases, leading to increased myocardial stiffness.[10,11] Diastolic heart failure is usually detected after exclusion of other possible reasons for heart failure symptoms.

New York Heart Association Classification System. The **New York Heart Association (NYHA) Classification system** is a simple and widely used tool that classifies patients with heart failure into one of four classes according to their degree of symptoms at rest and with activity. In the early stages of heart failure, the heart may function adequately both at rest and with activity. With progression of the disease, the heart will first not be able to meet the demands of the body with activity, and patients will begin to demonstrate clinical signs and symptoms with activity. With further progression of the disease, patients will demonstrate signs and symptoms of heart failure even at rest. The NYHA Classification system is the system most commonly used by physicians to prognosticate and monitor the effectiveness of treatment interventions in heart failure.[12] The classes used in this system, I to IV with I indicating less severity and higher numbers indicating greater severity, are described in Table 25-1. Classification is based on the patient's self-report of symptoms in response to activity. Patients can move between classes, either up or down, depending on the severity of their disease at the time.

◎ *Clinical Pearl*

The New York Heart Association Classification system for heart failure classifies patients into four classifications based on their self-report of symptoms in response to activity.

CHARACTERISTICS OF HEART FAILURE CONTRIBUTING TO EXERCISE INTOLERANCE

Regardless of etiology or classification, heart failure is characterized by the inability of the heart to meet the demands of the body. This results in the hallmark symptom of heart failure: Decreased exercise tolerance.

◎ *Clinical Pearl*

Many patients with significant heart failure tire with very low levels of exertion such as simply brushing their teeth or walking to the bathroom.

A normal exercise response requires the coordination of multiple systems, including the cardiac, pulmonary, vascular, and musculoskeletal systems. During exercise, **cardiac output,** which is heart rate multiplied by **stroke volume,** should be able to increase to four to six times its resting level. Patients with heart failure may only achieve half of this normal increase in cardiac output during exercise.[13]

Central hemodynamic characteristics of heart failure contribute to exercise intolerance. These include abnormal pressures within the heart, reduced left ventricular EF, reduced cardiac output, and increased pulmonary capillary wedge pressure. New evidence suggests that a number of additional peripheral factors, including alterations in sympathetic and other neurohormonal control mechanisms, as well as changes in skeletal muscle, pulmonary, and vascular function, may also contribute to the reduced activity tolerance seen in this population.

TYPICAL EXAMINATION FINDINGS

Examination of the patient with heart failure consists of a comprehensive patient history and a systems review, followed by the appropriate tests and measures. Factors that will vary the selection of procedures used in examination of the patient with heart failure may include age, social history, diagnosis of chronic or acute heart failure, time since onset of initial heart failure diagnosis, other current medical conditions, and patient goals.

PATIENT HISTORY

The examination includes a comprehensive patient history that can be gathered from the patient's inpatient or outpatient chart, as well as through direct interview with the patient or family members. In addition to general demographics, such as age, gender, and race, information about family and caregiver support for the patient is included. Heart failure is a progressive disease, often characterized by exacerbations that can be kept to a minimum with the support of family and friends reinforcing compliance with the medical regimen.

The patient history includes information about the patient's employment, home environment, equipment the patient is using, and health and social habits (e.g., compliance with medications, diet, exercise routine, medical follow-ups, smoking, and drug and alcohol use). The medical and surgical history; current medications; and clinical tests, including echocardiograms, cardiac catheterizations, exercise testing, laboratory tests, electrocardiograms, and radiographic imaging, are reviewed. Additionally, it should be determined if the patient has a pacemaker or implanted cardiac defibrillator (ICD) and any history of recent arrhythmias.

Finally, the patient's current functional status, complaints, and symptoms are thoroughly documented, including fatigue, shortness of breath, reduced exercise and activity tolerance, and peripheral edema; what kind and duration of activity brings on each of these symptoms; how long they last; and what relieves these symptoms. Common signs and symptoms seen in the patient with heart failure are included in Box 25-1.

TESTS AND MEASURES

Musculoskeletal. Musculoskeletal tests and measures include quantification of range of motion (ROM), flexibility, postural alignment, joint integrity, and mobility (see Chapter 4). Anthropometric characteristics relative to heart failure also include the determination of body mass index (BMI). BMI is based on the patient's weight

---

BOX 25-1	Common Signs and Symptoms in Patients with Heart Failure

- Dyspnea
- Fatigue
- Paroxysmal nocturnal dyspnea
- Peripheral edema
- JVD
- Rales
- Abnormal heart sounds (S3, S4)
- Ascites/liver congestion/hepatomegaly
- Decreased functional exercise capacity
- Angina
- Renal insufficiency/failure
- Hypotension
- Orthopnea
- Tachycardia

JVD, Jugular venous distention.

TABLE 25-2	Calculation and Classification of Body Mass Index (BMI)

BMI = Body Weight in Kilograms/(Height in Meters)²

Classification	BMI (kg/m²)
Underweight	<18.5
Normal	18.5-24.9
Overweight	25-29.9

Class of Obesity	
I	30-34.9
II	35-39.9
III	>40

Adapted from *Arch Intern Med* 158:1855-1867, 1998.

TABLE 25-3	Angina Scale

Stage	Description
1	Onset of angina; mild but recognized as the usual angina-of-effort pain or discomfort with which the subject is familiar.
2	Some pain, moderately severe and definitely uncomfortable but still tolerable.
3	Severe anginal pain at a level that the subject will wish to stop exercising.
4	Unbearable chest pain; the most severe pain the subject has felt.

From Allred EN, Bleecker ER, Chaitman BR, et al: *Environ Health Perspect* 91:89-132, 1991; Allred EN, Bleecker ER, Chaitman BR, et al: *N Engl J Med* 321:1426-1432, 1989.

TABLE 25-4	Dyspnea Index

Level	Description
0	Able to count aloud to 15 without taking a breath
1	Must take one breath to complete counting aloud to 15
2	Must take two breaths to complete counting aloud to 15
3	Must take three breaths to complete counting aloud to 15

From Watchie J: *Cardiopulmonary physical therapy: A clinical manual,* Philadelphia, 1995, WB Saunders.

and height. The formula for calculating BMI and the interpretation of its values are given in Table 25-2.

Neuromuscular. Aspects of the neuromuscular examination that are generally most important in patients with heart failure are measures of arousal, attention, cognition, and pain.

Arousal, Attention, and Cognition. Recent research suggests that some degree of cognitive dysfunction is commonly associated with heart failure. Cognitive deficits in patients with heart failure are thought to be caused by cerebral infarction and/or cerebral hypoperfusion. Although there is insufficient evidence to recommend specific tools to measure cognitive dysfunction in patients with heart failure,[14] it is important for clinicians to recognize the potential presence of these deficits and to adjust their interventions accordingly.

Pain. In patients with heart failure, symptoms of angina and dyspnea that may limit performance of functional tasks are measured. Perceived pain or breathlessness can be measured on a 0 to 10 scale (see Box 24-1). Angina can also be rated on a 1 to 4 scale (Table 25-3). For patients with ischemic heart disease, exercise should not precipitate symptoms exceeding a rating of 2/4 on the angina scale. Dyspnea can be rated on the Dyspnea Index, which is also rated on a 0 to 4 scale (Table 25-4). The Dyspnea Index score is the number of breaths required while the patient counts out loud from 1 to 15. Patients should also not exceed a score of 2/4 on the Dyspnea Index at any time during rehabilitation interventions.

Cardiovascular/Pulmonary. Most of the tests and measures performed in the examination of patients with heart failure focus on assessing circulation and aerobic capacity. As discussed previously, the clinical presentation of heart failure results from vascular, musculoskeletal, pulmonary, cardiac, and hematological abnormalities and can cause peripheral and **pulmonary edema,** dyspnea, **orthopnea, jugular venous distention (JVD),** abnormal heart sounds, and exercise intolerance. The examination therefore includes tests and measures of fluid accumulation, JVD, heart rate and BP, and lung and heart sounds to provide a baseline for comparison with later reexamination and an objective indication of a patient's response to treatment interventions.[15]

Circulation

Fluid Accumulation. When the heart cannot pump fluid through the vasculature adequately, fluid may accumulate in the periphery, centrally, and/or in the lungs. Therefore fluid status can be used to assess the severity of disease and the effectiveness of some treatment interventions in heart failure. Fluid status can be assessed by monitoring body weight, detecting JVD, and evaluating for the presence and degree of pulmonary and peripheral edema. Since short-term volume changes can readily be detected by measuring body weight with a scale, heart failure management guidelines recommend daily weight monitoring for patients with heart failure. Clinicians should pay particular attention to a patient's weight because a weight gain of 3 or more lb in 3 days can be a sign of decompensation.

○ *Clinical Pearl*

Heart failure decompensation can cause fluid retention that presents with weight gain of 3 or more lb in 3 days and symmetrical distal lower extremity edema.

Jugular Venous Pressure. Jugular venous pressure (JVP) is the pressure of blood in the jugular veins. JVP is elevated in patients with heart failure when they cannot pump blood out of the heart adequately, causing blood to accumulate in the venous system. JVP is examined by observing the height and characteristics of the pulse of the internal and external jugular veins with the patient lying at a 45-degree angle, with the head turned slightly to avoid compression of the vein by the sternocleidomastoid muscle.[16] The height of the pulsation above the sternal angle can be used to estimate mean **right atrial pressure**.[16,17] A height of 3 to 4 cm is normal, and a height of more than 4 to 5 cm from the sternal angle is consistent with JVD, elevated right atrial pressure, and fluid retention.

Heart Rate and Rhythm. Although heart rate should be assessed during the systems review for many patients, particular attention should be paid to specific examination of heart rate and rhythm in the patient with heart failure as these are often indicators of the patient's physiological status and prognosis and may predict the patient's tolerance for activity-based interventions (see Chapter 22 for detailed descriptions of methods of measuring heart rate and rhythm). Tachycardia is a common compensatory attempt to maintain cardiac output in patients with heart failure. Resting tachycardia in the absence of other causes can be attributed to a heightened sympathetic drive from poor ventricular performance.

Abnormal heart rhythms are called *arrhythmias* (or *dysrhythmias*). Arrhythmias can provide prognostic information in the heart failure population.[18] According to the Framingham study, the rate of sudden death (i.e., death caused by arrhythmia) is increased by nine times in heart failure. Approximately 50% of deaths in patients with heart failure are caused by arrhythmias, most commonly fast ventricular arrhythmias. Atrial arrhythmias, including atrial fibrillation and flutter, occur in 10% to 30% of patients with heart failure, and the incidence is proportional to the degree of heart failure.[19] Therefore it is important for therapists to monitor heart rhythm, on telemetry if available, at baseline, as well as during and after interventions.

Because of the risk of arrhythmias and sudden death, many patients with heart failure have pacemakers and/or ICDs. ICDs can recognize and terminate rapid heart rhythms. Patients are at risk for inappropriate firing of the ICD during exercise if the heart rate exceeds the programmed threshold. The threshold for ICD firing should be identified from the medical history to prevent inappropriate discharges from occurring during the interventions.

Blood Pressure. BP is used to assess systemic perfusion (see Chapter 22 for detailed descriptions of methods of measuring BP). BP must be measured at least at baseline, after each intervention, and if there are any signs or symptoms of decompensation. Both the underlying pathology of heart failure and the medications used to treat it can cause hypotension (low BP). The clinician should monitor each patient for signs and symptoms of hypotension intolerance, including cool, clammy extremities; complaints of dizziness, particularly when rising from supine or sitting; fatigue; and/or blurred vision.

Heart Sounds. Heart sounds are heard by auscultation of the heart through the chest wall with a stethoscope. Heart sounds generally reflect the closing of the heart valves and include normal and abnormal sounds.

Aerobic Capacity and Endurance

Lung Sounds. Lung sounds are assessed by chest auscultation (see Chapter 24). **Crackles** can reflect fluid

---

BOX 25-2	Indications for Terminating an Exercise Test for a Cardiac Patient

- Drop in systolic BP by >10 mm Hg from baseline
- Moderate to severe angina (level 3 or 4 on the Angina Scale)
- Ataxia, dizziness, or near syncope
- Cyanosis or pallor
- Subject's request to terminate the test
- Sustained ventricular tachycardia
- ST elevation >1 mm in leads without diagnostic Q waves
- Technical difficulties in obtaining ECG or BP readings

From Gibbons RA, Balady GJ, Beasley JW, et al: *J Am Coll Cardiol* 30:260-315, 1997.
BP, Blood pressure; *ECG,* electrocardiogram.

---

overload in the lungs because of an acute exacerbation of or onset of heart failure. However, crackles are neither sensitive nor specific signs of heart failure.

Measures of aerobic capacity and endurance are used to monitor and document the severity and progression of heart failure, including clinical exercise testing and the 6-minute walk test (6MWT).

Clinical Exercise Testing. The standard clinical method for assessing functional aerobic capacity and endurance is exercise testing. Exercise testing uses a bicycle or treadmill and gradually and progressively increases the workload until a maximum, symptom-limited, or submaximum level is reached. During the test, the patient's heart rhythm and rate, BP, and signs and symptoms are closely monitored. The test is terminated using specific guidelines as outlined in Box 25-2 (see also Chapter 23).[20]

Information obtained from exercise testing can be used to classify patients into functional classes and can be used to guide exercise using the work level the patients attained according to **metabolic equivalents (METs),** maximum heart rate, or maximum oxygen uptake ($\dot{V}_{O_{2max}}$).

One measure of functional capacity obtained by exercise testing is a MET level. One MET is equivalent to 3.5 ml oxygen/kg/min, which is the typical **oxygen consumption rate ($\dot{V}_{O_2}$)** of a healthy adult at rest. MET levels are independent of body weight and can be used for exercise prescription or to estimate energy requirements for specific activities. Energy expenditure in MET levels for various activities are well documented in published tables.[21,22] Sample MET levels for common activities of daily living (ADLs) are included in Table 25-5. Activities that require a greater MET level require more consumption of oxygen and energy. The information from Table 25-5 can be used to educate patients about activities that they can perform safely at home or at work. Patients with a maximum activity tolerance of less than 5 METs, as determined by exercise testing, have a worse prognosis than those who achieve more than a 5 MET level of exercise.[21,22] Most ADLs require a MET level of less than 5.

Ventilatory gas exchange can also be measured during exercise testing to provide additional information about

TABLE 25-5	Metabolic Equivalent Levels for Activities of Daily Living
Activity	**MET Level Range**
Sitting	1-2
Eating	1-2
Dressing	2-3
Toileting	2-3
Bathing/showering	2-4
Walking on level surfaces 2mph	2-3
Walking on level surfaces 3mph	3-4
Walking up a flight of stairs	4-7
Sexual intercourse	3-5
Shoveling snow	6-7
Vacuuming	3-4
Washing dishes	2-3
Gardening	2-4
Washing a car	6-7

Adapted from Ainsworth BE, Haskell WL, Leon AS, et al: *Med Sci Sports Exerc* 25:71-80, 1993.
MET, Metabolic equivalent.

functional capacity. Measures of gas exchange, including peak $\dot{V}_{O_2}$, **anaerobic threshold (AT),** and other ventilatory parameters, can be used to guide exercise prescription, prognosis, and treatment interventions. Oxygen consumption measurements are reliable and reproducible, provide an accurate assessment of functional capacity, and can help distinguish between pulmonary and cardiac causes of a patient's symptoms.[23-25] However, this type of testing may not be available at all facilities because it requires expensive equipment, personnel training, and time.

Six-Minute Walk Test. The 6MWT is a simple clinical tool that can be used by clinicians to assess submaximum exercise capacity. This tool is a useful measure for documenting baseline function and the effectiveness of therapy interventions, including exercise training. The 6MWT can be used more frequently than other types of exercise testing because it is quick and easy, requires minimal equipment, and is well tolerated by patients. For the 6MWT the patient is instructed to walk along a hallway as far as they can in 6 minutes.

Clinical Pearl

The 6MWT is a simple clinical tool to assess submaximum exercise capacity that can be easily performed in hospital corridors or therapy gyms and does not require any special equipment other than a stopwatch.

The 6MWT is easy to administer and well-tolerated and demonstrates good reproducibility in patients with heart failure.[26] However, it does not distinguish patients in NYHA class II and III as well as a graded exercise test, and it is less sensitive to changes than clinical exercise testing.[27]

Medical Tests for Patients with Heart Failure. Several medical tests can provide useful information about cardiac function in patients with heart failure. These tests include echocardiography and **heart catheterization.** Echocardiography uses ultrasound to image the heart in real time. It can provide information about the size of the heart chambers, the thickness of the heart walls, valve form and function, EF, relative pressures within the heart chambers, and wall motion. Catheters can be used to measure pressures at various sites in the heart and blood vessels. Right and left heart catheterization can provide important information about cardiac function and hemodynamics, including pulmonary artery pressure and pulmonary capillary wedge pressure, which have been shown to be predictors of outcome in patients with heart failure.[28]

Function. Quality of life (QOL) measures are often used to determine a patient's sense of the effects of a disease process on his or her life. Two disease-specific measures have been developed to assess QOL in patients with heart failure: the Minnesota Living with Heart Failure Questionnaire (LHFQ) and the Kansas City Cardiomyopathy Questionnaire (KCCQ). The LHFQ was developed to assess patient perceptions of the effects of heart failure and its treatment on daily life.[29] This questionnaire uses a 0- ("no") to 5-point ("very much") Likert scale to assess 21 limitations commonly reported by patients with heart failure. Scores are determined by summing the 21 responses for a maximum total score of 105. However, the LHFQ has been criticized for its poor discriminative ability in patients with moderate to severe heart failure (NYHA class II and III).[30,31]

Because of the limitations of the LHFQ, a second disease-specific QOL measure, the KCCQ, was developed.[32] This tool has 23 items within 8 domains: Physical status, symptoms, symptom stability, social limitations, self-efficacy, QOL, functional status, and clinical summary. This scale is recommended for detection of self-reported changes in QOL after interventions in patients with heart failure. A copy of the KCCQ can be found on the Evolve site that accompanies this book.

EVALUATION, DIAGNOSIS, AND PROGNOSIS

According to the *Guide,* most patients described in this chapter will be classified into the preferred practice pattern 6D: Impaired aerobic capacity/endurance associated with cardiovascular pump dysfunction or failure. It is anticipated that 80% of patients classified into this pattern with cardiovascular pump dysfunction will achieve optimal aerobic capacity and endurance and the highest level of functioning in home, work, community, and leisure environments over the course of 6 to 12 weeks, during a single continuous episode of care.

INTERVENTION

The mainstays of medical interventions for patients with heart failure are medications that optimize fluid balance and cardiac preload, afterload, and contractility. More recently, surgery, including heart transplantation and placement of left ventricular assist devices (VADs), has been successful in some patients with severe heart failure. Rehabilitation interventions for patients with heart failure focus primarily on different types of exercise. Appropriate exercise, in combination with optimal medical care, can

TABLE 25-6	Responses to Exercise in People with and without Heart Failure	
Measure	**Response in People without Heart Failure**	**Response in People with Heart Failure**
Cardiac output	Increased to 4-6 times resting level with maximum exercise.	Less than 50% of the increase seen in people without heart failure.
Heart rate	Linear increase in heart rate with a twofold to fourfold increase with maximum exercise.	The heart rate does not linearly increase to meet the demands of exercise, resulting in a blunted heart rate response.
Stroke volume	Increases by 20%-50%, at least 100 ml in response to maximum exercise.	Decreased stroke volume at rest. Peak stroke volume increase of 50-65 ml with exercise.
Cardiac contractility	Increased force of contraction.	No change in force of contraction.
$\dot{V}O_2$	Peak $\dot{V}O_2$ averages 30-40 ml/kg/min.	Peak $\dot{V}O_2$ averages 10-20 ml/kg/min.
Blood pressure	Systolic BP increases, diastolic BP changes minimally from baseline.	Both systolic and diastolic BP change minimally from baseline.
Peripheral vascular dilation	Vasodilation leads to decreased peripheral resistance.	No vasodilation.

Adapted from Pina IL, Apstein CS, Balady GJ, et al: *Circulation* 107(8):1210-1225, 2003.
$\dot{V}O_2$, Oxygen consumption rate; *BP*, blood pressure.

improve function, symptoms, and QOL in patients with chronic heart failure.[33-35] Exercise training provides benefit primarily by altering the peripheral factors that contribute to exercise intolerance rather than by changing left ventricular function. Functional and symptomatic improvements have been reported when training is performed consistently 3 times per week for 3 or more weeks for 20 to 40 minutes per session at an intensity of 40% to 70% of $\dot{V}O_2$, as determined by a graded exercise test.[13,36]

◎ *Clinical Pearl*

Rehabilitation interventions for patients with heart failure focus primarily on different types of exercise to alter peripheral factors and thereby improve function, symptoms, and QOL in patients with chronic heart failure.

In the past, patients with heart failure were instructed not to exercise for fear that this additional stress on an already failing heart would exacerbate their conditions. In addition, bed rest was recommended because it was theorized that the supine position would promote diuresis.[37] However, the many risks of inactivity, including deep vein thrombosis, pulmonary embolism, skin breakdown, muscle atrophy, and deconditioning, as well as advancements in drug therapy, prompted reconsideration of these restrictions. Furthermore, recent research has demonstrated that exercise can provide many benefits to this population.

During exercise, the heart maintains cardiac output by increasing heart rate and stroke volume. In people with good cardiac function, during the early phase of exercise, cardiac output is increased by rapidly increasing stroke volume and gradually increasing heart rate.[38] With continued exercise, stroke volume plateaus and any further need for a rise in cardiac output is met by increasing heart rate. In patients with heart failure, exercise is limited by an inadequate cardiac output response because of a reduction in both stroke volume and heart rate. These patients have a reduced stroke volume at rest as a result of a decreased EF and have a blunted stroke volume response to exercise. Patients with heart failure also often have a

high resting heart rate to compensate for their reduced stroke volume but are not able to further increase this rate in response to maximum workloads. The higher resting heart rate and lower peak exercise heart rate limit the heart rate reserve (HRR) substantially. The combination of limited responses in stroke volume and heart rate contribute to a decreased peak exercise response to exercise in patients with heart failure.[39] Table 25-6 summarizes the differences in exercise responses between people with and without heart failure.

Alterations in gas exchange also limit exercise tolerance in this patient population. Fluid accumulation in the lungs results in abnormal gas exchange and can cause shortness of breath. Patients with heart failure also have more vasoconstriction at rest because of elevated sympathetic tone, which further limits the delivery of oxygenated blood to the muscles. Reduced oxygen extraction combined with reduced cardiac output limits the delivery of oxygen to the working skeletal muscles. In addition, skeletal muscle changes in patients with heart failure, including reduction in the size of muscle fibers and change of muscle fiber types, can further contribute to early fatigue during exercise.[40]

Various pharmacological interventions are used to improve exercise tolerance in patients with heart failure, but these have met with limited success.[41-44] Therefore investigators have sought out alternative means, such as exercise therapy, to improve exercise and activity tolerance in the population with heart failure. Much of the research in this area focuses on trying to identify the optimal exercise regimen for patients with heart failure.

AEROBIC EXERCISE

Aerobic exercise is any continuous activity that involves rhythmic contraction of large muscle groups and increases the rate of aerobic metabolism. Since aerobic exercise was the primary type of exercise used in cardiac rehabilitation for patients after myocardial infarction, aerobic exercise was the first to undergo investigation for optimizing function in patients with heart failure. Potential benefits of aerobic exercise include improvements in central hemodynamics, such as increases in cardiac output, heart rate, and stroke volume during exercise, and decreases in cardiac demand at rest. Potential peripheral improvements include improved delivery of oxygen to the working muscles, improved oxygen extraction by the muscles, and improved skeletal muscle fiber function.[45]

Exercise prescription in heart failure can be challenging because many factors can limit exercise tolerance. Initially, exercise studies focused on patients with heart failure who were less debilitated (NYHA class I and II) because of concerns that exercise could have adverse effects in patients with more advanced disease.[36] More recently, studies have also demonstrated that exercise benefits patients with severely reduced left ventricular function (NYHA class III and IV).[13] These studies suggest that short bouts of moderate intensity exercise (a home walking program) are safe and effective for improving QOL, depression, and response to exercise.

Clinical Pearl

Appropriately selected aerobic exercise can be helpful for patients with all classes of heart failure if their heart failure is not decompensated.

Although the mechanisms for the benefits of exercise in patients with heart failure need further elucidation, the present evidence does support the use of aerobic exercise in patients with stable heart failure to improve exercise and activity tolerance, as well as QOL.

RESISTIVE TRAINING

Isometric resistance exercise should be avoided in patients with heart failure because it increases afterload on the heart. However, mild-to-moderate resistive training may be used in patients with heart failure with close monitoring for signs or symptoms of worsening heart failure, such as increased fatigue and dyspnea.[46]

Clinical Pearl

Isometric resistance exercise should be avoided in patients with heart failure.

Although studies suggest that moderate resistive training in combination with aerobic exercise may be safe in this population, firm recommendations on the use of resistive training in heart failure cannot be made until further studies assess the long-term effects of this type of intervention on cardiac function.

INTERVAL TRAINING

Interval training consists of short bouts of exercise followed by periods of rest applied in a repeated sequence. Interval training allows the muscles to work harder than they could with steady-state exercise without excessively stressing the cardiovascular system. Interval training with 30 seconds of exercise followed by 60 seconds of rest at an intensity of 75% of peak $\dot{V}o_2$ produced a lower **rate-pressure product,** lower **rate of perceived exertion (RPE),** and lower increases in plasma catecholamine levels than steady-state exercise at the same intensity.[47] The safety of this type of exercise makes it appealing for patients with heart failure.

Interval training may be performed using a stationary bicycle or a treadmill, and a variety of exercise-to-rest ratios may be used, including 15 seconds/60 seconds, 10 seconds/60 seconds, or 30 seconds/60 seconds for a total of 15 to 30 minutes.[48,49] Interval training may be gradually progressed in intensity by lengthening the exercise period or shortening the rest periods.

EXERCISE SAFETY IN HEART FAILURE

Despite the fact that evidence indicates that exercise can help patients with heart failure, there are still concerns about the safety of exercise training in this population. In standard outpatient cardiac rehabilitation programs, observational studies estimate the incidence of cardiovascular complications from exercise in patients with heart failure to be 1 for every 60,000 participant-hours.[50] In a review of the literature on exercise training in patients with heart failure, which included 20 studies with a combined sample of 467 patients, the AHA found only 19 reported adverse cardiac events, which included heart failure exacerbations, ventricular tachycardia, atrial fibrillation, hypotension, and exhaustion but no reported deaths.[51] They found that the three most important factors affecting the risk of exercise in patients with heart failure were the patient's age, the intensity of the exercise, and the presence of ischemic heart disease.

Based on this review, the AHA developed standards for exercise testing and training in patients with heart failure.[51] In their most recent recommendations, they encourage aerobic activity to improve activity and exercise tolerance, except during periods of decompensation, but advise patients with heart failure to avoid heavy labor or exhaustive sports.[52] However, neither the AHA nor any other group provides specific recommendations for exercise in this population, although the AHA's risk stratification system does provide some helpful guidelines for adjusting exercise intensity in patients with NYHA class I to III heart failure.[51-53]

Clinical Pearl

Exercise should be avoided during periods of heart failure decompensation.

Patients with decompensated heart failure should not exercise. Signs of decompensated heart failure that should exclude patients from participating in exercise include the acute onset of crackles, signs of worsening pulmonary edema, ventricular arrhythmias, uncontrolled atrial fibrillation, bradycardia, symptomatic hypotension, and dyspnea and fatigue at rest. Further contraindications and relative contraindications to exercise in the heart failure population are listed in Box 25-3.

EXERCISE PROGRAM FOR PATIENTS WITH HEART FAILURE

The AHA guidelines recommend clinicians individualize exercise prescription in patients with heart failure specifying the exercise mode, intensity, duration, and frequency.

Exercise Mode. The mode of exercise refers to the type of activity performed. At a minimum, the exercise prescription will include some form of aerobic exercise.

BOX 25-3 | Relative and Absolute Contraindications for Exercise for a Patient with Heart Failure

- Systolic BP >240 mm Hg or diastolic BP >110 mm Hg
- Decrease in systolic BP by more than 10 mm Hg from baseline
- Angina > level 2 on the Angina Scale
- Dyspnea ≥level 2 on the Dyspnea Index
- Symptoms of worsening failure such as pallor, excessive fatigue, or mental confusion
- ECG abnormalities such as second or third degree heart block, ventricular arrhythmias, acute ST changes, onset of left or right bundle-branch block, uncontrolled atrial fibrillation
- Resting systolic BP <80 mm Hg
- Decreased HR response to exercise
- HR elevation close to ICD firing threshold
- New onset of pulmonary rales
- New onset of S3 heart sound
- Borg RPE Scale rating of >13 on the 6-20 scale

Adapted from American College of Sports Medicine: *ACSM's guidelines for exercise testing and prescription*, Baltimore, 2000, Williams & Wilkins.
BP, Blood pressure; *ECG*, electrocardiogram; *HR*, heart rate; *ICD*, implanted cardiac defibrillator; *RPE*, rate of perceived exertion.

The exercise should include activities that are predominately aerobic in nature such as walking and/or stationary cycling. Cycle ergometry has the advantages of easy reproducibility, allowing exercise at a very low workload, and being safe for patients with deficits in dynamic balance. Because of fluctuations in the environment, outdoor cycling is recommended only for clinically stable NYHA class I and II patients and not for patients in class III or IV.[36] Cycling in a recumbent or semirecumbent position is generally discouraged, since it may limit exercise tolerance by increasing venous return and thereby pulmonary edema and by decreasing diaphragmatic excursion.[54]

Walking can be performed by a wide range of patients with heart failure because its speed can easily be varied. Patients with a documented peak $\dot{V}O_2$ of at least 13 ml/kg/min can generally tolerate treadmill speeds as high as 3.7 mph, with less fit patients (peak $\dot{V}O_2$ of 8 ml/kg/min) generally tolerating speeds of 1.9 mph or less.[55] Jogging is generally not advised because even a slow jogging speed of 3 mph is only tolerated in patients with a $\dot{V}O_2$ of 20 ml/kg/min or greater.[36]

Clinical Pearl

Brisk walking can elicit an adequate training effect in many patients with heart failure.

Exercise Frequency and Duration. In all patients with heart failure the clinician must monitor patients closely for any signs or symptoms of intolerance during or after exercise and should adjust exercise frequency and duration accordingly. Severely compromised patients may require a longer rest interval between exercise sessions, with a gradual progression to a frequency of 3 to 5 times per week, and/or shorter sessions initially with a gradual progression of duration over time.

The American College of Sports Medicine (ACSM) recommends that patients with a functional capacity of less than 3 METs (see Chapter 23) will generally tolerate multiple daily bouts of exercise lasting 5 to 10 minutes. Patients functioning at a 3 to 5 MET level will tolerate and benefit from 1 to 2 daily sessions of 15 minutes each and those with a functional capacity of greater than 5 METs are recommended to exercise 3 to 5 times per week for 20 to 30 minutes each session, with close monitoring for any signs or symptoms of intolerance.[20] Interval training may also be used in patients who do not tolerate sustained exercise throughout the exercise period.

Exercise prescription in all patients, particularly those with cardiac conditions, always includes adequate warm-up and cool-down periods. The warm-up period should include 5 to 10 minutes of intermittent or continuous low-intensity aerobic activity at approximately 25% to 50% of the patient's functional capacity. This phase can also include gentle stretching to reduce the risk of musculoskeletal injuries, especially in a deconditioned population.[56,57] In patients with heart disease, adequate warm-up is thought to reduce the risk of myocardial ischemia by promoting the opening of collateral vessels and preventing vascular spasm and redistribution of blood from areas at risk. After the warm-up, exercise can be progressed to the goal intensity level. The cool-down period should be similar to the warm-up period. This will allow the heart rate and BP to gradually return to preexercise levels. This will enhance venous return and decrease the risk of postexercise hypotension.[58] Patients with heart failure who do not adequately cool down are also thought to be at increased risk of arrhythmias because of myocardial irritability from the large volume of blood returned to the heart when exercise stops suddenly.

Clinical Pearl

A cool-down period after exercise is particularly important in patients with heart failure to control the risk of postexercise arrhythmias.

Exercise Intensity. As with other populations, the intensity of aerobic exercise in a patient with heart failure can be prescribed as a percentage of peak $\dot{V}O_2$, a percentage of peak heart rate, or according to the Borg RPE Scale (see Box 23-1). Generally, patients with heart failure can tolerate an initial intensity ranging from 40% to 70% of peak $\dot{V}O_2$, or an intensity corresponding to 10 beats per minute below the level where symptoms, such as shortness of breath or angina, occur. Because of the abnormal heart rate response to exercise and the frequent use of beta-blocker therapy in patients with heart failure, determining exercise intensity using heart rate can be difficult. Therefore the Borg RPE Scale is often recommended for setting exercise intensity in patients with heart failure. The Borg RPE Scale ranges from 6 to 20 and has a linear relationship to the heart rate response with increasing

TABLE 25-7	Exercise Progression for the Patient with Heart Failure*		
Stage	**Intensity**		**Duration†**
Initial	Low level 40%-50% of peak $\dot{V}O_2$		10-15 minutes
Improvement	Primary goal to increase intensity 50%-70% of peak $\dot{V}O_2$		15-30 minutes
Maintenance	Primary goal to maintain intensity 70% of peak $\dot{V}O_2$		30-35 minutes

Data from American College of Sports Medicine: *ACSM's guidelines for exercise testing and prescription*, Baltimore, 2000, Williams & Wilkins.
*First progress exercise duration, then frequency, then intensity.
†Not including warm-up and cool-down.
$\dot{V}O_2$, Oxygen consumption rate.

BOX 25-4	Sternal Precautions*

- No lifting >10 lb.
- No lifting of both hands above the head at the same time.
- No placing of both hands behind the back at the same time.
- No driving for 6-8 weeks or until surgeon provides clearance.
- No pushing or pulling anything >5-10 lb.
- Encourage splinted coughing techniques.

*Sternal precautions are facility dependent, and the reader is referred to the policies of the specific institution for further details.

---

intensity of exercise.[59] Exercising at a Borg RPE rating of 11 to 14 ("light" to "somewhat hard") on this scale corresponds to a heart rate response between 40% to 70% of peak $\dot{V}O_2$ and is generally appropriate for patients with heart failure.[59]

Exercise Progression. Progression of exercise depends on the patient's baseline functional status, activity tolerance, vital sign response, and subjective complaints. Patients with a low initial exercise capacity will generally make faster initial progress than those who start at a high functional capacity. Training can be considered as occurring in three stages: Initial stage, improvement stage, and maintenance stage.[20] Progression from one stage to another is based on the patient attaining specific intensity and duration goals. These three stages are outlined further in Table 25-7. Exercise should be progressed sequentially with adjustments first made to duration, then frequency, and finally intensity of the program.

HEART TRANSPLANTATION

Heart transplantation may be indicated in patients with end-stage heart failure that is refractory to optimal pharmacological support. Indications for transplant include NYHA class III or IV heart failure, cardiac index of less than 2.0 L/min/m², exercise capacity less than 14 ml/min/kg, age less than 70 years, and adequate psychosocial support. Contraindications include active sepsis, renal insufficiency, ongoing substance abuse, severe pulmonary disease, severe peripheral vascular disease or cerebrovascular disease, malignancy, human immunodeficiency virus (HIV) infection, morbid obesity, fixed **pulmonary hypertension,** and uncontrolled diabetes.[60]

Heart transplantation is the last resort for patients with heart failure because although it can produce good outcomes, it is fraught with complications, and the availability of hearts for transplantation is far less than the demand. According to the Organ Procurement and Transplantation Network (OPTN), in 2003 there were 4,200 patients waiting for a heart transplant, with 2,500 transplants performed each year. It is estimated that 30% of patients waiting for a heart transplant will die before receiving a heart because of the shortage of organs. One-year survival after heart failure is now 86%, with 75% of patients surviving for 5 years or more. Patients are listed and receive an organ for transplantation using a system established by the United Network for Organ Sharing (UNOS) that prioritizes patients according to disease severity and listing time. Once a patient reaches the top of the list, potential organs must be matched to the recipient's body size and blood type.

The transplant procedure is performed using a **median sternotomy** approach with anastomosis at the vena cava, aorta, and pulmonary arteries. The immediate postoperative care is similar to that provided after other open-heart procedures and generally includes observation of sternal precautions for 6 to 8 weeks after the procedure (Box 25-4). However, cardiac vagal denervation and side effects of antirejection medications can limit function and exercise tolerance. Cardiac output after heart transplant is approximately 25% to 30% lower than in the normal population. BP is typically elevated at rest, with a greater systolic BP response to exercise. Peak $\dot{V}O_2$ is also lower than in age-matched controls (usually 70% to 80% of age-matched controls).[61]

Exercise training is recommended as part of a comprehensive posttransplant management plan that includes proper nutrition, drug therapy, and frequent medical and surgical follow-up. The clinician must keep in mind that patients with heart transplants will respond differently because their heart is denervated. The loss of vagal input makes heart transplant recipients have an elevated heart rate at rest. Their heart rate will rise little if at all when exercise is started. With continued exertion, their heart rate will rise gradually and slightly to a lower peak during maximum exercise than in age-matched healthy people without heart transplants (Fig. 25-2). Because of this abnormal heart rate response, heart rate should not be used as a target for exercise prescription in patients with heart transplants. In this population, a target Borg RPE Scale rating of 12 to 14 can serve as a guide for exercise intensity.

Since some of the immunosuppressive agents used after organ transplantation increase the risk for bone density loss and osteoporosis, weight-bearing exercise, as well as resistive training, is recommended in this population (see Chapter 3). Outpatient cardiac rehabilitation, which is generally initiated 6 to 8 weeks after surgery once the sternum has healed, has been shown to improve exercise tolerance and QOL in patients after heart transplant.[45,62]

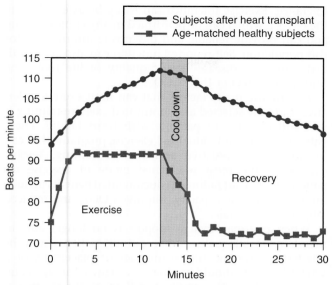

FIG. 25-2 Heart rate response to exercise in subjects after heart transplant and age-matched healthy subjects.

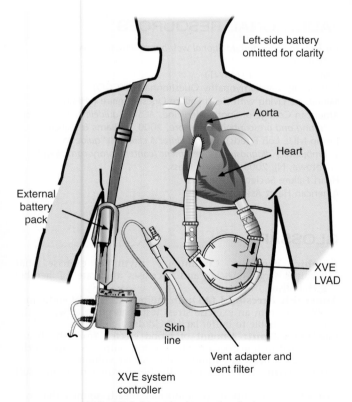

FIG. 25-3 Ventricular assist device.

MECHANICAL ASSIST DEVICES

Mechanical assist devices are devices that can be used to provide either temporary or permanent support for a failing heart. These devices include intraaortic balloon pumps (IABPs), VADs, and cardiopulmonary bypass machines (CPBs). VADs can provide support to either the right or the left ventricle or both (Fig. 25-3). Indications for mechanical assist devices include recovery after cardiac surgery or acute myocardial infarction, as a bridge to heart transplantation, or as destination therapy. Mechanical assist devices are implanted when cardiac output is insufficient to perfuse the vital organs despite maximum pharmacological support. The Food and Drug Administration (FDA) recently approved the HeartMate VAD for use as destination therapy, so that patients can have the device implanted permanently. Previously, VADs were only approved as a "bridge" for patients until a heart was available for transplant. Therapists may see patients with these devices in a variety of settings beyond the acute care hospital.

VADs are implanted using a median sternotomy, as with other types of cardiac surgery. Although many facilities follow sternal precautions for 6 to 8 weeks after median sternotomy (see Box 25-4), early progressive mobilization has been shown to improve outcomes in patients with left VADs (LVADs).[63] LVADs have also been shown to improve functional exercise tolerance in patients with heart failure.

NYHA CLASS III HEART FAILURE

Patient History

AT, a 58-year-old man, presents to the hospital with complaints of dyspnea and weight gain of 6 lb over the past 2 days. His history is significant for idiopathic dilated cardiomyopathy with NYHA class III heart failure. He had an ICD placed 2 years ago. He also has diabetes, hypertension, and hypercholesterolemia and was admitted from the emergency room to the coronary intensive care unit for diuresis, right heart catheterization, and possible initiation of new medications. AT is on disability because of his cardiac condition but was independent in all ADLs before this hospital admission. He reports frequent shortness of breath. His ICD threshold is set at 185 bpm, and the ICD has fired one time; he had blurred vision before the firing. A physical therapy consultation was requested.

Tests and Measures—Significant Findings
Musculoskeletal
- Upper and lower extremity strength and ROM grossly within functional limits. BMI was 28.

Cardiovascular/Pulmonary
- Heart rate 100 bpm, rhythm irregularly irregular (atrial fibrillation). BP 90/50 mm Hg. 2+ pitting edema in both ankles.
- Respiratory rate was 28 breaths/min, lungs were clear to auscultation. Dyspnea at rest 1/3 on the Dyspnea Index.
- 6MWT: Distance walked 850 feet, with 1 minute rest during the 6-minute time frame, heart rate ranged from 100 to 130 bpm, BP ranged from 92/50 mm Hg to 110/55 mm Hg during the test.
- Borg RPE Scale: Score ranged from 8 at rest to 13/20 with activity.
- Minnesota LHFQ: QOL score was 20/105.

Diagnosis

Preferred practice pattern 6D: Impaired aerobic capacity associated with cardiopulmonary pump dysfunction.

Interventions

Session 1 (Day 3 of Hospital Stay)
- Ambulation with close monitoring of vital signs, RPE, and Dyspnea Index.

Session 2 (Day 4 of Hospital Stay)
- Ambulation with close monitoring of vital signs, RPE, and Dyspnea Index.
- If patient reacts well to ambulation, light warm-up exercises to be added.
- If patient reacts well to above, light ambulation on a treadmill.

Session 3 to Discharge from Hospital
- Patient should progress using treadmill exercise. Begin progression with an increase in time, then an increase in speed. RPE rating should be less than 13.
- A home exercise program will be created for this patient, and he will be instructed on the proper way to use the Borg RPE Scale and the Dyspnea Index.

Role of the Physical Therapist Assistant
- Select and describe 3 lower extremity and 3 upper extremity light warm-up exercises that could be appropriate for session 2.
- Describe an appropriate ambulation program for session 2. How would you monitor the patient during this activity?
- Produce a written home exercise program for this patient.
- What warning signs should the patient watch for to indicate he should stop or modify his home exercise program?

Additional Information

For the full version of this case study, including detailed examination results, interventions, and outcomes, see the Evolve site that accompanies this book. A full case study for a patient after heart transplantation also appears on the Evolve site.

CHAPTER SUMMARY

Heart failure is a progressive disease that results from the heart's inability to pump blood to meet the demands of the body. Patients with heart failure commonly present with intolerance of ADLs and exercise. Heart failure is globally classified as either systolic or diastolic dysfunction, with both types presenting with similar symptoms of fatigue, dyspnea, and decreased exercise tolerance. The NYHA Classification system can be used to classify the severity of heart failure and its resultant functional limitations. Rehabilitation clinicians' comprehensive examination of patients with heart failure includes measurement of peripheral edema and JVP; auscultation of the heart and lungs; measurement of vital signs at baseline, during activity, and after all interventions; and assessment of exercise tolerance. Exercise tolerance can easily be assessed using the 6MWT, which can be performed in any clinical setting and can provide reliable and prognostic information for this population. Self-reported function can also be quantified using two disease-specific quality of life tools, the Minnesota LHFQ or the KCCQ.

Despite the many factors that can limit exercise tolerance, carefully selected and monitored exercise training is safe and effective in patients with heart failure. These patients require individualized exercise programs that can include aerobic, resistive, and interval training. Aerobic exercise is the most researched mode of exercise for patients with heart failure. Its documented benefits include improved exercise capacity, improved QOL, and reduced fatigue and dyspnea.

When pharmacological support is no longer able to maintain an adequate cardiac output, patients may be referred for cardiac transplantation or placement of a VAD. Clinicians should be able to recognize the signs and symptoms of rejection and be familiar with the mechanics of the assist devices when treating patients who have undergone these procedures.

ADDITIONAL RESOURCES

For links to these and additional web-based resources, see the Evolve site.

6-Minute Walk Test (6MWT)
Kansas City Cardiomyopathy Questionnaire (KCCQ)
Minnesota Living with Heart Failure Questionnaire (LHFQ)
American College of Sports Medicine: *ACSM's guidelines for exercise testing and prescription,* Baltimore, 2000, Williams & Wilkins.
Jessup MLL, Loh E (eds): *Heart failure: A clinicians' guide to ambulatory diagnosis and treatment (contemporary cardiology),* Totowa, NJ, 2003, Humana Press.
Heart Failure Society of America
American Heart Association

GLOSSARY

Aerobic exercise: Continuous, rhythmic exercise that involves large muscles and increases the rate of aerobic metabolism.

Anaerobic threshold (AT): An indirect measure of endurance obtained from an exercise stress test. The point at which the blood is unable to buffer lactic acid during exercise.

Cardiac output: Amount of blood ejected from the heart, expressed in liters per minute. Cardiac output is equal to the product of heart rate multiplied by stroke volume.

Cardiomyopathy: A disease of the heart muscle that can result in heart failure.

Crackles: Adventitious or abnormal breath sounds that can reflect acute fluid accumulation in the distal airways of the lungs.

Diastole: Period of the heart's pumping cycle in which the heart muscle relaxes to allow the heart to fill with blood.

Diastolic dysfunction: Decreased ability of the heart to accept blood.

Dilated cardiomyopathy: Disease of the cardiac muscle with dilation of the ventricles.

Dyspnea: Shortness of breath.

Echocardiography: Diagnostic test that uses ultrasound to assess structures and function of the heart.

Ejection fraction (EF): The percentage of end-diastolic volume ejected from the left ventricle with each heartbeat.

End-diastolic volume: The volume of blood in the left ventricle at the end of diastole.

Heart catheterization: Procedure performed under fluoroscopy in which a catheter is inserted into the left side or right side of the heart to measure pressures and/or assess the coronary arteries and heart valves.

Heart failure: Previously called *congestive heart failure*. Inability of the heart to pump enough blood to meet the demands of the organs.

Hypertrophic cardiomyopathy: Disease of the heart muscle that results in excessive thickening of the left ventricle.

Ischemic heart failure: Heart failure caused by an inadequate supply of blood to the heart muscle.

Jugular venous distention (JVD): Distention or stretching of the jugular veins because of fluid overload.

Median sternotomy: Surgical incision using a midline cut through the sternum.

Metabolic equivalent (MET): Energy requirement while resting, which is the energy used to burn 3.5 ml of oxygen per kilogram of body weight per minute.

Myocardium: Heart muscle.

New York Heart Association (NYHA) Classification system: System used to classify patients with heart failure according to subjective limitations in functional activities.

Orthopnea: Shortness of breath with lying supine.

Oxygen consumption rate ($\dot{V}o_2$): Amount of oxygen consumed while performing an activity, measured by exercise testing.

Pulmonary edema: Excessive fluid accumulation in the lungs.

Pulmonary hypertension: Abnormal elevation of the pulmonary artery pressure.

Rate of perceived exertion (RPE): Subjective rating of exercise intensity.

Rate-pressure product: Heart rate multiplied by systolic blood pressure. An index of myocardial oxygen requirement.

Restrictive cardiomyopathy: Disease of the heart muscle that is characterized by fibrosis of the ventricles and leads to diastolic dysfunction.

Right atrial pressure: Pressure of the blood in the right atrium.

Stroke volume: The volume of blood ejected from the left ventricle with each heart beat.

Systolic dysfunction: Inability of the heart to eject blood.

Chapter 26

Respiratory Failure

Robert L. Dekerlegand, Lawrence P. Cahalin, Christiane Perme

OBJECTIVES

After reading this chapter, the reader will be able to:
1. Describe the prevalence and incidence of respiratory failure and its economic impact on society.
2. Describe normal physiological processes associated with ventilation and respiration.
3. Describe pathophysiological processes leading to respiratory insufficiency and failure.
4. Classify types of respiratory failure.
5. Identify common diseases and diagnoses associated with respiratory failure.
6. Identify potential complications of respiratory failure and discuss their impact on rehabilitation and functional capacity.
7. Be familiar with commonly used rehabilitation tests and measures for individuals with respiratory failure.
8. Describe and apply rehabilitation interventions for individuals with respiratory failure and demonstrate understanding of their proposed mechanisms of action.

$\mathcal{R}$espiratory failure is caused by impairment of gas exchange between ambient air and circulating blood because of reduced intrapulmonary gas exchange or reduced movement of gases in and out of the lungs.[1] Breathing is a multistep physiological process with the vital purposes of delivering oxygen to and removing carbon dioxide from the human body. Efficient maintenance of appropriate blood gases is vital to survival and provides the energy needed for daily activities. By breathing, the lungs allow gases to be exchanged between the environment and the blood through the terminal airways known as the **alveoli.** Breathing involves two linked processes, **respiration** and **ventilation.** Respiration is the process of gas exchange between the alveolar air spaces and the blood, and ventilation is the movement of air in and out of the lungs. These processes interact and both need to function efficiently to balance oxygen (O_2) supply and demand and to eliminate metabolic waste products such as carbon dioxide (CO_2). The body relies on the cardiovascular system's ability to transport O_2 and CO_2 and on the tissue's ability to extract and utilize O_2 while producing and eliminating CO_2. Together, the respiratory and cardiovascular systems and the tissues' ability to extract and utilize O_2 make up the O_2 transport system (Fig. 26-1). Respiratory insufficiency and subsequent failure occur when the pulmonary system cannot maintain a steady state of gas exchange in response to the metabolic demands of the body, resulting in inadequate delivery of O_2 and/or inadequate elimination of CO_2.

Respiratory failure is a common and severe health problem. Acute respiratory failure has been shown to be associated with a 58% overall mortality in children.[2] In adults, respiratory failure is generally due to either acute respiratory distress syndrome (ARDS) or chronic obstructive pulmonary disease (COPD). The incidence of ARDS is 1.5 to 17.9 cases per 100,000, and approximately 24 million adults in the United States have evidence of COPD, as demonstrated by impaired lung function.[3] COPD is currently the fourth leading cause of death in the United States and predicted to be the third leading cause of death by the year 2020. COPD is also anticipated to be the fifth leading cause of disability in the world by 2020.[4] As respiratory failure becomes more common, rehabilitation professionals will play a growing role in providing preventive education and procedural interventions that help restore lost functional capacity and improve quality of life while containing costs associated with complications of respiratory failure.

Respiratory failure is a state or condition that may result from a disease, condition, or process. In general, respiratory failure can be caused by disorders of the airways, the lung tissue, or the skeletal, muscular, and neural components of the respiratory system. Regardless of the underlying pathology, the degree of resulting

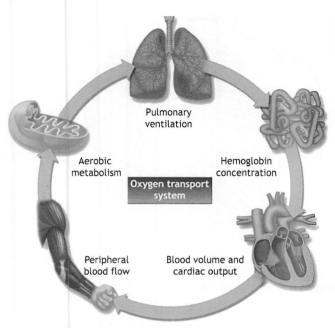

FIG. 26-1 The oxygen transport system mobilizes oxygen into the body and eliminates carbon dioxide. *From McArdle WD, Katch Fl, Katch VL: Exercise physiology: Energy, nutrition, and human performance, ed 5, Philadelphia, 2001, Lippincott Williams & Wilkins.*

BOX 26-1	Diagnoses Associated with Respiratory Failure (ICD-9 Codes)

- Poliomyelitis (045)
- Cystic fibrosis (277.0)
- Parkinson's disease (332)
- Huntington's chorea (333.4)
- Spinocerebellar disease (334)
- Amyotrophic lateral sclerosis (335.20)
- Multiple sclerosis (340)
- Quadriplegia (344.00)
- Guillain-Barré syndrome (357.00)
- Muscular dystrophy (359.1)
- Viral pneumonia (480)
- Bacterial pneumonia (482)
- Chronic bronchitis (491)
- Emphysema (492)
- Asthma (493)
- Bronchiectasis (494)
- Pneumothorax (512)
- Pulmonary edema (514)
- Lung involvement in conditions classified elsewhere (517)
- Inflammatory pulmonary fibrosis (515)
- Other disorder of the lung (518)
- Acute respiratory failure (518.81)
- Disorders of the diaphragm (519.4)
- Curvature of the spine (737)
- Burns (941-949)

ICD-9, International Classification of Diseases, ninth revision.

functional limitation will be assessed by the physical therapist to select the most appropriate interventions to progress the patient toward realistic goals. Box 26-1 lists diagnoses commonly associated with respiratory failure.[5]

◎ *Clinical Pearl*

Respiratory failure can be caused by disorders of the airways, lungs, or the skeletal, muscular, and neural components of the respiratory system.

The preferred practice patterns addressed in this chapter are 6E: Impaired ventilation and respiration/gas exchange associated with ventilatory pump dysfunction or failure and 6F: Impaired ventilation and respiration/gas exchange associated with respiratory failure.

PATHOLOGY

For the O_2 transport system to function effectively and efficiently, each component, as shown in Fig. 26-1, must work optimally. Although small deficiencies in one component may be compensated for by other systems, when deficiencies increase or are prolonged or demands increase, compensation generally fails and respiratory failure ensues. Since activity increases demands on the O_2 transport system, the rehabilitation professional may be able to compensate for reduced O_2 transport by curtailing the patient's activity level or intensity.

RESPIRATORY ANATOMY

The respiratory system can be divided into four components: The skeletal components, the muscular components, the lungs and airways, and the neural control centers.

Skeletal Components of the Respiratory System. The skeletal components of the respiratory system are the thoracic vertebrae, the sternum, and the ribs, which together make up the thorax (Fig. 26-2). The thorax contains and protects the heart, lungs, and major vessels. It provides a stable base for attachment of the muscles of respiration and allows for lung expansion. The upper portion of the rib cage is much less mobile than the lower portion. For optimal ventilation, the lungs and thus the thorax must be able to expand in all dimensions: Anterior-posterior, superior-inferior, and medial-lateral. This requires appropriate rib mobility. Limitations or restrictions in the ability of either the lungs or ribs to expand will increase the workload (O_2 demand) of the respiratory system, limit how much air can move into the airways, and may indirectly contribute to respiratory muscle fatigue and failure.

Muscular Components of the Respiratory System. The muscular components of the respiratory system consist of the primary breathing muscle, the diaphragm, and the accessory muscles of ventilation (Fig. 26-3). These muscles together affect the volume of air in the lungs and the flow of air through the airways.

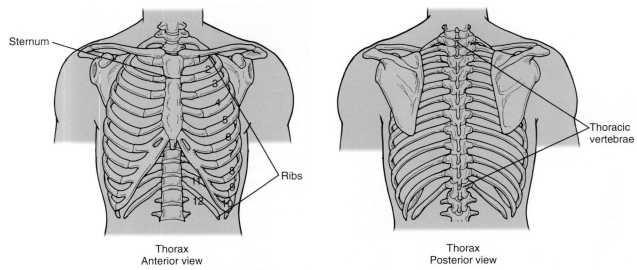

Thorax
Anterior view

Thorax
Posterior view

FIG. 26-2 The skeletal components of the respiratory system.

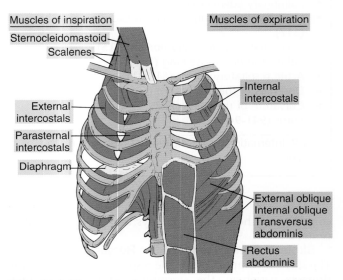

FIG. 26-3 The muscular components of the respiratory system.

Contraction of the respiratory muscles creates negative pressure to "pull" air into the airways. If at any time the diaphragm cannot sustain ventilation, the accessory muscles will assist. Any muscle that attaches directly to the thorax can act as an accessory muscle of ventilation. The accessory muscles are best understood by dividing them into muscles of inspiration and muscles of expiration as shown in Fig. 26-3.

The diaphragm is innervated by the phrenic nerve, which is composed of nerve roots from C3, C4, and C5. (Remember: "C3, 4, 5 keeps the phrenic nerve alive!") The diaphragm originates from the upper three lumbar vertebrae, the lower border of the rib cage, and the xiphoid process of the sternum. The fibers converge to form and insert on the common central tendon. The diaphragm is the only muscle that works in three dimensions and that

has a bony origin but does not have a bony insertion. At rest the diaphragm is elevated in a domed-shaped position that optimizes the length-tension relationship of the fibers and thus the efficiency of its contraction. In some disease processes, such as emphysema, the resting position of the diaphragm may change, creating a mechanical disadvantage that impairs muscle contraction force generation.[6] The position of the diaphragm also varies among normal individuals and is affected by age, weight, and thoracic dimensions.[7] As the diaphragm contracts, it flattens and lowers (Fig. 26-4), increasing thoracic volume and producing most (if not all) of the negative inspiratory pressure required to inhale air at rest. The diaphragm is primarily composed of slow-twitch oxidative muscle fibers (type I fibers) that are resistant to fatigue, but it also contains fast-twitch glycolytic muscle fibers (type II fibers) that are designed for strength.[8] This combination of fibers not only enables the diaphragm to sustain breathing day in and day out but also allows it to generate increased force when needed.

When the diaphragm initially contracts, it begins to flatten and descend, drawing air into the lungs and producing an observable rise of the abdomen.[9] As contraction progresses, the diaphragm continues to descend until it touches the abdominal contents. At this point, the central tendon becomes "fixed" or stationary. When the diaphragm contracts further, it pulls up on the ribs causing an observable expansion of the lower border of the rib cage. To achieve maximum lung expansion the accessory muscles of ventilation must expand the upper chest. The sequential abdominal rise, lateral costal expansion, and upper chest rise overlap to some degree, but all contribute to achieving optimal lung capacity during inhalation.[9] The rate of inhalation and control of breathing can also affect the penetration of air into the lungs. Controlled slow breathing may allow inhaled air to reach deeper within the airways.[10,11]

Lungs and Airways. The organs of respiration, the lungs, are located within the thorax. The two lungs, the

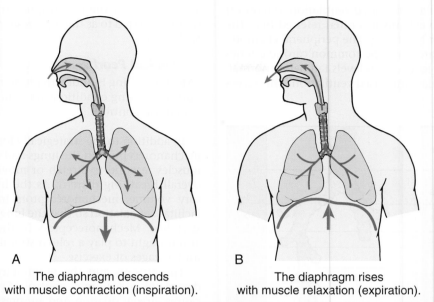

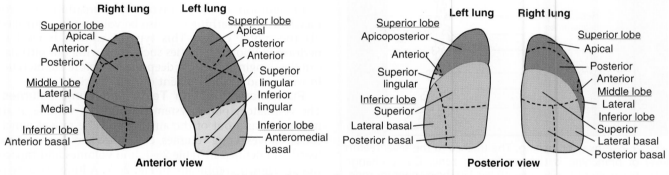

A The diaphragm descends with muscle contraction (inspiration).

B The diaphragm rises with muscle relaxation (expiration).

FIG. 26-4 The diaphragm is the primary muscle of respiration. **A,** The diaphragm descends with muscle contraction (inspiration). **B,** The diaphragm rises with muscle relaxation (expiration).

FIG. 26-5 The lobes and segments of the lungs.

left and the right, are each subdivided into lobes and segments (Fig. 26-5). Air enters the lungs via the trachea that branches into the left and right mainstem bronchi at the level of the sternal angle anteriorly and the spinous process of T3 posteriorly. The airways then continue to branch into the smaller lobar bronchi, followed by the segmental bronchi, and then into the bronchioles to finally reach the alveoli where gas exchange takes place (Fig. 26-6). There may be 23 to 25 levels of airway branching. The airways from the trachea down to approximately the seventeenth level of branching only conduct air to the **respiratory airways.** No gas exchange occurs in these **conducting airways.** The respiratory airways, or respiratory zones, in which gas exchange takes place, begin after approximately the seventeenth branching. These airways are characterized by the appearance of alveoli, with the number of alveoli increasing with further branching of the airways. The airways are protected primarily by the epiglottis and a functional cough that works to keep the airways clear of mucus and foreign material.

RESPIRATORY PHYSIOLOGY

Neural Control of Breathing. Breathing is designed to facilitate **alveolar ventilation** and is under both voluntary and involuntary control. The neural respiratory control center is located within the pons and medulla of the brainstem. It is here that information from the motor cortex, chemoreceptors in the periphery, and mechanoreceptors in the skeletal muscle and the lung tissues is integrated to produce efferent impulses that control the respiratory muscles to alter the rate and depth of breathing in response to the metabolic demands of the body.[12]

Most breathing is under involuntary control and responds to input from mechanoreceptors and chemoreceptors. Under normal resting conditions, breathing is primarily under chemical control.[12] Central and peripheral chemoreceptors sense levels of CO_2 and O_2, respectively, and determine respiratory drive. The central chemoreceptors in the brainstem respond to blood levels of CO_2 to provide the primary drive for breathing. As CO_2

levels rise, they stimulate increased ventilation to blow off the extra CO_2. This mechanism is often referred to as the hypercapnic drive for breathing. The peripheral chemoreceptors in the aortic arch and the common carotid arteries respond to blood O_2 levels. If O_2 levels fall below normal, these receptors stimulate increased ventilation. This serves as a back-up for the hypercapnic drive, and this response is often referred to as the *hypoxic drive* or the *secondary drive for breathing.*

Clinical Pearl

Most breathing is under involuntary control, and under normal resting conditions breathing is primarily under chemical control.

In addition to the strategically located chemoreceptors, mechanoreceptors in the lungs and the peripheral skeletal muscles respond to stretch or movement to regulate the overall breathing pattern. As the lungs near full inspiratory volume, mechanoreceptors inhibit inhalation and facilitate exhalation so that the lungs do not become overstretched. Mechanoreceptors in the skeletal muscles are also thought to play a role in stimulating breathing at the initial stages of exercise.

The airways and the pulmonary vessels are under a degree of autonomic control. Sympathetic activation causes airway dilation and suppression of secretion production, whereas parasympathetic activation has the opposite effect. The pulmonary vessels are primarily affected by their O_2 level and constrict in response to low O_2 levels. This phenomenon is known as *hypoxic vasoconstriction.*[13]

In addition to these involuntary breathing control mechanisms, breathing can also be voluntarily controlled via the motor cortex. This type of control is used to perform volitional activities such as blowing out birthday candles, singing, taking a deep breath before submerging in water, and to some extent during exercise.

Pulmonary Function Tests and Lung Volumes. The ventilatory pump system controls the volume of air moving in and out of the airways and the rate at which the air moves. Lung volumes, capacities, and flow rates are listed and defined in Table 26-1, and volumes and capacities are shown graphically in Fig. 26-7. A lung capacity is the sum of two or more volumes. Lung volumes and capacities vary in the normal individual based on body size, gender, height, and weight and can be compromised

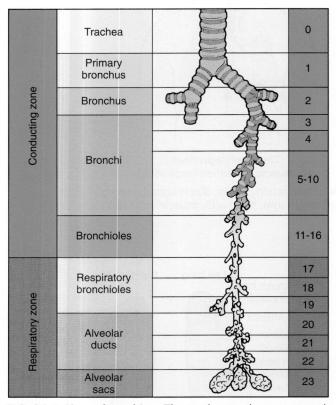

FIG. 26-6 Airway branching. The trachea to the seventeenth level of branching is the conducting zone. Gas exchange takes place after the seventeenth level in the respiratory zone. *From McArdle WD, Katch FI, Katch VL: Exercise physiology: Energy, nutrition, and human performance, ed 5, Philadelphia, 2001, Lippincott Williams & Wilkins.*

TABLE 26-1	**Lung Volumes Associated with Ventilation**
VOLUMES	**DEFINITIONS**
Total lung capacity (TLC)	Volume of air in the lungs at the end of maximum inspiration
Forced vital capacity (FVC)	Volume of air forcefully exhaled from maximum inspiration to maximum expiration
Residual volume (RV)	Volume of air in the lungs after maximum expiration
Inspiratory capacity (IC)	Volume of air from tidal expiration to maximum inhalation
Functional residual capacity (FRC)	Volume of air in the lungs after a tidal expiration
Inspiratory reserve volume (IRV)	Volume of air from end of tidal inspiration to maximum inspiration
Tidal volume (TV)	Volume of air inspired or expired per breath
Expiratory reserve volume (ERV)	Volume of air from end tidal expiration to maximum expiration
FLOWS	
Forced expiratory volume in 1 second (FEV_1)	Volume of air moved in the first second of an FVC maneuver
FEV_1/FVC ratio	
Peak expiratory flow (PEF)	Peak flow reached during an FVC maneuver

Figure labels (Fig. 26-6):

Conducting zone:
- Trachea — 0
- Primary bronchus — 1
- Bronchus — 2
- Bronchi — 3, 4, 5-10
- Bronchioles — 11-16

Respiratory zone:
- Respiratory bronchioles — 17, 18, 19
- Alveolar ducts — 20, 21, 22
- Alveolar sacs — 23

by pathology. Compromised lung volumes and capacities are often associated with restrictive lung diseases.

Clinical Pearl

Compromised lung volumes and capacities are often associated with restrictive lung diseases.

Measures commonly used to evaluate airway function are forced vital capacity (FVC) and forced expiratory volume in 1 second (FEV_1). FVC is the volume of air moved from maximum inhalation to maximum exhalation. To measure FVC the patient is asked to inhale maximally and then forcefully blow out into a measuring device or spirometer until their lungs feel completely empty. The total volume moved during this forced maneuver is the FVC. FEV_1 is the volume of air moved during the first second of the FVC maneuver and represents air movement through the larger airways. Compromised flow rates are often associated with obstructive lung diseases.

Clinical Pearl

Compromised flow rates are often associated with obstructive lung diseases.

Arterial–Alveolar Oxygen Difference. The difference in O_2 concentration between the arterial blood and the air within the alveoli is known as the **arterial–alveolar oxygen difference,** or gradient, and is abbreviated as $PAO_2–PaO_2$. This value reflects the adequacy of gas exchange within the lung. $PAO_2–PaO_2$ will widen if diffusion between the alveoli and the pulmonary circulation is impaired and less O_2 reaches the bloodstream from the alveoli. $PAO_2–PaO_2$ is normally less than 20 mm Hg but may be as low as 10 mm Hg in children and as high as 30 mm Hg in the elderly.[14]

Ventilation and Perfusion. Ventilation ($\dot{V}$) refers to the movement of a volume of air from the atmosphere in and out of the airways and greatly depends on the ability of the respiratory muscles to generate force to bring air into the lungs. **Minute ventilation (MV)** is the volume of air moved in 1 minute and is usually measured liters per minute (L/min). MV is equal to the tidal volume (TV) multiplied by the respiratory rate:

$$MV = TV \times RR$$

where:
MV = minute ventilation
TV = tidal volume
RR = respiratory rate in breaths per minute (breaths/min)

Maximal voluntary ventilation (MVV) is an individual's maximal MV and contributes to his or her overall functional aerobic capacity, which is also affected by the entire O_2 transport system. MVV can be measured with pulmonary function tests. MVV is rarely reached at maximum aerobic capacity and is not a limiting factor in individuals without pulmonary dysfunction. However, those with pulmonary disease may approach their MVV with certain activities or exercise.[15] When an individual's MV reaches about 50% of his or her MVV, he or she will feel short of breath.[16] At 70% of MVV, the respiratory muscles will begin to fatigue, and 90% MVV is only sustainable for a short period of time.[17] Ventilatory reserve (MVV—MV) is associated with outcome (progression to respiratory failure) in individuals experiencing COPD exacerbations.[18] Although rehabilitation professionals may not always have exact objective measurements of these values, these concepts should be considered when working with patients with respiratory compromise and when selecting exercise intensities.

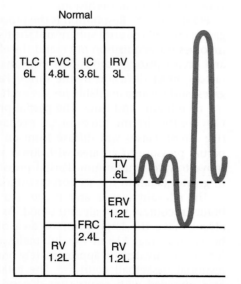

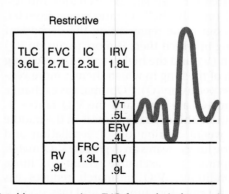

FIG. 26-7 Lung volumes and capacities. *TLC,* Total lung capacity; *FVC,* forced vital capacity; *RV,* reserve volume; *IC,* inspiratory capacity; *FRC,* functional residual capacity; *IRV,* inspiratory reserve volume; *TV,* tidal volume; *ERV,* expiratory reserve volume. *From Hillegass E, Sadowsky HS:* Essentials of cardiopulmonary physical therapy, *ed 2, Philadelphia, 2001, Saunders.*

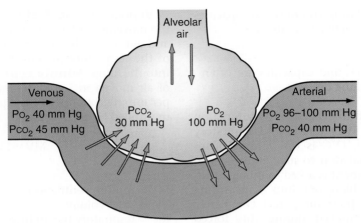

FIG. 26-8 Gas exchange occurs through diffusion in the alveoli.

When an individual's minute ventilation reaches about 50% of his or her maximal voluntary ventilation, he or she will feel short of breath.

Perfusion ($\dot{Q}$) of the lungs refers to the amount of blood flowing through the lungs. **Alveolar perfusion** has the greatest effect on respiration because only the blood that reaches the alveoli participates in gas exchange. The pulmonary circulation is primarily determined by the status and integrity of the cardiovascular system. Conditions, such as congestive heart failure, pulmonary embolism, and hypertension, may reduce pulmonary perfusion and thus interfere with respiration.

Ventilation and perfusion are not distributed equally through the lungs.[19-22] When an individual is upright, gravity causes more perfusion in the inferior portions and more ventilation in the superior portions of the lungs.[23] Therefore, because the dependent portions are less inflated, they have the greatest potential for expansion (i.e., they have the greatest amount of reserve volume). Thus, if ventilation is increased beyond normal levels, the extra ventilation will likely occur inferiorly.

Ventilation and Perfusion Matching. Ventilation and perfusion must match for adequate gas exchange and respiration to occur. Normally, the $\dot{V}:\dot{Q}$ ratio ranges from 0.6 to 3.0, with the lesser value representing the dependent portions of the lung in which there is more perfusion ($\dot{Q}$) and less ventilation ($\dot{V}$), and the higher value representing the upper portions of the lung in which there is more ventilation ($\dot{V}$) and less perfusion ($\dot{Q}$).[24] Optimal gas exchange occurs where $\dot{V}$ and $\dot{Q}$ are equal and the $\dot{V}:\dot{Q}$ ratio = 1. In the upright position, this exchange occurs in the middle lung zones. The overall distribution of ventilation and perfusion within the lungs creates an aggregate $\dot{V}:\dot{Q}$ match that allows for optimal gas exchange within the lungs under normal conditions. $\dot{V}:\dot{Q}$ mismatch reduces gas exchange and limits respiratory function and may occur if either ventilation or perfusion are impaired.

Dead space refers to areas within the lungs in which the air is not participating in respiration and thus breathing is impaired. Dead space can be anatomical (normal) or physiological (abnormal or pathological). Anatomical dead space consists of areas that normally have a high $\dot{V}:\dot{Q}$ ratio such as the conducting airways (i.e., the trachea through approximately generation 16 of the bronchi). It is normal for the air in these locations not to participate in gas exchange. Physiological or pathological dead space describes areas where air that should be participating in respiration does not do so because of a disease process or abnormal condition that limits perfusion but not ventilation. For example, physiological dead space may occur when a pulmonary embolism occludes blood flow (perfusion) to a given area of the lungs, limiting alveolar perfusion.

With **pulmonary shunt**, perfusion is greater than ventilation ($\dot{Q} > \dot{V}$). This may occur normally in the dependent portions of the lungs but can also be pathological. The classic example of pulmonary shunt is in areas of **atelectasis** (collapse of the airways) or consolidation (filling of alveoli with secretions). These conditions reduce ventilation but not perfusion.

Respiration. Respiration is the process of exchange of gases between the atmosphere and the tissues. This process involves the acquisition of O_2 and the elimination of CO_2 and occurs through diffusion in the alveoli. Four primary factors affect diffusion in the lungs: Partial pressures of gases, surface area available for gas exchange, thickness of the membrane, and time. The partial pressures of O_2 and CO_2 are the driving forces of gas exchange and diffusion (Fig. 26-8). Gases will diffuse from an area with higher partial pressure to an area with lower partial pressure to move toward equilibrium. Partial pressures are discussed in greater detail in the section on arterial blood gases.

The relevant surface area is the area of alveolar membrane in contact with air and blood. As an aggregate, the alveoli have the largest surface area of all the airways, being on average 118 m^2 in adult males and 91 m^2 in adult females, equivalent to approximately one-quarter of a professional basketball court.[25,26] The total alveolar surface area involved with respiration depends on the number and size of the alveoli and can be affected by various disease states and by the amount of ventilation. The alveolar membrane is made up of a single layer of endothelial cells, creating a very thin membrane through which gas

TABLE 26-2	Normal Arterial Blood Gas Values and Common Simplified Abnormalities*			
	pH	PaCO$_2$ (mm Hg)	PaO$_2$ (mm Hg)	HCO$_3$ (mEq/L)
Normal	7.35-7.45	35-45	>80	22-26
Respiratory acidosis	<7.35	>45	>80	22-26
Respiratory alkalosis	>7.45	<45	>80	22-26
Metabolic acidosis	<7.35	35-45	>80	>26
Metabolic alkalosis	>7.45	35-45	>80	<22

*These represent pure uncompensated states of either respiratory or metabolic acidosis/alkalosis and may or may not be associated with varying degrees of hypoxemia, depending on the severity of illness.

exchange can occur. Certain diseases and/or the presence of mucus may increase airway thickness or limit the number of alveoli participating in respiration. Infiltrates from pneumonia may reduce the number of alveoli available for ventilation, and emphysema will reduce alveolar surface area by destroying the alveolar walls. Both will ultimately limit alveolar gas exchange and impair respiratory function.

The final component that affects diffusion is the amount of time the gas is in contact with the alveoli. Alterations in gas partial pressures, alveolar surface area, or alveolar membrane thickness may potentially be compensated for by increasing the contact time for diffusion.

Arterial Blood Gases. Arterial blood gases (ABGs) are measures of the partial pressure of O$_2$ (PaO$_2$), partial pressure of CO$_2$ (PaCO$_2$), levels of bicarbonate (HCO$_3$), and the pH of arterial blood and are primary indicators of the respiratory and ventilatory status and overall physiological state of the body. Under normal circumstances, respiration balances O$_2$ supply and demand, as well as CO$_2$ production and elimination. The normal ranges for the components of the ABGs, along with common acid-base disorders, are summarized in Table 26-2. For an ABG to be considered normal, all values must be within normal limits.

Breathing primarily affects PaCO$_2$, pH, and PaO$_2$. Inadequate ventilation (hypoventilation) causes PaCO$_2$ to increase and PaO$_2$ to decrease by limiting respiration. The increase in PaCO$_2$ will cause pH to fall and make the blood more acidic. An increase in ventilation (hyperventilation) will cause PaCO$_2$ to decrease. The decrease in PaCO$_2$ will cause pH to rise and make the blood more alkaline. Hyperventilation generally does not significantly affect PaO$_2$ because this value is close to its maximum under normal conditions and cannot increase further.

Work of Breathing. **Work of breathing (WOB)** is the amount of energy or O$_2$ consumption needed by the respiratory muscles to produce enough ventilation and respiration to meet the metabolic demands of the body. Under normal resting circumstances, the WOB is about 5% of maximum O$_2$ uptake ($\dot{V}$O$_{2max}$).[27] In individuals with pulmonary problems, WOB may exceed 50% of $\dot{V}$O$_{2max}$, reducing their energy reserve and exercise capacity and stressing other systems to compensate.[28,29]

WOB is affected by various factors. The first factor is the metabolic needs of the body. As the body demands more energy, WOB needs to increase to provide adequate

ventilation. WOB is also affected by how much force the respiratory muscles must exert to overcome the resistance to airflow to move air in and out of the airways and maintain adequate lung volumes. The final determinant of WOB is the rate at which the muscles need to generate force, which is represented by the respiratory rate. WOB is determined by how hard and how fast the respiratory muscles must contract. $\dot{V}$:$\dot{Q}$ mismatching and impaired diffusion from various disease processes can also make the respiratory system inefficient, increasing ventilatory demands and the WOB.[28-30]

Airway Resistance. Airway resistance is the force opposing air flow in the airways. Airway resistance depends on the radius and length of the airway.

Anything that changes the radius or diameter of the airway will tremendously affect resistance to airflow. For example, bronchoconstriction as a result of asthma or airway obstruction as a result of mucus will cause the airway radius to decrease. The respiratory muscles will need to generate much more pressure to overcome this resistance and produce adequate airflow. Generating more pressure will require increased WOB and energy expenditure.

Clinical Pearl

Bronchoconstriction as a result of asthma or airway obstruction from mucus will increase airway resistance and increase the work of breathing.

Elasticity. **Elasticity** refers to the ability of the lungs and chest wall to recoil or deflate passively during exhalation. Since exhalation is normally passive at rest, it consumes no energy and therefore does not contribute to the overall WOB. The elastic recoil of the lungs and chest wall is similar to a balloon deflating without any external pressure when you let go of it after it is inflated. It deflates as a result of the elasticity, or passive recoil, of the balloon. Conditions that decrease the elasticity of the lungs may prevent passive exhalation. In this scenario, the accessory muscles of exhalation may need to contract and expend additional energy to maintain adequate ventilation and prevent hyperinflation of the lungs. The net result will be an increased WOB, which may eventually result in respiratory muscle fatigue or the inability to maintain adequate respiration.

If airway resistance increases, as with bronchoconstriction from asthma, passive elastic recoil may not generate enough force to overcome this resistance and empty the

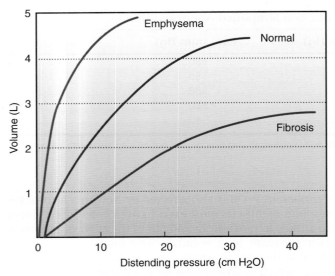

FIG. 26-9 Lung compliance is the change in lung volume per unit of pressure change. *From http://oac.med/jhmi.edu/res_phys/Encyclopedia/Compliance/Compliance.html.* Copyright 1995, Johns Hopkins University.

lungs. In this scenario, the body will need to use the accessory muscles of breathing to complete exhalation. This increase in muscle activity increases the WOB. This problem is exacerbated by the fact that when air is unable to get out, the trapped air functions as dead space and does not participate in respiration, making even less O_2 available to the body to produce energy.

Compliance. Lung **compliance** refers to the change in lung volume per unit of pressure change, and the standard compliance curve is shown in Fig. 26-9. Lung compliance affects the ability of the lungs to expand during inspiration. The less compliant the tissue, the more stiff or resistant to expansion it will be. Anyone who has attempted to blow up a balloon has experienced this concept. The initially low compliance of the balloon makes it very difficult to inflate. Thus high pressures and much energy are required to inflate the balloon. Efficient ventilation requires that both the lungs and the chest wall be compliant. The respiratory muscles will need to exert more inspiratory force if either lungs and/or chest wall compliance are decreased, thereby increasing the WOB.

A number of musculoskeletal, neurological, and pulmonary conditions can also affect lung or chest wall expansion. For example, severe scoliosis can significantly restrict thoracic expansion and thus limit lung expansion. Neurological conditions, such as cerebrovascular accidents, may increase muscle tone in the trunk restricting chest wall expansion.[30,31] Chest expansion may also be limited by neurological conditions that paralyze the respiratory muscles.[32] For example, individuals with mid- or high-cervical spinal cord injury may have paralyzed respiratory muscles that cannot generate force to draw air into the lungs and therefore limit chest wall and lung expansion.[33]

Surface Tension. The term *surface tension* refers to the cohesive state that occurs at a liquid-gas interface or liquid-liquid interface.[34] Within the lungs, this occurs at the interface between the alveolar membrane and the airway. Increased surface tension increases cohesion within the alveoli, pulling the alveoli closed. The alveolar cells produce a specialized liquid, **surfactant,** that decreases the surface tension in the airways, reducing the amount of energy required to expand the lungs.[35] When surface tension increases, more force is needed to expand the lungs, increasing the WOB. This occurs in respiratory distress syndrome in premature newborns because until around 36 weeks of gestation the fetus produces immature surfactant that inadequately reduces surface tension.[35] The resulting increased WOB causes most of these infants to initially need ventilatory assistance.

PATHOPHYSIOLOGY OF RESPIRATORY FAILURE

Respiratory failure refers to the inability of the body to maintain adequate gas exchange to meet its metabolic demands. Many factors affect gas exchange, but ventilation, diffusion, and perfusion are the primary contributors. Ventilation requires the respiratory muscles to produce sufficient force to sustain ventilation at all times and in response to a range of demands. If the WOB exceeds the capacity of the individual, fatigue and eventually respiratory failure will occur. Even if the muscles can generate enough force, diseases of the lung and airways may make this effort futile. Respiratory failure can be classified as being caused by hypoventilation, $\dot{V}:\dot{Q}$ mismatch, abnormal diffusion, or a combination of these factors.[36-38]

Hypoventilation. Hypoventilation refers to a state of decreased or inadequate ventilation. Many factors can contribute to hypoventilation. However, the primary causes of hypoventilation are central nervous system depression, neurological disease, or disorders of the respiratory muscles.[32,36]

Under normal circumstances, ventilation maintains a steady state between O_2 supply and demand and between CO_2 production and elimination. Tidal volumes exceed the volume of dead space in the conducting airways so that air reaches the alveoli for gas exchange to take place. Hypoventilation, which causes low tidal volumes, will decrease alveolar ventilation that in turn will decrease the potential for gas exchange. When gas exchange fails to keep the circulating concentrations of O_2 and CO_2 within the normal range, this indicates respiratory insufficiency and potential failure.

Ventilation-Perfusion Mismatch. Mismatching of ventilation and perfusion ($\dot{V}:\dot{Q}$ mismatch) is one of the more common causes of respiratory failure or inadequate gas exchange. As explained previously, ventilation-perfusion matching is determined by the distribution of air and blood flow in the lungs. Many factors, including diseases and body position, can affect the $\dot{V}:\dot{Q}$ ratio and lead to excessive dead space or areas of shunt.[19-21,36,39] In either case, the result of the $\dot{V}:\dot{Q}$ mismatch is impaired gas exchange in the affected areas of the lungs and a decreased ability to maintain a steady state of O_2 and CO_2 concentrations.

If $\dot{V}:\dot{Q}$ mismatching only occurs in part of the lungs, the body may be able to compensate by redistributing perfusion or increasing ventilation within the lungs to maintain appropriate $\dot{V}:\dot{Q}$ matching overall. Hypoxic vasoconstriction is a physiological reflex aimed at minimizing $\dot{V}:\dot{Q}$ mismatch to preserve respiration.[13] In response to low ventilation ($\dot{V} < \dot{Q}$) of an area, the body also decreases the perfusion ($\dot{Q}$) to this area through vasoconstriction to try to keep ventilation and perfusion matched and thus maintain gas exchange. This is an example of the cardiovascular components of the O_2 transport system attempting to compensate for pulmonary impairments at the expense of increased workload. This compensation may effectively keep circulating CO_2 and O_2 levels within normal limits. If it fails, CO_2 levels will rise, stimulating an increase in respiratory rate. This will increase the WOB and may eventually lead to respiratory fatigue or failure.

Diffusion Abnormalities. Gas exchange occurs at the alveolar level by diffusion and depends on alveolar surface area, partial pressures of O_2 and CO_2, the thickness of the alveolar wall, and time. Isolated abnormalities of diffusion are less common contributors to respiratory failure than $\dot{V}:\dot{Q}$ mismatching; however, impaired diffusion may result in $\dot{V}:\dot{Q}$ mismatching.[36] Inadequate diffusion increases the overall WOB by interfering with gas exchange. In the presence of other abnormal conditions, such as respiratory muscle weakness, the body may not be able to sustain the additional WOB and respiratory fatigue or failure may result.

Classification of Respiratory Failure. With inadequate respiration, O_2 levels decrease (**hypoxia**) and CO_2 levels increase (**hypercapnia**). The increase in CO_2 produces a decrease in blood pH. Respiratory failure can alter all aspects of the ABGs. The ABG criteria for respiratory failure are a PaO_2 of less than 60 mm Hg, a $PaCO_2$ greater than 50 mm Hg, or a pH of less than 7.3.[36,37]

Respiratory failure can be classified as primarily hypoxic (known as type I) or as primarily hypercapnic (known as type II). Hypoxic respiratory failure is primarily characterized by abnormally low PaO_2 and a normal or close to normal $PaCO_2$, whereas hypercapnic respiratory failure is primarily characterized by an abnormally elevated $PaCO_2$ that may or may not be associated with hypoxia.[37]

Respiratory failure can also be classified as acute or chronic depending on its time course. Acute respiratory failure occurs over a short period of time (minutes to hours), whereas chronic respiratory failure develops over a longer period of time (days to months). The patient history can help determine the acuity of respiratory failure, and ABGs can help distinguish between acute and chronic hypercapnic respiratory failure. With acute hypercapnic respiratory failure, CO_2 levels rise, causing a fall in arterial pH. Over time, the kidneys can compensate for this change by retaining bicarbonate (HCO_3) to bring the pH back toward normal. Thus, with acute hypercapnic respiratory failure, $PaCO_2$ is elevated and pH is low, whereas with chronic hypercapnic respiratory failure, $PaCO_2$ is elevated, but pH is almost normal. The acuity of hypoxemic respiratory failure cannot be determined from ABG values since

PaO_2 does not influence pH. Acute hypoxemia can be differentiated from chronic hypoxemia by the history and the presence or absence of clinical indicators of long-standing hypoxemia such as polycythemia (an increase in the number of red blood cells).

It is important to distinguish between acute and chronic respiratory failure because individuals in the acute stages of respiratory failure should limit their activity, since increasing the O_2 demand may worsen their condition. However, early mobilization, positioning, and breathing exercises can help these patients by improving ventilation, enhancing $\dot{V}:\dot{Q}$ matching, and stimulating respiratory drive. For individuals with chronic respiratory failure, or those at risk of developing failure, rehabilitation interventions should focus on improving breathing efficiency and improving overall conditioning through strength and aerobic training (see Chapter 23).

TYPICAL EXAMINATION FINDINGS

PATIENT HISTORY

The patient history contains a range of information, including what the patient understands to be the cause(s) of his or her respiratory failure and how his or her respiratory function has evolved over time. The patient's current and prior activity tolerance, as well as the need for supplemental oxygen is also included. In addition, for most patients with respiratory failure, the patient history component of the examination includes information about medications and other medical diagnoses such as heart failure, neuromuscular conditions, or depression.

SYSTEMS REVIEW

For the patient with respiratory failure the systems review includes examination of the level of consciousness and the ability to follow commands, as well as vital signs, ABG values, and results of cardiovascular tests such as cardiac catheterization, echocardiography, electrocardiogram (ECG), and cardiac enzymes.

TESTS AND MEASURES

Musculoskeletal. The primary musculoskeletal tests and measures for persons with respiratory failure are measurements of upper and lower extremity range of motion (ROM), strength and endurance, and joint integrity and mobility.

Neuromuscular. The primary neuromuscular tests and measures for persons with respiratory failure are measurements of cognition, reflexes, sensation, coordination, motor function, balance, and pain.

Integumentary. The integumentary system should be examined frequently in patients with respiratory failure who are bed bound (see Chapter 28).

Cardiovascular/Pulmonary

Ventilator Settings and Oxygen Requirements. For the patient on a ventilator, the ventilator settings and O_2 requirements are checked before other tests and measures are performed. Patients receiving more O_2 are likely to have poorer O_2 transport and a greater dependency on supplemental O_2. Supplemental O_2 can be provided with mechanical ventilation and is often described in terms of percentage of inspired O_2. Patients receiving a greater percentage of inspired O_2 have poorer O_2 transport and are in greater need of additional O_2.

Arterial Blood Gases, Oxygen Saturation, and Noninvasive Carbon Dioxide Measures. As discussed previously, ABG measures can be used to examine O_2 transport and respiratory performance.[40-42] When interpreting ABGs, one should first determine if the pH is greater (alkalosis) or less than 7 (acidosis).[39] With a primary respiratory acidosis as a result of hypoventilation, which often occurs with respiratory failure, the pH will be low and the $PaCO_2$ will be high. CO_2 levels provide specific information about alveolar ventilation. CO_2 levels are obtained with the ABGs and may also be measured transcutaneously, although this is thought to be less accurate, particularly in infants or children.[43,44]

Measures of O_2 saturation, as discussed in detail in Chapter 22, also provide information about respiratory performance and O_2 transport. O_2 saturation is the amount of O_2 saturating the hemoglobin molecule. Normal O_2 saturation is 95% or greater, mild hypoxemia is an O_2 saturation level between 90% and 95%, and moderate and severe hypoxemia are O_2 saturation levels between 80% and 90% and less than 75% and 80%, respectively.[41-43] O_2 saturation may be measured intermittently as a component of the ABG and continuously or intermittently with a pulse oximeter worn on the finger, earlobe, or other body part (see Chapter 22).

CO_2 levels provide specific information about alveolar ventilation. CO_2 levels are obtained with the ABGs and may also be measured transcutaneously.

Auscultation of the Heart and Lungs. Auscultation of the heart and lungs is performed in persons with respiratory failure. Chest auscultation may detect the presence of certain cardiac or pulmonary disorders, the presence or absence of retained pulmonary secretions, and if secretion removal techniques are needed and successful.

Cardiovascular Tests and Measures. The heart rate and blood pressure (BP) of a person with respiratory failure should be examined while the patient is resting lying down and in various body positions and during exercise or functional activities (see Chapter 22). In patients receiving mechanical ventilation, one should be aware that intrathoracic pressure may be increased by the positive pressure ventilation and this may reduce venous return, causing a decrease in BP. Therefore one should always examine for signs or symptoms of hypotension in persons receiving mechanical ventilation. Other common cardiovascular findings in persons with respiratory failure include faster resting and exercise heart rates, as well as more easily produced anginal symptoms because of more rapid heart rate with activity and poorer O_2 transport.

◎ *Clinical Pearl*

In hospitalized patients with respiratory failure, vital signs, including O_2 saturation, are usually monitored continuously by telemetry.

Chest Wall and Abdominal Motion. Chest wall and abdominal motion should be examined in patients with respiratory failure. This examination may be performed using observation, palpation, and measurement of chest expansion.

Observation. Observation of the breathing pattern includes comparison of the magnitude of upper chest movement (superior to the xiphoid process) and lower chest wall movement (abdominal area around the umbilicus) and determination of the synchrony of these motions.

Palpation. Movements of the upper and lower chest during inspiration and expiration are also examined by palpation to evaluate for areas of hypermobility or hypomobility and timing and coordination of the breathing pattern.

Measurement of Chest Expansion. A tape measure can be used to quantify chest wall excursion in different areas of the thorax. The amount of chest wall motion during normal breathing (which can be referred to as *tidal volume breathing*), as well as during a maximum inspiration, is recorded in centimeters or inches.

Respiratory Muscle Strength and Endurance. Respiratory muscle weakness is assessed using manual muscle testing, measurements of maximum inspiratory pressure (MIP) and maximum expiratory pressure (MEP), and tests of breathing muscle strength via weighted breathing (weights added to the abdominal area of a supine patient).

Function. The primary functional tests and measures used for the person with respiratory failure include measurements of bed mobility, transfer ability, sitting ability, standing ability, walking ability, and activities of daily living (ADLs). A variety of methods to examine each of these areas exists, and although patients with respiratory failure are frequently intubated or receiving noninvasive positive pressure ventilation (NIPPV), the same tests and measures used for other patients receiving physical therapy are applicable. It is important to frequently reassess each of these tests and measures so that a patient's rehabilitation program can be progressed optimally.

EVALUATION, DIAGNOSIS, AND PROGNOSIS

The initial physical therapy goals are generally directed toward preventing secondary complications of bed rest, whereas the ultimate goals of physical therapy for patients requiring prolonged mechanical ventilation are to minimize loss of mobility, maximize independence, and facilitate weaning. The outcomes for patients with respiratory failure who receive rehabilitation management and mechanical ventilation are listed in Box 26-2. They include both favorable and unfavorable outcomes.[45-58]

INTERVENTION

MEDICAL MANAGEMENT OF RESPIRATORY FAILURE

Medical interventions for patients with respiratory failure either treat the disease causing the failure or provide support to maintain ventilation and respiration when the cause cannot be eliminated. Interventions aimed at treating diseases that cause respiratory failure are described in

---

BOX 26-2 **Possible Outcomes for Patients Receiving Mechanical Ventilation**

Adverse Outcomes	Favorable Outcomes*
1. Infection	1. Improved survival by resolving respiratory failure
2. Deconditioning and muscle weakness	2. Improved pulmonary, cardiovascular, and multisystem function
3. Altered cardiovascular and pulmonary function	3. Rapid wean from mechanical ventilation
4. Greater dependency on anaerobic metabolism	4. Ability to exercise and increase functional activities
5. Poor nutritional status	5. Improved psychological function
6. Hypertension/hypotension	6. Exercise training adaptations
7. Anxiety/psychosis	a. Improved skeletal and cardiac muscle function
8. Depression	b. Lower resting heart rate and BP
9. Osteoporosis	c. Lower rate pressure product
10. Psychological dysfunction	d. Increased peak O_2 consumption
11. Physiological dysfunction after endotracheal intubation or tracheostomy	e. Increased lean muscle mass
12. Ventilator dependency	f. Decreased body weight and body fat
	g. Greater heart rate responsiveness during exercise
	h. Improved lipid and blood sugar profiles
	i. Decreased rate of bone mineral loss

*Many of the favorable outcomes can only be achieved with exercise training.

---

depth in a range of medical texts and are not discussed further here. Supportive measures, mechanical ventilation, and supplemental O_2 are discussed in the next section.

Supplemental Oxygen. Supplemental O_2 is indicated when the patient can sustain sufficient WOB to maintain ventilation independently but cannot maintain adequate levels of oxygenation. Supplemental O_2 can be delivered by a wide range of devices varying in complexity and the amount of O_2 they can deliver.

Oxygen Delivery Sources. All O_2 delivery systems consist of a supply source and a delivery device. O_2 may be supplied from a portable reservoir in the form of an O_2 gas tank or a liquid O_2 system. In hospitals, patients may receive O_2 from a fixed main hospital supply through a wall hook-up. To avoid confusion with other medical gases, all O_2 tanks and ports are colored green.

The amount of time a portable O_2 gas tank will last depends on its size, how full it is (measured as the pressure of the gas in pounds per square inch [psi]), and the flow rate.

Oxygen Delivery Devices. O_2 is usually delivered from the supply to the patient by a nasal cannula or a face mask. The nasal cannula is used most often. The amount of O_2 delivered to a patient by this device is affected by the concentration and rate of delivery, as well as the patient's respiratory rate, depth, and pattern of breathing. It consists of nasal prongs that sit in the patient's nasal passageway on one end and a connector that attaches to the O_2 source on the other end. It is recommended that at flow rates of more than 3 L/min a humidifier be used with this device to minimize drying of the nasal mucosa.

If adequate O_2 saturation cannot be maintained by the nasal cannula or if flow rates greater than 6 L/min are required, a face mask should be considered. Face masks vary in complexity and in the concentration of O_2 they can deliver for a given flow rate. The most commonly used masks are the simple mask, the venturi mask, the rebreather mask, and the nonrebreather mask (Fig 26-10).

Oxygen Dosage. Dosage, or the amount of O_2 delivered, can be expressed in terms of flow rate, generally in L/min, or in terms of concentration. O_2 concentration is expressed as the percentage of O_2 inspired (FiO_2). FiO_2 may range from 21% (the concentration of O_2 in room air) to 100%, depending on the device. When O_2 is delivered by nasal cannula the dosage is given in L/min, whereas when a face mask is used, the dose may be given in either form.

Oxygen Is a Medication. O_2 is classified by the Food and Drug Administration (FDA) as a medication. Therefore only a physician may prescribe the O_2 dosage and how it should be delivered, except in an emergency. In nonemergency situations, rehabilitation professionals should modify O_2 demand by altering patient activity or exercise intensity or adjust the O_2 supply if the physician orders titration of delivery to demand or within a given range. For example, a physician may request that O_2 be titrated up to 6 L/min via nasal cannula to keep O_2 saturation above 90%.

Mechanical Ventilation. Patients with respiratory insufficiency or failure who cannot sustain the necessary WOB independently can have their breathing supported by mechanical ventilation. Indications for mechanical ventilation include acute respiratory failure, impending respiratory failure, need for protection of the airway, secretion management, upper airway obstruction, and allowing for paralysis or sedation.[37] Mechanical ventilators are used most often in the intensive care unit (ICU) or a critical care setting. However, patients who are expected to need support from a mechanical ventilator for a prolonged period may be seen in a variety of settings, including inpatient rehabilitation facilities and at home.

A mechanical ventilator substitutes for or assists the patient's ventilatory pump to allow breathing to occur. Supplemental O_2 is usually administered in conjunction

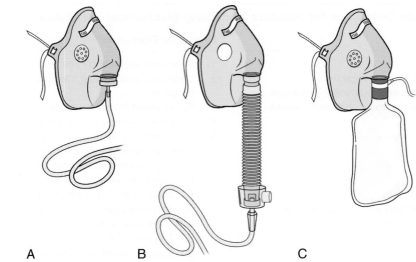

A   B   C

FIG. 26-10 Face masks. **A,** Simple. **B,** Venturi. **C,** Nonrebreather. *From deWit SC: Fundamental concepts and skills for nursing, ed 3. St. Louis, 2009, Saunders.*

with the mechanical assistance to maintain oxygenation. Ventilator design has progressed over time to better mimic normal physiological ventilation, with one major exception: mechanical ventilators support ventilation by applying positive pressure to the airways, "pushing" air with varying O_2 concentrations into the lungs, whereas normal physiological breathing is driven by negative pressure that essentially "pulls" air into the airways. This difference can cause complications.

Route of Intubation. The route of intubation is the way the patient is connected to the ventilator. There are four basic routes of intubation: Via nasopharyngeal airway, oropharyngeal airway, endotracheal tube (ETT), or **tracheostomy.** The first two are generally seen in emergent situations and occasionally in the ICU for short-term airway management but are generally not seen in the rehabilitation field. The latter two airways are more commonly seen in patients requiring prolonged mechanical ventilation.

In general, ET intubation, with an ETT (Fig. 26-11), is used for short-term intubation. A standard ETT is a long, flexible tube that is inserted through the mouth into the trachea. The distal end of the tube sits just above the level of the carina, just before the trachea bifurcates into the left and right mainstem bronchi. The cuff, which is at the distal end of the ETT, is inflated to hold the tube in place and maintain a seal to ensure that the breath enters the lungs and does not escape through the upper airways. The proximal end exits the patient's mouth and is connected to the ventilator through a series of tubing. This tubing and all its connections are called the *ventilator circuit.* ETTs come in various sizes based on the patient's size and age.

When an ETT is present, the rehabilitation professional must ensure that it does not dislodge or advance within the airways during activities because this may disconnect the patient from the ventilator or render the ventilator nonfunctional. If the rehabilitation professional suspects

Proximal end of ETT, connects to ventilation system

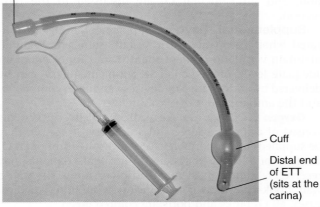

Cuff

Distal end of ETT (sits at the carina)

FIG. 26-11 Endotracheal tube.

that the ETT has moved, they should immediately alert the physician, nurse, or respiratory therapist to ensure appropriate tube placement.

Tracheostomy is indicated when long-term use of the ventilator is expected and consists of surgical placement of a tube in the trachea through an opening made at the level of the jugular notch, below the glottis and vocal cords. Tracheostomy tubes come in various sizes and types (Fig. 26-12). The tube prevents the patient from speaking or performing a functional cough unless it is fenestrated with an opening that allows air to flow out the upper airways and over the vocal cords. The distal end of the tube may or may not have a cuff as in the ETT, and the proximal end is attached to the ventilator circuit.

Some patients may be able to speak when off the mechanical ventilator by occluding the tracheostomy with a finger or a speaking valve. The rehabilitation

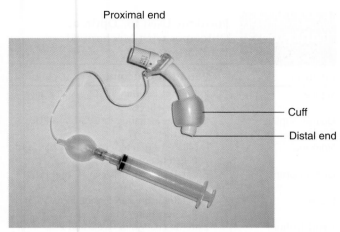

FIG. 26-12 Tracheostomy tube.

professional should consult with the physician and the speech therapist to determine who may tolerate this. However, whenever occluding the tracheostomy to facilitate speech, the cuff must be deflated.

Modes of Ventilation. The mode of ventilation determines whether the ventilator or the patient initiates breathing and which performs most of the work of breathing. Current ventilators allow for selection of various modes of mechanical ventilation.

Controlled Ventilation, Assisted Ventilation, and Assist Control. With controlled ventilation (CV) the mechanical ventilator controls all aspects of ventilation, including FiO₂, respiratory rate, and volume and pressure of each delivered breath, and the patient does not need to actively breathe at all. The patient may be completely paralyzed or sedated as the ventilator is doing all the WOB. With assisted ventilation (AV) the patient controls the rate and rhythm of breathing. When the ventilator senses negative pressure as the patient initiates a breath, it delivers a breath at a preset volume, pressure, or flow rate. With AV, the respiratory muscles are active and initiate the breath, but the ventilator is doing most of the work. If the patient does not initiate the breath, the ventilator will not be triggered. With the assist control (AC) mode, which combines CV and AV, the ventilator delivers the breath with the patient's inspiratory effort at a preset volume and/or pressure as in the AV mode, thereby allowing the patient to control the rate and rhythm if able. However, if the patient does not initiate a breath within a predetermined period, the ventilator still delivers the breath. This allows the patient to initiate breaths but provides the safety of delivering a breath if the patient fails to initiate breathing. With all of these modes, most if not all of the WOB is performed by the ventilator.

Synchronized Intermittent Mandatory Ventilation. Synchronized intermittent mandatory ventilation (SIMV) mode delivers a breath at a set volume and pressure and at a rate that coordinates with the patient's respiratory cycle. Although this mode has a set rate, it will not deliver a breath if the patient is exhaling and it will only deliver "mandatory" breaths if the patient-initiated breaths do not meet the minimum ventilator settings. In SIMV mode,

the patient and the ventilator contribute to the WOB to varying degrees, depending on the set rate, pressure, and volume. The higher the minimum settings (i.e., rate, pressure support, and TVs) on the ventilator the less likely the patient will achieve them and thus the ventilator performs more work. Similarly, the lower the minimum settings, the more WOB is performed by the patient.

Continuous Positive Airway Pressure. With continuous positive airway pressure (CPAP) mode, the patient controls the respiratory rate, rhythm, and volume, and the ventilator maintains positive pressure throughout inspiration and expiration to decrease the overall WOB. The amount of assistance given by the ventilator is directly related to the pressure setting on the ventilator. CPAP mode is frequently used when weaning a patient from a ventilator, since it allows the patient to breathe independently but provides enough assistance to overcome the resistance of breathing through a long narrow tube.

Complications of Mechanical Ventilation. Most of the complications associated with mechanical ventilation occur during intubation or as a result of the positive pressure ventilation. During insertion of an ETT, there may be tracheolaryngeal injury. This may only become apparent after extubation when the patient has a hoarse voice, cough, persistent sputum production, or **hemoptysis.**

The positive pressure can cause trauma because of overdistention of the alveoli, which can cause long-term fibrosis of the lungs that permanently limits ventilatory capacity. Positive pressure can also cause a **pneumothorax** as a result of alveolar rupture and in severe cases can cause the lung to collapse.

With prolonged use, the cuff at the distal end of an ETT or tracheotomy tube can cause tracheal necrosis. The presence of the artificial airway also increases the risk for pneumonia and promotes secretion production, which can worsen respiratory failure.[59]

Complications of mechanical ventilation are not confined to the pulmonary system. Cardiovascular complications of mechanical ventilation include pulmonary hypertension, decreased cardiac output, hypotension, and cardiac arrhythmias. Pressure ulcers are also common in ventilated patients because of immobility, loss of muscle mass, decreases in ROM, difficulty maintaining hygiene, and malnutrition.

One of the greatest challenges of prolonged mechanical ventilation may be the overall effect on the ventilatory muscles themselves. The mechanical ventilator is often used to assist the muscles of ventilation. However, assisting these muscles promotes disuse atrophy and when the artificial ventilation is removed, the respiratory muscles may not have the strength and endurance to sustain ventilation. In this circumstance, mechanical ventilation may need to be weaned gradually over time to allow the muscles to regain strength.[60-62]

◎ Clinical Pearl

When artificial ventilation is removed, the respiratory muscles may not have the strength and endurance to sustain ventilation. Mechanical ventilation may need to be weaned gradually over time to allow the respiratory muscles to regain strength.

Weaning from Mechanical Ventilation. Weaning from mechanical ventilation is the process of gradually decreasing ventilatory support until the individual can sustain spontaneous breathing. Weaning may be needed to allow the strength and endurance of the respiratory muscles to improve or to allow the underlying cause of the respiratory failure to resolve. When weaning, the energy demand of breathing at rest may compromise the ability to exercise. Under normal circumstances, only about 5% of the maximum energy available at rest is used to breathe, and the remaining 95% is potentially available to perform exercise or ADLs. When weaning from mechanical ventilation, more energy will be needed for breathing, leaving less of a reserve for other activities. If pushed too hard, the patient may fail the weaning process. However, if not pushed at all, the patient will probably get weaker. The rehabilitation professional must carefully select and monitor the level of activity for the optimal outcome.

The process of weaning from mechanical ventilation varies among patients, physicians, and facilities. Many hospitals have "weaning protocols" or pathways to help guide this process. Weaning is generally initiated when the patient shows signs of being able to breathe adequately without support by meeting "weaning criteria." Examples of weaning criteria are O_2 saturation maintained at greater than 92%, FiO_2 requirements less than 40% to 50%, respiratory rate less than 35, respiratory rate to TV ratio less than 100 breaths/min/L, and no signs of distress.[37] When these criteria are met, trials of breathing without support are attempted. If the patient is intubated for a prolonged period, these trials may be gradually increased in duration until the patient can breathe independently for 24 hours, at which time they are extubated. If the patient cannot be extubated after 3 months of weaning trials, the patient is generally considered ventilator dependent.

Noninvasive Mechanical Ventilation. Noninvasive mechanical ventilation is any form of assisted ventilation in which an ETT is not used. This type of assisted ventilation is usually provided via a face mask. Evidence suggests that the use of noninvasive mechanical ventilation in patients in the ICU may reduce the need for intubation or reintubation and that outpatients with COPD who receive noninvasive mechanical ventilation are able to exercise more than similar patients who do not receive this intervention.[63-70]

REHABILITATION INTERVENTIONS

New technologies in the areas of mechanical ventilation and critical care medicine have allowed many critically ill patients to survive and have led to a dramatic increase in the number of patients who are ventilator-dependent. Patients who require mechanical ventilation have limited mobility because of multiple medical problems, equipment, and weakness. The prolonged bed rest associated with a stay in the ICU can also lead to a significant loss of functional abilities. Patients requiring prolonged mechanical ventilation experience high morbidity, high costs of care, and poor functional outcomes. Rehabilitation programs for patients with respiratory failure are generally initiated in the ICU and focus on early mobilization and ambulation. Before returning home, these patients

TABLE 26-3	Positions Used for Optimal Outcomes with Mechanical Ventilation*
Position	**Potential Outcome**
Supine	Important position in SCI because of gravity effects
Quarter-supine	Facilitates a change in CVSC and PUL function
Sidelying	Facilitates a greater change in CVSC and PUL function
Quarter-prone	Facilitates a change in CVSC and PUL function
Prone	Facilitates a greater change in CVSC and PUL function
Trendelenburg	Extreme change in CVSC and PUL function
Reverse Trendelenburg	Extreme change in CVSC and PUL function
Semi-Fowler's position	Achieving more normal CVSC and PUL function
Fowler's position	Achieving more normal, functional CVSC and PUL function
Continuous rotation	Facilitates continuous change in CVSC and PUL function
Upright	Desired position for optimal CVSC and PUL function

*Moving patients in and out of these positions will help achieve outcomes as well as maintain optimal integumentary status.
SCI, Spinal cord injury; *CVSC,* cardiovascular; *PUL,* pulmonary.

will continue to benefit from a rehabilitation program and often spend extended periods of time in long-term acute care (LTAC) units or rehabilitation units.

Positioning and Adjunctive Techniques for Clearance of Secretions. The use of different body positions to achieve optimal outcomes has been considered one of several critical adjunctive interventions for patients in respiratory failure receiving mechanical ventilation. The primary goals of proper positioning include the reduction of pulmonary complications and skin breakdown and promotion of optimal cardiovascular and pulmonary function. A number of positions are typically used to achieve these key outcomes (Table 26-3).

The prone position and the upright body position, which replicates normal cardiovascular and pulmonary function during most functional activities, have been found to significantly improve cardiovascular and pulmonary function. However, not all patients receiving mechanical ventilation are able to attain a prone or upright position and therefore other positions are often used.

Clinical Pearl

Many of the beds used in the intensive care unit can be moved to support the patient in a sitting position, allowing the patient to sit upright before they can tolerate transferring to a chair.

Alternating right and left sidelying is commonly used. Positioning together with specific postural drainage positions may also improve cardiovascular and pulmonary function.[45-48,50]

Patients with respiratory failure receiving mechanical ventilation who also have neurological and/or musculoskeletal disorders may benefit from a positioning program to prevent the development of contractures and pressure ulcers (especially in the sacral and heel areas). An optimal positioning program should include training of patients, nurses, and family members in utilization of positions that are most effective for individual patients. Information sheets describing positions with schematics of body positions to be used may facilitate optimal outcomes for persons receiving mechanical ventilation in the hospital, home, or rehabilitation unit.[46,50]

Traditional secretion clearance techniques, as described in detail in Chapter 24, can also be used in patients with retained secretions who cannot mobilize them through the use of different body positions or active movement alone. Perhaps the most important of these techniques is deep breathing exercises followed by coughing or huffing.

Functional and Exercise Training. There is limited research on the effects of functional and exercise training in people with respiratory failure receiving mechanical ventilation.[45-48,50] Most of the support for this type of intervention is based on expert opinion and inferred from changes known to accompany exercise in healthy and diseased individuals.

A recent comprehensive overview on the effects of exercise and mobilization on acutely ill patients (including patients receiving mechanical ventilation) presented specific guidelines regarding safety and progression of exercise for patients in the ICU.[58] Patients receiving mechanical ventilation were considered appropriate for mobilization when (1) oxygenation, hypercapnia, and the breathing pattern were relatively normal or within acceptable limits, (2) they were able to tolerate more supportive ventilatory modes (pressure control ventilation or SIMV with high mandatory rates) during exercise, (3) they were alert and able to follow commands, and (4) the level of weaning from mechanical ventilation was such that mobilization did not induce excessive demand on the respiratory or cardiovascular systems. Caveats to these recommendations are that acceptable limits of oxygenation, hypercapnia, and breathing pattern may be patient specific and that although patients who require more supportive ventilatory modes during exercise are appropriate for exercise and mobility training, mobility training should generally be postponed in patients requiring high levels of ventilatory support at rest. Box 26-3 lists potential reasons for stopping or postponing exercise and mobility training in patients with respiratory failure.[58]

Overall, the evidence indicates that exercise may accelerate weaning, decrease hospital length of stay, and improve the sense of well-being in patients with respiratory failure receiving mechanical ventilation.

Inspiratory Muscle Training. Inspiratory muscle training (IMT) is a type of exercise that involves using a device that provides resistance to inspiration[71-79] (Fig. 26-13). If not using mechanical ventilation, the patient places their mouth around a mouthpiece and then breathes in and out of the device. If using mechanical ventilation,

BOX 26-3	Reasons for Stopping or Postponing Exercise and Mobility Training in Patients with Respiratory Failure

1. High level of ventilatory support required at rest.
2. Hypotension associated with fainting, dizziness, and/or diaphoresis.
3. Severe intolerable dyspnea during exercise.
4. Saturation less than 90% on supplemental O_2.
5. Significant chest pain or discomfort.
6. Extreme fatigue.
7. Patient wishes to stop exercise.

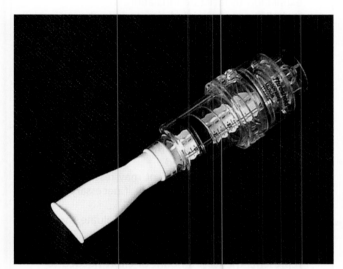

FIG. 26-13 Inspiratory muscle trainer. *From Frownfelter D, Dean E:* Cardiovascular and pulmonary physical therapy: Evidence and practice, *ed 4, St. Louis, 2006, Mosby.*

the IMT device can be used via the ventilator tubing.[78] Increasing inspiratory muscle strength and endurance may then increase function in patients with respiratory failure and assist in weaning from mechanical ventilation.[76,77]

A number of studies have evaluated the effectiveness of IMT. Overall, these studies demonstrate that IMT can improve pulmonary function, increase MIP, and decrease wean time from mechanical ventilation.[71-79] However, although IMT appears to be a beneficial adjunct for patients receiving mechanical ventilation, heart rate and O_2 saturation should be monitored during treatment sessions. In clinical practice, protocols for IMT vary. A suggested protocol for performing IMT with a patient using a typical IMT device is provided in Box 26-4.

Several studies suggest that relaxation biofeedback therapy can decrease weaning times in patients receiving mechanical ventilation.[80-83] In addition, the functional and exercise training methods discussed previously may also improve a patient's sense of psychological well-being by providing proprioceptive, visual, and general sensory

BOX 26-4 — A Typical Method for Performing Inspiratory Muscle Training

1. Obtain baseline pulmonary function tests including MIP, MEP, FEV_1, FVC, and TV with ventilated patients and MIP alone in nonventilated patients.
2. Position the patient supine or sitting. If the patient is supine, elevate the head of the bed at least 45 degrees. Have the patient's legs and arms in a relaxed position.
3. Set the IMT at 50% of the participant's baseline MIP measurement.
4. If necessary, give a gentle quick stretch in an inward and upward direction to the participant's abdomen (level of umbilicus and upper chest) at the end of exhalation to facilitate inhalation.
5. Verbally encourage inhalation to help the patient overcome the resistance felt during inspiration, and exhale along with the patient to ensure as much air as possible is expelled from the lungs.
6. Instruct the patient to breathe in and out as normally as possible despite feeling some resistance when breathing in. They should increase their effort to overcome this resistance and then breathe out with usual force.
7. The patient should perform 4-6 sets of 8 repetitions, or stop sooner if fatigued.
8. Between each set the patient may rest and be put back on mechanical ventilation if necessary until the training begins again.
9. The RPE scale should be used to evaluate the amount of effort the patient experiences. 0 represents no effort required with breathing, 1 represents the least amount of effort needed to breathe and 10 represents the most amount of effort needed to breathe with the trainer. After each set, the patient should grade his or her effort on the RPE scale. If the patient's RPE is between 1 and 5, increase the resistance by 1-2 cm H_2O. If the rating is 6-8, do not change the amount of resistance. If the rating is 9-10, reduce the resistance by 1-2 cm H_2O.

MIP, Maximum inspiratory pressure; *MEP*, maximum expiratory pressure; *FEV_1*, forced expiratory volume in 1 second; *FVC*, forced vital capacity; *TV*, tidal volume; *IMT*, inspiratory muscle training; *RPE*, rating of perceived exertion.

stimulation.* Accelerated weaning from mechanical ventilation may improve the ICU experience for patients and their families, as well as for the rest of the health care team.

Behavioral Interventions. Behavioral, emotional, and psychological issues affect many patients with respiratory failure receiving mechanical ventilation. Individuals constrained to a bed with very little movement or stimulation who depend on a mechanical device for every breath often find this experience psychologically stressful, resulting in emotions and behaviors that range from fear and complacency to anger and hostility.[86] A recent study of patients' recollections of their ICU experience during prolonged mechanical ventilation found that most patients remembered the majority of their ICU stay and most notably remembered the ETT.[87] Most recollections were of moderately to extremely bothersome experiences, including pain, fear, anxiety, lack of sleep, feeling tense, inability to speak or communicate, lack of control, nightmares, and loneliness.

CASE STUDY 26-1

BRONCHIOLITIS OBLITERANS ORGANIZING PNEUMONIA

Patient History

DN, a 42-year-old woman, was admitted to the hospital with end-stage bronchiolitis obliterans organizing pneumonia (BOOP). On the same day, she underwent bilateral lung transplantation. In the immediate postoperative period, DN developed hypoxemic respiratory failure as a result of pneumonia and required mechanical ventilation. The patient has had BOOP for several years and has been experiencing progressively greater difficulty breathing and performing functional tasks. She has been hospitalized 10 times over the past year with the last 2 hospitalizations lasting approximately 3 weeks each. Her past medical history is also significant for hypertension, Cushing's syndrome caused by chronic steroid use, osteoporosis, and osteopenic fractures of her thoracic vertebrae. DN was referred to physical therapy on the fifth day after her lung transplantation surgery. Since the patient was not able to talk, most of the patient history was obtained from her medical chart.

Tests and Measures—Significant Findings
Musculoskeletal
- Muscle strength is at least 3/5 in all four extremities, except both hips are 2/5.

Cardiovascular/Pulmonary
- Heart rate: 93 bpm, respiratory rate: 23 breaths/min, BP: 146/97 mm Hg, O_2 saturation: 92%
- Ventilator settings: SIMV: 8 breaths/min, TV: 450 ml, FiO_2: 0.6
- ABG: pH: 7.45, Pco_2: 40 mm Hg, Po_2: 65 mm Hg, O_2 saturation: 93%, base excess: 4 mEq/L, HCO_3: 27.9
- Chest x-ray: Bibasilar pulmonary parenchymal infiltrates

Function
- Supine-to-sit with maximal assistance; turning side-to-side with maximal assistance; unable to stand; bed-to-chair with maximal assistance.
- Patient is dependent for all ADLs.

*References 45-58, 63-70, 84, 85.

Diagnosis

Preferred practice pattern 6F: Impaired ventilation and respiration/gas exchange associated with respiratory failure.

Interventions

Special Intervention Notes

- Vital signs must be continually monitored over the course of treatment to ensure the patient is not responding negatively.
- As prescribed by the physician, O_2 saturation equal to or greater than 90% on supplemental O_2 was required throughout all physical therapy sessions.
- After physical therapy sessions, the patient should be placed in positions to modify her WOB and to optimize cardiovascular function and drainage of retained pulmonary secretions.

Initial Interventions

- Leg strengthening exercises using resistance from elastic bands. Begin with 3 sets of 10 reps, gradually increasing repetitions.
- Mobility training should be incorporated, including progression of activity from supine to sitting on the edge of the bed. Patient should be encouraged to sit on the edge of the bed for at least 10 minutes and perform one or a combination of the following activities: Leg exercises, trunk control, unsupported sitting, and ADLs.
- DN should also begin attempts to stand with a walker and assistance on a daily basis.
- If initial intervention attempts are not successful, the patient may benefit from increased ventilatory support and supplemental O_2 to tolerate increased levels of activity.

Progressive Interventions

- IMT with behavioral biofeedback training. Behavioral biofeedback training should consist of a mirror placed to allow the patient to observe her chest and abdominal area move during inspiration and expiration to help with control of breathing.
- When tolerable, the patient should begin ambulating short distances without ventilator support.
- Goals of progression should be to focus on increasing gait distance to improve endurance.
- If the patient has met previous rehabilitation goals, upper extremity exercises may be added.

Role of the Physical Therapist Assistant

- What kinds of strength and/or endurance training exercises would be helpful for this patient?
- How would you determine if the patient is ready to increase exercise intensity?
- What warning signs should you watch for that indicate too much intensity?

Additional Information

For the full version of this case study, including detailed examination results, interventions, and outcomes, see the Evolve site that accompanies this book.

CHAPTER SUMMARY

The primary function of the respiratory system is to bring O_2 into the body and release CO_2. The respiratory system can be divided into the musculoskeletal pump system, the gas exchange unit, and its neural control centers. Respiratory failure is a state or condition in which the respiratory system fails to meet the body's needs for gas exchange. When respiratory failure occurs, arterial CO_2 concentration will increase and O_2 concentration will decrease. Many pathological conditions can cause respiratory failure, but the physiological mechanisms causing failure include (1) diffusion abnormalities, (2) hypoventilation, and (3) $\dot{V}{:}\dot{Q}$ mismatching.[36]

Respiratory failure can be classified as either type I (hypoxic) or type II (hypercapnic), depending on the primary blood gas abnormality. Individuals may live in chronic states of respiratory failure or may experience sudden acute bouts of failure. Medical management is generally supportive in nature (i.e., mechanical ventilation and/or supplemental O_2). This chapter focuses on rehabilitation intervention for patients receiving mechanical ventilation. These interventions can be applied to other individuals with respiratory failure.

Rehabilitation of the individual with respiratory failure requiring mechanical ventilation is an area in need of further investigation. A limited number of studies have examined the rehabilitation of such patients. The most evidence-based areas of rehabilitation for such patients, with clinically applicable results, are in the areas of IMT and behavioral feedback as adjunctive methods for weaning patients from mechanical ventilation. Patients weaning from mechanical ventilation who perform IMT appear to have improved breathing muscle strength and endurance and some measures of pulmonary function and most importantly, are able to wean from mechanical ventilation when previously they had failed. Behavioral feedback and biofeedback mechanisms also improve several measures of respiratory function and hasten weaning from mechanical ventilation. Other rehabilitation efforts discussed in this chapter include positioning and adjunctive techniques, as well as functional and exercise training.

ADDITIONAL RESOURCES

For links to these and additional web-based resources, see the Evolve site.

DeTurk W, Cahalin L: *Cardiovascular and pulmonary physical therapy: An evidence-based approach,* 2004, McGraw-Hill.

Irwin S, Tecklin JS (eds): *Cardiopulmonary physical therapy: A guide to practice,* ed 4, Philadelphia, 2004, Elsevier.

American Association for Respiratory Care

American Thoracic Society

Cardiovascular and Pulmonary Section of the American Physical Therapy Association

GLOSSARY

Alveolar perfusion: The amount of blood flow that comes in contact with the alveoli and participates in respiration.

Alveolar ventilation: The amount of air flow that comes in contact with the alveoli and participates in respiration.

Alveoli: The distal terminal air sacs in the lungs where gas exchange occurs.

Arterial–alveolar oxygen difference (P_{AO_2}–Pa_{O_2}): The difference between the partial pressure of O_2 in the alveoli and the partial pressure of O_2 in the arterial blood.

Atelectasis: A collapsed airway or section of the lung in which air cannot move through the airways and participate in gas exchange.

Compliance: A measure of the ease of expansion of the lungs and chest wall.

Conducting airways: Airways within the lungs that serve as a conduit for air to travel down to the alveoli. Because of the absence of alveoli, gas exchange does not occur in these airways. These are found in the upper airways from generation 0-16.

Dead space: Air within the lungs that does not participate in respiration.

Elasticity: The ability of an object to return to its original state after being deformed.

Hemoptysis: Expectoration of blood.

Hypercapnia: An increased level of CO_2 in the circulating blood.

Hypoxia: A decreased level of O_2 in the circulating blood.

Maximal voluntary ventilation (MVV): The most amount of air an individual can move in and out of the airways over 1 minute. It is determined by the maximum respiratory rate and vital capacity.

Minute ventilation (MV): The amount of air moved into or out of the lungs over 1 minute.

Pneumothorax: Air in the pleural cavity.

Pulmonary shunt: Blood flow moving through the lungs that does not participate in respiration.

Respiration: The process of gas exchange between the atmospheric air and the pulmonary capillary bed.

Respiratory airways: The airways in the tracheobronchial tree in which gas exchange may occur because of the presence of alveoli. These airways generally begin at generation 17.

Surfactant: Substance produced by the alveolar cells that reduces surface tension in the airways.

Tracheostomy: A surgical incision in the trachea through which an artificial airway may be placed.

Ventilation: Air flow through the airways.

Work of breathing (WOB): The energy cost of breathing.

Chapter 27

Lymphatic System Disorders

Ahmed Samir Elokda

OBJECTIVES

After reading this chapter, the reader will be able to:
1. Understand the anatomy and the physiology of the lymphatic system.
2. Discuss the risk factors for pathologies associated with the consequences of lymphedema.
3. Be familiar with common examination techniques for a patient with lymphedema.
4. Use evidence-based interventions for patients with lymphedema.

Rehabilitation clinicians treat patients with a variety of systemic disorders, including disorders of the **lymphatic system.** This chapter discusses the rehabilitation of patients with lymphatic disorders who fall into the *Guide to Physical Therapist Practice*[1] preferred practice pattern 6H: Impaired circulation and anthropometric dimensions associated with lymphatic system disorders. Through discussion of anatomy and physiology of the lymphatic system, common classifications of lymphatic system disorders, examination findings, and interventions for patients with lymphatic system disorders, this chapter helps practitioners understand lymphatic system disorders and provides them with the tools to effectively treat patients presenting with disorders of the lymphatic system.

Although the lymphatic system includes both a circulatory and an immune function, **lymphedema** (which is caused by dysfunction of the lymphatic circulatory system) is the major focus of this chapter.

It is estimated that 250 million persons worldwide have lymphedema.[2] **Filariasis,** a disease involving infestation of the lymphatics with filarial worms, is the most common cause of lymphedema worldwide. The World Health Organization (WHO) estimates that 120 million people, including 40 million in Africa and 700,000 in the Americas, have lymphatic filariasis.[3] In the United States, however, lymphedema is usually iatrogenic and results from radiation and/or surgery used to treat breast cancer.[2] Among this population, 10% to 40% develop some degree of ipsilateral upper extremity lymphedema.[2]

> ### ◎ *Clinical Pearl*
> Radical mastectomy and modified radical mastectomy, both of which are treatments for breast cancer and involve removal of lymph nodes, are associated with the development of lymphedema.

Although lymphedema rarely impacts life expectancy, except when it affects the small intestine, if untreated or uncontrolled, it can impair quality of life by reducing mobility and activity and by predisposing the individual to infection.[4] Lymphedema can affect activities of daily living, recreation, and work, and it is estimated that 30% of people with lymphedema of the upper extremity have reduced shoulder and/or arm function.[5-8]

THE LYMPHATIC CIRCULATORY SYSTEM

The lymphatic system has two main functions. It transports **lymph** from the periphery to the venous system to maintain fluid balance, and it serves an immune function, helping to protect the body from infection. The lymphatic system is made up of lymph (i.e., lymphatic fluid), **lymphatic vessels, lymph nodes,** and the lymphatic organs: The spleen, thymus, and tonsils (Fig. 27-1).[9]

Lymph is a fluid that originates from the blood plasma and enters the capillaries from the arteries. When blood enters the capillaries, some of the intercellular fluid diffuses out of the blood circulation. Approximately 90% of

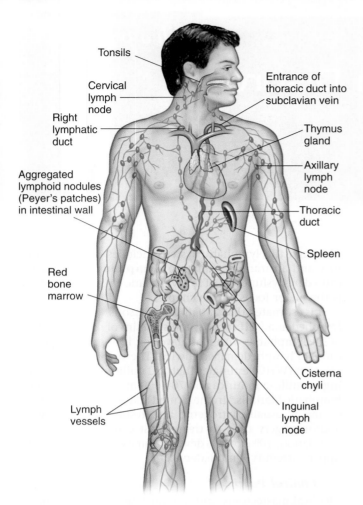

Tonsils

Cervical lymph node

Right lymphatic duct

Aggregated lymphoid nodules (Peyer's patches) in intestinal wall

Red bone marrow

Lymph vessels

Entrance of thoracic duct into subclavian vein

Thymus gland

Axillary lymph node

Thoracic duct

Spleen

Cisterna chyli

Inguinal lymph node

FIG. 27-1 The lymphatic system. *From Patton KT, Thibodeau GA:* Anatomy and physiology, *ed 7, St. Louis, 2010, Mosby.*

this fluid is reabsorbed by the venous system in the venous leg of the capillary loop. The remaining approximately 10% contains macromolecular proteins that cannot be reabsorbed by the venous system. This fluid and the proteins are returned to the circulation by the lymphatic system in the form of lymph.[9]

Lymph primarily contains proteins, immune cells, fat (which is present in intestinal lymph also known as **chyle**), and waste products. Lymph protects the body from foreign organisms and other materials by removing them from the interstitial fluid. Lymph tissue (the nodes and organs) contains macrophages, B- and T-lymphocytes, plasma cells, and reticular cells. Substances typically removed via lymph and the lymphatic system include excess interstitial fluid and normal by-products of cellular processes.[9,10]

Lymph flows through lymph-specific capillaries that run through both superficial and deep tissues. Protein-rich lymph collects at lymph nodes that filter and produce components of lymph. The nodes produce lymphocytes, particularly when an immune reaction is required, and they regulate the protein content of lymph. The average person has about 650 lymph nodes located in clusters or

chains around the lymphatic vessels (see Fig. 27-1). The size of lymph nodes can vary widely, from a few millimeters to 1 to 2 cm in diameter in their normal state and up to 8 cm in diameter, or more, when activated or diseased.[9]

Lymph moves through the body powered by intrinsic and extrinsic pumping mechanisms. Intrinsic pumping is provided by spontaneous contraction of lymphatic vessels. If this intrinsic pump fails, lymphatic circulation depends on extrinsic pumping by skeletal muscles to compress the lymphatic vessels. Arterial pulsations, respiration, and massage may also contribute in a small way to lymph propulsion.[10] The lymphatic circulation is a one-way transport mechanism that moves fluid from the interstitium to the blood circulatory system.[11]

The spleen and thymus have supportive immune functions. The spleen produces some lymphocytes and also destroys defective red blood cells and blood-borne pathogens. The thymus produces genetically imprinted T-lymphocytes prenatally until early adulthood. These lymphocytes participate in the humoral immune response. Collectors at the base of the tonsils collect lymphatic fluid from the head and neck.[9,12]

ANATOMY OF THE LYMPHATIC CIRCULATORY SYSTEM

The lymphatic circulatory system is made up of the lymphatic vessels and the lymph nodes. The vessels are organized into a superficial system (also known as *subcutaneous* or *epifascial*) and a deep system. The superficial system drains the skin and subcutaneous tissue, and the deep system drains the muscles, bones, joints, and viscera. Perforating vessels connect the two systems and can conduct lymph from the deep system to the superficial system.[9,13,14]

The superficial lymphatic circulatory system begins distally with very narrow lymphatic capillaries that have no valves. All the lymphatic vessels beyond the capillaries have valves to prevent fluid backflow. The capillaries empty into medium-sized precollector vessels. The precollectors flow into larger diameter collector vessels, which divide into several branches and transport lymph to regional lymph nodes. From the nodes, the lymph enters even larger diameter vessels, the lymphatic trunks.[9]

The deep lymphatic vessels run deep to the fascia, parallel to the major arteries and accompanying veins, and drain the muscles, bones, joints, and viscera of the entire body, except for the upper right quadrant and face. These vessels drain into deep lymph collectors that are similar to the superficial collectors, and these deep collectors then drain to lymph nodes and join with fluid from the superficial system to drain into the lymphatic trunks.[9,13,14] If the vessels or nodes of the deeper circulation are removed, all of the fluid may be forced to travel in the superficial circulation. This can lead to congestion, fluid extravasation, and edema.[9]

The lymph from the lower portion of the body collects in a dilated vessel in the lumbar region of the abdominal cavity, the cisterna chyli. The cisterna chyli extends for about 6 cm just to the right of the abdominal aorta, and

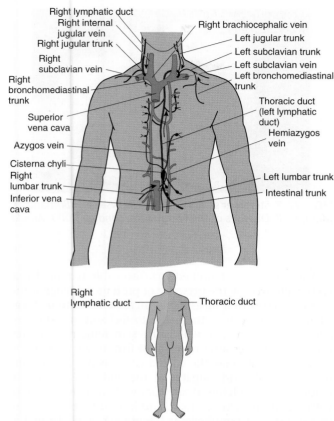

FIG. 27-2 Lymph drainage through the thoracic duct and the right lymphatic duct. *From Casley-Smith JR, Casley-Smith JR: Modern treatment for lymphoedema, ed 5, Adelaide, Australia, 1997, Lymphoedema Association of Australia.*

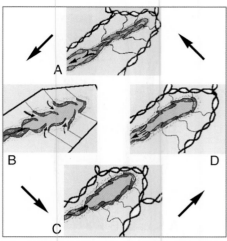

FIG. 27-3 Lymph formation. **A,** The initial lymph vessel is empty and collapsed. **B,** Filling phase. **C,** The initial lymph vessel is filled with lymph. **D,** The pressure inside the initial lymph vessels opens the valve to the precollector and thus the lymph flows toward the precollector. *From Földi M, Földi E, Kubik S:* Lehrbuch der Lymphologie, *ed 6, München, 2006, Urban & Fischer.*

at the level of the twelfth thoracic vertebra, it narrows to become the thoracic duct. Lymph from the rest of the body, except for the upper right quadrant, drains into the thoracic duct more cranially. The thoracic duct empties into the base of the left subclavian vein to be mixed with blood. Lymph from the lymphatic vessels in the upper right quadrant of the body empties into the right lymphatic duct and then into the base of the right subclavian vein (Fig. 27-2).

PHYSIOLOGY OF LYMPH TRANSPORT

The primary task of the lymphatic system is to transport interstitial fluid and its components from the interstitium back to the venous system. The endothelial cells that make up the lymphatic capillaries overlap to form "swinging flaps" (Fig. 27-3). When the pressure of fluid in the interstitium exceeds the pressure inside the capillaries, the flaps open and fluid moves into the lymphatic capillaries. This is known as the *filling phase*.[15] When the pressure in the capillaries equals the interstitial pressure, the swinging flaps close and the lymphatic capillaries open to the precollectors, allowing lymph to flow into them. This is known as the *emptying phase*.[15] Once the protein-rich lymph is in the precollectors, intrinsic and extrinsic pumps propel the lymph fluid to its final destination, the venous circulatory system.

PATHOLOGY

When functioning properly, anatomically and physiologically, the lymphatic circulatory system can accommodate a certain degree of variability in the amount of interstitial fluids and large molecular weight substances it transports from the periphery to the central venous system. If the lymphatic system becomes overloaded, either by an excessive increase in load or more commonly because of damage that limits its ability to accommodate, fluids and other substances may accumulate in the interstitium causing swelling known as *lymphedema*. As proteins in the accumulated fluid degrade, chronic inflammation and cell proliferation may then occur.

LYMPHEDEMA

Lymphedema is a symptom of lymphatic transport malfunction that occurs when the lymphatic load exceeds the transport capacity of the lymphatic circulatory system. Lymphedema presents clinically with swelling of the soft tissues because of accumulation of protein-rich fluid.

> **◎ Clinical Pearl**
>
> Lymphedema occurs when the lymphatic load exceeds the carrying capacity of the lymphatic circulation.

Once it occurs, lymphedema often progresses because the initial buildup of macromolecules in the interstitium causes an increase in interstitial osmotic pressure that "pulls" yet more fluid out of the vessels into the interstitium. The prolonged presence of swelling and proteins leads to inflammation and fibrosis and provides a suitable medium for repeated local infection of the lymph vessels **(lymphangitis)** and the surrounding soft tissues **(cellulitis).** Persistent dilatation of the lymphatics, in addition to incompetent valves, leads to further stagnation

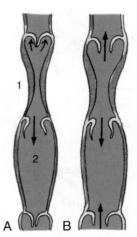

FIG. 27-4 Structure and function of the valve segments. **A,** Normal function. **B,** Dilated lymph vessel with valvular insufficiency and reflux. *1,* Contracted segment (emptying phase). *2,* Relaxed segment (filling phase). *From Földi M, Földi E, Kubik S: Lehrbuch der Lymphologie, ed 6, München, 2006, Urban & Fischer.*

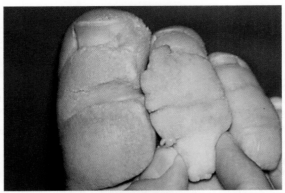

FIG. 27-5 Stemmer's sign. *From Browse N, Burnand K, Mortimer P: Diseases of the lymphatics, London, 2003, Arnold.*

(Fig. 27-4). Lymphedema most commonly occurs in the extremities but can also occur in the face, neck, abdomen, and genitalia.

Lymphedema may be classified according to its etiology as primary (also known as *idiopathic*) or secondary.[4]

Primary Lymphedema. Primary lymphedema is a benign condition that is generally caused by malformation of the lymph vessels and/or lymph nodes. Primary lymphedema may be congenital (present at birth) or may develop later in life. Primary lymphedema may develop later in life when local inflammation from a musculoskeletal injury, local infection, or insect bite causes an increase in fluid load in a person with a congenital anatomical predisposition. However, lymphedema that develops in adulthood is more likely to be secondary lymphedema.

Secondary Lymphedema. Secondary lymphedema is lymphedema that occurs in the absence of an anatomical malformation. Secondary lymphedema may develop at any age and may be caused by a malignant tumor obstructing lymph flow, a traumatic injury such as a fracture or injury to tissue surrounding a normal lymphatic flow, or by filariasis (filarial worm infestation that damages the lymph nodes or lymphatic vessels). Iatrogenic lymphedema may also occur as the result of medical interventions, such as radiation therapy or lymph node removal, that damage the lymphatic circulation while treating cancer, particularly breast cancer.[4]

Stages of Lymphedema. Untreated, both primary and secondary lymphedema progress through the following stages.

Stage 0. Stage 0 (latency/subclinical stage) lymphedema is characterized by reduction of the normal lymph transport capacity. During this stage, there is approximately 30% more fluid in the interstitium than normal and the patient may feel discomfort, heaviness, and aching in the affected limb, but there is no measurable increase in volume.

Stage I. Stage I lymphedema (reversible lymphedema) is characterized by the presence of protein-rich edema and is associated with a measurable increase in volume. Stage I lymphedema causes the tissue to feel soft and doughy, and pitting edema, in which the skin remains indented for a few minutes after removal of firm finger pressure, is present. At this stage the edema is reversible. The edema may be visible and palpable at the end of a day, but it reduces or completely disappears with rest overnight or with elevation. Activity, heat, and humidity may cause or increase stage I lymphedema. Stemmer's sign, defined as the inability to lift the thickened cutaneous folds at the dorsum of the toes or fingers, is negative or borderline positive in stage I lymphedema (Fig. 27-5).[16]

Stage II. Stage II lymphedema (spontaneously irreversible lymphedema) presents with increased volume, replacement of some of the protein-rich lymphatic fluid with tissue fibrosis, and a positive Stemmer's sign. The skin may thicken or break down, and there is a greater risk of recurrent infection because the lymph does not move. Pitting is also much more difficult to induce than with the stage I lymphedema because the tissue is stiffer and filled with more lymph fluid and interstitial fibrosis.[16]

Stage III. Stage III lymphedema (lymphostatic elephantiasis) is characterized by **subcutaneous fibrosclerosis** (hardening of the soft tissues under the skin) and severe skin alterations, including **hyperkeratosis** (a thickening of the outer layer of the skin) and papillomatosis (the development of numerous papillomas). In most but not all cases, there is more swelling in stage III lymphedema than in stage II.[16,17] Since grading is based on pathological and anatomical factors, a large volume does not necessarily imply a higher stage of lymphedema.

The stages of lymphedema are sequential, but their duration can vary and lymphedema may not progress through all the stages. Typically, tissue changes seen as lymphedema progresses or becomes more chronic include proliferation of connective tissue, increased production of collagen fibers, an increase in fatty deposits in the affected limb, and fibrotic changes.[15] Secondary skin changes can also occur in both primary and secondary lymphedema and may include development of cellulitis, hyperkeratosis, and fungal infections (Fig. 27-6).

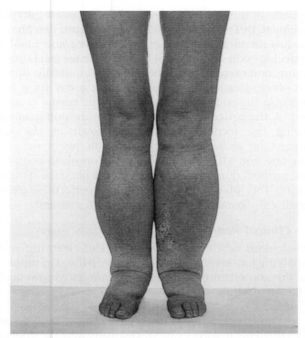

FIG. 27-6 Edema of both lower legs with early skin thickening and hyperkeratosis. *From Browse N, Burnand K, Mortimer P: Diseases of the lymphatics, London, 2003, Arnold.*

TYPICAL EXAMINATION FINDINGS

PATIENT HISTORY

The history for any patient with lymphedema covers patient demographics, including age, sex, and country or countries of residence; a complete medical history, including any history of cancer, peripheral vascular, thyroid, renal, or cardiac disease, as well as any history of local surgery or trauma; the progression, nature, and severity of the edema; and the nature and degree of functional limitations caused by the lymphedema, as well as the nature and effectiveness of any compensation or intervention the patient has tried to reduce symptoms and optimize function.

SYSTEMS REVIEW

The systems review is used to target areas requiring further examination and to define areas that may cause complications or indicate a need for precautions during the examination and intervention processes. Chapter 1 includes details of the systems review.

TESTS AND MEASURES

Musculoskeletal

Anthropometric Characteristics. Edema is the most characteristic sign of lymphedema. Edema is generally measured by water displacement using a volumeter or through girth or circumferential measures with a flexible tape measure.[18] Results of these tests should be compared with the uninvolved limb and over time. Girth measurements should be taken at consistent locations relative to anatomical landmarks for valid comparison.

Range of Motion. Range of motion (ROM) should be checked in all major joints in the affected and contralateral limb.

Muscle Performance. Since lymphedema can lead to disuse and thus generalized reduced strength in an affected limb, strength for movements in the primary planes of motion in the affected and contralateral limb should be estimated using manual muscle tests.

Neuromuscular

Pain. If the patient reports the presence of pain, the severity, nature, and location, as well as easing and aggravating factors, should be determined (see Chapter 22 for pain measurement tools).

Sensory Integrity. Should the patient report sensory changes, including numbness or tingling, or if they have a secondary medical diagnosis associated with sensory changes, such as diabetes or peripheral vascular disease, sensory testing is also performed.

Integumentary. The skin in the affected area is visually inspected and palpated. During the early stages of lymphedema the skin may thicken, obscuring milder swelling. With progression of lymphedema the skin develops creases, horny scale, and hyperkeratosis and later, papillomas and then fibrosis.

Function. When lymphedema affecting the lower extremity alters ROM and strength, gait and balance may also be affected and are therefore examined.

INTERVENTION

Interventions for patients with lymphedema focus on education and procedures to facilitate proximal flow of lymphatic fluid. Recommended procedural interventions include a variety of manual techniques, compression approaches, and exercise. Since all lymph fluid that returns from the interstitium ultimately enters the cardiovascular circulatory system, before initiating any lymphedema treatment the potential consequences to the cardiopulmonary system if lymphatic drainage is successful should be considered. Patients with known or suspected cardiac involvement are at greatest risk for adverse effects of treatment because any lymphatic fluid that may be removed from an edematous limb or body part will initially increase cardiac load. Furthermore, since the kidneys help to remove excess fluid from the circulatory system, in patients with reduced renal function, the additional circulatory load may overload the kidneys. If therapy is to be initiated, the patient's condition must be monitored for any untoward side effects that may suggest cardiac or renal overload. Should any new symptoms, particularly shortness of breath, chest pain, or diaphoresis, or changes in laboratory values (increased blood urea nitrogen or creatinine), indicating worsening kidney function, occur during treatment, the therapy should be immediately discontinued and the supervising physical therapist and the patient's physician should be notified. Further interventions should be postponed until the patient is evaluated and cleared by the physician and physical therapist for further treatment.

Several other medical conditions are contraindications to certain components of lymphedema therapy. Patients with an infection, a blood clot, or a malignancy in the involved limb should not receive compression or manual techniques because these may spread the problem through the circulatory system to other areas, most notably the heart and lungs.

EDUCATION

Patients with lymphedema are at risk for a worsening of their condition and for a number of complications, particularly infection. Therefore patients with lymphedema should be instructed to observe the following precautions[19] throughout their lifetime:

- No blood pressure measurements on the involved extremity.
- No needle sticks or blood draws on the involved extremity.
- Immediately treat all wounds on the affected limb, no matter how small (e.g., insect bites, paper cuts, or hangnail).
- Protect the hands and feet of the involved extremities from mechanical trauma and burns at all times.
- Avoid constricting jewelry and clothing.
- Avoid overheating local body parts or a rise in core body temperature.
- Avoid lifting heavy objects; no heavy handbags with over-the-shoulder straps.

Education may be provided verbally or in the form of written materials, including pamphlets or brochures.

PROCEDURES

The treatment of lymphedema can be difficult, costly, and time consuming and is generally best performed by a multidisciplinary team.[20-24] Procedures for the management of lymphedema include surgical and pharmacological interventions, as well as manual procedures typically performed by a rehabilitation professional.

Surgical Interventions. There are two general types of surgery for lymphedema, debulking (reduction surgery), which involves removing excess fluid and tissues, and physiological procedures that attempt to improve lymphatic circulation. Evidence indicates that debulking procedures are associated with significant adverse effects, including infection and poor wound healing, and these are therefore rarely performed.[25,26] Although physiological procedures are not associated with such adverse effects, their effectiveness is also limited.

Pharmacological Interventions. A number of pharmacological interventions have been suggested as adjunctive measures for the management of lymphedema, but none have been consistently safe and effective. Antibiotics are often used to treat acute and chronic infections associated with lymphedema, including cellulitis and lymphangitis.

Manual Interventions. Although a number of manual therapy approaches have been recommended for the treatment of lymphedema, the approach with the greatest support at this time is complete decongestive physical therapy (CDPT). This approach is divided into two phases. The first phase, also known as the *intensive phase*, involves meticulous skin care, manual lymph drainage (MLD), bandaging, and exercises with the bandage on. Ideally, during this phase, treatment is provided twice a day for 4 to 6 weeks. At the end of the phase, when the edema is under control, the patient is fitted with a compression garment. During the second phase, also known as the *self-management phase*, the patient performs his or her own skin care and MLD and applies a custom-sized compression garment during the day and wears a bandage at night. During this phase, the patient may perform exercises wearing the bandage or the compression garment.

◎ *Clinical Pearl*

Meticulous skin care, including careful cleansing and applying lotions and emollients to keep the skin supple, is the cornerstone of complete decongestive physical therapy (CDPT).

Meticulous skin care is the cornerstone of both phases of CDPT. This involves careful cleansing and the application of low-pH lotions and emollients to keep the skin supple.[27-29] Careful drying, particularly in areas of creases, is also essential to avoid topical fungal and bacterial overgrowth and infection.[30-34]

MLD is a generic term for the massage used to reduce lymphedema. MLD massage is intended to increase the movement of lymph and interstitial fluid. The basic hand positions used for MLD are based on the anatomy and function of the lymphatic system. The approach involves combining a number of strokes, described as stationary circles, pumping, scooping, and rotary strokes. Each stroke consists of a working (stretching) and resting phase, in which the pressure smoothly increases and decreases, respectively. Each stroke lasts at least 1 second and is repeated 5 to 7 times, and all strokes are applied in the direction of lymph flow. When there is congestion or obstruction caused by surgery, trauma, or radiation, strokes are applied toward the intact lymphatic pathways. The most proximal areas, which are those closest to the venous angle in which the lymphatics enter the venous system, should be treated first to clear the way for drainage from more distal areas. Thus, when treating lymphedema in the extremities, treatment begins proximally and continues distally. In general, each session lasts 40 to 90 minutes. MLD should not be performed in patients with acute kidney infections or renal failure, those with edema caused by heart failure, those with deep venous thrombosis (DVT), or pregnant women.

◎ *Clinical Pearl*

The pressure exerted during manual lymph drainage (MLD) is very light to avoid compressing and closing off the lymphatic channels.

Studies evaluating the effectiveness of MLD on patients with secondary lymphedema caused by breast cancer have found that MLD significantly reduces excess limb volume, as well as pain, discomfort, heaviness, fullness, and hardness of the affected limb. MLD is most effective when used in conjunction with compression bandaging and garments, exercise, and skin care. Unfortunately, most of the research on MLD is of low quality (rated level III or lower). Additional higher quality studies are needed to provide strong evidence-based recommendations for treatment.

Compression. Compression is applied by surrounding a limb with a device that can apply inwardly-directed pressure. Compression may be applied by a pneumatic pump, bandaging, or a garment.

Pneumatic Compression Pumping. A variety of pneumatic devices may be used to apply compression to treat extremity lymphedema.[35] A number of studies show that pneumatic compression pumping at low inflation pressures, compression times, and treatment durations can improve clinical outcomes, reducing girth and discomfort and improving function. The recommended treatment parameters for pneumatic compression for treatment of lymphedema are 30 seconds of compression followed by a 5-second rest period for the upper extremity or a 10-second rest period for the lower extremity, with pressure of 45 mm Hg for the upper extremity, 60 mm Hg for the lower extremity during compression, and at or near 0 mm Hg during the rest period to allow the vessels to refill. Multichambered, sequentially inflating sleeves that allow pumping to progress from distal to proximal may be more effective than single-chamber sleeves. Despite some favorable evidence, the use of pneumatic compression for the treatment of lymphedema is controversial, with some authors claiming that it is ineffective and that it worsens or accelerates the fibrosis associated with lymphedema.[36-38]

Treatment sessions should initially last 20 minutes, and patients should be closely monitored for any adverse reactions, particularly numbness or tingling caused by compression of sensory nerves or systemic side effects caused by fluid overload. If no complications arise, treatment duration may be increased by 10 minutes per day up to a maximum of 1 hour.[39] A second session may be added if patient improvement continues.[39]

There are a number of precautions and contraindications for pneumatic compression pumping. Precautions to treatment are the following:

- Decreased sensation in the proposed treatment area.
- Pain, redness, numbness, or tingling in the extremity after treatment.
- Lymphatic vessel dilation or becoming visible during or after treatment.
- Increase in swelling proximal to the sleeve.
- Changes in skin texture at the base of the limb.

If any of these occur during treatment, the treatment should be stopped and the supervising therapist consulted.

Contraindications to pneumatic compression therapy are as follows[37,40,41]:

- Brachial plexus lesions.
- Radical breast surgery with radiation.
- Bilateral mastectomy.
- After pelvic surgery, if proximal portions of lower extremities have begun to swell.

- Primary lymphedema.
- Swelling present in abdomen or genitalia.
- Lymphatic vessel dilated or visible before treatment.
- Lower extremity ankle-brachial index (ABI) of <0.8 (see Chapter 29).
- Suspected DVT in the limb.
- Infection in the limb.
- Malignancy in the limb or proximal to the limb to be treated.
- Ongoing radiation therapy for active cancer in the limb or surrounding area.
- Renal or cardiac insufficiency.
- Uncontrolled hypertension.

Compressive Bandaging. Compressive bandaging can reduce lymphedema and maintain reductions in edema achieved by other methods. Compressive bandaging for lymphedema should be applied using short-stretch bandage materials that generate low resting pressures and high working pressures. Resting pressure is the constant pressure exerted by a bandage when the individual is at rest and not moving. The more elastic a bandage is and the more initial tension applied to it, the more resting pressure it exerts. Working pressure is the pressure that is exerted when muscles inside a compressive bandage attempt to expand as a result of active contraction. This active muscle contraction increases the pressure in the tissue if the tissue is wrapped by a bandage. The more rigid (less compliant) the bandage material is, the more working pressure will develop in response to an active muscle contraction.

The amount of pressure exerted by a compression bandage is generally expressed in millimeters of mercury (mm Hg). Compression bandages should be applied so that they create a pressure gradient, with more compression distally than proximally to facilitate movement of fluid proximally. The bandage should be applied concentrically (Fig 27-7), with equal tension, and overlapping and slipping bandages should be avoided.

◎ *Clinical Pearl*

Compression bandages should be applied so that they create a pressure gradient, with more compression distally than proximally.

Clinically, one type of bandage or multiple layers of different types of bandages may be used. Multilayer bandaging takes advantage of the differing properties of different types of bandages, with some exerting more resting pressure and others exerting more working pressure. Several layers of nonextensible bandages generate higher working pressures while maintaining lower resting pressures.[41] Multilayer bandaging may reverse skin changes, stop lymphorrhea (the light amber-colored fluid that drains from open skin areas), and soften underlying fibrosis; however, its clinical efficacy has not been demonstrated in randomized controlled trials.[41]

Compression Garments. Compression garments may also be used for compression therapy and have been shown to effectively reduce lymphedema.[40,42] Garments are available for various body parts, including the legs,

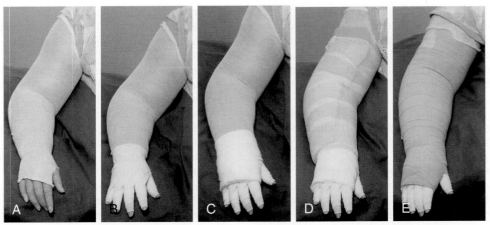

FIG. 27-7 Concentrically applied bandage. *From Browse N, Burnand K, Mortimer P:* Diseases of the lymphatics, *London, 2003, Arnold.*

arms, and trunk, and are available in different sizes and amounts of compression. Compression garments may be ready-made or custom-fit. The therapist must follow manufacturer recommendations for measuring patients for custom-fit garments to ensure proper fit and effective treatment.

The lightest compression garment is the surgical antiembolism stocking. This garment provides up to 17 mm Hg of compression and is only suitable for prevention of thromboses or emboli in immobile patients and not for the treatment of lymphedema.[43] Compression stockings suitable for the treatment of edema are available in four classes of compression and can be used in combination to exert even more pressure. Although recommendations vary, in general, 30 mm Hg of compression is appropriate for the upper extremity and 80 mm Hg is appropriate for the lower extremity.[20,36,42,44-46] The compression class, degree of compression, pressure provided, and indications for use for different compression garments are described in Table 27-1.

EXERCISE

Exercise is another essential component of CDPT. Exercise is thought to reduce lymphedema because skeletal muscle contraction increases pressure around the lymphatics, helping to push fluid proximally.[47] Exercise may also increase lymph vessel contraction, improve lymph circulation, enhance fluid transport by the thoracic duct by increasing deep breathing, and help normalize interstitial hydrostatic pressure.[28,48-52] Furthermore, exercise may help reduce ROM restrictions and weakness caused by disuse of the involved extremity.[47] Exercises of the involved extremity should be performed while wearing compressive bandaging or garments. It is suggested that limitations to mobility and muscular weakness be treated along with the lymphedema so the entire muscle chain and all associated joints can recover and be incorporated into the regimen of decongestive exercise therapy. Exercise for the patient with lymphedema should include a warm-up of stretching followed by strengthening, endurance, and coordination activities, as well as breathing exercises.[24,41,51,53,54]

TABLE 27-1	Compression Garments	
Compression Class	Degree of Compression	Pressure Provided
Antiembolism	Very light	Up to 17 mm Hg
1	Light	18-21 mm Hg
2	Medium	23-32 mm Hg
3	Strong	34-46 mm Hg
4	Very strong	>49 mm Hg

From Földi M, Földi E, Kubik S: *Lehrbuch der Lymphologie,* ed 6, München, 2006, Urban & Fischer.

CASE STUDY 27-1

EARLY STAGE I SECONDARY LYMPHEDEMA

Patient History

JS is a 65-year-old obese man who was referred to outpatient cardiac rehabilitation 3 weeks after a 3-vessel coronary artery bypass graft (CABG). His other medical problems include peripheral vascular disease, insulin-dependent diabetes mellitus, hypercholesterolemia, hyperlipidemia, and hypertension. His surgical history includes a femoral-popliteal bypass of the right lower extremity 4 months ago. The patient reported that he recently developed swelling of the lower extremities, abdomen, and scrotum. The lower extremity edema reduced slightly with elevation but returned rapidly after the legs were lowered. JS also has a nonhealing wound on the medial aspect of his left lower leg that has been present for more than 3 years and that did not improve with conventional wound care. Since JS does not have heart failure, his physician suspected that his swelling was caused by secondary lymphedema, as a result of removal of his saphenous vein and thus lymphatic overload, and referred him to a therapist for conservative management.

Tests and Measures—Significant Findings

Musculoskeletal
- JS is 5 feet 9 inches tall and weighs 260 lb.
- Edema was present in both legs. Girth was 15 inches around both ankles and 25 inches around both knees. Stemmer's sign was positive bilaterally.
- JS has limited active and passive ROM at the knees and ankles.

Neuromuscular
- Pain level is 5/10 in his lower extremities that reduced with rest and elevation.

Cardiovascular/Pulmonary
- Heart rate is 68 bpm and blood pressure is 160/90 mm Hg.
- Capillary refill at the nail beds of the toes and pedal pulses were minimally reduced.

Integumentary
- Pitting was easy to induce at the distal lower extremities. The skin on both legs appeared tight and shiny.
- Wound on the medial aspect of the left lower leg.
- The chest and leg incisions were clean with mild serosanguineous fluid draining from the leg incision.

Function
- JS's abdominal, scrotal, and lower extremity edema causes difficulty with donning clothes, toileting, and sitting.
- JS uses a straight cane when walking.

Diagnosis
Preferred practice pattern 6H: Impaired circulation and anthropometric dimensions associated with lymphatic system disorders.

Interventions
- Complete decongestive physical therapy treatment, including meticulous skin care, manual lymphatic drainage, compression bandaging, and active ROM exercises for his lower extremities with his legs elevated.
- Between therapy sessions the patient should bandage himself independently and perform a home exercise program.
- When girth measurements plateau, the patient should be measured for a full pantyhose compression garment with open toes for daytime wear and be instructed to bandage at night.
- He should also be instructed to elevate his legs when not ambulatory and to perform active ROM exercises when sitting for more than 20 minutes.

Role of the Physical Therapist Assistant
- What is the purpose of bandaging in this patient? How long is it likely he will need to keep wearing the bandages?
- What is the purpose of exercise in this patient? Describe three home exercises for him.
- How would you determine if the patient is ready to increase exercise intensity?
- How would you know if exercise intensity should be decreased?

Additional Information
For the full version of this case study, including detailed examination results, interventions, and outcomes, see the Evolve site that accompanies this book.

CHAPTER SUMMARY
This chapter focuses on the management of lymphatic system circulatory disorders. In North America and Europe, lymphatic system circulatory disorders are usually the result of lymph node or vessel damage or removal that occurs as a side effect of medical interventions for cancer. Lymph node or vessel damage can result in lymphedema, which is characterized by swelling of the extremity and risk for skin breakdown and infection, as well as soft tissue fibrosis. Optimal rehabilitation interventions for lymphedema involve an integrated in-clinic and home program of meticulous skin care, manual lymphatic drainage (MLD), compression, and exercise, in conjunction with patient education for ongoing management of this generally life-long disorder.

ADDITIONAL RESOURCES
For links to these and additional web-based resources, see the Evolve site.

The Lymphatic Research Foundation
British Lymphology Society
The Susan G. Komen Breast Cancer Foundation
National Breast Cancer Coalition

GLOSSARY
Cellulitis: Diffuse acute inflammation of the skin and subcutaneous tissue.

Chyle: The cloudy liquid product of digestion taken up by the small intestine, consisting mostly of emulsified fat. Chyle passes from the small intestine to the lymphatic system for transport to the venous circulation.

Filariasis: Disease caused by the presence of parasitic worms that occlude the lymphatic channels.

Hyperkeratosis: A condition marked by thickening of the outer layer of the skin that can result from normal use, chronic inflammation, or genetic disorders.

Lymph: The fluid that is collected from tissue throughout the body and that moves through the lymphatic vessels. Most of the cells in lymph are lymphocytes.

Lymph nodes: Small bean-shaped bodies located along the course of lymphatic vessels. Lymph nodes produce lymphocytes and monocytes. They act as filters keeping particulate matter, such as bacteria, from gaining entrance into the bloodstream.

Lymphangiography (lymphography): The x-ray examination of lymph glands and lymphatic vessels after an injection of contrast medium.

Lymphangitis: Inflammation of one or more lymphatic vessels.

Lymphatic system: The tissues and organs (including the bone marrow, spleen, thymus, and lymph nodes) that produce and store cells that fight infection and the network of vessels that carry lymph.

Lymphatic vessels: A body-wide network of channels that transports lymph to the immune organs and into the bloodstream.

Lymphedema: A disorder characterized by swelling caused by accumulation of lymph in soft tissues.

Subcutaneous fibrosclerosis: Hardening below the skin caused by abnormal formation of fibrous tissue.

Chapter 28

Tissue Healing and Pressure Ulcers

Rose Little Hamm

OBJECTIVES

After studying this chapter, the reader will be able to:
1. Discuss causative factors and risk factors for pressure ulcers.
2. Identify tissue and cellular changes that occur in pressure ulcers.
3. Identify patients at risk for developing pressure ulcers.
4. Understand the use of assessment and wound screening scales.
5. Be familiar with common examination techniques for patients with pressure ulcers.
6. Be familiar with staging of pressure ulcers according to stage and/or tissue involvement.
7. Implement effective interventions for prevention and treatment of pressure ulcers.

Impaired integumentary integrity resulting in acute and chronic pressure ulcers (PUs) is a concern for patients of all ages. A PU is "any lesion caused by unrelieved pressure resulting in damage of underlying tissue."[1] Rehabilitation professionals can help resolve and prevent PUs through patient mobilization, positioning, and family and caregiver education.

This chapter discusses the general management of chronic wounds, with a focus on PUs. This chapter provides information that applies to wounds in general and to PUs in particular. Chapters 29 to 31 refer to this chapter for general wound management.

EPIDEMIOLOGY

The **prevalence** and **incidence** of PUs depend on the patient population and the medical setting, ranging from as low as 0.29% in children to as high as 44% in adults who sustain spinal cord injuries (SCIs) during childhood.[2-11] The financial implications of PUs for the medical system are staggering and worsening as the median age of the population increases. In addition to the high financial cost of PU care, PUs can also have detrimental psychological and social effects for both patients and their families. PUs can cause pain, change in body image, patient and family stress, loss of work days, loss of functional mobility, and reduced ability to provide self-care.[12-14]

NATIONAL ORGANIZATIONS

The two major organizations in the United States advocating for research on, prevention of, treatment for, and education about PUs are the National Pressure Ulcer Advisory Panel (NPUAP) and the Agency for Health Care Policy Research (AHCPR), now known as the *Agency for Healthcare Research and Quality* (AHRQ). The NPUAP is an independent, nonprofit professional organization composed of a panel of experts whose mission is to "improve patient outcomes in PU prevention and management through education, public policy, and research."[15] The AHCPR is the primary Federal Agency charged with "enhancing the quality, appropriateness, and effectiveness of health care services."[1] The AHCPR supports research for improving the quality of health care, reducing medical costs, and broadening access to essential services.[16] In 1994, with seven NPUAP members contributing to the effort, the AHCPR published guidelines for the prevention and treatment of PUs.[1,17] These publications established the standards for PU wound description, evaluation, prevention, and medical treatment and also rated the strength of the evidence for the effectiveness of different wound care

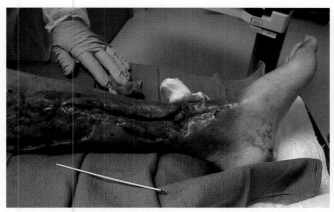

FIG. 28-1 A wound in the hemostasis phase of healing.

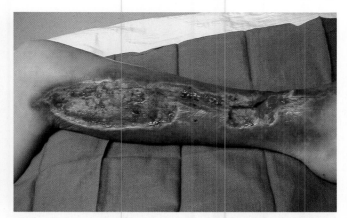

FIG. 28-2 A wound in the inflammatory phase of healing.

interventions.[1] The recommendations made in these guidelines are the basis for the interventions discussed in this chapter.

PATHOLOGY

Pressure ulcers usually occur over bony prominences (e.g., the sacrum, ischial tuberosities, greater trochanters, heels, malleoli, medial femoral condyles, elbows, scapular spine, vertebral spine, and occiput) in which the weight of the body is distributed over a small area, thereby producing high local pressure. This pressure reduces blood flow to the tissues, reducing oxygen and nutrient delivery to the skin and subcutaneous tissue, which causes the tissue to die. The body responds to this tissue **necrosis** by a sequence of events that can heal the wound. If the pressure is not relieved and the tissue damage exceeds the body's capacity for repair, a PU forms and over a period of time becomes visible as a chronic wound.

◎ *Clinical Pearl*

Pressure ulcers (PUs) usually occur over bony prominences where the weight of the body is distributed over a small area, producing high local pressure.

WOUND HEALING

Acute wounds, in which the tissue damage is recent and the healing environment is ideal, heal by a predictable and timely sequence of events that occur in a continuum traditionally characterized by five healing phases: Hemostasis, inflammation, proliferation, epithelialization, and remodeling.[18-20]

The first phase of healing, hemostasis, begins as soon as tissue destruction occurs (Fig. 28-1). Platelets rapidly aggregate and adhere to the exposed collagen in the injured tissue to slow or stop bleeding. Platelet aggregation also activates **Hageman factor** (clotting factor XII) to initiate clotting by converting prothrombin into thrombin, which then triggers the conversion of fibrinogen into fibrin. Fibrin forms the soft plug of a wound. The hemostatic phase lasts for about 30 minutes after the initial injury and prevents excessive bleeding, edema, and further tissue damage. During hemostasis, cells, proteins,

chemicals, and enzymes are also released or attracted to the wound site to initiate inflammation.

The second phase of healing, inflammation, is a complex sequence of events involving numerous cells and chemicals (Fig. 28-2). This phase lasts 3 to 7 days and begins with neutrophils, together with eosinophils, invading the injured area to lyse and clear away nonviable components, a process called **phagocytosis**. During early inflammation, platelets and neutrophils release growth factors needed for the next steps of tissue repair. At the same time, mast cells and basophils release histamine to increase vascular permeability and chemotactic factors to attract the next group of cells to the injured area. The next group of cells includes monocytes (which become macrophages when they leave the capillaries and enter the interstitial space) and lymphocytes (which regulate the body's immune response to microbes that enter the wounded area). The macrophages continue phagocytosis by producing enzymes, including **collagenases** and **proteases,** which promote autolytic **debridement.** During this phase, platelets, macrophages, fibroblasts, and keratinocytes also release growth factors that facilitate the synthesis of collagen. Macrophages, the regulatory cells of the inflammatory phase, also promote transition from the inflammatory phase to the proliferative phase.

Detectable signs of inflammation, which are redness, warmth, swelling, and pain, are caused by inflammatory factors released into the tissue during the inflammatory phase of healing. These factors include **prostaglandins, kinins** (e.g., bradykinin), and **anaphylatoxins.** Inflammation can reduce function in the area of the wound and in the patient overall. Patients with more severe wounds may also develop systemic fever during this phase. In the inflammatory phase, healthy systemic processes provide the cellular and chemical components necessary for healing. However, if the natural debridement or lysis process is not completed, the wound may become chronically inflamed, with persistent edema, erythema, and drainage. If chronic inflammation occurs, bacteria, necrotic tissue, and drainage must be managed effectively so that the wound can heal.

The third phase of healing is proliferation (Fig 28-3). The visible hallmark of the proliferative phase of healing is **granulation tissue.** Granulation tissue is made up

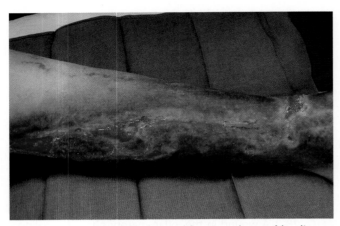

FIG. 28-3 A wound in the proliferative phase of healing.

of new capillaries and connective tissue. Endothelial cells produce the new capillaries, and fibroblasts (the most prevalent cells during proliferation) produce the collagen that forms the connective tissue that gives granulation tissue structure. During this phase, lymphocytes also produce antibodies to prevent wound infection and macrophages continue to phagocytose devitalized tissue and bacteria. If the granulation tissue grows without the development of a basement membrane, hypergranulation will occur preventing epithelial cells from migrating over the wound. Myofibroblasts, which contain actin (also responsible for muscle fiber contraction), are also prevalent in granulation tissue and can contract to bring the edges of the wound toward each other and reduce the wound size by wound contraction. A combination of growth factors, fibronectin, and **glycosaminoglycans (GAGs)** regulate the proliferative process in preparation for wound closure.

As with proliferation, the fourth phase of healing, epithelialization, involves tissue regeneration (Fig. 28-4). During this phase, beginning from the wound edges or from intact hair follicles and sweat ducts, epithelial cells migrate across the wound bed and produce a single-cell-thick layer to cover the granulation tissue (Fig. 28-5). This layer lies over the basement membrane, which is produced by basal cells that advance just a few cells ahead of the epithelial cells. Adhesive **glycoproteins,** such as fibronectin and laminin, adhere the new epithelial cells to the underlying lamina.

Remodeling, the fifth and final phase of wound healing, lasts from several weeks to 2 years after the initial tissue injury. During this phase, collagen in the dermal layer is reorganized to optimize tissue strength, maximize tissue mobility, and minimize scarring. Fibroblasts lay down new collagen fibers in some areas, while collagenase lyses excess collagen in other areas. When this deposition and lysis are balanced, they produce sufficient collagen fibers, with appropriate alignment, to withstand the forces applied to the tissue, and the collagen transitions from predominantly type III to the preinjury type I collagen. During remodeling, the skin also returns to its genetically determined color and the subcutaneous tissue returns to its normal vascularity, marking the end of the wound

healing process. Scar formation is a superficial sign of inner remodeling.

The entire area of a small wound may be in the same healing phase at any one time; however, in most wounds, especially PUs, different areas are often in different phases of healing. The phase of wound healing should be identified to allow for optimal clinical management.

The complete sequence of tissue healing just described occurs in response to acute wounds with full-thickness skin loss. Superficial wounds, in which only the epidermis is involved, do not require new collagen formation to close; therefore, after hemostasis and inflammation, they move directly to the epithelialization phase.

Clean full-thickness wounds with little or no tissue loss generally heal with minimal collagen deposition and thus minimal scarring, provided that the edges are kept approximated and secured during healing. This is termed *healing by primary intention.* In contrast, full thickness wounds with significant contamination or tissue loss may be left open to prevent accumulation of drainage. These wounds generally heal over a longer period with sufficient collagen production to result in a large scar. This is known as *healing by secondary intention.* If a wound cannot heal in the normal sequence in a timely manner, it is referred to as a *chronic wound.*

CHRONIC WOUNDS

Any of the phases of healing can be delayed or arrested, causing an acute wound to become chronic. In these circumstances, interventions are required to reinitiate or facilitate healing. Chronic wounds are defined as those that "fail to progress through a normal, orderly, and timely sequence of repair or wounds that pass through the repair process without restoring anatomic and functional results."[21] Without adequate treatment of the wound etiology and co-morbidities, the wound fluid will also develop properties that inhibit healing, such as increased **matrix metalloproteinases (MMPs)** and extracellular matrix, and decrease tissue protease inhibitors.[22] The primary factors that predispose wounds to chronicity are as follows[18]:

- Moderate-to-large amounts of necrotic tissue.
- High burden of microorganisms, with or without clinical infection.
- Chronic inflammation with persistently high numbers of neutrophils and macrophages.
- Impaired hemodynamics (e.g., hypoxia, ischemia, or edema).
- Senescent fibroblasts and keratinocytes that are unresponsive to growth factors; visible signs may include rolled edges or red, nongranulated tissue in the wound base.
- Abnormally high levels of growth-inhibiting proteases, especially metalloproteinases, that cause collagen degradation and can prevent development of a healthy extracellular matrix.
- Overgrowth of epithelium because of insufficient underlying connective tissue.

Because PUs develop insidiously rather than as the result of an isolated incident, they usually have many characteristics of chronic wounds by the time they reach the attention of the health care team and are evaluated. The exception would be the stage I ulcer that is treated early by effective removal of the causative factors. If there are no other impediments to healing, a stage I PU will heal quickly. However, with chronic PUs, changes in the interstitial fluid composition and the periwound fiber structure delay healing and weaken the periwound tissue.[23]

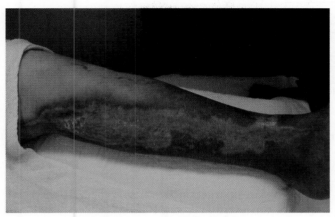

FIG. 28-4 A wound in the epithelialization phase of healing.

CAUSES OF PRESSURE ULCERS

There are four primary causes of PUs—shear, friction, pressure, and moisture (Fig. 28-6). Many other risk factors also predispose patients to PU formation. Determination and elimination of the causative factors, as well as evaluation and modification of risk factors, are integral to effective PU prevention and treatment.

> ### ◎ *Clinical Pearl*
> The four primary causes of pressure ulcers (PUs) are shear, friction, pressure, and moisture.

Shear. When skin is in contact with a support surface and the underlying tissue moves parallel to the support surface and the skin, shear forces develop in the subcutaneous fascia, muscle, and adipose tissue. For example, shear forces are exerted on the subcutaneous tissue at the spine and sacrum when a patient is in bed with the head elevated by as little as 10 degrees from horizontal or when the patient's cervical and upper thoracic spine is flexed.[24] A wheelchair-bound patient who slides forward and downward is also subject to destructive shear forces on the soft tissues overlying the sacrum. Shear forces compress, distort, or tear cutaneous and subcutaneous capillaries, resulting in tissue ischemia, initially in the deeper tissues and subsequently in the skin.[25] The resulting tissue destruction can cause deep tracts of necrosis along fascial planes

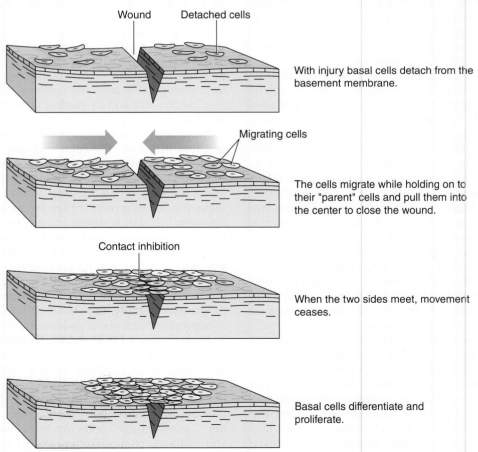

FIG. 28-5 Schematic diagram of epithelialization. *From Cameron MH: Physical agents in rehabilitation: From research to practice, ed 3, St. Louis, 2009, Saunders.*

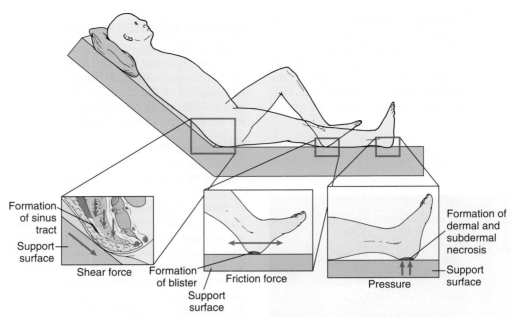

FIG. 28-6 Causes of pressure ulcers: Shear, friction, and pressure.

called *sinus tracts,* and these frequently become sites of infection. This type of damage may exist for quite some time before skin changes are visible. In addition to sinus tracts, PUs caused by shear forces have cratered walls and are round or oval shaped. Shear forces can be minimized by positioning the patient horizontally and by distributing forces on the support surface uniformly to reduce sliding movements that cause shear forces.[24,26,27]

Pressure. Pressure is the amount of force per unit area. When the external pressure applied to tissue exceeds the capillary closing pressure in that tissue, the capillaries become occluded, preventing blood flow and causing tissue hypoxia or anoxia and eventual cell death. Capillary closing pressure, defined as the pressure that occludes the smallest vessels, ranges from approximately 20 to 40 mm Hg. When a person lies in a standard hospital bed without a pressure-reducing surface, the pressure exerted on the greater trochanters and the heels is 50 to 95 mm Hg; when a person sits in a chair, the pressure exerted on the ischial tuberosities can be as high as 300 to 500 mm Hg.[28] If this much pressure is applied for a short period of time, the tissue can reperfuse when the pressure is relieved, preventing tissue damage; however, if this much pressure is exerted over a prolonged period, PUs may develop. The duration and amount of pressure that can be tolerated without cell death varies among patients and tissue type.[29] Therefore individual risk assessment, frequent skin inspection, and personalized turning schedules are recommended to reduce the risk of tissue damage.[11]

Friction. Friction occurs where two surfaces rub against each other (e.g., skin of the heels or elbows sliding on bed linens; see Fig. 28-6). Friction can destroy the superficial layers of the skin, including the epidermis and upper dermis, resulting in blisters, abrasions, or skin tears. A subsequent inflammatory reaction causes extrusion of watery transudate from the damaged area, further adding to skin destruction by causing maceration. These processes can eventually cause PUs. Unlike shear forces that cause ulcers to begin in deep tissue, wounds caused by friction begin with surface skin damage that then exposes subcutaneous tissue, making it more vulnerable to shear or pressure forces and bacterial contamination.[30] Wounds caused by friction tend to be painful because the nerve endings are exposed. Friction can be eliminated by lifting the patient slightly before repositioning; by protecting vulnerable areas with pillows, foam protectors, or rigid positioners; and by placing protective dressings over at-risk or damaged skin.

Moisture. Prolonged exposure of the skin to excessive moisture macerates the epidermis and increases the susceptibility of tissue to destruction from shear and friction, facilitates bacterial access to the subcutaneous tissue, and delays healing of an existing wound. Normal skin is slightly acidic to protect it from bacterial penetration and infection.[31] If skin is exposed to moisture from urinary or fecal incontinence, complications are more likely because this increases surface pH and bacterial exposure.[32] Excessive skin moisture can be prevented by use of moisture barrier creams; management of incontinence with catheters, fecal pouches, and use of bowel and bladder training programs (especially for patients with SCI); and placement of appropriate absorbent padding on the support surface.

Risk Factors for Pressure Ulcer Formation. Risk factors are circumstances that predispose patients to PU formation or to impaired healing when the skin and subcutaneous tissue are subjected to the causative factors just discussed. Risk factors for all populations may include immobility, joint contractures, decreased sensation, increased age, poor nutrition, incontinence (fecal and urinary), co-morbidities, altered mental status, and psychosocial factors.[17] PU risk factors may be classified as extrinsic or intrinsic. Extrinsic risk factors include

BOX 28-1	Extrinsic and Intrinsic Risk Factors for Pressure Ulcer Formation

Extrinsic	Intrinsic
• Older age	• Low body mass
• Poor family support	• Atrophy
• Psychosocial factors	• Medications, especially sedatives
• Use of braces, orthoses, or other semirigid support devices	• Immobility
	• Joint contractures
	• Paralysis
• Poorly fitting beds and wheelchairs	• Impaired sensation
	• Impaired circulation
• External devices such as catheters and tubes	• Co-morbidities
	• Confusion
	• Hypoalbuminemia
• Shear, pressure, and friction forces	• Urinary/fecal incontinence
	• Chemotherapy or radiation therapy
• Moisture against the skin	• Malnutrition
	• Low diastolic blood pressure
	• Fever

physical factors, such as equipment, orthoses, clothing, foreign objects, or medical apparatus, that can exert damaging pressure on patient skin and underlying tissue; intrinsic factors include patient co-morbidities or physical attributes, as well as medications that increase tissue vulnerability to PU formation (Box 28-1).[33] Effective treatment of PUs includes identifying and managing the risk factors while eliminating or reducing the causative factors.

Risk Assessment Scales. Several risk assessment scales have been developed to screen patients and determine their vulnerability to PU formation. Selection of a risk assessment tool involves consideration of the facility setting, the patient population, the raters using the tool, and the scale's validity and reliability within a given setting.[32] The Norton Scale,[17,34,35] the Braden Scale,[17,36-38] the Minimum Data Set (MDS),[39,40] the Outcomes and Assessment Information Set (OASIS),[41-44] and the Spinal Cord Injury Pressure Ulcer Scale (SCIPUS)[45,46] are the most commonly used PU risk assessment scales that have been tested for reliability and validity in various settings (Table 28-1). Copies of many of these scales, including examination forms and scoring details, can be found on the Evolve site that accompanies this book.

The Norton Scale and the Braden Scale. The Norton Scale and the Braden Scale (the Braden Scale for Predicting Pressure Sore Risk) are the PU risk assessment tools recommended in the AHRQ *Guidelines* because they have been extensively evaluated.[1,17] When using the Norton or Braden Scales, patients should be assessed at the time of admission and at frequent intervals thereafter because their condition may change over time. Preventive interventions are selected according to the noted impairments. When an ulcer occurs, it is recommended that the patient

be reassessed more frequently to monitor for risk of ulceration at other anatomical sites.[32]

The Minimum Data Set. All Medicare- and Medicaid-certified long-term care facilities are mandated to perform periodic comprehensive assessments of each of their residents, including assessment of PU risk. The Minimum Data Set (MDS), a component of the Resident Assessment Instrument (RAI), includes a tool for basic assessment of patients' clinical and functional impairments. Patients are assessed within 14 days of admission, quarterly, and on any change in medical status. Skin condition is one of 16 assessed aspects of patient well-being. The criteria for skin assessment can be used to establish an effective PU prevention program, and the entire data set is helpful for developing a comprehensive wound care plan.

Outcomes and Assessment Information Set. The Outcomes and Assessment Information Set (OASIS) is an extensive and comprehensive assessment form developed by the Health Care Financing Administration (HCFA) for use in the home health care setting. OASIS includes items specific to wounds, including the presence of PUs, tissue involvement, and the healing phase of existing ulcers. Although used primarily to establish reimbursement, the other areas, such as psychosocial support, sensory status, integumentary status, elimination status, cognitive functioning, toileting, transferring, and ambulation, included in this tool can assist the evaluator by identifying patients at risk for PUs and providing preventive information to patients and caregivers.

Spinal Cord Injury Pressure Ulcer Scale. The Spinal Cord Injury Pressure Ulcer Scale (SCIPUS) was developed for assessing PU risk in patients with SCIs. A follow-up study of patients with SCIs in the acute phase (within 30 days of admission) compared the reliability and sensitivity of various PU risk assessment scales *not* intended for use with patients with SCIs (Norton, Braden, Gosnell, and Abruzzese scales) with the SCIPUS, which was not intended for risk assessment during acute hospitalization.[46] Although the Braden Scale was found to be the most accurate of the general purpose scales, it was a poor overall predictor of PU formation in this patient population. Of the 226 patients studied, 97.3% had a Braden score of 18 or less. A cutoff score of ≤10 provided the highest balance of sensitivity (74.7%) and specificity (56.6%) for the Braden Scale. The authors concluded that if the Braden Scale is used for patients with SCIs, a score of ≤10 is most appropriate for identifying those at risk for PU formation.[46] As a result of this study, the original SCIPUS was modified for use with the patient with SCI during acute hospitalization. The authors recommend that the SCIPUS be used daily to assess all patients with SCIs in the acute care setting.

TYPICAL EXAMINATION FINDINGS

PATIENT HISTORY

Examination of a patient with a PU begins with a thorough history focused on the causes of wound formation, including onset, medical history, and functional status.

For hospitalized patients, long-term care residents, and especially cognitively impaired patients, much of this

TABLE 28-1	Pressure Ulcer Risk Assessment Scales		
Scale (Year Published)	**Recommended Population/Setting**	**Risk Categories Assessed**	**Scale Interpretation**
Norton Scale (1962)	Elderly in acute hospital setting	Physical condition Mental condition Activity Mobility Incontinence	Scale of 1-4; 1 highest Score range: 5-20 ≤ 16 = at risk <12 = at high risk
Braden Scale (1988)	Acute care Intensive care Nursing home Any patient regardless of skin color Older population	Sensory perception Moisture Activity Mobility Nutrition Friction and shear	Scale of 1-4; 1 highest Score range: 6-23 <12 high risk 12-14 moderate risk 15-16 mild risk 17-18 low risk
Minimum Data Set (MDS; 1987)	Long-term care facilities	Ulcers Type of ulcer History of resolved ulcers Other skin problems or lesions present Skin treatments Foot problems and care	Scale/score not provided for risk evaluation; used to determine payment category.
Outcomes and Assessment Information Set (OASIS; 1999 with ongoing revisions)	Home health care setting	Psychosocial support Sensory status Integumentary status Elimination status Cognitive function Toileting Transferring Ambulation	Scale/score not provided for risk evaluation; used to determine payment category.
Spinal Cord Injury Pressure Ulcer Scale (SCIPUS; 1996)	SCI patients in acute and long-term care settings	Extent of paralysis Level of activity Mobility Urinary incontinency Moisture Pulmonary disease Serum creatinine Albumin	Score 0-25 0-12 low risk 13-18 moderate risk 19-20 high risk 21-25 very high risk

SCI, Spinal cord injury.

information is obtained from the medical chart or during the functional assessment. Whenever possible, however, information regarding onset, pain, and aggravating and alleviating factors should be obtained directly from the patient. Components of the history that are usually obtained from the medical chart or from the referring physician include the medical and surgical history, medications, nutritional status, clinical tests, and detrimental environmental conditions.

Nutritional Status. The need for adequate nutrition to prevent and treat PUs is well documented. According to the National Pressure Ulcer Long-Term Study of 2,490 residents in 109 long-term care facilities, the two nutrition-related factors that most affect PU risk are involuntary weight loss of more than 10% of the total body weight (increased risk 74%) and dehydration (increased risk 42%).[47-49] In addition to adequate calories, wound healing requires sufficient protein intake. The caloric needs of wound and periwound tissue increases to 50% above baseline, and the protein requirement increases to 2 to 2½ times above baseline.[50] Clinical tests that are used to assess nutritional status are serum albumin and prealbumin levels. Albumin levels of less than 3.5 g/dl and prealbumin

levels of less than 20 g/dl are considered indicators of poor nutritional status.[51] Other nutritional components necessary for optimal wound healing include fats, fatty acids, and carbohydrates. In addition, vitamins A, B complex, C, and E and the trace elements zinc, copper, and iron influence PU formation and healing.[51,52]

Psychosocial Issues. Psychosocial assessment of a patient with a PU will include the patient's ability, willingness, and motivation to alter lifestyle habits, support system, stress level, depression, drug and alcohol abuse, and tobacco use of any form.[53]

SYSTEMS REVIEW

The systems review is used to target areas requiring further examination and to define areas that may cause complications or indicate a need for precautions during the examination and intervention processes. Chapter 1 includes details of the systems review.

TESTS AND MEASURES

The wound examination begins with observation to describe the wound tissue and drainage, skin color, edema, wound edges, and odor.

Tissue Description. Tissue description helps identify the depth of the PU and phase(s) of healing in the wound bed. When **eschar** is present, the tissue is described before and after debridement, and the wound is diagnosed or staged only after debridement. Estimating the amount of each tissue type as a percentage of the total wound area can also provide data for assessing change. Tissue types include the following:

- Eschar is black, brown, yellow, or grey tissue that may be dry and hard, or in the presence of an underlying infection, soft and "mushy." In PUs, the eschar may also have a rubbery texture. Eschar is composed of dead cells and should therefore be removed from most wounds to determine depth of tissue involvement, to facilitate healing, and to decrease risk of infection.
- Yellow **slough,** often visible under the eschar during the inflammatory phase of healing, is the softer and lighter necrotic debris that collects as the by-product of **autolysis.**
- Granulation tissue is the red, "beefy-looking" tissue that varies from an anemic salmon-color to a healthy, bright red, indicating that the wound is ready for surgical closure or that epithelialization can be supported. Granulation tissue is required for closure for any wound healing by secondary intention. It serves to fill in full-thickness wound cavities and matures into scar tissue during the remodeling phase of healing.
- Devitalized fascia is dull, fibrous connective tissue that can be tan or grey.
- Healthy muscle is striated, reddish, and sensate when pinched with forceps; devitalized muscle is brownish-grey and insensate.
- Healthy tendons are shiny, stringy, and covered with a fibrous sheath of connective tissue containing synovial or fatty fluid.
- Healthy bone is light tan with intact periosteum that gives it a moist appearance. Bone without periosteum is light-to-dark tan and very dry; necrotic bone is dark brown and requires surgical debridement.
- Fat, when healthy, appears as shiny globules. Fat has a poor vascular supply and therefore, when exposed, usually dies rapidly and shrivels.

Most wounds contain various tissue types that can be identified and quantified during the initial evaluation and periodic reassessment. Once the types of tissue present in a wound have been identified, all necrotic tissue should be removed and the healthy, vital tissue that provides the resources for new tissue to develop and for healing to progress should be protected.

Drainage. Drainage, a by-product of wound metabolism, is evaluated for quality and quantity (e.g., scant, minimal, moderate, or copious). Serous drainage is a clear, watery fluid that flows from blood vessels, collects in the extracellular spaces, and results in edema if the skin remains intact. If the skin is not intact, serous drainage appears as clear fluid seeping from the opening. If the fluid has a low protein concentration, it is termed *transudate*.[54] Sanguineous drainage is bloody drainage. Red sanguineous drainage occurs with recent bleeding, before hemostasis occurs, whereas brownish drainage is from old blood. Serosanguineous drainage is serous fluid with a slight bloody tinge. **Exudate** is pale yellow viscous drainage composed of serum, blood cells, plasma proteins, and lysed debris. Exudate is frequently present in the acute inflammatory stage of mild injuries.

Seropurulent drainage is slightly thicker and yellower than exudate and indicates colonization of the wound by bacteria but not necessarily active infection. In contrast, **purulence,** a thick necrotic drainage frequently accompanied by a foul odor, is a sign of infection. Odor can vary in type and severity. For example, green or greenish-blue drainage accompanied by a distinctive sweet odor is typical of *Pseudomonas* infection. A putrid foul odor is indicative of deep, chronic infection with anaerobic bacteria. Extensive necrotic tissue may have an odor that can only be described as that of nonviable tissue. Certain dressings can have a strong odor; therefore odor is assessed after removal of the dressing and thorough wound cleansing.

Periwound Skin Color. Periwound skin color can provide information about the type of wound and the status of the surrounding tissue. Any change in skin color and the extent of the change is documented because reduction or increase in the degree and size of color changes are indicators of improvement or decline in wound status. Skin color is presented here as it relates to PUs.

Erythema is redness of the skin that may result from an inflammatory response (reactive hyperemia), from underlying infection, or from unrelieved pressure. In darker-skinned patients, erythema may be more difficult to see; however, accompanying changes in warmth or texture may be detected. Erythema may be blanchable or unblanchable, meaning it does or does not pale with pressure. Normal skin pales when the blood is pushed out of the capillaries. Unblanchable erythema in the periwound area is a sign of the inflammatory response to healing or a sign of infection. Unblanchable redness or prolonged refill time in the foot indicates microvascular or small vessel disease. Dark-red discoloration, a result of repeated shear forces, may also be referred to as pre-ulcer or a purple ulcer. Blanched, white periwound skin is typical of maceration that occurs when moisture is inadequately managed. Darker skin tones around the periphery of an open PU are often an indication of extensive undermining.

Edema. Edema, caused by excess fluid in the interstitial tissue, can be multifactorial in origin and can occur with any type of wound. Edema in the area of a PU usually indicates infection or inflammation.

Wound Edges. The appearance of the wound edges can indicate the type of wound and the healing processes occurring within the wound site.

- Even edges are typical of arterial ulcers or surgically induced wounds.
- Irregular edges are typically seen in venous ulcers or PUs with undermining.
- Closed or rolled edges, which are signs of halted healing, appear curled or raised with epithelial cell migration stopping at the granulation edge. Rolled edges may require debridement to facilitate epithelialization.

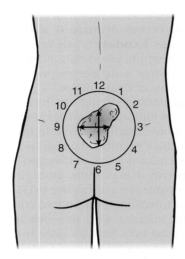

FIG. 28-7 Clockwise method of measuring pressure ulcer size.

- **Hyperkeratosis,** also termed *callus,* is overdevelopment of the horny cell layer of skin as a result of continuous tissue stress. The appearance is dry, thick, adhered epidermal tissue.
- Epithelialization is the migration of epithelial cells over granulation tissue.

Wound Size. The initial examination should also include a measure of wound size. In addition to dimensions, usually reported in centimeters, the measurement method and patient position should be documented to ensure valid and reliable assessment of progress. When using the perpendicular method, length (L) is the longest measurement of the wound regardless of orientation and width (W) is the longest distance perpendicular to the length. Measurements are documented as L × W, with length first. When using the clockwise method, length is the longest dimension along a 12:00 to 6:00 plane in an anatomical orientation (12:00 is cephalic and 6:00 is caudal) and width is the longest dimension on a 3:00 to 9:00 plane perpendicular to 12:00 to 6:00 (Fig 28-7).

Volumetric measurements, useful for small or cavity wounds, are estimated by multiplying the wound length by width by depth.[55]

Tracing, which provides an exact wound outline, may also be included in the documentation for later comparisons.

Technique for Tracing Wound Outline
- Place a clear film over the wound.
- Place a piece of clear acetate film with a measuring guide over the first layer of film.
- Trace the wound edges with an indelible pen on the top film layer.
- Note orientation, undermining, tunneling, bony prominences, or erythema.
- Label the tracing with the patient's name and measurement date.
- Discard the film that was next to the wound.

Photographs can also provide a visual description of the wound and complement documentation. If the photographs and measuring guides are gridded, surface area can be calculated. Care must be taken with photographing wounds to obtain consistent indicators of color and size.

Suggestions for Optimal Wound Photographs
- Position the patient with the wound easily visualized in the view box.
- Adjust the lighting for equal illumination throughout without shadows.
- Use blue or green towels around the wound to eliminate conflicting background and to absorb light, thereby minimizing glare.
- Close curtains or shades so that only fluorescent light exists in the room.
- Hold the camera at a 90-degree angle to the wound to avoid distortion of the shape.
- Take more than one photograph at different settings.
- Label photographs with the patient's name, medical record number, examination date, patient position, and wound location.

Subcutaneous wound extensions require probing and cleansing because they can conceal bacteria and facilitate infection. The size of wound extensions, as well as the size of the exposed wound, are indicators of wound severity and may be a measure of intervention efficacy. The four types of wound extensions are undermining, sinus tract, tunneling, and fistulas. Undermining, defined as a fan-shaped destruction of connective tissue between the dermis and subcutaneous tissue, may be indicated by red or brawny discoloration that extends beyond the wound edges. A sinus tract is a long, narrow opening along a fascial plane that may connect to an underlying, deeper abscess. Palpation of a hard, indurated area adjacent to an open wound may indicate the presence of an abscess. Tunneling is a tract that connects two open wounds. A fistula is tunneling that connects with a body cavity or organ (e.g., the small or large intestine). Undermining and sinus tracts are the types of subcutaneous wound extensions most frequently associated with PUs and occur most commonly in the areas of the sacrum and trochanters.

Undermining and tunneling are measured by slowly inserting a moistened sterile alginate or cotton-tipped applicator into the wound extensions and probing to the deepest parts for sinuses or abscesses. Alginate-tipped applicators are preferable to cotton ones because alginate fibers that adhere to the wound are absorbed, whereas if cotton fibers are left in the wound bed, they can irritate and provide a place for infection to start. Because the area being probed may not be visualized, probing should stop immediately when resistance is felt to avoid damaging tissue. The depth of the extension is marked on the applicator, measured with a graduated guide, and documented, along with the presence of any drainage, purulence, or blood on the applicator tip. The location of the extension is usually indicated according to the clockwise method of measuring or in relation to an anatomical landmark.[55]

Clinical Tests. In addition to the clinical tests that help determine a patient's wound healing potential based on nutritional status (serum albumin, prealbumin, and **body mass index [BMI]**), several other clinical tests are recommended in specific conditions (Table 28-2).

TABLE 28-2	Clinical Tests for Patients with Pressure Ulcers	
Test	**Normal Values**	**Interpretation of Abnormal Values**
Serum albumin	3.2-4.5 gm/dl	<3.5 gm/dl: Poor nutritional status 3.0-3.5: Mild 2.5-3.0: Moderate <2.5: Severe
Prealbumin	15-35 mg/dl	<5 mg/dl: Poor prognosis 5-10.9 mg/dl: Significant risk; aggressive nutritional support indicated 11-15 mg/dl: Increased risk; monitor status biweekly
BMI	20-25	<16: Severely underweight 16-19: Underweight 26-30: Mild obesity 31-40: Moderate obesity >40: Severe obesity
ABI	1.0	>1.2: Not reliable in diabetics because of arterial calcification 0.8-1.0: Mild PAOD 0.5-0.8: Moderate PAOD <0.5: Severe PAOD
Fasting plasma glucose	<110 mg/dl	110-126: Prediabetes >126: Diagnosis of diabetes >200: Impaired healing

BMI, Body mass index; *ABI,* ankle-brachial index; *PAOD,* peripheral arterial occlusive disease.

Ankle-Brachial Index. Determination of **ankle-brachial index (ABI)**, a measure of lower extremity arterial blood flow, is recommended for patients with diabetes or peripheral vascular disease who develop heel PUs. The values are used to determine healing potential, the safety of debridement, and the need for revascularization.

Blood Glucose Levels. Blood glucose levels should be checked in a patient with a chronic wound because approximately one-third of those who are diabetic are unaware that they have the disease.[56] See Chapter 30 for further information on chronic wounds associated with diabetes.

Cultures. Cultures are reserved for wounds with clinical signs of infection, which for PUs has been expanded beyond the classic signs of warmth, pain, erythema, and edema to also include purulent drainage, delayed healing, discoloration of granulation tissues, pocketing at the base of the wound, foul odor, and breakdown of recently formed new tissue.[57] All wounds have some bacteria present, and most chronic wounds are colonized with bacteria, meaning that organisms are present on the wound bed. In most cases, the host's immune system can manage the bacterial load without interfering with healing. In these situations, cultures are unnecessary and are not cost-effective.[58] If the organisms penetrate the wound tissue, infection occurs and the healing process is interrupted. Exactly when healing is affected depends on the type and amount of bacteria, as well as host immunity. If culturing the wound is essential to determine the amount and type of bacteria, the health care professional will determine the proper procedure for collecting the sample.

Pain. Pain assessment can indicate the cause and extent of a wound and the appropriate pain management approaches. The nature, onset, duration, and exacerbating and relieving factors, as well as pain severity, are aspects of pain to be considered. Pain caused by hypoxia or ischemia (see Chapter 29) is usually deep and cramping in quality, and pain that results from neuropathy (see Chapter 30) is usually burning, lancinating, or electric-like.[59] Pain severity can be assessed using a variety of scales as described in detail in Chapter 22.

Sensory Integrity. Testing for sensation is especially important in patients with chronic wounds and diabetic or peripheral neuropathies, SCI, or prolonged immobility. Sensation of light touch, pressure, temperature, vibration, and proprioception should all be tested. For patients at risk for PU formation, assessment of vulnerable areas (feet, sacrum, trochanters, or shoulders) can assist in selecting appropriate protective equipment. For patients with SCIs, the spinal level in which sensation stops should be determined, so the patient can be taught off-loading strategies to prevent wounds in insensate areas (see Chapter 20).

EVALUATION, DIAGNOSIS, AND PROGNOSIS

Any soft tissue wound may be classified according to the depth and type of tissue involved.[60] According to the classification scheme used by the *Guide to Physical Therapist Practice* (the *Guide*),[60] wounds can be classified according to depth into one of five preferred practice patterns. These patterns are 7A: Primary prevention/risk reduction for integumentary disorders; 7B: Impaired integumentary integrity associated with superficial skin involvement; 7C: Impaired integumentary integrity associated with partial-thickness skin involvement and scar formation; 7D: Impaired integumentary integrity associated with full-thickness skin involvement and scar formation; and 7E: Impaired integumentary integrity associated with skin involvement extending into fascia, muscle, or bone and scar formation. Partial thickness is defined as involving the epidermis and dermis; full thickness is defined as the complete destruction of the dermal layers and extending into the subcutaneous tissue.

The NPUAP published a staging system specifically for PUs in 1989 and revised this system in 1998. This system was adopted by the AHRQ and is universally used in the medical community to describe PUs. The staging system, intended for use with PUs only, is based on the deepest layer of tissue involvement at the time of the initial evaluation. The characteristics of the stages as revised in 1998 and the *Guide's* preferred practice patterns related to the integumentary system are shown in Table 28-3. Fig. 28-8 shows examples of the four NPUAP PU stages.

TABLE 28-3	National Pressure Ulcer Advisory Panel (NPUAP) Pressure Ulcer Stages Compared to the Guide's Integumentary System Preferred Practice Patterns

NPUAP Stage	Preferred Practice Pattern
No comparable stage	7A: Primary prevention/risk reduction for integumentary disorders
Stage I: Observable pressure-related alteration of intact skin whose indicators, as compared to adjacent or opposite area on the body, may include changes in skin color (red, blue, and purple tones), skin temperature (warmth or coolness), skin stiffness (hardness, edema), and/or sensation (pain).	7B: Impaired integumentary integrity associated with superficial skin involvement
Stage II: Partial-thickness skin loss involving epidermis and/or dermis. The ulcer is superficial and presents clinically as an abrasion, a blister, or a shallow crater.	7C: Impaired integumentary integrity associated with partial-thickness skin involvement and scar formation
Stage III: Full-thickness skin loss involving damage or necrosis of subcutaneous tissue that may extend down to, but not through, underlying fascia. The ulcer presents clinically as a deep crater with or without undermining of adjacent tissue.	7D: Impaired integumentary integrity associated with full-thickness skin involvement and scar formation
Stage IV: Full-thickness skin loss with extensive destruction, tissue necrosis, or damage to muscle, bone, or supporting structures (e.g., tendon, joint capsule).	7E: Impaired integumentary integrity associated with skin involvement extending into fascia, muscle, or bone and scar formation

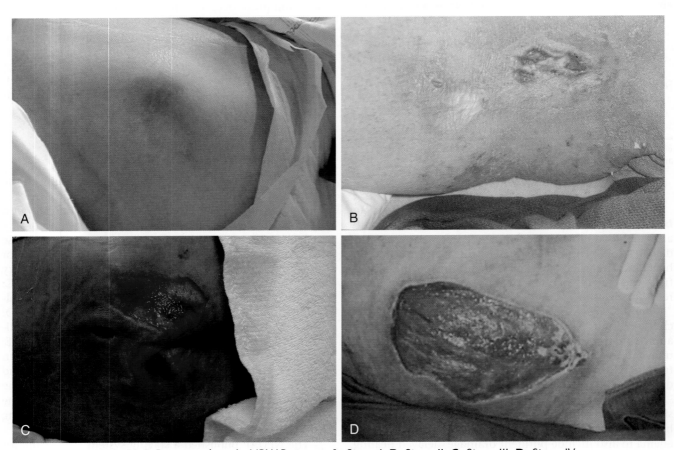

FIG. 28-8 Pressure ulcers in NPUAP stages. **A,** Stage I. **B,** Stage II. **C,** Stage III. **D,** Stage IV.

◎ *Clinical Pearl*

Pressure ulcers (PUs) should be staged after debridement because staging depends on identifying the type of tissue at the ulcer base.

Necrotic PUs are staged after debridement is completed because staging depends on identifying the type of tissue

at the ulcer base. Wounds are not staged in reverse when healing occurs. For example, a stage III does not become a stage II as the wound granulates, and a stage II does not become a stage I as it reepithelializes. The correct nomenclature would be a stage III PU in the proliferative phase or a stage II in the epithelialization or remodeling phase. Each wound is described according to the deepest layer of tissue involvement and the healing phase at the time of

TABLE 28-4	Guidelines for Pressure Ulcer Prevention Based on Risk Assessment[17]
For bed-bound individuals	• Reposition at least every 2 hours. • Use pillows or foam wedges to keep bony prominences from direct contact. • Use devices that totally relieve pressure on the heels. • Avoid positioning directly on the trochanter. • Elevate the head of the bed as little and for as short a time as possible. • Use lifting devices to move rather than drag individuals during transfers and position changes. • Place at-risk individuals on a pressure-reducing mattress. Do not use doughnut-type devices.
For chair-bound patients	• Reposition at least every hour. • Have patient shift weight every 15 minutes if able. • Use pressure-reducing devices for seating surfaces. Do not use doughnut-type devices. • Consider postural alignment, distribution of weight, balance and stability, and pressure relief when positioning individuals in chairs or wheelchairs. • Use a written plan.
Skin care	• Inspect skin at least once a day. • Individualize bathing schedule. Avoid hot water. Use a mild cleansing agent. • Minimize aggravating environmental factors such as low humidity and cold air. Use moisturizers for dry skin. • Avoid massage over bony prominences. • Use proper positioning, transferring, and turning techniques. • Use lubricants to reduce friction injuries.
Moisture/incontinence	• Cleanse skin at time of soiling. • Minimize skin exposure to moisture. Assess and treat urinary incontinence. When moisture cannot be controlled, use underpads or briefs that are absorbent and present a quick-drying surface to the skin.
Nutritional deficit	• Investigate factors that compromise an apparently well-nourished individual's dietary intake (especially protein or calories) and offer support with eating. • Plan and implement a nutritional support and/or supplementation program for nutritionally compromised individuals.
Education	• Etiology and risk factors for PUs. • Risk assessment tools and their application. • Skin assessment. • Selection and/or use of support surfaces. • Development and implementation of an individualized program of skin care. • Demonstration of positioning to decrease risk of tissue breakdown. • Instruction on accurate documentation of pertinent data.

From Pittman J: The chronic wound and the family, *Ostomy Wound Manage* 49 (2):38-46, 2003.
PUs, Pressure ulcers.

assessment. If a wound deteriorates during the period of intervention, at reassessment the stage can be advanced to reflect deeper tissue involvement.

INTERVENTION

PREVENTION BASED ON RISK FACTORS

Although labor intensive and costly, comprehensive PU prevention programs have been shown to decrease the incidence of PUs and are cost-effective in both acute and long-term care facilities (Table 28-4).

Some of the risk factors for PUs (e.g., older age, history of chemotherapy, and history of radiation treatment) are not modifiable. Other risk factors (e.g., confusion, poor family support, and psychosocial issues) necessitate referral to other professionals, including medical social workers, psychologists, psychiatrists, or other adult services. Fever, low diastolic blood pressure, medications, impaired circulation, and co-morbidities may require medical attention in addition to preventive measures. Some of the risk factors that can be addressed by rehabilitation interventions are impaired circulation (see Chapter 30), impaired sensation as it relates to the diabetic foot (see Chapter 31), and poorly fitting wheelchairs (see Chapter 33).

Most PU risk factors can be addressed by five specific interventions identified as effective in preventing PUs or in facilitating wound healing. These interventions are caregiver education, use of support surfaces, positioning, moisture control, and adequate nutrition. The AHRQ *Guideline* further states that the education should be structured, organized, and comprehensive; should be directed at all levels of health care providers, patients, family, and caregivers; and should include information about the other four interventions.[1]

Clinical Pearl

Interventions that can prevent pressure ulcers (PUs) or facilitate wound healing are caregiver education, use of support surfaces, positioning, moisture control, and adequate nutrition.

Support Surfaces. Support surfaces (including wheelchair cushions, bed overlays, and specialty mattresses) distribute pressure to decrease the amount of pressure over a body part at risk for PU formation. Support surfaces are divided into two categories: Pressure reducing, defined as a surface that inconsistently reduces the pressure below the capillary closing pressures in all positions,

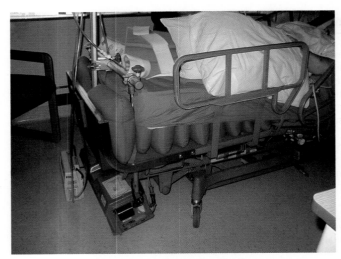

FIG. 28-9 Low-air-loss bed.

on all body locations (25 to 32 mm Hg), and pressure relieving, defined as a surface that consistently reduces the pressure below capillary closing pressures, in any position and in most body locations.

Interface pressure, defined as the pressure between a surface and the skin over a bony prominence, can be measured by a number of devices, ranging from hand-held sensors to large pressure-mapping devices. The ideal interface pressure would be lower than the patient's arterial capillary closing pressure, defined as the pressure that occludes the smallest vessels. The average capillary closing pressure in a healthy adult male forefinger is 32 mm Hg[61]; however, the values can vary, depending on body build, skeletal structure, amount of body fat, and the amount of soft tissue covering the bony prominences. Therefore all patient risk factors must be considered when selecting equipment for prevention or treatment of PUs. If pressure sensors are not available, the support surface can be checked for adequate off-loading by placing the hand between the support surface (mattress or cushion) and the base of the bed or wheelchair. If the bony prominence is palpable, the surface is said to have "bottomed out" and is not sufficiently reducing the interface pressure.

The low-air-loss (LAL) bed is intended to remove or reduce perspiration, provide localized cooling of the skin to prevent heat accumulation and thereby control the skin microclimate, and distribute the torso load (Fig. 28-9).[62] Lateral rotation beds that provide continuous side-to-side rotation have been shown to increase the oxygenation index (the ratio of arterial partial pressure of oxygen to fraction of inspired oxygen) and to decrease the incidence of ventilator-associated pneumonia.[63] The side-to-side rotation is not, however, sufficient off-loading to prevent PUs. Research for the optimal bed to prevent and treat PUs is ongoing, with new products continually being developed.

Wheelchair cushions, like beds, can be static or dynamic; nonpowered or powered; air, gel, or foam; and varied in size and shape. Unlike beds that distribute the weight over the entire body, cushions primarily protect the major weight-bearing surface in sitting (the ischial tuberosities) and transfer the weight to the area that is at least risk for PUs (the femurs). Some cushions are contoured to distribute the weight equally throughout the buttocks and posterior thighs; some are designed to eliminate pressure on the ischial tuberosities by providing a U-shaped pocket in which they are suspended (Isch-Dish, Span-America, Greenville, SC). Criteria for cushion selection are multifactorial and specific to each patient and can be found in Box 28-2.

Although no specific studies were found relating pressure reduction with doughnut-shaped cushions, it is generally accepted that these cushions are not effective in redistributing pressure on as much body surface area as possible, and they may contribute to ischemia in the tissue positioned inside the doughnut hole.

Clinicians have historically taught wheelchair-bound patients to do push-ups and weight shifts to allow reperfusion of the ischial and gluteal areas and thereby help prevent PU formation. A study of transcutaneous oxygen tension (TcPo$_2$) in the sitting (loaded) position and during pressure relief (unloaded) in patients with SCIs suggested that doing pressure lifts for 15 to 30 seconds is not sufficient to raise oxygenation to unloaded values.[64] The mean duration of pressure relief required to raise TcPo$_2$ to unloaded values was 1 minute 51 seconds. Therefore the authors recommend alternative methods of pressure relief.

Two specialty products designed for wheelchair pressure relief are the total contact seat (TCS) and the thoracic suspension orthosis (TSO). The TCS uses a prosthetic fitting technique to distribute sitting pressure and reduce resting pressure under the ischial tuberosities to below capillary pressure, presumed to be 1 pound per square inch **(psi).** A comparison of the TCS with three standard cushions showed significantly lower pressures at all times using the TCS with sustained pressures below the postulated threshold for tissue damage.[65] The TSO consists of a custom-molded thoracolumbosacral orthosis suspended from the wheelchair frame (also referred to as the *bucket design*) so that the body weight is supported primarily by the thorax, thereby off-loading the lower body pressure areas.[66,67] The TSO is recommended for patients with chronic PUs, chronic pain with sitting, severe scoliosis, or bilateral lower extremity amputation (Fig. 28-10). Three meta-analyses of randomized controlled trials assessing the effectiveness of pressure-relieving beds, mattresses, and cushions in the prevention and treatment of PUs summarized the high quality data in this area and reached the following conclusions[68-70]:

- Foam mattresses are more effective than standard hospital mattresses in moderate- to high-risk patients.
- Pressure-relieving overlays in the operating room reduced the incidence of postoperative PUs.
- Air-fluidized beds and LAL beds improve the rate of wound healing.
- Seat cushions and constant low-pressure devices have not been adequately evaluated.

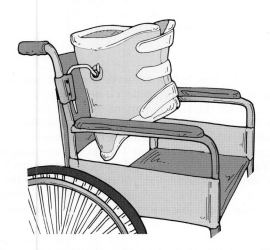

FIG. 28-10 Thoracic suspension orthosis is recommended for patients with chronic pressure ulcers, chronic pain with sitting, or bilateral lower extremity amputation. *Courtesy Fillauer, Inc, Chattanooga, TN.*

Positioners/Protectors. Positioners are support devices used to off-load bony prominences and to maintain optimal position of a body part, thereby reducing the risk of ulceration or promoting healing of an existing ulcer (Fig. 28-11, *A*). A positioner may also help prevent foot drop, maintain neutral hip position, keep the heels off the bed, or prevent ankles and knees from rubbing against each other. Positioners are constructed of rigid or semirigid frames with air, gel, foam, or lamb's wool padding. Semirigid frames are recommended if the patient does not have the range of motion (ROM) needed for equal weight distribution throughout the device. For example, the ankle should achieve 0 degrees dorsiflexion if a rigid boot is used, so that high pressures do not develop on the forefoot and Achilles tendon (Fig. 28-11, *B*). Other considerations in selecting a foot positioner are gait status (some styles have an ambulating surface, some do not), risk factors (e.g., fragile skin, insensate feet), and cost.

Protectors are soft devices that use foam, gel, air, fiber, or other pressure-absorbing materials to protect bony prominences (primarily on the heels and elbows) from shear and friction; however, protectors do not reduce pressure. Protectors are most useful when the patient has fragile skin and tends to slide against the linens or chair arms. The Rooke boot, an example of a substantial protector, is useful for the ischemic foot before surgery because it off-loads the heel, protects the toes, and maintains warmth. When a positioner or a protector is used on the heel, the lower leg should be elevated on a pillow to further reduce peak pressure where the heel touches the bed.

Clinical Pearl

When using a heel positioner or protector, place a pillow under the lower legs to off-load the heels (see Fig. 28-11).

Positioning. Although appropriate support surfaces can help prevent PUs and facilitate wound healing, they are only an adjunct to proper positioning and frequent turning. After identification of risk factors and inspection

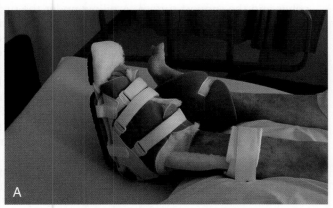

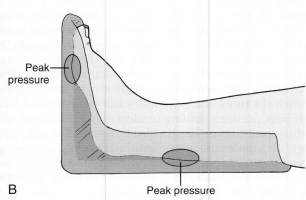

FIG. 28-11 **A,** Foot positioner and protector. Both require placement of a pillow under the calves for optimal off-loading of the heels. **B,** If the foot cannot be dorsiflexed to 0 degrees, the Achilles tendon and plantar metatarsal heads are at risk for increased soft tissue pressure and ulcer formation.

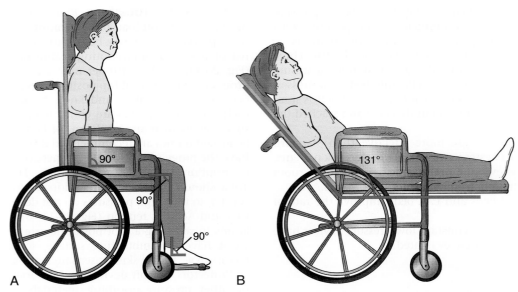

FIG. 28-12 A, The "90/90/90" sitting position in a wheelchair distributes body weight on the well-padded posterior thighs, off-loading the ischial tuberosities. **B,** Semi-reclining wheelchair position with the legs elevated on leg rests off-loads sacrum and prevents shear forces that occur with slumping positions.

of the skin, a turning schedule is instituted when indicated. Although most turning schedules are based on a 2-hour sequence,[32,71] patients at high risk may need to be repositioned more frequently or areas that are at high risk or with existing ulcers may require continuous off-loading, thereby eliminating a position from the sequence.[1] For example, if a patient has a stage III PU on the right greater trochanter, right sidelying would be eliminated or minimized, depending on the tissue integrity of the sacrum and left side. Having a written schedule posted in the patient's room facilitates involving all disciplines in the turning program and can improve compliance.

The ideal sitting position is one that distributes the body weight to nonbony areas (e.g., the posterior thighs) and that off-loads the bony prominences. The "90/90/90" position, with the hips, knees, and ankles flexed approximately 90 degrees, is often recommended (Fig. 28-12, A). In this position, the femurs are parallel to the floor with all but the distal 1½ to 2 inches supported on the sitting surface, the feet are supported on the floor or foot rests, the face is in a vertical position perpendicular to the floor, and the gaze is directed straight ahead. The weight is equally distributed on both sides, and the natural spinal curves are supported by the chair back or by cushions. The "90/90/90" position distributes body weight most equally through the trunk and extremities and reduces the risk of high peak pressures leading to ulceration. Additional off-loading in sitting can be provided by armrests of sufficient height to support the upper body weight without causing excessive shoulder elevation.[24] An alternative sitting position is with the wheelchair back semi-reclined, with the legs elevated on leg rests (Fig. 28-12, B).[72,73] Table 28-5 outlines common errant sitting patterns and positions and recommended remedies.

The ideal position for a supine patient is with the weight distributed as evenly as possible throughout the entire body. This is best achieved with the bed as flat as possible. However, this position is not always comfortable, especially for the elderly patient, nor is it ideal for some pathological conditions (e.g., patients on mechanical ventilation for whom a semi-recumbent position of 45 degrees is recommended to prevent ventilator-associated aspiration pneumonia).[74,75] Box 28-3 lists some strategies to consider when adjusting the patient away from the ideal position, and Table 28-6 lists common problems for recumbent positions, associated risks, and recommended solutions.

Two alternative positions for the bed-bound patient are 30- and 150-degrees sidelying. Both positions off-load the sacrum without increasing pressure to the greater trochanter, and both can be comfortable for the patient (Fig. 28-13, A). To maintain 30-degrees sidelying, a foam wedge or pillow roll is placed under one side of the shoulders and hips to form a 30-degree angle between the pelvis and the support surface. A pillow under the upper leg and between the knees prevents pressure on the inside of the knees and ankles. A pillow under the uppermost extremity also improves patient comfort. The 150-degrees sidelying position is maintained by placing a pillow or wedge under the chest, a pillow under the upper leg to prevent excessive hip internal rotation, and a small pillow or towel roll under the ankle of the lower leg (Fig. 28-13, B). Foam wedges with at least a 30-degree angle are excellent support devices and are available from commercial vendors.

The occiput is at risk for ulceration in the younger pediatric population,[3] especially if the head is larger than normal,[76] because at this age the occiput is proportionately the largest and heaviest bony prominence.[77] At around adolescence, pressure shifts from the occiput to areas typical for adults.[3,78] High occipital pressure was found to be consistently reduced with a 4-inch foam

TABLE 28-5	Causes and Solutions for Problematic Sitting Patterns	
Problematic Position	**Causes**	**Solutions**
Buttocks sliding forward in seat, face looking toward ceiling	<90° hip flexion	Recline the chair till face is vertical.
	Seat depth too short or too long	Modify to extend to within 1½ inches of popliteal fossa.
	Seat too high, feet do not touch the floor	Place cushion behind back.
		Use a drop-seat or foot rests.
		Minimize contact of the ball of the foot with foot rest.
	Increased trunk extensor tone	Use a lap belt or pommel cushion to hold hips back in the chair.
		Use a lower back rest.
		Change seat or back angle.
Forward trunk flexion, face looking at floor	Kyphosis >90° hip flexion contractures	Use a wedge cushion.
	Seat height too low	Add a seat cushion.
	Foot rests too high	Lower foot rests or add a cushion.
Weight unequally distributed side to side	Low trunk tone	Add trunk supports.
	Chair too wide	Use narrower chair.
	Structural deformity or post-surgical deformity	Use thicker cushion on the side with less weight or with lower pelvis.
	Poor femoral position	Use contoured cushion to support femurs.
		Use foam or towel roll between the chair and the lateral femur to maintain neutral hip.

Adapted from Hamm R, Behringer B: *The give and take of wound management: A guide to making clinical decisions,* Irvine, CA, 2004, ConceptMedia, Inc.
References: Rappl L: Management of pressure by therapeutic positioning. In Sussman C, Bates-Jensen BM (eds): *Wound care: A collaborative practice manual for physical therapists and nurses,* Gaithersburg, MD, 1998, Aspen.

BOX 28-3   Strategies for Tissue Protection in the Supine Position

- Test interface pressure between skin over bony prominences and support surface with commercial pressure sensor or by placing hand between mattress and overlay. If point of concern (e.g., sacrum, heel, greater trochanter) can be palpated or if there is less than 1 inch of support between the hand and bony prominences, support surface has "bottomed out" and is not effective.
- Use pillows or foam protective devices to protect bony prominences from rubbing against each other or against mechanical devices.
- Maintain head of bed lower than 30° except during meals. Increasing head elevation increases risk for shear forces over the sacrum. For patients who have NG feeding tube or have COPD, both requiring that head of bed be higher than 30°, maintaining it below 45° is advised.
- Off-load heels with pillows under calves, knees, and thighs (not under heels) or with heel protectors. After patient is positioned, check heel by placing hand underneath to ensure nothing is pressing on any side. Convoluted foam heel protectors require caution and frequent skin checks, especially if the foot and lower leg are edematous and skin is fragile. Raised points of foam on the inner surface of these devices can cause pressure points that lead to skin breakdown.
- Maintain <25° of knee flexion by supporting the knees with a pillow or by placing a bend in the bed if a hospital bed is used.

NG, Nasogastric; *COPD,* chronic obstructive pulmonary disease.

---

overlay.[78] There is little literature on effective methods to off-load the occiput; however, suggestions from caregivers include the use of a gel or air-cell pad or a rolled towel under the area just proximal to the occiput. Turning the head from side to side every 2 hours is also recommended.[79] The use of doughnuts is discouraged because they contribute to venous congestion and edema inside the ring[1] and may contribute to the formation of PUs.[80]

Patients who wear rigid cervical collars are also at risk for occipital PUs.[81] Risk factors associated with the collars are pressure, accumulation of moisture, and increased skin temperature.[82] As with any rigid orthotic device, the skin under the collar should be checked frequently, and the device should be adjusted for proper fit if any skin impairments are observed.

The amount of off-loading needed is different for every patient, depending on the impairments and the vulnerable areas of concern. After a thorough patient examination and evaluation, support surfaces and devices can be used creatively to establish an effective positioning and turning schedule specific for the patient. Through diligence and cooperation, members of the health care team can ensure

TABLE 28-6	Risks and Solutions for Problematic Recumbent Positions	

Problem	Areas at Risk	Solution
Exaggerated trunk extension	Occiput and heels	Support head with pillow and flex knees and hips to reduce tone.
Abnormal reflexes (e.g., tonic labyrinthine, asymmetrical tonic neck reflex)	Any bony prominence	Use firm support devices to reduce tone; avoid soft pillows that facilitate tone; use side-lying positions
Risk of aspiration; cardiopulmonary deficits; need HOB elevated >30°	Sacrum and heels	Off-load heels with pillows or protectors; limit time HOB is elevated >45°; keep below 30° if safe; sit in chair for meals if possible.
Kyphosis, prominent spinous processes	Spinous processes; sacrum; coccyx	Elevate HOB slightly and support head and neck with pillows; in severe cases, place small towel roll along each side of the spine.
Hip and knee flexion contractures (usually patient rolls to one side more than the other)	Inner knees, heels, greater trochanter, ischium, sacrum	Support the lower extremities in position of maximum extension; place a pillow between knees and ankles, turn side-to-side frequently.
Postsurgical incisions or scars	Ischemia around incision; dehiscence; ulcer recurrence	Position off the affected area; use support surface.
Foot drop	Heels	Use protective device; place a pillow under calf, knee, and thigh; use foam or pillows to support foot in neutral position.

Adapted from Hamm R, Behringer B: *The give and take of wound management: A guide to making clinical decisions*, Irvine, CA, 2004, ConceptMedia, Inc.
References: Rappl L: Management of pressure by therapeutic positioning. In Sussman C, Bates-Jensen BM (eds): *Wound care: A collaborative practice manual for physical therapists and nurses*, Gaithersburg, MD, 1998, Aspen; Rappl L, Hagler D: Prevention and treatment of pressure ulcers. In Kloth L, McCullough JM (eds): *Wound healing: Alternatives in management*, ed 3, Philadelphia, 2002, FA Davis.
HOB, Head of bed.

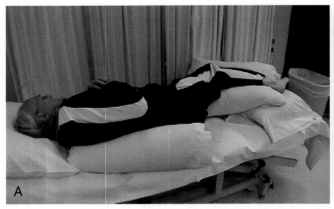 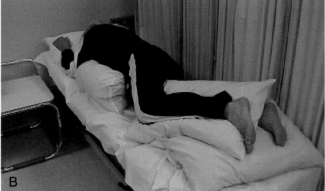

FIG. 28-13 **A,** Patient in 30-degree sidelying position to off-load the sacrum. **B,** Patient in 150-degree sidelying position to off-load the sacrum, greater trochanters, and scapulae.

that the care plan is adhered to by all therapies and the goals are shared by all disciplines.

Moisture Management. Although moisture management is traditionally considered a function of nursing care, understanding the following principles and strategies for the incontinent patient is helpful for all rehabilitation caregivers:

- Bladder training or prompted voiding.[83]
- Cleanse after each incontinent episode with no-rinse cleaner.
- Apply a moisture barrier ointment or cream after every cleansing.
- Use absorbent underpads or briefs.
- Avoid thin plastic-backed underpads that hold moisture and heat against the skin.

- Use a catheter for urinary incontinence and a fecal pouch or rectal tube for fecal incontinence.
- Place absorbent material in skinfolds where perspiration may accumulate and cause skin impairment.
- Wash wheelchair cushions after every incontinent episode and allow the cushion to fully dry before using it again.

Patients are significantly less likely to develop PUs if they wear disposable briefs, but if the patient is in a specialty bed designed to reduce skin moisture and temperature, pads or briefs that have plastic backing are contraindicated. These specialty beds are especially beneficial for patients at risk for skin maceration from excessive perspiration. If the patient has a sacral or trochanteric PU, fishnet surgical panties are recommended to hold dressings in place and allow free flow of air on the surrounding skin.

Nutrition. The goals of any nutrition intervention for patients with PUs are to provide sufficient calories, protein, fluid, vitamins, and trace elements to facilitate wound healing and closure.[50,51] For patients with nutritional deficits at risk for or with existing wounds, nutritional supplementation should be given orally if the patient can eat. If the gastrointestinal system is functioning, but the patient cannot swallow enough food to meet his or her nutritional needs, feeding of liquids may be provided temporarily by a nasogastric tube or by a feeding tube permanently inserted into the gastrointestinal tract by a percutaneous endoscopic gastrostomy (PEG) procedure. If the gastrointestinal system is not functioning, nutrition may be provided intravenously by total parenteral nutrition (TPN). All nonoral alternative feeding methods have associated risks and are not as effective at meeting nutritional needs as oral feeding. Nutritional interventions are ordered by the physician, generally in consultation with a registered dietitian.

> ### Clinical Pearl
>
> All nonoral alternative feeding methods have associated risks and are not as effective at meeting nutritional needs as oral feeding.

INTERVENTIONS BASED ON WOUND STAGE

After a PU has been debrided of necrotic tissue and staged (based on the amount of tissue loss as described), effective local interventions can be implemented (Table 28-7). The process of improving the wound to facilitate healing, termed *wound-bed preparation,* involves multiple interventions with the following goals: To remove devitalized tissue from the wound, including necrotic eschar and fibrinous tissue; to facilitate **angiogenesis** and thereby increase the amount of granulation tissue; to reduce the number of senescent cells (cells incapable of mitotic activity) in the wound bed and at the edges and thereby facilitate both angiogenesis and epithelialization; to decrease

TABLE 28-7	Intervention Based on Pressure Ulcer Stage
Stage	**Intervention**
Stage I	Determine the causative factors.
	Adapt seating and bed surfaces to reduce pressure, friction, or shear forces at the areas of concern.
	Protect macerated skin with a moisture barrier cream or ointment.
	Protect areas exposed to friction forces with a transparent film dressing.
	Encourage frequent changes of position.
Stage II	Consistently position the patient to reduce pressure at the areas of concern.
	Cleanse the wound and periwound tissue with normal saline or a wound cleanser.
	Remove any loose devitalized tissue.
	Cover with a transparent film dressing if there is no drainage or a hydrocolloid dressing if there is minimal-to-moderate drainage. Both dressings are semipermeable to prevent bacteria from entering the wound.
	Evaluate the need for an indwelling urinary catheter or absorbent pads to prevent skin exposure to excess moisture.
	Protect the periwound skin from maceration or friction.
Stage III and stage IV	Consistently position the patient to relieve pressure at the areas of concern.
	Use a pressure-relieving support surface.
	Debride the wound of all necrotic tissue.
	Culture for infection (if signs of infection are observed) and treat with appropriate antibiotics and local antimicrobial dressings.
	Irrigate the wound daily with pulsed lavage with suction to remove slough, to decrease the bacteria load, and to help manage drainage.
	Assess for negative pressure therapy after more than 70% of the wound is free of necrotic tissue.
	Use a dressing appropriate for the bacterial load and drainage (e.g., alginates, foam fillers, hydrocolloids, collagen matrix dressings, or nontoxic topical ointments).
	Assess nutritional status and supplement diet as needed.
	Evaluate the need for surgical closure.
Post-Surgery	Maintain bed rest in a low-air-loss mattress or air-fluidized bed for 2 to 4 weeks.
	Manage incontinence to keep flap dry and free of contaminants.
	Observe flap for changes that may indicate hematoma formation (dark red appearance), flap necrosis (black tissue), dehiscence (separation at suture site), seroma (pocket of clear fluid), or infection (white appearance under the skin).
Post-Healing	Assess for proper support surfaces to off-load the flap or graft.
	Monitor support surfaces for "bottoming out" phenomenon for at least 2 years.
	Monitor the skin of the flap or graft for at least 2 years.
	Rehabilitate the patient to maximum functional level.
	Educate the patient on the necessity to stop smoking to maintain tissue viability.
	Encourage continued good nutrition.

TABLE 28-8	Methods of Debridement
Type	**Methods**
Surgical	Performed in the operating room by a licensed physician, podiatrist, or physician's assistant. Not tissue-specific; removes all necrotic tissue down to and often including some viable tissue. Required in the following conditions: • The wound is life-threatening. • There is more necrotic tissue than can be removed at bedside. • The risk of bleeding is high and sutures or cauterization may be required. • Infected or necrotic bone is being removed. • Pain cannot be controlled by standard medications or topical anesthetics.
Sharp	Selective removal of necrotic, infected, or foreign tissue with sterile instruments (scalpels, scissors, tweezers, and forceps). Performed bedside or in an outpatient clinic. Requires a physician's referral when performed by allied health personnel.
Mechanical	Nonselective removal of devitalized tissue from the wound and periwound areas using friction or pressure. May be painful. Used for loose debris and exudate. Includes moist-to-damp dressings, abrasion, syringe irrigation, PLWS, and whirlpool.
Autolytic	Phagocytosis of necrotic tissue by white blood cells in natural body fluids. Facilitated by moisture-retentive dressings (e.g., transparent films, hydrocolloids, calcium alginates). Selective and pain-free. Effective for adhered superficial eschar; is inefficient for large amounts of eschar.
Enzymatic	Is the application of enzymes in a topical petrolatum-based ointment to facilitate the liquefaction and digestion of nonviable wound tissue. Selective and pain-free. Helpful adjunct to sharp and autolytic debridement. Currently limited to two preparations: • Papain-urea–based combinations. • Collagenase.

PLWS, Pulsed lavage with suction.

exudate and edema, both of which retard the healing process; and to decrease the bacterial burden.[84,85]

Wound-bed preparation begins with debridement, removal of the devitalized tissue, which may be accomplished by one or more techniques (Table 28-8). With debridement, much of the bacterial burden is removed; however, if clinical signs of infection (redness, drainage, edema, pain, odor, or warmth) are present, a culture is indicated, followed by appropriate systemic or topical antibiotics. The removal of bacteria, exudate, and edema can be facilitated by a variety of techniques, including advanced dressings and physical modalities. After necrotic tissue, exudate, and bacterial load have been removed, dressings that effectively manage drainage and maintain a warm, moist wound environment are applied.

Wound Dressings. Wound dressings are identified as primary or secondary. Primary dressings are applied directly to the wound bed and secondary dressings are used to anchor or contain the primary dressings. The function and selection of the primary dressing is based on the wound characteristics (e.g., tissue type, healing phase, and bacterial count). The function and selection of the secondary dressing is based on the purpose and consistency of the primary dressing and on the patient's functional status. The appropriate wound dressing will likely change as the needs of the wound change and may vary among different areas of a wound that are in different healing phases. The informed clinician, being resourceful with the available supplies, matches the primary dressing to the wound needs and the secondary dressing to the patient needs (Table 28-9).

Selecting the optimal dressing for a PU is based on a few basic principles. The dressing should keep the wound bed moist while keeping the periwound skin dry to protect it from maceration. If the wound bed tends to be dry, dressings that add moisture are advised. If there is drainage, the dressing should manage any excessive moisture. Periwound skin should also be protected with moisture barrier creams, protective films, or hydrocolloid dressings. When dressing a PU with a cavity, the cavity should be lightly filled with the dressing material so that there is no dead space to collect exudate and increase the risk of infection or abscess formation. Self-adhesive dressings are recommended to avoid applying tape to the periwound skin because removing tape can cause skin tears. Many of the advanced dressings can remain in place for 24 to 72 hours or longer, reducing caregiver time and facilitating wound healing by limiting wound bed disturbance, thereby decreasing the overall cost of treatment.

◎ *Clinical Pearl*

The appropriate wound dressing will keep the wound bed moist while keeping the periwound skin dry.

Topical Antibiotics. Topical antibiotics are not recommended for wounds that are responding to conservative treatment with risk factor management and dressings. However, when a clean PU is not healing or a wound has persistent exudate after 2 to 4 weeks of standard care, the AHRQ *Guidelines* recommend a 2-week trial of topical antibiotics.[1]

Silver, in the forms of dilute silver nitrate liquid, silver sulfadiazine cream, and **nanocrystalline silver** in a dressing, can be used as a topical antimicrobial medication for wound management.[86] Silver sulfadiazine cream also keeps the wound bed moist. Because the silver in silver nitrate liquid and silver sulfadiazine cream is released and absorbed quickly, these preparations must be applied twice daily, and an absorbent secondary dressing may be needed to manage exudates in moderate to heavily draining wounds. Nanocrystalline silver absorbent dressings can remain in place for 2 to 4 days.

Debridement. Debridement, the removal of nonviable tissue and foreign bodies from the wound bed, is an important part of wound-bed preparation. For stage IV wounds involving muscle, tendon, or bone, a surgeon may

TABLE 28-9 Dressing Categories

Dressing Category	Composition	Uses	Advantages	Disadvantages
Wound cleansers				
• Normal saline	0.9% saline, sterile water	Cleansing wound Moist to damp dressing	Inexpensive	Contains no preservatives, should be discarded 24 hours after opening
• Cleansing solutions	Surfactants in assorted bases	Cleansing wound Mechanical debridement	Helps disrupt bond between necrotic tissue and wound bed Neutral pH	Reduces frictional force of sterile gauze
Gauze	100% cotton or synthetic fabric	Cleansing wound Filling cavity and sinus wounds Anchoring primary dressings	Available in a variety of sizes and shapes Inexpensive Conforms to wound shape Absorbs exudate	Dries easily Destroys healthy tissue if allowed to dry Needs to be changed twice per day Does not contain exudate
Transparent film	Polymer sheet with adhesive layer on one side	Autolytic debridement Reduce friction over bony prominences Superficial wounds with minimal drainage Secondary dressing over foam or gauze	Conforms easily to any shape Impermeable to bacteria Reduces friction between wound bed and contact surfaces Waterproof Adheres well to dry skin Can stay in place 3-7 days Cost effective	Nonabsorbent May cause periwound maceration May tear fragile skin if removed improperly Will not stick to moist areas
Hydrogel sheets	Hydrophilic polymers entrap water to form solid sheet	Thermal burns and painful wounds	Promotes epithelialization Soothes inflamed tissue Protects granulation tissue	Slippery Requires a secondary dressing
Amorphous	Polymers and water in a gel form	Dry eschar wounds Clean granulating wounds Exposed tendon and bone	Maintain moist wound environment Assume shape of cavity wounds Promotes autolysis Noncytotoxic to granulation tissue Cost effective	Requires a secondary dressing May contribute to periwound maceration if applied too heavily
Hydrocolloids	Combination of adhesive layer, absorbent hydrocolloid layer, and semipermeable layer	Shallow full-thickness wounds with minimal to moderate exudate Stage II or III pressure ulcers Macerated tissue	Absorbent Promotes granulation and epithelialization Promotes autolysis Protects skin from friction May not require second dressing Can stay in place 3-4 days Available in variety of sizes and shapes and in combination with other dressings	May roll at the edges Moderately expensive May create an odor as it absorbs exudate May tear fragile skin if removed improperly
Foams	Polyurethane	Wounds with minimal to copious exudates Cavity wounds (chips and pillows)	Available in a variety of sizes and shapes Highly absorbent Do not adhere to the wound bed Painless to remove	Expensive May require secondary dressing May be bulky Difficult to conform to some areas
Calcium alginates	Calcium salts of alginic acid which have been spun into fibers	Wounds with moderate to copious drainage	Highly absorbent Conforms to wound shape May be bacteriostatic and mildly hemostatic Decreases odor	Requires secondary dressing Not advised over bone or tendon because of desiccation Difficult to remove if allowed to dry in wound bed

Continued

TABLE 28-9	Dressing Categories—cont'd			
Dressing Category	**Composition**	**Uses**	**Advantages**	**Disadvantages**
Collagen matrix	Collagen derived from bovine material with all cells extracted, freeze-dried, and shaped into sheets, particles, or gels	Any recalcitrant wound to facilitate collagen migration	Conforms to wound bed Promotes granulation and epithelialization	Expensive Requires secondary dressing
Gels and ointments	Water or petrolatum-based gels and ointments containing active ingredients; used as primary dressing on wound bed (antimicrobials, growth factors, silver, enzymes)	Wounds requiring topical medications Painful wounds (topical anesthetics)	Allows local application of antimicrobials without use of systemic antibiotics Maintains moist wound environment while delivering active ingredient to wound bed	Usually requires prescription depending on active ingredient Requires a secondary dressing Risk of allergic reaction to active ingredient Some may not be used simultaneously (e.g., enzymatic and silver sulfadiazine)
Small intestine submucosa (SIS) dressings	Collagen tissue extracted from porcine submucosa, processed to remove cells, and shaped into sheets	Full or partial thickness wounds of any etiology Autograft donor sites Second degree burns	Promote cell migration Present no risk of rejection Minimize scarring Reduce frequency of dressing changes (in place 5-7 days) Has long shelf life	Expensive
Living skin equivalents	Human fibroblasts embedded in a bovine collagen matrix and bioabsorbable scaffold	Full- or partial-thickness flat wounds	Promote epithelialization Noninvasive and painless May help avoid skin grafting Decrease scarring	Require fully granulated, infection-free wound bed Expensive Short shelf-life (5 days)

perform debridement under anesthesia to avoid pain during the procedure and to allow for ready control of bleeding should this occur. For stage II and III PUs, a physical therapist may perform selective sharp debridement at the bedside. Physical therapist assistants are generally not licensed to perform wound debridement but may assist the physical therapist with this procedure.

Debridement with tools may be augmented by use of topical enzymatic chemical debriders. Although these cannot substitute for surgical or sharp debridement when there is a large amount of necrotic tissue, they are effective for maintenance debridement or for removing adhered fibrous tissue that is difficult to debride with instruments.[87] The two active ingredient combinations currently used for enzymatic debridement are collagenase and a papain-urea combination. Collagenase ointment (Santyl) contains a partially purified preparation of collagenase enzyme that degrades nonviable collagen and converts it to gelatin, thereby facilitating the removal of the devitalized tissue.[88] The enzyme is selective for nonviable tissue and does not cause pain when applied. Papain-urea ointments (Panafil, Accuzyme) contain urea, which denatures protein and exposes the papain activators, allowing the papain enzymes to proteolyse the devitalized tissue. The papain-urea combination breaks down both viable and nonviable protein and may cause an inflammatory response and

pain.[88] Papain-urea is effective for debridement of eschar, dried fibrinous exudate usually found in chronic venous ulcers, and burn eschar. Collagenase is effective for burn eschar, heat-denatured collagen, and dermal ulcers.[89]

Clinical Pearl

Enzymatic debridement may be a useful adjunct for removing devitalized tissue; however, interventions for off-loading tissue, reducing bacterial load, and managing exudate are still essential for effective treatment of any pressure ulcer (PU).

Adjunctive Therapies. Physical modalities, including electric, light, sound, and mechanical energy to effect tissue changes at the cellular level, are used to promote soft tissue healing in a variety of conditions.

Physical agents are a "broad group of procedures using various forms of energy that are applied to tissues in a systematic manner and that are intended to increase connective tissue extensibility; increase the healing rate of open wounds and soft tissue; modulate pain; reduce or eliminate soft tissue swelling, inflammation, or restriction associated with musculoskeletal injury or circulatory dysfunction; remodel scar tissue; or treat skin conditions."[20] Electrotherapeutic modalities, as they relate to wound healing, are a broad group of agents that use electricity to

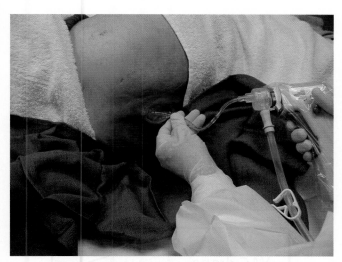

FIG. 28-14 Pulsed lavage with suction being used to remove debris, bacteria, and exudate from wound bed.

increase the rate of healing of open wounds, modulate or decrease pain, reduce bacterial load, and reduce or eliminate soft tissue swelling or inflammation. Negative pressure wound therapy (including pulsed lavage with suction and vacuum-assisted closure), electrical stimulation, ultraviolet C, and ultrasound are modalities that may be used for treatment of PUs; however, it is important to remember that they are adjunct therapies and not substitutes for standard care (i.e., tissue off-loading, debridement, and provision of a moist wound environment).

Pulsed Lavage with Suction. Given the fact that removal of bacteria, devitalized tissue, foreign bodies, and exudates facilitate wound closure, the clinician is faced with selecting the most effective method of removing these impediments. Pulsed lavage with suction (PLWS) combines low- or high-pressure irrigation of normal saline at a controlled pressure (measured in pounds per square inch [psi]) and suction at a controlled subatmospheric pressure (measured in mm Hg) to remove debris, bacteria, and exudate from the wound bed (Fig. 28-14). A pressure range of 4 to 15 psi will safely mechanically debride a wound, remove bacteria, and stimulate angiogenesis.[90]

Recommended Pressure Ranges (in psi) for Pulsed Lavage with Suction
- 4-6: For sensitive areas, sinus tracts, tunneling, and painful wounds.
- 8-15: To decrease bacterial load in infected wounds.
- 9-15: To remove necrotic tissue.
- 15 and above: Use only with physician present.

The PLWS unit may be plugged into a wall outlet or battery-powered and includes a hand piece with a trigger to control the pressure, a tip to deliver the water into the wound bed and suction away the contaminated fluid, and two tubes—one connected to the bag of sterile normal saline and one connected to a suction pump. Four systems, each with specific recommendations for providing patient care, are currently available. The Pulsavac System (Zimmer, Inc, Dover, OH) consists of a portable pump that can be transported to any patient care location and detachable,

disposable handgun and tips. The Simpulse VariCare System (Davol, Inc, Cranston, RI) consists of a battery-operated hand piece that can be cleaned and stored for multiple treatments with the same patient when used with a special diverter tip that prevents the contaminated saline from traveling through the hand piece. The Davol Simpulse Plus System (Davol, Inc) is powered by medical air or nitrogen. The InterPulse System (Stryker, Inc, Kalamazoo, Mich) has a battery-powered hand piece with trigger-controlled pressure and disposable diverter tips.

Advantages and Disadvantages. PLWS provides a higher pressure than syringe irrigation and delivers a larger amount of irrigating solution to the wound in a shorter length of time than bulb irrigation. PLWS can be used to treat bedridden and medically unstable patients (e.g., those in intensive care and cardiac care units) who cannot be transported to hydrotherapy for whirlpool treatment. It also enables treatment of isolated patients without risking exposure of other patients. Cross-contamination of multiple wounds on the same patient is reduced, and exposure to bacteria from other body parts, as may occur in full body submersion in a large whirlpool, is eliminated. The variable and controlled pressure and suction of PLWS allows adjustment to minimize pain. Treatment of foot ulcers with PLWS avoids the dependent position required for whirlpool treatment. In addition, PLWS is more time efficient than transporting patients to hydrotherapy and cleaning whirlpools. Specifically related to patients with PUs, PLWS enables patients to be treated in off-loaded positions and avoids transporting and treating patients with sacral ulcers in supine positions on hard surfaces.[91]

Indications and Contraindications. Indications for PLWS include stage III and IV PUs, especially those that are infected, draining, or necrotic. Irrigation performed before debridement facilitates sharp debridement by loosening slough and softening eschar. Long flexible tips are available to treat areas of tunneling or undermining, in which bacteria can colonize and exudate can collect. These tips deliver lower pressure and are safe to use in sinuses in which the base of the wound is not visible.

Special Precautions. Special precautions are recommended for some unusual or complex wounds such as tunneling wounds that cannot be observed or probed to the base, facial and groin wounds, wounds that expose major vessels, and wounds with excessive bleeding. Patients on anticoagulants, patients who are insensate, and patients who have pain not controlled by pain medications can also benefit from precautions. Precautionary measures include using lower pressure or different tips, lowering the suction to 60 to 80 mm Hg, or using a Yankauer suction tip rather than suctioning through the irrigation tip.

Method of Application. Depending on the size of the wound, 500 to 3,000 ml of sterile normal saline solution in intravenous-type bags is used for each treatment.

Suction pressure is adjusted to 60 to 100 mm Hg. In wounds that are sensitive, close to major vessels, or have soft tissue that is easily pulled into the tip shield, lower suction is advised. In wounds with fragile tissue, crevices, or undermining that is difficult to suction, a Yankauer suction tube can be connected to the wall canister and used in conjunction with any irrigation tip. The pressure is selected according to the treatment goals, exposed tissue, and patient pain levels.

Infection control with the use of PLWS is important because of the aerosol nature of treatment and the possible spread of microbes in the wound.[92] The Centers for Disease Control and Prevention has recently supported recommendations developed by Loehne,[93] including the wearing of personal protective equipment by all staff in the room at the time of treatment, providing treatment only in private patient or treatment rooms, strict disposal of contaminated waste in appropriate biohazard bags, and disinfection of horizontal surfaces after each treatment. Guidelines for disposal of body fluids in a biohazard bag state to include fluid in the suction canister and any dressing containing >20 cc drainage. To minimize contamination between treatments, reusable components of the PLWS system are stored between treatments, wrapped in sterile towels, sealed in a plastic bag, and labeled with the patient name, room number, and date of first use.

Outcomes. Expected outcomes of PLWS intervention include elimination of odor and exudate in 3 to 7 days, full debridement after 1 to 2 weeks, and advancement from the chronic to inflammatory phase in 1 week and to the proliferative phase in 2 weeks.[93] Treatment is discontinued after 1 week if no improvement is noted. Frequency of treatment initially is daily and may be decreased to 2 to 3 days per week to maintain a clean wound bed if surgical closure is expected. In stage III or IV PUs, once the wound bed is clean and more than 70% granulated, either advanced dressings that can be changed less frequently or vacuum-assisted closure is recommended.

Vacuum-Assisted Closure. The application of topical negative or subatmospheric pressure to open wounds was first reported in Europe in the early 1990s[94-96] and was introduced in the United States in 1997.[97] Early application involved the use of wall suction apparatus or surgical vacuum bottles; however, these systems lacked control and maintenance of required pressure levels.[98] Since that time, a purpose-designed vacuum-assisted closure (VAC) device (VAC, Kinetic Concepts, Inc, San Antonio, TX) that uses a microprocessor-controlled pump has become widely accepted as an adjunctive therapy for wounds of all etiologies. VAC application consists of filling or covering the wound with sterile polyurethane foam with pores ranging from 400 to 600 μm in size, inserting a suction tube into the foam, and connecting the tube to the pump that contains a collection canister. The foam, part of the tubing, and periwound tissue are then sealed with an occlusive sterile drape (Fig. 28-15). Continuous or intermittent suction, ranging from 50 to 200 mm Hg, creates a vacuum that reduces edema, exudate, and bacteria. In addition, the closed wound environment is kept moist, thereby promoting healing and preventing contamination.

The first article on VAC therapy reported that negative pressure increased local blood flow by up to 4 times baseline and increased the rate of granulation by 63% to 103%.[99] Based on these results, a protocol of using continuous pressure for the first 48 hours of treatment to decrease edema and using intermittent pressure thereafter

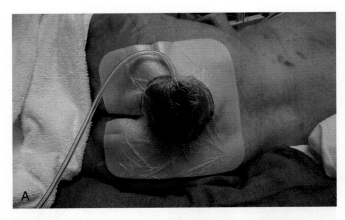

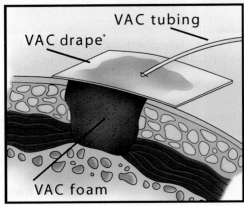

FIG. 28-15 A, Vacuum-assisted closure on a sacral pressure ulcer. **B,** A cross-section of a cavity wound illustrates the position of the foam and tubing. *Courtesy KCI, San Antonio, TX.*

to optimize granulation tissue formation was developed.[100] Studies suggest that treatment with the VAC is a cost-effective intervention for chronic wounds.

Many case studies and retrospective reviews of the use of the VAC for treatment of wounds of various etiologies have been published; however, there are few randomized controlled trials of this intervention in human subjects.

Advantages and Disadvantages. Advantages of VAC are the decrease in the number of dressing changes from 1 to 2 times per day to every 2 to 3 days and the ability of the occlusive drape to keep moisture (e.g., urinary and fecal incontinence, perspiration, and leaking exudates) away from the wound and periwound skin. The primary disadvantage is the expense with current estimates for pump rental of $75 to $125 per day, in addition to the supplies (packaged to include foam, drape, and tubing for each dressing change), which cost approximately $20 to $30 per application. Given the cost of one hospital day, however, cost savings are likely if use of this device shortens hospital stays.

Indications and Contraindications. VAC therapy is indicated for any cavity wound, dehisced or acute surgical wounds, skin grafts and flaps, traumatic wounds, and neuropathic stage III PUs or stage IV PUs, after adequate debridement has been achieved. It is contraindicated for wounds with more than 30% devitalized tissue, untreated osteomyelitis, wounds with cancerous or malignant tissue, and exposed blood vessels. Precautionary measures are recommended for wounds that have not achieved hemostasis or wounds that bleed easily because the patient is on anticoagulants. Precautionary measures include lowering the pressure or delaying initiation of therapy until active bleeding ceases. Wounds adjacent to major vessels or bypass grafts may be lined with nonadherent mesh under the polyurethane foam or dressed with denser, saline soaked foam available from the manufacturer. Wounds containing fistulas may require customized application of dressings and suction to adequately manage drainage.

Treatment Guidelines. The use of sterile technique and supplies are recommended for VAC application, although it is known that chronic wounds are generally not sterile. The entire cavity is filled with foam (including undermining and sinus tracks) to prevent accumulation of fluid in dead spaces—a condition that provides an environment for bacterial growth. Nonadherent mesh can be placed between the wound surface and the provided black foam to prevent granulation tissue from penetrating the foam, thereby decreasing destruction of new tissue and patient discomfort when removing the dressing. The foam should be cut and positioned so that some part of every piece touches another piece of foam. The occlusive drape needs to extend 3 to 5 cm beyond the wound edge to obtain a good seal and prevent leakage, and the suction tube needs to be embedded in the foam so that the drainage holes at the end of the tube are covered. Directions for starting therapy and changing the canister are included with every unit and are therefore not included here. The suction pressure should be set at between 50 and 125 mm Hg, according to patient comfort.

VAC dressings are changed as follows: Infected wounds, every 12 hours; heavily draining wounds, every 24 hours; clean wounds, every 48 hours; and meshed graft wounds, after 4 to 5 days. Full canisters can be changed without complete dressing changes. The wound is inspected daily, and the dressing is changed immediately if any of the following conditions are observed:

- Odor comes from the wound or canister, possibly a result of accumulation of blood in the foam.
- If hemostasis is not maintained in the wound bed and bleeding occurs, the negative pressure suctions blood and an alternative dressing is recommended.
- Foam is no longer tightly wrinkled, indicating the seal is lost and suction is insufficient.
- Suction is off for more than 2 hours. Accumulated drainage under the foam is an ideal environment for bacterial growth that may cause infection.
- Pain or discomfort under the foam is unrelieved by decreasing the pressure.
- Drainage accumulates under the adhesive drape. This may cause skin maceration.

Treatment with the VAC is usually discontinued when full granulation is achieved. Then another dressing that facilitates epithelialization or surgical closure should be considered. In summary, VAC is a versatile, effective adjunctive therapy for removal of edema, bacteria, and loose debris from wounds; for stimulating cell proliferation; and for providing protection from external contaminants.

Electrical Stimulation. Electrical stimulation (ES), with various treatment parameters, has been used for many years to facilitate tissue healing. The proposed rationales for applying electricity to facilitate tissue healing include the presence of an electrical charge in healing tissue, attraction of specific cell types by an applied electrical current (termed **galvanotaxis**), the stimulatory effect of electricity on cells to promote biosynthesis and replication, possible bactericidal effects of electricity, and effects of electricity on circulation and myofibroblast contraction.

The surface of intact human skin has a negative charge of approximately 23 mV, while the inner layers of the epidermis have a positive charge. When a dermal wound occurs, a Na ion flows from the deeper wound bed to the surface, attracting the cells required for tissue repair. The wound must stay moist for this current of injury to flow. The current of injury continues through all phases of healing until a wound closes. Once a wound is closed, there is no further current flow.

The current of injury is thought to cause charged cells to move toward the area of opposite charge. Applied electrical currents with a fixed polarity (i.e., monophasic currents) can also promote galvanotaxis.[101] In addition to attracting appropriate cells to an area, pulsed electrical currents can trigger calcium channels in fibroblast and lymphocyte cell membranes to open, increasing the level of intracellular calcium triggering increased synthesis of proteins by fibroblasts.

An electrical current can be applied to a wound by placing electrodes on or near the wound bed (Fig. 28-16). The polarity of the electrode at the wound site is selected, depending on the type of cells required to facilitate or advance a particular healing phase. The charge of each of the cell types involved in wound healing processes and the electrode to which they are attracted are listed in Table 28-10. Based on this information, the clinician can select the appropriate polarity for the active electrode according

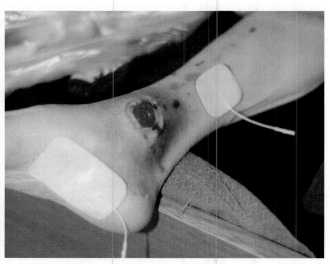

FIG. 28-16 Electrode placement to promote tissue healing.

TABLE 28-10	Cell Charge and Attracting Electrode		
Cell Type	**Healing Phase**	**Charge**	**Electrode that Attracts the Cell**
Platelets	Hemostasis and inflammatory	Positive	Negative
Macrophages	Inflammatory	Negative	Positive
Neutrophils	Inflammatory	Negative (with infection)	Negative
		Positive (without infection)	Positive
Mast cells	Inflammatory	Negative	Positive
Fibroblasts	Proliferative	Positive	Negative
Epidermal cells	Epithelialization	Negative	Positive

From Sussman C, Byl N: Electrical stimulation for wound healing. In Kloth L, McCullough JM (eds): *Wound healing: Alternatives in management,* ed 3, Philadelphia, 2002, FA Davis; Hamm R, Behringer B: *The give and take of wound management: A guide to making clinical decisions,* Irvine, CA, 2004, ConceptMedia, Inc.

to the presence or absence of infection and the healing phase of the wound.[101]

Indications and Contraindications. The effects of ES on wound and periwound tissue are related to the phase of wound healing rather than the wound etiology. Therefore, except for the listed contraindications, ES is considered safe for all types of wounds. Contraindications for ES include the presence of any neoplasm in or around the wound, untreated or nonresolving osteomyelitis in underlying bony structures, metal ions (e.g., silver from topical medications), any electronic implant that would be affected by the ES, and close proximity to any reflex center (carotid sinus, phrenic nerve, heart, or laryngeal muscles) that would be sensitive to ES. Therefore ES is not recommended on the chest or anterior neck.[102]

Treatment Guidelines. When using ES to treat wounds, the clinician selects the polarity of the active electrode (defined as the electrode on or in proximity to the wound), the type of electrodes and the conducting medium, the electrode placement, waveform, frequency, and the current amplitude. The polarity of the cells one wants to attract to the wound bed generally determines the polarity of the active electrode placed at the wound site. In general, the positive pole is used to promote epithelialization, autolysis, and reactivation of the inflammatory phase, and the negative pole is used to promote granulation and resolution of edema and inflammation. A high-voltage pulsed current (HVPC) waveform is used with a frequency of 30 to 120 pulses per second and daily treatments of 45 to 60 minutes duration.

The active electrode may be made of saline-soaked gauze, amorphous hydrogel, or a hydrogel sheet. For cavity wounds, the gauze is moistened with saline solution, fluffed, lightly packed into the wound cavity, covered with an aluminum foil electrode, and anchored with tape. A pre-gelled, self-adhesive electrode can be used for the dispersive electrode. After the ES treatment, an appropriate secondary dressing is applied over the gauze or hydrogel, or a new dressing is applied.

The active electrode may be placed directly over or just proximal to the wound, or two electrodes of the same polarity, each half the size of the wound area, may be placed on intact skin at either side of the wound (termed the *straddling technique*).[102] A dispersive electrode larger than the wound area is placed 15 to 30 cm proximal to the wound site. If the wound is deep, the dispersive electrode should be farther from the wound so the current will flow more deeply.

The current amplitude is adjusted to a level that causes the patient to feel a slight tingling without any motor activity. For the insensate patient, the amplitude is adjusted to a submotor level (i.e., it is increased until a contraction is seen and then decreased by approximately 10%). Additional recommendations for the application of ES for the treatment of chronic wounds include the following:

- Remove all topical dressing residue that may contain petrolatum or heavy metal ions (for example, iodine or zinc).
- Cleanse the skin that will be under the electrodes with normal saline or soap and water to remove oils or debris that can impede good current flow.
- Perform sharp debridement before application of ES. The conducting medium can then remain in the wound as a primary dressing, thereby reducing the amount of time the wound is exposed to air.
- If the patient complains of tingling or burning under the dispersive electrode, check for dryness or poor skin contact. If either condition exists, interrupt treatment to moisten the electrode and reapply with good contact.
- After each treatment, inspect the skin under both active and dispersive electrodes for any signs of irritation.

Ultraviolet C. Ultraviolet (UV) radiation is electromagnetic radiation with a frequency range of 7.5×10^{14} to 10^{16} Hz and with wavelengths of 400 to 100 nm. UV radiation is divided into three spectral bands, UVA, UVB, and UVC; UVA is the longest and UVC is the shortest at 290 to 100 nm. Only UVC is used to facilitate wound healing. UVC may facilitate healing in chronic wounds by stimulating fibroblasts to produce collagen, by killing bacteria and viruses, by causing vasodilation and thereby increasing capillary permeability and oxygen delivery to the affected tissue, by destroying senescent epithelial cells at the wound edge to enhance reepithelialization, by increasing production of growth factors, and by causing sloughing of necrotic tissue.[103] Wound contraction may also be facilitated by increased production of fibronectin in epithelial fibroblasts.[104]

Indications and Contraindications. UVC may be used for treatment of infected wounds, independent of etiology; however, any type of UV radiation should not be applied to the eyes and is contraindicated for a number of patients, including those with the following[105]:

- Acute onset of psoriasis, herpes simplex, or eczema in periwound skin
- Malignant wounds or cancer in periwound tissue
- Fever*
- Skin grafts
- Local erythema
- Acquired immunodeficiency syndrome (AIDS)/ human immunodeficiency virus (HIV) infection
- Pulmonary tuberculosis*
- Cardiac, renal, or liver disease*
- Severe diabetes*
- Systemic lupus erythematosus
- Hyperthyroidism*
- Deep x-ray therapy

Precautions are advised for patients with poor tolerance to sun exposure. Photosensitivity may also be increased by certain medications, including the antibiotics tetracyclines, sulfonamides, and quinolones; the phenothiazine antipsychotics; psoralens used for treatment of acute psoriasis; gold therapy used historically as an antiinflammatory agent in patients with rheumatoid arthritis; and the cardiac antiarrhythmic drugs, amiodarone hydrochloride and quinidine. Also, any recently irradiated tissue that is more susceptible to developing cancer should be treated with extreme caution,[100] although there have been no published reports of increased incidence of skin cancer with the use of UVC.[105]

Treatment Guidelines. Derma-wand (National Biological Corporation, Twinsburg, OH) is the only UVC device currently on the market in the United States. It is a relatively inexpensive, hand-held unit that is convenient to use for treatment of infected wounds (Fig. 28-17). Treatment with UVC should be preceded by a complete wound evaluation, sharp debridement of necrotic tissue, and removal of any residual dressing with normal saline. Both the patient and the therapist should avoid exposure of the eyes to UV radiation by wearing UV-blocking goggles. UV radiation therapy should be discontinued as soon as clinical signs of infections have resolved.

Procedure for Ultraviolet C Treatment of Infected Wounds

- Position the patient so the UV wand can be placed parallel to the wound bed and the rays can be transmitted perpendicular to the tissue to maximize energy delivery to the wound.
- Apply a UV-blocking agent with an SPF of 30, a thick layer of petrolatum, or a cotton drape over the periwound skin for protection.
- Position the UVC lamp 2.5 cm from the wound.

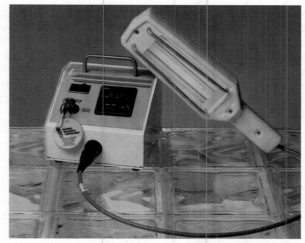

FIG. 28-17 Derma-wand is a hand-held ultraviolet C unit used to treat infected wounds. *Courtesy National Biological Corp, Twinsburg, OH.*

- Expose the wound to UVC according to the following guidelines:
  - Group A streptococcus (GAS) infection: 4 seconds, twice per day
  - GAS plus *Staphylococcus aureus:* 120 seconds, twice per day
  - Methicillin-resistant *S. aureus* (MRSA): 90 seconds, daily
  - Vancomycin-resistant *Enterococci* (VRE): 45 seconds, daily
  - Antibiotic-susceptible bacteria: 30 seconds, daily
- Apply the appropriate dressing to the wound as soon as possible to prevent drying and cooling of the wound tissue.
- Clean the equipment with an antiseptic solution after each use.

Ultrasound. Ultrasound (US) is sound waves with a frequency of greater than 20 kHz (20,000 cycles per second). Therapeutic US is generally in the 1 to 3 MHz (1 to 3 million cycles per second) frequency range. When US waves are absorbed by tissue, they cause a range of effects. Lower intensities of pulsed US do not cause measurable increases in tissue temperature but may promote tissue repair by nonthermal mechanisms. Nonthermal effects of US include cavitation, microstreaming, and acoustic streaming.

Cavitation is the production of small, gas-filled bubbles within conducting mediums and tissue fluids that absorb US. The intensities of US that can be produced by therapeutic US devices cause these bubbles to oscillate in size, becoming bigger and smaller. This is stable cavitation. Stable cavitation is thought to increase cell membrane permeability and diffusional properties. Much higher intensities of US can cause the bubbles to burst. This unstable cavitation can cause tissue damage but does not occur at the US intensities used in therapy.[106]

Microstreaming refers to microscopic fluid movements. US causes microstreaming next to cell membranes and around the bubbles produced by cavitation. Microstreaming is thought to enhance transport of ions and molecules

---

*UVC is contraindicated if used in conjunction with UVA or UVB to large body surface areas.

involved in tissue healing. Acoustic streaming is a larger scale flow of fluids produced in the US field. This flow is also thought to enhance the flow of ions and molecules involved in wound healing. Stable cavitation, microstreaming, and acoustic streaming are thought to underlie the following physiological changes associated with wound healing that have been observed with the application of US:

- Mast cell degranulation, resulting in a release of histamine and chemotactic factors into the periwound tissue and an initiation of the inflammatory healing phase.
- Increased vascular permeability, resulting in an increased flow of platelets, macrophages, leukocytes, and mast cells, all of which are active during the inflammatory phase of healing.
- Increased phagocytosis of hematoma material by macrophages and neutrophils.
- Stimulation of fibroblast activity, resulting in increased collagen synthesis, and in turn producing two positive healing effects—accelerated wound closure and stronger scar tissue.
- Stimulation of endothelial cell activity, resulting in accelerated dermal repair.[102]

Indications and Contraindications. The indications for the use of US in wound healing are acute wounds in the inflammatory healing phase (preferably within a few hours of onset), hematomas, bruises, and recalcitrant wounds. Contraindications are irradiated tissue; tumors or malignancies; pregnant uterus; deep venous thrombosis (DVT), emboli, or thrombophlebitis; ischemic or insensate tissue; pacemakers or implanted defibrillators; reproductive organs, eyes, stellate ganglion, central nervous system tissue; joint cement or plastic joint components. Precautions include use in hemophiliacs who are not receiving factor replacement, acute wound inflammation (avoid high-dose continuous US), bony prominences, and fractures (use lower intensity to avoid heating the periosteum or causing pain). US therapy should be discontinued if precautionary methods fail to eliminate pain.

Treatment Guidelines. The adjustable variables of US include frequency, duty cycle, intensity, coupling medium, size of the treatment area, and treatment duration. Control of each variable is determined by the intended effect and expected treatment outcome. As previously stated, the higher frequency of 3 MHz (which penetrates 1 to 2 cm) is used for shallow tissue, whereas 1 MHz (which penetrates up to 5 cm) is used for deeper tissue (Fig. 28-18). Pulsed-mode US with a 20% duty cycle is recommended for treatment of open wounds. In general, the recommended US intensity for wound healing is 0.5 to 1.0 W/cm^2.

A coupling medium is used between the sound head and the treatment tissue to eliminate air spaces that deflect the sound waves. Water, transmitting gels, hydrogel sheets, and transparent films are effective coupling mediums. When using a transmitting gel from a nonsterile container, a sterile transparent film between the wound bed and the gel reduces the risk of contamination. When using a transparent film, all air bubbles should be pressed

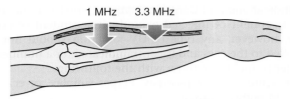

FIG. 28-18 Frequency controls the depth of penetration of ultrasound; 1 MHz ultrasound penetrates approximately 3 times as far as 3.3 MHz ultrasound. *Courtesy Mettler Electronics, Anaheim, CA.*

out before applying a thin layer of gel over the film. Hydrogel sheets used as a coupling medium can remain in place after US treatment and be used as a primary dressing. The coupling medium should extend several centimeters beyond the wound edge to enable treatment of periwound tissue. After treatment with US is complete, the hydrogel sheet should be trimmed to the size of the wound to avoid maceration of periwound skin. Water is used on distal areas over bony prominences and curved areas in which maintaining full contact between the sound head and the treatment area (such as ankles, heels, and elbows) is difficult. When water is the coupling medium, clean the container with antiseptic solution between treatments, use a container large enough to submerge the treatment area and the sound head, and fill the container with water several minutes before treatment so that air bubbles can dissipate. There are two guidelines for treatment times reported in the literature—1 min/cm^2 of treatment area or 5 minutes for each area that is 2 times the size of the sound head, with a recommended maximum time of 15 minutes.[107]

When applying US to a chronic wound using gel as the transmission medium, cleanse the sound head with an antiseptic agent before and after each treatment to prevent wound contamination, and warm the gel to approximately body temperature before putting it on the patient.

> ### Clinical Pearl
> Negative pressure wound therapy, electrical stimulation (ES), ultraviolet C (UVC), and ultrasound (US) are adjunctive interventions for pressure ulcers (PUs) and not substitutes for standard care, including tissue offloading, debridement, and provision of a moist wound environment.

CASE STUDY 28-1

STAGE IV SACRAL PRESSURE ULCER

Patient History

LM is a 44-year-old woman admitted to an acute care hospital with complaints of severe abdominal pain, diminished appetite with nausea, and diarrhea for 4 days. Past medical history includes end-stage liver disease secondary to amyloidosis, resulting in a liver transplant 4 years ago, end-stage renal disease with hemodialysis 2 times per week, hypertension, and a DVT with onset 4 months ago. LM has also had a sacral ulcer for 4 months. Her nutritional status is compromised because of her abdominal symptoms and liver disease. Blood cultures are negative.

Tests and Measures—Significant Findings

Musculoskeletal
- 2/5 gross lower extremity strength and 3/5 gross upper extremity strength.

Integumentary
- LM has impaired integumentary integrity and several risk factors, including diminished BMI, medications, impaired mobility, numerous co-morbidities, and poor nutritional status.
- Wound size: 3.7 × 3.4 cm with 2-3 cm of undermining from 10:00 to 2:00.
- Tissue type: 85% yellow rubbery eschar, 15% red granulation of poor quality.
- Drainage: Minimal serosanguineous drainage on the old dressing.
- Periwound skin color: Brawny discoloration of the periwound skin, proximal > distal.
- Sensation: Impaired to light touch.
- Braden Scale score: 9.

Function
- LM has been wheelchair bound for more than 2 years. Moderate-to-maximal assistance was required for all bed mobility and transfers.

Diagnosis

Preferred practice pattern is 7E: Impaired integumentary integrity associated with skin involvement extending into fascia, muscle, or bone and scar formation.

Interventions
- Planning appropriate interventions began with addressing each aspect of care recommended by the AHRQ *Guidelines*.
- LM was placed on a LAL bed, and a turning schedule was posted for all disciplines to follow. A chair-sized, air-cell cushion, to allow proper sitting position, was also provided.
- Sharp debridement of the eschar was performed at the bedside with sterile sharp instruments, followed by daily serial debridement of underlying devitalized tissue and slough.
- Periwound skin was covered with hydrocolloid strips.
- At each treatment session the wound was irrigated with PLWS using 1,000 ml of warmed normal saline, 6 to 12 psi pressure, and 80 mm Hg suction. Sterile technique was used with each treatment to reduce the risk of nosocomial infections.
- LM and her family were educated about the factors contributing to the ulcer formation, the optimal sidelying and sitting positions to off-load the sacrum, and the importance of keeping the head of the bed below 30 degrees.

Role of the Physical Therapist Assistant
- Why is it important for this patient to keep the head of her bed below 30 degrees?
- Write a paragraph describing the optimal sidelying and sitting positions to off-load the sacrum.
- What is the relevance of the Braden Scale score? Is it high? Low?
- What does the presence of yellow rubbery eschar indicate?

Additional Information

For the full version of this case study, including detailed examination results, interventions, and outcomes, see the Evolve site that accompanies this book. A full case study for a patient with a stage III and a stage IV PU also appears on the Evolve site.

CHAPTER SUMMARY

Pressure ulcers are wounds that occur as a result of sustained pressure, shear, or friction in an area over a bony prominence. In addition, prolonged exposure to moisture can cause skin maceration, thereby contributing to PU formation. PUs occur in a wide range of patients, particularly those with limited mobility, poor nutrition, and multiple co-morbidities. The first step to PU prevention is to identify risk factors and alter the patient's intrinsic and extrinsic environments to eliminate the circumstances that increase the risk for ulceration. Preventive strategies include pressure relief through modification of support surfaces and positioning, increasing mobility, optimizing nutrition, treating systemic disease processes, managing urinary and fecal incontinence, and educating patient and family members. Once a PU has developed, assessment of the patient's medical status and evaluation of the wound are used to determine appropriate interventions. Standard care consists of off-loading the affected area, frequent repositioning, debridement of devitalized tissue, and maintenance of a clean moist wound environment with appropriate dressings. Adjunctive modalities that may help facilitate wound healing include PLWS, negative pressure wound therapy, ES, UV, and US.

ADDITIONAL RESOURCES

For links to these and additional web-based resources, see the Evolve site.
Norton Scale
Braden Scale for Predicting Pressure Sore Risk
The Minimum Data Set (MDS)
Outcomes and Assessment Information Set (OASIS)
Spinal Cord Injury Pressure Ulcer Scale (SCIPUS)
National Pressure Ulcer Advisory Panel
National Institutes of Health information on pressure ulcers
UK National Health Service guidelines on pressure ulcer risk assessment and prevention
Cameron MH: *Physical agents in rehabilitation: From research to practice,* ed 3, St. Louis, 2009, Saunders.

GLOSSARY

Anaphylatoxins: Substances that induce the degranulation of mast cells, causing the release of histamine and increased vascular permeability.

Angiogenesis: New capillary formation.

Ankle-brachial index (ABI): The ratio of the systolic blood pressure at the ankle to the systolic brachial blood pressure. This number is used to assess the degree of peripheral vascular occlusion in the lower extremities.

Autolysis: The breakdown of necrotic tissue by the body's own white blood cells.

Body mass index (BMI): Weight in kilograms (kg)/height in meters squared (m^2).

Collagenase: An enzyme that catalyzes the hydrolysis of collagen.

Debridement: The removal of necrotic or nonviable tissue from a wound with sharp instruments, mechanical force, enzymes, or autolysis.

Eschar: Black, grey, brown, or yellow nonviable tissue, usually dry or rubbery, within a wound.

Exudate: Pale yellow fluid drainage composed of blood cells, serum, and lysed debris.

Galvanotaxis: The attraction of living cells to an electrical charge.

Glycoproteins: Carbohydrate-protein complexes that regulate collagen interactions that lead to fibril formation.

Glycosaminoglycans (GAGs): Polysaccharide chains, which form an inflexible gel that fills extracellular spaces. GAGs provide mechanical support to tissues while allowing diffusion of water-soluble molecules and migration of cells.

Granulation tissue: The matrix of collagen, hyaluronic acid, and fibronectin that contains new capillary growth during the proliferative phase of healing.

Hageman factor (clotting factor XII): The enzyme in blood that initiates clotting by converting fibrinogen into fibrin.

Hyperkeratosis: Overdevelopment of the horny cell layer of skin.

Incidence: The number of individuals who develop a disease or disorder during a specified time.

Interface pressure: The pressure between a support surface and the skin covering a bony prominence.

Kinins: Substances produced by plasma during the early phases of inflammation that cause an increase in the microvascular permeability.

Matrix metalloproteinases (MMPs): Enzymes that degrade proteins in the extracellular matrix.

Nanocrystalline silver: Slow-release silver ions used in antimicrobial dressings, referred to as *nanocrystalline* because their size is measured in nanometers (10^{-9} meter).

Necrosis: Tissue death.

Phagocytosis: The process by which macrophages and neutrophils lyse and carry away nonviable cellular and noncellular components during the process of wound healing.

Prevalence: The number of individuals who have a disease or disorder at a defined time.

Prostaglandins: Unsaturated fatty acids produced by all cells in the body and released in response to injury to increase vascular permeability, facilitate neutrophil chemotaxis, and induce pain.

Protease: A protein-splitting or proteolytic enzyme.

psi: Pounds per square inch; the unit of measurement for the pressure exerted by water on tissue during the irrigation process.

Purulence: Thick necrotic drainage frequently accompanied by a foul odor; may have a high bacterial count if associated with infection.

Slough: Nonviable tissue within a wound that is the result of autolysis of dead cells.

Vascular Ulcers

Bonnie J. Sparks-DeFriese

OBJECTIVES

After reading this chapter, the reader will be able to:
1. Describe the anatomy and function of the vascular system in the lower extremities.
2. Understand the etiology of different vascular ulcers.
3. Differentiate arterial from venous ulcers.
4. Implement a plan of care for vascular ulcer management.
5. Apply information learned regarding vascular ulcer management to presented case studies.

*P*eripheral vascular insufficiency, a dysfunction of blood flow, often leads to soft tissue **ischemia** and ulceration. Although peripheral vascular insufficiency may occur anywhere in the body, it is most common in the distal lower extremities where the vessels are the longest. Insufficiency of the venous system, the arterial system, or both, can result in skin and soft tissue ulceration. Such vascular ulcers are complex, requiring treatment of not only the area of soft tissue damage but also the underlying pathology, as well as consideration of the likely life-long lifestyle changes needed to heal the wound and minimize the risk of recurrence.

Lower extremity vascular disease (LEVD) may cause pain, tissue loss, and changes in appearance and function.

Venous ulcers are the most common of the vascular ulcers and generally have the best prognosis. In contrast, arterial ulcers are less common and have a much poorer prognosis; these ulcers often result in amputation. In some patients, both venous and arterial vessels are involved, presenting an even greater clinical challenge.

Differences in interventions and expected outcomes make it imperative that clinicians know the type of ulcer they are managing. A review of common tests, both non-invasive and invasive, is included in this chapter to guide the reader in accurately determining the etiology of a lower extremity ulcer and the status of the lower extremity blood vessels.

EPIDEMIOLOGY

Vascular ulcers can place great psychological, financial, and physical strain on patients and their families and thus adversely impact their quality of life.[1] Leg ulcers affect approximately 2.5 million people in the United States and approximately two million workdays are lost annually because of lower extremity vascular ulcers.[2] The average direct costs (for one patient with vascular ulcers) over a lifetime exceeds $40,000.[3]

Lower extremity ulcers may be caused by **arterial insufficiency, venous insufficiency,** or mixed vascular disease. Approximately 20% to 25% are caused by arterial or mixed disease, and the remainder are caused by venous disease.[4-9]

It is estimated that approximately 30% of people over the age of 66 have lower extremity arterial disease (LEAD).[2] In 1999 the Centers for Disease Control and Prevention (CDC) reported that 15.5 million people had **atherosclerosis.** Before the age of 70, **peripheral arterial disease (PAD)** is more common in men, but thereafter there is no gender difference in prevalence.[10] Intermittent **claudication** is the most common symptom of PAD and is experienced by 2% to 3% of men and 1% to 2% of women aged 60 years and older.[11,12]

The American Venous Forum estimates that, at any given time, one person in every 1,000 in the United States has an unhealed venous ulcer.[8] The Wound, Ostomy and Continence Nurses Society (WOCN) Guideline (2004) reported that LEVD is more common among the elderly and that 62% of patients with LEVD are female.[9]

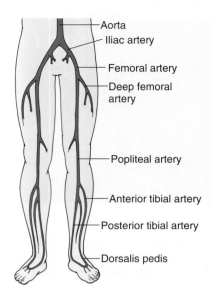

FIG. 29-1 The major arteries of the lower extremity.

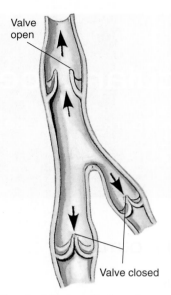

FIG. 29-2 Unidirectional valves in the veins prevent backflow of blood. *From Thibodeau GA, Patton KT:* Anatomy and physiology, *ed 5, St. Louis, 1999, Mosby.*

PATHOLOGY

VASCULAR ANATOMY

The lower extremity vasculature is comprised of arterial, venous, and lymphatic vessels. Figs. 29-1 and 29-3 show the major vessels of the lower extremity arterial and venous systems. The anatomy of arteries and veins is briefly described in the following section (see Chapter 27 for more information on lymphatic circulation).

Arterial System. Arteries are elastic, strong, muscular contractile vessels that convey blood from the heart to the periphery. The major arteries in the lower extremities are the iliac, femoral, popliteal, and tibial arteries (Fig. 29-1).

All arteries have three layers: The tunica intima, tunica media, and tunica adventitia. The tunica media includes smooth muscle that allows the artery to constrict or dilate. If the muscle in the tunica media is damaged, the vessel loses contractility and the rate of blood flow becomes fixed, preventing any increase in arterial blood supply in response to increased metabolic demand. Stenosis (narrowing) of the artery can also reduce blood flow. Downstream blood flow is reduced when there is 30% or greater stenosis of a peripheral artery and can reach a critical level when the arterial diameter is reduced by 50% or more.[13] Decreased flow can cause tissue ischemia, pain at rest, nonhealing wounds, and **gangrene.**[2]

Venous System. Veins, which convey blood from the periphery back to the heart, are made up of three layers that are similar to the arteries; however, the layers of the vein wall are thinner than in the arteries. The layers of the vein walls can be thin because the blood pressure in the veins is low.[14] The inner layer of smooth endothelium in the veins is folded at intervals to form unidirectional valves that prevent backflow of blood (Fig. 29-2). There are more valves in the leg veins than elsewhere because the blood often has to move against gravity to return to the heart.

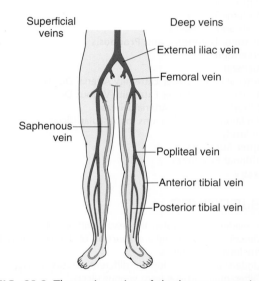

FIG. 29-3 The major veins of the lower extremity.

There are deep and superficial venous systems in the lower extremities (Fig. 29-3). The primary superficial vein of the lower extremity is the saphenous vein. The saphenous system is connected to the deep system by numerous perforator veins. The main deep veins are the external iliac, femoral, popliteal, and tibial veins. Distal to the tibial veins there are many smaller veins with numerous crosslinking branches.

The deep veins of the legs are surrounded by skeletal muscles that contract and relax during ambulation and other activities. When these muscles contract, they compress the veins, pushing blood back toward the heart (Fig. 29-4). This muscular pump is required for good return of venous blood to the heart. The deep veins (femoral, popliteal, and tibial) lie within the muscle compartment of the leg and are "milked" by muscle contractions. Venous

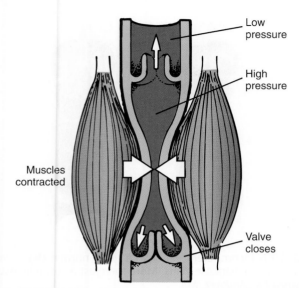

Low
pressure

High
pressure

Muscles
contracted

Valve
closes

FIG. 29-4 Muscle contractions compress the veins, pushing blood toward the heart. *From McCance K, Heuther S:* Pathophysiology, *ed 4, St. Louis, 2002, Mosby.*

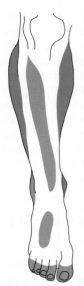

FIG. 29-5 Location of ulcers caused by arterial *(in red)* and venous *(in blue)* insufficiency.

insufficiency can occur if the vein walls, the valves, or the muscles do not function normally.

In the upright position, the blood pressure in the veins in the lower extremities is about 100 mm Hg. If this pressure is unopposed, it will cause significant venous hypertension and peripheral **edema.** Contraction of the gastrocnemius muscle compresses and empties the deep veins, which promotes venous return and reduces the ambulatory pressure within the venous and capillary systems to less than 20 mm Hg. Thus normal venous function is characterized by high "standing" pressures or "resting" pressures and low "walking" pressures.[1]

VASCULAR ULCERS

Arterial Ulcers. Arterial insufficiency occurs when the blood flow in the arteries is not sufficient to meet the needs of the skin, muscles, and nerves.[2] Arterial insufficiency can be caused by cholesterol deposits (atherosclerosis) or blood clots (emboli or thrombi) obstructing blood flow or by damaged, diseased, or weak vessels.[1,2] Arterial ulcers occur when there is an insufficient blood supply to the skin and subcutaneous tissues. An ulcer is usually precipitated by a combination of progressive arterial occlusion, increased external occlusive pressure (such as heel pressure in bed-bound patients), and an increase in local oxygen demand because of minor trauma.[15,16] Arterial ulcers generally do not heal unless tissue perfusion is restored.[17] If perfusion is not restored, amputation of an appendage and/or a limb is often necessary. The risk of amputation increases if the wound becomes infected and gangrenous.[17,18] Common locations for ulcers caused by arterial insufficiency are the anterior leg or tibial area, the lateral malleolus, the midfoot, and the tips of the toes (Fig. 29-5).[1,16]

Etiology of Arterial Insufficiency. LEAD, also known as peripheral vascular disease (PVD), peripheral arterial occlusive disease (PAOD), and PAD, is defined as

BOX 29-1	Risk Factors for Vascular Ulcers
Arterial	**Venous**
• Peripheral vascular disease • Smoking • Diabetes • Hyperlipidemia • Hypertension • Obesity • Physical inactivity • Male gender • Advanced age • Strong family history	• Thrombophilia • Deep venous thrombosis/ phlebitis • Trauma • Obesity • Sedentary lifestyle and occupation • Advanced age • High number of pregnancies • Varicose veins • Family history of venous disease

"atherosclerotic disease of the aorta and arteries of the lower extremity."[19] Approximately 90% of arterial problems in the legs are caused by atherosclerosis.[10] Atherosclerosis causes narrowing and hardening of the arterial vessels, which then results in increased resistance and decreased blood flow. The impaired blood delivery leads to inadequate nutrition and oxygenation of the tissues and over time, to cell death and tissue necrosis.[12]

Risk Factors for Arterial Ulcers. Risk factors for vascular ulcers, both arterial and venous, are listed in Box 29-1. Reversible risk factors for PAD include smoking, diabetes mellitus, hyperlipidemia, hypertension, obesity, and physical inactivity. Irreversible risk factors for PAD include male gender, advanced age, and a strong family history.[2,11,12,16,20]

The use of tobacco (smoked and smokeless) is the single most important preventable risk factor for arterial disease.

Smoking is associated with increased rates of PAD progression, increased amputation rates, lower success rates after vascular surgeries, and increased risk of myocardial infarctions, stroke, and death.[21] Smoking contributes to atherosclerosis by promoting lipid accumulation in the vessels and by promoting plaque enlargement. Smoking also impairs circulation by reducing or preventing nitric oxide–dependent vasodilation, causing vasoconstriction, and decreasing the oxygen-carrying capacity of red blood cells by loading them with carbon monoxide.[10] There is no evidence that low tar cigarettes decrease the effect of smoking on PAD risk.[12,22]

◎ *Clinical Pearl*

Tobacco use is the single most preventable risk factor for arterial disease.

Diabetes mellitus (DM) is associated with increased arterial plaque formation, increased blood viscosity, and hypercoagulability. It is not uncommon to find severe PVD before the age of 40 in patients with poorly controlled DM. More than 80% of patients with diabetes have some form of arterial disease within 20 years of their diagnosis, and approximately 75% of the deaths in patients with diabetes are due to arterial disease.[12] DM increases the risk of arterial disease by a factor of four.[21]

Hyperlipidemia contributes to PAD by causing an accumulation of lipids in the arteries, which causes narrowing of the vessels and reduced blood flow. How hypertension causes vascular injury is unclear. The damage may result from increased production of vascular smooth muscle, activation of the renin-angiotensin-aldosterone system, increased production of vasoconstrictive agents, and/or increased blood coagulability.

Venous Ulcers. Venous disease or insufficiency is a compromise in the venous circulation that can impair the return of blood from the periphery to the heart and cause congestion in the lower extremities. Venous insufficiency can be caused by incompetence of the venous valves (Fig. 29-6), deep vein obstruction or thrombosis, arteriovenous fistula, and/or calf muscle pump failure (caused by paralysis, decreased ankle range of motion [ROM], or ankle joint deformity).[15,23] Common locations for ulcers caused by venous insufficiency are the medial and lateral leg (the gaiter area) and the medial malleolus (see Fig. 29-5).

Etiology of Venous Ulcers. The progression of events from venous insufficiency to soft tissue ulceration is not completely understood, although it is known that factors that cause venous insufficiency are associated with an increased risk of ulcer formation.

Risk Factors for Venous Ulcers. The primary risk factors for venous ulcers are **thrombophilia** (a propensity to form blood clots), deep vein thrombosis/phlebitis, trauma, obesity, sedentary lifestyle and occupation, advanced age, high number of pregnancies, **varicose veins,** and a family history of venous disease (see Box 29-1).

Thrombophilia is present in as many as 41% of patients with venous ulcers.[16] Patients with thrombophilia should generally be treated with anticoagulant drug therapy. Deep venous thrombosis (DVT) with phlebitis is associated with a 60% to 90% risk of venous ulceration that may

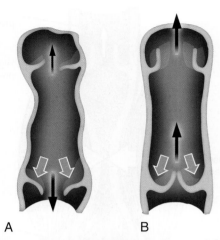

FIG. 29-6 Incompetent venous **(A)** and normal **(B)** valves. *Redrawn from* Varicose veins: More than just a cosmetic issue, *Diomed Inc, Andover, MA.*

occur up to 30 years after the DVT.[24] Trauma to the leg can initiate or exacerbate venous insufficiency in some patients.[3]

A sedentary lifestyle and occupations that require standing or sitting with the feet dependent for long periods of time (e.g., bank tellers and cashiers) are thought to reduce oxygen supply to the skin during periods of dependency. Obesity and the sitting position also impair venous blood flow because the abdomen exerts pressure on the central vascular system.[16,25]

Advanced age (peak prevalence between 60 to 80 years of age) is considered to be a risk factor for venous disease. However, it must be noted that 22% of venous ulcers develop in patients under 40 years of age and 13% develop in people under 30 years of age.[3]

For women, the number of pregnancies or closeness of pregnancies increases the risk for venous disease.[9,16] It is thought that distal venous pressures may increase because of the compression of the pelvic veins and inferior vena cava.[24] If untreated, varicose veins (Fig. 29-7) are associated with a 20% to 50% risk of lower extremity ulceration.

Mixed Arterial and Venous Disease. Patients may present with ulcers caused by a combination of arterial and venous insufficiency.[16] It is estimated that 21% to 25% of patients with a venous ulcer have some degree of coexisting arterial disease.[3,26] It is challenging to establish the diagnosis and design an effective plan of care for patients with such mixed disease.

TYPICAL EXAMINATION FINDINGS

PATIENT HISTORY

The patient history includes information about the patient's medical history, including risk factors (e.g., diabetes, atherosclerosis, trauma, coagulopathies, or history of DVT), previous surgical interventions, and the amount and duration of tobacco use, including tobacco products such as smokeless tobacco and nicotine patches. History of pain (amount, type, location, triggers, and reducers)

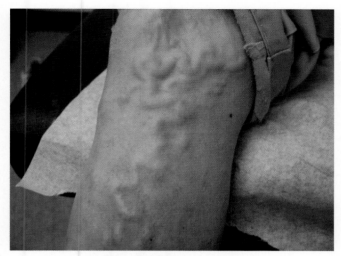

FIG. 29-7 Varicose veins.

and the ulcer's (or ulcers') onset and previous types of interventions used and their effects are also included. Ulcer duration and size are also important because they are indicators of healing potential. Chronic and larger ulcers are less likely to heal than more recent smaller ulcers.[9] Medications; laboratory test results, including lipid profiles and blood sugar levels; and nutritional status are also included because they may affect the potential for healing. Chapter 28 details other components included in the history of all patients with chronic wounds.

SYSTEMS REVIEW

The systems review is used to target areas requiring further examination and to define areas that may cause complications or indicate a need for precautions during the examination and intervention processes. Chapter 1 includes details of the systems review.

For patients with vascular ulcers, a basic review of the cardiovascular and pulmonary systems includes checking for edema; measuring heart rate, respiratory rate and pattern, and blood pressure; and assessing for history of lower extremity ulcers and for indicators of peripheral vascular status (lower extremity color, temperature, and pulses).[27]

TESTS AND MEASURES

Musculoskeletal

Range of Motion. ROM of the lower extremity joints is measured in all patients with lower extremity ulcers. A limitation in ROM of the lower extremity, especially dorsiflexion and plantarflexion at the ankle, may cause a dysfunctional gait pattern, including an ineffective foot or calf muscle pump, which may contribute to venous insufficiency.[28] ROM loss may be caused by structural or functional abnormalities, as well as by deposition of fibrotic tissue from venous insufficiency.[28,29]

Muscle Performance. A functional calf muscle pump plays a pivotal role in emptying the deep veins and reducing venous pressures, thus reducing the risk for venous ulceration and improving the prognosis for wound healing. Improving calf muscle strength may promote

healing and reduce ulcer recurrence in those with venous insufficiency.

Neuromuscular

Pain. Research has shown that many patients with wounds previously thought not to cause pain do report pain.[7,30] The pain may be constant or only occur with procedures or dressing change or when the patient is in certain positions.

Pain is typically an initial predictor of arterial disease, and patients with arterial insufficiency generally have less pain when their limb is in a dependent position. The location of the pain may indicate the area of arterial occlusion. More proximal involvement of the aortoiliac arteries causes pain that extends from the buttocks down the lower extremity to the calf, whereas superficial femoral artery involvement generally only causes pain in the calf. Ischemic foot pain in response to exercise generally indicates infrapopliteal artery involvement.[10] Depending on its severity, ischemia may cause intermittent claudication, nocturnal pain, or rest pain. Intermittent claudication is pain described as "cramping" or the "leg giving out" or "leg fatigue" that occurs only with activity and that is relieved by a few minutes of rest. As arterial occlusion and ischemia worsen, nocturnal pain develops. This is an aching pain that occurs at night (or when lying down) and that is relieved by putting the legs in a dependent position. Rest pain, a sign of advanced occlusive disease, feels like a "constant deep aching" and is present regardless of position or activity.[12,16] Since the pattern of pain indicates the severity of the ischemia, it also indicates the prognosis for healing of an arterial ulcer.

Pain caused by venous insufficiency is different from that caused by arterial compromise. Arterial insufficiency, as previously noted, causes pain early, and the pain is often worsened by activity and relieved by rest and dependency. In contrast, pain from venous insufficiency comes on later in the progression of the disease, and the discomfort, which generally worsens when the limb is down, is described as a feeling of fullness, swelling, tightness, aching, or heaviness in the leg. Venous insufficiency can also cause skin inflammation, leading to sensations of itching, soreness, or tenderness. Pain associated with venous insufficiency is typically worst at the end of the day after the person has been upright on his or her feet for a number of hours.[9] The tightness or pressure that people feel is caused by constriction of structures by edema. Some patients report having nocturnal leg cramps caused by irritability of the leg muscles. Since venous ulcers generally heal well, any of these types of symptoms indicate a better prognosis than the presence of symptoms associated with arterial insufficiency.

Sensory Integrity. Paresthesia (sensations such as numbness, tingling, or a "pins and needles" feeling) is one of the six "Ps" of arterial disease: Pulselessness, pain, pallor, poikilothermy (body temperature that varies with environmental temperature), paresthesia, and paralysis. Paresthesia and paralysis are signs of severe and potentially irreversible ischemia.[31]

Sensory loss is also common in patients with PAD, particularly those with neuropathy caused by diabetes. Since neuropathy and diabetes may go undiagnosed for many years, sensation is checked in all patients with lower extremity ulcers (see Chapters 18 and 30 for more information on diabetic neuropathy and ulcers related to diabetic neuropathy). In general, sensory testing includes at least an examination of light touch in all dermatomes and a check for protective sensation on both feet with nylon monofilaments.

Cardiovascular/Pulmonary

Circulation. In the evaluation and management of vascular ulcers, the value of vascular testing by pulse palpation, Doppler ultrasound, and other tests (noninvasive and invasive) cannot be overemphasized. This testing assesses the status and viability of the vascular systems, both arterial and venous, and determines healing potential, risk of recurrence, and complications.

Examination of circulation should include the color and temperature of the involved area(s) and the effects of limb elevation and dependency. Patients with PAD typically have a blue or dusky tone to the skin, pallor with elevation, and rubor with dependency. The presence, absence, and quality of pulses; measurement of ankle-brachial index (ABI) or toe-brachial index (TBI); and measurement of transcutaneous partial pressure of oxygen ($TcPO_2$) are also included in vascular assessment. Common findings for the patient with PAD include diminished or absent pulses, reduced ABI and TBI, and reduced $TcPO_2$ levels. Measurement of TBI is frequently recommended as an alternative to ABI in patients with diabetes because calcification of vessels, which generates an artificially elevated ABI reading, is common in these patients. Measurement of both venous and capillary filling times may also help the clinician differentiate arterial from venous disease. Venous and capillary filling times are both prolonged in arterial insufficiency and shortened in venous disease.

Limb Color. Both arterial and venous insufficiency may cause changes in limb color in response to changes in position. To examine for these changes, the patient is positioned supine and the leg is elevated at a 45- to 60-degree angle for 15 to 60 seconds. Elevational pallor of the foot (in patients with fair skin) or grey hues (in dark-skinned individuals) and rubor (purple-red discoloration) when the leg is returned to a dependent position suggest arterial insufficiency. Patients with mild disease develop pallor within 60 seconds of elevation, those with moderately severe disease develop pallor within 40 seconds, and those with severe occlusive disease develop pallor within 25 seconds.[15]

Skin Temperature. Skin temperature may be a physiological indicator or precursor to the development of leg ulcers in certain diagnostic groups. It is generally recommended that skin temperature of the involved limb be compared with the temperature of the uninvolved limb (if there is one) and that temperatures be compared along the limb, from proximal to distal. Differences in skin temperature may help identify pathology such as arterial compromise (which can cause a reduction in skin temperature distally, often with a sharp line of demarcation) and may also predict ulceration in the patient with venous pathology (temperature is increased in areas of ulceration). Temperature elevation can be associated with a local

TABLE 29-1	Interpretation of Ankle-Brachial Index Pressures
ABI	Interpretation
1.0-1.4	Normal
<0.9	LEAD
0.5-0.8	Moderate arterial insufficiency
<0.4	Severe ischemia

ABI, Ankle-brachial index; *LEAD,* lower extremity arterial disease.

inflammatory response or infection. Skin temperature gradients or differences may be estimated subjectively by the sensation in the dorsum of the clinician's hands or more objectively and quantitatively with an infrared thermographic scanner.

Lower Extremity Pulses. Palpation of lower extremity pulses is performed starting proximally and moving distally, and pulses are reported as "present" or "absent." Many clinicians believe that palpable distal pulses indicate normal vascular status; however, some authors suggest that the presence of palpable pulses does not rule out LEAD.[16,20,32]

Ankle-Brachial Index. The most common measure of lower extremity perfusion is the ABI, which is the ratio of the systolic pressure in the ankle relative to the systolic pressure in the brachial artery in the arm. The ABI, also called *ankle-arm index (AAI)* and *ankle pressure index (API),* is a reproducible, noninvasive test that helps clinicians objectify and quantify pulse values to determine diagnosis and assure appropriate intervention. In the 1980s, it was considered to be the most sensitive means for detecting large vessel arterial disease. Although invasive **angiography** is now considered to be a more sensitive test, ABI by Doppler is still 95% sensitive for diagnosis of PAD in comparison to the angiographic gold standard.[10,33] Therefore the ABI is still an excellent method for examining peripheral arterial circulation in most patients with lower extremity ulcers.

Normally, the blood pressure at the ankle should be equal to or slightly higher than the brachial pressure, producing an ABI of 1 to 1.4 (Table 29-1). An ABI of less than 0.9 indicates the presence of lower extremity arterial disease.[2] An ABI of 0.5 to 0.8 indicates moderate arterial insufficiency, and an ABI of less than 0.4 indicates severe involvement.[8] ABI readings of 0.5 to 0.8 are generally associated with intermittent claudication and an ABI of less than 0.3 is typically accompanied by rest pain and/or gangrene.[12,32] A decrease of 0.15 or more in the ABI is considered to indicate disease progression, whereas an increase of 0.15 or more indicates clinically significant improvement or response to therapeutic intervention.

Toe-Brachial Index. In patients with chronic DM or renal disease, it may be necessary to use toe pressures or the TBI rather than the ABI to evaluate perfusion because the ankle pressures may be falsely elevated as a result of vessel calcification.[16] Toe pressures are more reliable because digital vessels are rarely calcified. The TBI is calculated in a similar manner to the ABI, substituting the systolic pressure in the great or second toe for the ankle pressure.[34] A normal TBI is greater than 0.6, and a toe pressure of less than 40 mm Hg indicates poor perfusion and a low likelihood of wound healing. Pressures of less than or equal to 30 mm Hg predict failure to heal and indicate a need for revascularization.[2,9,21]

The ABI and TBI should be rechecked periodically (every 3 months) in patients with known vascular disease because they may worsen over time.[2]

Transcutaneous Partial Pressure of Oxygen Measurement. Another noninvasive method for assessing tissue perfusion is measurement of $TcPO_2$. $TcPO_2$ levels indicate healing potential and can be used to determine the appropriateness of aggressive debridement. $TcPO_2$ levels are commonly measured in the outpatient clinic or in a vascular laboratory and should be considered in the following situations:

- Nonhealing ulcer in patient with ABI <0.9 or toe pressure <30 mm Hg.
- Poorly compressible arteries at the ankle.
- Before amputation to determine the level at which healing is likely.[2]

This test is performed by placing an oxygen-sensing electrode directly on the skin of the lower extremity, often proximal to the ulcer. The electrode has a heating element that heats the skin to 41° C to facilitate oxygen transport from the capillaries to the skin. After approximately 20 minutes, a transcutaneous reading of the PO_2 is taken.[34]

A normal $TcPO_2$ value is 40 mm Hg, and values less than 40 mm Hg are associated with impaired healing[2] (Table 29-2). Values of less than 20 mm Hg generally indicate marked ischemia and an inability to heal.[15] Values between 20 and 40 mm Hg represent a "grey zone" in which healing is likely to be slow and uncertain, and additional interventions may be needed for a good outcome. If the $TcPO_2$ is greater than 30 mm Hg, debridement may be considered because although healing is impaired, it is possible. However, if the $TcPO_2$ is less than 30 mm Hg, debridement is not recommended.[34]

Venous Filling Time. Venous filling time can also be an indicator of venous or arterial disease. To determine venous filling time, the clinician should elevate the lower extremity above the level of the heart (≈75 degrees) and then rapidly move it to a dependent position. The time it takes for the veins of the dorsum of the foot to refill with blood is the venous filling time. If the venous valves are competent, the venous filling time will be longer than 20 seconds. If the valves are incompetent, indicating venous insufficiency, filling will occur much more quickly because of retrograde flow.[6,16] In addition, venous filling time will be prolonged by arterial compromise. A filling time of more than 30 seconds indicates fairly severe arterial occlusion.[2]

Capillary Refill Time. Capillary refill time is measured by pressing firmly with a finger against the toe pad to displace the contained blood and then determining how long it takes for blood to refill the area. A normal capillary refill time is 2 seconds. A delay in capillary refill (more than 3 seconds) indicates arterial insufficiency; however, capillary refill time may be normal in many patients with PAD because the emptied vessels may refill in a retrograde manner from surrounding veins.[2]

TABLE 29-2	Interpretation of Transcutaneous Partial Pressure of Oxygen Values
TcPO₂ Value	**Interpretation**
≥40 mm Hg	Normal cutaneous arterial supply.
20 to 40 mm Hg	Impaired cutaneous arterial supply. The patient may have problems with wound healing.
>30 mm Hg	Debridement may be considered.
<30 mm Hg	Debridement is not recommended.
<20 mm Hg	Marked ischemia.

TcPo₂, Transcutaneous partial pressure of oxygen.

Vascular Laboratory Tests. More detailed testing may be indicated to assess the presence, location, and severity of vascular disease. If any of these findings are noted, the patient should be referred back to the supervising physical therapist for possible referral to a vascular laboratory.

Integumentary. Skin integrity in the lower extremities may be impaired as the result of arterial and/or venous insufficiency. The integumentary system examination and testing includes a comprehensive wound assessment. This includes the same parameters as those identified for other chronic wounds (see Chapter 28), including wound location (specified according to anatomical landmarks); dimensions (length, width, and depth in centimeters and/or surface area in square centimeters); wound bed characteristics, appearance, and color (necrosis, slough, granulation, clean but nongranulating tissue, or epithelialization); drainage (amount, odor, color, and consistency); undermining, tracts, or tunnels (location and measurements); and the status of the wound edges (open or closed). Additional parameters include the status of the surrounding skin (erythema, induration, increased warmth, local edema, sensitivity to palpation, fluctuance, boggy tissue, and trophic changes); edema (presence, type, and severity); pain (severity, characteristics, triggers, or reducers), and signs of **osteomyelitis** or gangrene.

Ulcers caused by arterial and venous insufficiency have similarities and differences. The features that most often differ between arterial and venous ulcers can be found in Table 29-3.

Ulcer location and color and the volume of drainage are the most critical for differentiating between types of lower extremity vascular ulcers. Venous ulcers are typically located in the "gaiter" or medial malleolus area, whereas arterial ulcers are usually on the toes. The wound bed of a venous ulcer has a deep red color, whereas the less-perfused arterial ulcer has a necrotic, pale, or dusky blue color. Characteristically, the ulcer caused by venous insufficiency has a moderate to copious amount of drainage, whereas the arterial ulcer is often dry with little or no drainage.

Other indicators of venous insufficiency include lower extremity edema, hemosiderosis, venous **dermatitis, ankle flare,** and in the more advanced stages, **lipodermatosclerosis (hypodermitis sclerodermiformis).** Edema most often occurs at the site of greatest gravitational pressure, the ankle. This is also where hemosiderosis, a greyish-brown hyperpigmentation, can be seen (Fig.

TABLE 29-3	Typical Characteristics of Venous and Arterial Ulcers	
Characteristic	**Arterial**	**Venous**
Location	Usually distal, in between or on tips of toes, over phalangeal heads, over lateral malleolus, areas exposed to repetitive trauma (e.g., anterior tibia) and pressure (e.g., heels).	Typically around medial malleolus and the medial and lateral leg (the gaiter area).
Wound bed color	Ulcer bed usually pale, yellow or black; ulcer typically "dry" and granulation tissue minimal or absent.	Ulcer bed ruddy in color.
Drainage	Ranges from none to scant or minimal.	Typically moderate to copious.
Edges	Typically regular and "punched-out" in appearance; margins are distinct and often indolent.	Usually irregular.
Surrounding skin	Ischemic skin changes include atrophy of subcutaneous tissue, shiny, taut, thin, dry skin, hair loss, and dystrophic nails. Color changes with position changes include elevational pallor in the fair skin, greyness in the dark-skinned patient's limb, and dependent rubor in both.	Hemosiderosis is classic indicator; defined as increased deposition of iron; presents as grey-brown pigmentation also known as "hyperpigmentation" or "tissue staining" in the gaiter area.[3] Skin tends to be shiny, leading to taut and sclerotic; dermatitis is common; may appear itchy, erythematous, and weeping or dry, crusty, and scaly. High propensity for irritant dermatitis and contact dermatitis.[24]
Pulses	Perfusion diminished as indicated by ABI of <0.8 or a TBI <0.6.	Perfusion is adequate as indicated by palpable pulses (unless edema is significant), warm feet, and ABI often 1.0.
Pain	Severe and reported as sharp; can be exacerbated by elevation of leg.	Often mild and reported as "aching" at end of day. Pain is relieved by elevation.
Infection	Infection common but may not "appear" infected since compromised blood flow results in compromised immune response (inspect for faint halo of erythema, increased pain and tenderness).	
Edema	Not characteristic of arterial insufficiency unless venous component is present. If edema is noted in these patients, it is typically a result of other co-morbid conditions such as congestive heart failure, infections, or from long-standing dependent positioning to decrease pain.	Most often noted in site of greatest gravitational pressure, the ankle. Hemosiderosis can be seen. This tissue discoloration is the result of leakage of blood into the tissues where subsequent breakdown of red blood cells deposits pigment.

ABI, Ankle-brachial index; *TBI,* toe-brachial index.

29-8, *A*). This tissue discoloration is caused by blood leaking into the tissues in which the subsequent breakdown of red blood cells deposits pigment. Venous dermatitis, which makes the skin itchy, erythematous, and weeping or dry and scaly, is another common complication of venous insufficiency (Fig. 29-8, *B*). Contact dermatitis around a leg ulcer may also occur because of chemical or mechanical irritation. "Ankle flare," or "malleolar flare," a collection of small venous channels inferior to the medial malleolus and extending onto the medial foot, also often occurs in patients with a venous insufficiency (Fig. 29-8, *C*). In the later stages of the disease, lipodermatosclerosis (sclerosis of fat and dermal tissue layers) occurs as a result of protein (fibrin) deposits in tissues. The leg in the "gaiter (sock) area" becomes indurated and hyperpigmented. The surrounding tissue may become very edematous, causing a "bottle leg" shape (caused by edema above and below the gaiter area in conjunction with contraction of the tissues in the gaiter area).

Indicators of arterial insufficiency include trophic changes, such as thickened toenails, loss or thinning of hair, and shiny skin (due to loss of cellular nourishment), and absent or diminished pulses along with a low ABI and

TBI. In arterial insufficiency, Doppler examination reveals an ABI of ≤0.8 and a TBI of ≤0.6. Pain, often severe, is noted in the ischemic limb and may be less in a dependent position. Edema may be present if dependent positioning is frequently used to alleviate pain; otherwise edema is not characteristic.

Infection. Culturing of the wound bed (with sensitivity) is warranted to rule out infection if a wound fails to heal or there is deterioration and spreading erythema, an increase in the amount of drainage, onset of purulent drainage, increasing pain, or increased odor.[28] The classic signs and symptoms of invasive infection are characterized by induration, fever, erythema, and edema.[35] Indicators of critical colonization include sudden deterioration in the quality or quantity of granulation tissue, increased volume of exudates, and increased pain but no erythema, induration, edema, or warmth in the surrounding tissue.

Infection may be difficult to identify in patients with LEAD because the typical signs of redness, warmth, and swelling may be subtle or absent when there is reduced blood flow because of arterial insufficiency. In this circumstance, infection may be indicated by no change or an increase in wound size over a 2-week period or increased

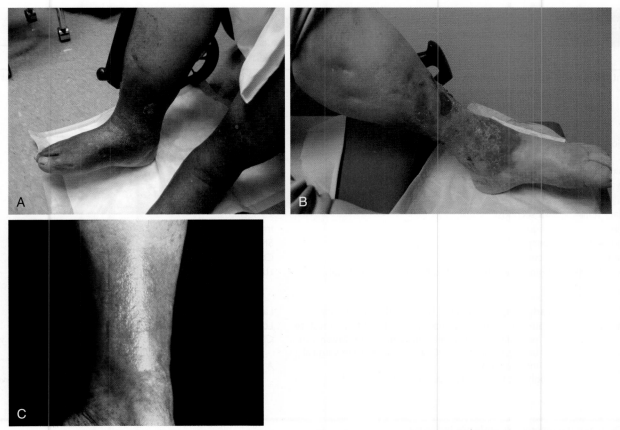

FIG. 29-8 Indicators of venous insufficiency. **A,** Lower extremity hemosiderosis and edema as a result of venous insufficiency and stasis. **B,** Venous dermatitis in an area of venous insufficiency. **C,** Ankle flare in an area of venous insufficiency.

drainage, pain, purulence, odor, or necrotic tissue.[2] Immediate referral to the appropriate physician (often vascular surgeons) for these infected wounds is imperative because of the potential for limb-threatening cellulitis and life-threatening sepsis.

Infection in the patient with LEVD may be confused with venous dermatitis or cellulitis. Characteristics of cellulitis include pain, edema, possible fever, and an increase in white blood cell count, whereas dermatitis typically causes a weepy, papular rash with **pruritus**.

Function

Gait. The absence of appropriate toe-off during terminal stance often indicates poor calf muscle function. This will impair the function of the calf muscle pump and thus reduce peripheral venous return.[36]

Assistive Devices. Assistive devices may be used to assist with independence in ambulation or to reduce pressure on a lower extremity ulcer, particularly those on the soles of the feet (see Chapter 33).

Self-Care and Home Management. Current and prior functional status in self-care and home management activities (including activities of daily living [ADLs]) that are examined in the patient with peripheral vascular disease include the patient's ability to follow care guidelines, access necessary equipment (running water, clean water source and supplies for wound cleansing, and furniture to elevate an edematous leg), and the availability and nature of social supports to assist the patient.

Safety is examined in patients with compromised lower extremity circulation because such patients are often at high risk for falls and soft tissue trauma. Any neuromusculoskeletal dysfunction (e.g., hemiparesis) may also hinder the patient's self-care and home management of a vascular ulcer. In addition, patients may adopt an unsafe compensatory gait (such as hopping on one leg) to decrease pressure and pain on the involved leg. These issues illustrate the importance of a comprehensive examination that includes the impact of the vascular ulcer on the patient's activities, as well as direct examination of the ulcer itself.

Work, Community, and Leisure. Patients with vascular ulcers may be incapacitated by their ulcer or by other symptoms of their underlying vascular disease (e.g., pain, edema, and drainage); because of this, many may lose work and income. Patients often report lifestyle issues and pain as their primary concerns rather than the healing of the wound.[37]

The occupation of the patient with vascular insufficiency may affect their symptoms. For example, edema caused by venous insufficiency may increase if the patient stands or sits for long periods with the legs in a dependent position. In contrast, the pain associated with arterial insufficiency will be worse if the patient has to walk long

TABLE 29-4	Common Examination Findings and Prognosis for Patients with Different Types of Vascular Ulcers	
	Arterial Ulcer	**Venous Ulcer**
Patient history	Cardiovascular disease, heart attack, hypertension, hyperlipidemia, diabetes mellitus,[21] stroke, increased pain with activity and/or elevation, intermittent claudication, tobacco use, traumatic injury to the extremity, vascular procedures/surgeries.	Previous DVT and varicosities, thrombophlebitis, reduced mobility, sedentary lifestyle, decreased ankle mobility, obesity, traumatic injury, heart failure, orthopedic procedures, multiple pregnancies.
Location	Distal, on or in area of the toes. Around the lateral malleoli. Areas exposed to pressure or trauma.	Medial aspect of the leg and ankle. Superior to the medial malleoli.
Edema	None.	Moderate to severe.
Pulses	Absent or diminished.	Normal.
ABI	<0.5	≥1.0.
Capillary refill	>3 seconds.	<3 seconds.
Borders	Regular.	Irregular.
Wound bed	Deep.	Shallow.
Drainage	Scant.	Copious.
Surrounding skin	Shiny, scant hair, cool to touch, thickened nails.	Hemosiderin staining, scarring from previous ulcers, dermatitis, lipodermatosclerosis, normal temperature or warm to touch.
Pain	Early symptom, aching, better with dependency.	Late symptom, tightness, worse with dependency.
Prognosis	Potential for healing depends on the ability to restore perfusion; wound will usually heal if perfusion can be reestablished; 20% of patients require surgical intervention.[21] High risk for limb loss because of ischemia.[12]	Long-standing wounds are less likely to heal. Chronic, large ulcers with a poor response to the first 3 weeks of therapy are unlikely to heal.[9] A history of vein stripping, or ligation, a total knee replacement, an ABI <0.8, fibrin on 50% or more of wound bed, and poor mobility are all indicators of a poorer prognosis.[48]

DVT, Deep vein thrombosis; *ABI,* ankle-brachial index.

distances, particularly walking up hills or stairs. Similarly, the patient's ulcer and associated problems, such as pain and exudate, may adversely impact leisure and/or socialization. The pain of intermittent claudication or edema may also limit walking.

A draining wound takes a toll on the patient, as well as his or her family. The wound can prevent socialization because its odor and the frequency of dressing changes or clothing changes to cover the wound are awkward or embarrassing for the patient. Activities that require prolonged sitting (e.g., flying on a plane) may also be difficult because the patient will have to change positions frequently to compensate for their circulatory compromise. For patients with venous insufficiency, performing ankle pumps when sitting at work and during travel or leisure activities may facilitate venous return.

EVALUATION, DIAGNOSIS, AND PROGNOSIS

Any soft tissue wound may be classified according to the depth and type of tissue involved.[27] According to the classification scheme used by the *Guide to Physical Therapist Practice* (the *Guide*),[27] wounds can be classified according to depth into one of five preferred practice patterns. These patterns are 7A: Primary prevention/risk reduction for integumentary disorders; 7B: Impaired integumentary integrity associated with superficial skin involvement; 7C: Impaired integumentary integrity associated with partial-thickness skin involvement and scar formation; 7D:

Impaired integumentary integrity associated with full-thickness skin involvement and scar formation; and 7E: Impaired integumentary integrity associated with skin involvement extending into fascia, muscle, or bone and scar formation. Partial thickness is defined as involving the epidermis and dermis; full thickness is defined as the complete destruction of the dermal layers and extending into the subcutaneous tissue.

The patient's prognosis for healing is determined by the type and severity of the vascular compromise. Table 29-4 lists the common examination findings and prognosis of arterial ulcers and venous ulcers. Ulcers that rapidly increase in size, present with atypical wound margins (rolled edges [epibole], cauliflower in appearance), fail to respond to treatment, or tend to bleed should be biopsied to rule out squamous cell carcinoma. Approximately one-third of chronic wounds are associated with malignancy.

INTERVENTION

GENERAL

All wound management interventions must start by considering the following priorities: (1) determining and correcting etiological factors, (2) addressing systemic factors, and (3) providing appropriate topical therapy.[15] In the case of vascular ulcers, wounds caused by arterial insufficiency are generally best addressed surgically by reestablishing circulation, whereas those of venous etiology are best addressed by enhancing venous return with compression.

For all types of ulcers, systemic support should be provided by addressing the patient's nutritional and hydration needs, maintaining tight glucose control, and providing topical therapy, including wound bed preparation, appropriate dressings, and adjunctive therapies such as physical agents and topical medications.

Wound bed preparation for vascular ulcers is similar to that for other chronic wounds (see Chapter 28) and includes cleansing, debridement of necrotic tissue, provision for moist wound healing, elimination of dead space, protection, and insulation. If the bioburden is high or infection is present, systemic antibiotics, topical antiseptics, or antimicrobial dressings may be prescribed by the patient's physician. If wound edges are closed but the wound is still open, the edges must be opened to allow healing to continue. General interventions for the patient with a wound may be found in Chapter 28; the selected interventions described in this chapter are specific to the vascular ulcer.

ARTERIAL ULCERS AND LOWER EXTREMITY ARTERIAL DISEASE

Interventions for the patient with arterial ulcers and LEAD are based on the severity, stage, and symptoms of arterial disease; the patient's general medical status; the goals of therapy; and the expected outcome or prognosis. The primary therapeutic focus in management of LEAD is to increase arterial blood flow and diminish pain. All interventions for LEAD initially focus on improving blood supply and decreasing pain. If this cannot be achieved with conservative or pharmacological intervention, surgical revascularization is considered. If surgery is not possible or would not be effective, then amputation must be considered.

Goals of nonoperative treatment focus on risk factor modification and control of disease progression, improvement of exercise tolerance, pain reduction, and prevention and/or treatment of complications. Smoking cessation, exercise, blood pressure control, dietary management, proper management of diabetes, use of physical agent modalities (e.g., electrical stimulation), and pharmacological therapy are the principal means to achieve these goals.[12,19] Meticulous foot care to decrease the risk of complications (e.g., trauma) is also important. Foot hygiene, daily inspection of feet and legs, and avoidance of harsh chemicals, extreme temperatures, and barefoot walking are recommended interventions for the patient with LEAD. Toenails should be trimmed by a professional health care provider because of the high risk for trauma to surrounding soft tissues.

Debridement. Debridement of an arterial ulcer is indicated only when there is adequate perfusion to support healing or when the wound is infected (to decrease bioburden). Debridement is recommended when an ulcer is infected, and surgical debridement is preferred in this situation[2] to minimize the risk of spreading the infection. However, debridement is contraindicated for a stable and severely ischemic wound because these wounds have poor healing potential. A stable wound is one with no induration, no erythema, no fluctuance, and no increased warmth. Thus debridement would generally be

contraindicated in a patient with an ABI of <0.5 (severe ischemia) who had an ulcer with no signs of infection.[2] If the clinician's examination indicates that nonviable tissue should be debrided, a carefully monitored trial of autolytic or enzymatic debridement is typically the initial approach of choice.[2]

> ### ◎ Clinical Pearl
>
> Debridement of arterial ulcers is indicated only if there is adequate perfusion or when the wound is infected.

Dressings. Most open, dry wounds should be managed according to the principles of moist wound healing. It is recommended that intervention for an arterial ulcer includes frequent assessment for evidence of developing infection or progressive ischemia.[2] In the acute care setting the ulcer should be assessed daily; in the home health care setting, assessment is routinely done at each nursing visit, which is usually 2 to 3 times per week. Occlusive and adhesive semiocclusive dressings should generally be avoided because they prevent frequent visualization of the wound. Nonadherent dressings (e.g., hydrogels), which are changed daily or every other day, are usually preferred for open wounds.[15]

However, in patients with significant arterial insufficiency and dry, noninfected necrotic wounds, it is currently recommended that the area be kept dry until the nonviable tissue separates naturally from the viable tissue.[4] A clinical solution to this difficult situation is to paint a topical antiseptic (e.g., povidone iodine) over the wound and allow it to dry.[2] It should be emphasized that this recommendation only applies to the stable wound with insufficient vascular supply to allow healing.

> ### ◎ Clinical Pearl
>
> Nonadherent dressings that keep the wound moist are usually the dressing of choice for arterial ulcers.

Pain Management. Pain management is important in patients with vascular ulcers because pain can severely and adversely impact the patient's quality of life and function and cause sympathetic stimulation and vasoconstriction, which can exacerbate arterial insufficiency.[16] Pain may be controlled with systemic analgesics, transcutaneous electrical nerve stimulation (TENS), visual imagery, or relaxation.

Exercise and Activity. To decrease the risk of ulceration, a graduated exercise program to increase perfusion in patients with LEAD is recommended. Generally, as long as arterial insufficiency is not severe, walking is well tolerated in patients with LEAD. Walking may improve LEAD by improving oxygen use at the cellular level, decreasing resting blood pressure, decreasing stress, and improving gait efficiency. Patients with intermittent claudication who participate in a regular walking program have been shown to increase their walking distance by 100% to 200%, suggesting that walking increases perfusion to the skin and soft tissues.[21]

However, walking programs are generally not effective or tolerated in patients with advanced arterial disease, including those who already have ulcers caused by arterial insufficiency and those who have pain at rest. For these patients, initial interventions are directed toward reducing tissue metabolic demands. This may necessitate a reduction in activity until the ulcer is healed.[12,38] Therefore it is recommended that activity, including walking and other exercise, be closely monitored and modified in patients with arterial ulcers to determine if the activity is facilitating or impairing tissue healing. In addition, if the patient is allowed to ambulate, it is imperative that the area of ischemia be protected either with protective footwear or by an assistive device.[38]

Electrotherapy. Electrical stimulation may be recommended for the treatment of wounds of various etiologies. Studies show that certain types of electrical stimulation may decrease pain from ischemia,[16] augment blood flow in lower extremities with an impaired calf or foot pump, and stimulate angiogenesis. See Chapter 28 for the mechanisms underlying the effectiveness of electrical stimulation for wound healing, further evidence about the effectiveness of this approach, and details of application technique.

Intermittent Pneumatic (Dynamic) Compression. Intermittent pneumatic compression consists of the alternating application and release of compression every few seconds for a total of 45 minutes to an hour for 3 to 4 or more hours each day. Although compression is generally reserved for the treatment of wounds caused by venous insufficiency, there is some evidence that patients with intermittent claudication and/or limb-threatening PAD for whom surgery is not feasible may benefit from intermittent pneumatic compression treatment.[2] Intermittent pneumatic compression is thought to increase blood flow by mimicking the calf muscle pumping that occurs during ambulation.[2]

Although more data are needed to determine the role of intermittent pneumatic compression in patients with LEAD, it appears that intermittent pneumatic compression may improve functional walking tolerance, blood flow, pain, and in some cases, ulcer healing.[2] It should be emphasized that this application of compression differs from the sustained, continuous compression recommended for the treatment of venous insufficiency, as described later in this chapter, and that any form of compression is contraindicated in severe arterial disease in which the ABI is <0.5 and when there is peripheral edema caused by congestive heart failure.[2,37]

> ### ◎ *Clinical Pearl*
> Any form of compression is contraindicated in severe arterial disease in which the ABI is <0.5 and when there is peripheral edema caused by congestive heart failure.

Hyperbaric Oxygen Therapy. Hyperbaric oxygen therapy (HBOT) involves the patient either breathing pure oxygen at high pressure or locally exposing the wound to oxygen at high pressure. The intervention is typically performed for 90 to 120 minutes either daily or twice daily for 10 days to 1 to 2 months. It is proposed that hyperbaric oxygen therapy may help patients with ischemic ulcers by increasing tissue oxygen perfusion. However, a systematic review of the literature performed in 2005 on HBOT for the treatment of chronic wounds found insufficient data to support this treatment for patients with venous or arterial ulcers.

Nutrition. Good nutrition is essential for patients with wounds because wound healing increases metabolic demand. Consultation by a dietitian is strongly recommended for any patient with a chronic wound with recent weight loss, low albumin or prealbumin levels, vitamin or mineral deficiencies, poorly controlled diabetes, obesity, or dehydration.[15] The dietitian will assess other essential nutritional components necessary for healing (e.g., fluids, proteins, calories, glucose levels, vitamins, minerals, and amino acids) and determine the need for supplementation.

Surgical Options. Surgical options for patients with arterial insufficiency include revascularization, angioplasty, debridement of necrotic tissue, and amputation.[2,21] Surgical revascularization to restore perfusion is preferred where possible. Surgery is indicated for patients with rest pain, tissue loss, or disabling claudication.[20,21] The vessel segment(s) to be treated are identified by angiography before surgery. Most commonly, the superficial femoral artery in the thigh is involved, although some patients have tibial or iliac artery involvement.[12] Revascularization is accomplished by bypass grafting or angioplasty.[12,16,20,21] Arterial bypass grafts may be accomplished by use of the saphenous vein, an upper extremity vein, or a synthetic graft.[4,12,16] Angioplasty is sometimes used for treatment of stenotic lesions in the iliac artery; this procedure is most effective for lesions <3 cm long.[12]

Surgical debridement of necrotic tissue may be necessary to rapidly remove infected tissue and reduce the risk of spreading an infection from an infected wound.[2]

Surgical amputation may be indicated if tissue loss has progressed beyond the point of salvage, if revascularization surgery cannot be performed or is too risky, if life expectancy is very low, or if functional limitations obviate the benefit of limb salvage.[20] The level of amputation is generally dictated by function and by the potential for healing at the amputation site. Generally, it is recommended that the amputation be performed at a level where preoperative $TcPO_2$ levels are greater than 20 mm Hg to ensure good potential for healing of the amputation site.[2]

Education. Education for the patient with vascular ulcers should include lifestyle modification measures to improve perfusion and minimize the risk of trauma. One of the most important "teaching points" is the negative impact of tobacco (in any form) on tissue perfusion and wound healing. Other key points to be included in patient education are included in Box 29-2. Patients with arterial insufficiency also need to maintain adequate hydration, control glucose, and see a professional for foot and nail care.

VENOUS ULCERS/LOWER EXTREMITY VENOUS DISEASE

Interventions for the patient with LEVD and venous ulcers should be based on the degree of venous insufficiency, duration of disease, and presenting complications. The desired outcome of interventions for patients with LEVD

BOX 29-2	Areas of Education for Patients with Lower Extremity Arterial Disease

- Chronic disease management (DM, HTN) and the effects of these diseases on LEAD.
- Reduction of hyperlipidemia and proper diet.
- Smoking cessation to slow progression of atherosclerosis and decrease the risk of cardiovascular events, including death.
- Compliance with medications.
- Neutral or dependent position for legs.
- Avoidance of chemical, thermal, and mechanical trauma.
- Routine professional nail and foot care.
- Use of properly fitting shoes and footwear.
- Wearing socks or hose with shoes.
- Pressure reduction for heels, toes, and bony prominences.
- Need for regular follow-up with health care provider.
- Importance of exercise.

Adapted from Bonham PA, Flemister BG: WOCN Clinical Practice Guideline Series: *Guideline for management of wounds in patients with lower-extremity arterial disease,* Glenview, IL, 2002, Wound Ostomy and Continence Nurses Society.
DM, Diabetes mellitus; *HTN,* hypertension; *LEAD,* lower extremity arterial disease.

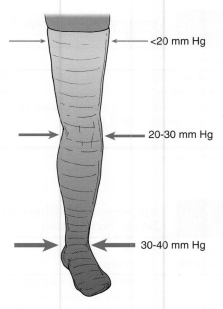

FIG. 29-9 Gradient compression from a compression bandage.

and venous ulcers is to decrease edema, prevent or resolve ulcers, return patients to an optimal level of functional activity, and educate patients and their families.

Compression Therapy. Compression is the most critical intervention for patients with venous insufficiency with and without ulceration because it supports venous return.[26] This intervention will be required for the patient's lifetime to prevent recurrence of ulcers because a compromised venous system does not recover.[8,16,24] Consistent compliance with **compression therapy** is crucial to good long-term outcomes. One study reported that in patients with lower extremity ulcers caused by venous insufficiency, 79% of those who did not adhere to compression therapy had wound recurrence as compared with only a 4% recurrence rate in those who continued with compression therapy.[39] Unfortunately, adherence to recommended compression therapy is generally poor. Without acceptance and understanding of the importance of compression therapy, patients often do not adhere to this key intervention, increasing their risk of ulcer recurrence.

Clinical Pearl

Compression is the most critical intervention for patients with venous insufficiency with or without ulceration.

Compression therapy addresses the changes caused by poor venous return by providing an external support (sustained or dynamic) to the calf muscle pump. The goal of compression therapy is to augment venous return

from the peripheral veins to the central circulation. Compression therapy increases interstitial tissue pressures by compressing the superficial tissues.[15] The amount of pressure underneath a bandage is governed by Laplace's law, which states that sub-bandage pressure is directly proportional to the tension and number of bandage layers and inversely proportional to leg circumference and bandage width[40-42]:

$$\text{Sub-bandage pressure (mm Hg)} = (\text{tension} \times \text{layers}) \div$$
$$(\text{circumference of leg [cm]} \times \text{width of bandage [cm]})$$

$$T = P \times R$$

where
T = tension
P = pressure
R = diameter

Thus an increase in tension and/or number of layers will increase the sub-bandage pressure; whereas an increase in leg circumference and/or bandage width will decrease the sub-bandage pressure. If bandage tension is consistent along the leg, the pressure will be greatest at the level of the smallest diameter, the ankle, and gradually decrease as one moves up the leg to just below the knee[8] (Fig. 29-9). Bandage or stocking compression pressure may range from less than 20 mm Hg, where the leg diameter is the greatest, to more than 60 mm Hg at the ankle, but generally 30 to 40 mm Hg of pressure at the ankle is recommended.[3,6,40] The current recommendation is that patients "should be offered the strongest compression with which they can comply."[9] Although adherence is better with medium compression than higher compression,[9] antiembolism stockings (e.g., TED hose), which provide approximately 13 to 18 mm Hg pressure compression, do not provide sufficient compression for the patient with venous insufficiency. Compression guidelines based on ABI can

TABLE 29-5	Compression Guidelines Based on ABI	
Compression		**ABI**
Standard (30-40 mm Hg)		ABI ≥0.8-1.0
Modified (23-27 mm Hg)		ABI 0.6-0.8
Elastic, multilayered bandages are contraindicated because force is exerted with ambulation and at rest.		
NO compression		ABI <0.6

ABI, Ankle-brachial index.

TABLE 29-6	Compression Guidelines Based on Clinical Presentation
Compression Pressure (mm Hg)	**Presentation**
20-30	Varicose veins, mild edema, leg fatigue
30-40	Severe varicosities or moderate CVI
40-50 and >60	Severe CVI and its complications

CVI, Chronic venous insufficiency.

be found in Table 29-5; compression guidelines based on clinical presentation are given in Table 29-6.

For some patients, especially those who are skeptical of wearing compression, afraid of claustrophobic symptoms, or uncomfortable with the idea of leaving one bandage on for a number of days, a lower to mid-level amount of compression may be used at first and then advanced to a higher level of compression as the patient's tolerance increases. Compression may be sustained (static) or intermittent (dynamic). Sustained compression may be applied with an elastic or inelastic device, and intermittent compression may be applied with a multichamber or single-chamber device.

Static Compression. Static elastic compression, as applied with bandages or stockings, has been shown to accelerate the healing of venous ulcers. Multilayered bandaging (Fig. 29-10) is more effective than single layer or inelastic bandaging. Elastic, rather than inelastic, bandaging is essential in patients who are not ambulatory because they provide higher resting pressure. High compression bandages are generally more effective than moderate compression bandages.

If a bandaging system is used, its application is key to safe, effective therapy. Some multilayered wraps have visual guides to direct how much stretch should be applied to produce the ideal amount of pressure (Fig. 29-11). Although application with too much pressure may cause ischemia,[43] more often too little pressure is used. In addition to the appropriate amount of tension, which should be based on the manufacturer's recommendations with regard to stretch, overlap, and wrapping style and be sufficient to wrap the limb snugly while maintaining palpable peripheral pulses, bony prominences should be padded and oversized footwear should be provided to accommodate the wrap.

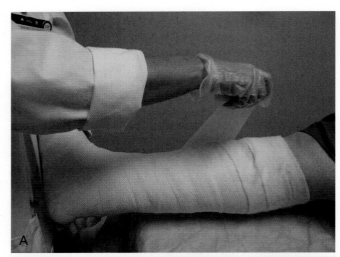

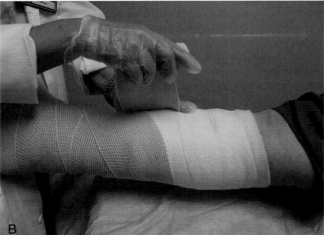

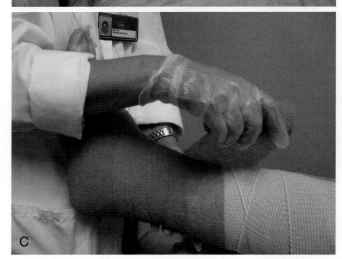

FIG. 29-10 Application of a 4-layer compression bandage.

Elastic wraps should be applied by a trained professional (Figs. 29-12 and 29-13). Stockings or removable orthotic devices may be applied by the patient if they have the physical skills to apply the wrap (adequate vision and manual dexterity) and if they can reach their feet, or by a caretaker, if the patient cannot reach their feet. Assistive devices, such as the stocking butler and rubber gloves, are also available to assist with donning compression stockings (Fig. 29-14).

Long-stretch elastic wraps (such as ACE bandages) are not recommended for compression in patients with venous ulcers because although they apply high resting pressure when the patient is not moving, they stretch too much when the calf muscle contracts and thus provide low compression when the patient walks.

Once the wound and the edema are stable, elastic stockings rather than bandage wraps should be used to provide static compression and prevent edema and ulcer recurrence. There are off-the-shelf compression stockings

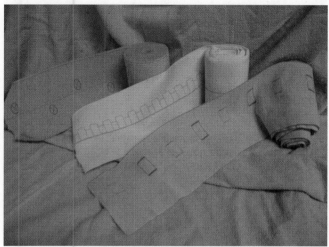

FIG. 29-11 Compression bandages with visual guides to direct how much stretch should be applied. With all of these, the bandage should be stretched until the boxes become square.

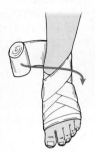 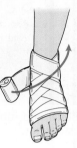 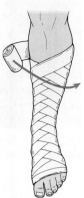

A The steep figure of eight turns aid the comformability of the bandage, accommodating contours in the leg.

B Maintain these turns.

C Finish the bandaging just below the knee.

FIG. 29-13 Applying an elastic bandage with a figure-8 wrap technique. *Redrawn from Morrison M, Moffatt C: A colour guide to the assessment and management of leg ulcers, ed 2, London, 1994, Mosby.*

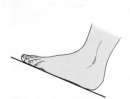 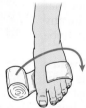 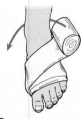

A Place the foot in a comfortable position, at a right angle to the leg.

B Begin by making two anchoring turns around the foot. Be sure to include the base of the toes.

C Next take a high turn above the heel.

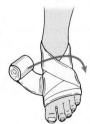 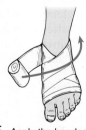 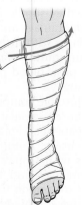

D Then fill the base of the foot with a low turn. From here, the bandage can be applied in a spiral as in this figure or in a figure of eight (see Figure 29-13).

E Apply the bandage in a spiral, ensuring there is a 50% overlap.

F Ensure the bandage is applied right up to the tibial tuberosity.

FIG. 29-12 Applying an elastic bandage with a spiral-wrap technique. *Redrawn from Morrison M, Moffatt C: A colour guide to the assessment and management of leg ulcers, ed 2, London, 1994, Mosby.*

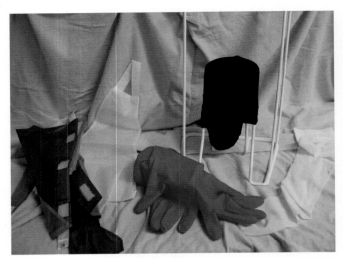

FIG. 29-14 Stocking butler and rubber gloves to assist with donning compression stockings.

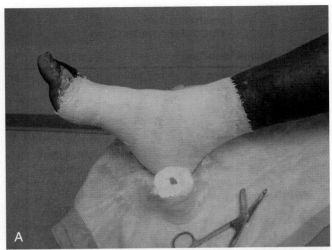

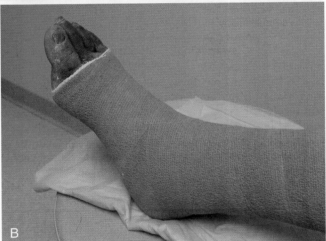

FIG. 29-15 Application of an Unna's boot.

available for the more common sizes and custom stockings are available for the "oddly" shaped or sized leg. It is recommended that the stockings be replaced every 6 months, since washing and use decreases their elasticity over time, even with the best care. These stockings are costly, poorly reimbursed, and too hot in some geographic areas during summer seasons. Often, patients think stockings are no longer needed once an ulcer has closed, but studies show a significant decrease in ulcer recurrence rate with continued wear.[27] However, there is no evidence that stockings that extend proximally beyond the knee are any more effective than knee-highs, and knee-highs tend to be better tolerated.[8,28]

Inelastic compression may be applied with an **Unna's boot,** short-stretch bandages (SSBs), or a removable compression orthotic. Unna's boots are similar to a cast (Fig. 29-15). They can be particularly helpful during initial edema management in the ambulatory patient because they provide high pressure during walking and do not stretch out with fluctuations in edema. However, because they are not easy to remove, they should not be used in patients with large amounts of drainage and poor hygiene habits.[8] SSBs, which are bandages with little to no elasticity, also produce high pressure during walking and low resting pressures, helping to push blood proximally and allowing for deep venous filling.

Readily removable and adjustable compression devices that fasten with Velcro straps are also available (Fig. 29-16). Although these can improve patient acceptance,[40] the ease of removal can also decrease usage. A number of studies have compared these devices with Unna's boots, below-the-knee stockings, 4-layer bandages, and SSBs and found them to be a viable and low-cost option for compression therapy.[44-47] They also require fewer provider visits because patients can often change their own dressings, whereas Unna's boots must be changed at least weekly by a professional.[44]

Dynamic Compression. Intermittent pneumatic compression pumps can be used to provide additional dynamic compression beyond the static compression provided by bandages or stockings, or as an alternative to bandages or stockings in nonambulatory patients (Fig. 29-17). Intermittent pneumatic compression is the application of controlled external pressure using compressed air and a pump, which cyclically inflates and deflates the chambers within a specially designed sleeve that envelops the extremity.[41] This cyclic inflation and deflation of intermittent pneumatic compression mimics calf muscle pump action and can promote venous return, reduce edema, stimulate fibrinolysis, and heal recalcitrant ulcers after other methods have failed.

Some but not all studies suggest that intermittent pneumatic compression may improve healing beyond the benefits provided by static compression. Therefore, until further research clearly determines the effect of intermittent pneumatic compression on the healing of venous leg ulcers, patients treated with intermittent pneumatic compression should still also receive static compression with a bandage or stockings for long-term control of venous insufficiency.

Intermittent pneumatic compression devices come with either single-chamber or multichamber sleeves. The

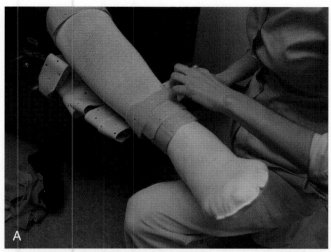

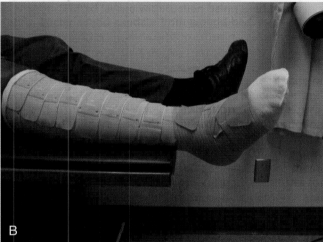

FIG. 29-16 A readily removable and adjustable Velcro-fastening compression device.

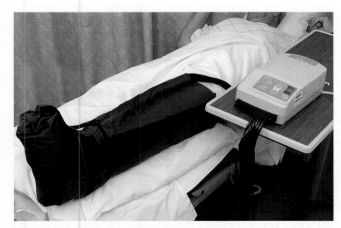

FIG. 29-17 Intermittent pneumatic compression. *From Pierson FM, Fairchild SL:* Principles and techniques of patient care, *ed 4, St Louis, 2008, Saunders.*

- Chronic disease management and the effects of these diseases on LEVD.
- Proper diet and weight control.
- Compliance with medications.
- Elevated position for legs.
- Avoidance of chemical, thermal, and mechanical trauma.
- Routine professional nail and foot care.
- Use of properly fitting shoes and footwear.
- Wearing socks or hose with shoes.
- Need for regular follow-up with health care provider.
- Importance of exercise.

LEVD, Lower extremity venous disease.

multichamber sleeve provides sequential compression intended to "milk" the fluid from distal to proximal, whereas the single-chamber sleeve inflates and deflates all at once. The multichamber sequential compression has been shown to be more effective in achieving venous return than the single-chamber compression.[8] For patients with venous insufficiency these devices are generally applied for 30 to 60 minutes twice per day at pressures of 30 to 50 mm Hg.

Contraindications and Precautions for Compression Therapy. All forms of compression are contraindicated in patients with symptomatic heart failure (because of the risk of system overload) and those with a thrombus (because of the risk of dislodgment) and may not be appropriate if an arterial revascularization has been performed on the involved limb.[8,48] In addition, the clinician must evaluate for the presence and severity of arterial insufficiency before compressing a limb. If the ABI is less than 0.5, all forms of static compression are contraindicated. If the ABI is greater than 0.8, standard or full compression (30 to 40 mm Hg) may be used. When the ABI is between 0.5 and 0.8, the compression pressure should be reduced to between 23 and 27 mm Hg.[2] If the patient also has neuropathy, careful monitoring is necessary because he or she may fail to recognize symptoms of ischemia such as pain, numbness, or tingling.[2,28]

Education. Box 29-3 provides guidelines for educating patients with LEVD. For the patient with venous insufficiency and resulting edema and wounds, it is important that elevation during the waking hours is emphasized and sitting with legs in a dependent position is avoided. One suggestion is to elevate the legs above the heart for 1 to 2 hours, 1 to 2 times each day, and at nighttime. Nighttime elevation can be accomplished by elevating the foot of the bed with blocks or an equivalent.[28]

Debridement. Nonviable tissue in the venous ulcer should be debrided. The type of tissue, the urgency of debridement, clinician preference, and the expected outcome and prognosis determine the method of debridement. The different methods of debridement (surgical, sharp, autolytic, enzymatic, and mechanical) are outlined in Chapter 28.

Dressings. Principles of moist wound healing are used with the venous ulcer in order to enhance healing and minimize complications. The venous ulcer tends to be highly exudative; therefore absorption of the excess moisture and elimination of pooled exudate will likely be the focus in dressing selection. Dressings, such as foams, alginates, or hydrofibers, should be considered because of their high absorption capacities. Protection of the surrounding skin from maceration caused by excess exudate may require application of a skin sealant (e.g., Skin Prep, Smith & Nephew, Largo, FL, or AllKare, ConvaTec, Princeton, NJ) to the wound edges, especially distal to the ulcer.[15] Once exudate has been minimized, a hydrocolloid may be considered for the wound dressing. The frequency of dressing changes is determined by the volume of exudate and the absorptive capacity of the dressing; the goal is to change the dressing frequently enough to prevent maceration and dermatitis caused by pooled exudate.

Providers should avoid excessive use of topical agents because patients may become sensitized or allergic to any agent used for prolonged periods.[28] One common problem in the management of venous ulcers is the high potential for contact dermatitis. If venous dermatitis (see Fig. 29-8, C) is present, low-dose topical steroids may be applied for short periods of time (2 to 6 weeks). Barrier ointments may be effective for xerosis (abnormal dryness); good choices include plain petrolatum or dimethicone products.[15] In addition to providing a moist wound environment, the wound dressing must be compatible with the chosen compression system. The dressing must continue to absorb effectively under the force of the compression and must be able to stay in place for the same amount of time as the compression system.

Skin Substitutes—Bioengineered Skin Equivalents. Studies have shown that bioengineered tissues may promote wound healing by releasing growth factors. These factors can convert a wound from a chronic, nonhealing state to actively healing[49]; however, because they are expensive, they should only be used for recalcitrant venous ulcers that fail to respond to standard therapy. Bioengineered skin equivalents, when used in conjunction with compression therapy, have been found to be an effective and cost-effective addition to compression therapy in patients with refractory venous ulcers.[6,9,50,51] Bioengineered skin equivalents should not be used if the patient has associated untreated dermatitis, infection, or exposed bone or tendon.[49]

Exercise, Activity, and Positioning. A walking and exercise program is important for the patient with venous insufficiency because this can improve calf muscle pump function. The key elements of such a program are described in the next section.

Exercise. Exercises that activate the calf muscle pump and assist with venous blood return should be performed frequently. These include (1) isometric contraction of the quadriceps and hamstrings, (2) active and active-resistive ROM for the lower extremities, (3) ankle pumps, (4) short arc quads, and (5) standing toe and heel raises.

In addition, aquatic therapy, swimming, and cycling may be encouraged.[36]

Gait Training. Gait training should focus on improving the heel-to-toe pattern during stance and toe-off in terminal stance to activate the foot and calf muscle pump. Patients should be encouraged to take walking and exercise breaks at work and at home.

Positioning. Lower extremity elevation is recommended for all patients with venous insufficiency and related edema. The current recommendation is to elevate the leg 6 to 9 inches above the level of the heart for 2 to 4 hours during the day and throughout the night. At night this can be accomplished by placing a 6-inch block at the foot of the bed to elevate the foot of the bed.[28]

Pain Management. As noted in the Typical Examination Findings section of this chapter, the pain reported by the patient with venous insufficiency is different from that caused by arterial compromise. In general, these patients do not have severe pain and their pain is worse when the lower extremity is dependent. Pain caused by venous insufficiency is managed primarily by addressing the etiology—venous congestion and edema. Interventions include elevation of the lower extremity (ankle above the heart), externally applied compression, wound dressings, and changes in ADLs and work patterns (e.g., decreased amount of sitting or standing and increased number of walking breaks).[9]

Ultrasound and Electrotherapy. There is some evidence that ultrasound and electrotherapy may help venous ulcer healing.[9] Chapter 28 includes a general discussion of the use of ultrasound and electrotherapy for promoting wound healing.

Nutrition. Careful attention to nutrition is paramount to the wound healing process. Nutrition is as critical to healing as perfusion.[15] A dietitian consult is strongly recommended for any patient with recent weight loss, low albumin or prealbumin levels, vitamin or mineral deficiencies, poorly controlled diabetes, or obesity.[28] The dietitian assesses other nutritional components necessary for healing (e.g., fluids, proteins, calories, glucose levels, vitamins, minerals, and amino acids) and determines the need and criteria for supplementation.

Surgical Options. Surgery for the patient with venous insufficiency and ulceration is generally considered only if the ulcer shows no signs of healing after 3 months of best-practice intervention (compression and good skin care). Surgery is an option when the valvular dysfunction involves the superficial or perforator veins. The procedure most commonly recommended for these patients is **subfascial endoscopic perforator surgery (SEPS)** during which incompetent perforator veins are clipped.[16,28,52,53] It is thought that the most important factor in venous insufficiency is malfunction of perforator veins and that the SEPS procedure removes these malfunctioning veins from the circulation.[54] This surgical technique has less postoperative morbidity than open surgical procedures. For best results, compression therapy should be applied immediately after the SEPS procedure.

Other surgical interventions for patients with venous ulcers include **vein stripping** and ablative surgery, saphenectomy, and free flap. Vein stripping and ablative surgery for superficial venous insufficiency and/or perforator vein incompetence helps reduce deep venous reflux and may help prevent ulcer recurrence.[8,28] Saphenectomy is used for isolated incompetence of the greater or lesser saphenous veins.[28] Excision of the ulcer and surrounding lipodermatosclerosis and placement of a free flap of muscle and skin or omentum is also used to promote the healing of wounds caused by venous insufficiency.[8]

MIXED VENOUS AND ARTERIAL DISEASE

Management of Edema. Whether compression should be used in patients with wounds and concomitant arterial and venous insufficiency with edema depends on the patient's ABI. Compression therapy should not be instituted if the ABI is less than 0.5. However, if the patient has moderate arterial insufficiency (ABI ≥0.6 and ≤0.8) and there is edema caused by venous insufficiency or dependent positioning (used for pain control), a trial of modified- or low-pressure compression of 23 to 30 mm Hg at the ankle may be used. If the wound does not improve with this intervention or the ABI is less than 0.5, a prompt consultation by a vascular surgeon is recommended.[2,9]

ADDITIONAL CONSIDERATIONS FOR VASCULAR ULCERS

If the physical therapist assistant has implemented appropriate therapy interventions and the wound does not start to heal or if the ulcer is atypical in appearance, he or she should consider referral back to the supervising physical therapist for further evaluation and possible referral for further evaluation by a physician. Biopsy may be performed because nonhealing chronic wounds may be caused by malignancy or may undergo malignant transformation.[2,16] Although rare, skin neoplasm (e.g., squamous or basal cell carcinoma) and certain inflammatory conditions (e.g., pyoderma gangrenosum) may also present with chronic soft tissue ulceration.[8,55]

CASE STUDY 29-1

VENOUS ULCER

Patient History

SB is a 51-year-old man with an open nonhealing wound on his right lower extremity. He also has pain, swelling, and skin discoloration of the right lower extremity. SB also has a long history of hypertension and has had two DVTs in his right leg since 2001.

Tests and Measures—Significant Findings
Musculoskeletal

Girth: 2 inches above lateral malleolus: Right: 24 cm, left: 18.7 cm. 4 inches below tibial plateau: Right: 35 cm, left: 26 cm.
- Ankle dorsiflexion ROM is decreased 20%, and plantarflexion is decreased 10% on the right compared to the left.
- Strength is grossly 2+/5 in the right ankle.

Neuromuscular
- Pain 5 to 9/10, worse at the end of the day and eases with rest and elevation.

Integumentary
- Wound locations: Medial aspect, gaiter area, right lower extremity.
- Wound dimensions: 2.0 × 1.5 cm; depth 0.5 cm.
- Wound bed: Dark red, 80% clean but not granulating, 20% adherent yellow slough.
- Drainage: Moderate to heavy, serosanguineous.
- No clinical signs or symptoms of local infection.

Cardiovascular/Pulmonary
- Pulses: Both dorsalis pedis and tibialis posterior pulses are palpable on the right and left lower extremities.

Function
- Independent in ambulation without an assistive device but with decreased heel-to-toe gait pattern.

Diagnosis

Preferred practice pattern 7D: Impaired integumentary integrity associated with full-thickness skin involvement and scar formation.

Interventions
- Wound cleaning, debridement, and dressing
- Compression
- Gait training
- Strengthening and stretching lower extremity exercises

Role of the Physical Therapist Assistant
- How would you clean this wound?
- What is the purpose of compression for this patient? What forms of compression could be used?
- What assistive device would you consider for gait training for this patient?
- Describe three strengthening and three stretching exercises appropriate for this patient.

Additional Information

For the full version of this case study, including detailed examination results, interventions, and outcomes, see the Evolve site that accompanies this book.

CHAPTER SUMMARY

PVD, both venous and arterial, commonly causes chronic open wounds. This chapter provides the reader with a foundation for building best practices in the management of the patient with a vascular ulcer. General anatomy and function of the lower extremity vascular system are reviewed, and pathology, examination, patient evaluation, characteristics of vascular ulceration, and interventions available for promoting healing of wounds caused by arterial and venous insufficiency are highlighted.

Examination follows three priorities in wound management: Determining etiology, addressing systemic factors, and providing appropriate topical therapy. Interventions can be as simple as elevation or as complex as surgical procedures (e.g., revascularization of a limb).

The clinician's management responsibilities also include patient and family education, physical and psychological assessment and preparation for possible limb loss, coordination of continuity of care, monitoring for complications, and provision of emotional support.

Vascular ulcers can be challenging for the patient, the patient's family, and the clinicians involved in the management of the ulcer. Accurate examination, evaluation, and management of the patient with a lower extremity vascular ulcer lead to the most effective comprehensive care and improve the quality of life for this patient population.

ADDITIONAL RESOURCES

For links to these and additional web-based resources, see the Evolve site.

Bonham PA, Flemister BG: Wound, Ostomy and Continence Nurses Society (WOCN) Clinical Practice Guideline Series: *Guideline for management of wounds in patients with lower-extremity arterial disease,* Glenview, IL, 2002, Wound, Ostomy and Continence Nurses Society.

Johnson J, Paustian C: Wound, Ostomy and Continence Nurses Society (WOCN) Clinical Practice Guideline Series: *Guideline for management of wounds in patients with lower-extremity arterial disease,* Glenview, IL, 2004, Wound, Ostomy and Continence Nurses Society.

Wound, Ostomy and Continence Nurses Society (WOCN)

American Physical Therapy Association, Section on Clinical Electrotherapy and Wound Management

GLOSSARY

Angiography: A procedure to view blood vessels by injecting a radiopaque contrast medium into them that can be seen on x-ray.

Ankle flare (malleolar flare): Visible capillaries caused by distention of small veins around the medial malleolar area.

Arterial insufficiency: Lack of sufficient blood flow in arteries to extremities. Can be caused by cholesterol deposits (atherosclerosis) or clots (emboli) or by damaged, diseased, or weak vessels.

Atherosclerosis: Plaques of cholesterol, fats, and other remains are deposited in the walls of large- and medium-sized arteries. The walls of the vessels become thick and hardened, leading to narrowing, which reduces circulation to areas normally supplied by the artery.

Claudication: Pain in the legs with cramps in the calves during walking that is relieved by rest. Caused by inadequate supply of blood to the legs.

Compression therapy: Application of sustained external pressure to the lower extremity to control edema and aid the return of venous blood to the heart, achieved by wraps, multilayer elastic compression therapy systems, or a pneumatic pump.

Dermatitis: Inflammation of the skin.

Edema: A localized or generalized abnormal accumulation of fluid in body tissues.

Gangrene (dry or moist): Death of tissue, usually the result of deficient or absent blood supply.

Ischemia: Inadequate blood supply to an organ or part, often marked by pain or organ dysfunction.

Lipodermatosclerosis (hypodermitis sclerodermiformis): The induration and hyperpigmentation of the lower third of the leg that often occurs in patients who have LEVD. This frequently causes the leg to have an "apple-core" or "inverted champagne bottle" appearance.

Osteomyelitis: Inflammation of bone and marrow, usually caused by microorganisms that enter the bone at the time of injury or surgery.

Peripheral arterial disease (PAD): Narrowing of the arteries that supply the extremities.

Pruritus: Sensation of itching.

Subfascial endoscopic perforator surgery (SEPS): A minimally invasive surgical technique for the ablation of incompetent perforator veins in the lower leg.

Thrombophilia: An increased tendency to form blood clots.

Unna's boot: Static inelastic zinc-impregnated bandage (with or without calamine) wrapped around the leg to provide compression.

Varicose veins: Swollen and twisted veins that appear blue and close to the surface of the skin. They may bulge, throb, and cause the legs to feel heavy and swell. Varicose veins may occur in almost any part of the body, but they are most often seen in the back of the calf or on the inside of the leg between the groin and the ankle.

Vein stripping: Surgical removal of varicose veins.

Venous insufficiency: Inadequate return of venous blood from periphery generally caused by poor venous valve function.

Chapter 30

Neuropathic Ulcers

Rose Little Hamm, Pamela Scarborough

OBJECTIVES

After reading this chapter, the reader will be able to:
1. Understand the pathology of neuropathic ulcers.
2. Compare and contrast normal physiology with pathological changes related to type 2 diabetes.
3. Identify causative factors for neuropathic ulcers.
4. Discuss the role of diabetes in ulcer formation.
5. Be familiar with common examination techniques for a patient with a neuropathic ulcer.
6. Implement a plan of care for a patient with a neuropathic ulcer.

Neuropathic ulcers (NUs) are wounds caused by mechanical stress and sensory loss and are generally associated with **diabetes mellitus (DM),** spina bifida, Hansen's disease, and in some cases, peripheral vascular disease (PVD) or other vascular pathologies. In addition, patients with central nervous system (CNS) disorders who have limited mobility and decreased sensation are at high risk for this type of wound. NUs are not only problems in and of themselves but also predispose patients to lower extremity amputation and systemic infection.

Clinical Pearl

Although neuropathic ulcers (NUs) occur in patients with a range of diseases, in the United States, most neuropathic ulcers are associated with diabetes.

Although NUs occur in patients with a range of diseases, reports of prevalence and incidence are primarily related to the population with diabetes. The American Diabetes Association (ADA) reports that 18.2 million people, 6.3% of the total population of the United States (US), have diabetes; 13 million of these are diagnosed and 5.2 million are undiagnosed.[1] The number of Americans diagnosed with diabetes is projected to increase by 65% over the next 50 years, from 11 million in 2000 (population prevalence of 4.0%) to 29 million in 2050 (population prevalence of 7.2%).[2] The largest percentage increase in diagnosed diabetes will be among those aged 75 years or older (Fig. 30-1).[2] Among certain ethnic groups, the prevalence of diabetes among people aged 20 or older can be as high as 14.5% (Table 30-1). Fifteen percent of people with diabetes will experience a NU during their lifetime, and 14% to 24% of all people with foot ulcers will require a lower extremity amputation.[3] NUs are one of the major risk factors for lower extremity amputation in patients with diabetes.[4] In 2001 and 2002, more than 82,000 amputations per year were performed on patients with diabetes, and diabetes was the cause of more than 60% of the nontraumatic amputations in the US over this period.[1] The factors most associated with foot ulceration are described in Box 30-1.[5] Because the majority of NUs occur in patients with **type 1** or **type 2 diabetes**, identifying and managing factors that contribute to plantar ulceration in patients with diabetes are the focus of this chapter.

PATHOLOGY

NUs most often occur on the feet of patients with DM because the feet are generally the first areas affected by peripheral **neuropathy** and because the feet often sustain abnormal mechanical forces or minor trauma during standing and walking. NUs usually form on the plantar surface of the foot, over the first and fifth metatarsal heads, or on the distal digits (Fig. 30-2). Bony

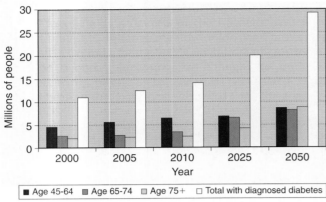

FIG. 30-1 Projections of the number of people with diagnosed diabetes by age group for selected years. *Data from American Diabetes Association:* National Diabetes Fact Sheet, *Alexandria, VA, 2005, The Association.*

TABLE 30-1	Prevalence of Diabetes by Race/ Ethnicity Among People Aged 20 Years or Older in the United States in 2002	
Race/Ethnicity	Number with Diabetes	Percent with Diabetes (%)
Non-Hispanic whites	12.5 million	8.4
Non-Hispanic blacks	2.7 million	11.4
Hispanic/Latino Americans	2 million	8.2
Native Americans/Alaska natives	107,775	14.5

BOX 30-1	Factors Associated with Foot Ulcers in Patients with Diabetes

- Elevated plantar pressures (>65N/cm²)
- History of amputation
- Presence of diabetes >10 years
- Foot deformities (hallux rigidus or hammer toes)
- Male gender
- Poor diabetes control (glycosylated hemoglobin >9%)
- One or more subjective symptoms of neuropathy
- Elevated vibration perception threshold (>25V)

Data from Lavery LA, Armstrong DG, Vela SA, et al: *Arch Intern Med* 158:157-162, 1998.

abnormalities, diminished or absent protective sensation, decreased tissue oxygen saturation, anhidrosis caused by **autonomic neuropathy,** and poorly fitting shoes may initially cause blisters, calluses, or minor traumatic wounds because of direct pressure, shear, or friction. The lack of protective sensation then causes the patient to be unaware of the wound, and any skin break becomes a portal for bacteria to enter the subcutaneous tissue. Because the high-risk individual usually has compromised healing

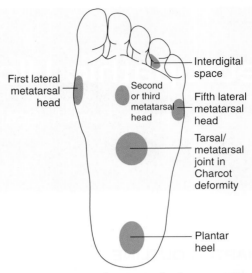

FIG. 30-2 Neuropathic ulcers usually form on the plantar surface of the foot, over the first and fifth metatarsal heads, or on the distal digits.

potential, complications from infection are common. Even a small neuropathic wound should be treated immediately to prevent increase in size, complications from infection, and the need for surgical intervention.

◎ *Clinical Pearl*

Neuropathic ulcers (NUs) usually occur on the plantar surface of the feet of patients with diabetes.

NEUROPATHY: SENSORY, MOTOR, AND AUTONOMIC

Diabetes and PVD are risk factors for distal symmetrical polyneuropathy (DSPN) (see Chapter 19). DSPN is a complex heterogeneous syndrome that includes sensory, motor, and autonomic neuropathies, all of which may be directly involved in the formation of NUs. In addition, diminished blood flow, as a result of occluded vessels, further impairs healing and immune function.

Sensory Neuropathy. Sensory neuropathy, caused by damage to the small nerve fibers, prevents patients from feeling the pressure of a callus or foreign body, the pain of minor trauma and puncture wounds, or the friction of poorly fitting shoes. Prolonged walking and standing under such circumstances can cause subcutaneous tissue damage. Because of sensory deficits, discomfort is not perceived until the tissue damage is deep, usually as a result of infection. Damage to the small nerve fibers, associated with a deficiency of nerve growth factors and diminished blood flow to the vasa nervorum, also causes a reduction in nerve conduction velocity. Both of these conditions occur with diabetes and are exacerbated by uncontrolled **hyperglycemia.**[6]

Motor Neuropathy. Motor neuropathy, caused by damage to the large fibers, results in the following sequence of events: Intrinsic muscles of the foot atrophy and weaken; force imbalances in the foot and lower extremity cause the tendons to pull in deviated alignment; and over time, structural deformities develop. Even during normal gait, these deformities produce abnormally high peak pressures over the bony prominences of the foot, increasing the risk for blisters and callus formation. The damaged cutaneous and subcutaneous tissue is the NU.

Autonomic Neuropathy. Autonomic neuropathy, caused by damage to the large nerve fibers and the sympathetic ganglia, decreases the production of sweat and oil in the skin, causing it to become dry and inelastic. Plantar fissures occur because of anhidrosis (lack of perspiration from the skin) in poorly vascularized areas of the foot, especially the heel. Fissures can deepen to result in full-thickness skin loss in which bacteria can enter and cause infection. The risk of ulceration and infection is increased in the presence of PVD because of reduced delivery of oxygen and nutrients, which are both needed for wound healing.

PATHOLOGY OF DIABETES MELLITUS

DM is a group of metabolic diseases characterized by hyperglycemia (elevated blood glucose) that results from defects in **insulin** secretion and/or action. Chronic hyperglycemia is associated with long-term damage, dysfunction, and failure of various organs, especially the eyes, kidneys, nerves, heart, and blood vessels.[7] The classic signs of acute hyperglycemia are increased urination, increased thirst, and unexplained weight loss. Prolonged hyperglycemia can also cause blurred vision, fatigue, musculoskeletal changes, balance and gait impairments, and gastrointestinal abnormalities. In many instances, patients are diagnosed with diabetes only when the long-term effects of poor glucose control result in a crisis or in chronic complications.

Two of the most common complications of hyperglycemia are impaired wound healing and suppressed immune responses. Hyperglycemia impedes wound healing by inhibiting phagocytic activity of leukocytes and macrophages and by slowing the migration of fibroblasts to the wound site, thereby impairing angiogenesis and limiting the delivery of nutrients to the area. Hyperglycemia also impairs the immune response by altering chemotaxis, phagocytosis, and superoxide anion production by neutrophils and macrophages.[8] In addition, **advanced glycation end-products (AGEs),** produced as a result of hyperglycemia, are detrimental to cell structure and formation.[9] A study on nondiabetic and diabetic animals supported the concept that hyperglycemia may impede wound healing by suppressing the activity of insulin-like growth factors (IGF) in the wound microenvironment.

Blood glucose levels are regulated by a balance between insulin and **glucagon** secretion and the amount and kinds of foods consumed, as well as the amount of daily activity performed by the individual. Insulin is a small protein hormone produced in the **beta cells** located in the **islets of Langerhans** of the **pancreas.**[10] Beta cells secrete insulin in response to rising levels of circulating blood glucose. Insulin binds to the insulin receptor in the plasma membrane of the responding cells (muscle, fat, and liver), causing tiny channels to open up and allow glucose into the cell. Insulin also activates transport of glucose to the cell nucleus and stimulates cells in the liver and skeletal muscle to convert glucose into **glycogen** for storage and stimulates fat cells to store fat.[11] All of these effects of insulin result in lower blood glucose levels.

Glucagon is produced by pancreatic **alpha cells** of the islets of Langerhans. It is a counter-regulatory hormone to insulin that increases circulating glucose levels. Glucagon stimulates the liver to release glucose (stored in the form of glycogen) and to produce glucose from precursors such as lactate and amino acids (known as *gluconeogenesis*).[12]

Type 1 Diabetes. Type 1 diabetes, previously termed *juvenile* or *insulin-dependent diabetes*, which has both genetic and environmental risk factors, is caused by progressive autoimmune destruction of the insulin-secreting beta cells in the pancreas. Once 80% to 90% of the beta cells are destroyed, hyperglycemia results and the patient can be diagnosed with diabetes.[13] The onset of type 1 diabetes is usually during puberty but can be as early as 9 months or as late as the fifth decade. Type 1 diabetes accounts for approximately 10% of all patients with diabetes.

Type 2 Diabetes. Type 2 diabetes, the most common form of diabetes in older adults, is generally caused by a combination of **insulin resistance** and beta-cell failure.[14] Insulin resistance, a decreased responsiveness of the cells to insulin, may begin years or even decades before the patient becomes hyperglycemic. Over time, the beta cells also progressively produce less insulin. Diabetes results when the body cannot compensate for combined defects in insulin action and secretion, resulting in elevated blood glucose levels (Fig. 30-3). The excess circulating glucose causes tissue and organ damage and thereby induces the long-term complications commonly seen in clinical practice, including NUs.

◎ *Clinical Pearl*

Type 1 diabetes is caused by autoimmune destruction of the insulin-secreting beta cells in the pancreas. Type 2 diabetes is caused by a combination of decreased responsiveness of all cells to insulin and reduced insulin production.

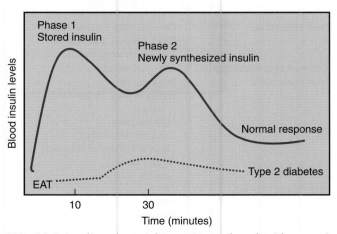

FIG. 30-3 Insulin release phases: Normal and with type 2 diabetes.

TYPICAL EXAMINATION FINDINGS

PATIENT HISTORY

The examination of a patient with a NU begins with a complete patient history. Chapter 28 includes elements to focus on in the patient with any type of chronic wound. Special attention is directed to recent minor trauma to the affected area, footwear, foot hygiene, co-morbidities, medications, and diet. Any reported incidents may give the examiner clues to the original etiology of the ulcer.

SYSTEMS REVIEW

The systems review is used to target areas requiring further examination and to define areas that may cause complications or indicate a need for precautions during the examination and intervention processes. Chapter 1 includes details of the systems review.

Diabetes can adversely affect every system in the body and crosses all four practice pattern categories in physical therapy. The data generated from the history and systems review aid the physical therapist (PT) in determining which tests and measures are appropriate for an individual patient and specifically for the patient with a NU. The systems review also assists the PT in identifying possible problems that require consultation with, or referral to, another provider.[15]

TESTS AND MEASURES

Tests and measures start with inspection of both feet, including the skin, nails, heels, areas between the toes, shoe fit, and inspection for foot deformities (Table 30-2).

TABLE 30-2	Inspection of the Neuropathic Foot
Inspection	**Things to Look for**
Skin inspection	Dry skin with or without fissures
	Thick calluses and blisters
	Discoloration in the dermal layer
	Loss of toe and dorsal hair
Nail inspection	Ingrown or poorly-cut toe nails
	Fungus growing beneath the nails
	Thick, cracking, malformed nails
Heel inspection	Dry skin with fissures
	Thick calluses and blisters
	Discoloration of the dermal layer
Between toes inspection	Skin maceration
Foot deformities	Pes equinus
	Hallux limitus, hallux rigidus, hallux valgus
	Hammer toes
	Cock-up deformity
	Varus deformity of the toes
	Tailor's bunion
	Charcot foot
Assessment of shoes	Fit
	Style
	Material
	Inserts
	Wear

Musculoskeletal. When assessing the patient with diabetes, it is sometimes difficult to differentiate abnormal findings caused by diabetes, aging, and other co-morbidities. Diabetes exaggerates the normal aging process and adds to the impairments and functional limitations associated with the aging musculoskeletal system. Specifically, AGEs affect joint mobility and range of motion (ROM), especially in the foot. AGEs act as "molecular glue" as a result of a chemical reaction that causes irreversible cross-linking between glucose and proteins.[11] When AGEs accumulate, they can cause tissues to become rigid and less functional. It is common for patients with diabetes to have decreased soft tissue extensibility and joint capsule mobility that cause decreased ROM and interfere with functional activities.

Patients with diabetes also frequently have multiple changes in the form and function of the foot and lower extremity. Sensory and motor neuropathies weaken the intrinsic foot muscles, causing muscle imbalances that may then result in one or more of the following deformities: Pes equinus, hallux limitus, hallux rigidus, hallux valgus, hammer toes, cock-up deformity, varus deformity of the toes, tailor's bunion, or Charcot foot (Table 30-3

TABLE 30-3	Foot Deformities Commonly Associated with Diabetes
Condition	**Characteristics**
Pes equinus	A shortening of the Achilles tendon so that there is no ankle dorsiflexion past the neutral ankle position.
Hallux limitus	Limited ROM of the great toe MTP joint, less than the normal ROM measurement of 0-50° dorsiflexion.
Hallux rigidus	Complete loss of range of motion in the great toe MTP joint; the IP joint of the hallux may be involved as well.
Hallux valgus	Lateral deviation of the hallux in relation to the first metatarsal shaft and head that may result in exostosis, defined as a bony prominence, over the medial metatarsal head.
Hammer toes	Extension of the MTP joint of the digit combined with flexion of the PIP joint, usually resulting in corn formation over the bony prominence of the PIP joint.
Cock-up deformity	Flexion of the great toe IP joint combined with extension of the MTP joint, this may result in ulceration of the callus on the dorsum of the IP joint.
Varus deformities of the toes	Medial drifting of the third, fourth, and fifth toes that may cause nails to impinge on adjacent toes, thus producing small interdigital ulcers.
Tailor's bunion	Exostosis of the lateral fifth metatarsal head often caused by fifth toe varus deformity.
Charcot foot	Collapse of the foot arch resulting in a rocker sole, frequently resulting in midsole ulceration.

MTP, Metatarsophalangeal; *ROM,* range of motion; *IP,* interphalangeal; *PIP,* proximal interphalangeal.

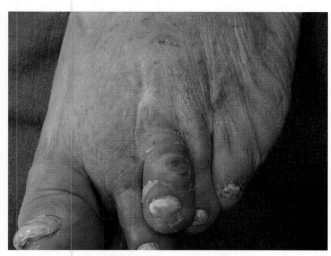

FIG. 30-4 Foot of person with diabetes.

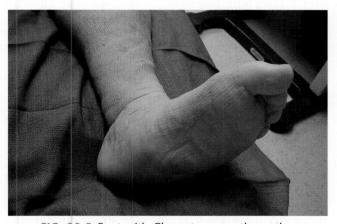

FIG. 30-5 Foot with Charcot neuroarthropathy.

and Fig. 30-4). Changes in foot muscle length and tension also contribute to thinning or shifting of the fat pad from under the metatarsal heads, leaving them unprotected.[16]

Changes in foot structure involving the joints associated with peripheral neuropathy are referred to as *neuropathic arthropathy* or *neuroarthropathy*. The most extreme example of neuroarthropathy is the Charcot foot, which is characterized by a collapsed arch with a rocker-bottom shape and shortened foot length (Fig. 30-5). These changes increase peak pressures on the plantar surface of the foot during gait, particularly at the apex of the rocker bottom, which is the most common site of ulceration. Prolonged weight bearing on the insensitive Charcot foot may also result in minor trauma that can cause hyperemia, edema, joint effusion, and increased tissue warmth, which in turn can cause bone resorption and fracture, a condition referred to as an *acute Charcot foot*.

ROM of the foot and ankle should be measured in patients with NUs because limited joint mobility in these areas can lead to increased plantar pressures and may be a risk factor for foot ulceration.[17,18]

Neuromuscular. Sensory and reflex impairments, as well as functional limitations in balance and gait, are commonly observed in patients at risk for or with NUs. Neuropathy may result in impaired joint proprioception, diminished skin sensation, paresthesias (e.g., burning, tingling), and gait and balance disturbances.

Observational gait analysis is used to examine gait in patients with NUs (see Chapter 32). Gait changes commonly observed in patients with or at risk for NU include a wide base of support, a "marching" gait, a "slap-foot" stepping pattern, and balance disturbances during transfers and gait. Sometimes, sensory "ataxia" is observed in patients with advanced neuropathy. Abnormal gait patterns, in addition to poorly fitting shoes, can contribute to the formation of NUs and delay the healing of existing ulcers.

Reflex Integrity. Diminished reflexes occur in patients with diabetic neuropathy because of large motor nerve involvement. These occur in a predictable pattern with the lower extremity reflexes being more involved than the upper extremity reflexes, distal reflexes more involved than proximal reflexes, and the responses being equal bilaterally. If the pattern is different from this, the deficits are probably not a result of diabetes and referral to a neurologist is recommended.[19]

Sensory Integrity. Sensation is tested using nylon **monofilaments** (Semmes-Weinstein monofilaments [SWM]) for pressure and a tuning fork for vibration. Both are useful for assessing protective sensation on the feet. The nylon monofilaments are a collection of graded filaments that apply a quantified amount of pressure to the skin. The test for protective sensation on the plantar surface of the foot uses the 5.07 filament that bends on 10 gm of pressure. This level of sensation is termed *protective sensation*. The inability to feel this monofilament on the plantar aspect of the foot has been shown to predict foot ulceration in persons with type 2 diabetes.[20]

Graded tuning forks or the 128 Hz tuning fork can be used to test vibratory sense and identify diabetic peripheral neuropathy.[21,22] The tuning fork is hit against a surface to make it vibrate and is then applied to the end of the great toe, the medial malleolus, or the tibial tuberosity. The tip of the fork handle is applied with firm pressure perpendicular to the body part being tested, and the patient answers "Yes" or "No" in response to "Do you feel the vibration?" Nonvibratory stimuli should also be included to ensure that the patient is responding to vibration and not just to touch.[23] This tuning fork test only provides information about the presence or absence of vibratory sensation. This test may be quantified to some degree by timing how long the patient can continue to feel the vibration, which should be 15 seconds in the normal healthy adult. Both the monofilament test and the vibratory test have been correlated to the presence of diabetic neuropathy and increased risk of ulceration.

Temperature. Measurement of plantar skin temperature is recommended to help locate infection, inflammation, or the fracture of an acute Charcot neuroarthropathy. Temperature discrepancies may initially be detected qualitatively by palpation. Quantitative measures can be made

BOX 30-2	System for Grading Pulses

0 Absent
1+ Faint
2+ Diminished
3+ Normal
4+ Bounding, abnormally strong

TABLE 30-4	Probability of Wound Healing Based on Toe Pressures

Absolute Toe Pressure (mm Hg)*		Probability of Healing (%)
With Diabetes	Without Diabetes	
<20	29	25
20-30	40	73
30-35	85	100
>55	97	100

From Carter SA: Role of pressure measurements. In Bernstein EF (ed): *Vascular diagnosis,* ed 4, St. Louis, 1993, Mosby-Year Book.
*Absolute toe pressure <30 mm Hg indicates that a person with ischemic tissue loss will need surgical revascularization for healing to occur.

with thermistors, thermocouples, or infrared scanners. An increase of 3° F above the surrounding area or a comparable area on the opposite foot indicates a problem.[24,25] If, in addition to the skin temperature discrepancy with the surrounding tissue or the opposite foot, the examiner can probe a wound to the bone, there is a high probability of osteomyelitis.[26]

Cardiovascular

Circulation. Ulcers caused primarily by vascular disease are discussed in detail in Chapter 29. Tests of peripheral vascular circulation are discussed briefly here because PVD is 4 to 6 times more common in people with diabetes than in the general population.[27] PVD may cause claudication (calf pain caused by inadequate oxygen supply to muscle tissue) at rest or with activity. Intermittent activity-related claudication is a sign of mild PVD, whereas claudication at rest suggests the presence of severe PVD. During the examination, the PT includes questions about claudication such as "Do your calves hurt during walking, when you are at rest, or during the night?" An affirmative answer to these inquiries indicates the possibility of arterial insufficiency and the need for referral for further vascular studies.

Pedal pulses are usually the first screening test for poor peripheral circulation. The dorsalis pedis and posterior tibialis pulses in the foot and ankle are palpated and graded according to the system for grading pulses in Box 30-2. If these are weak or absent, proximal pulses are palpated. Absence of a pulse indicates a more proximal complete or partial arterial occlusion. Faint or absent pulses are confirmed with a Doppler test; however, absent pulses audible with a Doppler are not graded but termed *positive Doppler signal.*

The PT often evaluates arterial circulation by measurement of the ankle-brachial index (ABI) at the first visit.[28] The ADA also recommends checking the ABI in all patients with diabetes, since PVD can be asymptomatic.[29] The ABI, a ratio of the ankle systolic blood pressure to the brachial systolic blood pressure, indicates the relative blood flow to the lower extremity and the amount of peripheral arterial disease present.

In patients with diabetes, the ABI may be falsely elevated with a reading of >1.3 because of calcification of the inner arterial walls. Since the digital arteries of the toes are generally not affected by calcification, great toe pressure should be checked to verify any ABI measured as >1.3.[30]

A number of other tests may also be used to evaluate peripheral circulation. These are described briefly here as they relate to the patient with a NU.

Capillary Refill Test. During the capillary refill test, the time required for the nail bed or toe tip to refill with blood after a blanching procedure is observed. The clinician presses on the nail to blanch the blood out of the nail bed, removes the pressure, and notes the time it takes for the nail bed color to return to normal. The normal refill time is less than 3 seconds. Longer capillary refill may indicate microvascular insufficiency, which is common in patients with diabetes.

Venous Filling Time. To test the venous filling time, the patient is supine and the extremity passively elevated 45 to 60 degrees above horizontal to drain the venous blood from the limb. After 1 minute, the patient is returned to sitting and the leg brought to a dependent position. The time in seconds required for the veins on the dorsal foot to fill is noted. Normal venous filling time is less than 15 seconds. A 15 to 40 second filling time indicates moderate arterial insufficiency; greater than 40 seconds indicates severe PVD.

Rubor of Dependency Test. To perform the rubor of dependency test, the patient is positioned supine and the extremity passively elevated 45 to 60 degrees. After 30 seconds of elevation the foot may blanche, especially in patients with diabetes. After 60 seconds of elevation, the foot is placed in a dependent position. Normal reperfusion is indicated by the return of pink color to the plantar surface in 15 seconds. If the color return is dark red (termed *rubor*) and takes 30 seconds or longer, the test is positive for arterial insufficiency.[46]

Great Toe Pressure. Great toe blood pressure is measured with a special mini-cuff designed especially to fit the great toe. The absolute toe pressure, usually 60% to 90% of the brachial systolic pressure, can be used to predict healing potential of patients with or without diabetes (Table 30-4). The normal toe-brachial index, also considered a reliable indicator of lower extremity vascular status, is 0.8 to 0.99.[31] If a patient is suspected of having PVD based on the above screening tests, referral to a vascular surgeon for further testing and possible revascularization surgery is indicated.

Transcutaneous Oxygen Tension. Transcutaneous oxygen tension (TcPO$_2$), a measurement of the oxygen delivery to the cutaneous capillaries, is helpful in determining the extent of microvascular disease and wound healing potential. The TcPO$_2$ probe has an oxygen sensor composed of two parts, an inner platinum cathode and an outer silver-chloride anode. A heating element in the sensor warms the underlying tissue to 43° to 45° C and dilates the cutaneous vascular bed for maximum oxygenation.

Systemic Blood Pressure. The ADA guideline for systemic arterial blood pressure in the patient with diabetes is less than 130/80 mm Hg, which is lower than that for the general population. If exercise is expected to be a part of the patient's interventions, screening for orthostatic hypotension is also recommended. The clinician can test for orthostatic hypotension by having the patient lie quietly in the supine position for approximately 5 minutes to allow the blood pressure to equalize. Blood pressure should be taken in both arms to identify the arm with the higher systolic pressure. The patient then stands and the blood pressure is taken in the arm with the higher pressure. Orthostatic hypotension is defined as a drop of more than 20 mm Hg in the systolic pressure or more than 10 mm Hg in the diastolic pressure.

Integumentary. Skin observation is an integral component of the examination of the patient with a NU. Anhidrosis (lack of sweating), a common result of autonomic neuropathy, contributes to dry skin as a result of loss of sweat and oil production, two processes that normally help protect the skin. The effects of aging on the skin (e.g., thinning) make the older patient with diabetes more susceptible to complications from integumentary insults.

Problems with healing any type of wound are common in patients with NUs, especially if they have poorly controlled diabetes or diminished blood flow because of PVD. Therefore traumatic wounds and incision sites should be observed for signs of complications with healing. The ADA recommends that patients with diabetes and neuropathy have a visual inspection of the feet at every visit with a health care professional. Areas of special concern include: Between the toes where maceration is common, under the metatarsal heads where callus formation is common, any areas of erythema or warmth, and cracks or fissures in the plantar heel. It is also suggested that both feet be examined as the patient may have undetected ulcers on the other foot.

Finally, a thorough wound assessment (including measurements, location, tissue type, and drainage) should be performed and infection confirmed or ruled out (see Chapter 28). The International Diabetic Foot Working Group and the Infectious Diseases Society of America Diabetic Foot Guidelines Group have agreed on the following definition of a foot infection: "the presence of either purulent secretions or two or more signs or symptoms of inflammation suggest that a wound is infected."[31] If there are clinical signs of infection, cultures are done to determine which organisms are present and which antibiotics are the most effective. If an ulcer can be probed to bone, there is a high probability of osteomyelitis (Fig. 30-6). Definitive diagnosis may be made by the physician using x-ray, bone scan, bone biopsy, or magnetic resonance imaging (MRI).[32]

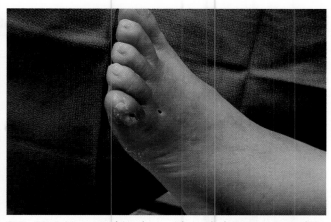

FIG. 30-6 Neuropathic ulcer with underlying osteomyelitis.

TABLE 30-5	Wagner Scale for Neuropathic Ulcers
Grade	**Characteristics**
0	Bony deformities, calluses, skin changes that are at risk for developing wounds, or postulceration that has healed.
1	Full-thickness skin loss with no infection, usually of neuropathic etiology.
2	Subcutaneous tissue involvement, infection, no bone involvement.
3	Deep ulceration, infection with cellulitis, osteomyelitis, or abscess formation.
4	Partial foot gangrene or necrosis.
5	Full foot gangrene.

EVALUATION, DIAGNOSIS, AND PROGNOSIS

The *Guide to Physical Therapist Practice* classification system for integumentary disorders based on patient risk and depth of tissue involvement can be used to diagnose NUs.[15] In addition, several other systems for classifying NU are discussed in the literature. The Wagner and the University of Texas (UT) scales are the most frequently used to diagnose and predict outcome of NUs in patients with diabetes. The Wagner scale, originally developed at Rancho Los Amigos in the 1970s, is the simplest and most frequently used diagnostic scale for NUs (Table 30-5). This scale has six classifications: The first four classifications are based on the extent of tissue loss in the foot; the last two are based on the degree of perfusion loss in the foot. Because depth of tissue loss and severity of ischemia present different problems in evaluating and treating NUs, the Wagner scale has been modified to allow separate evaluation of the wound and foot perfusion (Table 30-6).[33]

The UT Foot Classification System, developed by Armstrong, Lavery, and Harkless, has six categories intended to determine patient risk for ulceration and amputation (Table 30-7). In addition, treatment guidelines to lower the risk level for patients in each category are included.[34,35]

TABLE 30-6	Depth-Ischemia Classification of Diabetic Foot Lesions*
Grade/Definition	**Intervention**
DEPTH CLASSIFICATION	
0: The "at-risk" foot: Previous ulcer or neuropathy with deformity that may cause new ulceration.	Patient education, regular examination, appropriate foot wear and insoles.
1: Superficial ulceration, not infected.	External pressure relief: TCC, walking brace, special foot wear, etc.
2: Deep ulceration exposing a tendon or joint (with or without superficial infection).	Surgical debridement, wound care, pressure relief if the lesion closes and converts to grade 1 (antibiotics as needed).
3: Extensive ulceration with exposed bone and/or deep infection (e.g., osteomyelitis or abscess).	Surgical debridement; ray or partial foot amputation, intravenous antibiotics, pressure relief if wound converts to grade 1.
ISCHEMIC CLASSIFICATION	
A: Not ischemic.	Observation.
B: Ischemia without gangrene.	Vascular evaluation (Doppler, $TcPo_2$, arteriogram, etc), vascular reconstruction as needed.
C: Partial (forefoot) gangrene of the foot.	Vascular evaluation, vascular reconstruction (proximal and/or distal bypass or angioplasty), partial foot amputation.
D: Complete foot gangrene.	Vascular evaluation, major extremity amputation (TTA, TFA) with possible proximal vascular reconstruction.

TCC, Total contact cast; TTA, transtibial amputation; TFA, total foot amputation.
*Modification of the original Wagner classification.

Studies conclude that the UT classification system predicts ulceration and amputation and is an effective tool for identifying risks, planning interventions to lower risk, and for preventing lower extremity complications of diabetes.[36]

A study comparing the Wagner system with a variation of the UT system concluded that the risk of amputation increases significantly in the higher risk groups of both systems; however, the Wagner 3 classification was found to be a heterogeneous group that required more information to make a prediction and determine appropriate interventions. The authors concluded that the Wagner system is a "usable instrument in everyday clinical practice" but that the UT system provides more detailed information and may be preferable in multidisciplinary diabetic foot clinics and in multicenter research.

Another screening tool is the Neuropathic Disability Score (NDS) (Table 30-8). Studies show the NDS was the best clinical measure for detecting patients at risk for new ulcers. The NDS involves testing both feet with a **Neurotip,** a tuning fork, hot and cold rods, and a tendon hammer, scoring one point for each incorrect answer and an extra point if the Achilles tendon reflexes are absent even with reinforcement. The maximum score for each foot is 5 points, and a score greater than 6 out of 10 suggests neuropathy.[37]

INTERVENTION

Interventions for patients with or at risk for neuropathic foot ulcers can be divided into three stages: Prevention for the high-risk foot, treatment of the wound, and management of the foot after wound healing. During all stages, patients with diabetes should have good blood glucose control and all patients should have off-loading. Off-loading is the redistribution of foot pressures to eliminate areas of high peak pressure during weight-bearing activities.

PATIENT EDUCATION

One of the most important components for prevention of ulcers in patients with neuropathy affecting the foot is patient education. Education should cover blood glucose control, footwear, daily foot inspection, and good foot care.[38-40]

Patient education may have positive but short-lived effects on foot care knowledge and patient behavior. These positive effects may reduce foot ulceration and amputations, especially in high-risk patients.[41] However, patient education regarding care of the diabetic foot requires ongoing reinforcement and review.

◎ *Clinical Pearl*

Patient education regarding care of the diabetic foot requires ongoing reinforcement and review.

BLOOD GLUCOSE CONTROL

Good blood glucose control in conjunction with lifestyle therapy (medical nutrition therapy, physical activity, and oral and insulin medication when needed) is also important for preventing complications of diabetes, including NUs. Patient education should be initiated immediately when a diagnosis of diabetes is established, although approximately 50% of patients already have complications because of prolonged delay in diagnosis. Glycemic monitoring is used to assess the efficacy of interventions for diabetes and to adjust nutrition, exercise, and medication levels. The two techniques most frequently used are self-testing of capillary glucose levels by finger or forearm stick to obtain a measure of current blood sugar levels and laboratory or clinic testing of glycosylated hemoglobin (HbA1C) levels to indicate average blood glucose control over the preceding 2 to 3 months.

TABLE 30-7	University of Texas Diabetic Foot Classification System	
Category*	**Criteria**	**Treatment Guidelines**
0: No pathology	Patient diagnosed with diabetes mellitus. Protective sensation intact. ABI >0.80 and toe systolic pressure >45 mm Hg. Foot deformity may be present. No history of ulceration.	2-3 visits per year to assess neurovascular status, dermal thermometry, and foci of stress. Possible shoe accommodations. Patient education.
1: Neuropathy, no deformity	Protective sensation absent. ABI >0.80 and toe systolic pressure >45 mm Hg. No history of ulceration. No history of diabetic neuropathic osteoarthropathy (Charcot joint). No foot deformity.	Same as Category 0 plus: Possible shoe gear accommodation (pedorthic/orthotist consultation). Quarterly visits to assess foot wear and monitor for signs of irritation.
2: Neuropathy with deformity	Protective sensation absent. ABI >0.80 and toe systolic pressure >45 mm Hg. No history of neuropathic ulceration. No history of Charcot joint. Foot deformity present (focus of stress).	Same as Category 1 plus: Pedorthic/orthotic consultation for possible custom-molded/extra-depth shoe accommodation. Possible prophylactic surgery to alleviate focus of stress (e.g., correction of hammertoe or bunion deformity).
3: History of pathology	Protective sensation absent. ABI >0.80 and toe systolic pressure >45 mm Hg. History of neuropathic ulceration. History of Charcot joint. Foot deformity present (focus of stress).	Same as Category 2 plus: Pedorthic/orthotist consultation for custom-molded/extra-depth shoe accommodation. Possible prophylactic surgery to alleviate focus of stress (e.g., correction of bunion or hammertoe). More frequent visits may be indicated for monitoring.
4A: Neuropathic ulceration	Patient diagnosed with diabetes mellitus. Sensorium may or may not be intact. ABI >0.80 and toe systolic pressure of >45 mm Hg. Foot deformity normally present. No infected neuropathic ulceration. No acute diabetic neuropathic osteoarthropathy (Charcot joint) present.	Same as Category 3 plus: Off-weighting program instituted. Dressing change program instituted. Debridement program instituted. Dermal thermometric monitoring. Weekly to biweekly visits as needed. Possible prophylactic surgery.
4B: Acute Charcot joint	Patient diagnosed with diabetes mellitus. Sensorium absent. ABI >0.80 and toe systolic pressure of >45 mm Hg. Noninfected neuropathic ulceration may be present. Diabetic neuropathic osteoarthropathy (Charcot joint) present.	Same as Category 3 plus: Off-weighting program instituted; possible TCC. Weekly to biweekly visits (as per TCC regimen). Dermal thermometric and radiographic monitoring. If ulcer is present, treatment same as for category 4A.
5: Infected diabetic foot	Patient diagnosed with diabetes mellitus. Sensorium may or may not be intact. Infected wound. Charcot joint may be present.	Same as Category 4 plus: Debridement of infected necrotic tissue and bone. Possible hospitalization. Antibiotic therapy. Medical management. Contact casting generally contraindicated until diabetic category drops to 4.
6: Dysvascular foot	Patient diagnosed with diabetes mellitus. Sensorium may or may not be intact. ABI of >0.80 or toe systolic pressure of >45 mm Hg or pedal TcPo$_2$ of >40 mm Hg. Ulceration may be present.	Vascular consult, possible revascularization. If infection present, treatment same as for Category 5. Vascular consultation concomitant with control of sepsis. Contact casting generally contraindicated.

ABI, Ankle-brachial index; *TCC,* total contact cast.
*Categories 0-3 indicate risk factors for ulceration; Categories 4A-6, risk factors for amputation.

TABLE 30-8	Neuropathic Disability Score			
	Neuropathic Assessment	**Right**	**Left**	**Score**
Neurotip discrimination	Hallus-dorsal surface proximal to the toe nail			
Temperature discrimination	Hallus-dorsal surface proximal to the toe nail			
Reflexes	Achilles tendon			
128 Hz tuning fork	Pulp of hallux			

Score 1 point for each incorrect answer and an extra point if the Achilles tendon reflexes are absent even with reinforcement.

To optimize wound healing in patients with diabetes, blood glucose levels should be kept below 200 mg/dl.

Clinical Pearl

Blood glucose levels need to be kept below 200 mg/dl for optimal wound healing in the patient with diabetes.

EXERCISE

Along with eating correctly, exercise or regular physical activity is a primary means of blood glucose control for people with type 2 diabetes. Findings from the Third National Health and Nutrition Examination Survey (NHANES III) indicate that most adults with type 2 diabetes did not engage in recommended levels of physical activity nor did they follow dietary guidelines.[42] Individuals with low income, over age 65, women, minority groups, or those using insulin were more likely to report engaging in no physical activity.

Exercise, even in the absence of body weight loss, helps patients with diabetes because it reduces blood glucose levels.[43] After a bout of exercise, insulin sensitivity increases so that cells are better able to take up glucose from the blood. Younger people can maintain this higher insulin sensitivity for 3 to 4 days after an aerobic exercise session. However, this postaerobic exercise response only lasts for 1 day in older adults.[44] Therefore, for older people seeking to prevent or control diabetes through exercise, sessions must not only be regular but frequent to take advantage of exercise's direct effect on blood glucose levels.

Exercise has been shown to prevent and reverse some microvascular muscle changes in people with diabetes.[45] Maintaining adequate microvascular circulation, reducing hyperglycemia, and avoiding gait abnormalities may reduce the risk of NU development and improve healing if a NU does occur.

Stretching exercises are recommended if the ankle ROM is limited and causing increased plantar pressures. If the patient cannot tolerate the discomfort of stretching or if ROM goals are not achieved, then the contracture deformity can be attenuated by selecting shoes with a higher heel, using heel inserts, or building up an incline on the sole of the shoe to accommodate the shortened Achilles tendon.

ORTHOSES

An ankle-foot orthosis (AFO) may be indicated for a patient with peripheral motor neuropathy sufficient to cause foot drop (see Chapter 34). ROM and structure of the foot and ankle are assessed by the PT for fitting. The typical off-the-shelf AFO is usually fixed with a 90-degree bend at the ankle, assuming that the patient can achieve a neutral ankle position. If the patient has musculoskeletal impairments or swelling that prohibit dorsiflexion of the ankle to neutral, the AFO may not fit well, and if the patient also has peripheral sensory neuropathy, insults to the foot and ankle caused by the AFO may not be perceived. The outcome of a poorly fitted AFO may be breakdown of the skin with resulting wounds (Fig. 30-7).

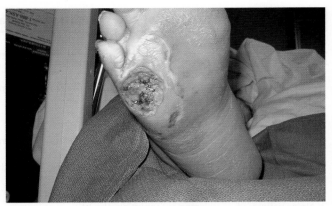

FIG. 30-7 Neuropathic ulcer on a diabetic foot as a result of a poorly fitting ankle-foot orthosis.

FOOTWEAR

Properly fitting shoes are less likely to cause blisters and calluses, thus decreasing the risk of ulceration.[46,47] The most difficult aspect of education on proper shoes may be getting the patient to accept that a good fit is more important than style or ease in putting on the shoe. Styles to avoid are platforms, high heels, pointed toes, flip-flops, stiff leather, plastic, or thin soles with no cushioning. These styles are more likely to produce mechanical friction or pressure over the bony prominences or weight-bearing surfaces of the foot. Purchasing shoes in the late afternoon when the feet are largest because of normal swelling is also advisable. Toe deformities, such as hammer or claw toes, may require extra-depth or custom-molded shoes with padded insoles to provide cushion and to improve plantar pressure distribution. Box 30-3 details important guidelines to use in assessing shoe fit. New shoes should be gradually broken in to avoid getting blisters, using the schedule in Box 30-4.

FOOT CARE

Patients with diabetes need to be instructed in daily foot inspection. Signs of potential problems the patient should look for include red areas over bony prominences, blisters, skin maceration between the toes, callus buildup, dry skin, cracks, subcutaneous hematomas, swelling, increased temperature, and minor cuts. The patient should be able to verbalize what he is looking for and should be able to see the plantar surface of the foot. The ability to see the plantar surface can be checked by placing a piece of tape on the bottom, writing a letter on it, and asking the patient to read the letter.[48] If the foot cannot be positioned for visualization of the plantar surface, a goose-necked mirror can be used or a mirror can be placed on the floor. If the patient is visually impaired or cannot achieve a position to see the plantar foot, a family member or caregiver needs to be instructed in how to perform the foot inspection or the patient can be instructed in tactile foot examination, feeling for calluses, maceration, or open wounds. The patient also needs to understand the importance of eliminating any source of irritation once problems arise and of seeking early medical intervention.

BOX 30-3	Guidelines for Assessment of Proper Shoe Fit

- The shape of the shoe must conform to the shape of the foot and should be evaluated in the standing position. To demonstrate shoe fit, have the patient stand barefoot on a piece of white paper and trace the foot. When the shoe is placed on top of the drawing, the patient can see where the vulnerable spots are and how well the shoe fits. The patient can use this tracing to test for fit when shoe shopping (see Fig. 30-3).
- There should be a ⅜-½ inch space between the end of the longest toe and the end of the shoe when the patient is standing.
- The widest part of the shoe should be at the first metatarsophalangeal joint.
- The toe box (front of the shoe that fits over the toes) should be deep enough to avoid rubbing on the joints of hammer or claw toes and wide enough to accommodate the spread of the foot in the standing and gait positions.
- The collar or back of the shoe should fit snug enough that it does not slide up and down on the heel.
- The insole should provide enough cushion that plantar abnormalities are not red or painful with the patient's maximum walking capacity.
- Laces or straps should be adjustable for a snug fit over the instep without causing friction across the top.
- There should be no areas of stitching over the forefoot of the shoe.

The shoes should be large enough to accommodate a thick white cotton sock.

BOX 30-4	Wearing Schedule for Breaking in New Shoes

- 1 hour in the morning and 1 hour in the afternoon for the first 3 days.
- 2 hours in the morning and 2 hours in the afternoon for the next 3 days.
- 3 hours in the morning and 3 hours in the afternoon for the next 3 days.
- When a total of 8 hours is reached, the patient can feel safe wearing the shoes for a full day.
- If there is any redness that does not disappear within 15 minutes after removal of the shoes, the shoes should not be worn again until adjustments are made to alleviate the pressure.

BOX 30-5	Guidelines for Care of the Diabetic Foot

- Avoid soaking feet in water because of the risk of burns, maceration, and fungal infections. Test water with hand or thermometer before getting into bath water.
- Never walk barefoot, including getting up at night to go to the bathroom. This is critical if the patient has loss of protective sensation.
- Keep feet away from hot surfaces (e.g., stoves, burners, heaters), chemicals, or extreme cold. Wear socks to keep feet warm; do not use heating pads or hot water bottles.
- Wash feet with nondrying soap and dry thoroughly, especially between the toes, with a clean towel.
- Lubricate skin with petroleum jelly or a non-perfumed cream at least once a day. Suggested brands include Eucerin (Beiersdorf, Inc, Wilton, CT), Sween Cream (Coloplast Corporation, Marietta, GA), or Vaseline (Kendall, Mansfield, MA).
- Do not use any adhesive on skin because removal pulls away the outer skin layer that is a natural barrier to infection and increases the chance of skin tears. This includes Band-Aids, tape, or self-adhesive pads.
- Wear thick white cotton socks. Thick is for cushion, white is for seeing signs of bleeding or drainage, and cotton is for absorbing moisture and preventing skin maceration.
- Cut nails straight across no shorter than the end of the toe, with care not to cut into nail bed or cuticle. Use a good pair of nail clippers and buff sharp edges; do not use sharp instruments. If poor eyesight makes cutting nails difficult, see a professional. Have thick nails, calluses, or corns removed by a foot care specialist who understands the complications of diabetes. Do not use chemical agents or strong antiseptic solutions on feet.
- Before donning shoes and socks, check them for foreign objects, torn linings, rough areas, or hard seams.
- Do not wear shoes without socks or stockings.
- Avoid high impact activities like jogging or aerobic exercises. Stretch the great toe and ankle to prevent friction at the end-range of motion in gait.

and reinforced with every resource available to the health care provider. The ADA web site (www.diabetes.org) has a wealth of information for both patients and health care providers. Consultations with certified diabetic educators are recommended for patients who are newly diagnosed with diabetes or who have difficulty maintaining acceptable blood glucose levels.

TREATMENT OF THE NEUROPATHIC WOUND

The six steps of treatment of the neuropathic ulcer are (1) treat infection, (2) revascularize if needed, (3) control

Proper foot care is an essential aspect of minimizing the risk of ulceration (Box 30-5). The ADA and many vendors have produced materials that can be used for patient education. Prevention is only as good as patient compliance. Good foot care should be reviewed at every foot screening blood sugars, (4) debride, (5) provide a moist wound dressing, and (6) off-load. If all of these components of treatment are adequately provided, NUs will heal as quickly as wounds in the normal population.[49] In addition, recent work indicates that growth factors can facilitate healing of NUs.

Treat Infection. Treatment by topical or systemic antibiotics, bone scraping, or surgical removal of infected necrotic tissue is determined on an individual basis and prescribed by the medical team.[50]

Revascularize if Needed. The need for revascularization is determined by the physician after vascular testing. Until the blood supply is adequate, the wound should not be debrided except to remove infected tissue or to open a pocket of purulence. Without sufficient blood supply and thus oxygen delivery, a debrided wound will become larger. Surgical revascularization may be performed using balloon angioplasty with or without stenting for focal superficial femoral artery lesions or with various by-pass procedures for iliac, long-segment superficial femoral artery, or tibial vessel lesions.[51] Controlling lower extremity edema after surgical revascularization is important for healing the NU and the surgical incision and to prevent incision dehiscence and infection.

Two interventions that may help reduce postoperative edema and facilitate healing are low compression or short-stretch bandages (these must provide less pressure than the diastolic blood pressure to avoid occluding the graft) and pneumatic foot compression. The use of intermittent pneumatic foot compression directly after revascularization surgery for patients with NUs can facilitate healing, most likely by improving periwound edema control.[52]

Control Blood Glucose Levels. As stated previously, blood glucose levels need to be kept below 200 mg/dl to optimize protein synthesis. Blood glucose levels tend to rise with any infection in patients with diabetes, thus additional medication may be needed to maintain control until the infection is effectively managed.

Debride. Once there is adequate circulation, the NU should be debrided of all necrotic tissue and periwound callus. Wound debridement may be performed by a suitably trained and experienced PT, but most states' licensing bodies do not allow PT assistants (PTAs) to perform wound debridement. In all circumstances, wounds should not be debrided until adequate blood supply is achieved.

> ◎ *Clinical Pearl*
>
> Wounds should not be debrided until adequate blood supply is achieved.

Provide a Moist Wound Environment. When all of the necrotic tissue has been removed, the wound should be dressed with a moist or occlusive dressing, depending on the amount of drainage and the wound depth. Special care should be given to the interdigital spaces where skin can easily become macerated. These spaces should be dried well after cleaning and separated with lamb's wool or cotton (Fig. 30-8). If there are open areas, an appropriate dressing should be applied first and then the toes adequately separated.

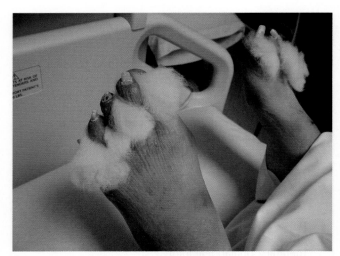

FIG. 30-8 Lamb's wool between the toes of a diabetic foot.

Off-Load. The purpose of any off-loading device is to distribute the plantar foot pressures and reduce the stress at the wound site.

Total Contact Casts. The gold standard for off-loading neuropathic wounds is the total contact cast (TCC); however, there are numerous orthotics, shoes, assistive devices, and materials that can be used if one's clinic is not equipped to do casting. It is generally accepted that even brief periods of bearing weight on a neuropathic wound, such as walking from the bed to the bathroom, will delay or prevent healing; therefore, the necessity of off-loading cannot be overstressed to the patient.

> ◎ *Clinical Pearl*
>
> The best treatment for off-loading neuropathic wounds is the total contact cast.

The TCC is indicated for any Wagner grade 1 or 2 plantar ulcer in the presence of insensitivity and is absolutely contraindicated for grade 3 to 5 ulcers with acute or active infection, sepsis, or gangrene. Relative contraindications for the use of TCC are ulcer depth greater than ulcer width, fragile skin, and excessive leg or foot edema (Box 30-6). Patient resistance to casting, the patient being unable to attend therapy for cast changes, or the patient being unsafe with transfers and gait while in TCC are also relative contraindications, as is an ABI <0.4.

The procedure for making a TCC is shown in Fig. 30-9. The procedure illustrated is used at the Diabetic Foot Clinic at the Hershey Medical Center, Hershey, PA. There are several variations of materials and techniques for making a TCC (e.g., using plaster of Paris casting rolls, placing felt pads over the malleoli, and using a rubber walking heel); however, the principles are the same: Pad the wound, protect bony prominences, maintain even and full contact, position the knee and ankle at 90 degrees, and stabilize the walking surface. If the ulcer is on the heel, positioning the ankle in slight plantarflexion may help further off-load the heel. The first cast is usually replaced after 3 to 10 days to allow for inspection of the skin and to assure that there are no pressure areas.

<table>
<tr><td>

BOX 30-6 | **Indications and Contraindications for the Use of Total Contact Casting**

Indication
- Wagner grade 1 and 2 plantar ulcer with loss of protective sensation.

Contraindications (Relative)
- Ulcer depth greater than ulcer width (risk of premature epithelialization).
- Fragile skin (risk of further ulceration).
- Excessive leg or foot edema (if edema fluctuates, TCC will fit poorly and require more frequent cast changes).
- If patient is resistant to casting or is unable to attend therapy for cast changes.
- Patient unsafe with transfers and gait while in TCC.
- ABI <0.4.

Contraindication (Absolute)
- Wagner grade 3-5; acute or active infection, sepsis, or gangrene

TCC, Total contact cast; *ABI,* ankle-brachial index.

</td></tr>
</table>

Thereafter the cast is replaced every 3 to 7 days (Hershey protocol) or every 1 to 3 weeks (Carville protocol).[53] A cast cutter is used to remove the TCC. The most common problem with the TCC is the formation of NUs over pressure points if the cast is not properly fitted and padded.[54] The cast can also be bivalved with a cast saw and held in place with Velcro straps or an elastic bandage. This permits more frequent inspection and dressing changes if infection is present, as well as removal for bathing or sleeping. The disadvantage is the patient can remove the cast, thereby reducing compliance.[55]

Cast Alternatives. Commercial or custom shoes and devices can be used to off-load a neuropathic wound and offer good alternatives when the TCC is not available (Box 30-7). Another option is to use adhesive felt padding as an adherent orthotic or accommodative dressing to off-load a plantar NU, a technique developed by James Birke.[56] The procedure for constructing the orthotic is described in Box 30-8.

One study compared the effectiveness of a wedge shoe, modified wedge shoes, a short leg walker, and a surgical shoe in reducing walking pressure over the area of previous great toe ulceration in individuals with diabetes. The authors concluded that while the TCC is the gold

---

BOX 30-7 | **Commercial Alternatives to Total Contact Cast for Off-Loading Neuropathic Ulcers**

- The DH Walker (Royce Medical, Camarillo, CA) and Diabetic Walker (AliMed, Dedham, MA) have soles made of small octagons of Velcro foam that can be removed under the wound. Good for small wounds; however, if too much foam has to be removed, foot bottoms out and patient walks on hard surface. Boot has rocker bottom for better gait; however, it is heavy and does compromise balance. Other disadvantages are that they do not distribute weight throughout entire lower leg like boot or TCC, foam can create a "doughnut" effect around a small wound, thereby decreasing oxygen supply to the wound, and foam may be inappropriate for heavier body weights.
- Charcot Restraint Orthotic Walker (CROW) is a custom-made, bivalved AFO composed of polypropylene outer shell, Plastazote lining, total contact molding, and rocker-bottom sole that is recommended for patients who need joint stability and alignment. Advantages are the ability to inspect wound and change dressings frequently, control edema, and ambulate. Risk of further skin damage is minimal. Disadvantages are decreased compliance, decreased ability to ambulate due to size and weight, vulnerability for skin breakdown, and need for frequent adjustments as edema abates.[11]
- Postoperative shoe is soft and comfortable, easy to don with Velcro straps, and can accommodate a bulky dressing. Inserts of dense, moldable foam or thick felt

can be used to redistribute pressure, and silicone gel "plugs" can be added by cutting out a part of the foam and inserting a circle cut from the gel sheet. This device, although comfortable for the patient, is not as effective at reducing pressure as the TCC or a DH Walker.
- D'Arco (D'Arco International, Huntington, WV) wedge shoe and the Integrated Prosthetic and Orthotic System (IPOS) (AliMed, Dedham, MA), used to off-load the forefoot, are recommended for forefoot wounds or recent digit amputations. Will compromise balance in some patients; thus an assistive device and thick-soled shoe for the unaffected extremity are recommended.
- PRAFO (Anatomical Concepts, Boardman, OH), Multi Podus boot (AliMed, Dedham, MA), and Heel Relief Orthosis (AliMed, Dedham, MA) off-load the heel. If patient is ambulatory, an appropriate walking sole must be part of the device. If used on patient while patient is supine, brace should be on 2-hour on/2-hour off schedule to avoid prolonged pressure on Achilles tendon, which is especially important if patient has plantarflexion contracture. If off-loading the heel is the only concern, a pillow under the calf (not heel) is effective, and use of the orthosis can be limited to when the patient is sitting or walking. If ankle stability is a concern, an alternating schedule is recommended and the Achilles tendon should be inspected with each change.

TCC, Total contact cast; *AFO,* ankle-foot orthosis.

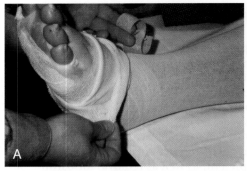

A, The wound is cleaned, debrided, and a saline-moistened gauze dressing applied to the open area. The gauze is anchored with a gauze roll and cotton or lamb's wool is placed between the toes. A bias stockinette is placed on the extremity from the toes to above the knee.

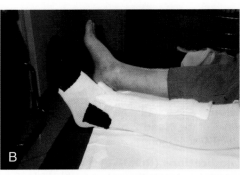

B, The toes and malleoli are covered with Sci-Foam pads to protect bony prominences, and a felt pad is placed along the tibial crest.

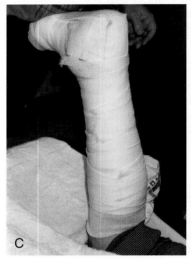

C, The patient is positioned in prone and cast padding is applied from the toes to just below the knee. The toes are totally covered to prevent trauma and maintain cleanliness.

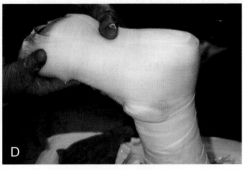

D, One person holds the extremity with the knee at 90 degrees of flexion and the ankle in a neutral position. A fiberglass cast is applied, first going around the foot and then from toe to knee, being careful to maintain full contact with minimal tension throughout the process. To create a smooth edge at the top, the excess stockinette is folded down before the final layer of casting material is applied.

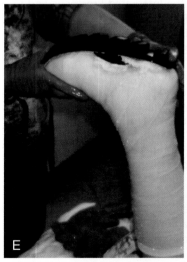

E, Plaster of Paris casting strips are used to even the plantar surface, a rocker bottom sole is positioned in the center, and another roll of fiberglass casting material is used to anchor the walking sole.

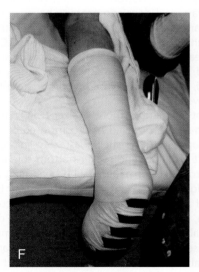

F, Completed contact cast.

FIG. 30-9 Total contact cast procedure.

BOX 30-8	Off-Loading Neuropathic Ulcers Using Adhesive Felt Pads

- Wound is cleansed and covered with transparent film dressing.
- Sole is cut from ¼-inch adhesive-backed felt.
- Smudge of lipstick is put on film at wound location.
- Patient stands on felt pad so that lipstick rubs off onto felt.
- Area of wound is cut from felt and edges that will be against the skin are beveled.
- Barrier film is applied to the sole of the foot.
- Position felt pad so it does not touch wound and is anchored with gauze wrap.
- Patient is instructed to wear the pad with a surgical or postoperative shoe.[1,12]

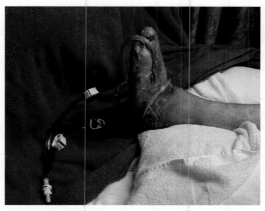

FIG. 30-10 Vacuum-assisted closure on a neuropathic ulcer after incision and debridement.

standard, a wedge shoe modified with relief under the lesion may be an effective, less expensive, and less time-consuming alternative for the management of NUs.[57]

During the time a patient is being treated for a NU on one foot, careful attention to the contralateral foot is imperative because of the increased demands placed on that foot during gait and because of the systemic nature of the risk factors for NUs. Proper shoes with total contact inserts, assistive devices, and meticulous skin care are recommended to prevent bilateral foot problems.

Assistive Devices. Walkers or crutches are useful for off-loading, especially in younger patients who have the balance to maintain non–weight-bearing status on the affected extremity during gait. Assistive devices are also recommended for patients with proprioception or balance deficits while adjusting to a cast or orthotic shoe. A shoe with a thick heel or sole worn on the unaffected foot is also helpful to minimize leg-length discrepancies and improve balance.

Vacuum-Assisted Closures. A retrospective study of 31 patients who were treated with negative pressure therapy, as provided by vacuum-assisted closure (VAC) (Fig. 30-10) after surgical debridement of NUs, was performed. Although the study supports the use of negative pressure therapy for indolent ulcers in patients at high risk for amputation, more studies are needed to establish a level of evidence.[58]

Growth Factors. The topical growth factor, becaplermin, which is recombinant human platelet–derived growth factor, is approved by the Food and Drug Administration (FDA) for treatment of NUs and is available commercially as Regranex (Ortho-McNeil Pharmaceutical, Inc., Raritan, NJ). Several studies report the efficacy of becaplermin for facilitating healing of NUs.[59-62]

Biological Skin Substitutes. Several biological skin substitutes, also known as *living skin equivalents* (LSEs), are available in both autograft and allogenic forms to facilitate closure of clean, granulating ulcers. Studies comparing the efficacy of advanced dressings and LSEs were not found.

Surgery and Amputation. Evidence thus far supports the value of conservative surgical intervention to treat both infected and noninfected NUs. A retrospective study of 58 patients hospitalized with diabetes and foot ulcers complicated by osteomyelitis evaluated the effectiveness of a conservative approach to treatment to avoid amputation or other aggressive surgery. Interventions included minimal bone resection and intravenous antibiotics during hospitalization, along with frequent dressing changes, debridement, and off-loading that was continued after discharge home. This study supports the trend to treat NUs complicated by osteomyelitis with early conservative surgery and long-term antibiotics rather than amputation, thereby conserving bony architecture and optimizing weight-bearing foot surfaces.[63]

A study that compared surgical (n = 24) with conventional nonsurgical management (n = 22) of noninfected NUs reported faster healing in the surgical group. The study concludes that although nonsurgical management is effective in many cases, surgical management may be more effective and facilitate faster healing.[64]

MANAGEMENT OF THE POSTAMPUTATION WOUND

The diabetic foot requires meticulous wound care after any surgical procedure. If the amputation site is left open to heal by secondary intention, the surgical dressings are removed on the first or second day postoperatively and the wound is irrigated to remove as much of the postoperative bleeding as possible. This may be accomplished with pulsed lavage using 3 to 6 psi pressure and gentle suction. The initial dressing can be a topical antimicrobial with an absorbent dressing to manage drainage, becaplermin, or collagen matrix dressings. Daily sharp debridement of devitalized tissue and dressing changes continue until the wound is granulated, at which time the dressing can be changed to one appropriate for the amount of drainage, or a negative pressure wound therapy device can be applied. Wound edges should be debrided regularly of periwound callus to prevent the epithelium from rolling under while waiting for the cavity to fill with granulation tissue. Orthoses and postoperative shoes (see Cast Alternatives section) are recommended to off-load the plantar surface of the amputation site.

BOX 30-9	Criteria for Eligibility for the Medicare Therapeutic Shoe Bill

- The patient must have diabetes mellitus.
- The patient must have at least one of the following conditions:
  - Previous partial or full foot amputation
  - History of previous foot ulceration
  - History of pre-ulcerative foot calluses, peripheral neuropathy with evidence of callus formation
  - Deformity of either foot
  - Poor circulation of either foot

MANAGEMENT OF THE POSTHEALING FOOT

Once a NU is healed, adequate protection must be provided to prevent ulcer recurrence. The Medicare Therapeutic Shoe Bill[65] mandates reimbursement for 80% of the cost of footwear and orthotics for patients with diabetes and associated foot problems. Specific eligibility criteria for benefits are listed in Box 30-9. Coverage includes one pair of custom-molded shoes with inserts and two additional pairs of inserts or one pair of extra-depth shoes and three pairs of inserts. Shoe modifications may be substituted for one pair of the inserts. The patient must be under the care of a physician who is providing comprehensive diabetic care and certifies need of diabetic shoes. The physician must write the prescription for the shoes and inserts; the provider furnishes the shoes and inserts and bills Medicare.

Several kinds of custom shoes are available for the patient with diabetes. Dense moldable foam (e.g., Plastazote, American Micro Industries, Chambersburg, PA; Zotefoams, Croydon, UK) may also be custom fit for protection of the vulnerable areas of the patient's foot. Correct fit is very important. The feet should be measured, rather than depending on the patient to give a size, and the shoes should be fitted to the larger foot. If the foot is misshapen (e.g., after a digit amputation or a Charcot foot), custom-molded shoes provide more protection than diabetic shoes with inserts.

Although a Cochrane Review found that there is limited evidence (because of poor quality of research in this area) to support or refute the effectiveness of pressure-relieving interventions for prevention and treatment of NUs, most of the published studies do support the use of therapeutic shoes.

Therapeutic shoes need to be worn at least 60% of the time to be effective. Poor compliance is often a result of dissatisfaction with style and fit of the shoes. The patient's perceived value of the shoes also has more influence on compliance than does the history of ulceration.[66]

In one study of the effectiveness of extra-depth shoes and insert combinations in preventing ulceration, the authors concluded that therapeutic shoes with inserts may be unnecessary for patients who do not have foot deformities and that careful attention to foot care may be more important than special footwear.[67]

Several studies have looked at the effectiveness of different types of socks in reducing plantar pressures and thereby reducing the risk of recurrent ulceration. These studies suggest that any socks with shoes may help distribute the plantar pressures along the plantar surface of the foot and reduce peak pressures in the metatarsal heads. No studies were done with diabetic socks with diabetic or molded shoes.[68,69]

Clinical Pearl

Therapeutic shoes, if worn at least 60% of the time and always with socks, can reduce the risk of pressure ulcer recurrence.

Other supplies that may help protect a diabetic foot are special socks with antimicrobial fibers or silicone gel bottoms, toecaps, toe separators, tubular foam, and hammertoe splints.

The preventive measures of good blood sugar control, good foot hygiene, daily foot inspections, and immediate medical care for any skin breaks, in addition to proper off-loading footwear, as described in the section on prevention for the high-risk foot, are even more important after NUs have healed because that patient has demonstrated high risk for ulcer formation and has more vulnerable tissue where the ulcer is remodeling.

CASE STUDY 30-1

PERIPHERAL VASCULAR DISEASE

Patient History

LC is a 73-year-old man with a history of PVD who presents with wounds on his left lateral foot, right heel, and right great toe. LC is currently unable to work because of the drainage from a right heel wound, inability to wear regular shoes, and inability to drive. LC's medical history includes coronary artery disease with history of coronary artery bypass graft and placement of pacemaker and defibrillator, left lower extremity bypass graft with delayed incisional wound healing, fall with a compound fracture of the right ankle requiring an open reduction with internal fixation (ORIF) and gastrocnemius flap to close the necrotic surgical wound (approximately 9 months before the current episode), and hypertension. LC just completed a course of systemic antibiotics (patient unable to identify which one). LC was also self-treating the wounds with bacitracin ointment.

Tests and Measures—Significant Findings
Musculoskeletal

- Both feet have evidence of motor neuropathy with claw toes, migrated fat pads, and dropped arches.
- Ankle ROM on the left: 0 to 50 degrees plantarflexion; on the right, 15 to 30 degrees plantarflexion.
- Ankle strength is grossly 3/5 and all other muscle groups grossly 4 to 4/5.

Neuromuscular

- Sensation is intact except for slight diminished light touch over the right lateral ankle muscle flap.
- Gait is characterized by bilateral flat-foot contact during weight acceptance phase, minimal toe push-off bilaterally, short stride length, and exaggerated lateral trunk sway to compensate for lack of ankle/knee flexion.

Integumentary

- Diffuse erythema with scaling skin and spotted weeping of serous fluid on both feet and ankles, right more than left. There is also a strong odor typical of fungal infection.
- Right fourth dorsal proximal interphalangeal (PIP) joint: 0.7 × 0.5 cm, 100% granulation, min+ serous drainage, mod+ edema and erythema extending to the metatarsophalangeal (MTP) joint.
- Right plantar heel: 3 × 1.5 cm, 100% dry black eschar over the calcaneus, unable to determine the depth until after debridement.
- Right medial heel: 1.2 cm area of soft callus with a 0.5 cm fissure.
- Left plantar first metatarsal: 1.5 × 1 cm, 100% dry brown eschar.
- Left lateral fifth metatarsal: 4.5 × 0.5 cm, 60% eschar, 40% fibrous slough, slight serous drainage, minimal erythema along lateral foot.

Diagnosis

Based on the information given, the patient had NUs as a result of motor, sensory, and autonomic neuropathy complicated by foot deformities and poorly fitting shoes, possible fungal infection of both feet, and lower extremity edema because of venous insufficiency as a result of removal of saphenous vein for bypass grafts or cardiovascular problems.

The physical therapy preferred practice pattern diagnosis of the five wounds was as follows:

- Right fourth toe: 7D: Impaired integumentary integrity associated with full-thickness skin involvement and scar formation.
- Right plantar heel: 7E: Impaired integumentary integrity associated with skin involvement extending into fascia, muscle, or bone and scar formation.
- Right medial heel: 7B: Impaired integumentary integrity associated with superficial skin involvement.
- Left plantar first metatarsal: 7C: Impaired integumentary integrity associated with partial-thickness skin involvement and scar formation or 7D (to be determined after debridement).
- Left lateral fifth metatarsal: 7C.

Interventions

- Referrals to an orthopedist to rule out osteomyelitis of the right heel and a cardiologist to rule out heart failure as a cause for lower extremity edema.
- Selective debridement of all necrotic tissue using antimicrobial topical dressings on the right heel and the right fourth toe. A petrolatum gauze dressing to be used on the left lateral foot and first metatarsal head. Moist wound dressings were continued to full closure of all wounds.
- The patient should use a foam reverse-wedge shoe (Darco wedge) on the right to off-load the heel and a front-wheeled walker to further decrease weight bearing.

Role of the Physical Therapist Assistant

- What symptoms would constitute "evidence of motor neuropathy"?
- What test might have been used to examine this patient's gait?
- Write a paragraph describing the process of debridement for this patient's wound.

Additional Information

For the full version of this case study, including detailed examination results, interventions, and outcomes, see the Evolve site that accompanies this book.

CHAPTER SUMMARY

Neuropathic ulcers (NUs) occur on the foot, usually the plantar surface or the digits, because of abnormal mechanical forces or minor trauma sustained during weight-bearing activities. They occur most frequently in patients with diabetes who are at risk because of motor, sensory, and autonomic neuropathies; diminished or absent protective sensation; and decreased tissue perfusion because of peripheral vascular disease. The components of NU prevention are good blood glucose control, proper footwear, daily foot inspection, and meticulous foot care. The six steps of wound management for the NU include treatment of infection with systemic and/or topical antibiotics, revascularization for the ischemic limb, maintaining blood glucose levels below 200 mg/dl, debridement of necrotic tissue, provision of a moist wound environment, and adequate off-loading (defined as redistribution of the plantar pressures to as large an area as possible). Periodic medical inspection, adequate protection of foot abnormalities with therapeutic footwear, and comprehensive patient education are required to prevent high risk for reoccurrence. Neuropathic ulcer care includes comprehensive care of the local and systemic factors contributing to the ulcer, meticulous wound management, and extensive patient education.

ADDITIONAL RESOURCES

For links to these and additional web-based resources, see the Evolve site.

Bowker JH, Pfeifer MA (eds): *The diabetic foot*, ed 6, St. Louis, 2001, Mosby

Veves A, Giurini JM, LoGerfo FW: *The diabetic foot: Medical and surgical management*, Totowa, NJ, 2002, Humana Press.

American Diabetes Association

American Association of Diabetes Educators

National Diabetes Information Clearinghouse

GLOSSARY

Advanced glycation (or glycosylation) end-products (AGEs): Produced in the body when glucose links with protein. They play a role in damaging blood vessels and can lead to the complications commonly associated with diabetes.

Alpha cell: Pancreatic cell that releases glucagon.

Autonomic neuropathy: Disease of the nerves that control autonomic functions, including sweat production, digestive function, bladder function, and cardiovascular function.

Beta cell: Pancreatic cell that releases insulin.

Blood glucose level: The amount of glucose in a given amount of blood measured in milligrams per deciliter (mg/dl).

Diabetes mellitus (DM): A condition characterized by hyperglycemia resulting from the body's inability to use blood glucose for energy.

Glucagon: A hormone produced by the pancreatic alpha cells that increases blood glucose.

Glycogen: The form of glucose found in the liver and muscles.

Hyperglycemia: Excessive blood glucose. Fasting hyperglycemia is blood glucose above a desirable level after a person has not eaten for at least 8 hours. Postprandial hyperglycemia is blood glucose above a desirable level 1 to 2 hours after a person has eaten.

Insulin: A hormone that facilitates utilization of glucose for energy; produced by the pancreatic beta cells.

Insulin resistance: The inability to respond to and use the insulin. Insulin resistance may be linked to obesity, hypertension, and high levels of fat in the blood.

Islets of Langerhans: Groups of pancreatic cells that make glucagons and insulin.

Monofilament: A short piece of nylon, like a hairbrush bristle, mounted on a wand and used to check sensitivity of the nerves in the foot or hand.

Neuropathy: Disease of the nervous system. The three major forms associated with diabetes are peripheral neuropathy (includes motor and sensory neuropathy), autonomic neuropathy, and mononeuropathy.

Neurotip: Monofilament calibrated at 40 gm force used to assess diminished sensation to sharpness and pain. The filament is placed in a hand-held pen for sensory testing.

Pancreas: The organ that produces insulin, glucagon, and digestive enzymes. The pancreas is located behind the lower part of the stomach and is about the size of a hand.

Type 1 diabetes: A disease characterized by high blood glucose levels caused by a lack of insulin. Occurs when the body's immune system attacks and destroys the insulin-producing beta cells in the pancreas.

Type 2 diabetes: A condition characterized by high blood glucose levels caused by either a lack of insulin or the inability to use insulin efficiently.

Burns

R. Scott Ward

CHAPTER OUTLINE

OBJECTIVES

After reading this chapter, the reader will be able to:
1. Describe the pathology associated with skin and soft tissue burns.
2. Explain interventions for patients with burn injuries, including those directed at wound healing and rehabilitation management.
3. Describe the consequences of and interventions for scarring after burn injury.
4. Presented with a clinical case and the therapist's evaluation, implement a plan of care for a patient with a burn.

*B*urn rehabilitation programs have traditionally been designed to maximize the restoration of health and function of individuals after burn injury.[1,2] Rehabilitation of a patient with burn injury begins at the time of admission and continues through the maturation of scar tissue. During this process, patients may require ongoing surgical intervention to aid wound healing and revision of scarring, as well as rehabilitation interventions aimed at care of the burn wound, managing edema, preserving and increasing mobility and strength, improving function, and controlling scar formation.

Clinical Pearl

Rehabilitation interventions after burn injuries are aimed at care of the burn wound, managing edema, preserving and increasing mobility and strength, improving function, and controlling scar formation.

Survival rates for patients with burns have increased steadily over the past several decades.[3] Patients are surviving because of improvements in fluid management, infection control, and emergency response, as well as more effective surgical interventions. With more patients surviving burn injury, there is a greater need for the services directed at improving their long-term outcomes. Such services often include physical therapy, occupational therapy, psychological counseling, and vocational rehabilitation. Given the many facets involved in the care of a patient with burns, from the time of injury throughout rehabilitation, and the many problems that might result along a course of recovery, optimal treatment requires a team approach.[4]

The American Burn Association (ABA) outlines factors influencing the severity of burn injury. All of these also influence prognosis. The criteria for burn severity are based on burn depth and size, the age of the patient, the anatomical area burned, and associated injuries. Box 31-1 provides an outline of the ABA's criteria for referral to a burn center, which reflects variables that contribute to the severity of a burn injury. These and other variables associated with burn injury, including other systems affected by the burn, edema, mobility, and strength, should be considered when examining a patient after a burn injury.

PATHOLOGY

Burn injury results from exposure of the integument to excessive temperatures. Burn etiology is variable, and causes include scald, flame, contact (including friction), chemical, flash (exposure to bursts of radiant heat), electrical, and other (e.g., radioactivity, irradiation).[5] Scald and flame injuries are the most common causes of burns.[5] Scald burns, caused by hot liquids (e.g., coffee, tea, water, oil),[6] are the most common pediatric burns in the United States.[7] Elderly persons are also at increased risk for scald injury.[8] Flame burns result from direct contact with flaming objects or clothing that have been ignited with a flame. Adult men between the ages of 16 and 40 years have the highest prevalence of this type of injury.[9] Contact burns occur when contact is made with a hot object, such as a radiator, iron, curling iron, or exhaust pipe, or when contact is made with a rapidly moving object (also referred to as a *friction burn*), such as a treadmill.[10-12] Contact burns most commonly involve the hands and are not usually life-threatening.[10,11] Chemical burns are often related to industrial accidents and tend to be deep. The extent of a chemical injury depends on the strength and concentration of the chemical agent and the duration of its contact with the skin.[13] Electrical injuries are not classic burn injuries.[5] There may be surface burns because of an associated flash, as well as entrance and exit wounds in which the current entered and exited the patient. Electrical burns can also injure deep tissues, including nerves, vessels, muscle, and bone, because resistance to current flow causes tissue heating. Electrical currents may cause cardiac arrhythmias, respiratory arrest that results from tetany of respiratory muscles, or fractures caused by skeletal muscle tetany.

After acute burn shock, the body is in a state of hypermetabolism and protein catabolism. It is thought that protein from muscle is used to fuel gluconeogenesis for increased energy needs in healing the burn. There is evidence to suggest that much of this activity is a result of hormonal changes related to the burn injury. Alterations in both the levels of circulating hormones and cellular hormonal receptors have been demonstrated after a burn.[14-18] All of these changes contribute to a severe catabolic state by changing or impairing metabolic activity. The hypermetabolic and catabolic state associated with burn injury causes loss of skeletal muscle and thus can impair strength.

TYPICAL EXAMINATION FINDINGS

PATIENT HISTORY

The history for a patient with a burn includes standard questions such as work, social, and medical history. In addition, the patient is asked where (e.g., home, work) and how the burn injury occurred and what caused the injury (e.g., flame, chemical, scald). The presence of an associated injury, such as an inhalation injury or fracture, may necessitate further testing.

SYSTEMS REVIEW

The systems review is used to target areas requiring further examination and to define areas that may cause complications or indicate a need for precautions during the examination and intervention processes. Chapter 1 includes details of the systems review. Although this chapter focuses on the injury to the integument caused by a burn injury, other systems included in a systems review for the patient with a burn generally include the cardiovascular/pulmonary system, the musculoskeletal system, and the neuromuscular system.

Associated injuries increase the severity of a burn injury (see Box 31-1) and influence the plan of care because they generally cause additional impairments. Trauma associated with burns can have many causes, including motor vehicle accidents, escaping a fire, or falling because of electrical shock, assault, or explosion.[19] Although any type of injury can accompany a burn, the most common is inhalation injury. Other injuries associated with burns that are particularly relevant to rehabilitation are fractures and peripheral nerve damage.

TESTS AND MEASURES

Musculoskeletal. The musculoskeletal system review includes examination of the gross range of motion (ROM) and strength of unburned areas, detailed examination of ROM and strength for any area directly affected by the burn injury, gross anthropometric symmetry, and height and weight.

Anthropometric Characteristics

Edema. Edema forms immediately after burn injury. Fluid from circulating plasma shifts to the interstitium because of increased capillary permeability (caused by inflammatory mediators) and changes in oncotic and hydrostatic pressures.[20] Because of the large shift of fluid out of the vessels that occurs with large burns, patients are treated with large volumes of intravenous fluid therapy to maintain perfusion of core organs. This fluid therapy, also referred to as *fluid resuscitation,* has decreased the incidence of vital organ failure after burn injury but has also increased the incidence of peripheral edema. Because the fluid shifts are so great, even when the fluid shifts back into the circulation there is often a noticeable residual edema. This may be worsened if the lymphatic vessels are damaged or blocked by fibrin or debris.[21] Persistent edema may adversely affect healing by impairing oxygen and nutrient delivery[22] and can also adversely affect mobility.

Edema is measured using any one of several standard measures such as volumetry, circumference measurements, or figure-of-eight measurements. These measures are commonly used in burn care settings and apply well to the measurement of burn-related edema. To avoid cross-contamination when measuring edema on a limb with an open burn wound, volumeters must be carefully cleaned after each use and measuring tapes must be disposed of or cleaned.

Range of Motion. Wound contraction, edema, and pain commonly cause restrictions of ROM in patients with burns. Wound contraction has beneficial and detrimental effects. On the positive side, it decreases wound size. On the negative side, wound contraction can impair mobility and function, and generally has poor cosmesis. If a wound heals with scarring, scar contraction creates nearly all of the late adverse sequelae of burns.[23]

Edema can limit motion because of its influence on the space within and around joints. The accumulation of exudate associated with edema may also lead to fibrosis, further impeding tissue mobility.[24,25]

Pain may inhibit motion simply because of a patient's avoidance of the painful motion or their anticipation of pain with movement.

Muscle Performance. Strength testing in patients with burns is performed similarly to other patients without burns. Manual muscle testing using standard grading (normal, good, fair, poor, trace, or the 0 to 5 scale) or using hand-held dynamometry is as reliable in patients with burns as it is in patients without burns.[26-28] Other strategies for testing muscle strength, such as isokinetic testing, can also be applied in this population (see Chapter 5).[29-31] The only special caution with this population is to avoid applying excessive force to a painful burn or to a site that is healing and has fragile new tissue. Testing that requires contact over these sites should be avoided until the tissue heals sufficiently for this to be safe. There should be few restrictions in testing for at least fair grade muscle strength, which only requires movement against gravity, except for a few days when immobilization is required after surgical skin grafting.

Patients with burns often have decreased strength overall because of the loss of lean body mass caused by the catabolism of muscle protein associated with burn trauma and healing.

Neuromuscular

Pain. Pain is a predictable result of a burn. The pain caused by a burn is generally described as "burning," "severe," or "acute."[32] Local pain is caused by the release of local inflammatory mediators and damage to nerve endings. Generalized pain is likely related to circulation of these inflammatory mediators, a patient's pain tolerance

or perception, and anxiety about the injury or care.[33] Superficial burns are very painful, and any large burn, including deep burns, will provoke continuous background pain that occurs at rest, as well as with activity. Certain care procedures, such as dressing changes and some exercises, can increase pain. This procedural-related pain generally declines over time.[33,34] Procedural pain is generally described as feeling different from the background pain associated with the burn wound. Procedural pain is often described as "stabbing," "severe," or "excruciating."[32]

Clinical Pearl

Superficial burns are very painful, and certain care procedures, including dressing changes and some exercises, can increase this pain.

Several common pain measures are used to assess pain in patients with burns. A visual analog scale (VAS) for pain can be used to rate the severity of the pain on a numeric scale (e.g., 0 to 10 where 0 is no pain and 10 is unbearable pain). Children and adults may prefer a scale with visual representation of pain with tools such as the faces pain scale (FPS) or a standardized color analog scale (see Chapter 22). Besides rating pain severity, the location of pain as related by the patient is also documented. Furthermore, it is important to measure pain at rest as well as during specific procedures or activities which may worsen the pain such as wound care sessions or tissue stretching. Knowing which activities produce more pain can help determine the type and timing of pain-relieving measures.

After the burn wound has healed, pruritus (itching) generally replaces pain as the predominant aberrant sensation in patients with burns. The severity of pruritus can be measured clinically with a VAS. The intensity of pruritus often diminishes as the remodeling phase of wound healing nears completion.

Peripheral Nerve Integrity. Peripheral neuropathy is the most common neurological complication of burn injury.[35] Neuropathy is most commonly caused by electrical burns but is also more likely in patients who chronically abuse alcohol or who are critically ill, severely burned, or elderly.[35] Over time, iatrogenic factors, such as improper limb positioning, improper application of compression dressings, or poorly fitted splints, can also contribute to the incidence of neuropathy.

Clinical Pearl

Peripheral neuropathy is the most common neurological complication after a burn injury.

Cardiovascular/Pulmonary. Direct cardiovascular and pulmonary responses to burn injury are mainly related to fluid moving from the blood vessels to the interstitium. This causes "burn shock" that is manifest by hypotension and relative hypothermia. Therefore blood pressure and body temperature are always checked in patients with burns (see Chapter 22). The fluid shifts and hypotension associated with burn shock can impair perfusion of core organs, including the heart, lungs, and kidneys. Decreased perfusion of the heart and lungs, along with pulmonary edema can cause pulmonary compromise, which in conjunction with bed rest and decreased pulmonary activity can increase the risk for pneumonia and respiratory failure.

Burn shock is also associated with decreased cardiac output.[36] This cardiac compromise may be a result of the vascular fluid shifts and/or decreased efflux of calcium from myocardial sarcoplasmic reticulum.[37] Once plasma fluid volumes are regulated, cardiac function can be expected to normalize.

Inhalation injury is often associated with burns that occur in enclosed spaces such as buildings. Inhalation injury is irritation or cellular damage to lung tissue caused by toxic gases, steam vapors, or chemicals in the air coupled with a burn event. Patients with inhalation injury are at increased risk for pneumonia and respiratory failure. Patients with burns who have an associated inhalation injury have a sixfold higher mortality rate than those without inhalation injury.[38]

Clinical Pearl

Patients with burns and an associated inhalation injury have a much higher mortality rate than patients with burns without inhalation injury.

Aerobic Capacity. The lungs are a target of the burn-related inflammatory response even if there is no inhalation injury. The inflammatory response can cause acute pulmonary edema that decreases diffusion of oxygen from the alveoli to the vascular system.[39] This situation contributes to decreased aerobic capacity. One report suggests that although pulmonary function improves after injury, decreased pulmonary function may last as long as 5 months after the actual burn injury.[40] Inhalation injury exacerbates cardiopulmonary problems in a patient with burns because of direct damage to lung tissue.

Loss of muscle caused by increased muscle catabolism and decreased activity after an acute burn leads to decreased activity. Decreases in physical activity may also contribute to decreases in aerobic capacity.

Standard physiological measures of blood pressure, heart rate, respiratory rate, oxygen saturation, and ratings of perceived exertion (RPE) for appraising aerobic capacity are generally used to measure cardiovascular function in patients with burns (see Chapters 22 and 26).

Integumentary

Burn Depth. The depth of a burn is related to the temperature and duration of exposure to extreme heat. The cause of the burn also affects wound depth because different materials have different maximum burning temperatures, specific heats, and thermal conductivity and certain chemicals are more caustic than others. If skin is exposed to temperatures of 60° C (140° F) for more than 1 second, epidermal loss causing a **partial-thickness burn** will occur. If the temperature is increased to 70° C (158° F), a **full-thickness burn** will occur after 1 second.[41]

Clinical Pearl

The depth of a burn is related to the temperature and duration of tissue exposure to extreme heat.

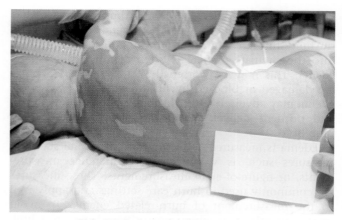

FIG. 31-1 A partial-thickness burn.

The depth of a burn is classified by the amount or type of tissue destroyed and can be determined by the presence of certain clinical findings.[1] The classification of depth of injury corresponds to the classifications of integumentary impairment provided in the *Guide to Physical Therapist Practice*.[42]

Superficial burns (preferred practice pattern 7B: Impaired integumentary integrity associated with superficial skin involvement, also referred to as *first-degree burns*) involve limited damage to the epithelial cells without exposure of dermal tissue. Sunburn is a common example of a superficial burn injury. A superficial burn is painful, dry, and erythematous and may exhibit some minor localized swelling. Superficial burns should heal in 3 to 5 days without scarring.[43]

Partial-thickness burns (preferred practice pattern 7C: Impaired integumentary integrity associated with partial-thickness skin involvement and scar formation, also referred to as *second-degree burns*) involve damage to the dermis and may be separated into subclassifications of superficial or deep partial-thickness burns (Fig. 31-1). Superficial partial-thickness burns exhibit destruction of the epidermis and minimal damage to the superficial layers of the dermis. Preservation of epidermal appendages, such as hair follicles and sweat glands, in this depth of burn allows for complete healing within 21 days with little or no scarring.[43] In deep partial-thickness burns, the epidermis and almost all of the dermis is destroyed, leaving very few epidermal appendages. Deep partial-thickness burns take longer than 21 days to heal and will heal with scarring. These wounds generally require skin grafting to close. All partial-thickness wounds are very painful, red, and weepy and have normal pliability. Blistering is associated with a partial-thickness burn.

Clinical Pearl

Partial-thickness burns are characterized by blister formation.

A full-thickness burn (preferred practice pattern 7D: Impaired integumentary integrity associated with full-thickness skin involvement and scar formation, also referred to as a *third-degree burn*) involve complete destruction of the epidermis and dermis (Fig. 31-2). These burns require skin grafting to heal functionally. If allowed to heal on their own, they may take several weeks to heal and will scar.[43] Full-thickness burns are usually not painful with palpation because the nerves are no longer intact. They may be a tan or yellowish-brown color and are generally leathery, with nonpliable skin.

Burn Size. The size of a burn injury is usually described as an estimate of the percentage of the total body surface area (%TBSA) that is affected. This estimate helps predict the magnitude of physiological response to the injury, including fluid loss and catabolism. The larger the burn injury, the larger the physiological responses will be. The two most common methods used to estimate burn size are the Rule of Nines and the Lund and Browder chart.[44] The Rule of Nines method estimates body surface area by dividing the body into 11 segments, each accounting for 9% of the surface area, plus another 1% for the genitals (Fig. 31-3). Charts with the body divided into these segments are often used to document and calculate burn surface area by this method. The Lund and Browder method uses a standard table for estimating surface area based on the part(s) of the body burned. Charts that include a body illustration on which the burn location is marked and a table to estimate burn size are often used for documentation when this method is used (Fig. 31-4). The Lund and Browder chart was initially published in 1944 and has since been modified to take into account proportional changes in the surface area of body parts that occur during growth and development.[45] This method for estimating burn size has been shown to be reliable when completed by experienced burn care providers.[44]

Scar. Although scars do not occur immediately after a burn, scarring is one of the most problematic late morbidities associated with burn injury and wound healing. Scar assessment is performed during reexamination of patients initially seen with acute burns whose wounds are now healing or healed, or during initial examination of a patient with healed burns. Scar assessment is performed mainly by observation and palpation. An actively

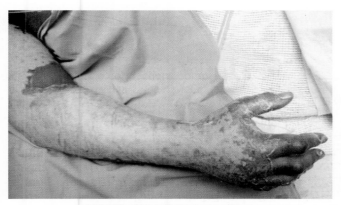

FIG. 31-2 A full-thickness burn.

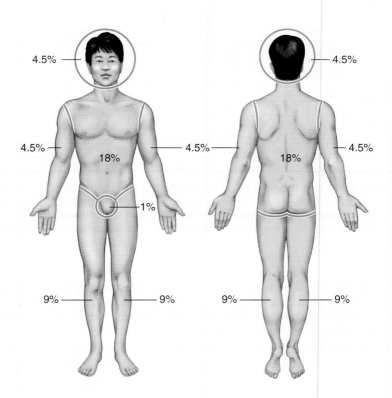

FIG. 31-3 Rule of Nines chart for estimating the surface area or size of a burn injury. The Rule of Nines divides the surface area of the body into 11 segments of 9% each, with the genitals equaling 1% of the body surface area. *From Patton KT, Thibodeau GA:* Anatomy and physiology, *ed 7, St. Louis, 2010, Mosby.*

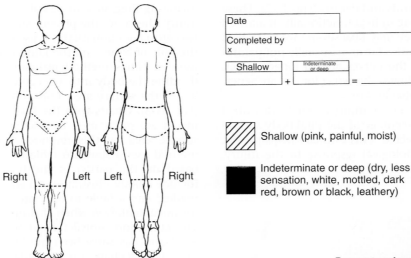

FIG. 31-4 The Lund and Browder chart for estimating the surface area or size of a burn injury. The Lund and Browder chart allows for estimation of the surface area of the burn injury through growth and development. *From Goodman CC, Boissonnault WG, Fuller KS: Pathology: Implications for the physical therapist, ed 2, Philadelphia, 2002, Saunders.*

maturing scar that is still forming is characterized by a rigid texture or lack of extensibility, an inflamed appearance (redness), some possible pigment changes (such as purple), and hypertrophy. It generally requires 6 to 18 months after the initial burn for a scar to "mature" or complete forming.[46]

Clinical Pearl

Scars do not form immediately after a burn. It generally takes 6 to 18 months after the initial burn for a scar to complete forming.

The most common variables used to quantify and document findings from examination of scar are the level of hypertrophy (height), the amount of redness or inflammation (vascularity), level of extensibility (pliability), and the amount of contraction.[1,47] The height of hypertrophy is generally measured with a ruler and the amount of redness is described qualitatively. Pliability is also generally described qualitatively; however, a device for quantifying pliability is available and may produce more accurate data for tracking changes over time.[48]

Two pathological types of scars can occur after burns. Burns generally cause **hypertrophic scars** (Fig. 31-5, *A*).

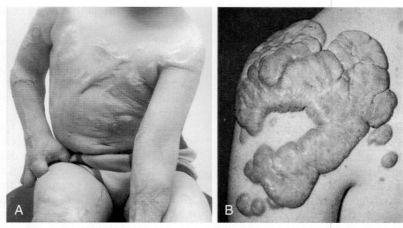

FIG. 31-5 Types of scars. **A,** Hypertrophic scar after burn. **B,** Keloid scar. *B from Patton KT, Thibodeau GA:* Anatomy and physiology, *ed 7, St. Louis, 2010, Mosby.*

TABLE 31-1	Scores Used in the Vancouver Burn Scar Scale to Assess Burn Scar			
Score	Height	Vascularity	Pigmentation	Pliability
0	Normal; flat	Normal; color closely resembles the color over the rest of the person's body.	Normal; color closely resembles the color over the rest of the person's body.	Normal.
1	Raised <2 mm	Pink.	Hypopigmentation.	Supple; flexible with minimal resistance.
2	Raised <5 mm	Red.	Hyperpigmentation.	Yielding; gives way to pressure.
3	Raised >5 mm	Purple.		Firm; inflexible, does not move easily, resistant to manual pressure.
4				Banding; tissue is rope-like and blanches when the scar is extended.
5				Contracture; the scar is permanently shortened producing a deformity or distortion.

Adapted from Sullivan T, Smith J, Kermode J, et al: *J Burn Care Rehabil* 11(3):256-260, 1990.

This type of scar is excessive but stays within the boundaries of the original wound. In contrast, **keloid scars** (Fig. 31-5, *B*), which are also excessive, extend beyond the boundaries of the primary wound. Both hypertrophic and keloid scars are prone to contraction.

Since 1990, the Vancouver Burn Scar Scale, or modifications of this scale, has been the most commonly used assessment tool for burn scars[47] (Table 31-1). The Vancouver Burn Scar Scale should be applied to the most severe parts of the scar being measured.

Function

Gait. Gait is examined and evaluated using standard measures (see Chapter 32) in patients with lower extremity burns. Gait deviations can be related to pain, alterations in ROM, wound or scar contraction, and changes in strength. Any associated injury that might affect gait is considered in the gait evaluation and any preexisting condition or associated injury that might affect balance and safety is considered when prescribing a locomotion program.

Self-Care and Home Management. There are no specific tests for the measurement of burn-related decreases in self-care and home management. The ability to carry out specific activities, such as feeding, dressing (e.g., buttoning, zipping, and tying), and hygiene activities (e.g., brushing teeth, combing hair, and toileting), are often documented and used to examine self-care in this population.

EVALUATION, DIAGNOSIS, AND PROGNOSIS

Burns over certain anatomical locations, such as joints, can cause crucial challenges in rehabilitation for the patient and the burn care provider. With increased burn size, burn-related impairments will generally also be greater, increasing the therapeutic needs of the patient. Impairments may be acute, secondary to pain or wound contraction in superficial-, partial-, and full-thickness burns. In addition, wound and scar **contracture** at a burn site can lead to chronic struggles with decreased function and disability, and with certain burn locations, poor cosmesis may have implications for long-term socialization of the patient with burns.

Burn wound depth also impacts prognosis. Superficial-thickness burns will heal within a few days with little if any risk for impairment. In the absence of wound complications, partial-thickness burns generally heal without scarring within 14 days. Full-thickness burns are generally treated with skin grafting to accelerate healing and decrease the risk for complications such as infection, fluid loss, and excessive scarring. Full-thickness wounds, if not skin grafted, can take several weeks to heal, and scarring can be severe. Scar contraction can occur at any time during the tissue remodeling phase, which lasts an average of 12 months, with ranges of at least 6 to 18 months.[46,49]

Some patients with burns may have long-term difficulties with self-care and home and work management. A report that included a literature review and a case series of 303 patients with burns found that patients stay off work for an average of almost 10 weeks after a burn.[50] This average time for returning to work was related to the size of the burn (larger burn → longer time off work) and the age of the patient (increased age → longer time off work). Also, in some cases, burns to the hand or upper extremity further delayed return to work. In this case series, a majority (55% to 90%) of the patients returned to some form of work by 6 to 24 months after the burn; however, at 24 months, only 37% of patients had returned to the same job with the same employer as before their burn. Others had taken new jobs with an old employer or simply taken different jobs altogether.

INTERVENTION

WOUND CARE

Care of burn wounds is determined primarily by the depth and location of the injury. Superficial burn wounds are typically treated with a lotion to increase moisture in the injured tissue and to enhance pliability of the damaged dry skin. Lotions without added perfume are recommended to decrease the risk of further irritating already inflamed skin.

Partial-thickness wounds are moist and should be kept moist. They can be gently cleansed using a mild soap and then dressed. Loose tissue should be debrided. Dressing should include a topical agent such as an antimicrobial ointment (e.g., bacitracin, combination bacitracin/polymyxin [Polysporin] or combination bacitracin/polymyxin/neomycin [Neosporin]) or an antimicrobial cream (e.g., silver sulfadiazine[51-53]). Chapter 28 provides general information on topical agents and dressings used in wound management.

Ointments and creams make the wound more comfortable and most include an antimicrobial agent to decrease local microbial growth. Ointments, which are typically used on partial-thickness wounds, are more lubricating and occlusive than other topical medications and are not water soluble, whereas creams are normally more soothing to the patient and are more easily washed off because they are water soluble. If an ointment is used to cover the wound, a dry gauze wrap should be used to cover the ointment. Creams should first be covered with a petroleum-impregnated gauze dressing, which is then held in place with a dry gauze wrap. Topical agents should be changed no less than once a day, with twice a day changes being optimal.

After cleaning and any necessary debridement of loose tissue, deep partial-thickness and full-thickness burns should be covered with a topical antimicrobial agent and dressings until surgery for skin grafting can be completed. The most common dressing protocol for these wounds is to apply an antimicrobial ointment, such as silver sulfadiazine, directly to the wound and cover it with a dry gauze sheet or wrap.

Deep partial-thickness and full-thickness burns have the best outcome when treated surgically. The most common surgery to treat these deep wounds is excision of the burn eschar and coverage of the excised wound with skin grafts. Surgical coverage of the burn wound decreases the risk of sepsis. Early surgical coverage also accelerates healing, which in turn leads to less scarring and thus greater probability of good functional and cosmetic outcomes.

After a skin graft, the graft must not be disturbed by movement or pressure until it becomes vascularized and adhered to the tissue bed. This generally takes at least 48 hours. Skin grafts to the lower extremities require caution when the leg is placed in a dependent position because of the risk of increased edema and pressure. Most clinicians therefore recommend supporting venous return in the lower extremity with some form of compression, such as elastic bandages, for the first 7 to 10 days after a graft procedure. If there is any concern that one wrap will not provide enough pressure support for a graft, a double wrap can be used.

> ### ◎ Clinical Pearl
>
> A skin graft should not be disturbed by movement or pressure for at least 48 hours until it is adhered to the tissue bed.

Moisturizers should be used on healed wounds to decrease itching and skin cracking associated with dryness. Lotions without added perfumes are suggested on newly healed tissue to decrease the likelihood of developing localized rashes or irritation.

EDEMA CONTROL

Edema control may be accomplished with various interventions. A positioning program, concentrating not only on preserving motion and proper joint position but also on elevation, is customary in the care of acutely burned extremities. Elevation of an extremity allows gravity to assist with draining excessive interstitial fluid from the limb and decreases hydrostatic pressure in the blood vessels.[54]

Burn-related edema is also treated with compression. Compression may support tissue hydrostatic pressure and facilitate venous and lymphatic flow.[55] Elastic wraps, self-adherent stretch and static wraps (such as Coban, 3M, St. Paul, MN), elasticized dressings, scar compression supports, and intermittent compression pumps are all used to provide compression in this population. Wraps that provide more consistent compression than intermittent pumps may better serve patients with burn-related edema. Many factors should be considered when applying compression wraps, including the amount of pressure, the direction of wrap, and the type of wrapping used. The amount of compression varies with the type of material being used and the force of application of the material. It is recommended that wraps be applied with gentle firmness and wrapped in a spiral or figure-of-eight pattern (to avoid a tourniquet effect) from distal to proximal on the digit or extremity. It should also be remembered that overlapping layers of compression material will provide more pressure in the area of overlap.

PAIN CONTROL

Pain experienced with wound care and other therapeutic procedures may be partially managed with medications. In addition, preparing the patient for the intervention (preparatory information), behavioral techniques, and cognitive techniques may also help alleviate pain during treatment sessions.[56]

◎ *Clinical Pearl*

Preparing the patient for a painful intervention by explaining what will be done and how it might make the patient feel can help to alleviate pain and anxiety associated with typically painful procedures.

Preparing a patient for the intervention should include an explanation of what will be done and how it might make the patient feel (procedural information and sensory information, respectively). For example, a patient could be told that as they sit by the side of a mat, their arm will be placed on the mat and their elbow will be stretched to try to straighten the elbow joint (procedural information). The patient can then be told that stretching the elbow may cause a feeling of tightness throughout the arm as the tissue stretches (sensory information). Reinforcement is the most common type of behavioral pain control strategy used in physical therapy. This involves encouraging the patient to focus on something other than the pain they feel and not allowing pain to become a determining factor in stopping a particular intervention. This technique requires that a preset criterion or "goal" for a specific intervention session is clearly outlined. The therapist and the patient work toward that "goal" and rewards, such as rest, are given related to the "goal" and not the amount of pain.

Distraction and reappraisal are examples of cognitive techniques frequently used to manage procedural burn pain. Distraction involves engaging the patient in thinking about something other than the painful intervention. Patients may be distracted in many ways, such as being asked to focus on a "relaxing" place, spelling words, or playing games. The therapist must be sensitive to the culture and capability of a patient to determine appropriate distraction techniques for individual patients. Reappraisal involves clarifying the purpose and benefits of an intervention. For example, when pain associated with dressing changes and stretching is interpreted by the patient as doing more harm than good, reappraisal would involve explaining to the patient that the pain caused by this procedure is not causing additional tissue injury and cannot be avoided. The patient may also accept that the pain may be a "good" sign of an appropriate, albeit possibly uncomfortable, tissue response.

Similar techniques can be used to help a patient manage pruritus. Additionally, systemic and topical medications, as well as standard moisturizers, may reduce pruritus.

STRENGTHENING EXERCISES

No evidence-based strengthening protocols exist for patients with burns. However, the indications for strengthening exercises are similar to those for any person with muscle weakness secondary to hypercatabolism and disuse. A program of progressive resistive exercise that addresses strength and mobility should be used.

Exercise activities and equipment that encourage mobilization of a joint or complex of joints should always be considered in an exercise program for patients with burns because they are at high risk for loss of motion because of scarring. A patient may be given any set of traditional exercises using any piece of equipment. Standard recommendations for resistance training can be followed (see Chapter 5). Exercises that train major muscle groups should be included along with exercises that focus on areas of weakness found in the examination. To increase strength, the exercises should be performed to the point of volitional fatigue at least twice a week through full available ROM.[57] A warm-up of up to 15 repetitions without weight with a rest period is also recommended.[57] There are no inherent contraindications to the prescription of strengthening exercises for patients with a burn injury. However, caution should be taken to avoid disrupting new skin grafts or sutures when exercising a patient after surgery, when exercising joints with associated exposed joint structure or tendons, and when exercising in the presence of a medical co-morbidity such as a significant cardiac or orthopedic condition.

RANGE OF MOTION EXERCISES

Passive ROM exercises are beneficial when soft tissue restricts motion and the patient has insufficient strength or endurance to overcome the force of the soft tissue restriction for a long enough time to elongate the tissue. This is also a useful technique when patients cannot move because of sedation or critical illness or, for some other reason, cannot respond, voluntarily move, or otherwise actively participate in their program. The motion should be performed slowly enough to allow for tissue elongation, the hold time should be tolerable for the patient, and the end-range should have a "leathery" or "tissue stretch" end-feel. After wound closure, this end-feel should be accompanied by visible blanching of the scar.

When end-range can be achieved actively, active-assistive and active ROM exercises are preferred to passive motion because this promotes greater patient independence. Patients should be instructed to hold the stretch for at least 30 to 60 seconds and should monitor their response to the stretch. Generally, a patient should feel only mild-to-moderate pain during a session and note increased mobility after stretching.

ROM exercises should be performed in anatomical planes and focus on opposing the direction of wound and

TABLE 31-2	Recommended Anticontracture Positions for Patients with Burns
Anatomical Area	**Preferred Position**
Neck	Slight hyperextension; no rotation
Shoulder	Abduction (90-110°); slight horizontal flexion
Elbow	Extension; supination
Wrist/hand	Slight wrist extension, slight MCP flexion, PIP and DIP extension, thumb abduction
Trunk	Straight postural alignment
Hip	Extension, abduction (20°), no rotation
Knee	Full extension
Ankle/foot	Neutral ankle (no plantarflexion), neutral toe position (no dorsiflexion or plantarflexion)

MCP, Metacarpophalangeal; *PIP,* proximal interphalangeal; *DIP,* distal interphalangeal.

scar tissue contraction forces. For example, if a wound is located over a flexor surface, the ROM exercises should emphasize extension. If joint motion is restricted and gains are not made with appropriate ROM exercises, joint mobilization can be considered. The tissue should be assessed before hand placement and implementation of joint mobilization to determine if the tissue will tolerate hand placement and any associated sheer forces.

It is recommended that ROM exercises be started early in care, and the exercises should remain consistent through progression from passive to active so that the performance of the ROM almost becomes "habitual" for the patient. This is important because of the extended period of time it takes the scar to remodel (see Evaluation, Diagnosis, and Prognosis section).

Positioning, also mentioned under interventions for edema, can be used to help preserve gains in ROM or to achieve gains in ROM.[58] Positioning is used to counteract wound contraction. Standard anticontracture positions are outlined in Table 31-2.

Splinting can be used to prevent deformity from contracture, to maintain or increase ROM, and to protect a fragile area of tissue.[59] Three common types of splinting interventions are used in burn care: Serial, static, and dynamic splinting. Serial splinting involves making a splint that positions the involved tissue at the limit of its current ROM and then successively remolding the splint toward greater ROM as ROM is increased by exercise, passive mobilization, or positioning. Static splinting immobilizes a joint to maintain its position. Dynamic splinting applies an ongoing, generally mild force to a body part to either mobilize it or to provide resistance for exercise.

Malleable thermoplastic material is most commonly used in burn care to fabricate individualized conforming splints for specific body parts and purposes. Splinting should be modified or discontinued if the patient develops skin or wound breakdown, pain, or other sensory impairments. Since splints frequently harbor microorganisms, they should be cleaned on a regular basis with an ammonia solution (1 fluid ounce per gallon of water).[60]

AMBULATION

Regardless of the location of the burn, patients with burns should be involved in a walking program to mitigate problems related to bed rest such as dependence, decreased ROM, diminished strength, and cardiopulmonary compromise including hypotension. An intervention program that includes ambulation may begin once the patient is medically stable, alert, and able to follow directions. Although burn care centers have many different protocols for ambulation after burn injury, most clinicians recommend starting ambulation as early as possible. Because of the cardiovascular consequences of the fluid shifts associated with large burns, physiological responses to ambulation should be monitored, particularly in the acute phase of care.

The effects of gravity may cause patients with lower extremity edema to feel pain and other sensations, such as tingling, when they first put their legs in a dependent position to prepare for walking. However, these sensations generally subside with ambulation as the muscle contractions help to pump fluid proximally. If the pain does not decrease with walking, supportive elastic bandage wraps that provide some vascular support will generally help decrease the pain.[61]

If there has been skin grafting of the lower extremities, the extremities should be wrapped with elastic bandage whenever they are in a dependent position for sitting or ambulation, until the graft has fully taken. This is to support the graft and prevent excessive vascular pressures that might lead to bleeding and pooling of blood between the graft and the tissue bed. Such bleeding and pooling can separate the skin graft from the vascular tissue bed to which it must adhere, causing graft disruption and failure. In burn centers, dependence of a grafted lower extremity is initiated with caution, starting with dangling the leg for a minute or two and then elevating the extremity, unwrapping it, and checking for bleeding and graft integrity. If the graft tolerated this, then the duration of dependence can be increased and the patient can try to ambulate. No standards exist for when ambulation may first be attempted after grafting, but it has been documented to occur as early as 1 day after surgery, with the average across the country being about 7 days after surgery.[62] Once the skin graft has taken, ambulation can occur without any graft-related restrictions.

Standard guarding techniques and assistive ambulation devices can be used if necessary. Open- or closed-chain exercises directed at specific limitations in gait should be considered as part of the intervention program.

AEROBIC CONDITIONING

Patients with burns need aerobic conditioning because of the catabolic nature of the injury and the disuse frequently associated with inactivity imposed by the injury or surgical interventions. The metabolic demand of burn wound healing can affect various physiological parameters, including heart rate and blood pressure,[63] body temperature,[64-68] respiratory rate and ventilation,[63,69] and RPE.[63,70] Therefore these signs should be monitored with any strenuous exercise but should not preclude aerobic exercise during burn rehabilitation. To accommodate the physiological stress produced by a burn, an RPE of 12 to 16/20 on the Borg scale has been recommended for aerobic conditioning in patients with burns.[71]

Standard protocols for aerobic conditioning can be applied to this population (see Chapter 23). The exercise intensity, duration, frequency, and mode should be selected and progressed according to the patient's tolerance. Progression should allow for adaptation to the program and take into consideration the likelihood of interruptions, or regression at times, if the patient has surgeries or other medical care needs or complications. Patients may generally begin with a program that lasts between 15 and 30 minutes 3 to 5 times per week and progress the exercise intensity and/or duration gradually over about a 3 to 6 week period. Some patients will need to start with shorter and more frequent periods of exercise.[71]

Exercise for aerobic conditioning should focus on large muscle groups and rhythmic activities such as cycling, walking, or running.[71] Standard aerobic exercise equipment, such as treadmills, upper and lower extremity ergometers, and stair steppers, can be safely used in the treatment of patients with burns. The only limiting factors for using any of these devices may be location of the burn and associated pain. Aerobic exercises may be combined with exercises intended to increase ROM. For example, cycling on an exercise bicycle may improve aerobic conditioning and increase knee flexion ROM.

SCAR MANAGEMENT

Since this chapter focuses on conservative rehabilitation management after burns, surgical and pharmacological interventions for scarring are not discussed. ROM exercises, positioning, and splinting may be used to preserve joint and soft tissue mobility that can be lost as a result of scarring. Although there is no evidence for this, it is generally assumed that lengthening scar tissue during the proliferation and remodeling phases of healing by moving it through its normal anatomical and functional range improves the alignment of the scar tissue being deposited. During remodeling, scar tissue is deposited in a disorganized fashion without specific alignment.[72]

Compression therapy is often recommended to minimize the formation of hypertrophic scars because it is thought to help the scar conform to the shape of the underlying tissue.[73] Compression may also alter scar hypertrophy by decreasing capillary flow to the fibroblasts (thereby decreasing collagen formation) or by decreasing edema or excess deposition of mucopolysaccharides in the tissue matrix.[72,74] The amount of pressure often recommended is 25 mm Hg, which is close to average capillary pressure.[75]

◎ *Clinical Pearl*

Compression garments or bandages can apply local pressure over a scar and minimize hypertrophic scarring. Compression garments should be worn 23 hours/day throughout the remodeling period for optimal outcome.

Pressure may be applied in a variety of ways. Standard elastic wraps and self-adherent wraps, such as Coban (3M, St. Paul, MN), and tubular cotton bandages, such as Tubigrip (SePro Healthcare, Morristown, NJ), are often used to apply pressure to control edema or prevent excessive scarring shortly after a burn injury and can also be used to apply pressure during later phases of scar treatment. Custom-fit pressure garments are most commonly used to apply pressure to areas with or at risk for hypertrophic scarring after a burn. These pressure support garments can be made to fit any extremity, the torso, the head, the face, and the hands. For optimal outcome, these garments should fit closely and apply even pressure to all areas of tissue injury. Follow-up visits should occur regularly to check and arrange for adjustment of the fit of the support if necessary.[74] These garments should be worn 23 hours a day throughout the remodeling period, which may be as long as 2 years after the initial injury. Pressure garments are available in various colors, which may help with patient self-esteem and compliance.[76]

Silicone gel sheets have been used to treat scarring after burns since the 1980s.[77-79] It has been shown that this intervention decreases hypertrophy and redness of the forming scar.[77-80] It is generally recommended that this be applied during scar remodeling, since later application is unlikely to change the scar.[81] The mechanism for the effects of silicone gel on scar formation is not known. However, as with pressure garments, silicone gel may exert its effect by increasing local temperature.[82] Silicone gel sheets are thin and pliable and are applied directly over the scar to be treated. They are typically used over smaller areas of scarring or in locations where adequate pressure is difficult to administer by other means. No specific guidelines exist for how long silicone gel should be applied. Most clinicians use the intervention until the scar has flattened and the vascularity has decreased. If signs of remodeling, such as redness or hypertrophy, reappear, the gel is reapplied. Complications of this intervention may include rash or skin breakdown. Typically, a rash related to silicone gel sheeting will clear after the removal of the product and once the rash clears, the product can be reapplied without reoccurrence.

IMPROVING FUNCTIONAL SELF-CARE AND HOME MANAGEMENT

Edema, pain, lack of mobility, and loss of strength after burn injury often combine to decrease a patient's ability to execute functional tasks. These impairments can range from simple but important self-care skills to more complex proficiency in home and work duties. Therefore exercises should address mobility and strength, as well as specific motor programming requirements for particular skills. Early in care, functional exercise may focus on basic self-care activities such as hygiene, feeding, and dressing. These activities can then be progressed to exercises that prepare the patient for jobs in the home and at work. Specific work-directed and work-hardening programs can be instituted at the judgment of the practitioner to prepare the patient to return to a particular work setting.

REHABILITATION FOR ASSOCIATED INJURIES

No specific rehabilitation intervention can be linked in the literature to inhalation injury. However, as the patient progresses through medical pulmonary care and therapy, working to increase ventilation through a program that increases general mobility and improves endurance will likely be beneficial (see Chapters 24 and 26).[83]

The functional consequences of peripheral neuropathy in patients with burns should receive similar interventions to those applied to other patients with peripheral neuropathy (see Chapter 18). Most importantly, efforts should be taken to prevent iatrogenic neuropathy that results from pressure or poor positioning. Patients who are positioned, splinted, or bandaged should be monitored frequently to assure that no symptoms of neuropathy, such as distal numbness, pain, or weakness, are present. Areas at increased risk for neuropathy are the shoulder (brachial plexus), the elbow (ulnar nerve), and the knee (peroneal nerve).[84] Edema may also increase the risk for a pressure-related nerve compression injury.

In children and adults with burns, fractures can be successfully managed with either internal or external fixation without necessarily increasing the risk for infection.[85-87] After fracture fixation, rehabilitation of fracture-related impairments in patients with burns can proceed as it would for any other patient (see Chapter 9).

CASE STUDY 31-1

FULL-THICKNESS BURN

Patient History

GR is a 23-year-old female college student with no significant past medical history. She sustained an 11% TBSA full-thickness scald burn to her right anterior thigh, anterior lower leg, and dorsal foot when she spilled hot soup on herself while cooking dinner. After evaluation of the wounds, she was scheduled for surgery to excise the burn eschar and skin graft the wound. Before the injury, she was independent in all activities and now she has difficulty walking. She was referred to physical therapy to help manage the wounds in preparation for surgery, control edema, control pain, and improve her mobility and gait.

Diagnosis

Preferred practice pattern: 7D: Impaired integumentary integrity associated with full-thickness skin involvement and scar formation.

Immediate Acute Phase (Presurgery)
Tests and Measures—Significant Findings
   Musculoskeletal
• Patient is 5 foot 6 inches tall and weighs 125 lb.
• Lower extremity girth: Midthigh: Right 50 cm, left 43 cm; midcalf: Right 41 cm, left 35 cm; foot (figure-of-8): Right 54 cm, left 45 cm.

• Muscle performance: Left lower extremity strength 5/5 throughout. Right knee flexion and extension 4/5. Right ankle plantarflexion and dorsiflexion 4/5 (tests may have been affected by pain or edema, patient was hesitant).
• ROM: Left lower extremity passive ROM WNL throughout. Right knee flexion 0 to 90 degrees; right ankle plantarflexion 20 degrees, dorsiflexion 5 degrees.
   Neuromuscular
• Pain in right lower extremity at rest 4/10, with movement 6/10.
   Cardiovascular/Pulmonary
• At rest: Heart rate (HR): 90 bpm, blood pressure (BP): 145/112 mm Hg, respiratory rate (RR): 21 breaths/min.
   Integumentary
• 11% TBSA, full-thickness burns to right anterior thigh, anterior lower leg, and dorsal foot.
   Function
• Ambulates independently 20 feet in 19.5 seconds; "step-to" gait (right to left); Tinetti Gait Assessment score 7/12.

Interventions
• Burn wounds to be washed with water and a mild soap twice a day followed by dressing change, including application of silver sulfadiazine as a topical agent covered by gauze wrap.
• Affected leg is to be elevated when resting to control edema.
• Ambulation will be encouraged for muscle pump activation.
• Active ROM exercises for the right lower extremity.
• Gait training to address gait deviations.

Role of the Physical Therapist Assistant
• How will activation of the muscle pump aid in controlling edema?
• Which members of the health care team are likely to be involved in GR's care? What is the role of physical therapy in her care? How might this vary between institutions?
• Do you need to use sterile procedures for the dressing changes? Why or why not?

Acute Postoperative Phase
Patient History
Skin grafting surgery was performed 4 days after admission.

Tests and Measures—Significant Findings
   Musculoskeletal
• Edema decreased but still present in right lower extremity: Girth midthigh 46 cm, midcalf 38 cm, foot 50 cm. Girth on left unchanged from admission.
• PROM: Right knee flexion 0 to 85 degrees, plantarflexion 15 degrees.
   Neuromuscular
• Pain in right lower extremity at rest 2/10, with movement 3/10.
   Cardiovascular/Pulmonary
• At rest: HR 88 bpm, BP 140/105 mm Hg, RR 19 breaths/minute.

- Immediately after ambulation on treadmill for 5 minutes: HR 108 bpm, BP 155/112 mm Hg, RR 28 breaths/min; oxygen saturation 94%; RPE 8/20.
  Integumentary
- Split-thickness autografts to right anterior thigh, anterior lower leg, and dorsal foot.
  Function
- Patient able to ambulate independently 20 feet in 14 seconds; Tinetti Gait Assessment score 9/12.

Interventions
- Affected leg to be elevated when patient is resting to control edema.
- ROM exercises for the right lower extremity.
- Gait training to address specific gait deviations once the patient is cleared for ambulatory activity.
- Measure and order burn scar supports (pressure garments) for her lower extremity.

Role of the Physical Therapist Assistant
- Which member of the clinical team will clear the patient for ambulatory activity?
- Describe three appropriate ROM exercises for this patient
- What is the purpose of the pressure garments?

Rehabilitative Phase (After Discharge)
Patient History
The patient was discharged from the burn center 14 days after admission. She now presents to outpatient physical therapy 1 month after her initial injury. She received her pressure garments but only wears them for 3 to 4 hours on some days.

Tests and Measures—Significant Findings
Musculoskeletal
- Girth: Right lower extremity midthigh 42 cm, midcalf 37 cm, foot 47 cm; left lower extremity unchanged.
- Muscle performance: Right knee flexion and extension 4/5; right ankle plantarflexion and dorsiflexion 4/5.
- ROM: Right knee flexion 0 to 140 degrees; right ankle plantarflexion 35 degrees, dorsiflexion 15 degrees.

Neuromuscular
- Pain in right lower extremity at rest 0/10, with movement 0/10; itching at the graft site varies from 3/10 to 7/10.

Cardiovascular/Pulmonary
- At rest: HR 74 bpm, BP 125/80 mm Hg, RR 15 breaths/min.
- Immediately after ambulation on treadmill for 15 minutes: HR 96 bpm, BP 152/110 mm Hg, RR 26 breaths/min; oxygen saturation 95%; RPE 7/20.

Integumentary
- Hypertrophic scarring on right anterior thigh, anterior lower leg, and dorsal foot.

Function
- Patient able to ambulate independently 20 feet in 4 seconds; Tinetti Gait Assessment score 11/12.

Interventions
- ROM exercises for the right lower extremity.
- Gait training.
- Strengthening exercises for the lower extremities.
- Aerobic conditioning exercises.

Role of the Physical Therapist Assistant
- What can the patient do at home to help reduce edema?
- What is the ideal wearing schedule for the patient's pressure garments? Why should she wear the pressure garments/what is the goal of this intervention? How could you encourage GR to wear her pressure garments as much as necessary to optimize her outcome?
- List three aerobic training exercises this patient will be able to complete at home.

Additional Information
For the full version of this case study, including detailed examination results, interventions, and outcomes, see the Evolve site that accompanies this book. A full case study for a patient with a flame burn also appears on the Evolve site.

CHAPTER SUMMARY
Rehabilitation of patients with burns provides a diverse array of challenges and requires a broad range of practice skills. Early burn rehabilitation focuses on interventions directed at managing tissue healing, edema, and pain. Later interventions focus on scar management, as well as regaining prior levels of mobility, strength, and aerobic conditioning. This chapter provides essential information related to the pathology of burns and the rehabilitation management of patients with burns.

ADDITIONAL RESOURCES
For links to these and additional web-based resources, see the Evolve site.
Ace Elastic Bandages: Becton Dickinson, Franklin Lakes, NJ
Flex-Wrap: Kendall, MA
Tubigrip: ConvaTec, Princeton, NJ
Tubiton: Medlock Medical, Cheshire, UK
Bio Concepts: Phoenix, AZ
Barton-Carey: Toledo, OH
Gottfried Medical: Toledo, OH
Medical Z Corporation: San Antonio, TX

GLOSSARY
Contracture: Permanent shortening (of muscle, tendon, or scar tissue) producing deformity or distortion.

Full-thickness burn (also third-degree burn): Severe burn characterized by destruction of the skin through the depth of the dermis and possibly into underlying tissues.

Hypertrophic scar: Connective tissue composed of fibroblasts and dense collagenous fibers that stay within the boundaries of the original wound.

Keloid scar: Scar that extends beyond the boundaries of the primary wound.

Partial-thickness burn (also second-degree burn): Burn marked by pain, blistering, and superficial destruction of dermis with edema and hyperemia of the tissues beneath the burn.

Superficial burn (also first-degree burn): Mild burn characterized by heat, pain, and reddening of the burned surface but not exhibiting blistering or charring of tissues, only affecting the epidermis.

Chapter **32**

Gait Assessment and Training

Robert Wellmon

CHAPTER OUTLINE

OBJECTIVES

After reading this chapter, the reader will be able to:
1. Describe the components of the normal gait cycle.
2. Describe how pathological processes can affect the normal gait cycle.
3. Identify and discuss the importance of the components of the gait examination.
4. Describe common interventions for individuals with gait dysfunction.

*W*alking is an important functional skill, and mastery of this skill impacts human development. Walking provides access to the environment, which can affect cognitive, emotional, psychological, and psychomotor development. Walking also allows a vast number of behavioral goals to be achieved and provides exercise that helps maintain cardiovascular fitness and prevents adverse effects of a sedentary lifestyle.

Gait deficits are associated with significant functional limitations.[1,2] Gait deficits can make it difficult for an individual to get into and move about their home. Community access requires not only the ability to walk but also the ability to manage a variety of terrains, including uneven surfaces, elevations, curbs, and ramps.

Clinical Pearl

Community ambulation requires the ability to walk and manage distractions, uneven terrain, ramps, stairs, curbs, and elevations.

Rehabilitation clinicians frequently treat patients who have difficulty walking. Difficulty with walking and the resultant functional limitations and disability can occur after a wide range of pathological processes. For example, after a stroke, gait disturbances are common because altered motor control can cause problems with weight bearing and balance.[3] In the elderly, gait changes often increase the risk of falling.[1] In addition, instability while walking may be the first indication of an undiagnosed disease process, particularly in the elderly.

Problems with walking can be caused by deficits in one or more body systems. Impairments in either the musculoskeletal or somatosensory systems can affect gait quality and efficiency.[4] Weakness can change the gait pattern and worsen movement quality by reducing control and stabilization of the lower limbs. Sensory deficits can alter movement quality by impairing localization of the extremity in space and the accuracy of limb placement.[5] Because inaccurate foot placement can reduce stability, the patient may try to compensate by increasing the force with which they make contact with the supporting surface to augment sensory feedback. Over time, these forces can traumatize the musculoskeletal system. To improve stability in the face of weakness or sensory loss, a person may also walk more slowly, reducing walking efficiency.[6,7]

Cardiac or pulmonary dysfunction can also limit walking distance and endurance, making timely and efficient completion of activities involving gait difficult. Although cognitive deficits do not directly affect the gait pattern, they can affect the patient's ability to attend to the surrounding environment and thus impair his or her safety while walking.

Given the impact of gait-specific impairments on patient function, rehabilitation specialists have an important role in treating mobility deficits associated with walking that arise out of disease processes affecting a number of organ systems. Gait-specific interventions address gait-specific deficits and help the patient achieve the maximum functional benefits from interventions that specifically target gait dysfunction.

PATHOLOGY

To understand and treat gait dysfunction, the clinician must first understand normal functional walking. Familiarity with the terminology used to describe gait is also essential. The terms associated with the gait cycle, many of which describe events that should occur during walking, allow for effective communication between health care professionals and with others such as third-party payers.

FUNCTIONAL WALKING

Successful walking requires maintaining upright alignment against a number of destabilizing forces. When walking, the person's weight is constantly being transferred from limb to limb. This transition requires aligning the body weight over one limb briefly during each step. Successful walking also requires movement efficiency. Normal gait is characterized by a smooth progression of the body's center of gravity (COG) and related limb segments as weight is shifted from one limb to the other, minimizing the associated energy demands. Gait must also be adaptable. People must be able to walk on a variety of surfaces under environmental conditions that can be

destabilizing. They must be able to manage raised surfaces, such as curbs, door jambs, or steps, and be able to change their path of travel by moving sideways or walking slower or faster to accommodate other people or obstacles in the environment.

Gait can also be described and examined in terms of the functional tasks that must be achieved. Three critical functional tasks for successful walking have been identified: Acceptance of weight by the supporting limb, a period of single limb support, and advancement of the limb.[8,9]

THE GAIT CYCLE

The **gait cycle** is the fundamental unit of walking. It is defined by the events that occur between the contact of one extremity with the supporting surface and the second contact of the same extremity with the supporting surface. The gait cycle is divided into two periods or phases, which are known as stance and swing. A single gait cycle is comprised of two swing and two stance phases with associated temporal and distance characteristics (Fig. 32-1). These characteristics can be described absolutely or as a percentage of the entire gait cycle. Describing the phases as percentages of the whole cycle controls for variations in time and distance associated with gender, age, or anthropometric factors.

Stance Phase. **Stance phase** is the period of the gait cycle during which the foot or supporting limb is in contact with the ground or other supporting surface. In nondisabled adults, stance phase typically lasts less than a second and comprises approximately 60% of the gait

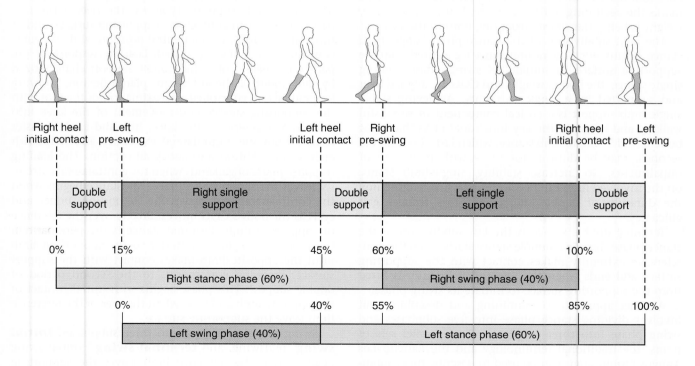

FIG. 32-1 Phases of the gait cycle. *Adapted from Inman VT, Ralston HJ, Todd F: Human walking, Baltimore, 1981, Williams & Wilkins. In Magee DJ: Orthopedic physical assessment, ed 5, St. Louis, 2008, Saunders.*

cycle. The amount of time spent in stance phase decreases as walking speed increases.

Swing Phase. Swing phase is the period of the gait cycle when the reference limb or foot is in the air or not in contact with the supporting surface. Swing phase ends just before the reference limb contacts the supporting surface. Typically, swing phase encompasses approximately 40% of the gait cycle. While one limb is in swing phase, the other (contralateral) limb is in stance phase.

> ◎ *Clinical Pearl*
>
> The gait cycle can be divided into stance phase, when the foot is in contact with the ground, and swing phase, when the foot is not in contact with the ground.

Subdivisions of the Gait Cycle. Stance and swing phase can be divided into several subdivisions. One approach is to divide stance phase into three subdivisions: (1) initial **double stance,** (2) single stance, and (3) terminal double stance. Initial and terminal double stance are also referred to as the *period of double support.* During double support, both feet are in contact with the supporting surface. The period of double support typically is 20% of the gait cycle. In dysfunctional gait, the period of double support often increases.

> ◎ *Clinical Pearl*
>
> Double-limb support time often increases in dysfunctional gait.

The initial double-stance period begins when the reference foot makes contact with the supporting surface. This marks the beginning of the gait cycle. During this period, weight is being transferred from one limb to the other.

The next subdivision of the stance phase, single-limb stance, begins when the nonreference leg is lifted from the supporting surface to initiate its swing phase. During single stance, the body's weight and COG are aligned over and supported by a single extremity. Achieving stable single-limb support is a critical component of successful walking and is one of the key functional tasks that must be achieved.[8,9] Single-limb stance, which lasts less than 0.5 seconds, may be difficult for those with pathology or impairments. To increase stability, single-limb stance on the involved limb can be shortened while lengthening the duration of double stance, but this reduces gait efficiency.

Terminal double stance is the last subdivision of the stance phase. Terminal double stance starts when the nonreference extremity makes contact with the supporting surface and ends when the reference extremity is lifted from the supporting surface to initiate its swing phase.

Another approach to examining and describing gait involves dividing stance phase into five subphases and swing phase into three subphases. Two parallel sets of terms, the traditional terminology and the Rancho Los Amigos terminology, can be used to describe these subdivisions. The clinician should be familiar with both sets of terms because both are commonly used in clinical practice and in the published literature. The traditional terminology, which is based on a description of normal gait, was developed first and can be useful for describing both

normal gait and many gait disturbances but is limited in some patients whose gait sequence deviates significantly from normal.

Traditional Gait Terminology. The components of stance in the traditional approach to gait are (1) **heel strike,** (2) **foot flat,** (3) **midstance,** (4) **heel off,** and (5) **toe off.** At heel strike, the reference limb makes contact with the supporting surface. Foot flat occurs immediately after heel strike and ends when the plantar surface of the foot makes contact with the supporting surface. The midstance phase of gait begins as the body's COG moves directly over the supporting limb. Heel off describes the period from midstance to when the heel of the reference limb leaves the supporting surface. Toe off describes the period from heel off to the beginning of the swing phase.

Swing phase is divided into three subphases: (1) acceleration, (2) **midswing,** and (3) deceleration. Acceleration begins when the toe of the reference limb leaves the supporting surface and ends when the extremity is directly under the body. Midswing is when the reference limb passes beneath the body. Deceleration starts after midswing when the tibia is no longer perpendicular to the ground and ends with the knee in maximum extension just before the foot contacts the supporting surface.

Rancho Los Amigos Gait Terminology. The five subphases of gait associated with stance are: (1) **initial contact,** (2) loading response, (3) midstance, (4) terminal stance, and (5) **preswing** (Table 32-1). Note that these terms do not identify which part of the foot contacts the floor. Initial contact begins when the foot first contacts the supporting surface and encompasses part of the period of initial double support. Typically, the heel is the first part of the foot to contact the supporting surface, and at this time the ankle is in a neutral position while the knee is extended and the hip flexed. Loading response is the part of the period of initial double support characterized by movement of the ankle into plantarflexion, allowing for gradual and controlled approximation of the foot with the supporting surface and movement of the knee into flexion. Movements at the knee, hip, and ankle transfer weight from the contralateral extremity and help with energy conservation and shock absorption. The loading response phase of gait ends when the contralateral extremity leaves the supporting surface. Midstance begins when the contralateral limb leaves the supporting surface and ends as the body's COG moves directly over the reference or supporting limb. Terminal stance is the period when the body's COG moves anterior to the supporting limb until the opposite limb makes contact with the support surface. Preswing corresponds to the second period of double support. This phase begins with initial contact of the opposite limb and ends when the toes of the reference limb leave the supporting surface.

Swing phase is divided into three subphases: **Initial swing,** midswing, and **terminal swing.**[9] Initial swing begins when the reference limb leaves the supporting surface and ends when the knee is in maximal flexion. The period from maximal knee flexion to the point where the tibia of the reference limb is perpendicular to the supporting surface is midswing. Terminal swing begins when the tibia is perpendicular to the supporting surface

TABLE 32-1	Critical Tasks and Rancho Los Amigos Terminology for the Gait Cycle						
← Stance Phase 60% →				← Swing Phase 40% →			
Weight Acceptance		Single-Limb Support		Swing-Limb Advancement			
Initial contact	Loading response	Midstance	Terminal stance	Preswing	Initial swing	Midswing	Terminal swing

and ends just before the foot contacts the supporting surface.

Functional Events of the Gait Cycle. Kinematic and kinetic events associated with the gait cycle can also be described by the functional tasks that must be accomplished. The three critical functional gait tasks are **weight acceptance,** single-limb support, and swing-limb advancement (see Table 32-1).[9] When examining gait in patients with problems walking, deficits could be classified as affecting one or more of these functional phases of gait. This approach will aid in both the diagnosis and treatment of gait dysfunction.

Weight Acceptance. Weight acceptance occurs during initial contact and the loading response of the stance phase of the gait cycle. During this time, the stance-phase limb must rapidly accept the body's weight and attenuate potentially destabilizing ground reaction forces, while relative movements of the various limb segments and the joints of the lower extremity and trunk smoothly move the body forward. At initial contact, ground reaction forces cause plantarflexion of the ankle and flexion of the knee and hip. Eccentric muscle activity at the ankle (pretibial), knee (quadriceps), and hip (extensors) contributes to limb stability and provides force attenuation.

Single-Limb Support. Single-limb support, which encompasses events associated with the single stance or support phase of gait, is characterized by progression of the body's COG over a single limb and includes midstance and terminal stance. The key goals of this functional task are maintaining forward momentum and stability while the body's weight is balanced on one limb.

Swing-Limb Advancement. Swing-limb advancement is the final functional task of the gait sequence and includes the events from preswing to terminal swing. The primary goal of swing limb advancement is to unload and move the reference limb forward, from behind the body to in front of the body, to prepare for the next functional phase of gait. This requires both clearing the foot and limb advancement.

Temporal and Distance Parameters of Gait. Temporal and distance parameters of gait are measured to compare an individual's performance with known norms and to track changes during rehabilitation. Normalization of **walking velocity,** step or **stride length,** increases in single-stance time, or decreases in double-support time generally indicate improvements in gait.

◎ *Clinical Pearl*

Improvements in gait are indicated by normalization of gait velocity, step or stride length, increases in single-stance time, or decreases in double-support time.

A single right step and a single left step (one gait cycle) make up one stride (Fig. 32-2). **Step length** is the distance between the point of initial contact of one extremity and the point of initial contact of the opposite extremity. Stride length is the distance between the point of initial contact of one extremity and the next point of initial contact of the same extremity.

Stride width, also called **base of support,** is the distance between the heels of the two feet during double stance. Stride width is measured either between the medial-most borders of the two heels or between lines through the midline of the two heels. Normal stride width for adults is between 1 to 3 inches (3 to 8 cm). Stride width often increases with gait instability.[10-12]

Walking velocity, also referred to as *speed,* is the distance covered per unit time. Walking velocity is measured in meters per second (m/sec) or miles per hour (mph). Average self-selected walking velocity in adults varies from 1.04 to 1.39 m/sec. The capacity to walk at different speeds to meet specific task and environmental demands is also important. For example, when crossing a street, one may need to walk faster to safely reach the other side, whereas when walking on a slippery surface such as ice, one may need to walk more slowly to maintain balance.

Cadence is the number of steps per unit of time. Typically, cadence is reported in steps per minute (steps/min). Cadence is fairly constant for nondisabled adults, at 100 to 117 steps/min when walking at preferred speeds on a level surface, but can vary with the demands of the task.[13] Once a mature pattern of gait is reached, cadence tends to be relatively stable across the adult lifespan.

Step time is the amount of time needed to complete a single step. **Stride time (stride/duration)** is the amount of time required to complete one stride. The time taken to complete a single stride should correspond to the time required to complete two steps. Swing time is the time that the foot is in the air. The amount of time when only one limb is in contact with the supporting surface is known as *single-support time.* The amount of time spent in **single support** is affected by a variety of factors, including limb strength,[14] balance confidence,[15] aging,[16] pain,[17-19] or the presence of pathology.[14,17,20] Single-support time decreases in the presence of weakness or pain on the support side. Step, stride, and swing time vary with gait velocity, anthropometric characteristics, and patient preference, as well as the type of task being performed. With increased gait velocity, step, swing, and stride times decrease; with decreased gait velocity, swing time increases.

Double-support time is the amount of time both lower limbs are in contact with the supporting surface and as with the base of support, increases with instability because the phase of double support is most stable.[15,20,21]

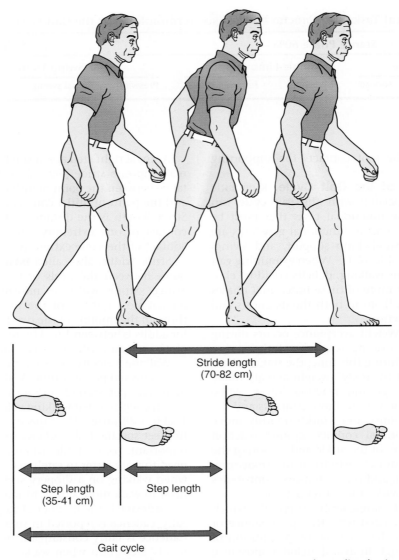

FIG. 32-2 The gait cycle: Step and stride length. *In Magee DJ:* Orthopedic physical assessment, *ed 5, St. Louis, 2008, Saunders.*

Double-support time generally increases in the presence of pathology and decreases when walking velocity increases to become almost zero during running.[15,20,22]

The temporal and distance measures associated with the swing and stance phases of gait are intimately related. Nondisabled gait is generally characterized by symmetry. Step length and time and stride length and time are roughly equal for both sides, and differences between the two sides in either temporal or distance measures are indicators of gait dysfunction. For example, after a stroke, individuals often have difficulty weight bearing on the paretic or involved limb. This reduces the corresponding single-support time and the step length of the opposite extremity and increases double-support time. Other factors, such as impaired balance, loss of sensation, alterations in motor unit recruitment, and increased tone in the lower limb or trunk, can also affect temporal and distance parameters of gait and cause asymmetry.

Temporal and distance measures of gait can also be used to track patient progress. With recovery and intervention, paretic lower extremity motor control should improve, resulting in increased weight-bearing capacity and thus increased single-support time, step length on the uninvolved side, and walking velocity, and decreased double-support time.

Limb and Trunk Kinematics During Gait. Kinematics describes movements of body parts in terms of velocity, acceleration, and displacement. Factors affecting the kinematics of gait include patient height, weight, age, balance abilities, force production capacity, flexibility, pain, speed of walking, and the presence of pathology.

Movements of the limb and trunk during gait allow a constant, rhythmic, and smooth forward progression of the body through space. As the body moves forward, the COG typically moves both vertically and laterally in a sinusoidal pattern. Limb segments primarily flex and extend to produce an average vertical displacement of about 5 cm.[23] The vertical movement upward, from the lowest point during double stance, uses metabolic energy and provides potential energy for doing work during the downward movement. When the body's COG reaches its highest point, during the midstance phase of gait, potential energy is the greatest. This potential energy is converted into kinetic energy with downward movement. Rotation and lateral listing of the pelvis, combined with knee flexion and movements of the ankle and subtalar joint, determine the vertical displacement of the COG.

Tables 32-2 and 32-3 describe the expected joint excursions of the trunk, pelvis, hip, knee, ankle, and foot during stance and swing phases of gait. For example, during

---

TABLE 32-2   Joint Excursion During the Stance Phase of Gait

Body Segment		Weight Acceptance		Single-Limb Support		
		Initial Contact	Loading Response	Midstance	Terminal Stance	Preswing
Trunk	Position	0° flexion/extension	0° flexion/extension	0° flexion/extension	0° flexion/extension	0° flexion/extension
Pelvis	Motion	5° forward rotation	5° forward rotation	0° rotation	5° backward rotation	5° backward rotation
Hip	Motion	Flexion	Flexion	Flexion to extension	Extension	
	Angle	Positioned in 30° flexion	30 → 25° flexion	25 → 0° flexion	0 → 10° extension	20 → 0° extension
	Muscle	Gluteus maximus, hamstrings, adductor magnus	Gluteus maximus, hamstrings			Iliopsoas
Knee	Motion	Extension	Flexion	Flexion to extension	Extension	Extension to flexion
	Angle	Positioned in 0° extension	0 → 15° flexion	15 → 5° flexion	5 → 0° flexion	0 → 30° flexion
	Muscle	Quadriceps, hamstrings	Quadriceps	Quadriceps	Gastrocnemius	Gastrocnemius
Ankle	Motion	Plantarflexion	Plantarflexion	Plantarflexion to dorsiflexion	Dorsiflexion	Dorsiflexion
	Angle	Positioned in 0° dorsiflexion/plantarflexion	0 → 15° plantarflexion	15° plantarflexion to 10° dorsiflexion	5 → 0° dorsiflexion	0 → 20° plantarflexion
	Muscle	Dorsiflexors	Dorsiflexors	Plantarflexors	Plantarflexors	Plantarflexors
STJ	Position	Inversion → eversion	~5° eversion	Eversion	~2° eversion	Neutral eversion and inversion
MTP	Angle	Positioned in 0° flexion/extension	Positioned in 0° flexion/extension	Positioned in 0° flexion/extension	0 → 20° extension	30 → 60° extension

STJ, Subtalar joint; *MTP*, metatarsophalangeal.

TABLE 32-3   Joint Excursion During the Swing Phase of Gait

Body Segment		Swing-Limb Advancement			
		Preswing	Initial Swing	Midswing	Terminal Swing
Trunk	Position	0° flexion/extension	0° flexion/extension	0° flexion/extension	0° flexion/extension
Pelvis	Motion	5° backward rotation	5° backward rotation	0° rotation	5° backward rotation
Hip	Motion	Flexion	Flexion	Flexion	Flexion
	Angle	20 → 0° extension	0 → 15° flexion	15 → 25° flexion	25 → 20° flexion
	Muscle	Iliopsoas	Iliopsoas		Extensors
Knee	Motion	Extension to flexion	Flexion	Extension	Extension
	Angle	0 → 30° flexion	30 → 60° flexion	60 → 25° flexion	20 → 5° flexion
	Muscle	Gastrocnemius	Hamstrings, sartorius, gracilis	Hamstrings	Hamstrings, quadriceps
Ankle	Motion	Dorsiflexion	Dorsiflexion	Dorsiflexion	Dorsiflexion
	Angle	0 → 20° plantarflexion	20 → 5° plantarflexion	0° plantarflexion/dorsiflexion	0° plantarflexion/dorsiflexion
	Muscle	Dorsiflexors	Dorsiflexors	Dorsiflexors	Dorsiflexors
STJ	Position	Neutral inversion and eversion	Neutral inversion and eversion	Inversion	Inversion
MTP	Angle	30 → 60° extension	Positioned in 0° flexion/extension	Positioned in 0° flexion/extension	Positioned in 0° flexion/extension

STJ, Subtalar joint; *MTP*, metatarsophalangeal.

initial contact, the trunk is in a neutral alignment, the pelvis rotates forward 5 degrees, and the hip is in 30 degrees of flexion. The knee and ankle are in neutral positions. At loading response, the hip moves toward extension, the knee moves from neutral to 15 degrees of flexion, and the ankle moves into plantarflexion to allow approximation of the foot with the supporting surface. The subtalar joint everts during loading response.

Patterns of Muscle Recruitment During Gait. Muscles generate the force needed to initiate and control the movements of the limb segments and trunk during gait. They control the acceleration and deceleration of the limb segments to produce smooth movement and protect body structures by counteracting gravity and ground reaction forces. Most of the muscle activity during walking produces eccentric or lengthening contractions to control the moments produced by contact of the limb with the supporting surface. Muscles also provide force for upward vertical movement during gait, performing the work needed to meet the energy demands of walking. Table

32-4 summarizes the muscles activated during stance phase of gait, and Table 32-5 summarizes the muscles activated during swing phase of gait.

TYPICAL EXAMINATION FINDINGS

PATIENT HISTORY

The patient history gives the therapist specific information about the person's symptoms or difficulties with walking such as pain with walking, loss of balance when ambulating on an uneven surface, or weakness or fatigue with walking.[24] After gathering and recording patient demographics, the patient's primary reason for seeking rehabilitative services is determined and then the time course or progression of the symptoms is ascertained. Finding out when the problem with walking first occurred begins to identify the historical progression of the symptoms and provides information about the stability of the gait changes. Changes in gait may reflect the progression of various disease processes.[25-30] For example, more frequent

TABLE 32-4	Muscle Activity During the Stance Phase of Gait*				
	Weight Acceptance		**Single-Limb Support**		
Muscle	**IC**	**LR**	**MSt**	**TSt**	**PSw**
Gluteus maximus	■	■	■		
Gluteus medius	■	■	■		
Hip flexors					
Adductors	■				■
Quadriceps femoris					
Hamstrings	■	■	■		
Pretibial/dorsiflexors†	■	■			■
Plantarflexors‡			■	■	

IC, Initial contact; *LR,* loading response; *MSt,* midstance; *TSt,* terminal stance; *PSw,* preswing.
*Shaded areas of the table indicate when muscle groups are most active during the stance phase of gait.
†Pretibial/dorsiflexors: Tibialis anterior, extensor hallucis longus, extensor digitorum longus.
‡Plantarflexors: Gastrocnemius, soleus, tibialis posterior, flexor hallucis longus, flexor digitorum longus, peroneus longus and brevis.

TABLE 32-5	Muscle Activity During the Swing Phase of Gait*			
	Swing Limb Advancement			
Muscle	**PSw**	**ISw**	**MSw**	**TSw**
Gluteus maximus				■
Gluteus medius				■
Hip flexors				
Adductors	■			
Quadriceps femoris				■
Hamstrings				■
Pretibial/dorsiflexors†		■	■	■
Plantarflexors‡				

PSw, preswing; *ISw,* initial swing; *MSw,* midswing; *TSw,* terminal swing.
*Shaded areas of the table indicate when muscle groups are most active during the swing phase of gait.
†Pretibial/dorsiflexors: Tibialis anterior, extensor hallucis longus, extensor digitorum longus.
‡Plantarflexors: Gastrocnemius, soleus, tibialis posterior, flexor hallucis longus, flexor digitorum longus, peroneus longus and brevis.

falls may be the first sign of Parkinson's disease or a consequence of a recent stroke.[26,31] Walking instability and falling are not an inevitable part of aging and both can be due to modifiable impairments.[25,32] Progressive worsening of gait also indicates a poor prognosis for rehabilitation.[33,34]

The therapist then determines when the problem is at its worst, how often the person experiences difficulty with walking, the specific functional activities that are limited, the degree of participation in the functional activity that makes the problem worse, and how the patient compensates for the identified problem with walking, as well as when and how often the person experiences difficulty with walking. To establish when the problem is at its worst, the therapist may ask "Does the problem occur more frequently at a particular time during the day, week, or month?" or "Tell me about your typical day." How long or how far the patient can walk before experiencing the symptoms may be used as a baseline against which progress can be evaluated.

How the patient compensates for problems with walking helps to identify factors that ease the problem or reduce symptoms. A variety of context-specific strategies may be used to compensate for difficulties with walking. For example, if the primary problem is endurance, the patient may compensate by limiting the distance walked or by resting frequently during activities. Depending on the patient's expected roles, this strategy may or may not be effective. Frequently, patients are discharged from rehabilitation unable to walk far enough to access community resources and will therefore either not have access to these resources or require assistance to access areas outside the home.[35]

Assistive devices may also be used to offset lower extremity weakness, problems with balance, or pain (see Chapter 33). The type of assistive device may vary with the environment. For example, a patient may use a walker for increased support in the community, but while at home, he or she may use a cane or no device.

The impact of a gait dysfunction on the person's ability to fulfill expected roles establishes the purpose and need for rehabilitative services. Weakness or limitations that do not impact function are generally not considered sufficient justification for physical therapy or other rehabilitative services.[36]

Information about the available social support may influence interventions and prognosis. The availability of someone to help at home and to bring the patient to therapy may determine whether a patient can go home to receive further care as an outpatient or must go to a facility where help is provided. After discharge from rehabilitation, patients will frequently require some level of assistance with activities of daily living (ADLs) that depend on ambulation. For some patients, although fully independent walking may not be a realistic goal, walking at home with assistance may be achievable. Interventions may include teaching the caregiver how to help the patient.

Questions about the home, community, and work environment are also included in the patient history. At home, the location of bathrooms and sleeping quarters, the number steps to enter and within the home, and the presence of rails to provide support when walking on steps may all be important. In the community, function may depend on the patient's ability to manage curbs, walk on uneven surfaces, or ascend and descend ramps. At work, function may depend on the physical structure and layout of that environment. Many patients need to walk at work or to access the job site. The patient's work and hobbies provide a context for understanding the level of disability being imposed by the impairments and functional limitations reported by the patient.

The patient history for a patient with a gait dysfunction also includes relevant information about the patient's past medical history, the effects of previous interventions for the current problem, social and health habits, and in some cases, information about the patient's family history. The patient's goals and expectations for the episode of care are also ascertained. Achieving consensus about realistic goals before starting therapy is likely to optimize patient satisfaction.

SYSTEMS REVIEW

The systems review is used to target areas requiring further examination and to define areas that may cause complications or indicate a need for precautions during the examination and intervention processes. Chapter 1 includes details of the systems review. The systems review for a patient with gait disturbances depends on their underlying problems.

TESTS AND MEASURES

The selection of tests and measures is based on ruling in or out hypotheses about possible sources of symptoms as derived from the patient history. The following section discusses tests and measures commonly applied to patients with gait dysfunction. Since abnormal gait patterns can arise from range of motion (ROM) restrictions,[37-40] weakness,[41-44] pain as a result of short- or long-term changes in the musculoskeletal system,[40,45] and postural alterations,[46] these aspects are the focus of this section. This is followed by a detailed discussion of gait-specific tests and measures.

Musculoskeletal

Anthropometric Characteristics. Increased joint girth, particularly from inflammation, can cause pain that limits the patient's desire to either move or bear weight on an extremity. Reduced limb girth is generally caused by muscle atrophy, which correlates with weakness.

Range of Motion. Excessive or limited ROM can adversely affect gait.[47-49] ROM may be altered by changes in ligamentous stability, loss of joint capsule integrity, or changes in the articular surfaces of the joint, as well as by alterations in muscle and tendon length or involvement of a neural structure crossing the joint. For example, iliopsoas tightness can limit the available hip extension ROM and alter the phases of the gait cycle when the supporting limb should be behind the body.[47] Table 32-6 summarizes the ROM required in the pelvis and lower extremities for normal gait.

Muscle Performance. Lower extremity strength affects gait in a variety of patient populations,[50-57] and weakness has been shown to impair motor performance and control

TABLE 32-6	Pelvis and Lower Extremity Range of Motion Required for Normal Gait	
Joint	**Stance Phase**	**Swing Phase**
Pelvis	0-5° forward and backward rotation	0-5° forward and backward rotation
Hip	0-30° flexion 0-10° extension	20-30° flexion
Knee	0-40° flexion	0-60° flexion
Ankle	0-10° dorsiflexion 0-20° plantarflexion	0° dorsiflexion/plantarflexion
STJ	0-5° eversion	

STJ, Subtalar joint.

during walking.[41,50,58-62] Therefore all patients with gait dysfunctions are screened for weakness of the muscles involved in gait.

Manual muscle testing (MMT) may be used to screen for weakness in patients with gait dysfunction. Walking at preferred speeds or slightly faster usually requires the ability to produce muscle force at a grade of 3 to 3+/5.

Isokinetic testing, which allows dynamic measurement of the strength, speed, and endurance of eccentric, concentric, and isometric contractions at any point in a joint's available ROM, can be a more precise and accurate indicator of force production problems related to gait than MMT. However, such testing is time consuming and may limit the number of muscles that are tested and the frequency of retesting. Isokinetic testing may also be inappropriate for patients with poor isolated control. Force deficits detected by isokinetic testing have been found to correlate with gait dysfunction[53,63-65] and with the risk for falls when walking.[52,53]

Joint Integrity and Mobility. Joint stability may be assessed by selective application of forces to the joint. These techniques can implicate potential hypomobile, hypermobile, painful, or inflamed structures that can affect functional gait.

Neuromuscular

Pain. Pain elicited with palpation can indicate a problem with one or more underlying soft tissue and/or osseous structures and can affect the pattern of movement during gait. Pain elicited with weight bearing is often a result of dysfunction in intraarticular structures.

Sensory Integrity. Sensory loss can alter gait biomechanics. Individuals with sensory loss are at greater risk for falling and for damage to the feet when walking.[5,27,66-69] When sensation is impaired, the patient often exerts more force during the weight-acceptance phase of gait, increasing the risk for skin breakdown and damage to joint structures.[5] Impaired sensation may also limit the types of orthotic or prosthetic interventions that may be implemented to address gait dysfunction.

Highly coordinated movements, including gait, can occur in the absence of sensory feedback because much of the programming of muscle recruitment for gait occurs within the spinal cord. There is evidence that humans and other organisms can produce gaitlike movement, although

of a different quality, in the absence of sensory feedback from peripheral limb and joint receptors.[9,70-72]

Cranial and Peripheral Nerve Integrity. Gait function can be affected by impairments of the cranial nerves (CNs) and/or spinal nerve segments. CNs II, III, IV, and VI have a role in vision and are examined whenever a patient reports difficulty with walking. The integrity of CNs III, IV, and VI, which are responsible for eye movements, affect the patient's ability to acquire information about the environment that is used to guide and plan motor output. CNs II and III affect the quality of the visual information gathered. The vestibular component of CN VIII affects balance while walking. The vestibular system provides feedback on the position of the head in space and movement of the body as it is being translated during walking. The functioning of peripheral sensory receptors, the visual system, and the vestibular system all affect balance during walking (see Chapter 13).

Although vision and the vestibular system provide a great deal of the information needed to control motor output for gait, the peripheral nervous system must also provide feedback about the position of the extremities and provide input to the muscles to produce muscle contractions. Peripheral nerve integrity is examined with motor and sensory tests, as described previously, and with electrophysiological testing.

Motor Function—Control and Learning. Several simple tests of motor control can provide useful information about the patient with gait dysfunction. Difficulties with reaching for and touching a target with the foot or performing rapidly alternating movements of the ankle or knee, all of which require the recruitment and relaxation of agonist and antagonist muscle groups, may indicate difficulty coordinating movement when walking, since walking requires the capacity to reciprocally and sequentially recruit and relax muscles.

The presence of atypical movement patterns are noted and explored. Atypical movement patterns reduce gait efficiency by altering the translation of the body's COG. Lesions in the brain, such as those caused by stroke, traumatic brain injury, multiple sclerosis, or Parkinson's disease, may disrupt supraspinal input and make muscles overactive, underactive, or recruited out of sequence, resulting in atypical movements during gait.[68,69,73,74] Abnormal tone can also affect movement control and adversely affect movement quality during gait. Tone may be measured with the Modified Ashworth Scale.

Cardiovascular/Pulmonary

Ventilation and Respiration/Gas Exchange. Respiratory rate at rest and during and after exercise will give an indication of the patient's activity tolerance. Monitoring of oxygen saturation with pulse oximetry is also recommended initially during gait training of patients with cardiovascular or pulmonary dysfunction. Oxygen saturation levels should generally be kept above 95% during gait training.

Aerobic Capacity and Endurance. Walking places a demand on the cardiovascular and pulmonary systems. Checking heart rate and blood pressure at rest, while the patient walks, and immediately after the patient stops walking will provide the clinician with information on how the patient's cardiovascular and pulmonary systems respond to functional ambulation (see Chapter 22). An increase in heart rate and blood pressure in response to ambulation is normal, but this increase will be more pronounced in deconditioned patients. A decrease in heart rate or blood pressure in response to walking is a sign of poor activity tolerance. Additional cardiovascular monitoring with telemetry is recommended for patients with more severe impairments in cardiac and pulmonary function such as those who have recently undergone cardiac surgery or those with a recent myocardial infarction.

Integumentary

Integumentary Integrity. The feet are inspected for signs of skin breakdown such as open wounds, areas of redness, and other indications of excessive pressure such as callus formation. Individuals with impaired sensory integrity, particularly those with diabetes, are at increased risk for skin breakdown and soft tissue ulceration on the plantar surface of the foot if they walk or increase their walking.[10] This occurs primarily because loss of sensation limits the person's ability to perceive trauma to the feet from walking (see Chapter 30).

Gait-Specific Tests and Measures. Gait-specific tests and measures are generally designed to examine either impairment or functional limitations. At a minimum, the therapist observes the patient walking from multiple perspectives and determines if the patient needs an assistive device and if the patient needs personal assistance with ambulation. Walking is observed in a variety of environments such as on a level surface; up and down a curb, ramp, or steps; and on uneven surfaces.

Selection of additional gait-specific tests and measures depends on the purpose of the test and its reliability and validity, sensitivity and specificity, responsiveness or capacity to detect change, and appropriateness for a particular population, as well as its ease of use. Each of the tests and measures discussed in this section was developed for a specific purpose. Some were developed to identify individuals at increased risk for falling when walking, whereas others, such as the Wisconsin Gait Scale, were developed for identification and description of gait dysfunction in a specific population. Certain measures primarily quantify the degree of functional limitation and focus less on quantifying the degree of impairment. For example, two items on the Functional Independence Measure (FIM), a tool used to predict burden of care, examine the level of functional independence for gait on level surfaces and when ascending stairs. The test indirectly captures impairments affecting gait.

Observational Gait Analysis. Observational gait analysis (OGA) is an approach frequently used for the examination and quantification of gait dysfunction in the clinical setting. OGA can be used to identify patients who would benefit from a more detailed examination and to qualitatively or quantitatively classify the degree of gait impairment. OGA is popular because it is relatively quick and easy to use, requires no equipment, and can be performed in any setting.

Observational Gait Analysis Procedure. The clinician observes the patient walking, looking from the right and left sides to focus on kinematic changes in the sagittal plane, including step and stride length; single- and double-stance times; vertical displacements of the body's COG; flexion and extension movements of the hip, knee, and ankle; and the position of the head and trunk. This is followed by observation from the front and back to appreciate kinematic changes in the frontal plane, including base of support during double stance, foot angle, lateral or horizontal displacements of the body's COG, varus and valgus deformities at the knee, alterations in normal hip abduction and adduction, and the position and movements of the subtalar joints.

During OGA, the examiner also monitors the movements of the various limb segments (tibia-foot complex, femur-tibia, femur-trunk), observing one joint at a time, starting where the patient reports symptoms or where earlier testing suggested that there are deficits. The primary goal of OGA is to identify primary and secondary gait changes caused by specific impairments. Secondary changes are those caused by a primary gait deviation. For example, decreased ankle dorsiflexion ROM will cause the primary gait deviation of reduced anterior movement of the tibia on the ankle-foot complex during weight acceptance. To compensate, there may be secondary changes such as increased knee extension or hip flexion during weight acceptance (initial contact and loading response).

Gait is observed at a variety of speeds. Although it is easiest to start with the patient's preferred walking speed, faster and slower walking speeds should also be observed. Some gait deviations may only be apparent at faster speeds because the patient's preferred speed is likely to be one that minimizes gait deviations. With patients who report difficulty with prolonged walking, the OGA may also need to include longer distances or durations for gait deviations to occur. Various speeds and inclines, as well as distances and durations of walking, may be simulated in the clinic using a treadmill.

Although OGA has many limitations, the simplicity and ready availability of the approach will likely result in its ongoing use in a variety of clinical and research settings. The findings may be used to direct care or to screen for dysfunction and direct the selection of other more reliable and specific tests and measures that can implicate specific system involvement, localize the impairments, and quantify functional gait deficits. The use of standardized instruments in conjunction with OGA can improve reliability and therefore provide better tracking of patient progress during an episode of care.

Videotaping of Observational Gait Analysis. Videotaping may enhance the reliability of OGA, particularly when a standardized measurement tool is used.[75-77] Videotaping also creates a permanent record of the client's walking, allowing for comparison of preintervention and postintervention performance and for repeated viewing of a walking trial, avoiding patient fatigue with repetition.

Clinical Pearl

Videotaping can enhance the reliability of observational gait analysis and allow for comparison of preintervention with postintervention performance.

Standardized Tests and Measures That Rely on Observational Gait Analysis. A number of standardized tests and measures have been developed to quantify the findings from OGA. These tests and measures include decision rules and standardized scoring systems for OGA. There is evidence that raters can reliably identify gait impairments in patients with cerebral palsy,[78] stroke,[77] and spinal cord injury[79] when using standardized scoring systems in conjunction with OGA.

Rancho Los Amigos Observational Gait Analysis System. A form was developed at Rancho Los Amigos Hospital to document the findings from OGA, and this form has since been used in a variety of settings and been refined many times over the years.[9] This instrument allows for consistent documentation of OGA; however, its reliability, sensitivity, and specificity and its capacity for detecting change have not been studied.

Wisconsin Gait Scale. The Wisconsin Gait Scale (WGS), developed in 1996, is a 14-item scale intended to measure clinically relevant components of gait in persons after stroke.[77] Asymmetries in step length and single-stance time, capacity for weight bearing on the involved extremity, base of support during double stance, and changes in joint excursions frequently occur after a stroke.[80] The WGS uses an ordinal scale to categorize the findings from OGA. Improvements in WGS scores were reported in patients after rehabilitation for stroke-related gait deficits, with improvements correlating positively with increased gait velocity.[81]

Gait Abnormality Rating Scale. The Gait Abnormality Rating Scale (GARS) is a scale for evaluating gait that was specifically developed to identify elderly adults at risk for falling in a nursing home environment, although it can be used to quantify various aspects of gait in a variety of populations.[82] A 0 to 3 ordinal scale is used to rate 16 aspects of gait noted during OGA. When scoring the items, 0 = normal, 1 = mildly impaired, 2 = moderately impaired, and 3 = severely impaired. The total score is the sum of scores for all items, with a higher score indicating greater impairment and fall risk.

Modified Gait Abnormality Rating Scale. The Modified Gait Abnormality Rating Scale (GARS-M), a variant of the GARS, is a 7-item scale developed to predict fall risk among community-dwelling, frail elderly adults.[83] The items are scored with the same 0 to 3 scale as the GARS.

Tinetti's Performance-Oriented Mobility Assessment. Tinetti's Performance-Oriented Mobility Assessment (POMA) is a commonly used clinical measure of both gait and balance that was developed specifically for use with older adults.[84] This instrument consists of 16 items, 7 related to gait and 9 related to balance. The POMA examines step length and height, gait initiation, step symmetry and continuity, straightness of the path of travel while trying to walk in a straight line, trunk position, and base of support during the period of double support. Performance on all items is scored from 0 to 1 or 2 for a maximum score of 28, with a higher score indicating better gait and balance. Low scores on the instrument have been shown to correlate with fall risk in elderly adults.[85,86] A total score of 19 or less indicates a high risk for falling and a score between 19 and 24 indicates a moderate risk.[84,87]

Dynamic Gait Index. The Dynamic Gait Index (DGI) is a gait-related tool developed to identify elderly adults at risk for falls. It rates tasks on a 0 to 3 scale. Lower scores indicate greater impairment. A score of 19 or less has been shown to be related to increased risk for falling, and scores have been shown to increase in adults undergoing rehabilitation for balance disorders because of central and peripheral nerve impairments.[88-91]

Standardized Tests and Measures Related to Gait That Do Not Rely on Observational Gait Analysis

Timed Up and Go Test. The Timed Up and Go (TUG) test is a performance-based measure of functional mobility that was initially developed to identify mobility and balance impairments in older adults.[92,93] The test requires the subject to rise from a chair, walk 3.0 m at a comfortable pace to a mark placed on the floor, turn around at the 3.0 m mark, walk back to the starting point, and return to sitting in the chair. The test's score is the time it takes the subject to complete the test.[93] Individuals who take longer than 30 seconds to complete the test need physical assistance with transfers and generally cannot manage steps.[92] Individuals who can complete the test in less than 20 seconds will likely be independently mobile and most can manage steps and walk outside the home.[92]

Berg Balance Scale. The Berg Balance Scale (BBS) is a performance-oriented measure of balance for use with elderly adults. It consists of 14 items scored on a 0 to 4 scale. The tool measures balance during mobility tasks that form the basis for walking, together with a number of other measures such as strength, integrative balance, flexibility, and cognition.

Activities-Specific Balance Confidence Scale. The Activities-Specific Balance Confidence (ABC) Scale is a 16-item questionnaire used to rate self-perceptions of mobility confidence for a variety of walking and standing activities. Each item is scored from 0% to 100% in 10% increments, with higher scores indicating greater confidence in mobility.[94,95] A score of 0% to 10% indicates no confidence in performing the activity, whereas 90% to 100% indicates complete confidence when performing the listed activity. The instrument captures the individual's perception of his or her abilities when performing a variety of functional tasks involving standing and walking.[95,96] Poor performance on this measure may indicate that the patient would benefit from interventions that increase their confidence in walking. Lack of confidence in walking has been shown to be related to changes in gait performance.[15,97]

Functional Independence Measure. The Functional Independence Measure (FIM) is an instrument that was developed as a measure of disability for a variety of populations.[98] The instrument includes measures of independence for self-care, including sphincter control, transfers, locomotion, communication, and social cognition. The locomotion scale examines walking ability on steps and level surfaces. Walking is scored according to the observed distance walked and the level of assistance required.

Stride Analysis, Gait Velocity, and Footfall Measurement Technologies. Various tools and devices can be used to measure temporal and distance parameters of gait. These range from simple, inexpensive, and easy-to-use tools, such as a stopwatch and tape measure, to complex and more expensive devices, such as instrumented walkways specifically designed to measure gait. The more complex devices provide more detailed and precise information allowing for closer monitoring of patient progress over time.

Hand-Held Stopwatch. The simplest way to determine gait velocity is to time the patient walking a measured distance. Gait velocity is an excellent global indicator of walking capacity.[99-102] Elderly adults who walk more slowly are more disabled, have lower self-efficacy or balance confidence, and have lower scores on the BBS.[103] Gait velocity, along with distance covered, is also related to perception of general health in elderly adults.[104] Changes in gait velocity can also predict functional dependence in elderly adults.[105] Decreased gait velocity has been linked to an increased risk of falling.[106,107] Individuals who walk at a speed of 0.57 m/sec or less have an increased fall risk and may benefit from rehabilitation services.[108] Improvements in motor control are associated with increased gait velocity, and gait velocity can be an indicator of the effectiveness of interventions.[41,101]

◎ *Clinical Pearl*

Gait velocity is an excellent indicator of walking capacity.

Six-Minute Walk Test. The 6-minute walk test (6MWT) requires the patient to walk for 6 minutes at his or her preferred pace. The patient is instructed to walk as long and as far as possible in the prescribed amount of time, and the test is scored by measuring the total distance walked. Rest breaks may be taken as needed. The test is stopped when the 6-minute time limit is reached or when vital signs or patient fatigue indicate a need to stop. Observational gait analysis can be completed during the 6MWT, and this test also allows for examination of the effects of fatigue on gait.

Inked Footprint Methods. Temporal and distance measures of gait can also be examined by applying inked moleskin to a patient's feet and then having him or her walk on a roll of paper.[109] The moleskin is first applied to the heel and toe of the patient's shoes (Fig. 32-3, *A*) and then ink is applied to the moleskin. The patient then walks on paper, leaving marks as they go (Fig. 32-3, *B*). Step length, stride length, base of support during double stance, and angle of **toe out** can then be measured. The inked footprint method provides a reliable, valid, and low-cost means to quantify gait function.[109] An even simpler alternative to using moleskin involves the attachment of felt-tipped markers to the heel of the shoe (Fig. 32-3, *C*). As the subject walks, marks made on the paper can be used to measure step and stride length (Fig. 32-3, *D*).

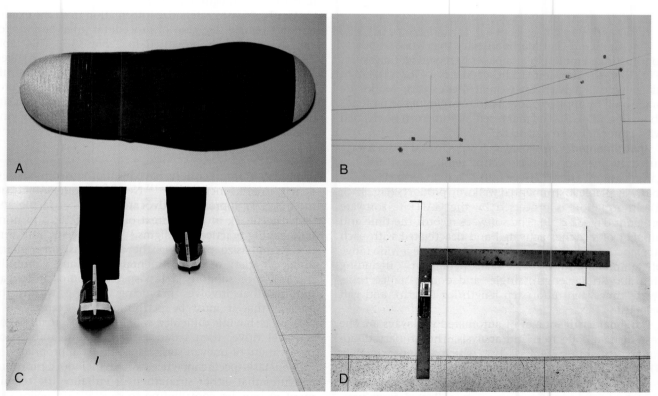

FIG. 32-3 Inked footprint methods for measuring gait. **A,** Moleskin attached to the heel and toe of the shoe. **B,** Measurement of selected gait parameters from footprints made with moleskin attached to the heel and toe of shoes. **C,** Felt-tipped markers attached to the back of the shoes. **D,** Measurement of step length from marks generated by the felt-tipped marker method.

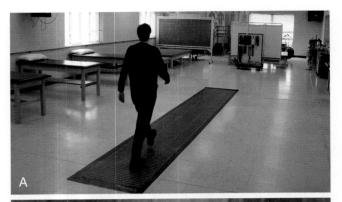

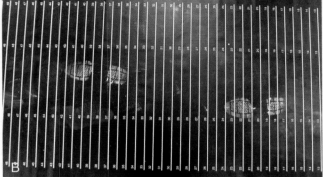

FIG. 32-4 A, Gait Grid Gait Mat. **B,** Marks left by powder on the sole of the shoe on the Gait Grid Gait Mat. **A** *courtesy Gait Rite, Tustin, CA.*

The Gait Grid Gait Mat is a device that works similarly to using inked moleskin and paper to record gait measures (Fig. 32-4, *A*). The Gait Grid Gait Mat is a 7.62 × 0.762 m naugahyde mat with lines on it 4 cm apart. Marks are made on it by applying powder to the soles of the patient's shoes (Fig. 32-4, *B*). The mat is reusable and can be cleaned with water between gait trials.

Instrumented Walkways. Instrumented walkways automate the process of collecting temporal and distance gait measures. The GAITRite Gait Mat is an example of the many available instrumented walkway products (Fig. 32-5, *A*). Information is processed by the GAITRite software program (Fig. 32-5, *B*). The software records the time and number of switches activated and deactivated with each step and from this information can compute a wide range of temporal and distance gait parameters, including step and stride length, single- and double-stance time, swing time, step ratio (step length/leg length), and gait velocity.

The major advantages of automated walkways are the ease of data collection and analysis. The primary disadvantage of this system is cost, which is approximately $10,000 to $15,000.

Stride Analyzers and In-Shoe Microprocessor Systems. Stride analyzers use data collected from pressure-activated microprocessor switches on an insole placed in the patient's shoes (Fig. 32-6, *A* and *B*). Stride analyzers can record and calculate gait velocity, cadence, stride length, single- and double-support time, swing and stance

time, and total gait cycle time (Fig. 32-6, *C*). This type of system has the advantage of allowing the patient to move about freely rather than being restricted to a straight walkway. However, these systems are expensive and for a similar cost to an automated walkway, provide less information about gait pattern.

EVALUATION, DIAGNOSIS, AND PROGNOSIS

Evaluation of the data from all components of the examination leads the physical therapist to a preferred practice pattern and prognosis. When evaluating the underlying causes of gait dysfunction, the clinical decision-making skill lies in the ability to classify the importance of and causal links between the problems observed during the examination. Primary problems are those that are thought to be the cause of other observed problems. These are the most appropriate target of procedural interventions. Secondary problems are problems that arise out of, or are a consequence of, the primary problems. Targeting a procedural intervention toward a secondary problem will generally be less effective in ameliorating the patient's problems with walking.

Diagnosis is the process of assigning meaning to the findings of the examination.[24,110] The *Guide to Physical Therapist Practice* recommends assigning the patient to one or more of the preferred practice patterns within the broad categories of musculoskeletal, neuromuscular, cardiopulmonary, and integumentary.[24]

Another way to categorize information from the examination to guide selection of procedural interventions for gait dysfunction is presented in Table 32-7. This table identifies impairment level causes of observed gait changes. Impairment level tests can thus be used to confirm or rule out a cause of an observed gait change and to direct procedural interventions. Other typical gait dysfunctions are described in Tables 32-8 and 32-9 with possible underlying causes identified.

INTERVENTION

A number of interventions have been proposed to address deficits in gait function.[32,111-115] Neurodevelopmental treatment (NDT) approaches advocate the use of tactile and verbal feedback in the context of task-specific and non–task-specific practice paradigms.[111] Task-specific interventions emphasize practicing the actual task of walking under a variety of environmental conditions. Currently, the evidence supports a task-specific approach to gait training that involves practicing walking within the context that it must be performed. For example, if a patient is having difficulty walking to the mailbox on a gravel drive, then balance training and ambulation on a variety of uneven surfaces would be appropriate.

Non–task-specific practice would include performing activities that either strengthen or enhance the recruitment of muscles contributing to gait[111,115] or repetitively practicing the problematic elements of walking outside the context of the actual task.[32,111] Although continuing to be popular clinically, there is little evidence to support the effectiveness of NDT approaches in improving measurable

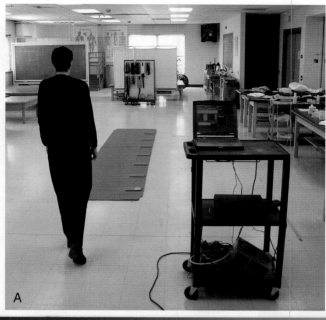

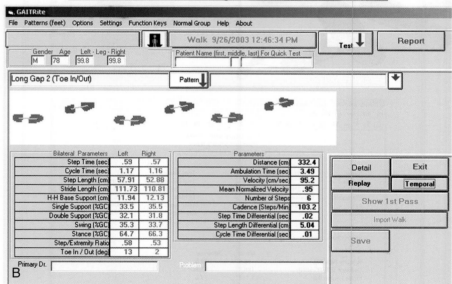

FIG. 32-5 GAITRite Gait Mat. **A,** System set-up. **B,** GAITRite Gait Mat screen shot of selected temporal and distance gait measures. *Courtesy Gait Rite, Tustin, CA.*

parameters of gait.[116] Non–gait-specific interventions that combine strengthening activities, balance training, and endurance training have also been shown to be effective in some cases.

◎ *Clinical Pearl*

Current evidence provides the most support for task-specific training (i.e., practicing walking within the context that it must be performed), as being effective for improving functional gait.

BODY WEIGHT–SUPPORTED TRAINING

Treadmill (Fig. 32-7, *A*) and overground body weight–supported training (Fig. 32-7, *B*) are promising interventions

that can accelerate the return to walking and improve ambulation in a variety of patients with gait dysfunction.[117-120] Body weight–supported training involves partially supporting the patient's body weight with a harness during walking. The harness is suspended from a ceiling, a supporting structure, or a mobile device with wheels. Supported walking is intended to increase the strength of muscles used for standing or walking, improve balance, allow for task-specific practice to facilitate the relearning of movement patterns, and enhance patterns of muscle activation or recruitment for standing and walking tasks. Gradually decreasing the amount of support and increasing the amount of weight being managed by the patient, while controlling the speed of walking, is thought to most effectively improve gait performance.

Text continued on page 524

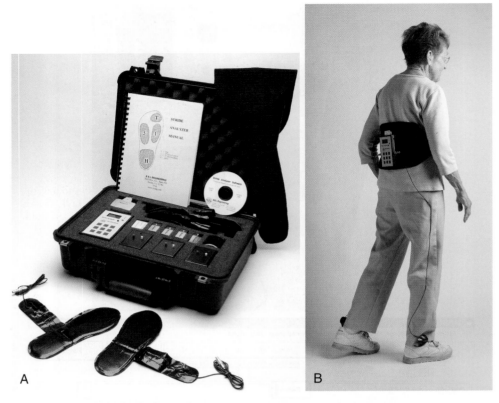

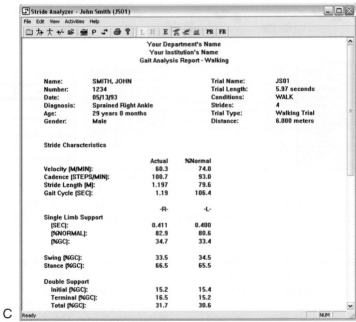

FIG. 32-6 Stride analysis system. **A,** Components. **B,** Stride analysis system on model. **C,** Stride analysis system computer screen shot. **A** *courtesy Gait Rite, Tustin, CA;* **B** *and* **C** *courtesy B & L Engineering, Tustin, CA.*

| TABLE 32-7 | Impairment Level Causes of Observed Gait Changes | | | |

Body Segment	Period	Observed Gait Problem	Phase of the Gait Cycle	Evaluation and Diagnosis
Trunk	Stance	Lateral lean	IC through PSw	Weak hip abductors Hip joint pain Leg-length discrepancy
		Backward lean	IC through PSw	Hip extensor weakness
		Forward lean	IC through PSw	Hip extensor weakness Inadequate lumbar flexibility Hip flexor or joint contracture
	Swing	Lateral lean	ISw through TSw	Compensation for weak hip abductors on the contralateral stance-phase limb
		Backward lean	ISw through MSw	Compensation to advance the involved limb through swing
Pelvis	Stance	Posterior tilt	Stance and/or swing	Inadequate lumbar flexibility Back pain Postural malalignment Tonal increases
		Anterior tilt	Stance and/or swing	Inadequate lumbar flexibility Hip flexor or joint contracture Back pain Impaired abdominal force production Postural malalignment
		Retraction	Stance and/or swing	Inadequate hip flexor or joint flexibility
	Swing	Pelvic drop	Stance	Force production deficit: Abductors
Hip	Stance	Inadequate flexion	IC to LR	Impaired force production: Hip flexors Decreased ambulation velocity Impaired motor control: Synergistic movement patterns Pain
		Excessive flexion	IC through PSw	Hip flexor contracture Joint contracture
		Inadequate extension	IC through PSw	Hip flexor contracture Joint contracture Pain
		Abduction	IC through PSw	Varus deformity Leg length discrepancy Joint contracture Pain
		Adduction	IC through PSw	Valgus deformity Adductor contracture Increased adductor tone/hypertonicity Impaired motor control associated with CNS impairments
	Swing	Excessive flexion	ISw through TSw in conjunction with increased knee flexion	Compensation for decreased dorsiflexion due to impaired force production of the ankle dorsiflexors
Knee	Stance	Inadequate flexion	During any of the stance phases, less than the expected amount of knee flexion is observed.	Inadequate knee extensor strength Contracture at the knee: Joint or muscle Pain Knee extensor hyperactivity Co-contraction: Knee flexor and extensor Inadequate ankle dorsiflexion Impaired proprioception
		Excessive flexion	During any of the stance phases, more than the expected amount of knee flexion is observed.	Inadequate knee extensor strength Contracture: Joint capsule, ligaments or muscle Knee flexor hypertonicity or hyperactivity Co-contraction: Knee flexors and extensors secondary to CNS dysfunction Pain Leg-length discrepancy on the contralateral side: Osseous changes or joint contracture (hip, knee, or ankle) Excessive ankle dorsiflexion Impaired proprioception

Continued

TABLE 32-7	Impairment Level Causes of Observed Gait Changes—cont'd			

Body Segment	Period	Observed Gait Problem	Phase of the Gait Cycle	Evaluation and Diagnosis
		Hyperextension or rapid movement of the knee into extension	IC to MSt	Inadequate knee extensor strength Contracture: Decreased dorsiflexion at the ankle Knee extensor hypertonicity or hyperactivity Contracture at the ankle: Limited dorsiflexion Impaired proprioception Mechanism for increasing limb stability
		Varus/valgus posture	IC through PSw	Knee joint or ligamentous instability Bone deformity or erosion Varus or valgus deformity at the hip
		Rapid knee flexion/buckling	LR through TSt	Knee extensor weakness Poor eccentric control of the gastrocnemius-soleus muscle group See Chapters 12 and 33 for the effects of orthotics and prosthetics
	Swing	Inadequate flexion		Contracture: Joint or muscle Knee extensor hypertonicity or hyperactivity Co-contraction: Knee flexor and extensor
		Excessive flexion		Limited dorsiflexion at the ankle
Ankle	Stance	Forefoot first contact	IC occurs with the ball of the foot.	Plantar flexion contracture Heel pain Excessive knee flexion at the end of swing
		Flat foot contact	IC occurs with the whole plantar surface of the foot.	Ankle joint contracture Limitations in force production at the knee Pain
		Foot slap	At IC leading into loading response, foot rapidly plantarflexes when contacting the supporting surface.	Weakness of ankle dorsiflexors Impaired proprioception
		Increased plantar flexion/decreased dorsiflexion	At LR, lack of mobility into dorsiflexion.	Plantar flexion contracture Increased tone in the plantarflexors Impaired proprioception
		Excessive inversion	At IC, foots lands on the lateral border in excessive inversion.	Overactivity of the tibialis anterior, tibialis posterior, or gastrocnemius-soleus muscles Plantarflexor contracture Internal tibial torsion Calcaneovarus deformity
		Lack of heel off	TSt	Gastrocnemius: Soleus weakness
		Early/rapid heel rise	MSt through PSw	Lack of dorsiflexion: Joint or plantarflexor contracture
		Delayed heel rise	MSt through PSw	Impaired force production: Plantarflexors
		Medial heel whip	Lateral movement of heel at terminal stance.	Lack of dorsiflexion: Joint or plantarflexor contracture
	Swing	Foot or toe drag	Contact of the toes or ball of the foot with the supporting for either a portion of or throughout swing phase.	Lack of dorsiflexion: Joint or plantarflexor contracture Increased tone in the plantarflexors Weakness of ankle dorsiflexors Inadequate hip flexion Inadequate knee flexion Somatosensory deficits: lack of awareness of the position of the foot in space
Foot	Stance	Excessive eversion or pronation	IC through PSw	Ligamentous laxity; compromised osseous integrity: Long-term musculoskeletal trauma Leg-length discrepancy Tibialis anterior weakness
		Excessive inversion or supination	IC through TSt	Overactive invertor muscles Overactive gastrocnemius-soleus Leg-length discrepancy
		Toe clawing	LR through PSw	Overactive toe flexors Increased toe flexor tone Reduced length of the toe flexors
	Swing	Excessive inversion	Swing	Overactive invertor muscles Underactive evertor muscles Overactive gastrocnemius-soleus

IC, Initial contact; *PSw,* preswing; *ISw,* initial swing; *TSw,* terminal swing; *LR,* loading response; *MSt,* midstance; *TSt,* terminal stance; *CNS,* central nervous system.

TABLE 32-8	Terms Used to Describe Gait Pathology		
Term	**Description**	**Phase of Gait Cycle**	**Evaluation and Diagnosis**
Antalgic	Difficulty or decrease in weight bearing on a limb during stance phase due to the presence of pain.	Stance	Pain caused by the compression of a joint or soft tissue structure when bearing weight.
Crouch-knee gait	Pattern of gait characterized by excessive flexion affecting both knees.	Stance	Tonal increases associated with CNS involvement; contracture involving either the joint and/or soft tissue structure crossing the joint
Early heel rise/premature heel rise	Premature rise of the heel during the stance phase of gait.	Stance	Ankle joint or soft tissue structure contracture; hyperactivity of the plantarflexors.
Gluteus maximus lurch	Posterior inclination of the trunk during the stance phase of gait as a compensation for weakness.	Stance	Gluteus maximus weakness.
Quadriceps avoidance pattern	A decrease in the typical amount of flexion seen during stance to prevent excessive anterior tibial translation.	Stance	ACL injury.*
Trendelenburg	Lateral inclination of the trunk during stance phase.	Stance	Weakness of the hip abductions.
Circumduction	Circular movement of the lower extremity into increased abduction.	Swing	Leg-length discrepancy arising from a hip, knee, or ankle joint or soft tissue structure contracture; osseous shortening or lengthening.
Hip hiking	Increased vertical translation of the pelvis.	Swing	Compensation for a leg-length discrepancy.
Scissoring gait	A gait pattern characterized excessive hip adduction.	Swing	Increased adductor tone or recruitment; synergistic pattern of recruitment.
Steppage gait	Excessive hip and knee flexion during the swing phase to allow increased clearance.	Swing	Excessive plantarflexion at the ankle because of a lack of recruitment or excessive tone.
Toe drag	Contact of the foot with the supporting surface throughout swing.	Swing	Impaired dorsiflexor force production; plantarflexor hypertonicity; ankle joint contracture; loss of sensation.
Ataxic	An uncoordinated pattern of gait that can be characterized by difficulty with stability of the trunk or achieving a smooth trajectory with the limb during swing.	Stance and swing	CNS dysfunction; impaired lower extremity sensation.
Stiff-knee gait	Decreased knee flexion	Stance and swing	Compensation for weak knee extensors; pain; increased knee extensor tone; synergistic pattern of recruitment.
Vaulting	Increased vertical translation of the body's center of gravity by plantarflexing at the ankle and increasing knee extension during stance.	Stance and swing	Leg-length difference caused by osseous tissue structure changes; inadequate hip or knee flexion during swing.

CNS, Central nervous system; *ACL,* anterior cruciate ligament.
*Data from Ferber R, Osternig LR, Woollacott MH, et al: *Clin Biomech* (Bristol) 17(4):274-285, 2002; Georgoulis AD, Papadonikolakis A, Papageorgiou CD, et al: *Am J Sports Med* 31(1):75-79, 2003.

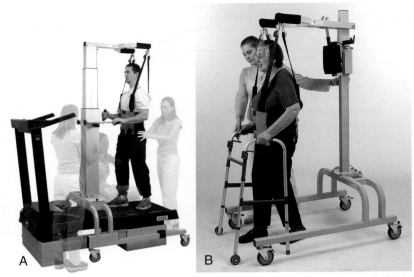

FIG. 32-7 A, Body weight–supported treadmill ambulation. **B,** Body weight–supported gait training with walker. *Courtesy LiteGait System, Mobility Research, Tempe, AZ.*

TABLE 32-9	Gait Dysfunctions and Possible Causes
Gait Dysfunction	**Evaluation and Diagnosis**
Decreased ambulation velocity	Lower extremity weakness
	Tonal increases
	Balance deficits
	Decreased mobility confidence
Asymmetrical step length	Lower extremity weakness
	Tonal increases
Reduced step length	Decreased ambulation velocity
	Reduced capacity for weight bearing on an involved limb
	Impaired lower extremity motor control
Asymmetrical stance and swing phase times	Lower extremity weakness
	Tonal increases
Increased base of support during double stance	Tonal increases
	Osseous changes at the hip or knee
	Valgus deformity at the knee
	Balance deficits
Increase toe in/toe out	Femoral or tibial medial or lateral torsion
	Retroversion or introversion of the hip
	Inadequate dorsiflexion: Joint contracture, gastrocnemius-soleus shortening

Much of the literature on supported ambulation focuses on patients with impairments and functional limitations as a result of central nervous system (CNS) pathology, although unweighting during gait training may also help patients with pain as a result of arthritis to exercise at a sufficient intensity to improve aerobic conditioning.[121] Support by the harness reduces joint loading and ensures patient safety when walking, allowing those who otherwise need a substantial amount of assistance from another person or a device to walk unassisted. Feedback via tactile cues or physical assistance with lower extremity placement can also be provided by the treating therapist.

Strength Training. Since weakness has been shown to affect gait, strength training has been used with the goal of improving gait.[50,122-124] Strength training has been associated with improvements in gait function for patients with a variety of diagnoses[10,16,122-134] and is frequently a component of interventions designed to improve walking performance.

Hip extensor strengthening may also improve walking capacity in elderly adults,[135] and lower extremity strengthening programs have been shown to improve gait function[136] and reduce fall risk in elderly adults.[137,138]

Neurodevelopmental Treatment Approaches. NDT approaches were developed for patients with CNS impairments such as stroke or cerebral palsy.[139] NDT emphasizes the use of verbal and tactile feedback in conjunction with functional retraining to help promote motor skill acquisition. Feedback can be provided either within the context of walking (task-specific training) or as a therapeutic pre-gait activity (non–task-specific training). The theoretical rationale to support the effectiveness of NDT is based on concepts of motor control from the 1950s, and the rationale has recently been updated to reflect a modern understanding of neurophysiology and principles of motor control and motor learning.[137,140]

There are no published randomized controlled trials (RCTs) supporting the effectiveness of NDT in treating individuals with gait dysfunction and non-RCTs have had mixed results. Despite the lack of supporting evidence, NDT approaches continue to be used clinically.

Motor Relearning Programme Approach. The Motor Relearning Programme (MRP) involves practicing the most difficult components of gait.[141] For example, if the patient has difficulty shifting weight onto a paretic limb when walking, then one would work on that element outside the context of gait. For example, in standing, the patient works on shifting weight from the noninvolved limb to the paretic limb.

Balance Training. Balance training has been proposed as an intervention for improving walking; however, there are no studies that indicate that practicing standing balance actually improves gait. This may be because balance control for walking is different from balance control for other activities such as standing.[142] During gait, large muscle groups must counteract the forces generated by movements of the body's COG, whereas in standing, only small muscles around the ankle and knee need to act to control small anterior-posterior perturbations.[142]

In contrast, working on balance within the context of walking may improve walking performance. Activities that may improve walking balance include walking on uneven surfaces, stepping up on to curbs, practicing directional changes, stepping over and around obstacles, and performing multiple tasks such as carrying objects in the upper extremities. Stepping over obstacles has been shown to improve walking speed, stride length, performance on the 6MWT, and the capacity for clearing obstacles, as well as improving the mechanics of walking and thereby reducing its energy demand.[143] Tai chi, which consists of slow, rhythmic movements that emphasize trunk rotation and weight shifting, has been reported to improve gait and reduce fall risk in elderly adults, although its reported effects on gait in healthy adults are mixed.[16,144-147]

CASE STUDY 32-1

GAIT DYSFUNCTION AFTER STROKE

Patient History

MM is a 40-year-old right-handed woman who reports difficulty walking outside of her home, managing steps, and using her right upper extremity for ADLs. She was diagnosed with Hodgkin's lymphoma approximately 2 years ago and was treated with radiation therapy that resulted in stenosis of the left carotid artery that subsequently caused a left-sided stroke 1 year ago. MM reports fatigue when walking more than one-half block, occasional tripping (no falls to date) when walking on uneven surfaces, and difficulty managing steps, particularly when leading up or down with the right lower extremity. MM feels unstable managing steps without a rail, and her maximum reported ambulation distance is one block.

Tests and Measures—Significant Findings
• Heart rate 70 bpm, blood pressure 100/70 mm Hg.

Musculoskeletal
• In standing without her ankle-foot orthosis (AFO) but with her assistive device, the right ankle is maintained in a supinated position with increased lateral weight bearing and the right toes are curled with a hammertoe deformity of the great toe.
• MM has a posterior pelvic tilt and holds her right elbow flexed approximately 20 degrees.

Neuromuscular
• She has occasional difficulty finding words because of mild expressive aphasia.
• Right upper extremity: Volitional control was characterized by a predominance of nonfunctional synergistic movements consisting of shoulder elevation and abduction (0 to 45 degrees) with elbow flexion and pronation or shoulder adduction and internal rotation with elbow extension. No active movement could be elicited at the hand. No isolated movement was noted. Velocity-dependent tonal increases noted for the following: Shoulder external rotation and elbow extension and flexion.
• Right lower extremity: Synergistic movements noted, which consisted of hip flexion and abduction, with knee extension and ankle dorsiflexion, or hip and knee extension with ankle plantarflexion. No isolated volitional movement was noted at any joint. Velocity-dependent tonal increases noted for the knee flexors and extensors. Tonal increases noted for the toe flexors of first digit.

Function
• A molded AFO (MAFO) is used when walking outside the home and in the community.
• MM states she occasionally uses a straight cane when walking outside of her home.
• Increased postural sway noted with the eyes closed while standing, no loss of balance (LOB).
• The following changes in gait were observed (without the use of the MAFO):
  • Unequal step length: Right greater than left.
  • Unequal single stance time: Left greater than right.
  • Decreased knee flexion during both swing and stance phase on the right.
  • Decreased hip extension during stance phase from midstance to preswing on the right.
  • Initial contact on the right occurs with a flat foot at the start of weight acceptance.
  • Increased right ankle inversion at initial contact with rapid pronation at loading response and decreased supination at terminal swing and preswing on the right.
  • Increased toe out and hip external rotation on the right during stance.
  • Delayed initiation of swing phase on the right.
  • Posterior pelvic tilt maintained throughout all phases of gait.
• With the MAFO, MM's pattern of gait was consistent with these observations except that ambulation velocity, step and stride length, and single-stance times were increased.
• 3-m ambulation velocity: 0.7 m/sec without the MAFO
• TUG: 10 seconds
• Wisconsin Gait Scale score (Table 32-10)
• GAITRite Gait Mat data (Table 32-11)

Diagnosis

Preferred practice pattern is 5D: Impaired motor function and sensory integrity associated with nonprogressive disorders of the central nervous system—acquired in adolescence or adulthood.

Interventions

- Task-specific gait training, including walking in an outdoor environment on a variety of surfaces to improve anticipatory control of gait to minimize the potential for tripping.
- Verbal feedback and tactile feedback at the knee and hip to improve swing and stance phase knee control, increase hip extension at terminal stance, and increase step length.
- Gait training on the treadmill (wearing the MAFO) with verbal feedback to emphasize longer step lengths, enhance motor recruitment and relaxation across a range of velocities, and promote improvements in endurance.
- Request consultation or referral for further modification to the MAFO to reduce the amount of plantarflexion in the orthosis.

Role of the Physical Therapist Assistant

- What is the TUG? How is it performed?
- How does the MAFO change this patient's examination results?
- What active means could you use to increase this patient's confidence in her mobility?
- List three additional activities or tasks she could do at home to help her progress.

Additional Information

For the full version of this case study, including detailed examination results, interventions, and outcomes, see the Evolve site that accompanies this book.

CHAPTER SUMMARY

Gait dysfunction, a common problem for patients in rehabilitation, can result from impairments in a variety of diagnostic categories. Systematic gait examination is used to identify the underlying source or cause of gait dysfunction so interventions can be directed to ameliorate the effects of impairment on function and disability. The patient history provides information for the selection of tests and measures. Findings from impairment level tests and measures are combined with information from qualitative or quantitative gait-specific tests and measures to determine a patient diagnosis.

Observational gait analysis is one of the most commonly used qualitative methods of screening for gait dysfunction. Quantitative information can be obtained with simple tools such as stop watch and a measured walkway. Gait velocity, a reliable and valid indicator of gait dysfunction and rehabilitation effectiveness, can easily be calculated and is a widely recognized indicator of performance and level of independence. Gait velocity may be the best measure of function given the ease of measurement, its capacity to objectively document progress, and the link to functional performance and outcomes in a variety of populations with disability. A variety of standardized tests are reliable and valid measures of functional walking and may provide indicators of rehabilitation effectiveness.

TABLE 32-10	Wisconsin Gait Scale Score for Patient in Case Study 32-1
Item	Score
1. Uses assistive device	1
2. Stance time	2
3. Step length	1
4. Weight shift	1
5. Stance width	2
6. Guardedness	2
7. Hip extension	2
8. External rotation in initial swing	2
9. Circumduction	1
10. Hip hiking	2
11. Knee flexion toe off to midswing	2
12. Toe clearance	3
13. Pelvic rotation	1
14. Initial foot contact	2
TOTAL	26

TABLE 32-11	GAITRite Gait Mat Data for Patient in Case Study 32-1				
	Without MAFO		**With MAFO**		
Parameter	Left	Right	Left	Right
Step time (sec)	0.48	0.68	0.42	0.67
Cycle time (sec)	1.16	1.16	1.11	1.09
Step length (cm)	36.08	37.90	48.87	60.24
Stride length (cm)	73.37	73.06	110.74	109.18
Base of support (cm)	11.59	11.55	16.55	17.52
Single support (% gait cycle)	42.2	28.6	43.9	32.6
Double support (% gait cycle)	29.0	28.9	22.1	20.3
Swing (% gait cycle)	28.6	42.4	32.1	44.6
Toe in/toe out (degrees)	8	16	1	4
Velocity (m/sec)	0.625		1.001	
Cadence (steps/min)	101.0		110.1	

MAFO, Molded ankle-foot orthosis.

A number of interventions may be used to address gait dysfunction. Intervention selection is determined in part by patient diagnosis and the experience and training of the clinician. Few RCTs exist to support the effectiveness of gait-directed interventions; however, task-specific gait training and interventions designed to improve lower extremity strength, balance, and cardiovascular endurance are most likely to be helpful. Body weight–supported training can also be effective, although at a greater cost than is possible in many settings.

ADDITIONAL RESOURCES

For links to these and additional web-based resources, see the Evolve site.

Activities-Specific Balance Confidence (ABC) Scale
Berg Balance Scale (BBS)
Dynamic Gait Index (DGI)
Rancho Los Amigos Observational Gait Analysis System
Tinetti's Performance-Oriented Mobility Assessment (POMA)
Wisconsin Gait Scale (WGS)
Craik R, Oatis CA (eds): *Gait analysis: Theory and application,* St. Louis, 1994, Mosby.
Inman VT, Ralston HJ, Todd F, et al*: Human walking,* Baltimore, 1981, Williams & Wilkins.
Perry J: *Gait analysis: Normal and pathological function,* Thorofare, NJ, 1982, SLACK.
Winter DA: *ABC of balance during standing and walking,* Waterloo, Ontario, 1985, Waterloo Biomechanics.
Alfred I. DuPont Gait Lab Online Clinical Cases
Gait and Clinical Movement Analysis Society
Journal of Biomechanics

GLOSSARY

Base of support: The distance between midpoint of the heel of one foot to the same point of the other foot.
Cadence: Number of steps taken in a minute (steps/min).
Double stance: Period of time when both feet are in contact with the supporting surface.
Foot flat: Point in time during the stance phase when the whole plantar surface of the foot is in contact with the supporting surface.
Gait cycle: The events between initial contact of the reference limb or extremity and the successive contact of the same extremity. A gait cycle consists of two successive steps—one right and one left.

Heel off: Point in time during the stance phase when the heel leaves the supporting surface in preparation for starting the swing phase of gait.
Heel strike: Traditional term referring to the moment of contact with the supporting surface at the beginning of the gait cycle.
Initial contact: The point in the gait cycle when the foot initially makes contact with the supporting surface. This represents the start of the stance phase of the gait cycle.
Initial swing: The period in the gait cycle that begins when the reference limb leaves the supporting surface and ends when the knee achieves maximal flexion.
Midstance: The portion of the gait cycle corresponding to the single stance phase of gait; begins when the contralateral limb leaves the supporting surface to begin swing and ends when the stance phase limb is under the body.
Midswing: The point during the swing phase of gait when the extremity passes directly beneath the body.
Preswing: The period of the gait cycle involving the terminal period of double support before the foot is lifted from the supporting surface.
Single support: Period of time when only one foot is in contact with the supporting surface.
Stance phase: The period or phase of the gait cycle that begins when one extremity contacts the ground (heel strike/initial contact) and ends when the same limb leaves the supporting surface (toe off/heel off); comprises approximately 60% of the gait cycle.
Step length: Distance between the point of initial contact of one extremity and the point of initial contact of the opposite extremity.
Step time: The amount of time needed to complete a single step.
Stride length: Distance between the point of initial contact of one extremity to the next point of initial contact of the same extremity.
Stride time (stride/duration): The amount of time required to complete one stride.
Swing phase: The period or phase of the gait cycle when the foot is not in contact with the supporting surface; comprises approximately 40% of the gait cycle.
Terminal swing: Period of the gait cycle that occurs just before contact of the foot with the supporting surface; marked by movement of the reference limb from a vertical position under the body and ends before contact of the foot with the supporting surface.
Toe off: Final phase of stance marked by the toe being the only aspect of the foot in contact with the supporting surface.
Toe out/toe in: Outward or inward angulation of the foot relative to the line marking the forward progression of the body.
Walking velocity: Distance covered per unit time.
Weight acceptance: Period of the gait cycle encompassing the initial contact and loading response phases.

Chapter 33

Assistive Devices for Mobility: Canes, Crutches, Walkers, and Wheelchairs

Joan E. Edelstein

OBJECTIVES

After reading this chapter, the reader will be able to:
1. Relate the patient's examination to selection of assistive devices for mobility.
2. Describe ambulatory and seated assistive devices.
3. Assist the physical therapist in the selection of assistive devices according to the patient's pathology, impairment, and functional limitation.
4. Fit ambulatory and seated assistive devices.
5. Recognize signs and symptoms of assistive device misfit.
6. Safely and appropriately progress devices, within the physical therapist's plan of care, based on the patient's abilities.

*B*eing able to interact with people and the environment is fundamental to quality of life. Bioengineers focused on adaptive or assistive technology have developed a wide range of devices to increase, maintain, or improve the functional capabilities of individuals with disabilities. Many assistive devices can now allow people with mobility impairments to move within the environment easily, efficiently, and safely. More people than ever before are using assistive devices for mobility. The number of people using these types of devices almost doubled between 1980 and 1990,[1] and in 2000, it was estimated that 6.8 million

noninstitutionalized Americans were using assistive **mobility devices** such as canes, walkers, wheelchairs, and scooters.[2]

To select the optimal device for an individual's needs, the physical therapist (PT) performs an examination to clarify the patient's pathology, impairments, and functional limitations, as well as their rehabilitative goals and preferences. The PT will also reexamine the patient over time to reassess the appropriateness of any device and to consider changes that could improve functional mobility and environmental access. The complexity and variability of funding sources and the constant addition of new products and features add to the challenge of selecting the ideal device to meet each individual patient's needs. This chapter outlines how to select, fit, and appropriately progress devices to assist ambulatory and seated mobility.

PATHOLOGY

More than 4 million Americans use canes, and over 1.5 million use walkers to improve their mobility.[3] Assistive devices can aid ambulation for patients with musculoskeletal and neuromuscular disorders. They can improve the comfort and function of people with a wide range of disorders, including osteoarthritis and rheumatoid arthritis,[4-7] hip and knee arthroplasty,[8-14] fractures,[15,16] and lower extremity amputations.[17] Adults and children with neuromuscular disorders, including stroke,[18-25] spinal cord injury,[26-32] cerebral palsy,[33,34] spina bifida,[35] peripheral neuropathies affecting the lower extremity,[36] post-poliomyelitis,[37,38] vestibular dysfunction,[39] Parkinson's disease,[40] and multiple sclerosis,[41] may also achieve greater mobility by using assistive devices. In addition, canes and walkers may be used by healthy elderly adults to reduce the risk of falling.[42-47]

For adults ages 18 to 64 years old, multiple sclerosis, paraplegia, and cerebrovascular disease are the leading conditions associated with the use of wheelchairs and scooters.[2] For those older than 65, osteoarthritis and cerebrovascular disease are the most common diagnoses related to the provision of wheeled devices.

TYPICAL EXAMINATION FINDINGS

PATIENT HISTORY

The patient history helps the clinician develop a broad understanding of the physical impairments causing the

The author would like to thank Steven Leonard for his consultation on this chapter.

need for an assistive device and the internal and external factors that influence the person's mobility needs.

Clinical Pearl

Selection of an assistive device for mobility should take into account expected changes in patient size and expected progression of disease and disability.

Areas addressed include the following:

Demographics What is the patient's age? Will an assistive device need to accommodate physical growth? Does the person attend school, work, or live in an institution?

Health/medical history What primary diagnosis has resulted in the patient's requiring a device? When did the disorder start, and what is the expected progression? Does the patient have any pertinent secondary diagnoses; how may these affect mobility needs? What surgery has the patient undergone, and what future procedures may affect the need for devices?

Psychosocial and cognitive status How important is the appearance of the device to the patient? The behavioral status of a patient influences device selection. The patient may need to understand safety precautions, the gait sequence, weight-bearing precautions, and the possible sequencing of device selection.

Self-management skills Can the patient conduct activities of daily living (ADLs) independently? Does the patient require a device to complete ADLs?

Current mobility equipment What is the patient currently using? Is the device effective? Is the patient satisfied? Should the patient change to a different device, or should the current device be modified? For example, modifying the grip portion of a cane may decrease hypertonic grip responses.

Home and environmental demands Is the device needed for indoor and/or outdoor use? Is the home environment suitable for the device, particularly floor surfaces, stairs, and width of doorways? Is a caregiver present to assist with use of the device?

Transportation What are the transportation needs of the patient? Does the patient need to disassemble the device to place it in a car? Does the patient have assistance with transportation?

Vocational demands What mobility requirements are imposed by the patient's vocational and avocational activities?

Ability to maintain the device Does the patient have the physical and cognitive ability to keep the device in safe working order? Is a caregiver able to maintain the device?

Funding Does the patient's insurance pay for durable medical equipment? Does the patient require assistance to locate funding sources? Recent Medicare regulations governing payment for powered wheelchairs specify that the candidate must be examined by the physician or treating practitioner and that pertinent parts of the medical record kept by the durable medical equipment supplier must be made available to the Centers for Medicare and Medicaid Services.[48]

TESTS AND MEASURES

Musculoskeletal

Posture. An assistive device should be selected and fit to optimize patient function. Optimal patient function will usually be achieved by promoting a more symmetrical, erect posture, although in some cases incorporating or accommodating an abnormal posture may allow the patient to be more independent. The patient's posture is examined as described in detail in Chapter 4. Observed deformities are assessed as either fixed or flexible. Fixed deformities are accommodated by the device selected. With flexible deformities, the device may help reduce the deformity or accommodate it.

Anthropometric Characteristics. When selecting and fitting an ambulatory assistive device, the patient's height and arm length is measured. For wheeled mobility devices, the patient's sitting breadth, thigh length (from buttock to popliteal crease), leg length (from popliteal crease to heel), and general body composition is assessed.

Range of Motion. Passive and active range of motion (ROM), as well as the assumed positions of the joints, will be measured. This component of the examination may be performed with the patient supine or sitting on a mat. ROM affects the selection, fitting, and modification of devices. For example, an individual with a fixed elbow flexion contracture who needs to use a cane, crutch, or walker will need a forearm platform. The position of the patient's joints when sitting on the mat may also give an indication of functional sitting ability to sit and the need for support in a wheelchair. For example, an individual with limited hip flexion who requires a wheelchair will need a back-to-seat angle of more than 90 degrees to accommodate this loss of range.

Muscle Performance. Strength, power, and endurance will be measured as described in detail in Chapter 5. Impairments of strength, power, or endurance are often major factors contributing to a patient's need for an assistive mobility device and affect which device is most suitable for an individual. Patients may need a variety of devices if their strength and endurance vary over time or are expected to worsen.

Joint Integrity and Mobility. Quantitative and qualitative changes in joint integrity and mobility can have substantial bearing on the clinician's final recommendation for a specific device. Impairments of joint integrity or mobility may exclude the use of certain devices or may require the clinician to balance the potential benefits of the device against the injury risk associated with its use. For example, a manually propelled wheelchair may not be suitable for the patient with shoulder joint dysfunction because of the stresses its use places on the shoulder complex.

Neuromuscular

Arousal, Attention, and Cognition. The level of arousal, attention, and cognitive ability affect the individual's ability to use an assistive device. This is particularly important when improper handling of the device may lead to injury to the user or others. Cognition and attention influence the patient's ability to solve logistical problems and learn to negotiate the environment with a new piece of equipment. Various members of the rehabilitation team, including the PT, occupational therapist, speech therapist, physician, and psychologist, may be involved in examining the patient's cognitive abilities.

Pain. Information regarding the location, quality, and intensity of pain can aid in the selection of an assistive device. Baseline data about pain from the initial examination can also be used to assess the effectiveness of a device.

Cranial Nerve Integrity. The cranial nerves (CNs) involved in vision and eye movements (i.e., CN II, III, IV, and VI) may be tested because visual perception can impact the safe operation of an assistive device. In addition, the function of CN VIII may be examined because this may affect balance and thus the need for and choice of a device.

Peripheral Nerve Integrity. Any history, such as numbness or weakness, that might indicate the presence of a neuropathy will be investigated, since weakness or sensory loss, particularly in the upper extremity, may prevent safe or effective use of many assistive devices.

Sensory Integrity. If the patient's history or systems review reveals sensory loss or dysfunction, then sensation will be tested thoroughly. Sensory modalities that may be examined include pain, temperature, touch, proprioception, and vision.

Cardiovascular/Pulmonary. A basic review of the cardiovascular and pulmonary systems, including checking for edema; monitoring heart rate, respiratory rate and pattern, and blood pressure (see Chapter 22); and assessing aerobic capacity and endurance (see Chapter 23), may be performed, since the use of most assistive devices increases energy demand.

Integumentary. The examination includes inspection of the skin, looking particularly for scars, open or healing wounds, grafts, and areas of pressure and any other potential sites of skin and soft tissue breakdown.

EVALUATION, DIAGNOSIS, AND PROGNOSIS

Most patients needing assistive devices for mobility have a range of abnormal examination findings, often including pain, weakness, restricted ROM, and edema from musculoskeletal disorders, and abnormal tone, weakness, and insensitivity from neuromuscular disorders.

Studies evaluating the effectiveness of assistive devices for patients with musculoskeletal and neuromuscular disorders have yielded varied results. People with osteoarthritis or arthroplasty of the hip or knee report that using a cane, particularly when held in the contralateral hand, helps to relieve pain.[5,12] One study reported that people with arthritis walk faster when using crutches than without assistance,[13] but another study found that although adults with hip arthroplasty who used forearm crutches took longer strides and had more symmetrical gait, they walked more slowly than when walking without crutches.[11] In addition, although studies show that assistive devices help reduce pain and improve function, many people do not use prescribed assistive devices,[7] although those who are older or in poorer health and those with greater pain or disability are more apt to use their prescribed devices.[4]

> ### Clinical Pearl
> A cane used in the hand opposite the affected lower extremity can relieve pain in people with osteoarthritis of the hip or knee and increase walking speed and stability in people with hemiparesis.

In patients with hemiparesis, use of a cane on the uninvolved side has been shown to reduce mediolateral and anteroposterior sway and increase walking speed and stability, as well as stance time on the affected leg.[23] Similarly, individuals with peripheral neuropathy affecting the lower extremities have better balance when walking with a cane,[36] and children with spina bifida have less pelvic motion with forearm crutches than without them.[35] People with vestibular disorders have reduced sway when using a cane,[39] and those with Parkinson's disease have less difficulty initiating gait and walk somewhat faster with a wheeled walker.[40] Assistive devices can also improve safety, reduce falls, and thus reduce health care costs in the frail, elderly population.[49]

Despite the documented improvements in function achieved with assistive devices, adults who walk with a cane are apt to be less active than adults of the same age who do not use assistive devices,[44,46] and hospitalized older people who require a cane or walker at the time of discharge have been found to have a higher risk of functional decline than those who were able to walk unaided.[50]

INTERVENTION

SELECTION OF ASSISTIVE DEVICES FOR AMBULATION

Assistive devices for ambulation include canes, crutches, and walkers. Selection is based on the ability of the patient to use the device safely and for the desired function. Additional factors considered in device selection are short- and long-term prognosis and co-morbidities. One or more of the following functions may be served by assistive devices for ambulation:

- Improve balance.
- Assist propulsion.
- Reduce load on one or both lower extremities.
- Transmit sensory cues through the hand(s).
- Enable the individual to obtain the physiological and psychological benefits of upright posture and to maneuver in places inaccessible to a wheelchair.
- Provide a safe environment for patients with cognitive impairment.
- Notify passersby that the user requires special considerations such as additional time when crossing streets or a seat on the bus.

> ### Clinical Pearl
> Selection of assistive devices for ambulation is based on the ability of the patient to use the device safely and the desired function.

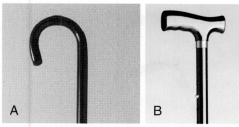

FIG. 33-1 Cane handles. **A,** Inverted U. **B,** Pistol grip. *Copyright Sunrise Medical, Carlsbad, CA.*

At any stage in the rehabilitation process, the clinician must consider the level of stabilization the patient requires for safe mobility. For example, immediately after lower extremity amputation, the patient may require maximal assistance to maintain standing balance because the loss of the limb deprives the person of weight bearing on the amputated side and shifts the center of gravity toward the intact side. Before gait training, the clinician may choose to initiate standing and weight-shifting activities in parallel bars, which provide more stability than crutches or walkers. As the patient gains stability and is able to walk in a protected environment, the clinician may then choose a walker. Later, the clinician may progress the patient to a large-base quadruped cane, then a single-point cane, and eventually walking with no assistive device if the patient can proceed safely. Some patients continue using a cane outdoors to signal others that they need extra time or assistance. When walking long distances, they may also use a cane to reduce load on the amputated side.

Canes. The simplest assistive device for ambulation is the cane. It offers balance or light support, as well as sensory feedback, from the walking surface. Canes are made from a variety of sturdy materials, such as walnut, oak, and other woods; metal, especially aluminum; and plastics, such as acrylics (e.g., Lucite), as well as fiberglass and carbon fiber. Canes can be decorated in many colors and patterns.

There are several kinds of cane handles (Fig. 33-1). The basic handle is an inverted U, which permits one to hang the cane over the forearm or the back of a chair when not walking with it. Other handle options include a pistol grip, handles designed to contact more of the hand to increase comfort, and a handle designed to keep the wrist in a neutral rather than an extended position.

Cane shafts may be solid, straight, offset, folding, or height adjustable (Fig. 33-2). Solid straight shafts are the least expensive and most durable. The SuperCane has an offset shaft with a higher hand grip for walking and a lower hand grip for coming to stand from sitting. Folding canes are easier to store; an adult-sized cane can be folded to approximately 1 foot in length. One type of cane has a force measuring device in the shaft and a feedback mechanism in the handle to let the user know how much weight they are transferring to the cane. This can be helpful for patients who need to limit loading on an affected lower extremity.

The base of the cane is usually a single rubber tip (Fig. 33-3). It should be broad with deep grooves and kept clean to provide maximum traction. Other designs include the

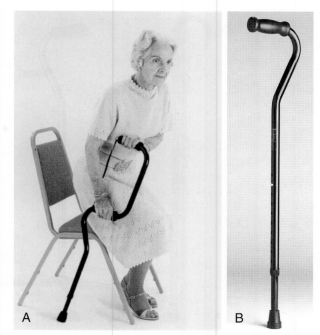

FIG. 33-2 Cane shafts. **A,** SuperCane. **B,** Offset shaft with adjustable height. ***A** courtesy Momentum Medical, Des Moines, Iowa; **B** copyright Sunrise Medical, Carlsbad, CA.*

standard or wide-based quadruped (quad) base, made of a rectangle with tips off each corner. Having these four tips increases the base of support but may not be any more effective than a standard single tip for improving balance or reducing pain.[51,52] More novel designs include the side walker/cane or hemi-walker, which has four widely spaced rubber tips to increase stability, especially when used unilaterally by a patient with hemiplegia. Another base has a spring-loaded tip to absorb shock at initial contact. The AbleTripod has a flexible triangular tip that maintains floor contact at a wide range of shaft angles; this tip also absorbs shock. To increase stability when the user walks on ice or snow, the cane may have a retractable metal spike. The Pilot Rolling Cane has an L-shaped base fitted with three **casters**, providing the user with the support of a **quad cane** without the need to lift the cane with each step. It also has a brake in the handle for added stability. The Pilot Step-Up Cane has a broad base with a flip-up platform that allows patients to maneuver over curbs and stairs without losing cane support. The user pushes a button on the handle to flip the hinged platform open to enable stepping half the distance of the conventional 8-inch step. With the step retracted, the cane functions as a standard quad cane. The cane also has a second handle farther down on the shaft to facilitate rising from toilets and other bench-type seats.

Several canes are specifically designed to allow adults with unilateral lower extremity amputation to ambulate without a prosthesis (Fig. 33-4). The iWALKFree has a platform on a vertical shaft to support the transtibial amputation limb; the patient supports weight through the thigh and knee. The iWALKFree can also be used in place of standard crutches for patients with non–weight-bearing lower leg injuries, including fractures, sprains, tendon

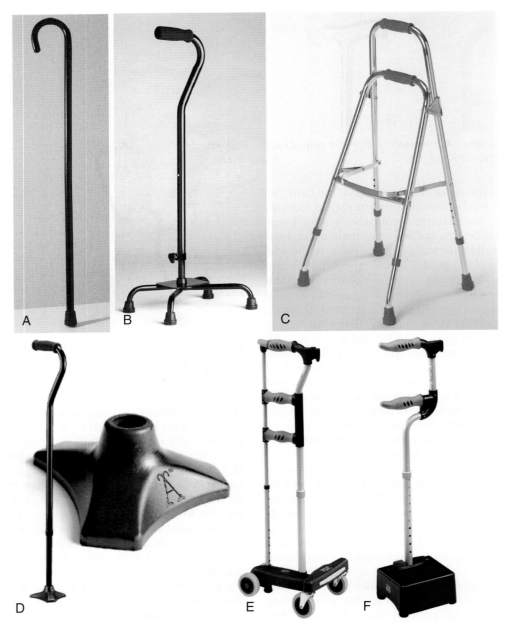

FIG. 33-3 Cane bases. **A,** Single tip. **B,** Quad. **C,** Side walker. **D,** AbleTripod. **E,** Rolling. **F,** Step-up. *A, B, and C copyright Sunrise Medical, Carlsbad, CA; D courtesy L.A. Care; E and F courtesy Full Life Products, Moorestown, NJ.*

damage, foot ulcers, or amputations. The ED Walker has a bicycle seat mounted on top of a vertical shaft and a second curved shaft with a platform for the amputation limb. Both of these devices have a stationary base. The Roll-A-Bout has four wheels. This folding device has a cushioned platform for the lower leg and a handle that the user holds while propelling with the opposite foot.

Most patients who use a cane to assist with ambulation use one cane, usually on the side opposite the affected lower extremity, although some people use a pair of canes for added stability. A few individuals may refuse to use a cane, regarding it as a sign of disability or senility. Some people with visual impairment use a long cane to transmit sensory cues through the hand. The lower portion of the shaft is painted red to alert passersby not to impede them (Fig. 33-5).[53-57]

Crutches. The four major types of crutches are the underarm or axillary, triceps, forearm **(Lofstrand crutches),** and platform crutches (Fig. 33-6). Crutches, regardless of design, are usually used in pairs.

Underarm Crutches. Underarm crutches, also known as **axillary crutches,** are made of wood, aluminum, or titanium (Fig. 33-6, *A*). Although they are called underarm or axillary crutches, patients should never support themselves on the crutch through the axilla because the crutch may impinge on superficial nerves and blood vessels. The top of the crutch should be held firmly against the side of the chest. The top of the crutch is usually covered with

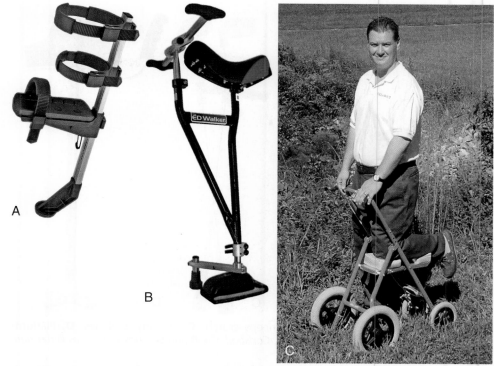

FIG. 33-4 Canes for people with lower extremity amputation. **A**, iWalkFree. **B**, ED Walker. **C**, Roll-A-Bout. **A** *courtesy Thomas Fetterman, Southampton, PA;* **B** *courtesy Hartford Walking Systems, Syracuse, NY;* **C** *courtesy Roll-A-Bout Corporation, Frederica, DE.*

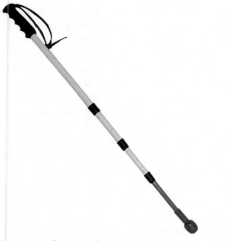

FIG. 33-5 Long cane for people with visual impairment. *Courtesy RehabMart, Winterville, GA*

sponge rubber to increase friction and cushion stress against the user's lateral chest or ribcage. The Easy Strutter Functional Orthosis System has a crutch top that includes, in addition to the underarm piece, a cushioned strap intended to go over the shoulder to distribute weight over a broad, pressure-tolerant area. This crutch also has two parallel struts that terminate in a broad, spring-loaded shock-absorbing base. When three-point gait with regular axillary crutches was compared to performance with the Easy Strutter Functional Orthosis System, the latter put less stress on the palms and subjects also reported feeling more secure on level surfaces and stairs with the novel crutches.[58]

> ### ◎ *Clinical Pearl*
> To avoid compression of nerves and vessels in the axilla, the top of an axillary underarm crutch should be held firmly against the side of the chest and never in the axilla.

The shape of the crutch handle does not appear to affect function or comfort.[59] The handle should have a resilient cover to cushion compressive stress on the palm. The shaft of a metal crutch has several spring-loaded detents to expedite adjusting length and hand-grip height. The traditional shaft bifurcates partway up from the base; however, streamlined single-shaft crutches are available. The usual crutch tip is rubber; however, many tips described for canes can also be used on crutches. Crutches can also have a spring-loaded mechanism at the distal end to absorb shock at impact. This type of mechanism was found in a limited trial to reduce shock waves and peak stresses.[60] Rocker-bottom crutches are also available. Studies conflict on whether this does[61,62] or does not[63] reduce energy consumption as compared with single-tip crutches.

Triceps Crutches. **Triceps crutches** are always made of aluminum (Fig. 33-6, *B*). Triceps crutches, sometimes known as Warm Springs crutches, were popularized at the Roosevelt Institute for Rehabilitation in Warm Springs, GA, during the poliomyelitis epidemic in the twentieth century. The crutch is intended for use by patients with

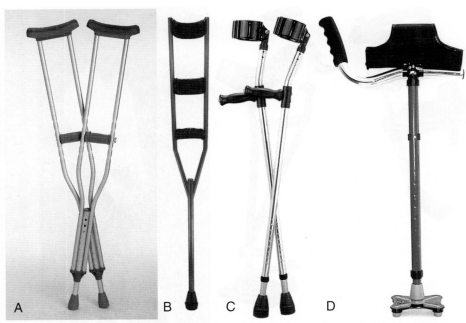

FIG. 33-6 A, Underarm crutches. **B,** Triceps crutch. **C,** Forearm crutches. **D,** Platform crutch. *A and C copyright Sunrise Medical, Carlsbad, CA; B and D courtesy Thomas Fetterman, Southampton, PA.*

paralyzed shoulder muscles. The proximal portion of each crutch has medial and lateral uprights joined by a pair of posterior bands that keep the elbow extended, mimicking the action of the triceps muscle. The distal part of the crutch is a single shaft with a rubber tip at the base.

Forearm (Lofstrand, Canadian) Crutches. Forearm crutches are made of aluminum or titanium with a vinyl-covered steel forearm cuff (Fig. 33-6, *C*). Forearm crutches provide more support than a cane but less trunk support than crutches and allow the patient to have their hands free when not needing support as may be the case when standing. Forearm crutches allow adjustment of length and cuff position. A folding model convenient for storage is also available. A less restrictive cuff known as the Kenny Armband, named after Sister Kenny, a pioneering clinician who treated patients with poliomyelitis, is available and is used by some individuals with post-polio syndrome and by some people with cerebral palsy.

Platform Crutches. Platform crutches have a horizontal support for bearing weight on the forearm (Fig. 33-6, *C*). These crutches are used by patients, such as those with upper extremity fractures, who cannot tolerate weight transmission through the hand, wrist, or forearm.

Walkers. Walkers are frames, usually made of aluminum, designed to provide support through both arms without the control needed to use a pair of canes or crutches. Walkers come in a variety of styles. The base may be fixed, requiring the patient to pick up the walker to move it, or wheeled, so it can be advanced by rolling. The uprights may be rigid, folding, reciprocating, or stair climbing. In addition, various hand grips and platforms, as well as accessories, such as a seat or a basket, can be added to many walkers.

Basic wheeled and pickup walkers are available in various sizes to accommodate a range of patient heights and trunk girths. Adaptations can be added to many walkers. For example, direct-forming thermoplastic can be added to the handles to improve conformation to the user's hand and reduce the risk of compression trauma. The child with cerebral palsy may walk with more erect posture with a walker fitted with hip guards or with a Rear Walker in which the walker is used posteriorly.[33,34,64] A motorized robotic walker is being developed by the Veterans Affairs Personal Adaptive Mobility Aid Laboratory for use by the elderly or adults with visual impairments.[65]

Pickup Walkers. **Pickup walkers** are the simplest walkers (Fig. 33-7), with four legs ending in rubber tips. They are stable and sturdy but must be lifted with each step. They are appropriate for patients with poor balance, patients who are non–weight-bearing on one lower extremity, and for use on high-friction surfaces such as carpet, grass, and gravel. Walker uprights may be height adjustable. The front uprights of the Rising Star Super-Walker are angled with upper and lower handles for the patient to use when rising from a chair and to provide stability when the patient is upright.

Rolling Walkers. Rolling walkers have two or more wheels at the base (Fig. 33-8). They can be pushed forward without having to pick up the walker and provide moderate stability and are suitable for use on smooth surfaces, such as hardwood flooring and vinyl tiles. Many rolling walkers have two front wheels and two rubber tips on the rear uprights. Tennis balls or other glides on the rear uprights reduce friction and may ease ambulation. The Strider and Wenzelite walkers have adjustable wheels and handles. The foldable Red Dot Walker has front swivel 5-inch wheels and rear glide brakes. The Walkabout has an upper portion that encircles the user's shoulders. It also has a built-in seat with a basket.[66] Other walkers with seats include the folding steel Merry Walker and the

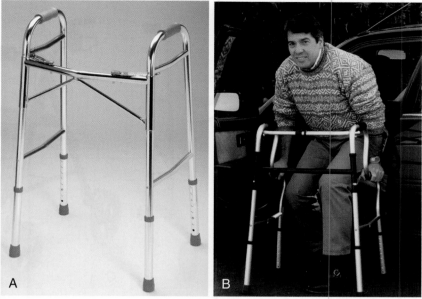

FIG. 33-7 Pickup walkers. **A,** Standard. **B,** Rising Star. *A copyright Sunrise Medical, Carlsbad, CA; **B** courtesy Momentum Medical, Des Moines, IA.*

polyvinylchloride Dura-Walker, both designed to provide a secure environment for patients with cognitive impairment; their bulkiness impedes passage through narrow doorways. The steel U-Step Walker has a padded seat, hand brakes, folding mechanism, and an optional laser light intended to encourage patients with Parkinson's disease to step forward. Some walkers have a reciprocating mechanism to facilitate stepping. The Universal Stair Climbing Walker is intended to aid the patient when climbing a staircase.

◎ *Clinical Pearl*

Tennis balls on the feet of the rear uprights of a front-wheeled walker can reduce friction and ease ambulation.

Three-Wheeled Walkers. Three-wheeled walkers have three angled uprights, each ending in a wheel; they are easier to maneuver in narrow corridors than traditional walkers with four uprights (see Fig. 33-8, *E*).

FITTING OF ASSISTIVE DEVICES FOR AMBULATION

An assistive device must fit properly for the patient to walk most comfortably and with the least effort.[47,67] A properly adjusted and positioned device keeps the patient's line of gravity within the base of support created by the device and the patient's feet.

◎ *Clinical Pearl*

Proper fit of an assistive device, keeping the patient's line of gravity within the base of support, is necessary for the patient to walk most comfortably and with the least amount of effort.

The height of any device and the position of the handles should be assessed when all accessories, such as rubber tips, hand cushions, and top pad, are installed and with the patient wearing the type of shoes they would usually wear when using the device. Measurements should be performed with the patient standing erect in a secure environment such as in parallel bars. The following guidelines apply for most circumstances but may need to be modified, depending on the patient's size, available joint excursion, and strength, as well as expected gait pattern.

Canes. When holding a cane by its handle, its height should allow the elbow to be slightly flexed, at less than 30 degrees, and the tip of the cane should be 6 inches out diagonally from the toes at a 45-degree angle.[68,69] If the cane is too long, the user may bend backward or place insufficient weight on the cane. If it is too short, the user will tend to bend too far forward. Canes with a broad base, rather than a single tip, should be positioned so that the edge that flares laterally faces away from the shoe to avoid the base hitting the ankle during the swing phase of gait.

Crutches

Underarm Crutches. A crutch should extend from a point approximately 2 inches (2 fingerbreadths) below the axilla to a point on the floor 6 inches out diagonally from the toes at a 45-degree angle.[70] The hand piece should generally be placed so that the elbows flex about 30 degrees and the hand is at the level of the greater trochanter.[71] The elbows should be flexed a little more if the patient will use a gait that requires raising both feet from the floor simultaneously such as the drag-to, swing-to, or swing-through patterns.

Forearm Crutches. The forearm cuff should lie on the proximal third of the forearm. The crutch tip should be 5 to 10 cm lateral and 15 cm anterior to the shoe when the patient is standing with the crutch hand piece adjusted to provide 15 to 30 degrees of elbow flexion.

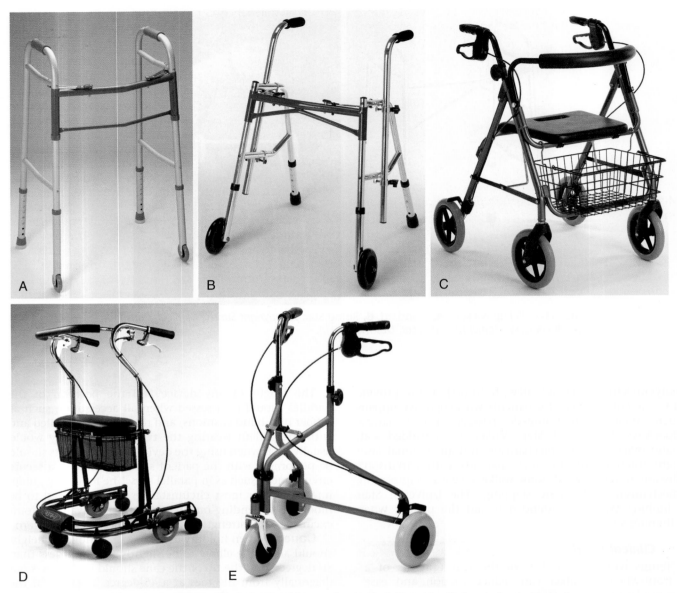

FIG. 33-8 Rolling walkers. **A,** Fixed front wheels. **B,** Adjustable. **C,** Four wheels. **D,** U step. **E,** Three-wheeled walker. *Copyright Sunrise Medical, Carlsbad, CA.*

Triceps Crutches. The upper cuff should contact the proximal third of the upper arm, approximately 5 cm below the anterior fold of the axilla. The lower cuff should lie 1 to 4 cm below the olecranon process, avoiding bony contact, yet providing adequate stability.[72]

Platform Crutches. The platform should be angled so that the forearm rests at a 90-degree angle to the upper arm, affording the greatest comfort and control of the crutch. The height should allow the person to stand upright with the shoulders relaxed. If platform crutches are too short, the user will have to lean forward. If they are too long, they can force the shoulders up and cause compression of the radial or suprascapular nerve.

Walkers. When holding a walker, the elbows should be flexed approximately 15 degrees.[39] Slight elbow flexion allows for some downward push on the walker, allowing the patient to bear some weight through the upper extremities. If the handles are too low, the patient may keep their elbows extended or bend too far forward, and if using a front-wheeled walker, they may push harder and hinder wheel rotation. Forward bending of the trunk can also inhibit hip extension during the stance phase of gait and by moving the center of gravity forward, can interfere with forward weight shifting, making it difficult to achieve adequate propulsion during terminal stance. If the handles are too high, the patient may need to flex the elbows more and lean excessively on the walker or push the walker farther forward from the trunk, increasing the risk of falling if this places the person's center of gravity behind the walker's base of support.

Complications of Assistive Device Use. It is not uncommon for musculoskeletal and neurovascular complications to develop when canes, walkers, and crutches are adjusted improperly or used incorrectly.[73] Problems can occur in the hand, arm, shoulder, or axilla. Injury to the radial,[74-76] ulnar,[77] median,[78,79] radial palmar,[80] and suprascapular[81] nerves have all been reported. Improperly fitted or used underarm crutches can cause axillary artery thrombosis.[82-84] Even when using properly adjusted crutches, some people develop painful abrasions of the lateral chest, shoulder pain, tenderness or bruising over the medial aspect of the arm, cramping of the triceps, or wrist osteoarthritis[85] or exert undue stress on the ulna.[86] Misuse of walkers has also been implicated in falls among some patients.[87]

WHEELCHAIR SELECTION

Although wheeled mobility can be achieved with many devices, such as scooters, adult tricycles, golf carts, hand-controlled cycles, sports wheelchairs, and standing motorized wheeled platforms, manual and powered wheelchairs are the most commonly used wheeled mobility devices. All wheelchairs enable the seated occupant to move or be moved about in the environment. Seated mobility is generally selected when the patient cannot ambulate safely or when the energy demands of ambulation limit functional ambulation distance. Many patients use a cane or a walker to assist with walking short distances and have someone push them in a wheelchair for longer distances. Wheelchairs can thus improve safety and participation.

> ◎ *Clinical Pearl*
>
> When the energy demands of ambulation are too great or when the patient cannot ambulate safely, seated mobility is an appropriate alternative.

Selection of a wheelchair should be based on a thorough examination of the patient's current and anticipated needs, as well as environmental, activity, and financial constraints. Although environmental constraints, such as narrow doorways or carpeted floor, can often be modified, an alternative wheelchair design or component may be more cost-effective. For example, wheelchair wheels with less camber or a narrowing device installed on the wheelchair may allow the chair to pass through a narrow doorway. A wheelchair with solid or semipneumatic tires is easier to propel over carpeted floors than one with pneumatic tires. Negotiating stairs and hoisting the wheelchair into an automobile require less strength and effort with a lightweight wheelchair, and a folding wheelchair can be transported more easily than one with a rigid frame.[88] Goals of wheelchair selection include the following:

- Providing comfort
- Supporting postural alignment to address:
  - Balance
  - Prevention or correction of flexible deformities
  - Accommodation of fixed deformity
  - Normalizing tone
  - Protecting skin integrity

- Facilitating function of:
  - Respiration
  - Swallowing and digestion
  - Circulation
  - Communication
  - Seated activities
  - Mobility

In addition to these goals, the wheelchair must allow for weight shifting and transfers. Patients must shift weight periodically while seated to avoid debilitating and sometimes life-threatening skin breakdown. This is usually done by transferring weight onto the patient's arms despite the fact that this places high loads on the shoulder and elbow joints,[89] especially for those with tetraplegia.[90] A firm cushion makes this type of weight shifting easier. In addition, the chair may have a seat-back tilt and recline mechanism to allow for weight shifting without weight bearing through the arms. How a patient is expected to transfer into and out of the wheelchair influences wheelchair selection and fitting, particularly seat height and angle, wheel and footrest placement, and armrest position.

WHEELCHAIR FEATURES

The basic wheelchair prescription should specify the following:

- Mode of propulsion
- Frame
- Seat, including seat cushion
- Backrest, including insert
- Armrests, including lapboard
- Front rigging (i.e., footrests and leg rests)
- Wheels, including tires, casters, hand rims, and brakes
- Support accessories

When feasible, the clinician should test wheelchair options by simulating various choices with a highly adjustable wheelchair. Many long-term users of manual and electrically powered wheelchairs have customized wheelchairs to optimize function, including posture and reach.[91] However, since customizing adds to cost, persons with limited funds, particularly the elderly, often do not have customizable wheelchairs.[92]

Mode of Propulsion

Dependent Propulsion. Dependent mobility is when the chair is propelled by someone other than the occupant (Fig. 33-9). Shower chairs, standing and seating systems, recliners, and tilt-in-space systems are often pushed by a caregiver. The frame of this type of chair usually does not fold, making it sturdy and relatively inexpensive but cumbersome to transport and store. One should always consider the physical capabilities of the caregiver who will assist the occupant of a wheelchair when selecting a chair for dependent propulsion. Caregiver training can improve use and safety, and as little as 50 minutes of wheelchair-handling skills training has been shown to carry over into skills that are retained for at least 6 months.[93]

Independent Manual Propulsion. Manual wheelchairs can be propelled by the patient independently using upper and/or lower extremity power (Fig. 33-10). Wheelchairs intended for independent manual propulsion have either

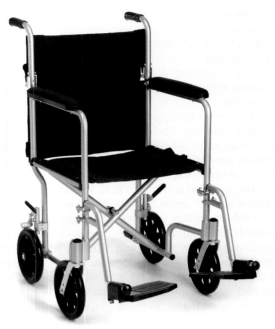

FIG. 33-9 Dependent propulsion wheelchair. *Copyright Sunrise Medical, Carlsbad, CA.*

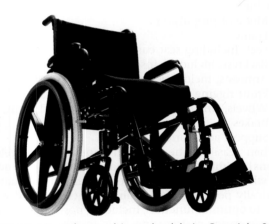

FIG. 33-10 Manual propulsion wheelchair. *Copyright Sunrise Medical, Carlsbad, CA.*

a folding or rigid frame and can be made of steel or other more lightweight materials. Aluminum, titanium, graphite, or magnesium wheelchairs weigh about half as much as a steel wheelchair.[94] Among able-bodied subjects, using a lightweight wheelchair reduces the frequency of collisions but increases the frequency of the front casters leaving the ground, as compared with using a standard-weight wheelchair.[95] It is recommended that patients with spinal cord injury use lightweight adjustable wheelchairs as these are associated with a lower incidence of upper extremity pain and injury.[96] The lightweight wheelchair is also easier for the patient and caregiver to lift when placing it in a car. Although a folding frame makes a wheelchair easier to transport, a rigid frame increases strength and durability while reducing weight and vibration.

The position and camber (angle) of the rear wheels, the size of the wheels or casters, and the type of hand rim can all affect the ease and efficiency of wheelchair propulsion. For most patients, positioning the rear axle as far forward as possible without compromising stability optimizes upper extremity propulsion. Using cambered wheels, which are closer together at the top than at the bottom, makes it easier to reach the top of the wheel while also increasing the stability of the wheelchair. But the greater overall width of the chair imposed by cambered wheels can limit access in narrow areas. Larger wheels and casters make it easier to propel the wheelchairs on carpet or rough ground. A hand rim with two driving rings can be placed on one of the wheels to allow for independent propulsion of the two rear wheels by the patient who can only use one hand.

A manual wheelchair may be propelled using the upper and/or lower extremities, depending on the individual's strength, ROM, and coordination, as well as his or her cardiopulmonary fitness. A manually propelled wheelchair is usually pushed by holding the hand rims on the wheels. Arm cranks and arm levers are also available, but these have not been shown to improve energy efficiency during wheelchair propulsion.[97]

The pectoralis major and anterior deltoid muscles are the primary muscles used for wheelchair propulsion.[98] They work together with the supraspinatus, infraspinatus, and the long head of the biceps to move the wheels and thus the wheelchair forward. The middle and posterior deltoid and the supraspinatus muscles contract to extend the arm during the recovery phase of propulsion.[99] Upper body strength training can improve wheelchair propulsion skill.[100] When using the lower extremities for wheelchair propulsion, using both legs is more energy efficient and quicker than using one leg, even in people with hemiplegia.[101]

Independent Powered Propulsion. When a patient does not have the physical capability to propel a manual wheelchair, an electrically powered wheelchair or scooter may be used to provide independent propulsion (Fig. 33-11). Changing from a manual to a powered wheelchair can often increase independence and improve occupational performance in patients with mobility limitations.[102] An electric wheelchair can be controlled and steered with a joystick if the user has good hand function. For those with limited manual dexterity, the chair can be adapted for control with virtually any other type of volitional action such as chin or head movement, sip-and-puff breathing, or visual scanning. Electrically powered wheelchairs vary greatly in their stability, braking, the user's energy consumption,[103] and durability.[104] Most powered wheelchair users consider reaching, moving in confined spaces, and avoiding collisions more important than speed and avoiding the need to drive backward.[105] Therefore patients with powered wheelchairs should be taught maneuvering skills as part of wheelchair training.

> ## ◎ *Clinical Pearl*
>
> Changing from a manual to a powered wheelchair can often increase independence and improve occupational performance in people with mobility limitations.

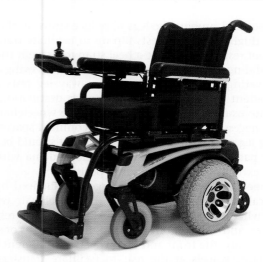

FIG. 33-11 Powered propulsion wheelchair. *Copyright Sunrise Medical, Carlsbad, CA.*

Combination Manual and Powered Wheelchairs. Hybrid manual and electrically powered wheelchairs usually have a motor on the rear wheels to supplement the force the user exerts on the hand rims of the chair's rear wheels. This decreases the workload for the user and may allow weaker patients to propel themselves independently.[106]

Frame. The basic wheelchair has a frame with vertical posterior uprights with push handles attached for a caregiver to use when the occupant is not propelling the wheelchair. Wheelchairs intended for patients with lower extremity amputations have the posterior uprights angled to position the rear wheels farther back than usual to increase stability, particularly when ascending ramps.

Seat. Most people who depend on a wheelchair for mobility are seated for extended periods every day. The basic leatherette sling seat typically found in a transportation wheelchair intended for occasional brief use is inexpensive and easy to fold but is not suitable for long-term use because it does not distribute pressure evenly and tends to maximize pressure on the tissue overlying the ischial tuberosities. Augmenting this sling seat with a solid, firm base with a cushion may be sufficient for patients who intend to use the wheelchair for short periods.

Seat Cushion. For patients expected to spend many hours each day in a wheelchair for months or years, a specialized seat cushion should be used. The cushion lies under the patient's buttocks and thighs and should distribute pressure widely while also dissipating moisture and heat and reducing shear. This improves comfort, reduces the risk of tissue breakdown, and contributes to postural control and stability. A wide range of wheelchair cushions are available and made of different materials and with different designs (see Additional Resources for wheelchair cushion manufacturers).

The cushion may be made of plastic or rubber foam. Foam cushions vary in density, thickness, memory (ability to return to their original shape), and cell type (open or closed). Thicker foam cushions have been found to decrease subcutaneous pressure more than thinner

cushions, but they can also increase subcutaneous shear stress.[107] Because foam is solid, it generally provides a fairly stable surface for postural control. It can also easily be carved or molded specifically for the individual to accommodate postural variation. Foam is flammable, which may be hazardous if the patient smokes.[108] In general, foam is relatively inexpensive and requires little maintenance except for changing and laundering the cloth cover when it becomes soiled.

Wheelchair cushions may also be made of a vinyl-covered viscous synthetic gel. This type of cushion can be used alone over a flat wheelchair seat or in combination with a rigid contoured seating surface if more stability is desired. **Gel cushions** require little maintenance, but the vinyl cover of the pack can tear, causing the gel to leak out. They are also heavier than foam cushions.

Cushions made of multiple air or fluid cells are also available. These types of cushions do not provide as much postural control and stability as solid cushions, but they distribute pressure very effectively. The air or liquid conforms to the bony prominences, equalizing pressure over the entire sitting surface. Air pressure between 17 and 42 mm Hg provides optimal reduction in interface pressure at the ischial tuberosities for patients with spinal cord injury.[109] This type of cushion needs to be looked after carefully because it is easily punctured.

Hybrid cushions made of more than one type of material are also available. These are intended to provide the desirable characteristics of each material. For example, a contoured foam cushion with a cut-out for placement of air cells under the buttocks may be used to give postural support while also distributing pressure at bony prominences.

To assess for adequacy of off-loading by a wheelchair cushion, place one's hand between the cushion and the seat of the wheelchair. If the bony prominence is palpable, the surface is said to have "bottomed out" and is not off-loading sufficiently.

Backrest. The backrest of a wheelchair is usually made of leatherette and attached to the frame. Backrests are available in various heights; for example, a patient with poor neck control may benefit from an extended high backrest (Fig. 33-12). Someone who needs to transfer backward from the wheelchair may require a backrest with a vertical zipper or snap fasteners. Backrest tilt-and-recline mechanisms can reduce fatigue by enabling the user to breathe more efficiently, improve pressure distribution to increase comfort and postural stability, and can enhance visual orientation. Backrest support may be increased by adding a solid insert with cushioning, although functional evaluation of 27 subjects with recent spinal cord injury tested with 4 different back supports found that for most activities, the type of back support did not affect activity participation.[110]

Armrests. Wheelchair armrests may be fixed, flip-away, or removable, with the latter facilitating transfers in and out of the wheelchair. The front of the armrests may be straight or desk style to allow them to fit under a desk (Fig. 33-13). Some armrests are adjustable to accommodate elbow flexion contractures. A tray may be added to the armrests to allow the user to eat and engage in other

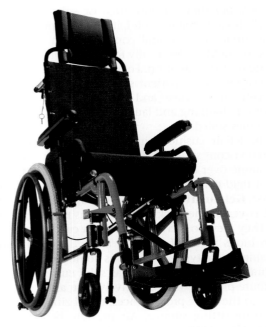

FIG. 33-12 Wheelchair with extended high backrest. *Copyright Sunrise Medical, Carlsbad, CA.*

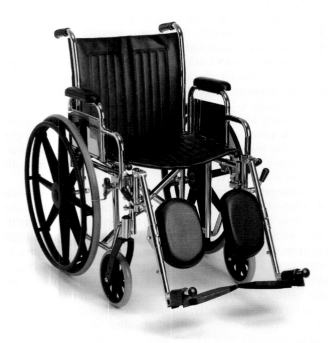

FIG. 33-13 Wheelchair with desk armrests and elevating leg rests. *Copyright Sunrise Medical, Carlsbad, CA.*

manual activities while sitting in the wheelchair. The tray can make it harder to get out of the chair, which may be cumbersome but may also improve safety in patients with poor safety awareness and standing balance who might otherwise try to stand up from the chair without assistance.

Front Rigging. There are many different types of footrests and leg rests. Footrests are used to keep the feet off the floor and support the legs to reduce stress on the posterior thighs. Most footrests flip up to facilitate transfers. The foot rests usually have a heel strap to prevent the feet from sliding backward. Leg rests may be fixed, swing away, or elevating (see Fig. 33-13). Swing-away leg rests allow the patient to get close to the transfer destination. Leg rests are usually detachable to reduce the wheelchair size when necessary for maneuvering in confined spaces. Elevating leg rests with a cushioned calf pad should be used if the patient would otherwise develop edema with the lower extremities in a dependent position.

Wheels. Wheel selection is largely influenced by the physical environment in which the wheelchair will be used, whether indoors or outdoors, with firm or resilient surfaces, and whether one needs to traverse curbs or stairs.

Generally, the front and rear wheels are different sizes, with large wheels at the rear to facilitate transfers and foster more erect sitting posture when the occupant propels the wheelchair. However, putting large wheels in the front makes it is easier to turn in confined spaces. In addition, moving the seat closer to the rear wheels reduces rolling resistance, making the wheelchair easier to propel.[111]

Large wheels have pneumatic or semipneumatic tires. Semipneumatic tires are recommended if the wheelchair will only be used indoors. Pneumatic tires are recommended if one wants to traverse soft or rough terrain. They should be inflated to 100 lb per square inch (psi) of pressure. Lower tire pressures will increase energy expenditure during wheeling.[112,113] The large wheels should have toggle or lever type brakes that should be engaged whenever the patient transfers to or from the wheelchair.

Smaller wheels are known as casters. Larger diameter casters make the ride smoother; smaller diameter casters provide for ease of maneuverability and mobility. Casters generally have solid rubber tires.

Hand rims are attached to the large wheels to allow the user to turn the wheels without soiling the hands. The hand rims are usually chrome plated, but vinyl coating, knobs, and projections are available to facilitate use by those with poor grip. The patient with unilateral upper extremity amputation or paralysis may benefit from a one-arm drive mechanism, in which both hand rims are placed on one side.

Support Accessories. Patients with poor trunk control, such as some individuals with cerebral palsy, muscular dystrophy, amyotrophic lateral sclerosis, or tetraplegia, may be more secure in a wheelchair equipped with supportive pads or other accessories. A medial thigh support (synonyms: Hip abductor, **pommel**, anti-adductor pad, abductor post, abduction wedge, or knee abductor) maintains the hips in the prescribed amount of abduction and prevents hip adduction. Lateral thigh supports (synonyms: Lateral knee adductor or adduction pads) prevent excessive or unwanted hip abduction and control hip external rotation. Lateral pelvic supports (synonyms: Hip support pads, lateral hip blocks, pelvic support, side cushions, or hip guides) maintain the lower trunk centered in the seat and provide counterforce to help control pelvic obliquity in conjunction with lateral thoracic supports. An anterior pelvic support (synonym: seat belt) prevents the occupant

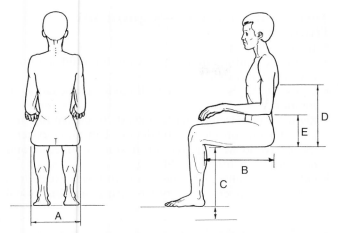

FIG. 33-14 General guidelines for wheelchair measurement. **A,** Seat width. **B,** Seat depth. **C,** Seat height. **D,** Backrest height. **E,** Armrest height. *Adapted from Wilson AB Jr: Wheelchairs: A prescription guide, New York, 1992, Demos Publications.*

from sliding forward on the seat. Seat belts are particularly important to prevent falls from electrically powered wheelchairs.[114]

⊚ Clinical Pearl

Supportive pads or other accessories can be added to a wheelchair to assist with positioning, particularly trunk and hip control.

WHEELCHAIR FITTING

Ideally, during wheelchair fitting, the patient is seated in an adjustable wheelchair in the most erect posture obtainable and wearing the shoes and orthoses he or she will use in the final wheelchair. If the person has extensive paralysis or very poor trunk control, then two or more people may need to support the patient while the lead clinician measures the person. Fig. 33-14 and the next section provide general guidelines for wheelchair dimensions. These may need to be modified for patients with special needs such as trunk deformity or unusual proportions.

Seat

Width. The width of the seat affects the occupant's comfort and posture, as well as which doorways and other narrow areas the wheelchair can pass through. The seat should be 1 to 2 inches wider than the widest part of the trunk in the frontal plane. The widest trunk measurement is usually the distance between the hips near the level of the greater trochanters in sitting. If the seat is too narrow, there will be too much pressure on the trochanters and lateral aspects of the thighs and squeezing the tissue will also be uncomfortable. It is also difficult to transfer into and out of an unduly narrow seat. If the seat is too wide, it will be hard for the patient to reach the hand rims of a manually propelled wheelchair, and the wheelchair may not pass through narrow doorways. The patient may also develop postural asymmetry if they lean to one side to support one forearm on an armrest. Asymmetrical posture can also interfere with respiration, speech, and

swallowing and may lead to high pressure concentration on the portion of the trunk in greatest contact with the backrest.

Depth. To ensure that the depth of the seat is correct, measure the longest body segment in a lateral view, usually from the back of the lower trunk to the popliteal fossa. Children should have seat depth approximately 1 inch shorter than this length. For adults, the seat depth should be approximately 2 inches shorter than this length. This will allow the seat to support the buttocks and thighs and avoid the front edge compressing the neurovascular structures in the popliteal fossa. Patients with significant kyphosis or who wear trunk orthoses may need extra seat depth. For patients with leg-length discrepancy, the depth of a sling seat should accommodate the length of the shorter leg. A solid seat can be modified to a different depth on each side; initially, the seat should suit the length of the longer leg.

A shallower seat should be used if the patient has tight hamstrings or intends to propel the wheelchair with the legs. However, in general, a shallow seat should be avoided because it reduces the area for pressure distribution and thus increases pressure on the ischial tuberosities and sacrum, increasing discomfort and the risk for tissue breakdown. A shallow seat also does not provide optimal distal lateral thigh stabilization and can cause the patient to sit with excessive hip abduction and external rotation. A seat that is too deep may impose excessive pressure on the popliteal fossa. The patient may compensate for this by tilting the pelvis posteriorly and adopting a kyphotic posture to prevent sliding forward. A wheelchair with excessive seat depth also reduces maneuverability in crowded areas.

Height. The distance from the footrests to the top of the seat cushion should equal the distance from the popliteal fossa to the base of the heel with the patient wearing typical footwear. For patients with plantarflexion contractures, use the distance from the popliteal fossa to the base of the toes. The height of the seat from the floor should allow the patient to place both feet completely on the floor when transferring and propelling the wheelchair with the feet when the leg rests are removed. With the leg rests installed, the footrests should be far enough off the floor to keep the feet from dragging.

If the seat is too low, the footrests may scrape the floor. Also, increased pressure will be placed on the ischial tuberosities because of inadequate lower extremity support. If the seat is too high, the patient may have difficulty transferring and may not be able to reach the ground for foot propulsion. A high seat can also lead to compensatory sliding into a posterior pelvic tilt. Seat height also affects wrist motion during wheelchair propulsion.[113]

Backrest

Width. For most patients, the width of the back of the chair should equal the width of the widest part of the patient's body in a frontal plane (facing the person). Patients with scoliosis may require a wider back to accommodate their spinal curvature. A wider-backed chair may also be needed if lateral thoracic supports are going to be placed in the chair. If the chair back is too narrow, there may be more pressure on sides of the trunk from the back canes and the patient may have inadequate trunk support. If the chair back is too wide, the patient may not be able to reach the wheels as readily and may have inadequate trunk support, which can lead to postural asymmetry.

Height. The backrest height should be determined with the seat cushion in place. The height of the backrest depends on the size of the patient and the amount of support needed. For full back support, the backrest height should equal the distance from the ischial tuberosities to top of the shoulders. If the patient does not require full back support, the backrest should extend from the ischial tuberosities only to the inferior angle of the scapulae to allow for greater upper extremity mobility. A backrest that is too low will not provide adequate support and may lead to compensatory kyphosis, which can contribute to fatigue or pain. If the backrest is too high, it may impede shoulder girdle mobility.

Armrests. Armrest height should be set to allow the patient to sit with the forearms supported and the elbows flexed 90 degrees. If the armrests are too low, the upper extremity may not be supported adequately, which may lead to shoulder subluxation and pain, particularly if the patient has a flaccid or hypotonic upper extremity. Unduly high armrests interfere with upper extremity function.

Complications of Wheelchair Use. Using a wheelchair can be associated with pain and injuries to the neck, back, shoulder, and buttocks.[115] The frequent and sustained extension of the neck caused by trying to look at the faces of people standing and the frequent rotation required to look around when turning the body are both thought to contribute to neck and back discomfort.[116] Shoulder injuries caused by overuse are common, particularly in those who began using a wheelchair in adulthood and did not develop the necessary strength and flexibility early on.[117] Buttock pain and pressure ulcers commonly result from the sustained pressure that occurs with prolonged sitting. The risk for pressure ulcers is greatest in patients, such as those with spinal cord injuries, who have reduced sensation and muscle mass in areas of pressure. Training in pressure relief, as well as scheduled periodic inspections of the wheelchair, can reduce the incidence of pressure ulcers.[118] Wheelchair inspections help with maintenance of safety features and can thus also contribute to injury risk reduction through accident prevention.

CASE STUDY 33-1

ASSISTIVE DEVICES FOR AMBULATION AND WHEELCHAIR AFTER TRANSTIBIAL AMPUTATION

Patient History

OB is a 75-year-old man who had a right transtibial amputation 6 weeks ago because of severe peripheral vascular disease, diabetes, and recurrent ulceration of his foot. He was fitted with a definitive prosthesis 2 weeks ago. He is now in a skilled nursing facility and will be discharged home next week.

OB is fearful of further amputation. He demonstrates limited understanding of diabetes control and has reduced his tobacco use and regulates his diet sporadically.

Tests and Measures—Significant Findings

Musculoskeletal
- Posture examination is significant for mild kyphosis with forward head.
- Trunk ROM is moderately limited, particularly in rotation.
- Right lower extremity passive ROM: 10-degree hip and knee flexion contractures bilaterally. Left lower extremity passive ROM: 5-degree hip flexion contracture and dorsiflexion is limited to 90 degrees.
- OB has generalized weakness in both lower extremities and trunk; upper extremity strength is within normal limits.

Neuromuscular
- OB complains of moderate pain in the residual limb; this pain resolves when the patient or clinician reapplies the prosthesis.
- OB has diminished tactile sensation on the dorsum and plantar surface of the left foot and moderate proprioceptive loss distal to the left ankle.

Integumentary
- A well-healed left plantar ulcer. No ulcerations on the amputation limb.

Function
- Limited standing balance on the left foot, and momentary standing balance on the right prosthesis. OB is fearful of falling.
- OB has difficulty donning his prosthesis correctly on a consistent basis.

Diagnosis

Preferred practice pattern 4J: Impaired motor function, muscle performance, range of motion, gait, locomotion, and balance associated with amputation.

Interventions
- OB will be fitted with a walker, cane, and manual wheelchair.
- Education in mobility and transfer training using the walker, cane, and wheelchair.
- Education in techniques of prosthesis donning and doffing and residual limb care.
- A bedside urinal will be recommended to reduce his need to ambulate to the toilet at night and risk falling.

Role of the Physical Therapist Assistant
- How can this patient increase his confidence in his mobility?
- What type of walker and wheelchair would you select for this patient? Why?
- Create a document that outlines for the patient the proper donning and doffing technique for his prosthesis.
- What precautions will help the patient avoid ulceration and amputation of his left foot?

Additional Information

For the full version of this case study, including detailed examination results, interventions, and outcomes, see the Evolve site that accompanies this book.

CHAPTER SUMMARY

Interacting with people and the environment is fundamental to quality of life. Assistive devices can increase, maintain, or improve the functional capabilities of individuals with disabilities. More people than ever are using assistive devices for mobility, particularly canes, walkers, and wheelchairs. Examination of the candidate for an assistive device should include medical history; demographics; psychosocial factors; self-management skills; current mobility equipment; home, environmental, and vocational demands; transportation requirements; and funding. Review of the musculoskeletal, neuromuscular, cardiopulmonary, and integumentary systems should focus on ROM, strength, and endurance.

Assistive devices for ambulation can improve balance, assist propulsion, reduce load on one or both lower extremities, transmit sensory cues through the hand(s), allow the individual to obtain the physiological and psychological benefits of upright posture and maneuver in places not accessible with a wheelchair, provide a safe environment for patients with cognitive impairment, and notify passersby that the user requires special considerations such as additional time when crossing streets. Canes, the simplest assistive device for mobility, offer a choice of handle, shaft, and base. Crutch designs include underarm, triceps, forearm, and platform. Walkers have various types of bases, uprights, hand grips and platforms, and accessories.

Wheelchairs can increase the user's comfort, support postural alignment, protect the skin, reduce energy consumption, improve safety, and facilitate function. The basic wheelchair prescription should specify the mode of propulsion, whether dependent, independent manual, or independent powered; frame; seat, including seat cushion; backrest, including insert; armrests, including lapboard; **front rigging** (i.e., footrests and leg rests); wheels, including tires, casters, hand rims, and brakes; and pelvic and thigh control accessories. Fitting assistive devices properly can prevent neurovascular compression and other complications of device misfit or misuse.

ADDITIONAL RESOURCES

For links to these and additional web-based resources, see the Evolve site.

ANSI/RESNA: *Wheelchair standards,* Arlington, VA, 1998, RESNA.

Axelson P, Chesney DY, Minkel J, et al: *The manual wheelchair training guide,* Minden, NV, 1998, PAX Press.

Axelson P, Minkel J, Perr A, et al: *The powered wheelchair training guide,* Minden, NV, 2002, PAX Press.

Cook A, Hussey S: *Assistive technologies: Principles and practice,* ed 2, Arlington, VA, 2002, RESNA.

Cooper RA: *Wheelchair selection and configuration,* New York, 1998, Demos Medical Publishing.

Croteau C: *Wheelchair mobility: A handbook,* Worcester, MA, 1998, Park Press.

Furumasu J (ed): *Pediatric powered mobility,* Arlington, VA, 1997, RESNA.

Karp G: *Choosing a wheelchair: A guide to optimal independence,* Sebastopol, CA, 1998, O'Reilly & Associates.

RESNA: *Resource guide for assistive technology outcomes,* Arlington, VA, 1998, RESNA.

ABLEDATA

Adaptive Device Locator System

Rehabilitation and Assistive Technology Society of North America (RESNA)

Thewheelchairsite (Comparison of different wheelchair manufacturers)

Refer to the websites of the various manufacturers mentioned in this chapter.

GLOSSARY

Axillary crutches: Underarm crutches.

Casters: Small wheelchair wheels, usually 5 or 8 inches in diameter.

Front rigging: Wheelchair leg rests and footrests.

Gel cushions: Wheelchair cushions filled with synthetic viscous material.

Lofstrand crutches: Forearm crutches.

Mobility device: Device that improves the user's ability to move within the environment, including canes, walkers, crutches, and wheelchairs; sometimes the term is used also to encompass adapted automobiles.

Pickup walker: Walking frame with four metal posts, each ending in a rubber high-traction tip.

Pommel: Wheelchair accessory located between the thighs to provide medial thigh support.

Quad cane: A cane with a base with four distal projections, each ending in a rubber high-traction tip. Also known as quadruped cane.

Triceps crutches: Crutches with top cuffs resting on the middle-third of upper arm. Also known as Warm Springs crutches.

Chapter 34

Orthotics

Joan E. Edelstein

CHAPTER OUTLINE

OBJECTIVES

After reading this chapter, the reader will be able to:
1. Identify the biomechanical principles underlying the design and prescription of orthoses.
2. Compare the characteristics of materials used in the construction of orthoses.
3. Describe the main components of lower extremity, trunk, and upper extremity orthoses.
4. Identify the principal features of lower extremity, trunk, and upper extremity orthoses assessed during the examination and evaluation process.
5. Recognize the role of the rehabilitation clinician in management of clients fitted with lower extremity, trunk, and upper extremity orthoses.

The word **orthosis** derives from the Greek expression "making straight." An orthosis is an orthopedic appliance used to support, align, prevent, or correct deformities of a body part or improve the function of movable parts of the body. The term **brace** is synonymous with orthosis. A **splint** is a temporary orthosis. Although "orthotic" is an adjective, the term is sometimes used to designate a foot orthosis. An **orthotist** is the health care practitioner who designs, fabricates, and fits patients with orthoses for any portion of the body. A **pedorthist** designs, fabricates, and fits patients with foot orthoses. Orthotics refers to the field of knowledge relating to orthoses and their use.

Physical therapy should have an integral role in patient management that includes orthotic prescription. Physical therapists (PTs) examine and evaluate the **strength,** range of joint motion, skin condition, and functional status of their patients and must also be knowledgeable about the patient's risk of developing contractures. They set short- and long-term goals for patients as part of

treatment planning. This information, combined with familiarity regarding contemporary orthoses, equips the therapist to recommend specific othotic designs. This chapter describes the common orthoses used by patients in multiple practice patterns.

 Clinical Pearl

Orthoses are devices that support or correct musculo-skeletal deformities or improve the function of movable parts of the body.

PATHOLOGY

Orthoses may be part of the treatment plan for patients who fall into a wide range of preferred practice patterns. These patients may have musculoskeletal disorders, neuromuscular disorders, integumentary disorders, and/or cardiopulmonary disorders. Orthoses are often helpful for patients with weakness, postural abnormalities, and poor control of motion. Lower extremity orthoses are commonly indicated for individuals with gait deviations.

DESIGN FACTORS

Orthosis Function. Orthoses apply forces to the body to resist motion, assist motion, or transfer force from one area to another. For example, a trunk orthosis with pads strategically placed to resist motion may be used to prevent a thoracic scoliosis from increasing. A person with quadriceps paralysis may wear a knee-ankle-foot orthosis (KAFO) that has a mechanical lock to resist knee flexion and maintain knee extension. Motion resistance is sometimes referred to as support. Two closely related functions are maintaining a particular alignment and protecting a body part from unwanted motion. For example, a KAFO may prevent the knee of an older adult with post-polio syndrome from hyperextending and a wrist-hand orthosis (WHO) may protect the joints of a patient with rheumatoid arthritis from pain and development of deformity.

The use of an orthosis to assist motion is illustrated by an ankle-foot orthosis (AFO) that assists dorsiflexion in the patient with foot drop. This orthosis may have a plastic or metal spring at the ankle area that compensates for the impairment by assisting ankle dorsiflexion during swing phase of gait. A foot orthosis that shifts load from subluxed metatarsal heads to the heel is an example of an orthosis that transfers force.

Comfort. Regardless of its purpose, an orthosis must be comfortable. An uncomfortable orthosis will probably not be worn and if it is worn, it may cause skin irritation or breakdown and may injure underlying structures. A major element in ensuring comfort is minimizing **pressure** by maximizing the area covered by the orthosis. The amount of subcutaneous fat and muscle tissue also influences orthotic fit and comfort. Therefore the individual with atrophy will need an orthosis that covers a wider area than the person who has a normal amount of soft tissue. Covering a large portion of the body can also cause some discomfort because the skin under the orthosis cannot readily dissipate heat or perspiration. Another way to improve comfort is to make the orthosis longer to provide greater leverage for the longitudinal segments of the orthosis to apply force through, but the orthosis must not be so long that it impinges on adjacent joints.

Some portion of an orthosis always touches the body. This contact should be snug but not constricting. An overly tight **band** will compress superficial blood vessels, causing pain and potentially tissue breakdown. Equally important, the contact should not be too loose, as this will likely result in friction with movement and may thus also cause skin irritation and breakdown. For example, a loose calf band on an AFO will rub on the calf and irritate the skin as the individual passes through the stance phase of gait.

Pressure Systems. Supportive systems involve a series of forces and counterforces, known as *pressure systems.* The basic pressure system for an orthosis is the three-point force system. A principal force acts in one direction, and two counterforces located proximal and distal to the principal force act in the opposite direction. For example, a man with genu valgum (knock-knee deformity) will have the deformity controlled by wearing an orthosis that exerts laterally directed force on the medial aspect of the knee and medially directed counterforces on the lateral aspect of the thigh and leg (Fig. 34-1).

The ground-reaction force may also be used strategically to help an orthosis perform its function. The ground-reaction force is the force exerted on the body by the floor in response to the force that the person exerts on the floor. All lower extremity orthoses interact with ground-reaction forces when the wearer stands or is in the stance phase of gait.

© *Clinical Pearl*

Even if an orthotic improves function, it will generally not be worn if it is not comfortable.

MATERIALS

Many materials are used to make contemporary orthoses. These materials differ in strength, flexibility, ease of forming, weight, and appearance. Certain principles should be used when selecting a material to achieve the purpose of the orthosis. Generally, thicker material will be less flexible, heavier, and bulkier. Materials can be strengthened by corrugation, curving, rolling the edges, or by

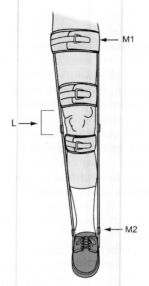

FIG. 34-1 Three-point force system to control genu valgum. *From Edelstein JE, Bruckner J:* Orthotics: A comprehensive clinical approach, *Thorofare, NJ, 2002, Slack.*

reinforcement with a stronger material such as carbon fiber. A given material shaped with an acute angle will bend and break more readily than will the same material with a wider angled curve. Thus breakage is more apt to occur at the site of a nick or hammer mark than in a smooth portion.

Material Properties—Strength (Stress Resistance), Strain, Stiffness, and Elasticity. The ability of a material to resist forces is known as its *strength*. Strength is measured by **stress** resistance, which is the amount of force that can be resisted per unit area. When a high force is applied over a small area, as occurs with a narrow band, particularly with a heavy patient, high local stress occurs. To avoid breakage, either the contact area must be increased or a very strong material must be used.

Compressive stress occurs when force squeezes a material; for example, the patient compresses the shoe heel during the early stance phase of walking. Tensile stress involves pulling the material, as in the case of a coiled spring in an AFO that pulls the toes upward during the swing phase of gait. The third type of stress is **shear,** which occurs when planes of the material slide over each other; the components of an overlapping joint in a WHO exert shear stress on one another.

Strain is the change in shape of a material as a result of stress. **Stiffness** is the amount of stress that must be applied to a material to cause strain, whether for intentionally shaping or unintentionally deforming or breaking the material. A brittle material breaks when relatively low force is applied. Metal becomes more brittle when cold, thus the patient is more likely to damage a brace in the winter than in the summer. Fatigue resistance is the ability of the material to withstand cyclic loading. An active child, for example, will subject his orthosis to frequent repetitive loading that may cause it to eventually fail because of material fatigue.

Elasticity is the ratio of stress to strain and thus represents the ability of a material to recover its original dimensions. **Plasticity** characterizes a material that changes shape without cracking; a malleable material reshapes under compression, whereas a ductile material alters under **tension.** Corrosion resistance refers to the extent to which materials deteriorate when exposed to chemicals. Some materials, particularly certain metals, are vulnerable to corrosion by urine and perspiration.

Specific Materials—Plastics, Metals, and Others. Plastic and metal components predominate in contemporary orthoses, although some orthoses have leather, rubber, wood, or cloth elements. The physical and aesthetic properties of each material influence orthotic design, durability, and cost, as well as the patient's acceptance of the device.

Plastics are synthetic, organic (carbon-containing) materials. The enormous variety of plastics results from the myriad ways in which molecules can be combined. Molecular arrangement dictates the properties of the plastic. As a group, plastics are relatively lightweight, easily shaped, strong, easily cleaned, corrosion resistant, and available in many colors.

Thermoplastics are popular materials for orthoses. When heated, thermoplastics become malleable and can be reshaped and then retain the new shape on cooling. Usually, thermoplastics can be reheated and reshaped indefinitely, allowing the orthotist to alter the fit of the appliance by heating the plastic, as well as by removing or adding material. The temperature at which thermoplastics become malleable varies. Many WHOs are formed from plastics that become malleable when immersed in warm water. The warm plastic is then molded directly on the patient. Unfortunately, if the person who wears a WHO made of such plastic washes dishes in hot water, the orthosis may also change shape. Thermoplastics that require a high temperature to become malleable are usually formed over a plaster model of the body part. Many thermoplastics are relatively weak, stain easily, and are flammable.

Alternate molecular arrangements produce **thermosetting plastics** such as polyester. Under most circumstances, thermosetting plastics cannot be reshaped after they are molded and the chemical reaction is complete. An orthosis made of thermosetting plastic cannot be reshaped by heating but can be altered by removing plastic or by adding pads or other material.

A metal is a chemical element that is lustrous, opaque, fusible, and ductile. Most metals used in orthoses are alloys, which are a combination of elements at least one of which is a metal. Combining a metal with other elements usually improves strength, wear resistance, and corrosion resistance. The mechanical properties of metals depend on their chemical structure. As a group, metals are strong, stiff, fatigue resistant, and impervious to the effects of environmental heat.

When steel is used in an orthosis, it is usually stainless steel. Stainless steel is heavier, stiffer, and stronger than most other materials. Because it is radiopaque, steel is undesirable if the patient requires radiographs to assess alignment while wearing the orthosis, for example, when

a trunk orthosis is worn by someone with scoliosis. Aluminum alloys are often used in orthoses. Aluminum is radiolucent, more malleable, and much lighter but also weaker than steel. To achieve the same rigidity as steel the aluminum components of an orthosis need to be thicker but are still lighter than steel parts. Aluminum is not suitable for hinges in orthoses because it is subject to fatigue failure. Titanium is as strong as steel while also being much lighter and corrosion resistant. However, it is much more expensive than steel or aluminum.

Some elements, such as carbon and silicone, have properties that are similar to both metals and nonmetals and are known as *metalloids.* Silicone offers little friction resistance and therefore provides an excellent interface between an orthosis and tender portions of skin. Carbon is stiff, light, and strong but not very malleable and is often used to reinforce an orthosis made primarily of other weaker materials.

Leather is animal skin that has been chemically treated by tanning to toughen the skin and make it more flexible, stronger, and more porous. The specific skin and the type of tanning determine the flexibility, durability, and appearance of the leather. The chemicals used for tanning can cause skin allergies in some patients, but a patient who is allergic to one particular type of leather may not react to another type of leather. Alternatively, a fabric or plastic interface may be placed between the patient's skin and the leather to prevent an allergic reaction caused by contact. Leather is porous and incompressible and can be molded over a model of a body part.

Cowhide is an exceptionally strong type of leather and is therefore frequently used for straps and the upper portion of shoes. Horsehide frequently lines bands, such as a calf band or thigh band, because its texture is particularly comfortable next to the skin. Kidskin and deerskin are very soft and may be used in shoe **uppers** for patients who have hammertoes and other tender areas on the dorsum of the foot.

Cork, which is made of the bark of the cork oak tree, is the most common wood used in orthoses. Cork is exceptionally lightweight and resilient and is used primarily for shoe lifts and arch supports.

Rubber is the sap of rubber trees that has been cured. Rubber has considerable elasticity, shock absorbency, and toughness. Synthetic rubber, such as neoprene, is less expensive and more resistant to corrosion but may be less elastic than natural rubber. Whether natural or synthetic, rubber provides excellent traction on shoe soles and is a good padding material. Open-cell (sponge) rubber recovers quickly when compressive stress is removed and is washable, soft, and very resilient. The cells, however, compress permanently after a relatively brief period of use. Closed-cell (expanded) rubber has excellent shear force and moisture resistance and responds more slowly than open-cell rubber to compressive stress.

Cotton, wool, and various synthetic fabrics are also commonly used in the manufacture of orthoses. Cotton is strong, absorbs perspiration readily, and is hypoallergenic. Consequently, cotton canvas is often used for sturdy abdominal fronts on trunk orthoses. Cotton flannel is a good padding material, particularly for the metal components of a trunk orthosis. Knitted cotton conforms readily to the body and is often used as a liner worn under an orthosis.

Wool has excellent resilience. Wool felt is used in certain foot orthoses and cervical orthoses. Felt is made of wool and other fibers matted together by steam and pressure. The higher the wool content the more durable the felt. Felt is lightweight and porous but compresses readily.

Polyester and nylon are synthetic fabrics that can be used in orthoses. Polyester fibers may be combined with cotton to create a relatively inexpensive material that is strong and dries easily. A **corset** made of polyester and cotton will not retain perspiration as much as one made entirely of cotton. A very popular use of nylon is hook and pile fasteners (Velcro) that are easier to engage than buckles, snaps, buttons, or laces.

> ### ◎ *Clinical Pearl*
>
> The selection of materials for an orthotic is influenced by the physical and aesthetic properties of different materials, as well as their durability and cost.

ORTHOSES

Lower Extremity Orthoses. Lower extremity orthoses include foot orthoses (FOs), which may be an insert worn inside the shoe, an internal modification glued inside the shoe, or an external modification secured to the shoe sole or heel. AFOs cover some portion of the foot and leg. Knee orthoses (KOs) extend from the distal thigh to the proximal leg. KAFOs encompass the thigh, leg, and foot. Hip orthoses (HOs) surround the hip. A hip-knee-ankle-foot orthosis (HKAFO) originates on the pelvis and terminates at the foot. A trunk-hip-knee-ankle-foot orthosis (THKAFO) encircles the trunk, both thighs and legs, and ends at the feet.

Shoes and Foot Orthoses. The foundation for nearly all lower extremity orthoses is the shoe. Each part of the shoe contributes to the efficacy of orthotic management and offers many options for selection. Shoes transfer body weight to the ground and protect the wearer from the bearing surface and the weather. The ideal shoe should distribute bearing forces to preserve optimum comfort, function, and appearance of the foot. For the individual with a musculoskeletal or neurological disorder, footwear may serve two additional purposes: (1) reducing pressure on sensitive deformed structures by redistributing weight toward pain-free areas and (2) being the foundation of AFOs or other more extensive bracing. Unless the shoe is correctly fitted and appropriately modified, the alignment of any attached orthosis will not provide the intended pattern of weight bearing. The major parts of the shoe are the upper, sole, heel, and reinforcements (Fig. 34-2). These features are found in both the traditional leather shoe and the contemporary athletic sneaker.

The upper is the portion of the shoe over the dorsum of the foot. If the shoe is to be used with an AFO that has an insert as its distal attachment, then the upper should extend to the proximal portion of the dorsum to secure the orthosis high onto the foot and the upper should have

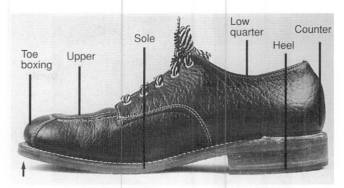

FIG. 34-2 Parts of a shoe. *From O'Sullivan S, Schmitz T (eds): Physical rehabilitation: Assessment and treatment, ed 4, Philadelphia, 2001, FA Davis.*

a separation at the distal margin of the lace stay to allow the foot to easily enter the shoe and for adjustability of fit. An extra-depth shoe with the upper contoured to have extra vertical space may be needed to accommodate an insert.

The sole is the bottom portion of the shoe. If the shoe is intended to accommodate a riveted metal attachment from an orthosis, it needs an outer and an inner sole, both made of leather or rubber with a metal reinforcement to receive the rivets. This type of shoe is heavier than one with a single sole. Except for a slight upward curve at the distal end, the outer sole is usually flat. The sole may be modified with a convex rocker bar to facilitate late stance or a **metatarsal bar** to transfer force posteriorly from painful metatarsal heads and reduce irritative motion.

The heel is the portion of the shoe adjacent to the outer sole and under the anatomical heel. A broad low heel provides the greatest stability and distributes force evenly between the back and front of the foot. For adults, a 2.5-cm (1-inch) heel tilts the center of gravity slightly forward, which aids transition through stance phase, while not disturbing knee and hip alignment significantly. A higher heel places the ankle in greater plantarflexion and forces the tibia forward. A high heel also transmits more stress to the metatarsals while reducing tension on the Achilles tendon and other posterior structures and accommodating a rigid pes equinus. Most heels are made of firm material with a rubber plantar surface; however, a compressible heel can be used to allow slight plantar-flexion if the ankle cannot move because of orthotic or anatomical limitation.

Reinforcements preserve the shape of the shoe. **Toe boxing** in the upper also protects the toes from horizontal trauma (e.g., stubbing) and vertical trauma and should be high enough to accommodate hammertoes or similar deformities. The **shank piece** is a longitudinal plate that reinforces the sole under the midfoot between the anterior border of the heel and the widest part of the sole at the metatarsal heads. A corrugated steel shank is necessary if a riveted orthotic attachment is to be used. The **counter** stiffens the posterior portion of the upper and usually terminates at the anterior border of the heel.

FOs are appliances that apply forces to the foot. The shoe itself may serve as a foot orthosis. Other FOs include

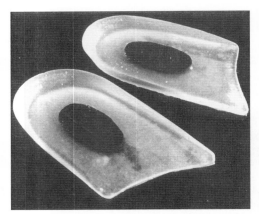

FIG. 34-3 Silicone heel cushions.

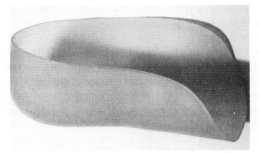

FIG. 34-4 University of California Biomechanics Laboratory foot orthosis.

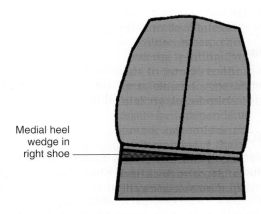

FIG. 34-5 Medial heel wedge. *From Edelstein JE, Bruckner J: Orthotics: A comprehensive clinical approach, Thorofare, NJ, 2002, Slack.*

an **insert** placed in the shoe, an **internal modification** affixed inside the shoe, or an **external modification** attached to the sole or heel of the shoe. FOs can enhance function by relieving pain and improving the wearer's transition during stance phase.[1] Pain may be lessened by modifications that transfer weight-bearing stresses to pressure-tolerant sites and by protecting painful areas from contact with the shoe and with adjacent portions of the foot. FOs may also improve gait and lessen back pain by equalizing foot and leg lengths[2] and by altering the rollover point in late stance.[3-5] Comfort and mobility can also be improved by correcting alignment of a flexible segment[6] or by accommodating a fixed deformity. In many instances, a particular therapeutic aim can be achieved by various devices.

Inserts and internal modifications are widely used because they are inconspicuous and may have a more direct effect on the foot than external modifications. Mass-produced inserts are also relatively inexpensive. Biomechanically, inserts and internal shoe modifications are identical. An insert can be transferred from one shoe to another, as long as the shoes have the same heel height, whereas internal shoe modifications are fixed to the specific shoe. Most inserts terminate just behind the metatarsal heads; thus they may slip forward, particularly if the shoe has a relatively high heel. Some inserts extend the full length of the sole, preventing slippage, but occupying the often-limited space in the anterior portion of the shoe. A heel insert (also known as a *heel cup*) extends from the back of the shoe to the midfoot (Fig. 34-3) and slopes anteriorly to reduce load on the painful heel and may have a concave relief to minimize pressure on the tender area.

Internal modifications are fixed to the shoe's interior, guaranteeing the desired placement, but limiting the patient to the single pair of modified shoes. Both inserts and internal modifications reduce shoe volume, so proper shoe fit must be judged with these components in place. Inserts made of soft materials such as viscoelastic plastic reduce shear and impact shock, thus protecting painful or sensitive feet.[7-9] A randomized controlled trial (RCT) on the effects of flexible inserts issued to military recruits found that those who wore these orthoses had less leg pain and no training injuries.[10] Inserts can also be constructed of semirigid or rigid plastics, rubber, or metal, often with a resilient overlay. These more rigid inserts can exert greater force and thus provide more support than compressible orthoses (Fig. 34-4). Obese patients may need rigid inserts to provide support when weight bearing.

The **metatarsal pad** is intended to transfer stress from the metatarsal heads to the metatarsal shafts. The pad has a convexity with its apex under the metatarsal shafts, and it may either be incorporated into the design of an insert or be a separate component that is glued to the inner sole of the shoe.

An external modification will not reduce internal shoe volume and ensures that the patient wears the appropriate shoes, but will be eroded by external elements as the patient walks and is somewhat conspicuous. In addition, the client is limited to wearing the modified shoe, rather than being able to choose from a wider selection of shoes. A heel wedge is a frequently prescribed external modification. A medial heel wedge (Fig. 34-5) applies laterally directed force and can aid in realigning flexible pes valgus or can accommodate rigid pes varus by filling the void between the sole and the floor on the medial side. A cushion heel is made of resilient material to absorb shock at heel contact. A cushion heel should be used when the patient wears an orthosis with a rigid ankle to allow some plantarflexion.

A metatarsal bar is a flat strip of leather or other firm material placed on the sole posterior to the metatarsal heads. At late stance, the bar transfers stress from the metatarsophalangeal joints to the metatarsal shafts. A rocker bar is a convex strip affixed to the sole proximal to the metatarsal heads. It shifts load from the metatarsophalangeal joints to the metatarsal shafts. The rocker bar also improves late stance by transferring the point of heel off posteriorly; thus the wearer can substitute trunk momentum for triceps surae muscle contraction to generate propulsive force.

◎ *Clinical Pearl*

A foot orthosis (FO) built into the structure of a person's shoe (external or internal modifications) ensures appropriate placement but limits the person to wearing only the one pair of modified shoes; inserts allow for modification of more than one pair of shoes.

Ankle-Foot Orthoses. The components of an AFO are a foundation, ankle control, and a superstructure, and in some cases, foot control.

The foundation consists of the shoe and a plastic, carbon fiber or metal component. An insert foundation is generally used because it facilitates donning the orthosis as the shoe can be separated from the rest of the brace,[11] and it can be used with various shoes, as long as they have the same heel height. Sneakers can be worn because the insert foundation is not riveted to the shoe. The orthosis with an insert is relatively lightweight because the insert is usually made of a thermoplastic, such as polyethylene or polypropylene, or from carbon fiber. Internal modifications can be incorporated into the insert.

An orthosis with insert foundation should consistently be worn with shoes with the same height heel. If the heel is too low, the **uprights** will incline posteriorly, increasing the tendency of the wearer's knee to extend. Conversely, if the orthosis heel is too high, the knee may not extend sufficiently and may be unstable. Inserts reduce interior shoe volume and thus must be used with a suitably spacious shoe.

Ankle control involves limiting plantarflexion and/or dorsiflexion or assisting ankle motion. The patient with dorsiflexor weakness or paralysis is likely to drag the toes during the swing phase of gait. An AFO can help in this circumstance, either by assisting dorsiflexion with a spring or by resisting plantarflexion with a rigid **stop.**

Foot control involves limiting mediolateral motion. Both **solid-ankle AFOs** and hinged AFOs have rigid sides that restrict transverse, sagittal, and frontal plane motions of the foot (Fig. 34-6, *A*). A metal-leather orthosis with a leather **valgus (or varus) correction strap** can also be used to control foot motion. The valgus correction strap is sewn to the medial portion of the shoe-upper, near the sole, and buckles around the lateral upright, exerting a laterally directed force to restrain pronation (Fig. 34-6, *B*). The varus correction strap has opposite attachments and force application. Either strap, although adjustable, complicates donning.

The superstructure of an AFO is the proximal portion, consisting of uprights and a **shell** and/or brim. Plastic AFOs usually have a single upright or shell. Solid-ankle

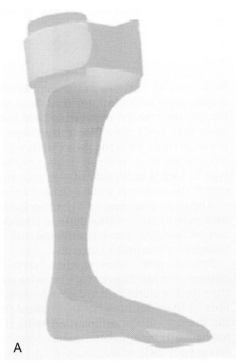

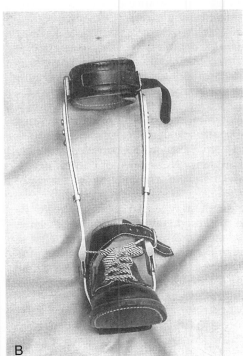

A   B

FIG. 34-6 **A,** Semisolid ankle-foot orthosis. **B,** Valgus correction strap on a left ankle-foot orthosis. **B** *from Edelstein JE, Bruckner J:* Orthotics: A comprehensive clinical approach, *Thorofare, NJ, 2002, Slack.*

and hinged AFOs both have a posterior shell extending from the medial to the lateral midline of the leg to maximize mediolateral control. The broad surface of the shell minimizes pressure. The **posterior leaf spring AFO** has a single posterior upright that therefore does not contribute to frontal or transverse plane control. The spiral AFO is made of nylon acrylic or polypropylene with a single upright that spirals from the medial aspect of the foot plate around the leg, terminating medially in a proximal band. The spiral orthosis controls but does not eliminate motion in all planes. Orthoses with plastic shells or uprights are molded over a cast of the patient's leg and should fit snugly for maximal control and minimal conspicuousness. Such AFOs are contraindicated for the individual whose ankle and leg volume fluctuates markedly because the orthosis cannot be readily adjusted.

Carbon fiber AFOs have become popular because carbon fiber is a very strong material, allowing the orthosis to be small and light. However, carbon fiber AFOs are more expensive than plastic AFOs and cannot be molded to fit an individual person.

A posterior calf band made of plastic or leather-upholstered metal is used to secure the orthosis to the patient's leg. The further the band is from the ankle joint, the greater the leverage of the orthosis on the ankle joint; but the band must not be so proximal that it compresses the peroneal nerve. If the AFO is intended to reduce the amount of weight transmitted through the foot, it may have a brim resembling a transtibial (below-knee) prosthetic socket (see Chapter 12).

Recent research indicates that adults with hemiparesis walk faster at less energy cost[12-15] and feel more confident[13] when wearing an AFO. They also have more dorsiflexion in early stance,[16] longer single-stance time on the paretic foot, and greater quadriceps activity.[17]

◎ *Clinical Pearl*

An ankle-foot orthosis (AFO) is used to assist with ankle dorsiflexion during swing phase of gait and to prevent knee hyperextension during stance phase of gait.

Knee-Ankle-Foot Orthoses. KAFOs consist of a shoe, foundation, ankle control, knee control, and superstructure (Fig. 34-7). They often also include a foot control. The shoe, foundation, ankle control, and foot control of the KAFO may be selected from the components already described for AFOs.

A hinge is the simplest type of orthotic knee joint. Hinges attached to the uprights on either side of the knee provide mediolateral, rotational, and hyperextension restriction while permitting knee flexion. An offset joint is a hinge placed posterior to the midline of the leg so that the patient's weight is anterior to the joint. This stabilizes the knee during the early stance phase of gait when the wearer is on a level surface and does not hamper knee flexion during swing or sitting. The joint may, however, flex inadvertently when the wearer walks down a steep ramp.

The most common knee control is the **drop ring lock.** When the client stands with the knee fully extended, the ring drops, preventing the uprights from bending.

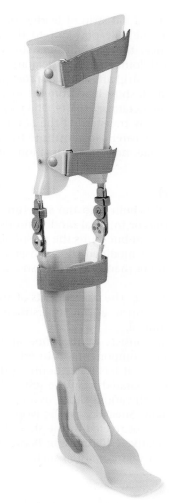

FIG. 34-7 Knee-ankle-foot orthosis. *Courtesy Becker Orthopedic, Beaverton, OR.*

Both medial and lateral joints should be locked for maximum stability but a pair of drop ring locks is inconvenient because the user has to hold both rings up at the same time to be able to flex the knee. An alternative to the drop ring lock is the **pawl lock** with bail release. This mechanism locks both uprights simultaneously, but this type of lock is bulky and may release the locks unexpectedly if the wearer is jostled against a rigid object.

The basic drop ring and pawl locks should not be used by a patient with a knee flexion contracture because the contracture will prevent aligning the orthotic uprights straight for the lock to engage.

Several new developments have the potential to improve the function of patients who wear KAFOs. Rather than steel or aluminum uprights, some KAFOs have carbon fiber or titanium uprights that reduce the weight but not the strength of the orthosis, allowing the person to walk further and be more comfortable.[18] In addition, the stance-phase knee lock, which locks in late swing and unlocks at the beginning of the next swing phase (heel off), allows free swinging of the knee during swing phase and stability during stance phase.

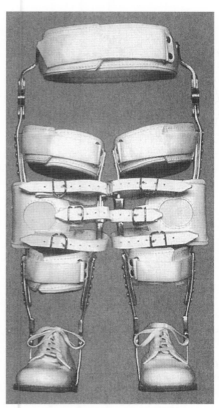

FIG. 34-8 Hip-knee-ankle-foot orthosis.

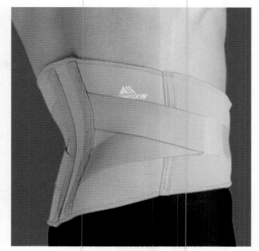

FIG. 34-9 Elastic lumbosacral binder.

Hip-Knee-Ankle-Foot Orthoses. A HKAFO is a KAFO with a **pelvic band** and hip joints (Fig. 34-8). The usual hip joint is a metal hinge that connects the lateral upright of the KAFO to a pelvic band. The joint prevents hip abduction, adduction, and rotation. An upholstered metal band is used to anchor the HKAFO to the trunk. This band should lodge between the greater trochanter and the iliac crest on each side. HKAFOs are not used very often because they are much more difficult to don than KAFOs, and if the hip joints are locked, they restrict gait to the swing-to or swing-through pattern. The pelvic band is also often uncomfortable when the wearer sits.

Trunk-Hip-Knee-Ankle-Foot Orthoses. A THKAFO incorporates a lumbosacral orthosis attached to a KAFO. The pelvic band of the trunk orthosis serves as the pelvic band used on HKAFOs. A THKAFO may be used by a patient with spinal cord injury to allow them to experience orthotically assisted ambulation. Because the THKAFO is very difficult to don and is heavy and cumbersome, it is seldom worn after the client is discharged from the rehabilitation program.

Trunk Orthoses. Trunk orthoses are usually named for the section of the torso encircled, as well as the type of control provided. These orthoses support the trunk to control spinal motion. They may be prescribed to reduce the disability caused by low-back pain, neck sprain, scoliosis, or other musculoskeletal or neuromuscular disorders. In patients with spinal cord injury, trunk orthoses control motion of the spine and compress the abdomen to improve breathing.[19,20] Individuals with cervical spinal cord lesions may also need to wear an orthosis that restrains neck motion until stability is achieved by surgery or spontaneous healing. There are also special trunk orthoses designed for children and adolescents with scoliosis.

Corsets and Lumbar Supports. A corset or lumbar support is a fabric orthosis without horizontal rigid structures, although it may have vertical rigid reinforcements (Fig. 34-9). A corset may cover only the sacroiliac or lumbosacral regions or may extend superiorly to the thoracic region. The primary effect of a corset is to compress the abdomen to increase intraabdominal pressure. Greater pressure increases spinal stability[21,22] and reduces stress on posterior spinal musculature.[23] Although temporary reduction of abdominal and erector spinae muscular activity may be therapeutic,[24] long-term reliance on a corset can promote muscle atrophy and contracture, as well as psychological dependence on the orthosis.

> ⊙ ***Clinical Pearl***
>
> Lumbar corsets can reduce abdominal and erector spinae muscle activity. This can be helpful temporarily after a muscle injury, but long-term use is not recommended because it can promote muscle atrophy and psychological dependence on the orthosis.

Rigid Lumbosacral and Thoracolumbosacral Orthoses. Lumbosacral orthoses (LSO) and thoracolumbosacral orthoses (TLSO) may include a corset or a fabric abdominal front that compresses the abdomen (Fig. 34-10, *A*) or more commonly are made of molded plastic (clam shell) (Fig. 34-10, *B*). These rigid types of braces are most commonly used after spinal surgery to provide stabilization during recovery.

Cervical Orthoses. Cervical collars encircle the neck with fabric, resilient material, or rigid plastic. A few collars also encompass the chin and posterior head for slightly greater restraint. The most common collar is made of soft material and provides minimal restraint (Fig. 34-11, *A*). It is usually used for support and comfort and does not restrict movement. A rigid collar made of foamed polyethylene reinforced with a rigid anterior strut is intended for use by

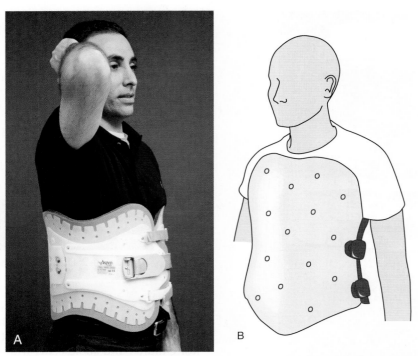

FIG. 34-10 **A,** Lumbosacral orthosis. **B,** Thoracolumbosacral orthosis. *A from Browner BD: Skeletal trauma, ed 4, St Louis, 2007, Mosby;* **B** *from Goodman CC: Pathology: Implications for the physical therapist, ed 3, St. Louis, 2009, Saunders.*

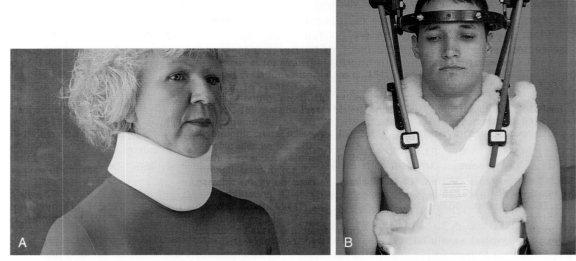

FIG. 34-11 Cervical orthoses. **A,** Soft cervical collar. **B,** Halo vest orthosis. *A courtesy Trulif;* **B** *from Harkreader H: Fundamentals of nursing: Caring and clinical judgment, ed 3, St. Louis, 2008, Saunders.*

patients with cervical fractures. This collar surrounds the neck and covers the lower portion of the jaw and the occipital area of the skull to prevent movement of the neck and cervical cord injury. Maximum orthotic control of the neck is generally achieved with a **halo vest** orthosis (Fig. 34-11, *B*). The halo vest orthosis has a circular band of metal that is fixed to the skull by four screws. Uprights connect the halo to a vestlike thoracic orthosis.

Orthoses for Patients with Scoliosis. Children and adolescents with thoracic, thoracolumbar, or lumbar scoliosis may be fitted with a TLSO that applies forces intended to maintain alignment of or realign the

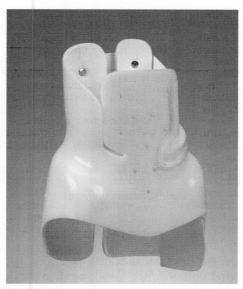

FIG. 34-12 Boston scoliosis orthosis. *Courtesy Boston Brace International, www.bostonbrace.com.*

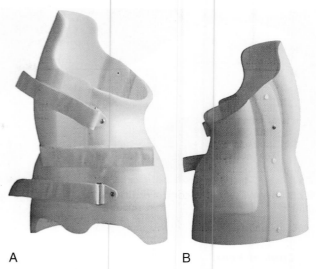

A   B

FIG. 34-13 Charleston bending brace. **A,** Anterior view. **B,** Posterior view. *Courtesy Spinal Technology, Inc, www.spinetech.com.*

vertebral column and thoracic cage. This orthosis usually prevents the curve from increasing beyond its original contour.[25-27]

The **Milwaukee orthosis** is a type of TLSO often prescribed for patients with scoliosis. This orthosis consists of a frame composed of a pelvic girdle, two posterior uprights, an anterior upright, and a superior ring. The current version features a superior ring that lies on the upper chest rather than just below or on the chin as with older models, allowing it to be hidden by most clothing. Various pads are strapped to the frame to apply corrective forces. The **Boston orthosis** is an alternative to the Milwaukee. It usually does not extend as high as the Milwaukee, and its foundation is a mass-produced plastic module that the orthotist alters to meet the needs of the individual (Fig. 34-12). A retrospective study of 151 patients who wore the Boston orthosis confirms that this orthosis can prevent curve progression.[28] It is most effective if worn for at least 18 hours a day,[29,30] and when the strap tension is between 20 and 40 N.[31]

The **Wilmington orthosis** is another contemporary design of TLSO used to treat scoliosis. It consists of a custom-made TLSO jacket intended to guide the trunk to straighter alignment and thereby avoid exaggeration of the scoliotic curve.[32] The **Charleston bending brace** and the **Providence orthosis** provide overcorrection of the spinal curve and have also been shown to control relatively slight scoliotic curves (Fig. 34-13).[33-36]

Orthoses for patients with scoliosis are most effective when the patient has an immature spine and moderate vertebral curves in the midthoracic or more inferior portions of the trunk.[37] The classic protocol required the orthosis to be worn 23 hours each day.[38] Today, to improve adherence, many recommend that the orthosis only be worn in bed when the effects of gravity are minimized.

Upper Extremity Orthoses. Orthoses for the upper extremity include appliances for the shoulder, elbow, wrist, and hand. Upper extremity orthoses may be assistive or substitutive, protective, or corrective. Assistive or substitutive orthoses are indicated for patients with paralysis. They augment residual motor power or substitute mechanical joint motion and stabilization for absent anatomical function. Protective orthoses either shield the affected joint from developing contracture or reduce painful motion. Corrective orthoses are used to increase joint range of motion (ROM) in the presence of contracture.

Wrist-Hand Orthoses

Assistive and Substitutive Wrist-Hand Orthoses. Assistive and substitutive WHOs are used primarily for people with weakness due to nerve damage. Assistive orthoses position the hand so that the patient can make maximum use of the residual motor power. Substitutive orthoses enable the patient to achieve prehension by moving the wrist or a more proximal body segment to cause finger movement.

The **basic opponens orthosis** is one of the simplest assistive WHOs. Also called the *short opponens splint*, it keeps the thumb pad beneath the palmar surfaces of the index and middle fingers, helping the patient use residual motor power to achieve palmar prehension. Its dorsal and palmar bars support the transverse palmar arch, protecting it from flattening. The abduction bar keeps the thumb abducted, preventing thenar web contracture and placing the thumb in a suitable position for opposition. The opponens bar prevents the first metatarsal from migrating to the plane of the other fingers. This orthosis is useful for the patient with median neuropathy who is in jeopardy of developing thenar contracture and a flat hand posture and who needs assistance for prehension.

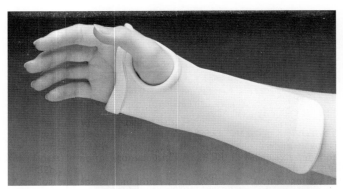

FIG. 34-14 Wrist flexion control orthosis (also called a cock-up splint).

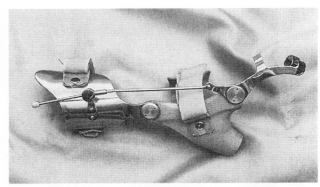

FIG. 34-15 Wrist-driven prehension orthosis.

Clinical Pearl

The short opponens splint keeps the thumb pad under the palmar surface of the index and middle fingers to help the patient achieve palmar prehension.

A forearm bar added to the basic opponens orthosis creates the opponens WHO with wrist control, also known as the *long opponens splint.* The forearm bar may be located on the palmar, dorsal, radial, or ulnar aspect of the wrist and forearm. The forearm bar maintains the wrist in a fixed position, preventing the hand from dropping into palmar flexion.

A **metacarpophalangeal-extension stop** can also be added to the basic opponens orthosis. The stop, sometimes called a *lumbrical bar,* is secured to the palmar bar and applies palmar-ward force to the proximal phalanges to resist metacarpophalangeal hyperextension. This component aids prehension by protecting the hand from forming a claw hand deformity, which is a risk with ulnar or combined median and ulnar neuropathy, thereby aiding prehension.

The wrist flexion control WHO, also called a *cock-up splint* (Fig. 34-14), is another assistive orthosis. This design features a palmar hand bar and forearm bar with straps to secure the orthosis to the extremity. The orthosis prevents the wrist from dropping into palmar flexion, thereby assisting the median- and ulnar-innervated muscles by placing them in a more functional position. The same orthosis is often used to protect the wrist from repetitive motion stress from prolonged typing.

Prehension orthoses are examples of substitutive appliances. They are especially suited to the patient with tetraparesis or tetraplegia. The orthoses enable the wearer to grasp an object, hold it, and release it voluntarily. The wrist-driven prehension WHO was originally called the *flexor hinge orthosis* because it has a hinge between the forearm bar and the finger stabilizer (Fig. 34-15). The orthosis includes a bar and a band to stabilize the first interphalangeal joint and a separate bar and band unit to prevent motion of the second and third proximal and distal interphalangeal joints. The two stabilizers pivot on a palmar and dorsal hand-bar assembly, and there is a second pivot at the junction between the hand and forearm bar. Wrist dorsiflexion causes the finger stabilizers

to approach the thumb stabilizer, enabling grasp. The user must maintain active dorsiflexion to retain the held object. Some prehension orthoses have a locking mechanism to relieve stress on the dorsiflexors. Most also have a mechanism to allow the wearer to select the size of grasp relative to the angle of wrist dorsiflexion. For grasping a piece of paper, the wearer adjusts the mechanism so that a small arc of wrist motion achieves finger closure. For grasping a thicker object, the wearer adjusts the mechanism so that the same small arc of wrist dorsiflexion achieves closure. The object is released when the wearer relaxes the dorsiflexors, allowing the wrist to passively palmar flex. The patient with C6 tetraplegia can use this type of orthosis only with the forearm pronated. If the forearm is supinated, the wearer could achieve grasp and holding but could not release the object voluntarily because of lack of control of the palmar flexors. Despite these limitations, the wrist-driven prehension WHO is a relatively useful device, facilitating hygiene, writing, and feeding.

The person with C4 or C5 tetraplegia lacks sufficient control of the wrist dorsiflexors to use a wrist-driven prehension WHO and therefore requires a different type of orthosis. The electrically driven prehension WHO is sometimes prescribed for these patients. The rigid parts of this orthosis are similar to those of the wrist-driven model but instead of a linkage between the hand and forearm components, the electrically driven orthosis has a steel cable secured to the finger stabilizer. The proximal end of the cable terminates in a rod linked to a battery-operated motor. To achieve grasp, the patient moves an actuator, usually located over the contralateral shoulder. Shoulder elevation triggers a microswitch, which turns on the motor that pulls the cable proximally. Cable movement causes the finger stabilizer to approach the thumb stabilizer. Holding occurs when the patient keeps the motor in the neutral position. Release is attained by voluntary shoulder pressure on a second microswitch in the actuator that reverses the direction of the motor, relieving tension on the cable. A spring located on the finger stabilizer is then able to recoil, opening the fingers. Usually a relatively large arc of shoulder elevation causes grasp and a smaller arc triggers the releasing microswitch. The battery and motor for this device are relatively heavy and bulky, making the orthosis awkward for an ambulatory patient but practical for transport on a wheelchair for a

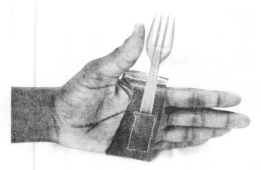

FIG. 34-16 Universal cuff.

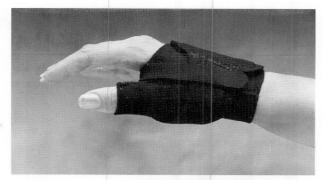

FIG. 34-17 Thumb-stabilizing orthosis.

wheelchair user. As with all battery-powered motors, the battery in the orthosis must be recharged periodically. Many patients eventually opt for a much simpler, lighter orthosis, such as those described in the next section, to perform grasp functions.

The **utensil holder,** sometimes called a *universal cuff,* is an orthosis that is usually mass-produced and consists of a spring clip or elastic webbing that wraps around the hand, across the palm (Fig. 34-16). The palmar or dorsal side of the cuff has a pocket into which one may place a pen, spoon handle, or other objects of appropriate size. This orthosis may have a forearm bar to prevent unwanted wrist motion and keep the hand in a more functional position.

◎ *Clinical Pearl*

The utensil holder (universal cuff) wraps around the hand and has a pocket into which the handle of various utensils can be placed for functional use.

Protective Wrist-Hand Orthoses. There are many mass-produced protective WHOs available, although nearly all the designs can be custom-made of plaster or plastic sheeting. The wrist–hand-stabilizing orthosis, also termed a *resting splint,* is a molded sheet of semirigid plastic formed to fit the palmar surface of the hand and forearm. The sheet extends from the distal tips of the fingers to the middle third of the forearm and is curved to support the palmar arch and cradle the forearm. Straps secure the plastic to the hand and forearm. Some wrist stabilizers also include a thumb component for thumb stabilization. Patients with inflammatory arthritis have been shown to have significantly less pain after 4 weeks of wearing a protective WHO.[39,40]

Thumb and Finger Orthoses. A thumb-stabilizing orthosis without a wrist-stabilizing component (Fig. 34-17) can be used to prevent movement of the first interphalangeal and metacarpophalangeal joints in patients with arthritis and in those with burns who are vulnerable to flexion contractures. This orthosis has a longitudinal bar along the length of the thumb, with stabilizing straps or a sleeve on the thumb and a strap around the hand.

Finger stabilizers are used by some patients to stabilize or correct a boutonnière deformity (hyperflexion of the proximal interphalangeal joint). This orthosis includes a band that applies palmar-directed force at the proximal interphalangeal joint. This force is opposed by two bands that apply dorsally directed forces to the proximal and middle phalanges.

A corrective WHO that applies a low, constant force with appropriate counterforces to reduce contracture can be used to correct extension contractures of the metacarpophalangeal joints. This device, known as a **finger flexor WHO** or a *knuckle bender,* has a dorsal plate over the metacarpals and another plate over the proximal phalanges linked to a palmar rod. Springs or rubber bands apply tensile force to the orthosis. If worn for a sufficient period of time, the orthosis will cause the metacarpophalangeal joints to yield. Care must be taken, however, to avoid skin breakdown and ulceration from undue pressure. The finger extensor hand orthosis, also called the *reverse knuckle bender,* has an opposite force system to the knuckle bender. It has a palmar-located bar linked to two dorsal bars. Tension is exerted by rubber bands or springs. Versions of these corrective orthoses are also available to correct extension and flexion deformities of the interphalangeal joints. Corrective WHOs were associated with improved grip strength and finger mobility in patients with rheumatoid arthritis and finger flexion contractures.[41] Among patients with traumatic upper extremity injury, those who wore a corrective WHO for 6 to 12 hours per day achieved significantly greater joint excursion than those who wore the orthosis for less than 6 hours daily.[42]

Forearm and Elbow Orthoses. A few patients benefit from protective or corrective elbow orthoses and a very few tolerate assistive or substitutive elbow orthoses. Forearm cuffs are readily available orthoses intended to reduce stress on the forearm extensor muscles and tendons in patients with lateral epicondylitis. The typical cuff is made of sturdy fabric with hook and pile closure. Some cuffs have reinforcing bars.

The elbow extensor orthosis is intended to increase elbow extension in the presence of an elbow flexion contracture. This type of device is intended for continuous wear and has a three-point pressure system, with anteriorly directed force near the olecranon and posteriorly directed counterforces at the distal forearm and proximal upper arm. Most models allow the clinician to increase the angle between the forearm and upper arm as the flexion contracture reduces. Others have a spring mechanism that is designed to maintain maximum separation between the cuffs. Some do not have an adjustable joint or spring but

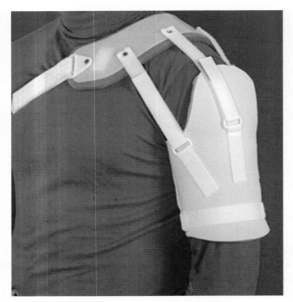

FIG. 34-18 Shoulder orthosis.

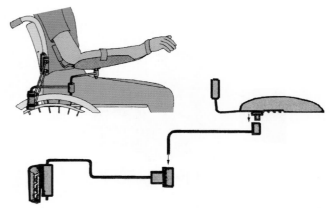

FIG. 34-19 Balanced forearm orthosis. *From Edelstein JE, Bruckner J:* Orthotics: A comprehensive clinical approach, *Thorofare, NJ, 2002, Slack.*

are designed to be remolded periodically as the contracture reduces.

Elbow assistive and substitutive orthoses are intended for patients with paralyzed elbow flexors or extensors. Lacking voluntary control of the elbow, the individual would have a limited work area in which to use the naturally or orthotically powered hand. The simplest orthosis is the elbow-stabilizing orthosis that maintains the elbow at 90 degrees of flexion and the forearm in moderate pronation, thereby placing the hand in a position to perform tabletop functions. The orthosis has no moving parts, making it durable and relatively inexpensive. However, the elbow is kept flexed, which is awkward when the individual walks or dons clothing.

Shoulder Orthoses. Most shoulder orthoses (SOs) are intended to protect the glenohumeral joint from subluxation caused by flaccid hemiplegia or injury to the shoulder joint capsule (Fig. 34-18). The simplest and most widely used SO is a sling. Although there are many sling designs, the most common are single-strap, multiple-strap, and humeral-cuff slings. The typical single-strap sling has a canvas forearm support to which is sewn a strap that is worn over the contralateral shoulder. The forearm support may be a continuous piece of fabric or may be divided into proximal and distal forearm sections. The single-strap sling supports the weight of the forearm, wrist, and hand. The sling reduces the risk of shoulder subluxation in patients with shoulder muscle flaccidity and can protect the upper extremity from swinging and inadvertently bumping into objects. The single-strap sling is easier to don than other models.

Clinical Pearl

Most shoulder orthoses (SOs) are used to prevent shoulder subluxation.

Multiple-strap slings have two or more straps. The forearm support has proximal and distal straps. The proximal strap passes over the ipsilateral shoulder, whereas the distal strap goes over the opposite shoulder. In the back, the two straps may be sewn to another oblique strap that maintains the appropriate distance between the two vertical straps. Because this sling has a strap lying vertically over the ipsilateral shoulder, it directly resists downward shoulder subluxation. As with single-strap slings, multiple-strap slings also support the weight of the forearm and hand to prevent the extremity from swinging into objects. Biomechanical analysis demonstrated that single- and multiple-strap slings were more effective than an axillary roll or a lap tray in supporting the flaccid shoulder.[43]

Humeral cuff slings do not support the forearm. Instead, they have a broad cuff that encircles the upper arm. Vertical straps extend from the anterior and posterior proximal margins of this cuff to a horizontal strap that encircles the chest. Some models have a pad over the shoulder to disperse pressure. Humeral cuff slings prevent shoulder subluxation without encumbering the elbow or forearm. Consequently, the wearer can conceal the sling under a shirt. One version of a humeral cuff sling has cuffs on both upper arms. The cuffs are joined posteriorly by a strap. Tightening the strap pulls both upper arms posteriorly, helping the humeral heads to lodge firmly in their respective glenohumeral fossae. Radiographic evidence confirms that the humeral cuff is significantly more effective than the single-strap sling in reducing subluxation.[44] However, a meta-analysis of RCTs involving the use of slings in hemiplegic patients with shoulder subluxation did not find any particular sling design to be significantly more effective than any other in reducing subluxation-related pain.[45]

A shoulder-stabilizing orthosis with a metal or rigid plastic frame for the upper arm joined to a trunk orthosis may be used for patients with good hand and elbow function who have lost shoulder control to allow for better use of the hand. This type of orthosis usually has a friction shoulder joint that keeps the shoulder where the wearer moves it.

The **balanced forearm orthosis** (BFO) is a practical orthosis to assist shoulder and elbow motion (Fig. 34-19). The BFO is sometimes referred to as a feeder because it facilitates the shoulder and elbow motions needed for feeding. This is a mass-produced appliance that is usually bolted to a person's wheelchair. The BFO consists of a proximal arm that fits into a ball-bearing receptacle attached to the wheelchair or other support and a distal arm that fits into a second ball-bearing receptacle between the proximal and distal arm. The distal arm is attached to a pivoting rocker arm mechanism to which the forearm trough is screwed. By adjusting the tilt and rotational position of the proximal and distal arms, one can assist or resist shoulder flexion, extension, and rotation. The first mechanical principle governing the BFO is that objects move down a slope. The second principle is that of the first-class lever exemplified by the action of the forearm trough. If the proximal portion of trough is screwed into the pivoting mechanism, elbow extension is aided. Locating the screws toward the distal end of the trough assists elbow flexion. The BFO is a relatively inexpensive orthosis that enables the user to move the arm horizontally and vertically. It is usually employed with a wheelchair to enable the patient with tetraparesis to accomplish many daily activities, such as feeding, facial hygiene, writing, keyboard operation, and painting, if the patient retains natural or orthotically assisted prehension.

CASE STUDY 34-1

ANKLE-FOOT ORTHOSES FOR A PATIENT WITH MULTIPLE SCLEROSIS

Patient History

EA is a 48-year-old mail delivery clerk in a large medical center. Two years ago, EA started to have difficulty focusing on the television and noticed tingling in both his feet. Some days he was so fatigued that he had to rest while delivering mail. At other times, he could drive to see his grandchildren and engage them in vigorous play. After he stumbled twice in the same week and then dropped a sack of mail in front of his supervisor, he sought medical attention. He was diagnosed with multiple sclerosis. Medications were partially effective in controlling his symptoms, but he was referred to physical therapy for assistance with functional mobility.

Tests and Measures—Significant Findings
Musculoskeletal
- Ankle dorsiflexion is limited to the neutral position bilaterally. Both feet exhibit mild pes varus.
- Bilaterally, dorsiflexors 3/5; plantarflexors 4/5; invertors 4/5; evertors 2/5; quadriceps 3/5; hip extensors 3/5; hip flexors 4/5.

Neuromuscular
- Mild clonus elicited in both ankles.
- EA complains of numbness on the plantar surface of both feet.

Integumentary
- EA has bruises from recent falls on both lateral thighs. Feet show abrasions on the medial portion of the dorsum where the feet have been rubbing on the margin of the shoes.

Diagnosis
Preferred practice pattern 5E: Impaired motor function and sensory integrity associated with progressive disorders of the central nervous system.

Interventions
- Hinged AFOs fitted bilaterally to control pes varus and drop foot.
- Shoes with rubber soles to increase traction and pliable leather uppers to minimize irritation on medial aspect of feet.
- Cane to assist with balance; trial with cane in either hand to determine best use.
- Orthosis donning, balance, and gait training with emphasis on safe performance and increased endurance.
- At work, request wheeled cart to reduce need to carry mail sacks.

Role of the Physical Therapist Assistant
- What types of activities would be involved in gait training for this patient?
- How would a hinged AFO control pes varus? How would it control drop foot?
- List three activities EA could do with his grandchildren to improve his endurance.

Additional Information
For the full version of this case study, including detailed examination results, interventions, and outcomes, see the Evolve site that accompanies this book. Full case studies describing the management of a child with scoliosis using a thoracolumbosacral orthosis and for the selection of upper extremity orthoses for a patient with a cervical spinal cord injury are also included on the Evolve site.

CHAPTER SUMMARY

Orthoses are appliances that apply forces to support, align, prevent, or correct deformities of a body part or improve the function of a movable part of the body. Orthotic selection and fitting are influenced by the functional purpose of the orthotic, the forces required to achieve the desired outcome, comfort, and cosmesis. Orthotic support involves force systems, usually a three-point system consisting of a principal force and two counterforces. There are orthoses designed for the lower extremities, upper extremities, trunk, and cervical spine. This chapter reviews general principles of orthotic design, including the different materials used to make orthoses, and describes commonly used orthoses for different body parts.

ADDITIONAL RESOURCES

For links to these and additional web-based resources, see the Evolve site.

Coppard BM, Lohman H: *Introduction to splinting: A clinical reasoning and problem-solving approach*, St. Louis, 2001, Mosby.

Edelstein JE, Bruckner J: *Orthotics: A comprehensive clinical approach*, Thorofare, NJ, 2002, Slack.

Edelstein JE, Bruckner J: *Orthotics: A comprehensive interactive tutorial CD ROM,* Thorofare, NJ, 2003, Slack.

Goldberg B, Hsu JD (eds): *Atlas of orthoses: Rehabilitation principles and application of orthotic and assistive devices,* ed 3, St. Louis, 1996, Mosby.

Lusardi MM, Nielsen CC (eds): *Orthotics and prosthetics in rehabilitation,* Boston, 2000, Butterworth Heinemann.

Redford JB, Basmajian JV, Trautman P (eds): *Orthotics: Clinical practice and rehabilitation technology,* New York, 1995, Churchill Livingstone.

Seymour R: *Prosthetics and orthotics: Lower limb and spinal,* Philadelphia, 2002, Lippincott Williams & Wilkins.

Shurr DG, Michael JW: *Prosthetics and orthotics,* ed 2, Upper Saddle River, NJ, 2002, Prentice Hall.

American Academy of Orthotists and Prosthetists

American Orthotic and Prosthetic Association

Association of Children's Prosthetic-Orthotic Clinics

GLOSSARY

Band: Rigid horizontal component in a lower extremity or trunk orthosis.

Basic opponens orthosis: Hand orthosis that includes an opponens bar, thumb abduction bar, and dorsal and palmar hand bands; maintains the thumb in opposition.

Balanced forearm orthosis: Mass-produced orthosis that assists shoulder and elbow motion, usually mounted on a wheelchair.

Blucher: Shoe upper design in which the distal margins of the lace stays are separate.

Boston orthosis: Plastic thoracolumbosacral orthosis that controls scoliosis. Made of a mass-produced module custom fitted to the patient.

Brace: Orthosis.

Charleston bending brace: Plastic thoracolumbosacral orthosis that controls scoliosis; intended to be worn by a recumbent patient, usually at night.

Corset: Trunk orthosis that has no rigid horizontal components but may have rigid vertical components.

Counter: Posterior reinforcement of a shoe upper.

Drop ring lock: Metal rectangle that, when engaged, prevents movement of orthotic uprights.

Elasticity: Ratio of stress to strain in a material; the ability of a material to recover its original dimensions.

External modification: FO consisting of material added to the exterior of the shoe, usually the sole.

Finger flexor WHO: Orthosis that applies forces to flex the metacarpophalangeal joints.

Halo vest: Rigid circular ring secured to the skull by four screws. Provides superior attachment points for posts in a cervicothoracic orthosis.

Insert: Removable foot orthosis that fits inside the shoe.

Internal modification: Foot orthosis that is attached to the interior of the shoe.

Metacarpophalangeal-extension stop: Band on a WHO that resists extension of the metacarpophalangeal joints.

Metatarsal bar: External foot orthosis located on the sole posterior to the metatarsal heads.

Metatarsal pad: Internal foot orthosis with apex located posterior to the metatarsal heads.

Milwaukee orthosis: Plastic cervicothoracolumbosacral orthosis that controls scoliosis. Pelvic girdle connected to neck ring by one anterior and two posterior uprights; control pads are attached to the uprights.

Orthosis: Orthopedic appliance used to support, align, prevent, or correct deformities of a body part or to improve the function of movable parts of the body.

Orthotist: Health care practitioner who designs, fabricates, and fits patients with orthoses.

Pawl lock: Knee lock, including a spring-loaded projection that fits into a notched disk.

Pedorthist: Health care practitioner who designs, fabricates, and fits patients with foot orthoses and shoes.

Pelvic band: Rigid portion of a lower extremity or trunk orthosis that fits over the posterior portion of the lower trunk.

Plasticity: Property of a material that changes shape without cracking.

Posterior leaf spring AFO: Plastic or carbon fiber orthosis consisting of a foot plate to which a posterior upright is attached, terminating in a calf band and anterior strap.

Pressure: Force applied per unit surface area.

Providence orthosis: Plastic thoracolumbosacral orthosis that controls scoliosis; intended to be worn by a recumbent patient, usually at night.

Shank piece: Shoe reinforcement located beneath the midfoot.

Shear: Stress occurring when force causes planes of a material to slide over each other.

Shell: Rigid plastic posterior portion of an AFO or KAFO.

Solid-ankle AFO: AFO with trimlines anterior to the malleoli.

Splint: Temporary orthosis.

Stiffness: Amount of stress that must be applied to a material to cause strain.

Stop: Rigid restraint in an orthotic ankle joint that resists dorsiflexion.

Strain: Change in shape of a material as a result of stress.

Strength: Ability of a material to resist forces.

Stress: Force applied per unit of area.

Tension: Stress occurring when force pulls on a material.

Thermoplastic: Plastics that become malleable when heated and retain the new shape on cooling.

Thermosetting plastics: Plastics that retain their shape on completion of the original chemical reaction.

Toe boxing: Anterior reinforcement of a shoe upper.

Upper: Portion of a shoe located above the sole.

Upright: Rigid vertical component of a lower extremity or trunk orthosis.

Utensil holder: WHO that includes a pocket on the palm; utensils can be inserted into the pocket.

Valgus (or varus) correction strap: Leather strap attached to the medial (lateral) portion of the shoe; strap buckles around the lateral (medial) upright of the AFO.

Wilmington orthosis: Plastic thoracolumbosacral orthosis that controls scoliosis.

Index

A

Abdominal bracing, in spinal stabilization exercises, 108, 109f
Abdominal motion, in respiratory failure evaluation, 408
Abduction, 35-36
Abnormal synergy, definition of, 263
Acapella device, for airway clearance dysfunction, 377-378, 377f
Accessory bone(s), 115
  definition of, 129
Actin, 43f
  definition of, 55-56
Action potential, 278, 279f
  definition of, 55, 292
  in muscle contraction, 43
Active assisted range of motion (AAROM), in soft tissue surgery rehabilitation, 158
Active cycle of breathing technique (ACBT), for airway clearance, 372-373
Active range of motion (AROM) exercises, in contracture prevention
  after amputation, 170
  after burn, 501-502
Active sitting, 31, 32f
  definition of, 40-41
Activities of daily living (ADLs), metabolic equivalents for, 390t
Activities-Specific Balance Confidence (ABC) Scale, 516
Activity-focused intervention(s)
  definition of, 247
  for pediatric nonprogressive CNS disorders, 238-240
Acute inflammatory demyelinating polyneuropathy (AIDP), definition of, 301-302
Acute respiratory distress syndrome (ARDS)
  incidence of, 398
  respiratory failure from, 398
Adaptation exercises, in vestibular adaptation, 201-202, 201f, 201t-202t
Adaptive devices. See also Assistive/adaptive devices.
  in muscle weakness evaluation, 47
  for pediatric nonprogressive CNS disorders, 242-243, 242f
Adhesive capsulitis, of shoulder, 80, 81t
Advanced glycation end-products (AGEs)
  definition of, 491-492
  in hyperglycemia, wound healing and, 477
Aerobic capacity
  in airway clearance dysfunction evaluation, 372
  in burns, 496

Aerobic capacity (Continued)
  in deconditioning evaluation, 361-363
  definition of, 384
  in gait deficit evaluation, 514-515
  in heart failure evaluation, 389-390
  impaired, in airway clearance dysfunction, 368
  in muscle weakness evaluation, 47
  in nonprogressive spinal cord disorder evaluation, 310
Aerobic conditioning/reconditioning
  for adult nonprogressive CNS disorders, 258-259
  for airway clearance dysfunction, 378
  in burn care, 502
  in fracture management, 124, 125f
Aerobic energy sources, for muscle rehabilitation, 47-48
Aerobic exercise
  for deconditioning, 363-366
    in acute care inpatient setting, 363-364
    duration and frequency of, 365-366
    intensity of, 364-365
    in outpatient setting, 364
  definition of, 391-392, 396-397
  in heart failure, 391-392
  in progressive CNS disorder management, 270
  in rheumatoid arthritis management, 71
Afferent, definition of, 292
Afferent pathways, of peripheral nervous system, 276
Age
  fracture healing and, 120
  intervertebral disc changes related to, 93-94
  muscle performance and, 44
Agency for Health Care Policy Research (AHCPR), 426-427
Agility training
  for adult nonprogressive CNS disorders, 259-260
  in fracture management, 124
  in progressive CNS disorder management, 270-272
Aging, deconditioning from, 360
Agonistic reversals
  definition of, 263
  as proprioceptive neuromuscular facilitation technique, 256t
Air splint, in postamputation edema control, 171
Airway clearance, in nonprogressive spinal cord disorders, in acute phase, 313-314
Airway clearance dysfunction, 368-384
  adverse outcomes of, 368
  airway clearance techniques for, 373-378
    breathing strategies as, 373-374. See also Breathing strategies for airway clearance.

Airway clearance dysfunction (Continued)
    manual and mechanical, 374-375
    mechanical devices for, 376-378
      assistive, 378
      high-frequency chest wall oscillation device as, 376, 376f
      positive expiratory pressure device as, 376-378, 377f
      vibratory positive expiratory pressure devices as, 377-378, 377f
  breathing patterns in, 371t
  in chronic bronchitis, case study of, 383-384
  communication on, 372
  examination findings in, 368-372
  functional training in, for self-care and home management, 382
  interventions for, 372-383
    coordination of, 372
    documentation of, 372
  mechanical ventilators for, 383
  oxygen sources and delivery devices for, 382-383, 382f-383f
  pathology of, 368
  patient/client-related instruction for, 372-373
  patient history in, 368-369
  postural drainage with chest percussion, vibration, and shaking for, 374
  systems review in, 369
  tests and measures for, 369-372
    cardiopulmonary, 369-372
    functional, 372
    musculoskeletal, 369
    neuromuscular, 369
  therapeutic exercise for, 378-382. See also Therapeutic exercise, for airway clearance dysfunction.
Airway resistance, 551
  definition of, 405
Airways
  anatomy of, 400-401
  branching of, 400-401, 402f
  conducting, 402f
    definition of, 416
    function of, 400-401
  respiratory, 402f
    definition of, 416
    function of, 400-401
  surface tension in, 406
Akinesia
  definition of, 275
  description of, 268t
  in Huntington's disease, 265-266
  in progressive CNS disorders, 269
Alberta Infant Motor Scale (AIMS), 214-215, 214f-215f
Alcohol abuse, skeletal demineralization and, 21
Alcoholic neuropathy, 297
  definition of, 301

Page numbers with "t" denote tables; those with "b" denote boxes; and those with "f" denote figures.